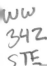

DVD Contents

DVD running time approximately 64 minutes

CATARACT
SURGERY

Commissioning Editor: *Russell Gabbedy*
Development Editor: *Alexandra Mortimer*
Editorial Assistant: *Poppy Garroway*
Project Manager: *Elouise Ball*
Design: *Charles Gray*
Illustration Manager: *Gillian Richards*
Illustrator: *Laurel Cook Lhowe*
Marketing Manager(s) (UK/USA): *Clara Toombs/Helena Mutak*

CATARACT
SURGERY

THIRD EDITION

Editor

ROGER F STEINERT MD

Professor and Chair of Ophthalmology
Professor of Biomedical Engineering
Director, Gavin Herbert Eye Institute

University of California Irvine
California
USA

Associate Editors

DAVID F. CHANG MD

HIROKO BISSEN-MIYAJIMA MD PHD

I. HOWARD FINE MD

HOWARD V. GIMBEL MD MPH

DOUGLAS D. KOCH MD

STEPHEN S. LANE MD

RICHARD L. LINDSTROM MD

THOMAS NEUHANN MD

ROBERT H. OSHER MD

SAUNDERS

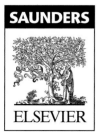

ELSEVIER

SAUNDERS
ELSEVIER

SAUNDERS is an imprint of Elsevier Inc.

© 2010, Elsevier Inc. All rights reserved.

First edition 1995
Second edition 2004

Copyright for figure 2.5 Lens Opacities Classification System, version III (LOCS III) is retained by the author Dr Leo T. Chylack Jr. (15 Bradford Road, Duxbury, MA, USA)

ISBN 978-1-4160-3225-0

Library of Congress Cataloging in Publication Data
A catalog record for this book is available from the Library of Congress

Notice

Knowledge and best practice in this field are constantly changing. As new research and experience broaden our understanding, changes in research methods, professional practices, or medical treatment may become necessary. Practitioners and researchers must always rely on their own experience and knowledge in evaluating and using any information, methods, compounds, or experiments described herein. In using such information or methods they should be mindful of their own safety and the safety of others, including parties for whom they have a professional responsibility.

With respect to any drug or pharmaceutical products identified, readers are advised to check the most current information provided (i) on procedures featured or (ii) by the manufacturer of each product to be administered, to verify the recommended dose or formula, the method and duration of administration, and contraindications. It is the responsibility of practitioners, relying on their own experience and knowledge of their patients, to make diagnoses, to determine dosages and the best treatment for each individual patient, and to take all appropriate safety precautions. To the fullest extent of the law, neither the Publisher nor the authors, contributors, or editors, assume any liability for any injury and/or damage to persons or property as a matter of products liability, negligence or otherwise, or from any use or operation of any methods, products, instructions, or ideas contained in the material herein.

The Publisher

Printed in China

Last digit is the print number: 9 8 7 6 5 4 3 2

Contents

Contents

Preface

The preface to the second edition, published in 2004 but written and edited in 2002-03, paid special tribute to the pioneers of phacoemulsification and intraocular lens implantation who founded and nurtured the American Society of Cataract and Refractive Surgery. ASCRS became a force that overcame tradition and regulation, launching a revolution in cataract surgery and vastly improving the quality of life of cataract patients world-wide. Special recognition was given to the singular contributions of Charles Kelman, MD.

In the following years, we have lost the ultimate innovator in our specialty. Highly controversial in his younger years, Charlie, as he was known to thousands of friends and colleagues, lived long enough to know that his contributions were universally recognized. He was always supportive of younger surgeons striving to make further progress. We all miss you, Charlie, and we are the poorer for your early passing.

This third edition follows the mission that this textbook has always followed: to be comprehensive, thorough, and balanced. While the chapters stand on their own, extensive references also assist the reader in pursuing a subject further. The rapid pace of innovation continues, and the reader must always follow recent advances that will not be reflected in these pages.

The third edition is thoroughly updated, and several new chapters have been added as well as extensive revisions of the previous edition. One completely new teaching medium has been added: a DVD collection of relevant operative video clips to illustrate the surgical techniques already captured in the written word and figures. Thirty-seven separate video segments illustrate many maneuvers, ranging from the basics through the most advanced.

Roger F. Steinert, MD
Irvine, CA

Contributors

RICHARD L. ABBOTT MD

Thomas W. Boyden, Endowed Chair
Health Science Clinical Professor of
   Ophthalmology
Research Associate
   Francis Proctor Foundation
UCSF Department of Ophthalmology
Beckman Vision Center
San Francisco
CA
USA

ANTHONY AGADZI MD

Redwood Eye Centre
Vallejo
CA
USA

DAVID J. APPLE MD

Professor of Ophthalmology and Pathology
   Director of Research
Pawek-Vallotton Chair of
   Biomedical Engineering
Former Professor and Chairman
Storm Eye Institute Medical University of
   South Carolina
Charleston
SC
USA

MARTIN S. ARKIN MD, PHD

Bay Eye Associates
Traverse City
MI
USA

SHALEEN BELANI MD

Kaiser Permanente
Mid Atlantic States
USA

C. DAVIS BELCHER III MD

Deceased, Formerly Harvard Medical School
Tufts Medical School
Ophthalmic Consultants of Boston
Boston
MA
USA

HIROKO BISSEN-MIYAJIMA MD PHD

Professor of Ophthalmology
Department of Ophthalmology
Tokyo Dental College Suidobashi Hospital
Tokyo
Japan

SCOTT E. BURK MD PHD

Cincinnati Eye Institute
Cincinnati
OH
USA

DAVID F. CHANG MD

Clinical Professor
University of California, San Francisco
Los Altos
CA
USA

LEO T. CHYLACK JR. MD

Director of Research
Center for Ophthalmic Research
Boston
MA
USA

ROBERT J. CIONNI MD

Cincinnati Eye Institute
Cincinnati
OH
USA

JOHN S. COHEN MD

Cincinnati Eye Institute
Cincinnati
OH
USA

ALAN S. CRANDALL MD

Professor and Senior Vice Chair of Ophthalmology
    and Visual Sciences
Director of Glaucoma and Cataract
John A. Moran Eye Center
University of Utah
Salt Lake City
UT
USA

ANDREA P. DA MATA MD

Research Ophthalmologist
Cincinnati Eye Institute
Cincinnati
OH
USA

ELIZABETH A. DAVIS MD FACS

Adjunct Clinical Assistant Professor
University of Minnesota
Partner
Minnesota Eye Consultants
Bloomington
MN
USA

BRIAN M. DEBROFF MD FACS

Associate Clinical Professor
Department of Ophthalmology and
    Visual Science
Yale University School of Medicine
Director of Pediatric Cataract Surgery
Yale University School of Medicine
Eye Surgery Associates, LLC
Stratford
CT
USA

H. BURKHARD DICK MD PHD

Chairman and Professor
Center of Vision Sciences and
    Department of Ophthalmology
Ruhr University
Bochum
Germany

KENDALL DONALDSON MD MS

Assistant Professor of Ophthalmology
Corneal and External Disease Service
Bascom Palmer Eye Institute
Miami
FL
USA

JAY S. DUKER MD

Director New England Eye Center
Chairman and Professor of Ophthalmology
Tufts Medical Center
Tufts University School of Medicine
Boston
MA
USA

JENNIFER A. DUNBAR MD

Director of Pediatric Ophthalmology
Ophthalmology
Loma Linda University
Loma Linda
CA
USA

DAVID A. EICHENBAUM MD

Retina Vitreous Associates of Florida
Clearwater
FL
USA

JARED EMERY MD

Professor of Ophthalmology
Emeritus
Baylor College of Medicine
Great Barrington
MA
USA

I. HOWARD FINE MD

Clinical Professor of Ophthalmology
Oregon Health & Science University
Drs Fine, Hoffman & Packer LLC
Eugene
OR
USA

WILLIAM J. FISHKIND MD FACS

Director
Fishkind, Bakewell, Maltzman
Eye Care and Surgery Center
Tucson, Arizona
Clinical Professor of Ophthalmology
The University of Utah
Salt Lake City, Utah
Clinical Instructor of Ophthalmology
The University of Arizona
Tucson, Arizona, USA

HOWARD V. GIMBEL MD MPH

Professor and Chair, Department of Ophthalmology, Loma Linda University, Loma Linda, California
Clinical Associate Professor, Department of Surgery, University of Calgary, Calgary, Alberta
Clinical Professor, Department of Ophthalmology, University of California, San Francisco, CA, USA
Executive Medical Director
Cataract and Refractive Surgeon
Gimbel Eye Centre
Alberta
Canada

ROBERT C. HAMILTON MB BCH FRCPC

Canmore
Alberta
Canada

DAVID R. HARDTEN MD FACS

Director of Refractive Surgery
Adjunct Associate Professor of Ophthalmology
University of Minnesota
Minnesota Eye Consultants
Minneapolis
MN
USA

KENNETH J. HOFFER MD FACS

Clinical Professor of Ophthalmology
Jules Stein Eye Institute
University of California
Los Angeles
CA
USA

RICHARD S. HOFFMAN MD

Drs Fine, Hoffmann & Packer LLC
Eugene
OR
USA

JAMES W. HUNG MD

Ophthalmic Consultants of Boston
Boston Eye Surgery & Laser Center
Boston
MA
USA

ALEX P. HUNYOR MB BS FRANZCO FRACS

Vitreoretinal Surgeon
Chatswood Retina Service
Sydney Eye Hospital
Chatswood
Australia

ANUP K. KHATANA MD

Cincinnati Eye Institute
Cincinnati
OH
USA

CHRISTOPHER KHNG MD

Cincinnati Eye Institute
Cincinnati
OH
USA

DOUGLAS D. KOCH MD

Department of Ophthalmology
Baylor College of Medicine
Houston
TX
USA

BARUCH D. KUPPERMANN MD PHD

Associate Professor of Ophthalmology
University of California Irvine
Irvine
CA
USA

STEPHEN S. LANE MD

Adjunct Clinical Professor
Department of Ophthalmology
University of Minnesota
Associated Eye Centre
Stillwater
MN
USA

RICHARD L. LINDSTROM MD

Founder and Attending Surgeon: Minnesota Eye Consultants, P.A.
Adjunct Clinical Professor Emeritus
Department of Ophthalmology
University of Minnesota
Minnesota Eye Consultants PA
Minneapolis
MN
USA

DENNIS C. LU MD

Minneapolis
MN
USA

MARTIN A. MAINSTER PHD MD FRCOPHTH

Luther L. Fry Professor of Ophthalmology
Department of Ophthalmology
University of Kansas School of Medicine
Kansas City
KS
USA

NICK MAMALIS MD

Professor of Ophthalmology and Visual Sciences
John A. Moran Eye Center
University of Utah
Salt Lake City
UT
USA

SAMUEL MASKET MD

Clinical Professor
David Geffen School of Medicine; UCLA
Los Angeles
CA
USA

MARIANNE B. MELLEM KAIRALA MD

Bascom Palmer Eye Institute
Miami
FL
USA

ANNE M. MENKE RN PHD

Risk Manager
OMIC
San Francisco
CA
USA

RANDALL E. NACKE MD

Adjunct
Washington University of St. Louis
Premiere Eye Associates
Crystal City
MO
USA

RAJA NARAYANAN MD

Consultant
Smt. Kanuri Santhamma Retina
Vitreous Center
LV Prasad Eye Institute
Banjara Hills
Hyderabad
India

THOMAS F. NEUHANN MD

Alz Augenklinik München
Munchen
Germany

BHARTI R. NIHALANI MD

Research Associate
Children's Hospital
Harvard Medical School
Boston
MA
USA

KENNETH D. NOVAK MD

Eye Associates of Utica
Utica
NY
USA

ROBERT H. OSHER MD

Cincinnati Eye Institute
Cincinnati
OH
USA

MARK PACKER MD FACS

Clinical Associate Professor of Ophthalmology
Oregon Health & Science University
Drs Fine, Hoffman & Packer LLC
Eugene
OR
USA

ROBERT I. PARK MD

Carolina Ophthalmology PA
Hendersonville
NC
USA

RICHARD K. PARRISH II MD

Associate Dean for Graduate Medical Education
University of Miami Miller School of Med
Anne Bates Leach Eye Hospital
Miami
FL
USA

MICHAEL B. RAIZMAN MD

Associate Professor of Ophthalmology
Tufts University School of Medicine
Ophthalmic Consultants of Boston
Boston
MA
USA

CHRISTOPHER D. RIEMANN MD

Cincinnati Eye Institute
Cincinnati
OH
USA

BRADFORD J. SHINGLETON MD

Assistant Clinical Professor of Ophthalmology
Harvard Medical School
Ophthalmic Consultants of Boston
Boston
MA
USA

RICHARD J. SIMMONS MD

Harwich
MA
USA

MICHAEL E. SNYDER MD

Consultant Ophthalmologist
Cincinnati Eye Institute
Volunteer Assistant Professor of Ophthalmology
University of Cincinnati
Blue Ash
OH
USA

TERRENCE S. SPENCER MD

Ophthalmologist
Spivack Vision Center
Centennial
CO
USA

ROGER F. STEINERT MD

Professor and Chair of Ophthalmology
Professor of Biomedical Engineering
Director, Gavin Herbert Eye Institute
Department of Ophthalmology
University of California Irvine
CA
USA

GEOFFREY TABIN MA MD

Professor of Ophthalmology and Visual Sciences
John A. Moran Eye Center
University of Utah
Salt Lake City
UT
USA

TREXLER M. TOPPING MD

Ophthalmic Consultants of Boston
Boston
MA
USA

PATRICIA L. TURNER MD

Clinical Associate Professor of Ophthalmology
Department of Ophthalmology
University of Kansas School of Medicine
Prairie Village
Kansas
USA

LI WANG MD PHD

Department of Ophthalmology
Baylor College of Medicine
Houston
TX
USA

MITCHELL P. WEIKERT MD

Department of Ophthalmology
Baylor College of Medicine
Houston
TX
USA

LILIANA WERNER MD PHD

Associate Professor
John A. Moran Eye Center
Salt Lake City
UT
USA

Dedication

To our parents
For nurturing our development and imbuing fundamental values

To our families
For your support, your encouragement, your tolerence every day

To our teachers
We try to honor you by building on your foundation

To our residents and fellows
You are the future; learn, then lead

To our patients
In return for entrusting us with the most precious of senses, we commit to an unrelenting pursuit of excellence

Acknowledgments

The revision of a major textbook is, strangely perhaps, more challenging than an entirely new endeavor. While authors can retain some prior words and figures, the painstaking re-working and revision is a complex endeavor for both primary authors and the editors. The first major thank you, therefore, is to the many contributors of chapters and to the Associate Editors who have worked for three years, from initial concepts to final page proofs. Assembling the video clips has been an added major effort, since most of us did not have tightly edited clips with voice over narration already produced that matched the chapter content.

The second major acknowledgment is to all the wonderful people who support the authors and editors. From office assistants who organize schedules, respond to emails, type, and coordinate manuscripts fragments, through residents, fellows, technicians, and nurses, and ending with family who tolerate and support the authors, we are grateful and thank you for the key roles you have played in bringing our teaching to successful conclusion. I am particularly grateful to my wife, April, who not only supported me as a loving spouse, but also served as the US based Managing Editor, serving as the contact point and coordinator for the UK based Elsevier team.

At Elsevier, many people have helped bring the third edition to fruition. My principal contacts have been Russell Gabbedy, Commissioning Editor, Alex Mortimer, Development Editor, and Elouise Ball, Production Manager. You have worked long and hard, through hundreds of emails and a dozen meetings, with patience and professionalism. In addition, many thanks to other key personnel: Fraser Johnston, Multimedia Producer, and Charles Gray, Book Designer.

Finally, in the third edition as was the case in the first two editions, Laurel Cooke Lhowe has maintained her uniquely clear style of ophthalmic art. She has an amazing ability to communicate with multiple authors and translate crude sketches and vague words into unfussy, eminently effective figures.

Roger F. Steinert, MD
Irvine CA

part i

EVALUATION

The Pathology of Cataracts

Terrence S. Spencer, MD and Nick Mamalis, MD

CONTENTS

CHAPTER HIGHLIGHTS

>> Development of the lens
>> Pathologic correlation of clinical cataracts

LENS EMBRYOLOGY

Knowledge of the embryology of the lens helps one better understand its normal anatomy and the nature of cataracts. Lens cells form early during embryogenesis from surface ectoderm. The optic vesicles (neuroectodermally derived outpouchings of the diencephalon) enlarge to come in contact with the surface ectoderm which thickens to form the lens plate. At the same time, the optic vesicle begins invaginating and an indentation called the lens pit forms in the lens plate. The lens pit continues to invaginate as surface ectoderm cells multiply. Eventually, a sphere of cells called the lens vesicle breaks off from the stalk which kept it connected to the remainder of the surface. The lens vesicle at this point contains a single layer of cuboidal cells within an outer basement membrane. The outer basement membrane forms the lens capsule.

The posterior cells of the lens vesicle begin to elongate anteriorly to become the primary lens fibers (Figure 1-1). These primary lens fibers meet the anterior lens cuboidal cells, obliterating the lumen of the lens vesicle. The primary lens fibers make up the embryonic nucleus, and the anterior lens cuboidal cells are now referred to as the lens epithelial cells. The layer of lens epithelium maintains its presence anteriorly and just posterior to the equator, but no epithelial cells are normally present in the posterior part of the lens.

Secondary lens fibers form from lens epithelial cells near the equator, which begin to multiply and elongate anteriorly under the lens epithelium and posteriorly under the lens capsule. These secondary lens fibers form the fetal nucleus during gestation and continue to grow in this manner adding new layers. As the lens fibers grow, they extend from the equator to meet anteriorly and posteriorly, forming Y-shaped sutures where they meet during fetal growth. During childhood and early adolescence, lens fibers surround the fetal nucleus to become the juvenile or infantile nucleus. Further growth of these lens fibers eventually forms the adult nucleus. Subsequent lens fibers grow to surround the entire nucleus, forming lens cortex.

During fetal development the lens nucleus becomes enveloped within the tunica vasculosa lentis, a nutritive support structure supplied by the hyaloid artery. This structure atrophies and usually disappears by birth.

NORMAL ANATOMY OF THE LENS

The lens is normally a clear, biconvex structure (Figure 1-2). Viewed from the side, it has an elliptical shape, measuring about 3.5–4.0 mm A–P by 9.0–10.0 mm in diameter. It is located posterior to and loosely apposed to the iris. Lens transparency is a function of regular cell shape, regular cell volume, minimal extracellular space, and minimal scatter elements.[1]

The lens is held in place by the zonules, which attach it to the ciliary body. The zonular fibers arise from the basement membrane of the non-pigmented epithelium of the ciliary body and attach just anteriorly and posteriorly to the equator of the lens. Tension on the zonules is reduced by contraction of the ciliary muscle, allowing the lens to become more spherical in shape for accommodation.

The lens is lined on its outer surface by the lens capsule, which is responsible for elasticity, allowing the lens to accommodate. The

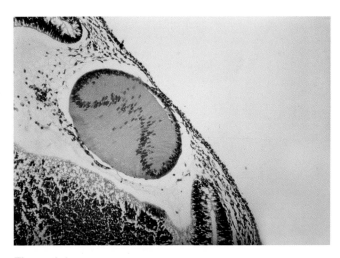

Figure 1-1 Embryo lens. Posterior epithelial cells of the lens vesicle elongate to become lens fibers. (Hematoxylin and eosin [H & E] stain; X10.)

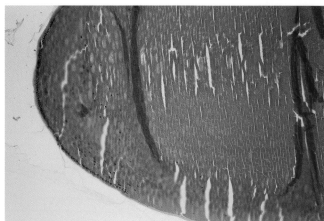

Figure 1-3 Lens bow. Lens epithelial cells elongate from the equator to form new lens fibers. The nuclei appear to "fan out" from the edge of the lens seen in cross section. There are no epithelial cells beneath the posterior surface of the lens capsule. (Hematoxylin and eosin [H & E] stain; X10.)

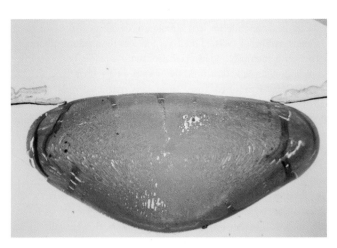

Figure 1-2 Normal lens. This histologic section of a normal lens from an enucleated globe showing artefactual clefts and folds. (Hematoxylin and eosin [H & E] stain; X2.)

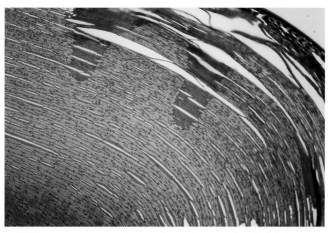

Figure 1-4 Lens substance. Normal fibers appear in layers at the periphery of the lens. The clefts are artifacts from histologic sectioning. (Trichrome stain; X20.)

lens capsule varies in thickness and is thinnest at the posterior pole. Histologically, the lens capsule stains positive with PAS stain since it is a true basement membrane of the lens epithelial cells.

Lens epithelial cells are arranged in a single row of cuboidal cells along the anterior surface of the lens and ending at the lens bow where new lens fibers are produced. Nutrients and waste products pass through the lens capsule by diffusion and active transport from the anterior epithelium. The equatorial bow region of the lens (Figure 1-3), just posterior to the equator, is where lens epithelial cells elongate to form lens fiber cells. Normally, there are no lens epithelial cells along the posterior pole of the lens capsule.

The cortex and nucleus make up the substance of the lens. The fibers derived earliest lie centrally and form the embryonic, fetal, juvenile and, finally, adult nucleus. The lens cortex is formed from the most peripheral fibers found between the nucleus and capsule (Figure 1-4). As more cortical fibers are produced at the periphery, inner fibers are added to the defined adult lens nucleus.

Studies of the morphology of differentiated lens fiber cells in all regions of normal adult human lenses have been performed.[2] The percentages of the lens thickness that is accounted for by the embryologic nucleus was found to be 4%, this was followed by 49% of the lens thickness made up of the fetal nucleus, 9% juvenile nucleus, 21% adult nucleus and, lastly, 17% the cortex. Evaluation of the morphology of lens fibers by electron microscopy showed that the cells in the embryonic and fetal nucleus were rounded with variable area. Adult nuclear cells were found to be more flattened with a relatively intricate, membranous interdigitation. Cortical cells evaluated by electron microscopy were irregularly hexagonal in shape.

INTRODUCTION TO CATARACT PATHOLOGY

The term cataract refers to any opacity of various degree of the crystalline lens, which is normally almost completely transparent. There are a variety of methods to classify cataracts clinically, but pathological examination of cataracts may be difficult. The lens tends to survive fairly well post-mortem because it does not have its own blood supply, but it does not have the same gross appearance as its clinical appearance in vivo. Hardness of the explanted lens correlates highly with clinical grading of nuclear sclerosis, but not with cortical or subcapsular opacities.[3,4] One problem with pathological examination of a cataract is the alteration in the appearance of the lens when it is placed in fixatives for the purpose of preservation of tissue. The microscopic alterations that are seen on histologic sections do not necessarily correlate with the severity of cataract and visual dysfunction seen clinically. When the lens is processed and sectioned for histologic examination, numerous artefacts appear in its structure.

With normal aging, the lens increases in overall size and loses its ability to accommodate. Continued growth of lens fibers with aging causes the nucleus to become compressed and less pliable (nuclear sclerosis).[3,5] Nuclear lens proteins aggregate and are chemically modified to produce pigmentation, decreasing transparency. The increase in pigmentation causes the lens nucleus to appear yellow, or with excess pigmentation, brown (brunescent cataract). Proteins within the cytoplasm of lens cells are modified in such a manner that scatters visible light, resulting in opacification.[6] A decrease in metabolic transport of antioxidants in an aging lens, as a consequence, may allow oxidation of nuclear components.[7] Hydrogen peroxide (H_2O_2), one oxidant, is found at elevated concentrations in some patients with maturity-onset cataract. The activities of glutathione peroxidase, the major enzyme which metabolizes H_2O_2, and other antioxidant enzymes may be reduced in older individuals.[8] The oxidative damage is thought to start in the nucleus of the lens where metabolic activities would be lowest and where modified proteins, susceptible to oxidation, would accumulate with age.[9]

Changes within the lens nucleus are usually accompanied by changes in other parts of the lens. Aging causes nuclear, cortical, and posterior subcapsular cataracts, each to varying degrees. When these changes cause a cataract in the lens, the patient may experience visual impairment, loss of contrast, dulling perception of color, and may also become increasingly myopic. In addition to loss of visual acuity, cataract development may be associated with visual abberations such as monocular double or triple vision.[10] Clinically mature or "ripe" cataracts may result in total opacification and liquefaction. A hypermature or "overripened" cataract sometimes progresses from the stage of morgagnian cataract (see below) to a shrunken membranous cataract after spontaneous loss of liquid protein and resorption of liquefied cortex.

Cataracts are clinically classified in different manners according to location, age of onset, appearance, or cause. The other sections of this book will thoroughly cover the etiology of cataracts related to disease and medications. At this point we will focus our chapter primarily on the histopathologic features of cataracts based mainly on location of the cataract within the lens.

■ CONGENITAL CATARACTS ■

Congenital cataracts are present at birth or noted shortly afterwards. The morphology of congenital cataracts can be helpful in establishing their etiology and prognosis.[11] They are usually bilateral and may occur in association with other medical problems. The insult to the developing lens is often mild enough that the resultant opacity does not interfere with vision.

Congenital zonular cataracts are characterized by opacities situated in one layer of the lens and surrounded by clear lens.

A central nuclear cataract from an insult early in development of the lens would be displaced deeper into the lens substance as new fibers grow throughout life.[12] An *embryonal nuclear cataract* results from an injury to the lens during the first 2 months of gestation and would be seen as a small central opacification. A *fetal nuclear cataract* (Figure 1-5) results from an insult at about the 3rd month of gestation and would lie between the level of the anterior and posterior Y-sutures or at the sutures (*sutural cataract*). Sutural opacities with secondary arborization or branching signify a teratologic insult later in gestation. A *perinuclear or lamellar zone* from a later insult would be arranged concentrically to the lens capsule with the cataractous layer surrounding the nucleus. The lamellar cataract takes its name from the laminar or sheet-like anatomy of the lens and is surrounded by the more peripheral clear cortical layers of the lens.[13,14]

Polar cataracts are opacities located on the anterior or posterior pole. Fibrous metaplasia of the anterior lens epithelium causes an *anterior polar cataract* (Figure 1-6). When caused by hyperplasia of the embryonal pupillary membrane, a conical mass of connective tissue (pyramidal cataract) protrudes into the anterior chamber. Histologically, a localized loss of epithelial cells with an

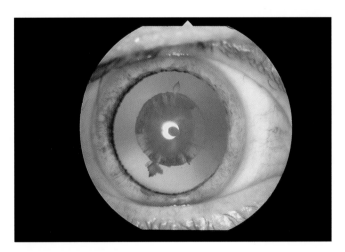

Figure 1-5 Fetal nuclear cataract. Clinical appearance of a central cataract surrounded by normal lens tissue.

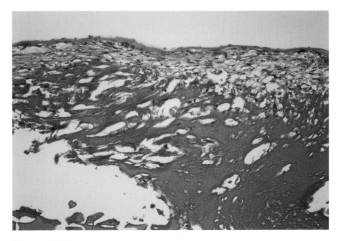

Figure 1-6 Anterior polar cataract. The lens epithelium has been replaced by fibrous metaplasia. (Hematoxylin and eosin [H & E] stain; X20.)

anterior subcapsular plaque is seen (see also anterior subcapsular cataract later in this chapter).

A *posterior polar cataract* is a larger disc-shaped opacity resulting from persistent hyperplastic primary vitreous, and can result in degeneration of the posterior subcapsular cortex with progressive opacification. A hyaloid vessel remnant, called a *Mittendorf dot*, is a small, dense white spot on the posterior surface of the lens and is clinically insignificant.

■ NUCLEAR CATARACTS ■

The most common age-related opacity of the lens is the nuclear sclerotic cataract (Figure 1-7). Increased compaction of nuclear fibers in age-related cataracts may be a contributing factor for excessive scatter in nuclear opacification.[15] Clinically, cataractous lens nuclei have decreased transparency in addition to the increased amount of pigmentation often found in normal aging. The lens nucleus normally appears histologically to have cellular laminations, which become more compact with aging. Lenses with nuclear sclerotic cataracts are characterized histopathologically by subtle changes with a dense homogeneous appearance (Figure 1-8). The laminations fade,

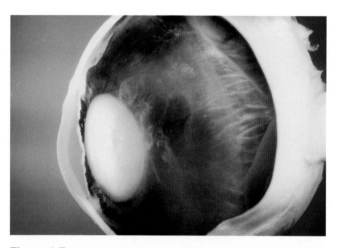

Figure 1-7 Cataractous lens. This enucleated globe is sectioned sagittally to show the gross appearance of a cataractous lens.

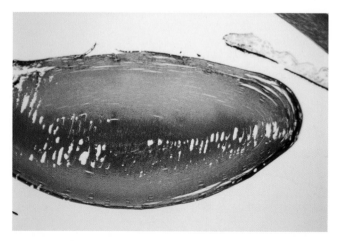

Figure 1-8 Nuclear sclerotic cataract. The nucleus from this post-mortem globe with a senile cataract takes on a dense homogenous appearance. Changes are often subtle, as in this specimen. (Trichrome stain; X2.)

and the nucleus becomes amorphous, taking on a more uniform eosinophilic staining characteristic. In an isolated nuclear sclerotic cataract, the surrounding cortical fibers would microscopically retain visible outlines of the cytoplasmic membranes. The increase in lens pigmentation seen clinically is not usually evident by histopathologic examination, but crystalline deposits are sometimes observed.[16]

■ CORTICAL CATARACTS ■

Aging changes in the lens cortex result in cortical cataracts. Cortical cataracts begin with relatively sharp clear fluid clefts which result in opaque spokes or can have more clear lamellar separations resulting in cuneiform-type opacities.[17] Lens epithelium likely plays a role in the loss of transparency of the cortex.[18] Insoluble proteins are assumed to be characteristic of cortical cataractous epithelium, which is also accompanied by various morphological abnormalities such as spokes or rosettes (Figure 1-9A, B).[19] Histopathologically, accumulation of eosinophilic fluid between lens cells with displacement and degeneration of bordering cells characterize cortical cataracts (Figure 1-10). Clefts seen microscopically correspond to visible changes observed clinically by slit-lamp examination. Spherical droplets or globules of released protein from the breakdown of cortical cell walls are called *morgagnian globules* (Figure 1-11). Encountering these droplets during surgical cataract excision may release milky fluid. These globules may accumulate and may eventually replace the entire cortex and result in a mature morgagnian cataract.[20] The central dense nucleus at this point would become gravity dependent often displaced inferiorly to the lower equatorial region of the lens (Figure 1-12).

The deep cortex of some lenses has been found to have crystalline deposits, which can appear as a "Christmas-tree cataract."[21] The crystals may be formed from cholesterol, lipids, calcium, or other compounds and in many cases does not decrease visual acuity unless other forms of cataracts coexist, but these crystals can be associated with phacolytic glaucoma.[22] Some forms of crystals are visible on histologic examination by use of cross-polarized filters.

In addition to various biochemical changes which may be related to the formation of cortical cataracts, physical forces must also be considered. An increase in nuclear lens hardening may lead to disaccommodation in older lenses which can theoretically develop mechanical sheer stresses between the soft cortex and the hard nuclei. These sheer stresses may be significant in the different cortical ruptures with a radial direction of sharply limited choroidal spokes or parallel micro-ridges at the area of lamellar separations which may explain some of the histopathologic changes seen in cortical cataracts. Various mechanical sharp limited cortical ruptures are caused by a combination of predisposing and sheer forces. The sheer forces occur during disaccommodation between the soft outer and the increasingly harder central lens layers.[17]

■ POSTERIOR SUBCAPSULAR CATARACTS ■

Clinically visible opacification located just anterior to the posterior lens capsule may be formed idiopathically or after an injury to the posterior area of the lens. In addition, posterior subcapsular cataracts may form secondary to multiple medications, such as

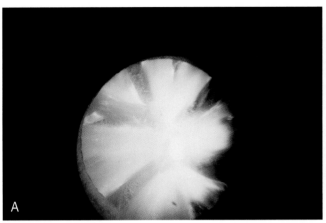 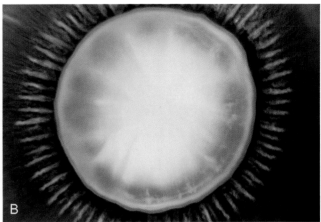

Figure 1-9 Cortical cataract. **A,** Clinical photograph of a senile cataract with cortical fluid clefts. **B,** Posterior view of an enucleated globe with cortical spokes.

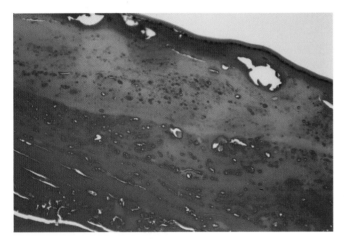

Figure 1-10 Cortical cataract. Histologic section of an early cortical cataract with accumulation of eosinophilic fluid between lens fibers. (Hematoxylin and eosin [H & E] stain; X10.)

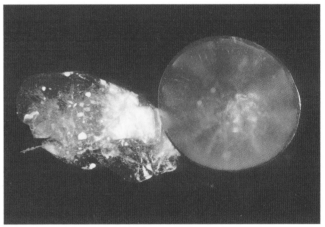

Figure 1-12 Morgagnian cataract. Gross appearance of a dense lens nucleus and its associated capsule in a mature morgagnian cataract.

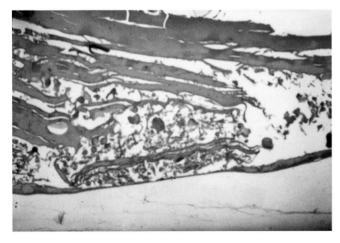

Figure 1-11 Morgagnian globules. Advanced cortical cataract with breakdown of lens proteins, histologically appearing as eosinophilic-staining spheres. (Hematoxylin and eosin [H & E] stain; X10.)

corticosteroids, and in association with various systemic conditions. These posterior subcapsular cataracts appear as focal dot-like granular areas or plaques in the posterior subcapsular cortex (Figure 1-13). This type of cataract is associated with degeneration of subcapsular posterior cortical cells followed by proliferation of peripheral lens epithelial cells, which migrate posteriorly beyond the lens bow at which it normally terminates.[23] The posterior migration of lens epithelial cells possibly represents an attempt to replace the degenerate, sometimes liquefied, lens substance in the cataractous lens and can be seen in diverse cataract conditions. The abnormally positioned epithelial cells enlarge and are called bladder or Wedl cells.[24] The nuclei of the bloated bladder cells are visible in histologic sections (Figure 1-14).

ANTERIOR SUBCAPSULAR ABNORMALITIES

Subepithelial lens opacities have been observed following an attack of acute glaucoma, and, when such an association exists, are described as *Glaukomflecken*. The severe elevation of

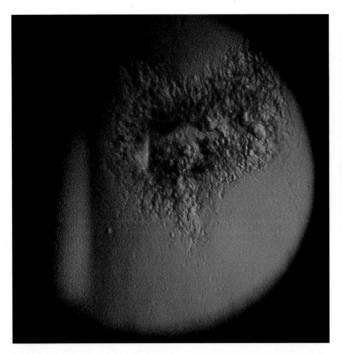

Figure 1-13 Posterior subcapsular cataract. Clinical photograph of a focal granular area in the posterior subcapsular cortex.

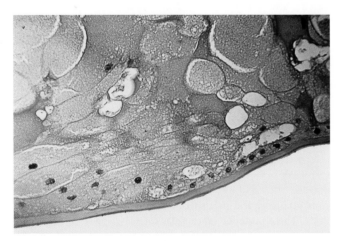

Figure 1-14 Bladder cells (Wedl cells). Lens epithelial cells have become swollen after abnormally migrating to the posterior pole of the lens. (Hematoxylin and eosin [H & E] stain; X20.)

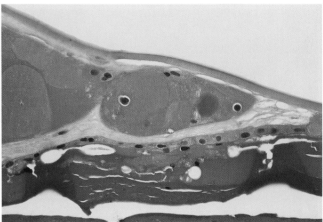

Figure 1-15 Anterior subcapsular cataract. Epithelial cells appear posterior to an abnormal fibrous plaque. (Hematoxylin and eosin [H & E] stain; X20.)

intraocular pressure may form grayish opacities localized beneath the anterior lens capsule, which histologically appear as focal areas of epithelial cell necrosis.[25] Epithelial cell degeneration can be in response to other insults, such as radiation and inflammation.

An *anterior subcapsular plaque* can form from proliferation and subsequent degeneration of lens epithelial cells leading to opacities. This type of cataract is usually the result of irritation, from uveitis, or disruption from trauma (discussed later in this chapter). Histologically, the plaque of the anterior or equatorial lens epithelium appears as a thin layer of fibrous tissue (fibrous metaplasia).[26] Multiple layers of such plaques may be laid down with intervening layers of normal cortex to form a reduplication cataract (Figure 1-15).

Anterior subcapsular cataracts have an accumulation of extracellular matrix that also contains lens epithelial cells which have fibroblast-like appearances. Studies of these various matrix components reveal them to be comprised of collagen, fibronectin, and fibrillin, as well as multiple different growth factors which may be responsible in helping to either signal or activate the lens epithelial cells in these types of cataracts.[27]

■ TRAUMATIC CATARACTS ■

Contusion of the eye may be severe enough to cause deposition of iris pigment on the lens capsule (Vossius ring). A Vossius ring is an imprint of the pupillary margin of the iris, and the pigment may resolve with time. Severe enough blunt force may cause formation of a cataract, which initially appears stellate with opacities lying in the cortex or capsule. Disruption of the lens zonular fibers due to injuries can cause the lens to be dislocated or partially dislocated (subluxated). Some blunt traumas cause both cataract formation and dislocation of the lens. The dislocation may be in any direction. Changes leading to lens opacity in traumatic cataracts appear to involve epithelial and subsequent cortical fiber deterioration.[28] In a contusion-type injury to the lens, traumatically induced dysfunction of lens epithelium may lead to edema of the superficial cortical lens fibers that subsequently undergo degeneration and produce a localized and permanent lamellar zone of vacuolization. With time and the formation of new clear lens cells, this layer becomes gradually compressed and displaced deeper into the cortex.[29]

Laceration or perforation of the lens capsule from trauma results in a localized opacity usually progressing to opacification of the entire lens. Histologically, the ruptured capsule typically appears as a wrinkled membrane. Opacities from small capsular injuries may remain stable as a focal cortical cataract, but exposed cortex often swells, expanding through the capsular tear. This process may induce a granulomatous inflammatory response of the remaining lens nucleus. Retained metallic foreign bodies within the lens may cause focal rusty appearing opacities (siderosis lentis).

The lens is susceptible to damage induced by ionizing radiation, with cataract formation often occurring many years after the initial exposure. Cataracts induced by radiation are usually observed in the posterior region of the lens, often in the form of a posterior subcapsular cataract.[30] There is a cumulative effect to radiation exposure of the lens, but large doses can cause sudden injury to lens epithelial cells and subsequent opacity of the entire lens. Infrared radiation and intense heat exposure to the lens, as seen in glass blowers, has caused cobweb-like cortical opacities and changes in the lens capsule.

When only a small portion of lens epithelial cells and cortical material remain in the periphery of the capsule following trauma or cataract extraction, a *Soemmerings' ring* cataract may form (Figure 1-16). The epithelial remnants undergo proliferation or fibrous metaplasia to form a doughnut-shaped ring. A histologic examination of the Soemmerings' ring would reveal a barbell-shaped cross-section with a residual lens capsular membrane forming the shaft that connects a bulbous prominence of retained lens cortex at one or both equators [31] (Figure 1-17).

Lens epithelial cells displaced through the capsule by accidental or surgical trauma can regenerate and proliferate in an abnormal location to form *Elschnig pearls*. Microscopically, the pearls resemble clusters of the bladder cells (Wedl cells) found in the posterior aspect of a cataractous lens, except they are found in the anterior chamber on the lens surface or iris stroma.

■ PSEUDOEXFOLIATION AND TRUE EXFOLIATION ■

Exfoliation syndrome (pseudoexfoliation) is a different entity to *true exfoliation*.[32] True exfoliation is a rare delamination of the lens capsule, which peels off in outward curling scrolls. Most patients with true exfoliation have a history of exposure to intense heat or infrared radiation. Histologically, the lens capsule appears thickened, and the outer portion may peel away from the intact layer closest to the lens epithelium. The peripheral portion of lens capsule often appears normal.[33]

In contrast, the more common pseudoexfoliation material is believed to be basement membrane material arising within the anterior chamber and appearing on the lens, iris, corneal endothelium, and trabecular meshwork. The material, initially believed to be a deposit on the lens,[32] is synthesized from lens epithelial cells, and by cells of the iris and ciliary epithelium.[34] Clinically, the deposit appears on the anterior lens capsule as a central disc surrounded by a relatively clear zone, surrounded by peripheral granular area. Pseudoexfoliation can cause secondary open-angle glaucoma called *glaucoma capsulare*. Weakening of the zonular fibers can complicate cataract surgery in these patients. Histopathologically, the lens capsule surface appears to have straight deposits resembling iron filings aligned on a magnet (Figure 1-18). The material may also be found on or within the iris, trabecular meshwork, and the corneal endothelium.

■ CONCLUSION ■

In conclusion, cataracts can present with a large variety of histopathologic changes. These cataractous changes can involve any of the structures of the lens including the nucleus and the cortex,

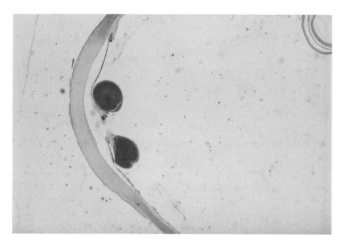

Figure 1-16 Soemmerings' ring cataract. The Soemmerings' ring in this eye formed after traumatic rupture of the capsule and loss of most of the lens contents. (Hematoxylin and eosin [H & E] stain; X2.).

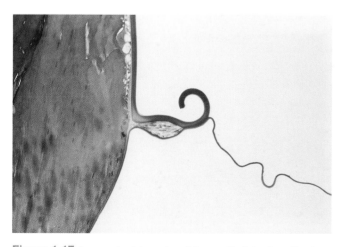

Figure 1-17 Soemmerings' ring cataract. Lens epithelial cells proliferate in the periphery of the lens capsule. (Trichrome stain x 40.)

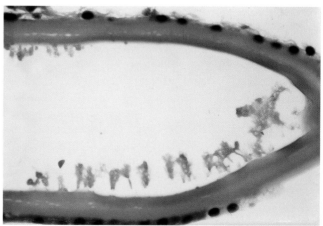

Figure 1-18 Pseudoexfoliation. This curled up piece of anterior lens capsule removed during cataract surgery shows deposits lined up resembling iron filings on a magnet. The outer surface of the lens capsule is opposite the remaining lens epithelial cells. (Hematoxylin and eosin [H & E] stain; X100.)

CONCLUSION

as well as anterior and posterior subcapsular areas. A thorough understanding of the pathology of various types of cataracts will allow the surgeon to more adequately prepare for the removal of a cataractous lens.

References

[1] Garner MH, Kuszak JR. Cations, oxidants, light as causative agents in senile cataracts. P R Health Sci 1993;12:115–122.

[2] Taylor VL, Al-Ghoul KJ, Lane CW, et al. Morphology of the normal human lens. Inv Oph & Vis Sci 1996;37:1396–1410.

[3] Heyworth P, Thompson GM, Tabandeh H, McGuigan S. The relationship between clinical classification of cataract and lens hardness. Eye 1993;7:726–730.

[4] Assia EI, Medan I, Rosner M. Correlation between clinical, physical, and histopathological characteristics of the cataractous lens. Graefes Arch Clin Exp Ophthalmol 1997;235:745–748.

[5] Duncan G, Wormstone IM, Davies PD. The aging human lens: structure, growth, and physiological behaviour. Br J Ophthalmol 1997;81:818–823.

[6] Clark JI, Clark JM. Lens cytoplasmic phase separation. Int Rev Cytol 2000;192:171–187.

[7] Truscott RJ. Age-related nuclear cataract: a lens transport problem. Ophthalmic Res 2000;32:185–194.

[8] Spector A. Oxidation and aspects of ocular pathology. J CLAO 1990;16:S8–10.

[9] Augusteyn RC. Protein modification in cataract: possible oxidative mechanisms. In: Duncan G, editor. Mechanisms of cataract formation in the human lens. London: Academic Press; 1981, p. 72–111.

[10] Campbell C. Observations on the optical effects of a cataract. J Cataract Refract Surg 1999; 25:995–1003.

[11] Lambert SR, Drack AV. Infantile cataracts. Surv Ophthalmol 1996;40:427–458.

[12] Eagle RCJ, Spencer WH. Lens. In Spencer WH, editor. Ophthalmic pathology: an atlas and textbook, 4th ed., vol. 1. Philadelphia: WB Saunders Company; 1996, p. 372–437.

[13] Grottrau PD, Schlotzer-Schrehardt U, Dorfler S, Naumann GOH. Congenital zonular cataract: clinicopathologic correlation with electron microscopy and review of literature. Arch Ophthalmol 1993;111:235–239.

[14] Potter WS. Pediatric cataracts. Ped Clin North Am 1993;40:841–851.

[15] Al-Ghoul KJ, Nordgren RK, Kuszak AJ, Freel CD, Costello MJ, Kuszak JR. Structural evidence of human nuclear fiber compaction as a function of aging and cataractogenesis. Exp Eye Res 2001;72:199–214.

[16] Zimmerman LE, Johnson FB. Calcium oxalate crystals within ocular tissues. Arch Ophthalmol 1958;60:372–383.

[17] Pau H. Cortical and subcapsular cataracts: significance of physical forces. Ophthalmologica 2006;220:1–5.

[18] Worgul BV, Merriam GRJ, Medvedovsky C. Cortical cataract development – an expression of primary damage to the lens epithelium. Lens Eye Toxic Res 1989;6:559–571.

[19] Kalariya N, Rawal UM, Vasavada AR. Human lens epithelial layer in cortical cataract. Indian J Ophthalmol 1998;46:159–162.

[20] Bron AJ, Habgood JO. Morgagnian cataract. Trans Ophthalmol Soc UK 1976;96:265.

[21] Shun-Shin GA, Vrensen GFJM, Brown NP. Morphologic characteristics and chemical composition of Christmas tree cataract. Invest Ophthalmol Vision Sci 1993;34:3489–3496.

[22] Flocks M, Litwin CS, Zimmerman LE. Phacolytic glaucoma: a clinicopathologic study of one hundred thirty-eight cases of glaucoma associated with hypermature cataract. Arch Ophthalmol 1955;54:37.

[23] Eshaghian J, Streeten BW. Human posterior subcapsular cataract, An ultrastructural study of the posteriorly migrating cells. Arch Ophthalmol 1980;98:134–143.

[24] Wedl C. Atlas der pathologischen Histologie des Auges. Leipzig: Wigand; 1860–1861.

[25] Anderson DR. Pathology of the glaucomas. Br J Ophthalmol 1972;56:146–157.

[26] Font RL, Brownstein S. A light and electron microscope study of anterior subcapsular cataracts. Am J Ophthalmol 1974;78:972–984.

[27] Ishida I, Saika S, Okada Y, Ohnishi Y. Grown factor deposition in anterior subcapsular cataract. J Cataract Refract Surg 2005;31:1219–1225.

[28] Rafferty NS, Goossens W, March WF. Ultrastructure of human traumatic cataract. Am J Ophthalmol 1974;78:985–995.

[29] Asano N, Schlotzer-Schrehardt U, Dofler S, Naumann GOH. Ultrastructure of contusion cataract. Arch Ophthalmol 1995;113:210–215.

[30] Lipman RM, Tripathi BJ, Tripathi RC. Cataracts induced by microwave and ionizing radiation. Surv Ophthalmol 1988;33:200–210.

[31] Apple DJ, Rabb MF. Lens and pathology of intraocular lenses. In Klein EA, editor. Ocular pathology, 3rd ed. St. Louis: Mosby; 1985, p. 118–159.

[32] Dvorak-Theobald GD. Pseudo-exfoliation of the lens capsule. Am J Ophthalmol 1954;37:1–12.

[33] Callahan A, Klien BA. Thermal detachment of the anterior lamella of the anterior lens capsule: a clinical and histopathologic study. Arch Ophthalmol 1958;59:73–80.

[34] Eagle RCJ, Font RL, Fine BS. The basement membrane exfoliation syndrome. Arch Ophthalmol 1979;97:510–515.

CONCLUSION

Surgical Anatomy, Biochemistry, Pathogenesis, and Classification of Cataracts

Leo T. Chylack, Jr., MD

2

CONTENTS

CHAPTER HIGHLIGHTS

>> Correlation of anatomy and surgery

>> Lens biochemistry, physiology, and metabolism

>> Lens opacity classification system (LOCS)

>> Mechanisms of cataract formation

>> Epidemiology of cataract

In the United States today, surgical extraction of the age-related cataract is the most frequently reimbursed operation in patients older than 65 years of age.[1] More than 1.4 million extractions per year are performed to restore visual function to older Americans. The technology supporting this procedure has evolved rapidly over the past 25 years as ophthalmic surgeons shifted from intracapsular to extracapsular techniques and as intraocular lenses (IOLs) replaced contact and spectacle lenses. The technology continues to evolve as new techniques and materials reduce costs and surgical complexity, and improve the optical quality of IOLs and the functional end results. In developing countries, modern techniques are being adapted by surgeons serving huge numbers of patients with cataract-related blindness. Age-related cataract (Figure 2-1) is the leading cause of visual impairment in the world today; more than 50 million individuals have cataract-related visual impairment.[2]

The timely dissemination of up-to-date surgical knowledge is one way in which skilled surgeons can address the worldwide problem of cataract-related visual impairment and blindness. This chapter focuses on the evaluation and surgical care of individual patients and thus may be more useful to the young surgeon beginning his or her training in cataract surgery or the older surgeon contemplating a change in surgical technique than to the public health official charged with organizing the treatment of cataract in millions of indigent patients. However, the most modern surgical techniques are being applied successfully even in the most primitive settings to alleviate visual loss, and we hope that this text facilitates the transfer of surgical knowledge to those areas of the world where it is badly needed.

SURGICAL ANATOMY OF THE LENS

The crystalline lens grows throughout life; changing its shape from a slightly rounded ovoid in childhood to a more flattened ovoid in old age. After the filling of the lens vesicle with lens fiber cells and the beginning of cortical fiber formation, the lens always contains a capsule, an anterior and equatorial layer of epithelium, a peripheral cortical region, and an inner nuclear core. In children and young adults with visually disabling cataracts, the capsule is strong, the vitreous is firm, and the ease with which the cortex and nucleus are removed is equal. In contrast, for older adults with age-related cataracts the surgeon must deal with an increasingly fragile capsule, a syneretic vitreous body, and a nucleus that may behave more like a piece of stone than a piece of living tissue. Knowledge of the surgical anatomy of the lens and of the changes that each region undergoes with age helps the surgeon to plan and execute a successful procedure regardless of the age of the patient.

CAPSULE

The capsule originates as the basement membrane of the epithelial cells of the embryonic lens vesicle, which it encapsulates in its entirety. As the posterior vesicle cells elongate anteriorly and fill

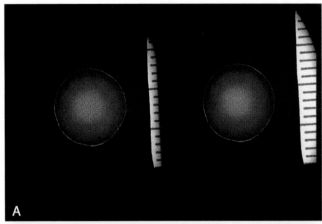

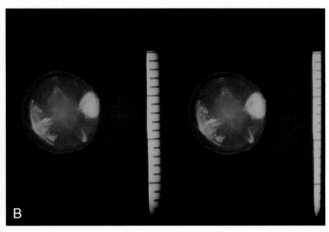

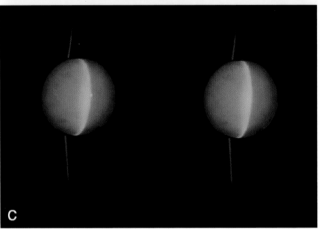

Figure 2-1 **A,** Minimal age-related nuclear cataract in an intracapsularly extracted lens. **B,** Moderately advanced mixed corticonuclear age-related intracapsularly extracted cataract. **C,** Hypermature age-related cataract.

the vesicle, the capsule assumes an anterior and posterior aspect. The anterior capsule remains a basement membrane for the epithelial cells, but the posterior capsule is now a thin membrane that is merely adherent to the fiber cells growing along its inner surface. A twofold increase in anterior capsule thickness occurs with age;[3] the capsule is always thinnest posteriorly.[4]

For more than a century accommodative changes in the lens have been attributed to the intrinsic elasticity of the capsule. It has been assumed that relaxation of lens zonules allowed capsular elasticity to deform (round up) the lens and increase accommodative power. However, more modern techniques have shown that the capsule distributes other forces on the lens (i.e., from the ciliary body) but does not act primarily to deform the shape of the lens. Mathematical modeling[5] of accommodation of the human lens has progressed and now is able to characterize some of the age-associated changes in this process.[6]

The surgeon performing neodymium:yttrium-aluminum-garnet (Nd:YAG) laser capsulotomy knows that the intrinsic elasticity or scrollability of the capsule is responsible for the expansion of the opening made by the laser pulse, and the scrolling usually occurs along the external surface of the capsular bag, suggesting that greater stress acts on the outer rather than the inner filaments of the capsule. The elastic characteristics of the capsule change with secondary cataract formation as a layer of epithelial and fibrous cells are laid down on the inner surface of the capsular scaffold. Less tendency to scroll externally exists;

often, cut flaps remain protruding stiffly into the optical zone. The formation of a capsular opacity may simply represent the continuation of the sliding movement of epithelial cells along the capsule that occurs normally in the lens. On the inner surface of the anterior capsule of the intact lens, the anterior epithelial cells move from the midperiphery to the equatorial region, where they differentiate into fiber cells. Lacking a cortical region to join, the cells may continue to move posteriorly along the intact capsule and form balloon cells, and fibrous or glassy plaques.

The expenditure of funds to cover the costs of treating posterior capsule opacification (PCO) is exceeded only by the cost of cataract surgery,[7] so there has been considerable interest in understanding the mechanism by which PCO occurs and in devising treatments for it. Many articles have emphasized the reduction in incidence of PCO if foldable acrylic IOLs are used.[8,9] It may be possible to reduce (or eliminate) PCO by developing improved IOL design, but a great deal of effort has been invested in studying the cell biology of this process using a variety of experimental systems (cultured human capsular bags obtained postmortem, cell culture systems, in vivo animal model systems, and in situ human observation).[10] Human lens epithelial cells can survive and multiply in serum-free cell culture, so there are intrinsic mechanisms sustaining these cells. If serum is added, however, the replication rate increases dramatically. This has led to the search for paracrine factors (proteins from other cells), and a number of candidates have been found (transferrin, basic fibroblast growth factor, epithelial growth factor, and transforming growth factor beta [TGF-β]) that either accelerate proliferation or stimulate transdifferentiation of epithelial cells into fiber cells. Also, autocrine factors (transferrin) and other cytokines have been found.[11,12] Simply performing a capsulorrhexis will stimulate epithelial cell proliferation[13] compared with the rate in the intact lens.

In a recent study of the effects of TGF-β2 on lens epithelial cells in capsular bag cultures, Wormstone et al[14] showed that a human monoclonal antibody CAT-152 (lerdelimumab) completely neutralized the effect of the TGF-β2-induced effects on the lens epithelial cells leading to PCO. Other approaches to preventing or minimizing PCO involve the addition of cytotoxins to the haptics and/or the IOLs, but in these cases, toxicity to other intraocular cells (particularly the corneal endothelium) is a major concern. These are all well reviewed in Wormstone's article.

A point about the anterior capsule that has surgical relevance is that it is thickest in the midperiphery. More peripherally the capsule thins considerably. This may be part of the reason why a capsulorrhexis placed too far peripherally extends into the equatorial region. The capsule tears easily as a circular disc if the tear is kept within the thicker zone.

EPITHELIUM

With age, the height of the epithelial cells decreases and the width increases. Some studies have shown that a decrease in the number of epithelial cells occurs with cataract formation; other studies have been unable to find decreased numbers of cells. No anatomic features of the epithelium exist that influence surgical technique, but all ophthalmic surgeons recognize that the epithelium is exquisitely sensitive to trauma; its key metabolic role makes it the "Achilles' heel" of the lens.

In addition to the accelerated proliferation of lens epithelial cells in response to paracrine, autocrine, and mechanical factors, these same cells may undergo apoptosis (programmed cell death) in response to oxidative stress and TGF-β2. Oxidative stress in a well-known risk factor for age-related cataract, and TGB-β2 is a growth factor associated with the cellular changes underlying PCO. It may be possible, however, to use this growth factor to increase apoptotic death of cells remaining on the posterior capsule after cataract surgery.

An excellent review of aspects of the lens epithelium that make it generally interesting to biologic scientists (no tumors were found in lens epithelium, and it is an excellent model for the effects of age on epithelial cell function) has been published.[15]

Another publication reveals the dramatic changes that occur in the lens epithelium with age,[16] showing that many "black holes" are apparent representing large areas of severely attenuated epithelial cells. In some areas there is no coverage of the overlying lens capsule. Other features (furrows, and cloudlike stuctures) are found in the aged epithelium, but none of these is associated with the type or severity of age-related cataract. It was hoped that noncontact specular microscopy could be used to identify patients at risk for cataract formation, but the changes noted are more a manifestation of aging than opacification.

CORTEX

The three-dimensional structure of the fiber cells in the developing lens has been published by Shestopalov and Bassnett.[17] Using

expression of green fluorescent protein in cells transfected by two different methods, they were able to show that the formation of the anterior and posterior sutures is asynchronous and that the disorganization of deep nuclear fiber cells seen in the aged lens is actually characteristic of the primary lens fibers in the embryonic lens and not a consequence of aging.

Several anatomic terms are used today to describe the different regions of the adult lens cortex:

- Peripheral cortex is just beneath the anterior epithelium or the posterior capsule.
- Supranuclear cortex is adjacent to the adult nucleus.
- Epinucleus is equivalent to the supranuclear region.
- Sutures are the lines formed by abutting ends of lens fibers.

Kuszak et al[18] have demonstrated in several studies the complex anatomy of human lens sutures (Figure 2-2). The dendritic suture structure of the adult cortical cataract often outlines the opaque cortical spoke.

Additional layers of cortical fibers are added throughout life, but the posterior cortex is always thinner than the anterior cortex.

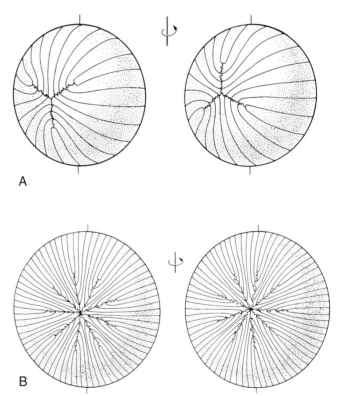

Figure 2-2 **A**, Scale computer-assisted drawings of the Y suture seen in normal human lenses at birth and in the fetal nucleus of senescent lenses. Left, Anterior Y suture. Right, Posterior inverted Y suture. Compare and contrast the irregular ends of secondary fiber cells overlapping to form suture branches with the regular and orderly juxtaposition of fiber cells along their length. The anterior and posterior suture patterns are directly offset as a result of opposite fiber cell end curvature. **B**, Scale computer-assisted drawings of the star suture seen in the cortex of normal, young adult human lenses and in the adult nucleus of normal, noncataractous, senescent lenses. Left, anterior; right, posterior. (From Kuszak JR, Deutsch TA, Brown HG: Biochemistry of the crystalline lens. In Albert DM, Jakobiec FA, editors: Priniciples and practice of ophthalmology, vol 1, Philadelphia, 1994, WB Saunders, p 569.)

What was the subcapsular region in the young child is the supranuclear or epinuclear region in the adult.

An interesting difference exists in the relationships among the capsule, the anterior epithelial cells, and the posterior lens fibers. The posterior fibers peel off easily from the capsule during stripping and aspiration, possibly because a potential space (the embryonic lens vesicle) exists between the posterior fibers and the posterior capsule. The anterior epithelial cells remain adherent to the anterior and equatorial capsule during stripping, perhaps because the capsule is part of the cell itself (its basement membrane) and not just a structure adjacent to it.

One may see the term followability in descriptions of the technique of aspirating lens cortex. It refers to the ease with which the cortex follows the aspiration tip as it strips the cortical fibers off the posterior capsule. Also, it means easily "aspiratable." Soft cortex is "followable;" stiff nuclear material is not.

NUCLEUS

Several anatomic terms refer to different concentric layers of the nucleus (Figure 2-3):

- Epinucleus is the outermost nucleus or innermost cortex.
- Adult nucleus is the next innermost layer.
- Fetal nucleus corresponds to the cotyledonous areas of light scattering in the clear adult lens.
- Embryonal nucleus is the innermost core of nucleus.

Surgically, the nucleus is characterized by a densely sclerotic posterior third, a slightly less sclerotic central core, and a softer peripheral shell. Occasionally in older patients, even the outermost nuclear shell is very rigid.

Nuclear sclerosis is an ambiguous misnomer often used inconsistently by clinical ophthalmologists to describe the yellowing and opacification of the nucleus with age. Modern systems of cataract classification identify the features of color change (brunescence) and opacification (opalescence) separately.

The term sclerosis is reserved for describing a tactile property of the nucleus – the increasing rigidity of the nucleus with age. This occurs as more cholesterol is incorporated into the

phospholipids of the lens membranes. The cholesterol-to-phospholipid ratio is a measure of capsular elasticity; it increases steadily with age and even more sharply after age 60 years.[19] Increasing nuclear sclerosis is responsible, in part, for the loss of the lens's focusing power on near subjects – a clinical age-related condition called presbyopia. Advanced sclerosis is also a major obstacle to phacosonication of the nucleus. If it is too sclerotic, the nucleus must be removed intact (as in a planned extracapsular extraction).

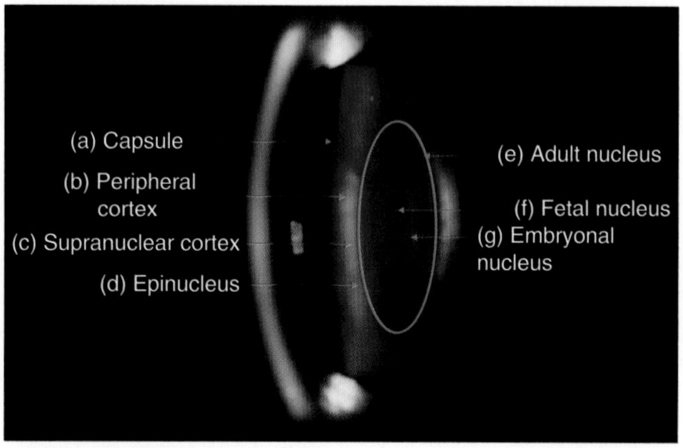

Opacification (or opalescence) of the nucleus is caused by the formation of light-scattering foci either in the nuclear fiber cytoplasm or on the nuclear plasma membranes. Light is scattered by huge protein aggregates that are formed as sulfhydryl (-SH) groups are oxidized to form protein-protein disulfide (-SS-) bonds and by larger molecular aggregates that have higher refractive indices than the monomeric proteins.[20]

The nucleus also changes color with age. The fetal lens is just a faintly perceptible yellow color; in the aged lens the nucleus may be golden yellow, orange, reddish brown, or black. This change in color is called brunescence (Figure 2-4). The change is distinct from the age-related increase in the light scattering (opalescence) of the nucleus. It is due to the accumulation of oxidized tryptophan (N-formylkynurenine), nonenzymatically glycated protein, and other chromophores. Moderate amounts of brunescence may be beneficial because chromophores absorb blue light and reduce glare. However, advanced brunescence causes a reduction in high-contrast acuity and contrast sensitivity independent of the opalescence of the nucleus.[21,22]

Good clinical correlation exists between the intensity of the brunescence and the hardness of the posterior nucleus. The intensity of the light scattering (opalescence) is also well correlated to the hardness of the nucleus.

OPTICAL BASIS OF TRANSPARENCY OF THE NORMAL LENS AND LIGHT SCATTERING IN CATARACT

The transparency of the normal lens is derived from its regular fiber arrangement and the minimal spatial variation in the index of refraction relative to the wavelength of incident light.[23,24]

In the cataractous lens, more abrupt changes occur in the index of refraction because of (1) the accumulation of fluid with a low index of refraction between fiber cells in cortical and subcapsular cataracts, (2) the formation of very high-molecular-weight cytoplasmic protein aggregates in nuclear cataracts, and (3) the binding of high-molecular-weight aggregates to cellular membranes in all forms of cataracts.[25–27]

BIOCHEMISTRY

The structural proteins of the lens are divided into three main groups (alpha, beta, and gamma crystallins) in order of decreasing molecular weight. Most of the enzymes are the size of beta-crystallins. They compose the pathways of aerobic metabolism in the organelle-rich epithelium and most superficial cortical fiber cells and anaerobic metabolism in the organelle-free fiber cell cytoplasm. The main metabolic substrate of lens is glucose derived from the aqueous humor, and the energy derived from

Figure 2-3 Color slit-lamp photograph of a clear lens showing the different cortical and nuclear layers.

(a) Capsule
(b) Peripheral cortex
(c) Supranuclear cortex
(d) Epinucleus
(e) Adult nucleus
(f) Fetal nucleus
(g) Embryonal nucleus

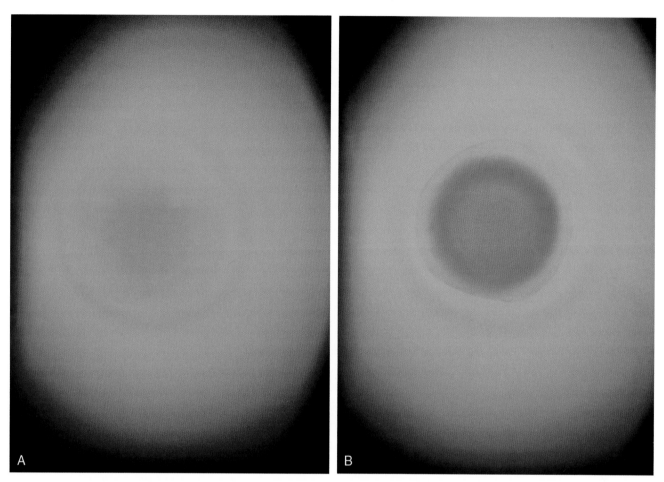

A   B

Figure 2-4 **A,** Minimal nuclear brunescence in an intracapsularly extracted lens photographed against a white background. **B,** Advanced nuclear brunescence in an intracapsularly extracted lens photographed against a white background.

glucose is used in protein-lipid synthesis, active transport of ions and amino acids, and maintenance of normal lens hydration. Kador[28] has provided an excellent summary of lens biochemistry and metabolism.

PHYSIOLOGY

Active transport mechanisms are found predominantly in the epithelium, and they are involved in the movement of ions, amino acids, and other metabolites. The movement of water in the lens is governed by the movement of ions or osmotically active substances, and a disruption of the normal movement of water in the lens can lead to acute cataract formation. In patients with insulin-dependent, acidotic diabetes who are brought back to euglycemia too rapidly, a mature or hypermature cataract occasionally forms within a few hours. The cataract is caused by the rapid movement of water into the lens to neutralize the hyperosmolarity in the fiber cytoplasm resulting from the abundant sorbitol (an impermeable sugar alcohol) found there. Sorbitol is the sugar alcohol of glucose; as it accumulates in the cytoplasm, it renders the cytoplasm hypertonic relative to the extracellular space, and water moves rapidly into the fiber cell. The abrupt lowering of the index of refraction of the cytoplasm as water enters the cell results in light scattering. Trauma may

disrupt epithelial active transport and water flux and result in rapid loss of lens clarity.

Although it has been known for decades that ascorbic acid is actively transported into the lens, only recently have the transport proteins been identified.[29] The specific ascorbic acid transporter SVCT2 was found in an epithelial cell line, and its gene expression was upregulated by oxidants and other cytokines. This paper suggests that such a transport system and the important antioxidant ascorbic acid may respond to the level of ambient oxidative stress.

Rae[30] provides an excellent review of lens physiology.

MECHANISMS OF CATARACT FORMATION

The following sections discuss the known mechanisms of cataract formation.

OSMOTIC STRESS

Osmotic stress in the diabetic cataract has been discussed previously. A similar mechanism is believed to apply in the human galactosemic cataract. In both the galactosemic and diabetic cataract, sugars are converted to their respective sugar alcohol by the enzyme aldose reductase in what is called the sorbitol pathway. The sorbitol pathway is composed of the enzymes aldose reductase and polyol dehydrogenase (iditol dehydrogenase). Like sorbitol, galactitol (dulcitol) cannot pass through plasma membranes, and once formed, it remains in the cytoplasm. Water enters the cell to neutralize the hyperosmolarity of the cytoplasm, and the epithelial and fiber cells swell. Also, low-index refraction fluid accumulates between fiber cells in sugar cataracts. Both intracellular and intercellular changes combine to create light-scattering foci and lens opacification.

The role of the sorbitol pathway in human, diabetic, age-related cataract is uncertain; there is not a lot of aldose reductase activity in the human lens epithelium and even less in the fiber cell cytoplasm of the cortex and nucleus.

When performing intraocular surgery, it is important to maintain the proper tonicity (ion concentration) and osmolarity of fluids infused into the eye. Before the introduction of salt solutions with the proper tonicity, osmolarity, and nutrient content, osmotically induced secondary cataracts were a frequent intraoperative or post-operative complication in vitrectomy surgery. In fact, the clear lens was often removed prophylactically during vitrectomy, because post-operative osmotic secondary cataract formation was seen so often.

PROTEIN AGGREGATION

None of the individual crystallin proteins in the clear lens is large enough to scatter light. In the aging lens and in the nuclear cataract, however, the different crystallins combine to form huge aggregates that are large enough to scatter light. The aggregation of millions of light-scattering foci in the lens constitutes a cataract. These aggregates may exist free in the cytoplasm (in nuclear cataracts) or may be bound to cell membranes (in cortical and posterior subcapsular cataracts).

OXIDATIVE STRESS

Oxidative stress denotes the adverse effects of oxygen and its various redox forms on the constituents of the lens. Oxygen can exist as hydrogen peroxide, singlet oxygen, hydroxyl radical, and superoxide. There are enzyme systems in the lens that produce and destroy these redox species. The relative balance between systems that produce and systems that destroy these oxidants determines whether or not the lens suffers oxidative damage. If the defense mechanisms are deficient, hydrogen peroxide can accumulate and (1) deactivate sulfhydryl-dependent enzyme systems, (2) aggregate proteins by forming protein–protein disulfide bridges, (3) change lens color by forming chromophores, or (4) disrupt membrane structure.

An excellent brief review of glutathione (GSH), an important antioxidant in the lens, has been published.[31] GSH participates in a redox cycle in the lens and is able to detoxify hydrogen peroxide, hydroxyl radical, and dehydroascorbic acid. Loss of GSH is associated with membrane damage and protein aggregation – factors underlying early opacification.

POSTTRANSLATIONAL PROTEIN CHANGES

In addition to oxidative damage, other changes in lens proteins occur after the protein is formed; these constitute posttranslational changes and include nonenzymatic glycosylation, racemization, and aggregation.

PHASE SEPARATION

One reversible mechanism of aggregation is phase separation.[32] As the temperature drops, certain protein molecules form large groups; although the individual protein molecules are not covalently bound together, the size of the group is large enough to scatter light. This mechanism applies to the cold cataract often seen in cooled calf lenses. Its relevance to human cataract is yet unknown. Whether or not phase-separated proteins are more likely to form covalently bound aggregates remains to be determined.

■ METABOLISM ■

Aberrant lens metabolism is suspected as a causative mechanism in many cataracts, but there is little evidence supporting this suspicion in humans. When specific abnormalities have been sought in cataractous lens epithelium, surprisingly normal metabolic activity has often been found. In the older human lens, there is little metabolic activity in the cortex and nucleus, even in the clear lens. Except for the declining ability of the lens to metabolically resist oxidative damage, there is little evidence that cataract formation is a metabolic event.

Of particular interest is the ability of the lens to accumulate dietary antioxidants. A recent study of one of the dietary carotenoids, lycopene, showed that this substance reduced the osmotic effects associated with galactose exposure and the extent of oxidative damage.[33] This report suggests that this dietary carotenoid can get into the lens where it does help to offset osmotic and oxidative stress.

■ CATARACT CLASSIFICATION ■

RATIONALE

Until recently, there has been little need to accurately classify cataract type or severity. Traditionally, clinicians have used anatomic (cortical, nuclear, etc.) or etiologic (radiation, steroid, etc.) terms to describe the type of cataract. Descriptors of cataract severity have been based on coarse, subjective scales and have included terms such as immature, advanced immature, and mature. As basic scientists developed means of identifying and quantitating mechanisms of human cataract formation, it became necessary to more accurately and consistently describe or classify cataracts.[34–37] Also, as pharmaceutical companies encountered drugs with cataractogenic toxicity and as epidemiologists began to study the risk factors of human cataract formation, better systems of cataract classification were needed. Several have been developed, and they include the Lens Opacities Classification System, versions I to III (LOCS I to III);[38–40] the Oxford Cataract Classification System;[41,42] the Wilmer System;[43,44] and the Wisconsin System.[45] The World Health Organization (WHO), in collaboration with many of the originators of the other cataract classification systems, sponsored the development and testing of a "simplified" cataract grading scheme which was published in 2002.[46] The simplification refers to the ability to use this system in the field and the reduced number of standards needed to grade the severity of cataract. The WHO anticipates using this system to estimate the type and severity of cataracts in patients who are blind from cataract. Such data will help host countries to plan their programs to care for these patients and for patients likely to soon become cataract blind. The reduced number or standard images in the WHO's system may reduce the applicability of this system to studies aimed at detecting the smallest amount of cataractous change in the shortest possible period (e.g., assessing the cataractogenic potential of new system drug candidates or measuring the impact of nonsurgical treatments of age-related cataract in the shortest possible time).

■ LENS OPACITIES CLASSIFICATION SYSTEM ■

A purposely degraded image of the set of LOCS III standards is reproduced in Figure 2-5. This figure is to be used only to understand the general format of the LOCS III standards. The images in Figure 2-5 should not be used for grading cataracts in patients because the image quality has been purposely degraded.[40] Non-degraded LOCS III standard images are available from the author. In the LOCS III system, the grader, working at the slit-lamp microscope with a set of standards on a nearby light box, estimates separately the extent of cortical and subcapsular cataract, the intensity of light scattering in the nucleus, and the color of the nucleus. Grades are in decimal form; for example, a cortical cataract, the severity of which is judged to be intermediate between cortical standards 2 and 3, would be graded 2.5. Similar grades could be generated for different degrees of nuclear opalescence and nuclear color. The LOCS II and III systems have been validated[47] and used widely in pharmaceutical trials, natural history studies, and other epidemiologic studies.

There has been some interest in using the LOCS II and III systems in clinical practice. It has been considered helpful in following the severity of a cataract and communicating information about cataract type and severity to patients. It has also been used to grade the intensity of nuclear opalescence and color in planning phacoemulsification surgery.[48] The greater the LOCS III grade for nuclear opalescence and nuclear color, the more likely it is that the nucleus will be sclerotic. Little apparent correlation exists between the ease of aspirating an opaque cortex or subcapsular lens fibers and the LOCS III grade. Clear cortex can be aspirated as easily as opaque cortex.

OBJECTIVE DOCUMENTATION OF CATARACT

Even finer grading of cataract severity is possible with standardized lens photography and techniques of image analysis. Such techniques include measurement of nuclear density,[49,50] the area of cortical or subcapsular opacity,[51,52] or the color of the nucleus[53,54] using Scheimpflug slit images, retroillumination images, or color slit images, respectively. These techniques allow measurement of the rates of change in cataract severity in different populations.

■ EPIDEMIOLOGY, RISK FACTORS, AND MEDICAL TREATMENT OF CATARACT ■

EPIDEMIOLOGY AND RISK FACTORS OF AGE-RELATED CATARACT

Many risk factors of age-related cataract have been identified during the past 20 years.[55-57] Factors that increase the risk of age-related cataract include female sex, smoking, heavy alcohol intake, limited education, use of corticosteroids, increased sun exposure, black race, dehydrating diarrhea, myopia, protein-deficient and specific amino acid-deficient diets, and diabetes mellitus. Factors that lower the risk of cataract include the use of multivitamin supplements and, possibly, aspirin.[58,59]

MEDICAL TREATMENT OF CATARACT

Many surgeons have expressed their conviction that surgery is the only appropriate treatment of cataract-related visual loss or blindness. In many parts of the world, however, there are too few surgeons and too many patients with visually disabling cataract. In these situations, the ability to address the age-related cataract problem with a medical, nutritional, or environmental approach would greatly reduce suffering and the need for medical and surgical care. Viewing cataract-related blindness from a worldwide perspective places the nonsurgical management of cataract in the proper context.

In many parts of the world, drugs with alleged anticataract efficacy are marketed widely and enjoy huge sales. None of these preparations has been shown to be effective through rigorous clinical investigative methods. Until recently, many countries were allowed to market drugs proved safe even though they were not proved effective. In countries in which medical practitioners are unable to offer cataract surgery to patients with cataract-related visual loss, use of preparations with purported anticataract efficacy and positive placebo effects might be understandable. However, the economic cost of using these nostrums is high, and such economic resources might be better spent on improving the surgical care delivered to such patients.

A National Eye Institute-sponsored 5-year study of the natural history of age-related cataract formation (the Longitudinal Study of Cataract) has been completed.[60,61] This study measured the rates of cortical, nuclear, and posterior subcapsular cataract formation and rates of nuclear brunescence. It also related personal, environmental, occupational, and nutritional data to these rates and provided insights into nonsurgical methods of intervening to slow the rates of age-related cataract formation (e.g., decrease smoking, use multivitamin antioxidants, avoid high body mass index [obesity]).

Two prospective, randomized, placebo-controlled clinical trials of the effect of antioxidant vitamins on the rate of age-related cataract have been published.[62,63] Interestingly, the Roche European American Cataract Trial (REACT) showed that a micronutrient mixture containing vitamin C, vitamin E, and beta-carotene was able to produce a small deceleration of progression of age-related cataract. The Age-Related Eye Disease Study (AREDS) trial using a similar mixture, but with lower dosages, showed no beneficial effects on cataract progression. Knowing whether or not these vitamins and beta-carotene slow age-related cataract will have to await the completion of a third randomized, placebo-controlled trial.

Unfortunately, at present, few additional medical anticataract agents have potential. In the United States, a phase separation inhibitor was tested as a means of slowing or preventing the nuclear cataract that follows vitrectomy and was found to have no beneficial effect. At present, it is particularly frustrating to have the technology to test anticataract drug efficacy but few anticataract agents to test.

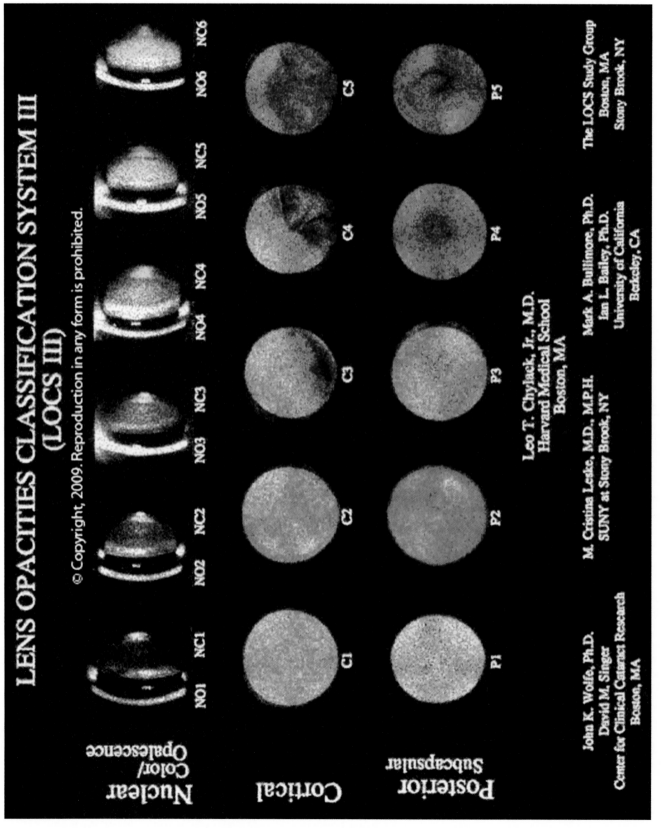

Figure 2-5 Lens Opacities Classification System, version III (LOCS III). Note: This figure illustrates only the format of the LOCS III standards: these standard images should not be used for grading cataracts in patients as the image quality of all standards has been purposely degraded. LOCS III consists of six standards to grade nuclear opalescence (NO) and nuclear color (NC), five to grade cortical cataract (C), and five to grade posterior subcapsular cataract (P). (Copyright 1992 retained by Leo T. Chylack, Jr, MD. Reprinted with permission from Archives of Ophthalmology.) Non-degraded standard images are available from the author.

Fortunately, in countries with great shortages of surgical practitioners, there are now low-cost, modern, surgical options for caring for patients with cataract-related blindness. From the cataract camps in India to the technician-staffed operating rooms in Africa, one sees ingenious ways of providing surgical care for patients with cataract where it is most needed.

References

[1] Stark WJ, Sommer A, Smith RE. Changing trends in intraocular lens implantation. Arch Ophthalmol 1989;107:1441.

[2] International Agency for the Prevention of Blindness. World blindness and its prevention. New York: Oxford University Press; 1980.

[3] Tripathi RC, Tripathi BJ. Lens morphology, aging, and cataract. J Gerontol 1983;38:258.

[4] Fincham EF. The mechanism of accommodation. Br J Ophthalmol 1937;8:5.

[5] Koretz JF, Handelman GH. A model for accommodation in the young human eye: the effects of elastic anisotropy on the mechanism. Vision Res 1983;23:1679.

[6] Burd HJ, Judge SJ, Cross JA. Numerical modeling of the accommodating lens. Vision Res 2002;42:2235.

[7] Bertelmann E, Kojetinsky C. Posterior capsule opacification and anterior capsule opacification. Curr Clin Ophthalmol 2001;12:35.

[8] Apple DJ, Peng Q, Visessook N et al. Eradication of posterior capsule opacification: documentation of a marked decrease in Nd:YAG laser posterior capsulotomy rates noted in an analysis of 5416 pseudophakic human eyes obtained post-mortem. Ophthalmology 2001;108:505.

[9] Javdani SM, Huygens MM, Callebaut F. Neodymium:YAG capsulotomy rates after phacoemulsification with hydrophobic and hydrophilic acrylic intraocular lenses. Bull Soc Belge Ophtalmol 2002;283:13.

[10] Wormstone M. Posterior capsule opacification: a cell biological perspective. Exp Eye Res 2002;74:337.

[11] Majima K. Human lens epithelial cells proliferate in response to exogenous EGF and have EGF and EGF receptor. Ophthalmic Res 1995;27:356.

[12] Wormstone IM, Tamiya S, Marcantonio JM et al. Hepatocyte growth factor and c-Met expression in human lens epithelial cells. Invest Ophthalmol 2000;41:4216.

[13] Rakic JM, Galand A, Vrensen GF. Separation of fibers from the capsule enhances mitotic activity of human lens epithelium. Exp Eye Res 1997;64:67.

[14] Wormstone IM, Tamiya S, Anderson I et al. TGF-beta2-induced matrix modification and cell transdifferentiation in the human lens capsular bag. Invest Ophthalmol Vis Sci 2002;43:2301.

[15] Bhat SP. The ocular lens epithelium. Biosci Rep 2001;21:537.

[16] Balaram M, Kuszak JR, Ayaki M et al. Noncontact specular microscopy of human lens epithelium. Invest Ophthalmol Vis Sci 2000;41:474.

[17] Shestopalov VI, Bassnett S. Three-dimensional organization of primary lens fiber cells. Invest Ophthalmol Vis Sci 2000;41:859.

[18] Kuszak JR, Bertram BA, Macsai MS et al. Sutures of the crystalline lens: a review. Scanning Electron Microsc 1984;3:1369.

[19] Li LK, So L, Spector A. Age-dependent changes in the distribution and concentration of human lens cholesterol and phospholipids. Biochim Biophys Acta 1987;917:112.

[20] Siezen RJ, Owen EA. Physicochemical characterization of high-molecular-weight alpha-crystallin subpopulations from the calf lens nucleus. Biochim Biophys Acta 1983;749:227.

[21] Chylack Jr LT, Padhye N, Khu PM et al. Loss of contrast sensitivity in diabetic patients with LOCS II classified cataract. Br J Ophthalmol 1993;77:7.

[22] Chylack Jr LT, Jakubicz G, Rosner B et al. Contrast sensitivity and visual acuity, as functions of cataract type and extent. J Cataract Refract Surg 1993;19:399.

[23] Benedek GB. Theory of transparency of the eye. Appl Opt 1971;10:459.

[24] Trokel S. The physical basis for transparency of the crystalline lens. Invest Ophthalmol 1962;1:493.

[25] Tripathi RC, Tripathi BJ. Morphology of the normal, aging, and cataractous human lens. II. Optical zones of discontinuity and senile cataract. Lens Res 1983;1:43.

[26] Harding CV, Maisel H, Chylack Jr LT et al. The structure of the human cataractous lens. In: Maisel H, editor. The ocular lens: structure, function and pathology. New York: Marcel Dekker; 1985.

[27] Vrenson G, Willekens B. Biomicroscopy and scanning electron microscopy of early opacities in the aging human lens. Invest Ophthalmol Vis Sci 1990;31:1582.

[28] Kador PF. Biochemistry of the lens: intermediary metabolism and sugar cataract formation. In: Albert DM, Jakobiec FA, editors. Principles and practice of ophthalmology (basic sciences). Philadelphia: WB Saunders; 1994, p. 146.

[29] Kannan R, Stolz A, Ji Q et al. Vitamin C transport in human lens epithelial cells: evidence for the presence of SVCT2. Exp Eye Res 2001;73:159.

[30] Rae J. Physiology of the lens. In Albert DM, Jakobiec FA, editors: Principles and practice of ophthalmology (basic sciences). Philadelphia: WB Saunders; 1994, p. 123.

[31] Giblin FJ. Glutathione: a vital lens antioxidant. J Ocular Pharmacol Ther 2000;16:121.

[32] Clark JI, Benedek GB. Phase diagram for cell cytoplasm from the calf lens. Biochem Biophys Res Commun 1980;95:482.

[33] Mohanty I, Joshi S, Trivedi D et al. Lycopene prevents sugar-induced morphological changes and modulates antioxidant status of human lens epithelial cells. Br J Nutr 2002;88:347.

[34] Marcantonio JM, Duncan G, Davies PD et al. Classification of human senile cataracts by nuclear color and sodium content. Exp Eye Res 1980;31:227.

[35] Chylack Jr LT, Lee MR, Tung WH et al. Classification of human senile cataractous change by the American Cooperative Cataract Research Group (CCRG) Methods I: instrumentation and technique. Invest Ophthalmol Vis Sci 1983 1983;24:424, 1983.

[36] Chylack Jr LT, White O, Tung WH. Classification of human senile cataractous change by the American Cooperative Cataract Research Group (CCRG) Methods II: staged simplification of cataract classification. Invest Ophthalmol Vis Sci 1984;25:166.

[37] Chylack Jr LT, Ransil BJ, White O. Classification of human senile cataractous change by the American Cooperative Cataract Research Group (CCRG) Methods III: the association of nuclear color (sclerosis) with extent of cataract formation, age and visual acuity. Invest Ophthalmol Vis Sci 1984;25:174.

[38] Chylack Jr LT, Leske MC, Sperduto R et al. Lens Opacities Classification System. Arch Ophthalmol 1988;106:330.

[39] Chylack Jr LT, Leske MC, McCarthy D et al. Lens Opacities Classification System II (LOCS II). Arch Ophthalmol 1989;107:991.

[40] Chylack Jr LT, Wolfe JK, Singer DM et al. The Lens Opacities Classification System, Version III (LOCS III). Arch Ophthalmol 1993;111:831.

[41] Sparrow JM, Bron AJ, Brown NAP et al. The Oxford clinical cataract classification and grading system. Int Ophthalmol 1986;9:207.

[42] Sparrow JM, Ayliffe W, Bron AJ et al. Inter-observer and intra-observer variability of the Oxford clinical cataract classification and grading system. Int Ophthalmol 1988;11:151.

[43] West SK, Taylor HR. The detection and grading of cataract: an epidemiological perspective. Surv Ophthalmol 1986;31:175.

[44] Taylor HR, West SK. The grading of lens opacities. Aust NZ J Ophthalmol 1989;17:81.

[45] Klein BEK, Magii YL, Neider MW et al. Wisconsin system for classification of cataracts from photographs. NTIS Accession No. PB 90-138306. Available from National Technical Information Service, 5285 Port Royal Rd., Springfield, VA 22161.

[46] Thylefors B, Chylack Jr LT, Konyama K et al. A simplified cataract grading system. Ophthalmic Epidemiol 2002;9:83.

[47] Maraini G, Pasquini P, Tomba MC, et al., The Italian-American Cataract Study Group: An independent evaluation of the Lens Opacities Classification System (LOCS II). Ophthalmology 1989;96:611.

[48] Davison JA, Chylack Jr LT. Clinical application of the lens opacities classification system III in the performance of phacoemulsification. J Cataract Refract Surg 2003;29:138–145.

[49] Chylack Jr LT, Mantel G, Wolfe J et al. Monitoring cataract with LOCS II and counterpart objective measures: lovastatin and the human lens, results of a two year study. Optom Vis Sci 1993;70:937.

[50] Chylack LT, McCarthy D, Khu P. Use of Topcon SL-45 Scheimpflug slit photography to measure longitudinal growth of nuclear cataracts in vivo. Lens Res 1988;5:83.

[51] Wolfe JK, Chylack Jr LT. Objective measurement of cortical and subcapsular opacification in retroillumination photographs. Ophthalmic Res 1990;22:62.

[52] Wolfe JK, Chylack Jr LT. Differentiation between cortical and posterior subcapsular cataract using pattern matching in computerized image analysis. Invest Ophthalmol Vis Sci 1989;31:353.

[53] Herzberg S, McCarthy D, Kansupada K et al. Positional dependence of objective measures of nuclear color in the lens: correlation with LOCS II score. Invest Ophthalmol Vis Sci 1989;31:352.

[54] Chylack Jr LT, Wolfe JK, Friend J et al. Quantitating cataract and nuclear brunescence: the Harvard and LOCS systems. Optom Vis Sci 1993;70:886.

[55] Leske MC, Chylack LT, Suh-Wuh W et al. The lens opacities case control study: risk factors for cataract. Arch Ophthalmol 1991;109:244.

[56] The Italian-American Study Group. Risk factors for age-related cortical, nuclear, and PSC cataracts. Am J Epidemiol 1991;133:541.

[57] Harding JJ, van Heyningen R. Epidemiology and risk factors for cataract. Eye 1987;1:537.

[58] Cotlier E, Sharma YR. Aspirin and senile cataracts in rheumatoid arthritis. Lancet 1981;1:338.

[59] Seddon JM, Christen WG, Manson JE et al. Low-dose aspirin and risks of cataract in a randomized trial of US physicians. Arch Ophthalmol 1991;109:252.

[60] Leske MC, Chylack Jr LT, Wu SY et al. Incidence and progression of nuclear opacities in the Longitudinal Study of Cataract. Ophthalmology 1996;103:705.

[61] Leske MC, Chylack Jr LT, He Q et al. Incidence and progression of cortical and posterior subcapsular opacities: the Longitudinal Study of cataract. Ophthalmology 1997;104:1987.

[62] Chylack Jr LT, Brown NP, Bron A et al. The Roche European American Cataract Trial (REACT): a randomized clinical trial to investigate the efficacy of an oral antioxidant micronutrient mixture to slow the progression of age-related cataract. Ophthalmic Epidemiol 2002;9:49.

[63] AREDS Research Group. A randomized, placebo-controlled, clinical trial of high-dose supplementation with vitamins C and E and beta-carotene for age-related cataract and vision loss: AREDS Report No. 9. Arch Ophthalmol 2001;119:1439.

EPIDEMIOLOGY, RISK FACTORS, AND MEDICAL TREATMENT OF CATARACT

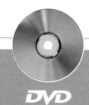

Preoperative Evaluation of the Patient with Visually Significant Cataract

Samuel Masket, MD and Shaleen Belani, MD

3

CHAPTER HIGHLIGHTS

>> Factors that influence endophthalmitis

>> Reduction of intraocular inflammation

>> Intraocular pressure fluctuations after cataract surgery

Preoperative evaluation of patients with visually significant cataracts is threefold. It includes an appreciation of the severity of the cataract, an assessment of the overall visual prognosis after cataract extraction, and a determination of preoperative conditions that may complicate surgery. The latter, in particular, includes the now well described intraoperative floppy iris syndrome (IFIS) associated with the use of alpha blocking agents, originally described by Chang and Campbell.[1]

Advanced cataract formation produces a characteristic symptom, profound visual loss, which may be deduced from the patient's medical history. Likewise, the physical findings of a well-developed cataract can be determined during a basic ocular examination, which includes simple tests of visual function. Cataracts in earlier stages or in eyes with concomitant disease, however, require a greater degree of diagnostic skill and clinical investigation to determine the visual significance of the cataract and how to best advise and treat the patient in question.

Until recently, the only device used to assess the loss of visual function associated with cataract formation was Snellen acuity testing developed by Dr. Hermann Snellen during the middle of the nineteenth century. Snellen testing employs high-contrast familiar letter optotypes. As such, it is a measure of the optical resolving power of the ocular system. Moreover, Snellen testing is performed under the controlled lighting conditions (generally darkened) of the refracting lane and therefore does not simulate the varied visual challenges of daily life. Patients with certain types of cataract in relatively early stages often note diminished visual function, although good Snellen acuity may be maintained.[2,3,4,5]

Given that "real-life" conditions present a far more complex series of visual clues to interpret than does Snellen testing, there has been an interest in and a need for the development of additional methods for testing visual function. Such devices have been referred to as tests of "functional vision," which are designed to simulate the visual disability induced by ocular disease and its impact on the visual tasks presented under conditions of daily life. Two general categories of functional vision testing devices have been developed; one system tests for glare disability, or diminution of vision induced by ambient light, and the other evaluates contrast sensitivity function (CSF), which tests visual recognition of varying target sizes against backgrounds of differing contrasts. Although the two testing systems have significant overlaps and a reduction in one function often leads to a diminution of the other, they are distinctly different, but vital, aspects of functional vision evaluation. They are useful in assessing the visual loss attributed to cataract and other ocular diseases when good Snellen acuity is noted despite significant visual complaints offered by the patient. Tests of visual function are designed to aid in the determination of the visual significance of cataract formation; they are not intended to be used as screening devices or to induce patients without functional complaints to have surgery.

Preoperative evaluation of the patient with cataract additionally requires an appreciation of the visual prognosis for surgery, or potential visual acuity. This is particularly valuable for patients with ocular disease occurring in association with cataract formation. Several methods are available to help determine the potential postoperative vision.

During the last decade, the Agency for Health Care Policy and Research, a previous arm of the Department of Health and Human Services, performed a comprehensive review of cataract care and issued a set of guidelines outlining suggested preoperative, intraoperative, and postoperative management of the adult with cataract.[6] They were a framework on which a paradigm (see further on) was constructed for the evaluation of the adult with cataract. Included in the guidelines, among other material, was a review of the ophthalmic literature regarding preoperative functional vision testing. The guidelines recognized that functional vision loss may be noted with certain cataract types and good Snellen acuity. Recently, The American National Standards Institute (ANSI) designated linear sine-wave gratings as the standard for measurement of contrast sensitivity. A survey of members of the American Society of Cataract and Refractive Surgery in 1998 indicated that 65% of the respondent members employed either glare disability testing or CSF in evaluating the patient with cataract.[7]

On the other hand, advanced cataracts, those that prohibit adequate ophthalmoscopy, require to be evaluated for the potential visual benefit of their removal because the integrity of the retina and optic nerve cannot be assessed by routine means.

Finally, the preoperative evaluation should include an assessment of conditions that may complicate surgery. This includes as assessment of pupillary dilation and zonular support. It is especially important to review the medication history for the use of alpha-1 blocking agents as preoperative and intraoperative measures can be utilized to adequately control complications arising from intraoperative floppy iris syndrome (IFIS).

■ GLARE DISABILITY ■

Glare may be considered a subjective visual response to light. In the absence of significant ocular disease, bright light may induce discomfort glare before retinal photic adaptation; visual function, however, is unimpaired by discomfort glare. Conversely, disability glare implies that there is a reduction in visual function caused by the scattering of incoming light by inhomogeneity of the ocular media. As in other ocular diseases that induce partial opacification of the ocular media, cataracts disperse incoming light, creating forward light scatter and a "veiling luminance" that interferes with the perception of the visual object of regard. More commonly, this phenomenon is called glare disability (Figure 3-1).[4] In general, opacities of the anterior segment (cataract being the most typical) are associated with glare disorders, whereas posterior segment abnormalities are less likely to induce disabling glare. The closer the media opacity is to the retinal image plane, the less the geometric opportunity for light scattering and obscuring of the image. Therefore, corneal edema is a more likely source of glare than is macular edema.[8] Cataracts disperse incoming light and are anterior in the path of light. Therefore, patients with cataracts may exhibit marked disability glare while retaining good visual acuity under favorable lighting conditions, such as the darkened refracting lane. Cortical and posterior subcapsular cataracts generally cause daytime glare more readily than do nuclear cataracts, which are more prone to cause nighttime glare.[9] Glare disability, therefore, is a common cataract-related symptom, and testing for glare should be sufficiently sensitive to correlate well with patient complaints and adequately specific to avoid confusion with posterior segment disorders.

Several useful devices for determining and measuring glare disability have been employed in clinical practice (Table 3-1). These devices, which may be in short supply today, are generally

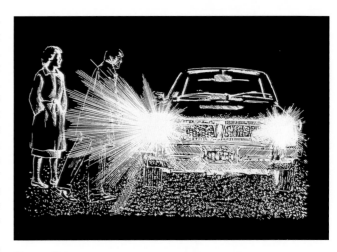

Figure 3-1 Glare resulting from oncoming car headlight hinders the ability to view pedestrians, as the dispersed light veils the objects. Glare loss is inversely related to the distance between the glare source and the object of regard. The pedestrian nearer the headlight is obscured more than is the pedestrian farther from the light. (From Koch DD: Glare and contrast sensitivity testing in cataract patients, *J Cataract Refract Surg* 15:158–164, 1989. Copyright Elsevier 1989.)

designed to test a function of vision with and without the addition of an offending light or glare source. The difference in visual function with and without the glare source is attributed to glare disability. However, each testing system uses a different glare source (central or peripheral point light sources, diffuse background illumination, and so on) and test of visual function (letter optotypes, sine wave gratings, Landolt ring, and so on). The brightness acuity tester (BAT) (Figure 3-2)[10] is in common use because it is readily portable, compact, and relatively inexpensive and may be used in conjunction with the Snellen chart of the refracting lane. The BAT offers three levels of background illumination in a small hemispheric bowl held near the eye. As a result, one possible source of error is pupil constriction by the illuminator; certain patients with cataract will perform better with pupil constriction, thereby giving a false-negative test. Conversely, the third level of brightness is dazzling, inducing false-positive results. Moreover, because no point source of light is used, the BAT does not simulate night-driving conditions.

Another popular device is the Miller–Nadler glare testing device (Figure 3-3).[11] This unit relies on a modified tabletop slide projector to provide diffuse background illumination against which the patient views one of a series of 20/400-sized Landolt rings that sit on a constant-contrast background circle. The rings vary in contrast to the background. Because the Miller–Nadler system employs background glare with a contrast test, it may be useful in simulating daytime glare disability but has been faulted for offering only one object size.[12]

As noted in Table 3-1, other automated devices have been developed and marketed. Moreover, simple, albeit noncalibrated, methods may also be used to assess glare disability. One simple means is to measure Snellen acuity indoors and then retest the patient outdoors with the chart positioned in front of the direct sunlight. Another method is to direct a penlight obliquely toward the pupillary margin while Snellen testing is underway; the difference between the Snellen acuity with and without the penlight is attributed to glare disability.[13]

Table 3-1 Automated instruments for measuring glare disability

Instrument	Manufacturer	Test Format	Glare Light
BAT	Mentor	Letter acuity	Background
Eye Con 5	Eye Con	Letters	Background
IRAS GT	Randwal Instrument Co	Sine wave acuity	4-point
MCT 8000	Vistech	Sine wave contrast	Points or background
Miller-Nadler	Titmus Optical	Landolt C contrast	Background
TVA	Innomed	Letter acuity	Point

From Ocular surgery news, Stack, Inc, Thorofare, NJ.

■ CONTRAST SENSITIVITY

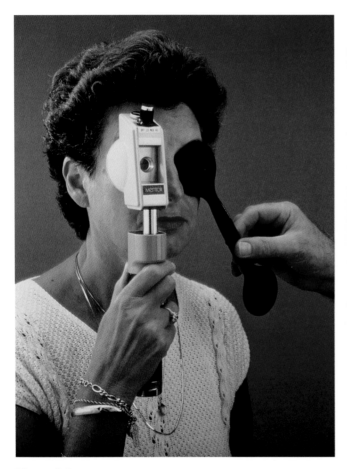

Figure 3-2 Brightness acuity tester (BAT). Handheld device allows patient to view distance charts. The bowl presents diffuse background illumination at three levels of light intensity. (Courtesy Mentor O & O, Santa Barbara, Calif.)

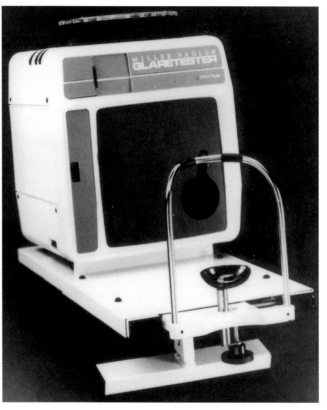

Figure 3-3 Clinical model Miller–Nadler glare tester. The unit is a modified tabletop projector. Glare is induced by the background illumination of the projector. The chin rest support system maintains consistent testing distance. (From Masket S: Reversal of glare disability after cataract surgery, *J Cataract Refract Surg* 15:165–168, 1989. Copyright Elsevier 1989.)

No uniform standards have been established for glare testing devices, a fact that limits their acceptance by rigidly scientific criteria. Nevertheless, it appears that measurement of disabling glare is most useful because it correlates well with cataract symptoms and is reversible with successful cataract surgery.[14–16]

■ CONTRAST SENSITIVITY ■

Activities of daily living, such as driving an automobile, confront the individual with an ever-changing set of visual targets, luminances, and contrasts that require rapid visual interpretation. CSF evaluates the patient's ability to perceive a variety of coarse, intermediate, or fine details at differing contrasts relative to the background (Figure 3-4). In such fashion, contrast testing seeks to objectively assess the equivalent of the patient's visual function in daily life.

Contrast sensitivity testing is somewhat analogous to audiometry, which measures hearing threshold sensitivity to audible tones of differing intensities and audio frequencies. Snellen testing of visual acuity, which is performed only at high contrast, is similar to audiometry performed at only one volume, or much like

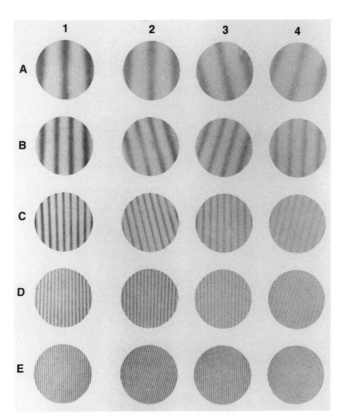

Figure 3-4 Representative portion of preprinted contrast sensitivity test plates. Note varied orientation of contrast bars. (Courtesy Vistech, Inc., Dayton, Ohio.)

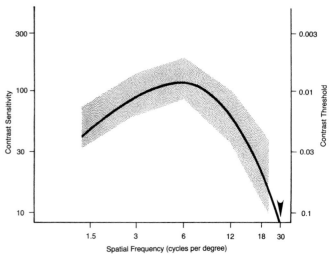

Figure 3-6 CSF curve typical for the normal eye depicted as solid line with surrounding gray area that corresponds to two standard deviations of the normal mean. Note that peak sensitivity occurs near six cycles per degree of subtended retinal arc. The arrow denotes the portion of the curve that corresponds to 20/20 Snellen acuity. (From Masket S: Glare disability and contrast sensitivity function in the evaluation of symptomatic cataract, *Ophthalmol Clin North Am* 4:365–380, 1991. Copyright Elsevier 1991.)

listening to music in which all notes are played at maximum loudness. Therefore, contrast sensitivity testing is a much more complete form of vision analysis than is Snellen testing.[17] Nevertheless, because different object sizes are tested in both systems, a clear relationship exists between visual acuity and contrast sensitivity. The 20/20 "E" optotype subtends a total of 5′ arc on the retina, with each arm and each space accounting for 1′. As noted in Figure 3-5, a contrast grating pattern correlates to the arm and space of the letter "E." One dark and one light bar together equal one cycle. Thirty cycles per degree (or 60′) of retinal arc, therefore, correspond to the spacing of a 20/20 optotype. It follows then, that just one point, 30 cycles degree, on a contrast sensitivity curve (Figure 3-6) at high contrast corresponds to the 20/20 line of Snellen testing. The typical human

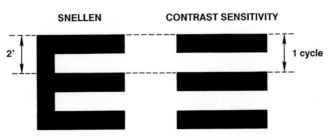

Figure 3-5 Comparison between 20/20 letter "E" optotype and contrast sensitivity bars. Note that the arm and space of the letter subtend 2′ arc and are equal in size to a contrast bar and space at 30 cycles per degree. Therefore, at high contrast the 30 cycles per degree bar is equivalent to 20/20 Snellen acuity. (From Masket S: Glare disability and contrast sensitivity function in the evaluation of symptomatic cataract, *Ophthalmol Clin North Am* 4:365–380, 1991. Copyright Elsevier 1991.)

contrast sensitivity curve, noted in Figure 3-6, reveals that the peak contrast sensitivity of the visual system occurs at image sizes near six cycles per degree as subtended on the retina. An object that subtends six cycles per degree on the retina corresponds in size to a 20/100 optotype. This indicates that the human visual system requires higher contrast for perception at higher spatial frequencies. Therefore, it is possible that the eye may perceive small target sizes at high contrast while not recognizing larger objects at reduced contrast levels. This concept offers an explanation for the visual complaints of patients who retain reasonably good Snellen acuity yet express difficulty in "real-life" visual function.

Given that CSF is analogous to a greatly expanded form of Snellen testing, it stands to reason that reduced contrast function will occur at high spatial frequencies when visual acuity is reduced for any reason, including uncorrected refractive errors and a number of anterior segment abnormalities, for example, keratoconus and pterygium.[18] CSF, therefore, is quite sensitive but not as specific as disability glare testing when evaluating symptomatic cataract.[19] It has been reported that early cataracts reduce contrast sensitivity primarily at high and intermediate frequencies (Figure 3-7),[20,21] whereas optic neuropathies are purported to reduce contrast sensitivity at low frequencies. Early PSC and cortical cataracts have the greatest effect on reducing CSF at intermediate frequencies, while early nuclear cataracts primarily reduce CSF at high spatial frequencies.[22] Reduced CSF has also been noted and reported in a host of posterior segment disorders, including macular degeneration and diabetic retinopathy.[18]

In addition, interest has centered on the effect of monocular cataract on binocular visual function. By means of CSF testing, it has been established that at high spatial frequencies, binocular contrast sensitivity decreases to a level below that of the cataractous eye alone. This demonstrates binocular visual inhibition and indicates that a patient with one cataract may suffer significant visual disability, even when the noncataractous eye has normal monocular vision.[23,24] Furthermore, this information suggests that correcting

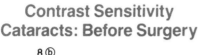

Contrast Sensitivity
Cataracts: Before Surgery

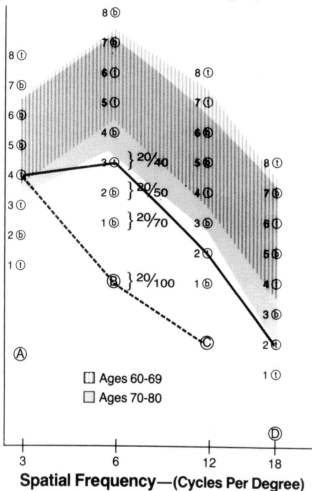

Spatial Frequency—(Cycles Per Degree)

Age: 76
— OD: 20/30
--- OS: 20/30

Figure 3-7 Typical CSF curve of the presurgical cataract patient. Note that the CSF curve of both eyes falls below the range of the accepted norm (90th percentile). The left eye (broken line) has markedly diminished contrast sensitivity yet the same high-contrast Snellen acuity as the right eye. (Courtesy Vector Vision, Inc., Dayton, Ohio.)

only one eye in a patient with binocular cataracts may not fully improve functional vision; often the second eye will require surgery for the patient to gain the benefits of cataract rehabilitation. Moreover, a patient's perceived visual disability with cataract may correlate better with tests of binocular contrast sensitivity than with any of the monocular tests of visual function.[25]

■ MEASUREMENT OF CONTRAST SENSITIVITY FUNCTION ■

The determination of a CSF curve for the eye requires measurement of two separate functions: (1) the perceived contrast threshold between the object and the background and (2) the target size of the object subtended on the retina and measured in cycles

per degree. Originally used as a research tool in the evaluation of ocular and neural diseases, early contrast testing systems used a series of sinusoidal (sine wave) grating patterns (Figures 3-4, 3-8, and 3-9). Currently, the familiar letter optotype contrast charts (Table 3-2) designed by Terry (Figure 3-10), Pelli-Robson (Figure 3-11), and Regan are used as clinical alternatives to sine wave gratings, and CSF is often measured in a fashion similar to Snellen testing, with the patient reading letter charts of differing contrasts. The Regan charts each employ log MAR optotypes between 20/200 and 20/20 at varying contrasts of 96%, 50%, 25%, 11%, and 4%. The 25% and 11% Regan contrast charts have been found particularly useful in evaluating cataract patients.[26] Because the Regan charts present letter targets of differing sizes at varied contrasts, they can be used to establish a true CSF curve for the eye, whereas the Pelli-Robson and Terry charts offer only one size of letter targets.

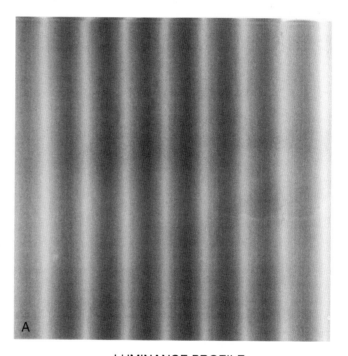

LUMINANCE PROFILE

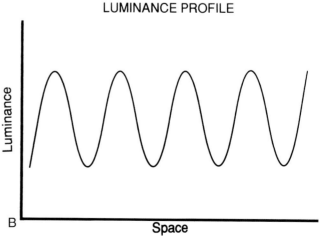

Figure 3-8 A, Sinusoidal grating pattern used in testing contrast sensitivity. B, Luminance versus spatial relationship in sinusoidal grating patterns. (From Jindra LF, Zermon V: Contrast sensitivity testing: a more complete assessment of vision, *J Cataract Refract Surg* 15:141–148, 1989. Copyright Elsevier 1989.)

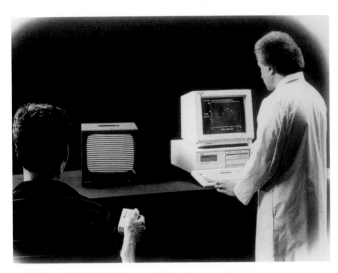

Figure 3-9 Computerized contrast sensitivity apparatus used for determining CSF. Contrast patterns are presented on a video display terminal as generated by the computer. (From Jindra LF, Zermon V: Contrast sensitivity testing: a more complete assessment of vision, *J Cataract Refract Surg* 15:141–148, 1989. Copyright Elsevier 1989.)

Both attempt to evaluate the most sensitive part of the contrast sensitivity curve, near six cycles per degree. Without targets of varied sizes, a complete contrast curve for the eye cannot be determined.

When contrast sensitivity is measured with letter charts, the room and chart illumination must be standardized. Self-contained tabletop vision testing devices offer the possible advantage of uniform internal illumination for enhanced reproducibility. Table 3-3 lists the available automated devices for evaluating CSF. Unfortunately, as in the case of glare disability testing, there has been no consensus on the appropriate standards for contrast sensitivity testing, and a number of devices are available to determine CSF, with each of them employing a somewhat different manner.

Advances in CSF include digital-image-processing software which translates contrast-sensitivity data into modified pictures that represent what the patient actually sees.[27] These images closely represent the quality of vision and can be used to evaluate visual function before and after surgery as well as compare IOL designs with respect to CSF.

In addition to light-scatter, loss of contrast sensitivity induced by cataract formation is also due to optical aberrations induced by lens changes, which can be measured using wavefront aberrometry.[28] Developed primarily for corneal refractive surgery, wavefront aberromety may be a useful method of detecting early lenticular changes in patients with subjective complaints and good Snellen acuity. In one study,[29] higher order aberrations of the whole eye and cornea alone were compared in eyes with nuclear and cortical cataract and eyes without cataract formation. While corneal higher-order aberrations were statistically equivalent between the three groups, patients with lenticular opacities had more higher-order aberrations than normal eyes and the polarity of the aberration depended on the nature of the cataract. In this study, nuclear cataracts induced negative aberrations while cortical cataracts induced positive aberrations. In another study, higher order aberrations were three times greater in eyes with nuclear sclerosis and two times greater in eyes with cortical cataracts compared to normal eyes.[28]

COMBINATION OF GLARE AND CONTRAST SENSITIVITY TESTING

It has been well established that glare disability reduces the contrast sensitivity of the visual system.[30] Therefore, certain glare testing systems, such as the Miller–Nadler glare tester, evaluate the effect of a glare source on contrast targets to determine glare disability. Testing of CSF or low-contrast visual acuity in the presence of glare is superior to the testing of disability glare with high-contrast targets in assessing cataract patients with essentially normal neuroretinal function.[31] It has become common practice to evaluate visual function when combining the BAT as a glare source with the Regan or Pelli–Robson contrast sensitivity charts.[25] This form of testing has been adopted by the United States Food and Drug Administration as requisite for determining visual function after placement of multifocal lens implants. Conversely, separate glare or contrast tests may have specific value for assessing other neural-visual conditions.[12] Given that high-contrast testing alone is of limited value in simulating the visual complaints of the patient with cataracts, it is likely that clinicians will accept into daily practice the combination of low-contrast visual acuity testing with an added glare source as the most effective means to quantify cataract-induced visual symptoms. A simple and gross system employs a penlight as a glare source in combination with Pelli–Robson contrast charts.[32] Hopefully, standard means for combining glare and contrast testing for the evaluation of patients with symptomatic cataract will be established and widely accepted among academicians, clinical practitioners, and regulating organizations.

INTRAOPERATIVE FLOPPY IRIS SYNDROME

In 2005, Chang and Campbell[1] described what is now increasingly recognized and commonly known as intraoperative floppy iris syndrome (IFIS). This condition is associated with the systemic use of alpha 1A blocking agents such as tamsulosin (Flomax, Boehringer Ingelheim Pharmaceuticals, Inc.) for the non-surgical management of benign prostatic hyperplasia. It is important to recognize the potential for IFIS in the preoperative

Table 3-2 Letter optotype charts for contrast sensitivity testing

	Pelli-Robson	Regan	Terry
Contrast range	1–100%	4%, 11%, 25%, 50%, 96%	2.5–80%
Letter sizes	20/80	20/20–20/200	20/70
Testing distance	10 ft	10 ft	10 ft

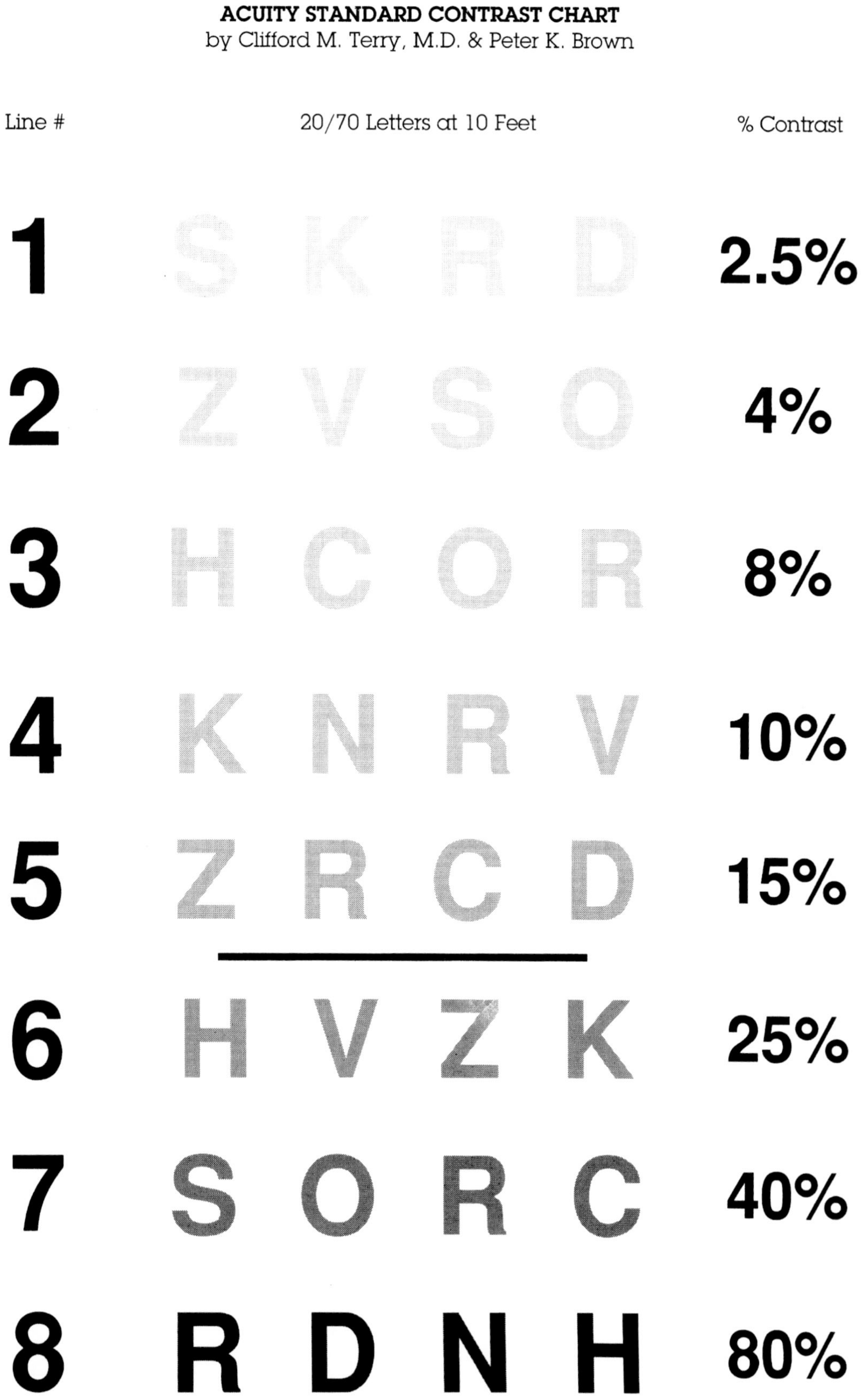

ACUITY STANDARD CONTRAST CHART
by Clifford M. Terry, M.D. & Peter K. Brown

Line #	20/70 Letters at 10 Feet	% Contrast
1	S K R D	**2.5%**
2	Z V S O	**4%**
3	H C O R	**8%**
4	K N R V	**10%**
5	Z R C D	**15%**
6	H V Z K	**25%**
7	S O R C	**40%**
8	R D N H	**80%**

Figure 3-10 The Terry acuity standard contrast chart. Letter optotype chart with contrast between letters and background varying between 2.5% and 80%. Letter size is equal to 20/70 optotype viewed at 10 ft. Nighttime driving may be hazardous for the patient who cannot read line 5 or above. This chart is for demonstration purposes only. (From Masket S: Glare disability and contrast sensitivity function in the evaluation of symptomatic cataract, *Ophthalmol Clin North Am* 4:365–380, 1991. Copyright Elsevier 1991.)

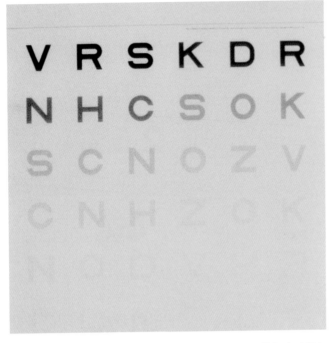

Figure 3-11 A portion of the Pelli–Robson letter contrast sensitivity chart. Note that the letters are of equal size but differ in contrast. (From Pelli DG, Robson JG, Wilkins AJ: The design of a new letter chart for measuring contrast sensitivity. In *Clinical vision science*, vol 2, Oxford, 1988, Pergamon Press, Ltd, p 187. Copyright Elsevier 1988.)

evaluation of the cataract patient. Its manifestations include iris floppiness or instability, poor pupillary dilation, progressive intraoperative miosis, and billowing of iris tissue in the presence of routine irrigating currents. Previous reports indicated increased complication rates in the presence of IFIS, including posterior rupture; however, identifying these patients preoperatively and applying preventative strategies can reduce or eliminate these complications. Standard methods for dealing with small pupils, such as pupil stretching maneuvers, do not help in the management or prevention of this condition.

Appropriate strategies include pharmacologic stimulation of the iris dilator muscle and blockade of the pupil sphincter, mechanical enlargement of the pupil with hooks or other devices, altered fluidic parameters during the phacoemulsification process, use of highly cohesive OVDs, or a combination of any or all of these modalities. Since there is considerable heterogeneity in the behavior of the iris in these patients, a tailored approach should be used in each patient.

Pharmacologic stimulation of the weakened iris dilator muscle with preservative-free, buffered intracameral epinephrine in a 1:2500 dilution has been shown to be safe and effective.[33] This approach helps to stabilize the iris, improves pupillary dilation and reduces iris floppiness. There may also be a synergistic benefit of using preoperative atropine 1% 2 days prior to surgery in addition to intraoperative intracameral epinephrine.[34] Atropine sulfate, as the strongest available pupiloplegic agent is a logical approach for pupillary dilation and preventing intraoperative miosis. Intracameral phenylephrine has also been reported to successfully reverse pupillary constriction and stabilize the iris intraoperatively in patients with IFIS.[35]

Though tamsulosin has the highest affinity for the alpha 1A receptor, it is important to perform a thorough medication history on these patients in order to determine if they are on any alpha 1A blocking agents besides tamsulosin. IFIS has also been reported with the use of alfuzosin[36] (Uroxatral, Sanofi-Aventis) and naftopidil[37] for benign prostatic hyperplasia and doxazosin for the treatment of systemic hypertension.[38] It has also been reported in a patient taking labetolol, which has predominantly beta-blocking effects, but some alpha-blocking effects as well.[39]

It is important that patients suffering from benign prostatic hyperplasia do not stop their alpha 1A blocker, especially when preoperative atropine is used, as acute urinary retention or systemic hypertension may ensue. Preoperative identification of patients on alpha 1A blockers and using appropriate strategies to deal with this condition can eliminate its potential complications.

■ ASSESSMENT OF POTENTIAL VISUAL FUNCTION FOLLOWING CATARACT REMOVAL ■

Patients with symptomatic cataract formation and otherwise normal ocular examinations can anticipate amelioration of their diminished vision with successful cataract removal. However, patients with cataract and concomitant ocular disease, for example, macular degeneration, may present a dilemma in

Table 3-3 Contrast sensitivity testing devices

Device	Manufacturer	Format	Target Type
B-VAT II	Mentor	Computer screen	Sine wave
CSV 1000	Vector Vision	Illuminated wall chart	Sine wave
Eye Con 5	Eye Con	Computer screen	Letters
MCT 8000	Vistech	Tabletop view box	Sine wave
Optec 1000	Stereo Optical	Tabletop view box	Sine wave
Optec 2000			
TVA	Innomed	Computer screen	Square wave
VCTS	Vistech	Near-far charts	Sine wave

From Ocular surgery news, Stack, Inc, Thorofare, NJ.

management because ophthalmoscopy may be misleading or particularly difficult with advanced cataracts. Often, the patient and surgeon are reluctant to consider cataract surgery when the prognosis for return of visual function is limited. Nevertheless, in some cases of multiple ocular disease, cataract rehabilitation may prove significantly beneficial to the patient. Determination of the expected visual improvement after surgery may allow the patient to arrive at an appropriate decision for or against surgery. Toward that end, a few devices for the determination of potential retinal function or visual return have been brought to the clinical arena (Tables 3-4 and 3-5).

Testing devices for the determination of potential visual acuity attempt to project visible targets through the cataract, in order to reach the retina for subjective interpretation. One system, the Guyton–Minkowski potential acuity meter (PAM),[40] is temporarily attached to a slit lamp and uses a reduced Snellen chart that is projected through a pinhole aperture onto the macular region; refractive errors may be compensated for by the apparatus. The principle of using a pinhole aperture to assess the potential visual acuity after proposed cataract surgery has been further adapted in the potential acuity pinhole test.[41] In this method, the increased depth of focus afforded by pinhole apertures is combined with bright light from a transilluminator to assess potential vision in the presence of a cataract. It is reported to be more accurate than the PAM.[42] The second type of potential acuity apparatus uses laser-generated interference stripes or fringes that are projected onto the retinal surface through the ocular media; the width of the fringes, corresponding to acuity, is variable.[43–46] Refractive errors need not be corrected with interferometry testing because projection of the laser images on the retina is not affected by ametropia.

The potential acuity devices – whether the Snellen chart, the PAM or the interferometry fringes – are subjective methods that require an alert and cooperative patient, in addition to a skilled

Table 3-4 Devices for determination of potential visual acuity

Guyton-Minkowski Potential Acuity Meter (Mentor)	Reduced Snellen chart
Lotmar Visometer (Haag-Streit)	Laser interferometer
Rodenstock (Rodenstock)	Laser interferometer
IRASInterferometer (Randwal)	Laser interferometer

Table 3-5 Methods for determination of retinal function-integrity

Blue-field entoptoscopy (Mira)	Foveal capillary net
Visual evoked potential	Evoked cortical responses
Electroretinography	Electroretinography
B-scan ultrasonography	Imaging
Pinhole acuity	Potential acuity
Penlight entoptic phenomena	Purkinje images
Maddox rod	Gross macular function
Two-point discrimination	Gross retinal function
Color perception	Gross macular function

and compassionate examiner. Moreover, these tests are of greatest value when the cataract has not advanced past the 20/200 level, because very dense lens opacities may yield false-negative results. A clinical rule of thumb indicates that a predicted improvement of four lines of vision by the acuity tester suggests a good prognosis for cataract surgery. Typically, if a patient's best corrected visual acuity is recorded at 20/70, a 20/30 potential acuity response is considered indicative of significant visual improvement with surgery. Caution must be exercised in interpreting the results of potential acuity testing because some cases of maculopathy may yield a false-positive response, whereas extremely dense cataracts may produce false-negative results.

In addition, simple and less expensive clinical tools may be useful in determining the visual prognosis after cataract removal in cases of suspected macular disease. One method is the yellow filter test suggested by Koch.[47] In this system, when a transparent yellow filter is placed over reading material, it is noted to worsen vision in the presence of a significant cataract but might be noted to improve vision if the macular degenerative process is more significant than the cataract.

Occasionally, a cataract or other media opacity may be sufficiently dense to preclude any view of the posterior segment; in such cases, the prognosis for return of vision cannot be assessed by the aforementioned testing devices. A number of alternative means to determine gross potential acuity in patients with markedly advanced cataracts have been developed over time and may be useful. Two-point discrimination, penlight-generated entoptoscopy, gross color perception, blue-field entoptoscopy, and Maddox rod testing are among the available tests of certain value (see Table 3-5). Standard B-scan ultrasonographic imaging and electrophysiologic studies, such as electroretinography and the visual-evoked potential, may provide useful information when considering an eye with totally opaque media, but these methods may be too costly for routine use in determining indication for cataract surgery.

In two-point discrimination testing, two light sources of equal intensity are held about 25 inches (or 62 cm) from the patient. If the patient can correctly identify the two lights, retinal function is assumed to be grossly intact. No information is learned about macular potential. This test is most useful in cases of fully mature cataracts or otherwise dense ocular media. Similarly, gross color perception may be useful as a tool to establish general retinal integrity; the cobalt blue light source or the green filter (red-free source) of the slit lamp may be useful for this purpose.

Tests of entoptic phenomena have also been used to assess the function of the retina. A penlight or transilluminator may be placed over the closed lid or directly on the globe to stimulate perception of the Purkinje vascular tree images. Although some patients may observe and describe the retinal vasculature, optic nerve, and macular region accurately, other patients, even with intact retinas, cannot observe the Purkinje images. Therefore, the test is most useful in comparing the two eyes of one patient, assuming that one eye is normal and the involved eye has opaque media. In patients with one normal eye and one eye with densely opaque media, testing for an afferent pupillary defect may also be beneficial, because at virtually all stages of development cataracts do not induce abnormal pupillary reactions.

Blue-field entoptoscopy is more specific for macular function and is based on the ability of the patient to observe the flow of white blood cells in the parafoveal capillaries. Blue light is absorbed by the red blood cells but not the white blood cells. As a result, with proper filters and an appropriate bright light source, the patient can observe "flying corpuscles" or white blood cells if the fovea is functionally intact. Unfortunately, the test requires a special apparatus, relies on a carefully discerning patient as observer, and may yield false-negative results with dense cataracts.

A Maddox rod may be used as a simple test of macular function in patients in whom the ocular media is not totally opaque. The Maddox rod is held in front of the eye to be tested, and a light source is held approximately 14 inches (or 35 cm) away. If the patient observes an unbroken red line, one may assume macular integrity. A discontinuity of the red line suggests a macular lesion. A totally opaque cataract or vitreous will not allow perception of the Maddox rod.

Imaging with B-scan ultrasonography may be helpful to determine the presence of vitreous hemorrhage or retinal detachment in cases of mature cataract. However, little to no information about macular function can be learned from imaging, whereas simple clinical testing (light projection, two-point discrimination, etc.) may offer an impression sufficient to determine an indication for surgery.

Electroretinography, which estimates overall rod function, is of little value in determining postoperative vision potential. Although evaluation of visual-evoked potential is more specific for macular function than is electroretinography, simpler clinical tests are generally as valuable in establishing a surgical indication, given the high success rate and low complication rate associated with modern cataract surgery.

Scanning laser ophthalmoscopy, a relatively new testing tool, is capable of imaging the retina in the presence of a significant cataract.[48] However, the cost of the device makes it impractical to use for the sole purpose of presurgical screening.

A PARADIGM FOR THE CLINICAL EVALUATION OF THE PATIENT WITH CATARACT

At present, there is no single, specific, valid, objective test of visual function to indicate the presence of an operable cataract. Rather, new testing tools add to the battery of ocular function tests and, when combined with a careful analysis of patient symptoms, physical findings, and assessment of potential visual function, they offer a rational means of determining an indication for cataract surgery.

Above all, and central to the issue of appropriate indications for cataract surgery, is the patient's history of visual disturbance and what impact the visual deficit has on the patient's daily tasks of life. A history of significant functional impairment may make it appropriate to remove a posterior subcapsular cataract despite distance Snellen acuity of 20/25 or better, if near vision is reduced or disabling glare is present. Conversely, an asymptomatic sedentary individual with a dense uniocular brunescent nuclear cataract may not perceive a significant benefit from surgery if visual symptoms are not noted. An old clinical adage suggests that it is impossible to help an asymptomatic patient; that concept remains valid today. Written entries in the patient's medical record should clearly state the patient's symptoms and the effect they have on activities of daily living. An activities-of-life scale, with written record for documentation, has been proposed as a means of evaluating the subjective significance of a patient's cataract.[49] Moreover, the patient's symptoms should correspond to the vision loss associated with cataract formation, whereas the progressive inability to see traffic signs under night lighting or against background glare could certainly be induced by evolving cataracts.

The objective ocular examination of the patient with cataract must be comprehensive to establish the absence or presence of concomitant ocular and systemic disease that might also produce visual symptoms or bear on the prognosis for recovery of vision. In addition, contraindications for surgery, such as untreated active blepharitis or uncontrolled intraocular pressure, should also be ascertained.

Best (spectacle) corrected acuity for distance and near vision should be determined; meaningful refractive changes might be significant because nuclear cataracts often induce a myopic shift. Given that cataract extraction with lens implantation is the most common procedure performed under Medicare coverage and accounts for $3 billion of health care expenditures, patients, third-party payers, and regulatory agencies have an understandable interest in the appropriateness of cataract surgery. As a result, certain agencies (e.g., State Professional Standard Review Organizations) have set limits of visual acuity (generally 20/50 spectacle corrected distance acuity) as appropriate for cataract surgery. However, it has long been well established that Snellen visual acuity alone is not an adequate means to establish indication for surgery.

Consideration of compromised near vision is often overlooked by review organizations. Posterior subcapsular cataracts are noted for their deleterious effect on reading acuity well in advance of marked reduction in distance acuity. Unfortunately, there are no governmentally ordained minimum requirements for near vision. Conversely, posterior subcapsular (and cortical) cataracts tend to induce symptoms of daytime glare with attendant visual disability. Although no specific glare testing device has received the tacit approval of review organizations, the clinician can employ any of the appropriate methods (see Table 3-1) to measure glare disability to establish documentation for proposed cataract surgery deemed necessary by patient symptoms. Daytime glare disability is best simulated by tests that use a diffuse background glare source.

Nuclear cataracts ordinarily reduce distance vision more than they do near vision. As a result, patients who are visually symptomatic with nuclear cataracts are more likely than patients with posterior subcapsular cataract to fall within review organizations' guidelines for surgical indications. This may be particularly true for some patients with opalescent (oil droplet appearance on retinoscopy) nuclear cataracts who may experience early loss of distance acuity. However, in some cases, advanced nuclear brunescence may be observed without a marked loss in Snellen acuity; the patients, however, are likely to complain about difficulty with nighttime vision, particularly while driving. Moreover, color perception may be significantly hampered by dense brunescent nuclear cataracts. If patients offer significant complaints regarding visual function in the presence of a nuclear cataract yet retain better than 20/50 Snellen acuity, it is likely that CSF will be reduced. In addition, tests of glare disability that simulate nighttime glare (peripheral or paracentral light spots rather than diffuse background illumination) are likely to demonstrate significant abnormality. Combinations of glare and contrast testing are certain to be best in documenting loss of vision function associated with nuclear cataracts.

Assuming that the patient's history suggests a significant visual deficit and that the physical findings support the presence of cataract formation commensurate with the functional vision loss, cataract surgery may be entertained. The patient must be the final arbiter in the decision to have cataract surgery. Moreover, it is essential to determine the prognosis for return of vision with the proposed cataract surgery. Tests of potential visual acuity must be entertained when the ocular findings include other pathologic features, particularly macular degeneration or optic neuropathy. When pupillary reactions are normal (no afferent defect) and the view of the fundus is sufficient to determine the lack of pathologic condition, specific tests of potential acuity are not necessary. However, if optic neuropathy is suspected, visual field studies should be performed. Moreover, in cases of macular degeneration, in which subretinal neovascularization may be considered, fluorescein angiography may be a useful diagnostic adjunct, although its quality is limited by media opacification. When employed in cases of questionable prognosis, specific tests of potential visual function may provide important information for clinician and patient. Given that the PAM, laser interferometers, and the potential acuity pinhole test can bypass some corneal disease, irregular astigmatism, and refractive errors, they are otherwise useful guides when the relative visual significance of a cataract is difficult to measure in view of concomitant disease of the posterior pole. In cases of extraordinarily dense or mature cataracts, one might consider the use of B-scan ultrasonography in addition to tests of entopic phenomena and so on.

Once the diagnosis of a visually significant, surgically remediable cataract has been established, the patient (and family members, as appropriate) should be counseled in regard to the findings and prognosis for return of vision. It is almost exclusively a patient-oriented decision whether to have surgery, as is the timing for the procedure. Assuming the patient chooses corrective surgery, it is then incumbent on the practitioner to ascertain the social and supportive needs of the patient during the perioperative period. Can the patient comply with the instructions for postoperative use of eyedrops or other medications? How will the patient be transported for surgery and postsurgical care? What assistance might the patient need for preparing meals early after surgery? These are a few of the pertinent questions.

When planning surgery for any given patient after determining that it is appropriate for and commensurate with the needs of the patient, a careful assessment of the eye to be operated on should be performed and a surgical plan established. The patient may wish to share in deciding the expected postoperative refraction, which is a particularly important consideration in cases of high preoperative ametropia. Presurgical planning should also consider corneal astigmatism and wound placement and construction. Size and type of intraocular lens might also be affected by the desired spherical and astigmatic results of surgery.

The comprehensive examination should also uncover potentially complicating factors, such as medication allergies, uncontrolled intraocular pressure, corneal endothelial compromise, a narrow chamber angle, a poorly dilating pupil, pseudoexfoliation, lens subluxation, posterior capsular defects (as in patients with posterior polar cataracts), a vitreoretinal pathologic condition with lattice peripheral retinal degeneration, and open retinal tears. In the days just before surgery, an external examination is helpful to rule out conjunctivitis or active blepharitis.

Requirements for presurgical medical evaluation may vary from region to region. However, elderly patients with cataract are subject to a range of general medical disorders. It may be beneficial to include the primary care physician in surgical planning, giving careful consideration to certain conditions, including diabetes, systemic hypertension, cardiovascular disease, pulmonary disorders, hyperthyroidism, anticoagulation, and long-term corticosteroid use.

In summary, the presurgical evaluation of the patient with a symptomatic cataract can be a significant and cognitive exercise. Depending on the density of the cataract and the degree of visual symptoms, the clinician must decide what tests are appropriate and necessary to fully evaluate the patient. After a thorough examination process, the patient can be informed of the findings and can make an educated selection from the options for care. If surgery is indicated and entertained, the patient's general medical and social conditions must also be explored before determining the best course of action.

References

[1] Chang DF, Campbell JR. Intraoperative floppy iris syndrome associated with tamsulosin. J Cataract Refract Surg 2005;31:664–673.
[2] Hess RF, Woo GC. Vision through cataracts. Invest Ophthalmol Vis Sci 1978;17:428–435.
[3] Cinotti AA. Evaluation of indications for cataract surgery. Ophthalmic Surg 1979;10:25–31.
[4] Jaffe NS. Glare and contrast: Indications for cataract surgery. J Cataract Refract Surg 1986;12:372–375.
[5] Koch DD. Glare and contrast sensitivity testing in cataract patients. J Cataract Refract Surg 1989;15:158–164.
[6] Cataract Management Guideline Panel. Cataract in adults: management of functional vision impairment. Clinical Practice Guideline, Number 4, Rockville, MD: US Department of Health and Human Services, Public Health Service, Agency for Health Care Policy and Research, AHCPR Pub No. 93–0542, February 1993.
[7] Koch DD, Liu JF. Survey of the clinical use of glare and contrast sensitivity testing. J Cataract Refract Surg 1990;16:707–711.
[8] Carney LG, Jacobs RJ. Mechanisms of visual loss in corneal edema. Arch Ophthalmol 1984;102:1068–1071.
[9] Neumann AC, McCarty GR, Steedle TO et al. The relationship between cataract type and glare disability as measured by the Miller–Nadler glare tester. J Cataract Refract Surg 1988;14:40–45.
[10] Holladay JT, Prager TC, Trujillo J et al. Brightness acuity test and outdoor visual acuity in cataract patients. J Cataract Refract Surg 1987;13:67–70.
[11] Hirsch RP, Nadler PM, Miller D. Clinical performance of a disability glare tester. Arch Ophthalmol 1984;102:1633–1636.
[12] Elliot DB, Bullimore MA. Assessing the reliability, discriminative ability, and validity of disability glare tests. Invest Ophthalmol Vis Sci 1993;34:108–119.
[13] Maltzman BA, Horan C, Rengel A. Penlight test for glare disability of cataracts. Ophthalmic Surg 1988;19:356–358.
[14] Masket S. Reversal of glare disability after cataract surgery. J Cataract Refract Surg 1989;15:165–168.
[15] Cink DE, Sutphin JE. Quantification of the reduction of glare disability after standard extracapsular cataract surgery. J Cataract Refract Surg 1992;18:385–390.
[16] Rubin GS, Adamsons IA, Stark WJ. Comparison of acuity, contrast sensitivity, and disability glare before and after cataract surgery. Arch Ophthalmol 1993;102:56–61.
[17] Jindra LF, Zemon V. Contrast sensitivity testing: a more complete assessment of vision. J Cataract Refract Surg 1989;15:141–148.
[18] Masket S. Glare disability and contrast sensitivity function in the evaluation of symptomatic cataract. Ophthalmol Clin North Am 1991;4:365–380.
[19] American Academy of Ophthalmology. Contrast sensitivity and glare testing in the evaluation of anterior segment disease (ophthalmic procedures assessment). Ophthalmology 1990;97:1233–1237.
[20] Adamsons I, Rubin GS, Vitale S et al. The effect of early cataracts on glare and contrast sensitivity: a pilot study. Arch Ophthalmol 1992;110:1081–1086.
[21] Drews-Bankiewicz MA, Caruso RC, Datiles MB et al. Contrast sensitivity in patients with nuclear cataracts. Arch Ophthalmol 1992;110:953–959.
[22] Chua B, Mitchell P, Cumming R. Effects of cataract type and location on visual function: The Blue Mountains Eye Study. Eye 1994;18:765–772.
[23] Pardhan P, Gilchrist J. The importance of measuring binocular contrast sensitivity in unilateral cataract. Eye 1991;5:31–35.
[24] Taylor RH, Mission GP, Moseley MJ. Visual acuity and contrast sensitivity in cataract. Eye 1991;5:704–707.
[25] Elliot DB, Hurst MA, Weatherill J. Comparing clinical tests of visual function in cataract with the patient's perceived visual disability. Eye 1990;4:712–717.
[26] Regan D. The Charles F. Prentice Award Lecture 1990: specific tests and specific blindnesses: keys, locks, and parallel processing. Optom Vis Sci 1991;68:489–512.
[27] Ginsburg A. Contrast sensitivity: determining the visual quality and function of cataract, intraocular lenses and refractive surgery. Curr Opinion in Ophthalmology 2006;17:19–26.
[28] Sachdev D, Ormonde S, Sherwin T et al. Higher-order aberrations of lenticular opacities. J Cataract Refract Surg 2004;30:1642–1648.
[29] Kuroda T, Fujikado T, Maeda N. Wavefront analysis in eyes with nuclear or cortical cataract. Am J Ophthalmol 2002;134:1–9.
[30] Abrahammson M, Sjostrand J. Impairment of contrast sensitivity function (CSF) as a measure of disability glare. Invest Ophthalmol Vis Sci 1986;27:1131–1136.
[31] Elliot DB, Hurst MA, Weatherill J. Comparing clinical tests of visual loss in cataract patients using a quantification of forward light scatter. Eye 1991;5:601–606.

[32] Williamson TH, Strong NP, Sparrow J et al. Contrast sensitivity and glare in cataract using the Pelli–Robson chart. Br J Ophthalmol 1992;76:719–722.

[33] Shugar J. Use of epinephrine for IFIS prophylaxis. J Cataract Refract Surg 2006;32:1074–1075.

[34] Masket S, Belani S. Combined Pre-Operative Topical Atropine Sulfate 1% and Intracameral Non-preserved Epinephrine HCL 1:2500 for Management of Intraoperative Floppy Iris Syndrome. J Cataract Refract Surg 2007; In press.

[35] Manvikar S, Allen D. Cataract surgery management in patients taking tamsulosin staged approach. J Cataract Refract Surg 2006;32:1611–1614.

[36] Settas G, Fitt AW. Intraoperative floppy iris syndrome in a patient taking alfuzosin for benign prostatic hypertrophy. Eye 2006;20:1431–143.

[37] Oshika T, Ohashi Y. Incidence of intraoperative floppy iris syndrome in patients on either systemic or topical alpha(1)–adrenoceptor antagonist. Am J Ophthalmol 2007;143:150–151.

[38] Muqit M, Menage M. Intraoperative floppy iris syndrome. Ophthalmol 2006;113:1885–1886.

[39] Calotti F, Steen D. Labetalol causing intraoperative floppy-iris syndrome. J Cataract Refract Surg 2007;33:170–171.

[40] Minkowski JS, Palese M, Guyton DL. Potential acuity meter using a minute serial pinhole aperture. Ophthalmol 1983;90:1360–1368.

[41] Hofeldt AJ, Weiss MJ. Illuminated near card assessment of potential acuity in eyes with cataract. Ophthalmol 1998;105:1531–1536.

[42] Meliki SA, Safar A, Martin J, Ivanova A et al. Potential acuity pinhole: A simple method of measure potential visual acuity in patients with cataracts: comparison to potential acuity meter. Ophthalmol 1999;106:1262–1267.

[43] Faulkner W. Laser interferometric prediction of postoperative visual acuity in patients with cataracts. Am J Ophthalmol 1983;95:626–636.

[44] Tabbat SE, Lindstrom RL. Laser retinometry versus clinical estimation of media: a comparison of efficacy in predicting visual acuity of patients with lens opacities. J Cataract Refract Surg 1986;12:140–145.

[45] Goldstein J, Hecht SD, Jamara RJ et al. Clinical comparison of the SITE IRAS hand held interferometer and Haag–Streit Lotmar visometer. J Cataract Refract Surg 1988;14:208–211.

[46] Bernth-Petersen P, Naeser K. Clinical evaluation of Lotmar visometer for macula testing in cataract patients. Acta Ophthalmology 1982;60:525–532.

[47] Koch P. Testing useful for cataract/macular disease patients. Ophthalmology Times 1992;17:1, 30.

[48] Kirkpatrick JN, Manivannan A, Gupta AK et al. Fundus imaging in patients with cataract: role for a variable wavelength scanning laser ophthalmoscope. Br J Ophthalmol 1995;79:892–899.

[49] Mangione CM, Phillips RS, Seddon JM et al. Development of the "activities of daily vision scale." A measure of visual functional status. Med Care 1992;30:1111–1126.

Intraocular Lens Power Calculation

Kenneth J. Hoffer, MD, FACS

4

CONTENTS

CHAPTER HIGHLIGHTS

>> Alternatives and advantages of different methods of biometry

>> Determination of corneal curvature

>> Anterior chamber depth determination

>> Personalized surgeon formulas

>> Management of special cases and exceptions

INTRODUCTION

Since Sir Harold Ridley experienced a 21 diopter "surprise" in lens power calculation on his first two cases in 1949–50, we have been seeking ways to calculate intraocular lens (IOL) power with greater accuracy (Figure 1-1). The science is rather dry and does not stimulate great interest on the part of the majority of cataract surgeons. To make the subject more understandable, it would be advantageous to break it down into its component parts.

The three major components of IOL power calculation are (1) biometry, (2) formulas, and (3) clinical variables. *Biometry* can be divided into its components needed to calculate IOL power: the axial length, the corneal power, and the IOL position. *Formulas* can be divided into their generations, their usage and their personalization. I will divide *clinical variables* into the topics: patient needs and desires, special circumstances, and problems and errors.

When the human lens is replaced with an IOL, the optical status becomes a two-lens system (cornea and IOL) projecting an image onto the fovea. The distance (X) between the two lenses affects the refraction as does the distance (Y) between the two-lens system and the fovea. X is defined as the distance from the anterior surface (vertex) of the cornea to the effective principle plane of the IOL in the visual axis. Y is defined as the distance from the principle plane of the IOL to the photoreceptors of the fovea in the visual axis. It is easy to see that X+Y is equal to the visual axis axial length of the eye (A). Therefore, knowing X and A will allow the calculation of Y (Y = A−X).

Also to calculate the IOL power (P), we must know the vergence of the light rays entering the cornea (refractive error (R)). For emmetropia, R is zero. The relationship of these factors (X, Y (A−X), P, K, R) is such that a formula can be written to describe it. Knowing the values of any four of these variables will allow for the calculation of the fifth.

BIOMETRY

AXIAL LENGTH

If the crystalline lens (cataract) is to be removed, obtaining an accurate axial length (AL) is mandatory. If the lens has already been removed (aphakia/pseudophakia) or will not be removed (phakic IOL), an AL is not always necessary because the correct implant lens power can be calculated using a refraction formula (see below). Because this formula requires an accurate vertex distance, it is not dependable in cases of aphakia where errors in the vertex distance of a high-powered refraction can have a significant effect.

The important considerations for obtaining accurate ultrasound AL are listed in Table 4-1.

Axial Length Instruments

Up to 1999, all axial length measuring instruments have been A-scan ultrasound units. There are many A-scan instruments available and it is important to make sure the unit that you are using has been calibrated and is capable of accurate measurements. It is important to be sure that the instrument has a true analog screen such that true echo spikes are observed in determining axiality. Instruments that merely report a numerical reading of the AL ("black box" or spike simulation) do not allow clinical decision making during the examination and are fraught with potential errors. A major step in improving accuracy would be to replace such an instrument with one that has an oscilloscope screen.

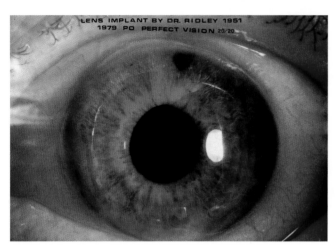

Figure 4-1 Uncorrected 20/20 vision in an eye with a Ridley posterior chamber IOL implanted by Harold Ridley in 1951. (Photo by author in 1979)

Table 4-1 Considerations for obtaining accurate measurements (in order of importance)

A. Ultrasound Axial Length	B. Corneal Power
A-scan ultrasound instrument	Instrumentation
Real-time oscilloscope screen	Contact lens wear
Immersion technique	Astigmatism
Experienced technician	Previous refractive surgery
Appropriate ultrasound velocities	Corneal transplant eyes
B-scan backup	

A newer methodology for axial length was introduced in 1999 by Carl Zeiss Meditec (Figure 4-2). It uses laser coherent interferometry to measure AL. The instrument, called the IOLMaster® performs four functions: (1) it measures the AL, (2) it measures the corneal power (K or r), (3) it measures the anterior chamber depth (ACD) (the latter two by optical means), and (4) it performs the formula IOL power calculations using four modern 3rd generation theoretic formulas. The author has performed side-by-side analysis of the accuracy of this instrument compared to our standard immersion A-scan technique and found the instrument to be comparable to immersion ultrasound. A multitude of reports in the literature conclude that the IOLMaster® cannot obtain results in from 10–17% of eyes because of either posterior subcapsular cataracts (PSC) cataract, the density of a cataract, or the patient's inability to fixate. Our results are similar. We have so far noticed considerable difficulty obtaining an AL measurement in eyes with PSC cataracts but have been impressed with the results up to this point and especially its ease of use and repeatability.

WARNING: *Be sure the Index of Refraction in the IOLMaster is set to 1.3375 in the Setup screen of the computer for the Hoffer® Q formula to operate accurately.*

Immersion Ultrasound Technique

The immersion technique of Ossoinig[1] has been shown to be more accurate than the standard applanation contact technique in several studies[2,3] over the past 15 years. They report a mean average shortening of the AL of 0.25–0.33 mm using applanation compared to immersion. If this shortening error by applanation were a consistent one it could be compensated for by the addition of a correction constant or by IOL power formula personalization. Unfortunately, this is not possible since the error varies from eye to eye.

Arguments against using the immersion technique are that it is time-consuming, more expensive, messy and requires the patient to be totally supine. On the contrary, the examination can be performed in a standard ophthalmic examination chair reclined back at a 45° angle with the headrest set back so that the patient's AL is perpendicular to the floor (Figure 4-3). To maintain a non-leaking fluid bath in the Ossoinig scleral shell (Hansen Ophthalmic Development Labs, 745 Avalon Place, Coralville, IA 52241, 319-338-1285 *www.HansenLab.com*), we use a 50/50 dilution of

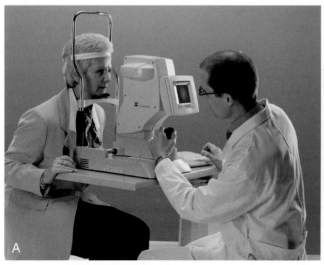
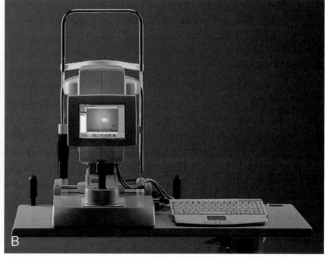

Figure 4-2 The Zeiss IOLMaster® laser tomography axial length measurement instrument. **A.** Side view, **B.** Front view.

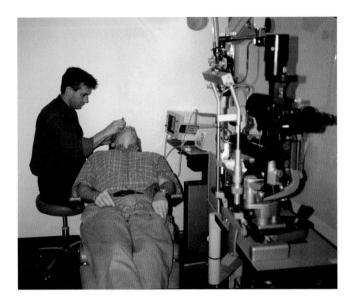

Figure 4-3 Immersion ultrasound technique setup for patient in normal ophthalmic examination chair.

2.5% hydroxypropyl methylcellulose (Goniosol®) in Dacriose® solution. Once the eye is anesthetized topically, the scleral shell is gently placed between the lids and filled 3/4 full with the solution. Any air bubbles should be vacuumed with a short silicone tube attached to a syringe. The latter can also be used to remove the solution at the completion of the procedure. The ultrasound probe is placed into the solution and positioned parallel to the axis of the eye (Figure 4-4). Axiality is judged by watching for the correct spike patterns on the oscilloscope screen as the probe position is adjusted. First the corneal and retinal spikes must be identified and "equally" maximized. An undilated pupil aids the examiner by the fact that eliminating the iris spikes improves the chances of being more axial; a dilated pupil eliminates this advantage.

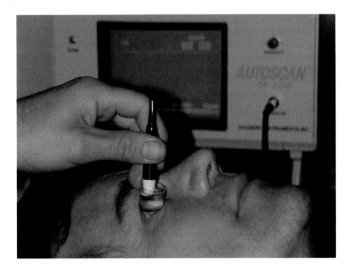

Figure 4-4 Immersion ultrasound technique showing the probe in the Ossoinig shell filled with 50/50 Goniosol/Dacriose solution.

Many find the Prager Shell (ESI, Inc., 2515 Everest Lane North, Plymouth, MN 55447, 763-473-2533, *tab@eyesurgin. com*) easier to use for immersion and studies appear to indicate it being accurate. The author has no experience with it.

WARNING: *Measuring the AL of BOTH eyes is prudent and customary.*

WARNING: *If the AL is very difficult to obtain and the eye appears to have a length greater than 25 mm, suspect a STAPHYLOMA. Use the IOLMaster or the Shammas method: By direct ophthalmoscopy (with patient fixating on the cross-hair target), measure the distance from the target (macula) to the edge of the optic nerve (in disc diameters). A B-scan exam is then performed to measure the AL at that distance from the edge of the optic nerve shadow (Figure 4-5).*

WARNING: *When measuring an eye containing an IOL, ignore multiple reduplication echoes caused by the IOL seen in the vitreous space.*

WARNING: *If planning silicone oil injection into the vitreous space, perform an accurate AL measurement before doing so and make this information available to the patient. It is practically impossible to measure a silicone oil eye (try using a velocity of 1000 m/s). The Zeiss IOLMaster® is the only way to get an accurate measurement in silicone oil-filled eyes. Alternatively, consider performing a secondary IOL after the aphakic refraction is obtained.*

Always measure AL to the nearest hundredth of a millimeter and record it carefully. Errors in AL are the most significant and amount to ~2.5 D/mm in IOL power, but it is important to be aware that this error drops to ~1.75 D/mm in very long eyes (30 mm), but jumps to ~3.75 D/mm in very short eyes (20 mm). Greater care must be taken in measuring short eyes.

Ultrasound Velocities

The ultrasound velocity[4,5] for the various parts of the eye, intraocular lens materials and average pseudophakic velocities that I have calculated are shown in Table 4-2.

WARNING: *Measuring an eye containing a silicone IOL with standard phakic velocity (1555 m/s) can amount to an error of 3–4 D.*

The nominal average velocity for the normal range AL eye is 1555 m/s. Because of the inversely proportional change in the axial ratio of solid to liquid as the eye increases in length, the average phakic velocity of a short 20 mm eye is 1560 m/s and that of a long 30 mm eye is 1550 m/s (Figure 4-6). This factor only amounts to a small (0.25 D) error in the extremes of AL, but it can be corrected for. The inversely proportional relationship is greater in pseudophakic eyes but is not a factor at all in aphakic eyes (1534 m/s).

If an eye has been measured using the wrong velocity, it can be easily corrected without remeasuring the eye by using the following formula:

$$AL_{CORRECTED} = (AL_{MEASURED}) \times (V_{CORRECT}) \div V_{MEASURED}$$

where V = ultrasound velocity

This is because the instrument does not measure length or distance (d) directly. Instead it measures the time (t) it takes the sound to traverse the eye and converts it to a linear value using the velocity (V) formula where d = V × t.

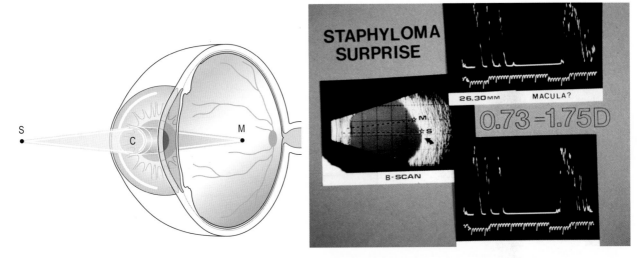

Figure 4-5 Staphyloma. B-scan (left) demonstrates staphyloma. A-scans show shorter reading at macula (upper) than at posterior pole (lower).

Table 4-2 Ultrasound velocities[4,5] (at body temperature)

A. From the following sound velocity values[4,5]

Cornea & lens	1641 m/sec
Aqueous & vitreous	1532 m/sec
PMMA IOL	2660 m/sec
Silicone IOL	980 m/sec
Acrylic IOL	2026 m/sec
Glass IOL	6040 m/sec
Silicone oil	987 m/sec

B. I calculated average sound speeds[4] for various conditions of a 23.5 mm eye

Phakic eye	1555 m/sec
Aphakic eye	1534 m/sec
PMMA pseudophakic	1556 m/sec
Silicone pseudophakic	1476 m/sec
Acrylic pseudophakic	1549 m/sec
Glass pseudophakic	1549 m/sec
Phakic silicone oil	1139 m/sec
Aphakic silicone oil	1052 m/sec

Optional CALF Method

Holladay[6,7] has offered an optional method to measure the AL which attempts to decrease the error inherent in changes in average velocity due to the length of the eye. The reasoning behind this method is that, if an "average" eye velocity is incorrect, it affects the entire AL measurement. However, if the estimate of the CALF value is wrong, it only affects a small percentage of the overall AL, i.e. only the lens portion. The method involves measuring all eyes, regardless of status, at a sound velocity of 1532 m/s (as if the eye was a bag of water) and to this value is added the Corrected AL Factor (CALF). The CALF value represents the thickness of a lens in the eye whether it is the crystalline lens or IOL(s). The formula for the CALF of any lens (including the cornea or IOL) is:

$$CALF = T_L \times (1 - 1532/V_L),$$

where T_L = the axial thickness of the lens and V_L = the sound velocity through that lens.

Holladay computes the thickness of the human cataractous lens using:

$$T_L = 4 + Age/100,$$

and the sound velocity through the cataract using:

$$V_L = 1659 - [(Age - 10)/2]$$

Substituting the above two formulas into the CALF formula above, the CALF formula for the crystalline lens yields:

$$CALF = \left[4 + \frac{Age}{100}\right] \times \left[1 - \frac{1532}{\left(1659 - \left(\frac{Age-10}{2}\right)\right)}\right]$$

The CALF for the cataractous lens is, therefore, calculated using only the age of the patient. Holladay recommends using a CALF value of 0.28 (value for a 70-year-old) for all ages because the value for a 1-year-old is 0.306 and that for a 100-year-old is 0.224. The maximum error in CALF for those younger than 70 years is 0.026 (0.07 D) and for those older than 70 years is 0.056 (0.14 D).

His formulation, however, ignores the factor of the corneal thickness (0.55 mm). To correct this, I recommend using a CALF of 0.32 (0.28 + 0.037). The correction for the cornea is calculated in Table 4-3B. A similar method can be used for pseudophakic eyes using CALF = $T_L \times (1-1532/V_L)$ and the known V_L for each IOL material (Table 4-3A). Knowing the thickness of the implanted IOL, the formulas in Table 4-3C can be used. If the IOL thickness cannot be obtained, Holladay[7] published a table to use. The AL of an eye containing two IOLs of different materials can be obtained using the formula in Table 4-3C.

Biphakic Eyes (Phakic Eye with a Phakic Intraocular Lens)

The problem here is eliminating the effect of the sound velocity through the phakic lens when measuring the AL using ultrasound. I published a method[8] to correct for this potential error by using the following formula:

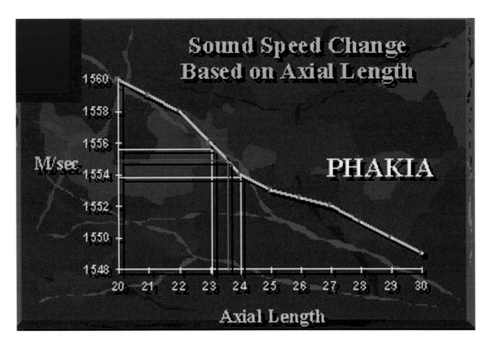

Figure 4-6 Phakic velocity. Graph of decline in average sound velocity of a phakic eye as the axial length increases.

Table 4-3 Formulas for calculating biometric parameters

A. CALF factors for pseudophakic eyes (using CALF = T_L *(1–1532/V_L) where V_L = the sound velocity for the IOL material in the eye

$\text{CALF}_{\text{PMMA}} = T_L * (1 - 1532/2660) = +0.424 * T_L$
$\text{CALF}_{\text{Silicone}} = T_L * (1 - 1532/980) = -0.563 * T_L$
$\text{CALF}_{\text{Acrylic}} = T_L * (1 - 1532/2026) = +0.243 * T_L$

B. The correction for the cornea:

$\text{CALF}_{\text{Cornea}} = T_C * (1 - 1532/1641) = 0.55 * (0.066423) = 0.037$

C. Knowing the thickness of the implanted IOL*, the following formulas can be used:

PMMA eye	$AL = AL_{1532} + 0.424 * T_L + 0.037$
Silicone eye	$AL = AL_{1532} - 0.563 * T_L + 0.037$
Acrylic eye	$AL = AL_{1532} + 0.243 * T_L + 0.037$
Piggyback IOLs	$AL = AL_{1532} + T_1 * (1 - 1532/V_1) + T_2 * (1 - 1532/V_2) + 0.037$, where T_1 and T_2 are the thickness and V_1 and V_2 are the velocity of each IOL.

*The IOL thickness can be obtained from the manufacturer.

$$\text{AL}_{\text{CORRECTED}} = \text{AL}_{1555} + (C \times T)$$

where AL_{1555} = the measured AL of the eye at the sound velocity of 1555 m/s, T = the central thickness of the phakic IOL and C = the material specific correction factor of +0.42 for PMMA, −0.59 for silicone, +0.11 for collamer and +0.23 for acrylic.

The publication[7] contains tables showing the phakic IOL central thickness of each dioptric power for each phakic IOL on the market today.

Retinal Thickness Factor

Some formula writers add a value to the ultrasonic AL measurement to take into account the additional distance from the surface of the retina to the level of the receptive end of the retinal cones. This value has been estimated to be 0.20–0.25 mm and is automatically added to the AL in some formulas (Binkhorst, Holladay) and not used at all in others (Colenbrander, Hoffer® Q).

CORNEAL POWER

The first lens in the eye's optical system is the cornea. We usually think of corneal power in terms of diopters of optical power but really we are measuring the radius of curvature of the anterior surface and making assumptions regarding the curvature of the back surface based on the Gullstrand eye. As newer instrumentation evolves, such as the Pentacam (Oculus, Inc USA, Woodenville, WA 888-284-8004 *www.oculus.de*), we may be able to use Scheimpflug photography to measure the posterior surface of the cornea and, thus, the true total optical effect of the cornea. It has been proposed by many that we should convert to using the radius of curvature (r) rather than diopters (D), but that may take a long time, especially in America.

The important factors to consider in obtaining accurate corneal power are listed in Table 4-1B.

Instrumentation

A manual keratometer measures only the front surface of the cornea and converts the radius (r) of curvature obtained to diopters (K) using an index of refraction (IR) of 1.3375 (some units use a different IR). The formula to change from D to r is (r = 337.5/D)) and from r to D is (D = 337.5/r). Many postulate that this index is too high and Holladay[6] recommends using 4/3 instead. To make this correction, one can simply multiply the K reading obtained (in D) by the factor 0.98765431. This will result in ~0.54 D decrease in corneal power (range; 0.43 D for 35 D cornea to 0.62 D for 50 D cornea). Use the formula 1/3/(IR-1) if your keratometer uses a different index of refraction (IR).

WARNING: *Before using this refractive index correction factor clinically, test it on a series of previously operated eyes to see what effect it would have had on your accuracy.*

To assure accuracy it is important to calibrate all keratometers (including the IOLMaster®) on a regular schedule.

WARNING: *Be sure the Index of Refraction is set to 1.3375 in the Setup screen of the computer on the IOLMaster® for the Hoffer® Q formula to operate properly.*

Corneal topography units also supply simulated corneal power values. I performed a prospective comparison study of the manual keratometer (B&L) with one such unit (TechnoMed C-Scan, Tubinger, Germany, *www.tmed.com*) on 172 cataract eyes. The mean of the central (3 mm zone) readings was 0.24 D flatter with the topography unit (43.55 D vs. 43.79 D), which may be explained by the index of refraction discussed above. When personalization was performed on both instrument data sets, however, IOL power calculation accuracy was statistically equal.

WARNING: *Hard contact lenses (including gas permeable) should be removed permanently for at least 2 weeks prior to measuring corneal power for IOL power calculation.*

Astigmatism

Regular astigmatism is not a factor in IOL power calculation because the goal is to predict the postoperative spherical equivalent refractive error. Therefore, the average of the two K readings is the only value used and should result in mixed astigmatism. If a myopic cylinder were desired, the flattest K reading could be used instead of the average. If astigmatism is surgically corrected at the time of lens implantation, it would be important to know the effect of this surgery on the final average corneal power and adjust the K reading used to calculate the IOL power accordingly. Due to the coupling ratio, this effect is usually zero but an analysis of your previous cases would be useful. Some have reported higher errors in eyes with severe astigmatism.

Keratoconus Eyes

Because a cornea with keratoconus can become very steep, it is important to consider the fact that formulas that use the K reading to estimate the IOL position or effective lens position (ELP) may overestimate this actual postoperative position. One should be aware that the K reading has less of this effect in the Hoffer® Q formula than the other modern theoretic formulas. It is not a factor at all with the Haigis formula since it does not use the K reading at all in estimating the ELP.

Previous Corneal Refractive Surgery

Previous corneal refractive surgery changes the architecture of the cornea such that standard methods of measuring the corneal power cause it to be underestimated (myopia) and overestimated (hyperopia). This was first reported by Koch[9] in 1989. Radial keratotomy (RK) causes a relatively proportional equal flattening of both the front and back surface of the cornea leaving the index of refraction relationship the same. On the other hand, photorefractive keratectomy (PRK), laser-assisted intrastromal keratomileusis (LASIK) and laser-assisted epithelial keratomileusis (LASEK) flatten only the front surface. In myopic eyes, this changes the refractive index calculation creating an underestimation of the corneal power by about one diopter for every seven diopters of refractive surgery correction obtained.

The major cause of error is the fact that most keratometers measure at the 3.2 mm zone of the central cornea, which often misses the central flatter zone of effective corneal power; the flatter the cornea, the larger the zone of measurement. There are at least seven methods to more accurately estimate the corneal power in these refractive surgery eyes. There are also seven methods to adjust the target IOL power. To calculate the target IOL power P_{TARG}. Many of these methods require knowledge of some of the following biometric information:

- The planned postoperative refractive error desired Rx_{TARG}
- Refractive surgery preoperative corneal power (K readings) K_{PRE}
- Refractive surgery preoperative refractive error (spherical equivalent) R_{PRE}
- Refractive surgery postoperative refractive error (spherical equivalent) R_{PO}.

Methods to Estimate True Postoperative Corneal Power

Clinical History Method[10–16]

This method is based on the fact that the final change in refractive error the eye obtains from corneal surgery was due only to a change in the effective corneal power. If this refractive change is added to the presurgical corneal power, we will obtain the effective corneal power the eye has now.

WARNING: *All patients having corneal refractive surgery should be given the following data to maintain in their personal health records: (1) preoperative corneal power, (2) preoperative refractive error, and (3) postoperative healed refractive error (before lens changes affect it).*

They should be told to give these data to anyone planning to perform cataract/IOL surgery on them.

All attempts should be made to obtain the above information from the refractive surgeon's records. Odenthal et al,[17] in 2002, discovered that, although it is optically correct, it is not beneficial to vertex correct the spectacle refraction as was originally recommended. Most recommend not vertexing the refractions because it causes underestimation of the K reading.

For this method, the estimated effective corneal power (**K**) can be calculated using the following formula:

$$K = K_{PREOP} + R_{PREOP} - R_{PO}$$

where:

R = refractive error
$PREOP$ = preoperative
PO = postoperative.

Contact Lens Method[10–19]

The contact lens method was first described in 1948 by Englishman Frederick Ridley[18] (the inventor of NaOH IOL sterilization), taught by Joseph Soper[19] in 1974 and popularized by Holladay in the 1990s. This method is based on the principle that if a hard PMMA (not rigid gas permeable) contact lens (**CL**) of plano power (**P**) and a base curve (**B**) equal to the effective power of the cornea, is placed on the eye it will not change the refractive error of the eye. That is, the difference between the manifest

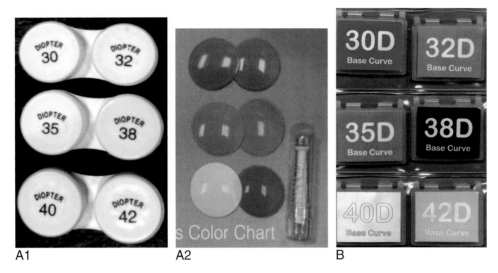

A1   A2   B

Figure 4-7 Hard polymethyl methacrylate (PMMA) contact lens kits in plano powers for the contact lens method. **A,** Ocusoft Kit. **B,** Eye Scan Consulting Kit.

refraction with the contact lens (R_{CL}) and without it (R_{NoCL}) is zero. The formula to calculate the estimated corneal power is:

$$K = B + P + R_{CL} - R_{NoCL}.$$

where:

B = base curve
CL = contact lens
P = power of CL
R = refractive error
NoCL = bare refraction.

Again, it is not presently recommended to vertex-correct the refractive errors to the corneal plane. Several computer IOL power calculation programs calculate these two methods automatically when needed (Hoffer® Programs and Holladay® IOL Consultant). There are commercially available hard PMMA CL sets in plano powers with appropriate base curves from Ocusoft (Figure 4-7A) and Eye Scan Consulting (Figure 4-7B) (Decatur, GA, 404-286-9067, *eyescan@comcast.net*).

Maloney Corneal Topography Method[20]

Based on his analysis of corneal topography central Ks (Kt) on LASIK eyes, Robert Maloney[20] developed a formulation in 1998 to predict true corneal power using only the Kt. The formula is:

$$K = Kt \times (376/337.5) - 5.5 \text{ or,}$$
$$K = 1.1141 \times Kt - 5.5$$

where Kt is postoperative topography central K.

Koch Modification of Maloney Method[21]

In 2003, Douglas Koch[21] analyzed several of these methods and obtained the best results using the Maloney method but only after increasing the constant from 5.5 to 6.1. The formula is:

$$K = Kt \times (376/337.5) - 6.1 \text{ or,}$$
$$K = 1.1141 \times Kt - 6.1$$

where Kt is postoperative topography central K.

He reported on series of eyes where the best results were obtained using this K estimation and the Aramberri Double-K method with a 3rd-generation formula. He also offered a second method to calculate estimated corneal power if the change in refractive error (RC) of the patient known. The formula is:

$$K = Kt - (0.19 \times RC)$$

where:

Kt = central average K from corneal topography
RC = refractive change in refractive error from the surgery.

Ronje Method[22]

The Ronje[22] Method proposes that the corneal power can be estimated by simply adjusting the flattest postoperative manual keratometry (K_{POFLAT}) by 25% of the change in the spherical equivalent refractive error (**RC**) that occurred from the corneal refractive surgery.

For example:

R_{PRE} − 5.00 R_{PO} plano; thus RC = −5.00 K_{POFLAT} 42.00

$$K = K_{POFLAT} + 0.25 * RC$$
$$= 42.00 + 0.25 * (-5.00) = 42.00 - 1.25 = 40.75$$

where:

R_{PRE} = refractive surgery spherical equivalent
R_{PO} = post refractive surgery spherical equivalent
K_{POFLAT} = flattest measured postoperative manual keratometry.

Shammas No History Method[23]

Another interesting proposal is by Shammas[23] who studied a series of eyes that have had LASIK. His results led him to propose a formula, in 2003, to predict the effective power of the cornea without needing any of the patient's clinical history, only the postoperative K reading obtained with manual keratometry. The formula is:

$$K = 1.14 \times K_{PO} - 6.8$$

where:

K = predicted corneal power

K_{PO} = the average corneal power obtained with manual keratometry after corneal refractive surgery.

Instruments: Topographers and Pentacam

The first instruments to measure corneal power by topography were the Eyesys, Technomed C-Scan and Humphrey units. Holladay developed the "Diagnostic Summary" for the Eyesys unit (Figure 4-8), but still, most of these measurements fall down in post-refractive-surgery eyes.

The next instrumentation developed was the Orbscan (Bausch & Lomb), but the difficulty with this unit has been in the post LASIK or PRK cornea. Here the Orbscan has a tendency to overestimate the elevation of the posterior cornea giving an artifactual ectatic appearance[24] (Figure 4-9). Additional error may be induced by a relatively long acquisition time allowing patient movement as the image is being taken.[25] There have also been documented inaccuracies in measurement of the posterior curvature in control standards.[26]

That brings us to the latest and most promising technology, the Oculus Pentacam, which images the anterior segment of the eye using a rotating Scheimpflug camera measurement providing three-dimensional images (Figure 4-10). These images provide a topographic analysis of the corneal thickness, its front surface and most importantly its back surface curvature. In conjunction with software provided by Holladay, the Pentacam is touted to have the ability to generate what they call a "TrueNetPower" map of the cornea and measure the power of the post-refractive-surgery cornea within ±0.55 D. This may provide a better estimation of the true corneal power but it has not yet been tested in a large randomized clinical trial.

Holladay has reported an analysis of the comparison of the postoperative Pentacam reading at 4 mm zone to the calculated postoperative power in a series of LASIK eyes. The calculated power was obtained by subtracting the change in refractive error (vertexed to zero) from the pre-refractive-surgery Eyesys Sim-K. The correlation resulted in an R2 of 0.9631 and y of 0.9555 indicating excellent correlation. He then recommended converting the True Net Power of the Pentacam to the Equivalent Sim-K of the Eyesys (e.g. 44.25 D = 45.00 D). The report provides the "Sim-K" and the "Equivalent K Reading."

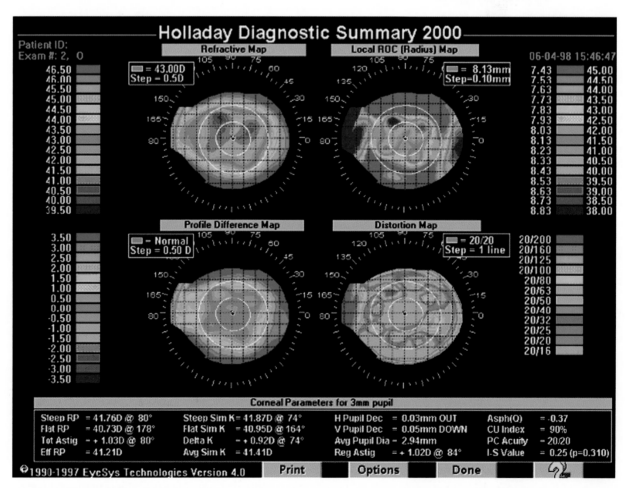

Figure 4-8 Eyesys Holladay Diagnostic screen showing corneal power.

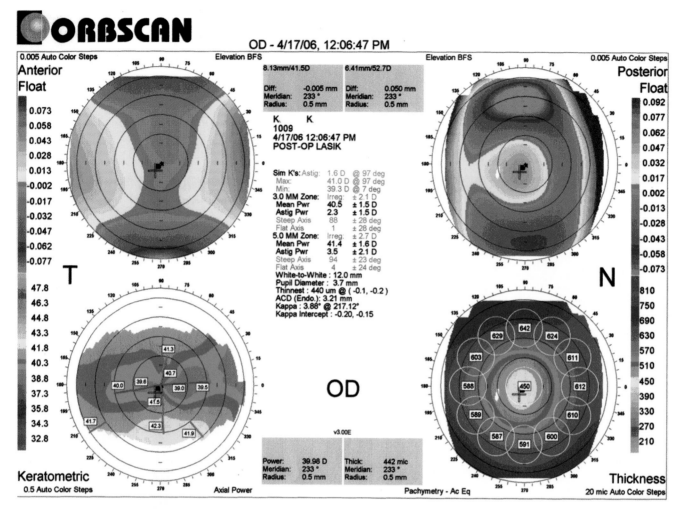

Figure 4-9 Orbscan screen showing corneal power maps.

Corneal Power Estimation Summary

In summary, if the results of the above K estimation methods differ, use the lowest estimated corneal power (highest for hyperopic refractive eyes). Rarely are such eyes myopic after IOL surgery. Obviously, some methods cannot be used if the historical data is not available and the CL method is impossible if the cataract precludes performing a refraction. In such cases, it might be wise to delay the IOL implantation and calculate the secondary IOL power using the aphakic refractive error in the refraction formula or use a piggyback lens or phakic refractive lens to correct any deficiency. However, there are other methods available.

METHODS TO ADJUST/CALCULATE THE TARGET INTRAOCULAR LENS POWER

Aramberri Double-K Method[27]

Once you have decided on the "best" estimated preoperative K, there is one more consideration. It is the "Double-K" method, one of the most important developments to improve the prediction of corneal power in eyes that have had refractive surgery. It was proposed in 2001 by Aramberri[27] of San Sebastian, Spain.

His proposal makes eminent sense. The modern theoretic formulas (except the Haigis) use the corneal power for two purposes; the first is to predict the ultimate position of the IOL (ACD or ELP) and the second (along with AL, target refraction and ELP) is to calculate the power of the IOL. The formulations and algorithms used to predict the ELP are based on the anatomy of the anterior segment which has not been changed by corneal refractive surgery (only the center is flattened and thinned). Therefore, if the postoperative refractive surgery K reading (which is significantly flatter) is used to calculate the ELP it will produce an erroneous ELP value. Since the anatomy has not changed, Aramberri recommends the use of the preoperative K reading to calculate the ELP. The IOL power is then calculated using the postoperative K reading, thus the "Double-K." His analysis of a small series of eyes proved the benefit of this idea. This method is available for the SRK/T, Holladay and Hoffer® Q formulas on the Hoffer® Programs computer system (see Figure 4-12).

Feiz Method[28,29]

This method was first described in 2001 by Feiz et al.[28] Their formula was developed by comparing manual keratometry values after LASIK and using the SRK/T formula, the IOL power calculated

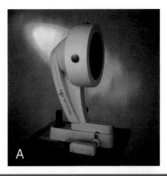

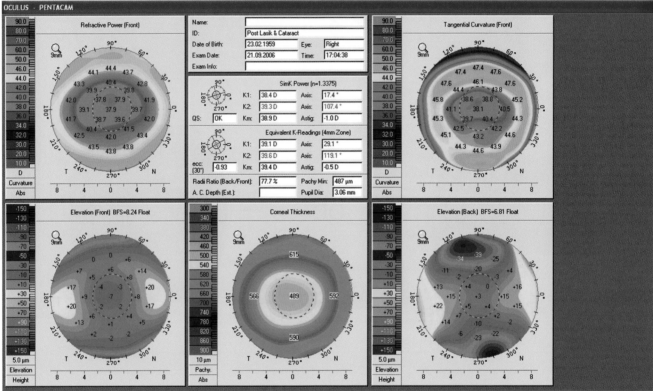

Figure 4-10 **A,** Oculus Pentacam instrument. **B,** Oculus Pentacam Holladay Power Map screen showing Sim-K and Equivalent K Reading (EKR).

(Continued)

using the historical method, and what they termed the vertexed IOL power method. In this method two assumptions were made. The first was that to achieve emmetropia, the change in spherical equivalent induced by keratorefractive surgery had to be balanced by the change in IOL power. The second assumption was that for every diopter of change in IOL power, only 0.7 D of change will be seen at the spectacle plane. This assumption is not true in all axial lengths.

Performing a linear regression analysis of the vertex IOL power compared to standard keratometry, they developed two linear regression formulas; one for myopic LASIK corneas and the second for hyperopic LASIK corneas:

For myopic LASIK corneas:
$$P = P_{TARG} - 0.595 * RC - 0.231$$

For hyperopic LASIK corneas:
$$P = P_{TARG} - 0.862 * RC + 0.751$$

where:

P = required IOL power

P_{TARG} = the IOL power calculated for the desired postoperative Target Rx using the AL and measured (unadjusted) K reading

RC = the change in refraction (spherical equivalent) caused by the refractive surgery.

In 2005, they reported a comparison of all three methods for IOL calculation[29] in 19 eyes after myopic LASIK or PRK, which resulted in consistently higher IOL powers using their formula compared to using the post LASIK measurements and the historical method. It still resulted in 16% of eyes being either moderately over- or under-corrected. The hyperopic formula has not undergone any reported study demonstrating its validity.

Below are example calculations (Table 4-4).

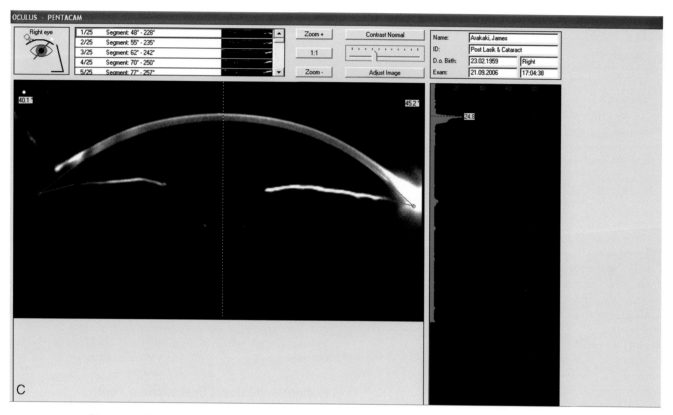

Right eye	1/25	Segment: 48° - 228°
	2/25	Segment: 55° - 235°
	3/25	Segment: 62° - 242°
	4/25	Segment: 70° - 250°
	5/25	Segment: 77° - 257°

Zoom + | Contrast Normal | Name: Arakaki, James
1:1 | | ID: Post Lasik & Cataract
Zoom - | Adjust Image | D.o. Birth: 23.02.1959 Right
Exam: 21.09.2006 17:04:38

Figure 4-10, cont'd C, Scheimpflug photograph of anterior segment by Pentacam.

Table 4-4 Feiz Method example calculations

Myopic Eye	Hyperopic Eye
SRK/T calculates 16.0 D IOL	Hoffer Q calculates 22.0 D
Change in Rx = −6.0 D	Change in Rx = +3.0 D
−0.595*(−6) −0.231 = +3.34	−0.862*(+3) + 0.751 = −1.84
P = 16.0 + 3.34 = 19.34 D	P = 22.0 − 1.84 = 20.16 D

From their formulae, they produced a nomogram for both types of eyes which might be easier for those without a calculator handy (Table 4-5):

Latkany Method[30]

The first proposal by Latkany's group[30] uses the manually measured flattest K of the postoperative cornea in the SRK/T formula. The resulting IOL power is then adjusted by the following formula:

$$P = P_{FlatK} − (0.47 * PRx + 0.85)$$

where:

P = required IOL power

P_{FlatK} = the IOL power calculated by SRK/T for desired postoperative Rx using the AL and the measured flattest K reading (unadjusted)

PRx = the preoperative refractive surgery spherical equivalent.

The study reported this method to be equal to the historical method for calculation of corneal power. Below is an example calculation (Table 4-6).

Table 4-5 Feiz Method nomogram

Feiz[29] Nomogram	Adjustment to Target IOL Power	
D Change in Rx from LASIK (X)	Myopic Eye [−0.595*x−0.231]	Hyperopic Eye [−0.862*x+0.751]
1.00	+0.36	0.00
2.00	+0.96	−0.97
3.00	+1.55	−1.84
4.00	+2.15	−2.70
5.00	+2.74	−3.56
6.00	+3.34	−4.42
7.00	+3.93	−5.28
8.00	+4.53	−6.15
9.00	+5.12	−7.00
10.00	+5.72	−7.87

Masket Refractive History Method[31]

In 2005, Masket[31] proposed yet another method which adjusts the power of the IOL calculated using the measured IOLM-master data. The formula to adjust the IOL power is:

Table 4-6 Latkany Method example calculations

Myopic Eye
SRK/T calculates 22.91 D IOL using Flattest K 42.00 D
Pre-LASIK Rx = −5.0 D
−(0.47*(−5) + 0.85) = +1.50
P = 22.91 + 1.50 = 24.41 D

IOL: intraocular lens; D: diopter.

$$P = P_{EMM} - 0.323 * RC + 0.138$$

where:

P = required IOL power

P_{EMM} = the IOL power calculated for emmetropia using the AL and measured (unadjusted) K reading

RC = the change in refraction (spherical equivalent) caused by the refractive surgery.

He recommends using the SRK/T formula for myopic ALs and the Hoffer® Q for hyperopic ALs. Here are example calculations (Table 4-7):

In a series of 28 post-LASIK eyes, he reported 43% of the eyes obtaining a postoperative refractive error of plano, 95% being within ± 0.50 D of prediction and a total error range from −0.75 D to +0.50 D. These early results in a small series by the author of the method are surprisingly impressive.

Wake Forest Method[32]

In 2005, Michael Gagnon[32] presented an alternative calculation method by the group at Wake Forest University, which has been discussed by others over the years. This method simply uses the patient's preoperative refraction before LASIK as the target or "desired" postoperative refraction in the calculation, and the measured AL and K readings without modification.

Ianchulev Intraoperative Aphakic Refraction Method[33]

In 2003, Sean Ianchulev[33] proposed calculating IOL power by performing an aphakic refraction on the operating table immediately after the cataract has been removed using a handheld automated refractor. The resultant refraction is modified by the following formula:

$$P = 2.02 \times AR + (A - 118.4)$$

where:

P = emmetropic IOL power

Table 4-7 Masket Refractive History Method example calculations

Myopic Eye	Hyperopic Eye
SRK/T calculates 16.0 D IOL	Hoffer Q calculates 22.0 D
Change in Rx = −6.0 D	Change in Rx = +3.0 D
−0.323*(−6) + 0.138 = +2.076	−0.323*(+3) + 0.138 = −0.82
P = 16.0 + 2.0 = 18.0 D	P = 22.0 − 1.0 = 21.0 D

AR = automated refraction

A = IOL A constant.

His early results are quite promising. This method would completely eliminate the need for axial length and corneal power measurements, in addition to the problems with LASIK and silicone oil-filled eyes. However, it would require a large inventory of IOL powers available in the OR.

Following on this idea, in 2006, Mackool[34] published a small series of patients who had cataract extraction without IOL implantation under topical anesthesia. Thirty minutes after the surgery, an aphakic manifest refraction was performed at a vertex distance of 12 mm. The following formula was then used to calculate IOL power:

$$P = 1.75 \times AR + (A - 118.84)$$

where:

P = emmetropic IOL power

AR = aphakic refraction

A = IOL A constant.

After the IOL calculation was carried out, the patient was immediately returned to the operating room for IOL implantation using the calculated power. Using the above formula in 12 eyes, he reported a mean absolute refractive error of 0.30 D, and an average refractive error of −0.18 D. However, having two separate surgeries would seem to be inconvenient.

Hoffer/Savini Excel Spreadsheet Tool

In 2006, it became obvious that there were so many methods to perform these calculations that it was becoming very confusing. This author in collaboration with Giacomi Savini of Italy decided to place all the various calculations on one Microsoft Excel spreadsheet so it would be easy to see what data needed to be collected (Figure 4-11). Once all or most of the data are entered into the appropriate cells, the calculations are performed automatically. Then the results of all the methods are displayed side by side allowing the surgeon to select the most appropriate calculation. Anecdotally, the first use of this spreadsheet (Figure 4-12) led to a 2-month postoperative refractive error of −0.25 D (SE) when the target Rx was −0.50 D (UCVA 20/25; BCVA 20/20). The tool is free and downloadable at www.EyeLab.com.

Retinal Detachment Eyes: Hoffer Double-Axial Length Method

Just as the Double-K method uses two K readings because the formulas use the K reading to predict the ELP, this method, proposed by the author in 2000, instead uses two ALs. The postoperative retinal detachment (RD) AL of the eye is used to calculate the IOL power. Since most post-encircling band RD eyes have a 1.0 mm increase in AL, and the ACD is not affected by the encircling band, it would be best to use the AL-1 in the part of the formula that calculates the predicted ELP. This method results in making the IOL a little weaker than would be predicted using all the modern formulas. Alternatively, one would just lower the recommended IOL power in such RD eyes.

Corneal Transplant Eyes

A problem also arises when attempting to predict what the corneal power will be after corneal transplantation. Some have suggested using the corneal power of the other eye (if it is

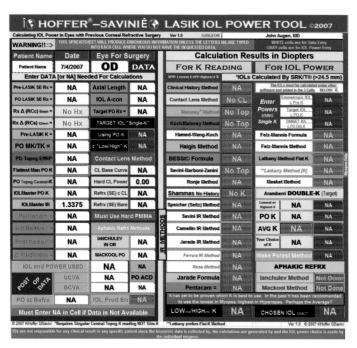

Figure 4-11 Hoffer/Savini LASIK IOL Power Calculation Spreadsheet organizer before data entry.

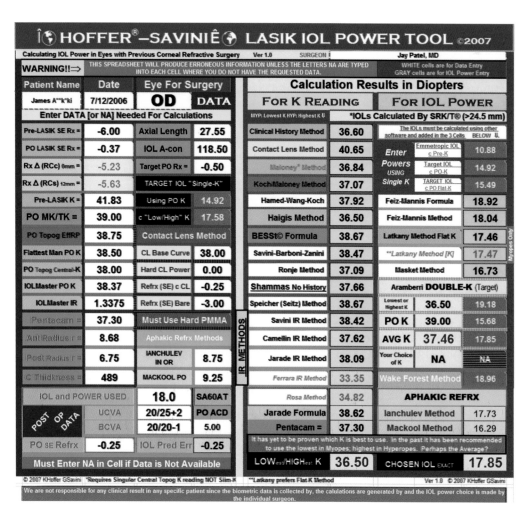

Figure 4-12 Hoffer/Savini LASIK IOL Power Calculation Spreadsheet organizer showing all data and postoperative results.

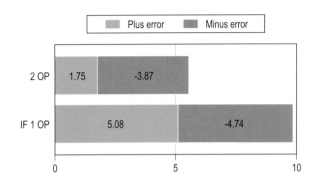

Figure 4-13 Corneal transplants. Dramatic decrease in range of IOL prediction error when IOL is implanted secondarily after transplant heals (5.62 D) vs. a triple procedure (9.82 D).

available) or using an average of one's post-transplant corneal powers, but published reports show a very large range of prediction and refractive errors using these attempts. Performing the IOL implantation after the corneal transplant has settled down was suggested by this author[35] in 1986 and in 1990, Geggel[36] reported excellent refractive results (Figure 4-13) using this two-stepped approach (66% 20/40 or better acuity without correction). A secondary piggyback toric IOL or toric phakic IOL is another alternative to correct residual ametropia.

Corneal Scar Eyes

The problem of getting an accurate corneal power measurement in eyes with corneal scarring and irregular astigmatism has not received much attention. Cua et al[37] studied this in two eyes needing IOL exchange due to large "IOL surprises" of +5 and −7.5 D. They compared six methods to ascertain the corneal power and found the hard contact lens over refraction method to be the most accurate; decreasing the error they would have obtained with the manual keratometer of +4–5 D to −0.4–1.6 D. This may be a useful clinical tool in such cases.

INTRAOCULAR LENS AXIAL POSITION

This factor was historically referred to as the anterior chamber depth (ACD) because the optic of all IOLs in the early era was positioned in front of the iris, in the anterior chamber. Because most IOLs today are positioned behind the iris, new terminology has been offered, such as effective lens position (ELP) by Holladay[6] and actual lens position (ALP) by the FDA.

ACD is defined as the axial distance between the two lenses (cornea and lens or IOL) or, more exactly, the distance from the central front surface (anterior vertex) of the cornea to the effective principle plane of the IOL (or front surface of the crystalline lens). This value is required for all formulas and it is incorporated into the A constant specific to each IOL style for regression formulas or as an ACD, both supplied by the manufacturer. Some have proposed that it would be useful to measure the preoperative anatomic ACD (corneal epithelium to anterior capsule) either with an A-scan unit or by optical pachymetry.

The author performed such a comparison study on 44 eyes and showed that the optical method resulted in a mean 0.20 (±0.35) mm deeper ACD than obtained by ultrasound using 1548 m/s (3.14 vs.2.93 mm).

The IOL position has been considered the least important of the three variables as a cause of IOL power error, but in 1998, the author saw an early postoperative IOL patient with a shallowed ACD and myopia of −2.50. After 3 days, the chamber deepened by 2.0 mm and the refractive error changed to plano. IOL position has received the most attention from formula writers over the past 10 years. The major effort has been toward better prediction of where the IOL will ultimately rest. A recent study by the author on a series of 270 eyes receiving a silicone plate haptic lens showed that the IOL shifted a mean of 0.06 mm posteriorly (ACD deepened) at 3 months, compared to its position on the first day after surgery. This was commensurate with a mean 0.21 D shift toward hyperopia.

WARNING: *An IOL intended for capsular bag placement should be decreased by 0.75–1.25 D (depending upon the IOL power) when placed in the ciliary sulcus.*

■ FORMULAS ■

GENERATIONS

First Generation

The first IOL power formula was published by Fyodorov[38] in 1967. Colenbrander[39] wrote his in 1972, followed by the Hoffer[40] formula in 1974. Binkhorst[41] published his formula in 1975, which became widely used in America. In 1978, first Lloyd and Gills[42,43], followed by Retzlaff[44] and, later, Sanders and Kraff[45] each developed a regression formula based on analysis of their previous IOL cases. This work was amalgamated in 1980 to yield the SRK I formula.[46] All these formulas depended on a single constant for each lens that represented the predicted IOL position (ACD).

Second Generation

In 1982, at the Welsh Cataract Congress in Houston, the author[47,48] demonstrated a direct relationship between the position of a PMMA posterior chamber IOL and the axial length, and presented a formula to better predict ACD. Others (Binkhorst[49], SRK II[50] (1988)) developed different mechanisms to apply this predictive relationship which Holladay defined as the second generation.

Third Generation

In 1988, Holladay[51] proposed a direct relationship between the steepness of the cornea and the position of the IOL. He modified the Binkhorst formula to incorporate this as well as the axial length relationship. Instead of ACD input, the formula would calculate the predicted distance from the cornea to the iris plane (using a corneal height formula by Fyodorov) and add to it the distance from the iris plane to the IOL. The latter he called the surgeon factor (SF) and it is specific to each lens. Retzlaff[52] followed suit and modified the Holladay I formula to allow use of A constants calling it the SRK/T theoretic formula in 1990. It was intended to replace the previous SRK regression formulas that 50% of American surgeons still use despite this. In 1992, Hoffer developed the Q formula[53] using a tangent function to accomplish the same effect.

Fourth Generation

In 1990, Olsen et al.[54] proposed using the preoperative ACD and other factors to better estimate the postoperative IOL position and published algorithms for this approach. After several studies showed that the Holladay I formula was not as accurate as the Hoffer® Q in eyes shorter than 22 mm, Holladay used the preoperative ACD measurement, as well as corneal diameter, lens thickness, refractive error and age, to calculate an estimated scaling factor (ESF) that multiplies the IOL-specific ACD. This Holladay II formula has been promulgated since 1996 but has yet to be published.

In 1999, Wolfgang Haigis[55] proposed using three constants based on the characteristics of the eye and the IOL to predict the position of the IOL. The formula calculates the predicted postoperative ELP by:

$$ELP = a_0 + a_1 * ACD + a_2 * AL$$

where:

ELP = predicted IOL position
a_0 = a lens-specific constant
a_1 = a constant to be effected by the measured preoperative ACD
a_2 = a lens-specific constant to be effected by the measured preoperative axial length
ACD = the measured axial distance from the corneal apex to the front surface of the lens
AL = axial length.

As in the Holladay formula, the constants must be optimized (personalized) to each IOL style and surgeon. Single optimization only optimizes the a_0 and creates accuracy equal to the Hoffer® Q and Holladay, but triple optimization of all three constants creates additional accuracy. The problem is that triple optimization requires a series of 500–1000 cases of one lens style and the eyes in the series must statistically cover all axial lengths from very short to very long. This may be quite difficult to achieve for the average surgeon.

Refraction Formula

Holladay[56] published a formula in 1993 to calculate the power of an IOL for an aphakic eye or ametropic pseudophakic eye (piggyback IOL) or a refractive lens (PRL) for a phakic eye. It does not need the AL, but does require the corneal power, preoperative refractive error and desired postoperative refractive error, as well as the vertex distance of both. The author does not recommend its use in aphakic eyes because the vertex distance is difficult to measure accurately and, owing to the high power of their refractive error, greater errors can result. It is, however, a good check against the AL formula calculation.

USAGE

Based on Axial Length

My study[53] of 450 eyes (by one surgeon using one IOL style) (Figure 4-14) showed that in the normal range (72%) of axial length (22.0–24.5 mm) almost all formulas function adequately, but that the SRK I formula is the leading cause of poor refractive results in eyes outside this range. It also showed that the Holladay I formula was the most accurate in medium-long eyes (24.5–26.0 mm) (15%) and the SRK/T was more accurate in very-long eyes (>26.0 mm) (5%). In short eyes (<22.0 mm) (8%) the Hoffer® Q formula was most accurate and this was confirmed ($P>0.0001$) in an additional large study of 830 short eyes as well as in a multiple-surgeon study by Holladay. Holladay has postulated that the other formulas overestimate the shallowing of the effective lens position (ELP) in these very short eyes.

A more recent study[57] performed by the author on 317 eyes, showed that the Holladay II formula equaled the Hoffer® Q in short eyes but was not as accurate as the Holladay I or Hoffer® Q in average and medium-long eyes (Table 4-8). Eyes shorter than 19 mm are extremely rare (0.1%) and may well be benefited by using the Holladay II formula. It appears that in attempting to improve the accuracy of the Holladay formula, the addition of more biometric data input has improved the Holladay II formula in the extremes of axial length but deteriorated its excellent performance in the normal and medium-long range of eyes (22.0–26.0 mm), which accounts for 82% of the population.

Methodology

There are several means by which to use these newer formulas including A-scan instruments, handheld calculators, and computer programs that run on DOS, Windows and Macintosh systems, as well as for the palm PDA operating system (Figure 4-15). You can also adapt the published ones yourself to a spreadsheet program. It is important to check the errata in references 41 and 42.

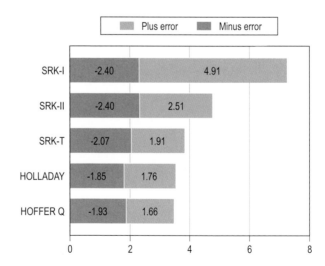

Figure 4-14 Error range. Range of intraocular lens power error in 450 eye study using regression formulas compared to modern theoretic formulas.

Table 4-8 Results of accuracy of four theoretical formulas on 317 eyes using the Holladay IOL Consultant for analysis [Shaded = recommended formulas][46]

| Formula | Mean Absolute Error | | | | | | All 317 Eyes | |
	Short <22.0	Normal 22.0–24.5	M-long 24.5–26.0	V-long >26.0	Long <24.5	All eyes	Max Error	>± 2 D error
Holladay 2	0.72	0.56	0.51	0.49	0.50	0.55	−1.60	0%
Holladay 1	0.85	0.42	0.37	0.56	0.43	0.43	−1.44	0%
Hoffer Q	0.72	0.43	0.47	0.58	0.50	0.45	−1.61	0%
SRK/T	0.83	0.46	0.35	0.44	0.36	0.44	−1.45	0%
AVERAGE	0.78	0.47	0.42	0.52	0.45	0.47		
BEST	H–Q H–2	H–Q H–1	S/T H–1	S/T	S/T			

Where M-long = medium long, V-long = very long, Long = all long eyes, Max = maximum.

The most popular commercial programs are the Hoffer® Programs System* (the first computer program for IOL power in 1994) and the Holladay® IOL Consultant* (1997), which include several formulas that can be personalized and provide routines to deal with odd clinical situations.

*Available from EyeLab, Inc. 1605 San Vicente Blvd, Santa Monica, CA 90402, 310-451-2020, *KHofferMD@AOL.com*.

PERSONALIZATION

The concept of personalizing a formula based on a surgeon's past experience and data was introduced by Retzlaff[52,58] using the A constant to refine the formula. Holladay incorporated this concept into backsolving for the Surgeon Factor and Hoffer backsolved for his personalized ACD. Several studies have proved that formula personalization definitely improves formula accuracy significantly.

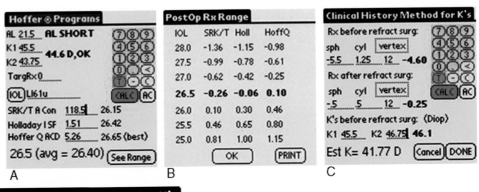

Figure 4-15 Hoffer® IOL power program on a palm personal digital assistant. **A,** Main calculation screen using Hoffer Q®, Holladay and SRK/T formulas. **B,** Next screen showing refractive results of different intraocular lens (IOL) powers. **C,** Clinical history method screen. **D,** Contact lens method screen. **E,** Personalization screen for adding new postoperative eyes. **F,** Personalization screen for various IOLs.

The following parameters are required from postoperative eyes:

1. Axial length (preoperative)
2. Corneal power (preoperative)
3. IOL power
4. Postoperative refractive error (stable).

The eyes should all contain the same lens style by one manufacturer that has been implanted by one surgeon. The same biometry instruments and technician should also have been used. Eyes with postoperative surprises or acuity worse than 20/40 should not be included in the analysis; this is due to poor accuracy in obtaining refractive error. Personalization involves backsolving for the exact IOL position that would produce the resultant refractive error with that IOL power, AL and K. Then all the "ideal" IOL positions are averaged to arrive at the personalized value to use in the future. Personalization can be easily performed using the Hoffer® Programs or Holladay® IOL Consultant computer programs.

■ CLINICAL VARIABLES ■

PATIENT NEEDS AND DESIRES

Most surgeons have developed their own plan for deciding on the clinical needs of their patients. It has often been recommended to aim patients for mild postoperative myopia (-0.5 to -1.5 D), so if the error is on the plus side, they will be emmetropic and if on the minus side, they will have reading vision. This is necessary because of the larger range of IOL power errors generally experienced. When the bell-shaped curve of prediction error is squeezed down to 67% within ±0.50 D, it is then possible to aim most patients for emmetropia. This is even more important when implanting a multifocal IOL. Senior citizens are much more active today then in the past and in emergency situations it would be a lot safer if they were emmetropic.

There are several exceptions, however. Patients who have been life-long myopes are never happy being hyperopes postoperatively. Patients that would wind up with a large anisometropia should be stimulated to be fitted with a contact lens in the other eye prior to deciding on an emmetropic IOL. Monocular contact lens wearers are more successful than binocular. It is wise to document all discussions in unusual situations.

SPECIAL CIRCUMSTANCES

Monocular Cataract in Bilateral High Ametropia

The dilemma is whether to make the ametropic eye emmetropic or to match the large ametropia of an eye that may never need surgery. Up until now, the author has convinced most patients to accept a monocular contact lens or ignore the unaffected eye and go for the "brass ring" of emmetropia. In the future, those that can't tolerate contact lenses could have a phakic IOL either placed in the unaffected eye or placed over the IOL to eliminate aniseikonia and have it removed should the affected eye ultimately need surgery.

Pediatric Eyes

Children have always posed a dilemma[59] in IOL power selection in that the eye will grow in length and become more myopic if a fixed emmetropic power is implanted. The study of pediatric eyes by Gordon and Donzis[60] shows a steep axial length growth rate from premature babies to age 2 years, increasing by 6 mm ($\sim$20 D), while corneal power drops from 54 D to 44 D offsetting 10 D. If IOLs are used in this age group it might be best to place piggyback lenses with the more posterior IOL having the average adult emmetropic power and the anterior IOL being the added power needed to reach emmetropia now. As the child grows, they can be corrected with myopic glasses until they are old enough to have the anterior IOL removed.

Between the ages of 2 and 5 years growth slows to about 0.4 mm per year and between the ages of 5 and 10 years the total growth is only another 1 mm, while corneal power remains stable. From age 2 to 10, it might be wise to aim for 1.5–2 D of hyperopia postoperatively, which allows for reasonable uncorrected vision and light spectacle correction in amblyopia treatment. When they mature, they will wind up emmetropic or mildly myopic, depending on the age at implantation. Growth slows after age 10–15 and emmetropia can be the aim. Future use of implantable phakic refractive lenses over the top of IOLs may be very helpful in these children since they can easily be exchanged as the eye grows, keeping them emmetropic throughout life.

Plager et al.[61] reported on 38 eyes of 27 subjects who had received an IOL in childhood. Based on their results, they recommend the following scheme for the refractive age-dependent goal for children (Table 4-9).

Multifocal Intraocular Lens

In 1991 the author[62] reported that to obtain -2.75 D myopia (reading at 14–16 inches) the IOL power in the near vision region must be about 3.75–4.00 D stronger than the emmetropic power. It was also shown that the amount of this additional power in a bifocal IOL is not affected at all by the axial length and very little by the corneal power. It is affected, however, by the IOL position and an AC lens needs less add power than a PC lens. Obviously, to negate the need for any glasses, it is important to aim for emmetropia, but mild postoperative hyperopia is far better than even the mildest myopia. The distance vision will be reasonable in the former (the patient can easily obtain readers if necessary); while in the latter it will not. Bifocal IOL patients with myopia are not happy

Table 4-9

Age	3	4	5	6	7	8	10	13
Goal	+5.00	+4.00	+3.00	+2.25	+1.50	+1.00	+0.50	Plano

and everything should be done to avoid this situation, since minus power "readers" are not readily available. A phakic IOL could be implanted over the top of the bifocal to make the eye emmetropic.

Silicone Oil Refractive Effect

The second problem that arises when the vitreous is replaced with silicone oil is that the refractive index of the oil is much less than that of the vitreous and it acts as a negative lens in the eye, which must then be offset with more power in the IOL. This effect is dependent upon the shape factor of the back surface of the IOL, such that a biconvex IOL creates the worst problem and a concave posterior lens (no longer commercially available) has practically no effect. In between the two is the plano-posterior lens, which is recommended in these cases. With a plano-convex lens, 2–3 D must be added to the IOL power to compensate for this silicone effect, but much more is needed for biconvex lenses.

Piggyback Lenses

Either piggyback lenses can be placed primarily or the second lens placed secondarily over a previously healed IOL. In the former, the anterior IOL forces the posterior IOL more posteriorly; a distance equal to the central thickness of the anterior lens. This causes the posterior lens (whose focal point is moved more posteriorly) to require more power to maintain the same focus. This effect diminishes the thinner (lower power) the anterior lens is and a thinner lens is easier to remove if that should be necessary. Primary piggyback lenses need special calculations to adjust for the posterior lens shift. One can simply add one-half the central thickness of the anterior IOL to the ACD being used by the formula.

Secondary lenses can be calculated using the refraction formula or by a more simple formulation based on the fact that the healed primary IOL is more stable. Because of the differences in the effects on vertex power changes between plus and minus lenses, the following formulation works well:

$$\text{Hyperopic}: \text{Piggyback IOL} = 1.5 \times Rx_{ERROR}$$
$$\text{Myopic Error}: \text{Piggyback IOL} = 1.0 \times Rx_{ERROR}$$

where Rx = PO spherical equivalent refractive error.

PROBLEMS AND ERRORS

The major problem is an unacceptable postoperative refractive error. The sooner it is discovered, the sooner it can be corrected. Therefore, it is wise to perform K readings and a manifest refraction on the first postoperative day. The author has long recommended immediate surgical correction[63] (24–48 h); this allows easy access to the incision and the capsular bag, one postoperative period, and excellent uncorrected vision. The majority of medico-legal cases today are due to a delay in the diagnosis and the treatment of this iatrogenic problem. Up until now, we could only correct this problem by lens exchange, which creates the dilemma of determining which factor created the IOL power error: axial length, corneal power or mislabeled IOL or a combination of all three. Today, with the advent of low-powered IOLs,

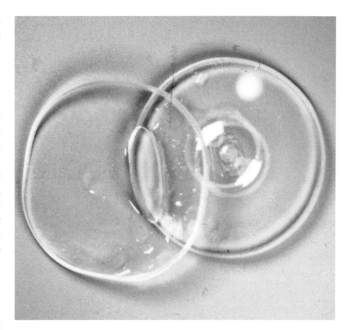

Figure 4-16 McReynolds intraocular lens power analyzer used in standard clinical lensometer.

the best remedy may be a piggyback IOL. When using a piggyback IOL, it is not necessary to determine what caused the error or to remeasure the axial length of the freshly operated pseudophakic eye. It is possible to confirm the power of an explanted IOL by using the McReynolds lens analyzer (Figure 4-16) (Vision & Hearing Center, PO Box 488, 1111 Main St. Quincy, IL 62301, 217-222-6656).

It is important to remember that a shallow AC can lead to as much as 3 D of myopia (depending on the power of the IOL), which will disappear when the AC reforms. An RK eye has a propensity for the cornea to flatten postoperatively causing large hyperopic surprises. It may take up to 3 or 4 months for the cornea to re-steepen, therefore, surgical correction should not be attempted until then.

Handling the Intraocular Lens Power Surprise

An inappropriate postoperative refractive result is disappointing to both the patient and the surgeon. It is often difficult to determine what caused this prediction error.

1. According to most studies, the most common cause is an error in measuring **axial length**:
   a. This is most commonly seen in eyes longer than 25 mm that have a higher incidence of **staphyloma**. The problem with staphylomas is that they can vary in size and position. If the macula is located at the deepest end of the staphyloma, the anatomical AL will equal the visual AL. Most often the macula lies somewhere else along the slope of the staphyloma and the ultrasound measures the anatomical AL which is longer than the true visual AL. Usually these errors are ones of too long AL and too weak an IOL power (hyperopic error).

b. Contact applanation ultrasound artificially shortens the AL and this built in variable error is worse as the AL becomes shorter. Though this fact has been well-accepted, still 70% of clinicians use this procedure and add a fudge factor to correct for it. This would be acceptable if the amount of artificial shortening was approximately the same for every eye, but it is not. Some eyes are shortened by as much as a 1 mm and others are not shortened at all. This leads to a too short AL and too strong IOL power (myopic errors).

c. Technician inexperience or a straightforward error is another cause for incorrect AL measurements.

d. Using the wrong average ultrasound velocity is another cause of measurement errors. Often an average velocity of 1550 m/s is used, which is incorrect. As proven by Hoffer,[42] the correct value for an average phakic cataractous eye is 1555 m/s. The problem is that the average speed for a short 20 mm eye is 1560 m/s and 1550 m/s for a long 30 mm eye.

e. Poor IOLMaster® readings that are not recognized by the examiner also cause errors in AL and are more common if the cataract's density is increased or the patient is not able to fixate properly.

f. Silicone-oil filled eyes are an especially vexing problem since the ultrasound wave is slowed so much in crossing the posterior segment that it is often impossible to obtain a reading. It is also difficult to determine what percentage of the vitreous body is filled and through which parts the beam is traveling. The IOLMaster must be used.

g. Lastly, there is the problem of the eye that "JUST CAN'T BE MEASURED"! This situation is a rare but unfortunate reality. No one has offered a complete explanation for this.

2. Incorrect measurement of the **corneal power** is the second most common reason for IOL power error:

a. Overestimation of the corneal power (K) is the rule in eyes that have had previous corneal refractive surgery. This is due to the fact that there has not yet been a keratometer or keratometer attachment that will allow the measurement of the true central effective corneal power in these eyes. Two factors are at play here: the first is the fact that most keratometers measure at the central 3.2 mm (wider if the cornea is flatter) of the cornea and are unable to measure the more central flat area that is being used by the eye; the second is the change in the refractive index of the cornea, which is difficult to correct for in any individual eye because it is dependent upon the amount that cornea has been flattened.

b. It is important to have a schedule of calibrating all keratometers to prevent errors in measurement.

c. The IOLMaster® has a setup screen that allows the operator to change the index of refraction (IR). Most users are unaware of this. The manufacturer did this to allow the instrument to produce K readings equivalent to that obtained by the manual keratometer used in the clinician's office. American keratometers are set at an IR of 1.3375

and European ones at 1.332. Hoffer recently discovered that if the IOLMaster® IR is not set for 1.3375, the Hoffer® Q formula will be in error.

d. In cataract patients that wear contact lenses, there is a corneal warping factor that produces incorrect K readings compared to those without the contact lens (the state in which the eye will probably be after IOL surgery). This is especially true in cases of patients wearing a hard contact lens. This can be corrected by asking the patient to remove the contact lens for two weeks in the eye to be operated.

e. Corneal scarring, especially in the center, can cause a great problem in measuring the corneal power.

f. Eyes that will need corneal transplantation also pose a problem in predicting preoperatively what the ultimate healed corneal power will be.

3. The third and least effective factor in prediction error is the healed **effective position of the IOL** in the eye. This is referred to as the A constant, the surgeon factor (SF) or the Hoffer anterior chamber depth (ACD). Holladay instituted the replacement term, effective lens position (ELP), since most IOLs today are not in the anterior chamber:

a. Errors may occur if the IOL settles in a deeper or shallower position than that predicted by the formula or what would be expected in an eye with that particular IOL, AL and K. Sometimes this can be a temporary situation in the early postoperative period.

b. Another cause of error is when the ACD constants have not been personalized to the individual IOL style, surgeon and clinic.

4. The use of **formulas** is a cause of IOL power error, especially regression formulas, for example the SRK I regression formula, when used in eyes outside the normal AL range of 22–24.5 mm. This has been shown in so many studies[14] over the past 12 years, it would be impossible to reference them all here.

5. There are other **miscellaneous** causes for IOL power errors that can be just as serious as those mentioned above. A rare manufacturer labeling error can be very serious and very difficult to pick up before the patient is discharged from the facility. If the operating room nurse hands the surgeon the wrong IOL power during the surgery this may not be easily recognized in time to correct the error. Lastly, transcription mistakes can cause some of the largest errors seen.

Prevention of Common Errors

- Use the IOLMaster® or immersion A-scan to measure the AL.

- Suspect a staphyloma in eyes >25 mm: use IOLMaster and/or Shammas A/B-scan technique.

- Use CALF method: measure eye using 1532 m/s and add +0.32 mm to the result to correct for any error in sound velocity.

- Employ a well-trained, experienced technician.
- Regularly calibrate manual keratometers.
- Carefully evaluate the IOLMaster® scan for reliability.
- Keep contact lenses out for 2 weeks prior to keratometry (at least in one eye.)
- Silicone-oil eyes need IOLMaster® if possible or ultrasound AL times 0.71.
- Use the Hoffer® Q formula in eyes <22 mm and in post-refractive surgery eyes.
- Use the Holladay® I formula in eyes 24.5–26 mm in length.
- Use the SRK/T formula in eyes longer than 26 mm.
- *Never use the SRK Regression formulas (SRK I or II).*
- Personalize your ELP factors in the formulas.
- Surgeon should personally select the IOL power for the individual patient.
- Prepare a sheet with all IOL powers that may be needed and place it on the wall and also on the microscope in the OR for the surgeon and OR nurse to verify the correct IOL power. Use red paper for right eyes and yellow paper for left eyes.
- Be sure to set the IR to 1.3375 in the setup screen of the IOLMaster®.
- Use the 'clinical history and contact lens methods' (have PMMA CLs in the clinic) for postrefractive surgery corneas and use the lowest calculated K (highest for hyperopes):
  - Consider the Shammas "No History" Formula: $K = 1.14 * K_{PO} - 6.8$ or the Maloney or Koch Corneal topography methods
  - Use the Aramberri double K: calculate the ELP using the preoperative K and the IOL power using the postoperative K
  - Consider using the Masket Method
  - Consider using the Haigis formula.
- Consider delaying the IOL implantation until the cornea has healed after a penetrating keratoplasty rather than performing a "triple procedure."

Suggestions for Diagnosing and Treating Intraocular Lens Power Surprises

- Make it a routine to perform a manifest refraction on postoperative day 1 so as to discover the problem early enough to take the patient back to the operating room and correct the problem in the first 48 h. The patient is immediately pleased and medico-legal actions are completely eliminated.
- Consider the use of a piggyback IOL or phakic IOL if the eye has healed beautifully and removal of the errant IOL would be more traumatic to the eye. For myopic error use 1 times the error and for hyperopic errors, use 1.5 times the error (or the Shammas Formula).
- Consider a minimal four-incision RK if repeat intraocular surgery is not possible.
- Measure the power of a removed IOL using the McReynolds Analyzer (William McReynolds 217-222-6656) or ask a manufacturer to be present in the operating room to do it.

■ CONCLUSION ■

Simple steps and attention to detail can be very useful in preventing IOL power errors and recent advances in IOL power range availability has made this problem more easily corrected. Since performing the first American ultrasound IOL power calculation[64] in 1974, the past 32 years have seen great improvement in the accuracy of postoperative refractive prediction. Future improvements may some day eliminate the problems we have left.

References

[1] Ossoinig KC. Standardized echography: basic principles, clinical applications, and results. Int Ophthalmol Clin 1979;19:127.

[2] Shammas HJF. A comparison of immersion and contact techniques for axial length measurements. Am Intra-Ocular Implant Soc J 1984;10:444–447.

[3] Schelenz J, Kammann J. Comparison of contact and immersion techniques for axial measurement and implant power calculation. J Cataract Refract Surg 1989;15:425–428.

[4] Hoffer KJ. Ultrasound speeds for axial length measurement. J Cataract Refract Surg 1994;20:554–562.

[5] Mark HF, Bikales N, Overberger CG et al. Encyclopedia of polymer science & engineering. Vol. 1. New York: Wiley and Sons; 1989.

[6] Holladay JT, Prager TC. Accurate ultrasonic biometry in pseudophakia. Am J Ophthalmol 1989;107:189–190.

[7] Holladay JT. Standardizing constants for ultrasonic biometry, keratometry, and intraocular lens power calculation. J Cataract Refract Surg 1997;23:1356–1370.

[8] Hoffer KJ. Ultrasound axial length measurement in biphakic eyes. J Cataract Refract Surg 2003;29:961–965.

[9] Koch DD, Liu JF, Hyde LL, Rock RL, Emery JM. Refractive complications of cataract surgery after radial keratotomy. Am J Ophthalmol 1989;108:676–682.

[10] Holladay JT. IOL calculations following radial keratotomy surgery. Refract Corneal Surg 1989;5:36A.

[11] Hoffer KJ. IOL power calculation in RK eyes. Phaco & Foldables 1994;7:6.

[12] Hoffer KJ. Calculation of intraocular lens power in post-radial keratotomy eyes. Ophthalmic Practice (Canada) 1994;12:242–243.

[13] Hoffer KJ. Ways to calculate IOL power in RK eyes. Refractive Surgery Update (Thornton). Ocular Surg News 1995;13:86.

[14] Hoffer KJ. Intraocular lens power calculation for eyes after refractive keratotomy. J Refract Surg 1995;11:490–493.

[15] Hoffer KJ. How to do cataract surgery after RK. Review of Ophthalmol 1996;20:117–120.

[16] Hoffer KJ. Intraocular lens power calculation for eyes after refractive keratotomy. Consultation Section. Ann Ophthalmol 1996;28:67–68.

[17] Odenthal MT, Eggink CA, Melles G, Pameyer JH, Geerards AJ, Beekhuis WH. Clinical and theoretical results of intraocular lens power calculation for cataract surgery after photorefractive keratectomy for myopia. Arch Ophthalmol 2002;120:431–438.

[18] Ridley F. Development in contact lens theory. Trans Ophthalmol Soc UK 1948;68:385–401.

[19] Soper JW, Goffman J. Contact lens fitting by retinoscopy. In: Soper JW, editor. Contact lenses. New York: Stratton Intercontinental Medical Book Corp; 1974. p. 99.

[20] Smith RJ, Chan WK, Maloney RK. The prediction of surgically induced refractive change from corneal topography. Am J Ophthalmol 1998;125:44–53.

[21] Koch D, Wang I. Calculating IOL power in eyes that have had refractive surgery. J Cataract Refract Surg 2003;29:2039–2042.

[22] Ronje LJ. Avoid IOL surprises in refractive patients. Eyenet 2004;XX:23–24.

[23] Shammas HJ, Shammas MC, Garabet A, Kim JH, Shammas A, LaBree L. Correcting the corneal power measurements for intraocular lens power calculations after myopic laser in situ keratomileusis. Am J Ophthalmol 2003;136:426–432.

[24] Nawa Y, Masuda K, Ueda T, Hara Y, Uozato H. Evaluation of apparent ectasia of the posterior surface of the cornea after keratorefractive surgery. J Cataract Refract Surg 2005;31:571–573.

[25] Wilson SE. Cautions regarding measurements of the posterior corneal curvature. Ophthalmology 2000;107:1223.

[26] Oshika T, Tomidokoro A, Tsuji H. Regular and irregular refractive powers of the front and back surfaces of the cornea. Exp Eye Res 1998;67:443–447.

[27] Aramberri J. Intraocular lens power calculation after corneal refractive surgery: double-K method. J Cataract Refract Surg 2003;29:2063–2068.

[28] Feiz V, Mannis MJ, Garcia-Ferrer F et al. Intraocular lens power calculation after laser in situ keratomileusis for myopia and hyperopia: a standardized approach. Cornea 2001;20:792–797.

[29] Feiz V, Moshirfar M, Mannis MJ et al. Nomogram-based intraocular lens power adjustment after myopic photorefractive keratectomy and LASIK: a new approach. Ophthalmology 2005;112:1381–1387.

[30] Latkany RA, Chokshi AR, Speaker MG, Abramson J, Soloway BD, Yu G. Intraocular lens calculations after refractive surgery. J Cataract Refract Surg 2005;31:562–570.

[31] Masket S, Masket SE. Simple regression formula for intraocular lens power adjustment in eyes requiring cataract surgery after excimer laser photoablation. J Cataract Refract Surg 2006;32:430–434.

[32] Walter KA, Gagnon MR, Hoopes PC, Dickinson PJ. Accurate intraocular lens power calculation after myopic laser in situ keratomileusis, bypassing corneal power. J Cataract Refract Surg 2006;32:425–429.

[33] Ianchulev T, Salz J, Hoffer KJ et al. Intraoperative optical intraocular lens power estimation without axial length measurements. J Cataract Refract Surg 2005;31:1530–1536.

[34] Mackool RJ, Ko W. Intraocular lens power calculation after laser in situ keratomileusis: Aphakic refraction technique. J Cataract Refract Surg 2006;32:435–437.

[35] Hoffer KJ. Triple procedure for intraocular lens exchange. Arch Ophthalmol 1987;105:609.

[36] Geggel HS. Intraocular lens implantation after penetrating keratoplasty: improved unaided visual acuity, astigmatism, and safety in patients with combined corneal disease and cataract. Ophthalmol 1990;97:1460–1467.

[37] Cua IY, Qazi MA, Lee SF, Pepose JS. Intraocular lens calculations in patients with corneal scarring and irregular astigmatism. J Cataract Refract Surg 2003;29:1352–1357.

[38] Fyodorov SN, Kolonko AI. Estimation of optical power of the intraocular lens. Vestnik Oftalmologic (Moscow) 1967;4:27.

[39] Colenbrander MC. Calculation of the power of an iris-clip lens for distance vision. Brit J Ophthalmol 1973;57:735–740.

[40] Hoffer KJ. Intraocular lens calculation: the problem of the short eye. Ophthalmic Surg 1981;12:269–272.

[41] Binkhorst RD. The optical design of intraocular lens implants. Ophthalmic Surg 1975;6:17–31.

[42] Gills JP. Regression formula. Amer Intra-Ocular Implant Soc J 1978;4:163. [editorial].

[43] Gills JP. Minimizing postoperative refractive error. Contact and Intraocular Lens Med J 1980;6:56–59.

[44] Retzlaff J. A new intraocular lens calculation formula. Am Intra-Ocular Implant Soc J 1980;6:148.

[45] Sanders DR, Kraff MC. Improvement of intraocular lens power calculation: Regression formula. Am Intra-Ocular Implant Soc J 1980;6:263.

[46] Sanders DR, Retzlaff J, Kraff MC et al. Comparison of the accuracy of the Binkhorst, Colenbrander and SRK implant power prediction formulas. Am Intra-Ocular Implant Soc J 1981;7:337–340.

[47] Hoffer KJ. Biometry of the posterior capsule: a new formula for anterior chamber depth of posterior chamber lenses. In: Emery JC, Jacobson AC, editors. Current concepts in cataract surgery (Eighth Congress). New York: Appleton-Century Crofts; 1983. p. 56–62.

[48] Hoffer KJ. The effect of axial length on posterior chamber lenses and posterior capsule position. Current Concepts in Ophthalmic Surg 1984;1:20–22.

[49] Binkhorst RD. Biometric A-scan ultrasonography and intraocular lens power calculation. In: Emery JE, editor. Current Concepts in cataract surgery: selected proceedings of the Fifth Biennial Cataract Surgical Congress. St. Louis: Mosby; 1987. p. 175–182.

[50] Sanders DR, Retzlaff J, Kraff MC. Comparison of the SRK II formula and the other second generation formulas. J Cataract Refract Surg 1988;14:136–141.

[51] Holladay JT, Prager TC, Chandler TY, Musgrove KH. A three-part system for refining intraocular lens power calculations. J Cataract Refract Surg 1988;14:17–24.

[52] Retzlaff J, Sanders DR, Kraff MC. Development of the SRK/T intraocular lens implant power calculation formula. J Cataract Refract Surg 1990;16:333–340. [Errata: 16:528, 1990].

[53] Hoffer KJ. The Hoffer Q formula: a comparison of theoretic and regression formulas. J Cataract Refract Surg 1993;19:700–712.

[54] Olsen T, Oleson H, Thim K, Corydon L. Prediction of postoperative intraocular lens chamber depth. J Cataract Refract Surg 1990;16:587–590.

[55] Haigis W. The Haigis Formula. In: Shammas HJ, editor. Intaocular lens power calculations. Thorofare, NJ: Slack Inc; 2003. p. 41–57.

[56] Holladay JT. Refractive power calculation for intraocular lenses in the phakic eye. Am J Ophthalmol 1993;116:63–66.

[57] Hoffer KJ. Clinical results using the Holladay II intraocular lens power formula. J Cataract Refract Surg 2000;26:1233–1237.

[58] Retzlaff J. Calculating the surgeon's personal A-constant. In: Retzlaff J, Sanders DR, Kraff MC, editors. Lens implant power calculation manual. 3rd ed. Thorofare, NJ: Slack Inc; 1990. p. 12–13.

[59] Hoffer KJ. Selection of lens power for implantation in infants and children. Am Intra-Ocular Implant Soc J 1975;1:49.

[60] Gordon RA, Donzis PB. Refractive development of the human eye. Arch Ophthalmol 1985;103:785–789.

[61] Plager DA, Kipfer H, Sprunger DT, Sondhi N, Neely EN. Refractive change in pediatric pseudophakia: 6-year follow-up. J Cataract Refract Surg 2002;28:810–815.

[62] Hoffer KJ. Lens power calculation for multifocal IOLs. In: Maxwell A, Nordan LT, editors. Current concepts of multifocal intraocular lenses. Slack, Inc; 1991. p. 193–208.

[63] Hoffer KJ. Early lens exchange for power calculation error. J Cataract Refract Surg 1995;21:486–487.

[64] Hoffer KJ. The history of IOL power calculation in North America. In: Kwitko ML, Kelman CD, editors. The history of modern cataract surgery. The Hague, Netherlands: Kuglen Publications; 1998. p. 193–208.

CONCLUSION

Intraocular Lens Power Calculations after Refractive Surgery

Li Wang, MD, PhD and Douglas D. Koch, MD

CONTENTS

CHAPTER HIGHLIGHTS

>> Understanding sources of error in post-refractive surgery eyes

>> Alternative methods to improve accuracy in intraocular lens (IOL) power determination

>> Pearls to improve IOL power accuracy

It is difficult to determine the intraocular lens (IOL) power in eyes that have undergone corneal refractive surgery.[1,2] IOL power errors in these eyes can be attributed primarily to two factors: (1) inaccurate determination of the true corneal refractive power, and (2) incorrect estimation of the effective lens position (ELP) by the third- or fourth-generation IOL power-calculation formulas when the postoperative corneal powers are used. Several methods have been proposed to improve the accuracy of the IOL power calculation in eyes following corneal refractive surgery.

This chapter will discuss the factors causing the IOL power errors, the methods and techniques available to improve the accuracy of the IOL power calculation in these eyes, and pearls in selecting IOL power in these challenging cases.

◼ FACTORS CAUSING INTRAOCULAR LENS POWER ERRORS ◼

INACCURATE DETERMINATION OF THE TRUE CORNEAL REFRACTIVE POWER

Corneal powers are routinely measured using keratometers or computerized videokeratography (CVK). Keratometry is accurate for measuring normal unoperated corneas, but it is inaccurate for eyes that have undergone corneal refractive surgery. These errors are caused primarily by two issues: (1) inaccurate measurement of anterior corneal curvature, and (2) inaccurate calculation of the net corneal refractive power.

Inaccurate Measurement of Anterior Corneal Curvature

Corneal refractive surgery alters corneal asphericity and induces wider ranges of curvature values within the central 5 mm zone. Standard keratometry or simulated keratometry from CVK measures only four points on the anterior cornea in a paracentral region, which misses the region where dramatic corneal curvature changes exist (Figure 5-1).

Mean values for central corneal powers overcome the limitation of measurements by the four points. Some CVK devices provide mean values over certain central areas, such as the EffRP (effective refractive power) displayed by the EyeSys Corneal Analysis System (Houston, TX). These central corneal values can be used in eyes that have undergone radial keratotomy (RK), but they are inaccurate in eyes following ablative corneal refractive surgery due to the inaccuracy of using 1.3375 as a standardized value for corneal refractive index, which is discussed below.

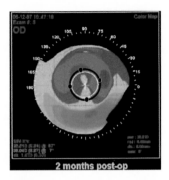

Figure 5-1 A map displays the four points in a paracentral region measured by standard keratometry or simulated keratometry from CVK. Central area with dramatic corneal power changes has been missed by the four points.

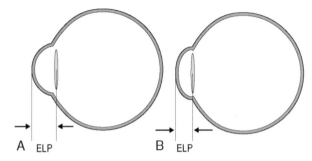

Figure 5-2 Some of third- and fourth-generation IOL power calculation formulas predict the effective lens position (ELP) based on the corneal power (A). In eyes following myopic surgery, if the flattened postoperative corneal power is used to calculate the ELP, the predicted ELP will be falsely shallow and result in underestimated IOL power (B).

Inaccurate Calculation of Total Corneal Refractive Power

In order to compensate for posterior corneal curvature, keratometers and CVK use a standardized index of refraction to convert measurements of anterior corneal curvature to the refractive power of the entire cornea. In most keratometers and CVK devices, a value of 1.3375 is used. Because ablative corneal refractive surgery (e.g., excimer laser photorefractive keratectomy (PRK) or laser in-situ keratomileusis (LASIK)) alters the relationship between the front and back surfaces of the cornea,[3] use of the standardized index of refraction of 1.3375 is no longer valid.

This problem will ultimately be solved by the development of devices that directly and accurately measure anterior and posterior corneal curvatures or, perhaps preferably, actual corneal refractive power. One currently available technology is Scheimpflug imaging. Studies have shown that posterior corneal curvatures cannot be reliably measured with the Orbscan system (Bausch & Lomb, Inc.).[4] Early data from studies of the Pentacam (Oculus, Inc.) are promising,[5] but we are unaware of peer-reviewed studies evaluating the accuracy of this and a new device, the Galilei dual scheimpflug analyzer (Ziemer Ophthalmic Systems, Port, Switzerland), in measuring posterior corneal power in post-LASIK eyes.

Tang and colleagues[6] investigated the repeatability of a high-speed corneal and anterior segment optical coherence tomography (OCT) prototype in measuring anterior and total corneal powers in 32 eyes before and 3 months after myopic LASIK. They found that the repeatability of the anterior corneal power measurement using the OCT was worse than that using the corneal topography (Atlas) in both unoperated corneas and corneas following LASIK (0.79 D and 0.73 D with the OCT, vs. 0.24 D and 0.28 D with the topography for virgin corneas and post-LASIK corneas, respectively). For total corneal measurements, the repeatability with OCT was 0.71 D preoperatively and 0.66 D postoperatively; the repeatability with the hybrid method, which combined the anterior corneal map from Placido ring corneal topography and corneal thickness map from OCT, was 0.24 D and 0.26 D, respectively.

INACCURATE ESTIMATION OF EFFECTIVE LENS POSITION

Third- and fourth-generation formulas have greatly improved the accuracy of IOL power calculations, particularly in atypical eyes. Most of these formulas predict the postoperative location of the lens or ELP based on the corneal power (one exception being the Haigis formula). If postoperative corneal power is used to calculate the ELP, then the calculated lens position will be more anterior than will likely occur. This will cause the formula to select an IOL of insufficient power, resulting in postoperative hyperopia (Figure 5-2).

Aramberri[7] proposed the so-called double-K method to overcome this problem. In this method, the preoperative K reading is used to predict the ELP and the postoperative K reading is used in the vergence formula to calculate the IOL power. Clinical case series have demonstrated that hyperopic surprises have been dramatically decreased with the double-K version of the IOL formulas.[7–9] This approach had previously been incorporated by Holladay in the Holladay II formula.

In previous studies, we investigated the ELP-related prediction error of SRK/T, HofferQ, Holladay I and Holladay II formulas. The magnitude of this error varies according to the particular formula, the amount of refractive correction, and the axial length (AL).[10,11] In general, a greater ELP-related prediction error is found for the SRK/T formula than for the Holladay I and Hoffer® Q formulas. The error increases linearly with increasing myopic and hyperopic corneal refractive surgical correction.

We have developed nomograms to adjust the IOL power when the modified corneal powers and the standard Holladay I, Hoffer® Q and SRK/T formulas are used (Tables 5-1 and 5-2).[11] With the Holladay II formula, one can check the "Previous RK, PRK or LASIK" box, and either enter the K reading before corneal refractive surgery or use the formula's default K value (43.86 D) to predict the ELP.

▪ APPROACHES IMPROVING THE ACCURACY OF INTRAOCULAR LENS POWER CALCULATION ▪

Various methods and techniques have been proposed to improve the accuracy of the IOL power calculation in eyes following corneal refractive surgery. These methods can be categorized into three groups:

1. Methods relying entirely on historical data

2. Methods using historical data and current corneal measurements

3. Methods only using current measurements.

Table 5-1 Nomogram for IOL power adjustment (D) following myopic surgery

Refractive correction (D)	Axial length (mm)											
	19	20	21	22	23	24	25	26	27	28	29	30
2	0.7	0.7	0.7	0.7	0.7	0.7	0.7	0.6	0.6	0.5	0.4	0.3
	0.5	0.4	0.4	0.3	0.3	0.2	0.2	0.2	0.1	0.1	0	0
	0.4	0.5	0.5	0.5	0.5	0.5	0.5	0.4	0.4	0.3	0.2	0.1
3	1.0	1.0	1.0	1.0	1.1	1.1	1.0	1.0	0.9	0.8	0.7	0.6
	0.7	0.6	0.5	0.5	0.4	0.3	0.3	0.3	0.2	0.2	0.1	0
	0.7	0.7	0.7	0.7	0.7	0.7	0.8	0.7	0.6	0.4	0.3	0.2
4	1.3	1.3	1.3	1.4	1.4	1.4	1.4	1.3	1.2	1.1	0.9	0.8
	1.0	0.8	0.7	0.6	0.5	0.5	0.4	0.3	0.3	0.2	0.1	0
	0.9	0.9	0.9	1.0	1.0	1.0	1.1	0.9	0.8	0.6	0.5	0.4
5	1.7	1.7	1.7	1.7	1.7	1.8	1.7	1.6	1.5	1.4	1.2	1.1
	1.2	1.0	0.9	0.8	0.7	0.6	0.5	0.4	0.4	0.3	0.2	0
	1.1	1.2	1.2	1.2	1.2	1.3	1.3	1.2	1.0	0.8	0.7	0.5
6	2.0	2.0	2.0	2.0	2.1	2.1	2.1	2.0	1.8	1.7	1.5	1.4
	1.4	1.2	1.0	0.9	0.8	0.7	0.6	0.5	0.5	0.4	0.3	0.1
	1.4	1.4	1.4	1.5	1.5	1.6	1.6	1.5	1.2	1.0	0.8	0.7
7	2.3	2.3	2.3	2.4	2.4	2.5	2.4	2.3	2.2	2.0	1.8	1.7
	1.6	1.4	1.2	1.1	0.9	0.8	0.7	0.6	0.6	0.5	0.3	0.1
	1.6	1.6	1.7	1.7	1.8	1.8	1.9	1.7	1.5	1.2	1.0	0.9
8	2.6	2.6	2.6	2.7	2.7	2.8	2.8	2.6	2.5	2.3	2.2	2.0
	1.8	1.6	1.4	1.2	1.1	1.0	0.8	0.7	0.7	0.6	0.4	0.2
	1.8	1.9	1.9	2.0	2.0	2.1	2.2	2.0	1.7	1.5	1.2	1.0
9	2.9	2.9	2.9	3.0	3.1	3.2	3.1	3.0	2.8	2.7	2.5	2.3
	2.0	1.7	1.5	1.3	1.2	1.1	1.0	0.8	0.8	0.7	0.5	0.2
	2.1	2.1	2.2	2.2	2.3	2.4	2.5	2.3	2.0	1.7	1.4	1.2
10	3.1	3.2	3.2	3.3	3.4	3.5	3.4	3.3	3.1	3.0	2.8	2.6
	2.2	1.9	1.7	1.5	1.3	1.2	1.1	1.0	0.8	0.7	0.6	0.3
	2.3	2.4	2.4	2.5	2.6	2.7	2.8	2.6	2.2	1.9	1.7	1.4

For third-generation formulas, nomogram for IOL power adjustment (D) in eyes following myopic surgery when modified corneal powers are used to calculate IOL power. The numbers in the first, second and third rows of each cell represent the amounts that need to be added to the IOL power calculated using the SRK/T, Hoffer Q and Holladay 1 formulas, respectively.
Reprinted from Koch DD, Wang L: Calculating IOL power in eyes that have had refractive surgery, *J Cataract Refract Surg* 29:2039–2042. Copyright (2003) Elsevier. With permission from Elsevier.

To illustrate these methods, an example of IOL power calculation in an eye following myopic LASIK will be used, and in Table 5-3 each of the methods will be applied to these data.

APPROACHES THAT RELY ENTIRELY ON HISTORICAL DATA

Methods relying entirely on historical data are entirely dependent on the accuracy of the prior data and in our experience are often less accurate than the other two approaches (described below). The problem is twofold: (1) historical data were typically acquired elsewhere and, therefore, may not be accurate, and (2) there is a one-to-one error if any datum is incorrect, including the pre-LASIK/PRK data and the post-LASIK/PRK refraction. To maximize accuracy, one should validate the historical data and use the most recent refraction obtained before the cataract began to develop.

Clinical History Method

The clinical history method requires pre-LASIK/PRK keratometry, pre-LASIK/PRK refraction and post-LASIK/PRK stable refraction. Using this method, the corneal refractive power is derived by subtracting the change in refraction at corneal plane from the preoperative keratometric value:

$$\text{Corneal power} = \text{Pre-LASIK/PRK K} - \text{RC}$$

where:
LASIK = laser in-situ keratomileusis
PRK = photorefractive keratectomy
RC = the amount of refractive correction induced by the surgery (prior to the development of the cataract).

This approach has been tentatively confirmed by studies involving small numbers of eyes and has been used as gold standard in studies comparing the accuracy of different methods

Table 5-2 Nomogram for IOL power adjustment (D) following hyperopic surgery

Refractive correction (D)	Axial length (mm)											
	19	20	21	22	23	24	25	26	27	28	29	30
2	0.7	0.7	0.7	0.7	0.7	0.7	0.7	0.6	0.5	0.4	0.2	0
	0.5	0.4	0.4	0.3	0.3	0.2	0.2	0.1	0.1	0.1	0	0
	0.4	0.4	0.4	0.4	0.4	0.5	0.5	0.4	0.3	0.2	0	0
3	1.1	1.1	1.1	1.1	1.1	1.1	1.0	0.9	0.7	0.5	0.2	0
	0.8	0.7	0.5	0.5	0.4	0.3	0.2	0.2	0.1	0	0	0
	0.6	0.6	0.6	0.7	0.7	0.7	0.7	0.5	0.3	0.2	–	–
4	1.4	1.4	1.4	1.4	1.4	1.5	1.4	1.2	0.9	–	–	–
	1.1	0.9	0.7	0.6	0.5	0.4	0.3	0.2	0.1	0	0	0
	0.9	0.9	0.9	0.9	0.9	0.9	0.9	0.6	0.4	0.4	–	–
5	1.8	1.8	1.8	1.8	1.8	1.9	1.8	1.7	–	–	–	–
	1.4	1.1	0.9	0.7	0.6	0.4	0.3	0.2	0.1	0	0	0
	1.1	1.1	1.0	1.0	1.0	1.0	1.0	0.7	0.3	–	–	–
6	2.2	2.2	2.2	2.2	2.2	2.5	–	–	–	–	–	–
	1.7	1.3	1.1	0.9	0.7	0.5	0.3	0.2	0	0	0	0
	1.1	1.1	1.1	1.1	1.1	1.1	1.1	0.7	0.3	–	–	–

For third-generation formulas, nomogram for IOL power adjustment (D) in eyes following hyperopic surgery when modified corneal powers are used to calculate IOL power. The numbers in the first, second and third rows of each cell represent the amounts that need to be subtracted to the IOL power calculated using the SRK/T, Hoffer Q and Holladay 1 formulas, respectively.
The corresponding formula is not applicable.
Reprinted from Koch DD, Wang L: Calculating IOL power in eyes that have had refractive surgery, *J Cataract Refract Surg* 29:2039-2042. Copyright (2003) Elsevier. With permission from Elsevier.

for IOL power calculation in eyes with prior corneal refractive surgery. However, studies involving cases following cataract surgery and IOL implantation have shown that the accuracy of this method varied largely, primarily due to less accurate historical data. In a previous study,[8] with the double-K Holladay I formula, the mean arithmetic IOL prediction error was -0.67 ± 1.53 D (range -3.50–2.38 D) with the clinical history method, compared to -0.62 ± 0.87 D (range -1.87–0.56 D) with the adjusted EffRP; note the higher standard deviation and range with the clinical history approach. In another set of cases, with the double-K Holladay I formula, the mean arithmetic IOL prediction error was -0.65 ± 1.05 D (range -3.30–0.36 D) with the clinical history method, -0.37 ± 0.74 D (range -1.97–0.56 D) with the adjusted EffRP, and $+0.06 \pm 0.69$ D (range -0.96–1.31 D) with the modified Maloney method (unpublished data).

Feiz–Mannis Method

The Feiz–Mannis method requires pre-LASIK/PRK keratometry and the amount of refractive correction.[12] With this technique, the IOL power is first calculated using the pre-LASIK/PRK corneal power and currently measured axial length as though the patient had not undergone keratorefractive surgery. This pre-LASIK/PRK IOL power is then increased by the amount of refractive change at the spectacle plane divided by 0.7, by assuming that every diopter of change in IOL produces 0.7 D of change in refraction at the spectacle plane. The formula is:

$$\text{Post-LASIK IOL power} = \text{Pre-LASIK/PRK IOL} + \text{RC}/0.7$$

where:
IOL = intraocular lens
LASIK = laser in-situ keratomileusis
PRK = photorefractive keratectomy
RC = the amount of refractive correction induced by the surgery (prior to the development of the cataract).

An advantage of this method is that it overcomes the problems of both inaccurate corneal power measurement and ELP estimation when the post-LASIK/PRK keratometric values are used. However, in a study that compared several techniques for calculating IOL power in 10 eyes after LASIK, this method was found to be less accurate than clinical history method or contact lens method.[13] In another study of 11 eyes after myopic LASIK, this method had the largest variance in the IOL prediction errors.[8]

Corneal Bypass Method

The corneal bypass method proposed by Walter and coauthors[14] requires pre-LASIK/PRK keratometry, pre-LASIK/PRK refraction and post-LASIK/PRK stable refraction. Using the current axial length and pre-LASIK/PRK keratometry, the IOL power calculation is targeted as the pre-LASIK/PRK refraction or the net refractive correction if the post-LASIK/PRK refraction is not plano.

Like the Feiz–Mannis method, this approach avoids the problems of both inaccurate corneal power measurement and

Table 5-3 Case example of intraocular lens power calculation in an eye with prior myopic LASIK from the authors' clinical series

Pre-cataract surgery data:	Adjusted EffRP:

Pre-cataract surgery data:

Pre-LASIK data:

Pre-LASIK refraction: −4.75 D

Pre-LASIK mean keratometry: 43.40 D

Post-LASIK data:

Post-LASIK refraction: plano

EffRP: 40.03 D

Central topographic power (Humphrey Atlas): 39.90 D

IOLMaster mean keratometry: 40.00 D

Flat K value with Humphrey Atlas: 40.00 D

Post-cataract surgery data:

IOL implanted: Alcon SN60WF lens with power of 21.0 D

Refraction after cataract surgery: −1.00 D.

Corneal refractive power estimation:

Clinical history method:

Refraction correction at corneal plane (vertex distance: 12.5 mm):
$0 − (−4.75) / \{1− [0.0125 \times (−4.75)]\} = 4.48$ D

Corneal power = 43.40 − 4.48 = 38.92 D

Adjusted EffRP:

Adjusted EffRP = 40.03 − 0.15 × 4.48 − 0.05 = 39.31 D

Modified Maloney Method:

Corneal power = 39.90 × (376/337.5) − 5.51 = 38.94 D

IOL power calculation with the Holladay 1 formula except Haigis-L formula (aiming at refraction of −1.00 D):

Clinical history method:

IOL power using corneal power obtained from the clinical history method and the double-K Holladay 1 formula: 21.56 D

Adjusted EffRP:

IOL power using Adjusted EffRP and double-K Holladay 1 formula: 21.00 D

Modified Maloney method:

IOL power using corneal power obtained from the Modified Maloney method and double-K Holladay 1 formula: 21.54 D

Feiz-Mannis IOL power adjustment method:

IOL power using pre-LASIK K: 14.81 D

IOL power after LASIK: 14.81 + 4.48 / 0.7 = 21.21 D

Masket IOL power adjustment method:

IOL power using post-LASIK IOLMaster K: 19.08 D

IOL power after LASIK: 19.08 + 4.48 × 0.326 + 0.101 = 20.64 D

Corneal bypass method:

IOL power using pre-LASIK K and pre-LASIK refraction: 21.16 D

Latkany formula:

IOL power for flat Humphrey Atlas K: 19.08 D

IOL power with Latkany formula = 19.08 − [0.47 × (−4.75) + 0.85] = 20.46 D

Haigis-L formula:

IOL power after LASIK: 20.97 D

IOL power prediction error using different methods (Implanted − Predicted):

Double-K clinical historical method:	−0.56 D
Double-K Adjusted EffRP:	0.00 D
Double-K Modified Maloney method:	−0.54 D
Feiz-Mannis IOL power adjustment method:	−0.21 D
Masket IOL power adjustment method:	+0.36 D
Corneal bypass method:	−0.16 D
Latkany formula:	+0.54 D
Haigis-L formula:	+0.03 D

A 54-year-old lady underwent cataract extraction and posterior-chamber IOL implantation in her right eye. (Since Pentacam data were not obtained, methods using this device are not illustrated.)

ELP estimation when the post-LASIK/PRK keratometric values are used. In nine eyes that had cataract surgery after LASIK, Walter and colleagues[14] found that this method consistently chose the most accurate and precise IOL power compared with other methods. Further studies are desirable.

APPROACHES THAT USE A COMBINATION OF PRIOR DATA AND CURRENT CORNEAL MEASUREMENTS

Some methods use current corneal measurements and then modify the measured corneal power or calculated IOL power based on the amount of refractive correction. The modifiers for the corneal powers range from 15% to 24% of refractive correction, and for the IOL powers 33% to 47%. Therefore, the errors due to incorrect historical data are significantly reduced compared to the one-for-one error involved in the approaches relying entirely on historical data.

Modified Computerized Videokeratography

There are several approaches to modifying current post-LASIK/PRK corneal power measurements:

• *Adjusted EffRP*: The EffRP is displayed on the Holladay Diagnostic Summary of the EyeSys Corneal Analysis System. This value samples all points within the central 3 mm and takes into account the Stiles–Crawford effect. The adjusted EffRP can be obtained using the following formulas in eyes after myopic LASIK/PRK or hyperopic LASIK/PRK, respectively:[3,15]

Adjusted EffRP in myopic LASIK/PRK eyes
= EffRP − 0.15 RC − 0.05

Adjusted EffRP in hyperopic LASIK/PRK eyes
= EffRP + 0.162 RC − 0.279

- *Adjusted K*: If the EffRP or other CVK values are not available, for myopic LASIK/PRK eyes, the current keratometry readings may be modified by a modifier of 24% of the refractive correction: [3]

Adjusted K = Keratometry − 0.24 RC + 0.15

Because of the aforementioned poorer accuracy of K readings in these eyes, the adjusted K approach is not as accurate as the adjusted EffRP method.

- *Adjusted Annular Corneal Power*: Some topography devices provide values for corneal power at incremental annular zones, e.g., 1 mm, 2 mm, etc. The accuracy of corneal power estimation in hyperopic LASIK/PRK eyes can be improved by adjusting the annular corneal power by a modifier of 19% of refractive correction:[15]

Adjusted AnnCP = AnnCP + 0.19 RC − 0.396,

where AnnCP is the average of powers at the center and the 1, 2 and 3 mm annular zones from the numerical view map of Humphrey Atlas device.

Latkany Formula

This method requires pre-LASIK/PRK manifest refraction. With the SRK/T formula, IOL power is first calculated using the current flat K reading or average K reading, and then adjusted using the following formulas:[16]

Adjusted IOL for flat K = −(0.47 × Pre-LASIK/PRK refraction + 0.85)

Adjusted IOL for average K = −(0.46 × Pre-LASIK/PRK refraction + 0.21)

Masket Formula

With this approach,[17] in both myopic and hyperopic LASIK/PRK eyes, IOL power is calculated in the standard way and then modified by around 33% of the refractive correction. In the study in which this method was developed, the IOL master K values were used:

Adjusted IOL = (RC × 0.326) + 0.101

APPROACHES THAT REQUIRE NO PRIOR DATA

Ideally, the optimal techniques for IOL power calculation in eyes following corneal refractive surgery are those that do not require prior data, eliminating the concern about accuracy or availability of historical data. Several methods have been developed:

Contact Lens Over-refraction

With this method, manifest refraction is performed first; a hard contact lens of known base curvature and power is then placed over the eye, and refraction is repeated. The corneal power is estimated as the sum of contact lens base curvature, contact lens

power and the difference between the refractions with and without the contact lens.

Zeh and Koch[18] evaluated this method in cataract patients who had normal corneas and found acceptable accuracy for eyes with Snellen visual acuity of 20/70 or better. Recent studies suggest that the hard contact lens method is less accurate than other approaches.[8,19] Contact lens designs with posterior curvatures that better fit the surgically modified corneal surface may improve the accuracy of this method. [20,21]

Modified Maloney Method

In this approach, the central corneal power measured by the Humphrey Atlas topographer is converted back to the anterior corneal power by multiplying this value by 376.0/337.5 or 1.114. The central corneal power is obtained by placing the cursor at the exact center of the axial map. An assumed posterior corneal power of 5.51 D is then subtracted from the anterior corneal power to yield the total corneal power. Corneal power is, therefore, calculated as follows:

Post-LASIK corneal power = Central power × (376.0/337.5) − 5.51

When used with either the Holladay II formula or third-generation formulas combined with the "double-K method," this technique produced significantly smaller variances in IOL prediction error than did the clinical history method, indicating that this method may produce more consistent results. In the previous study,[8] we proposed a posterior corneal power of 6.1 D to eliminate any hyperopic surprises following cataract surgery in eyes with prior myopic LASIK/PRK. In a separate series of 11 cases that had cataract surgery with prior myopic LASIK, as expected, this technique produced myopic outcome in 10 out of 11 eyes, with average refractive prediction error of −0.57 D (unpublished data). A posterior corneal power of 5.51 D would give a mean refraction error of zero, and we, therefore, recommend use of this value in this formula. Again, the modified Maloney method yielded more consistent results than did the clinical history method.

Haigis-L Formula

The Haigis-L formula is implemented in the Zeiss IOL Master. This formula uses a regression approach to adjust corneal power values measured by the IOLMaster® based on corneal powers derived from the history method. With this modified value, IOL power is calculated with the Haigis formula, and a small correction factor is then applied (*www.augenklinik.uni-wuerzburg.de/kurse/ascrs2006/haigis-l.pdf*).

Performance of the Haigis-L formula was evaluated in 77 cases from 30 surgeons (*www.augenklinik.uni-wuerzburg.de/kurse/ascrs2006/haigis-l.pdf*). The mean absolute refractive prediction error was 0.62 ± 0.55 D (range 0.01–2.40 D), and 51.9% of eyes were within ±0.50 D, 79.2% within ±1.0 D, and 96.1% within ±2.0 D of prediction error.

Intraoperative Refraction

Two approaches have been proposed to do intraoperative refraction in these challenging eyes:

- *Optical refractive biometry method*: With this technique, after the removal of the cataract and just prior to implanting IOL, aphakic retinoscopy is performed with a portable autorefractor. The IOL power is then calculated based on the intraoperative refraction:[22]

IOL power = 2.01 × intraoperative refraction

Axial length and K reading are not required by this method. Although early data on six post-LASIK eyes were promising, further studies are desirable.

- *Aphakic refraction technique*: After removal of the cataract, the patient is removed from the operating room. Manifest refraction is performed 30 min later, and the IOL power is then determined using the following formula:[23]

IOL power = 1.75 × Aphakic refraction.

We believe that larger studies are required before these approaches are more widely applied; we have seen a hyperopic surprise of 1.75 D with the second approach, and, because of the multiplier, both are subject to large errors if the refraction is not correct.

Gaussian Optics Formula

The Gaussian lens formula can be used to calculate the total corneal power when the anterior and posterior corneal powers are available. Using the Pentacam device, equivalent K-readings for central 4 mm zone and the BESSt formula are proposed to estimate the total corneal power:

- *Equivalent K-readings (4 mm zone)*: On the Holladay report display of the Pentacam system, equivalent K-readings for the central 4 mm zone can be used for IOL power calculation in eyes following corneal refractive surgery. We are unaware of studies evaluating the accuracy of these values in IOL power calculation in these eyes.

- *BESSt formula*: In 143 eyes that had wavefront-guided myopic LASIK or LASEK, Borasio and colleagues[24] developed the BESSt formula to estimate the total corneal powers in eyes after corneal refractive surgery. In 143 virgin corneas, they found that the corneal power produced by the Gaussian optics formula consistently underestimated topographic keratometry values (Topcon), and the BESSt_vc (vc = virgin corneas) formula for virgin corneas was obtained by compensating for these discrepancies. Using the clinical history method as gold standard, postoperative corneal powers estimated with the BESSt_vc formula were refined against the corneal powers calculated with the clinical history method to develop the BESSt formula. The formulas are:

K-values BESSt = 7.8385 + 0.7458 × K-values BESSt_vc

K-values BESSt_vc = 0.2431 + 0.9942 × K-values Gaussian optics

where K-values Gaussian optics are K values obtained with the Gaussian optics formula.

The accuracy of the BESSt formula was then tested in 13 eyes that had cataract surgery with prior keratorefractive surgery. The target refractions calculated with the BESSt formula were significantly closer to the refraction following cataract surgery than those calculated with double-K history method and contact lens method, with 46% of eyes within 0.5 D and 100% within 1.0 D of intended refraction.

■ PEARLS IN SELECTING INTRAOCULAR LENS POWER ■

When calculating IOL powers in eyes that had undergone corneal refractive surgery, we recommend that surgeons use several methods.

ESTIMATE CORNEAL POWERS WITH VARIOUS APPROACHES

- Adjusted EffRP with the EyeSys topography
- Modified Maloney method with the Humphrey Atlas topographer
- Clinical history method if historical data are available.

CALCULATE INTRAOCULAR LENS POWERS WITH DIFFERENT TECHNIQUES

- Masket formula
- Latkany formula
- Haigis-L formula
- Feiz–Mannis method
- Corneal bypass method
- Double-K method with the estimated corneal values. When modified corneal values are used to calculate the IOL power, the double-K version of the IOL power calculation formulas is required. With the SRK/T, HofferQ and Holladay I formulas, the calculated IOL powers should be modified by referring to the double-K tables (Tables 5-1 and 5-2). With the Holladay II formula, check the "Previous RK, PRK or LASIK" box, insert the pre-LASIK/PRK keratometry or the default average preoperative K value (43.86 D) can be used to predict the ELP.

In our practice, we use some of these methods as primary approaches and some as back-up options:

Primary Approaches

- Adjusted EffRP
- Modified Maloney method
- Clinical history method
- Masket formula.

Back-up Options

- Feiz–Mannis method
- Corneal bypass method
- Contact lens over-refraction.

■ POST-RADICAL-KERATOTOMY EYES ■

Since the RK procedure does not remove corneal tissue, eyes that have previously undergone RK experience flattening of both the anterior and posterior corneal radii. The relationship between the anterior and posterior corneal powers in virgin eyes may be applied in these post-RK eyes. Therefore, any map that provides a representative average of anterior corneal power over the central 2–3 mm gives a fairly accurate estimation of corneal refractive power. Examples include the EffRP from the Holladay Diagnostic Summary of the EyeSys Corneal Analysis System and averaging the 0 mm, 1 mm and 2 mm annular rings of the Numerical View of the Zeiss Humphrey Atlas topographer.

It is important to note that compensation for potential errors in ELP is still needed by using the Holladay II formula or the double-K approach with third-generation formulas as described above. Unfortunately, even with these measures, refractive surprises can still occur. We suspect that this is because there are some posterior curvature changes that deviate from those estimated by using the standardized index of refraction. Because of this relative inaccuracy of IOL calculations in post-RK eyes and their tendency to experience a long-term hyperopic drift, we usually target IOL power calculations for -1.00 D.

■ PATIENT EDUCATION ■

It is important to explain to patients that IOL power calculations following all forms of corneal refractive surgery are problematic. Patients should be warned of reduced accuracy of IOL power calculation and of the possible need for additional surgery. Additional surgeries include LASIK or PRK enhancement, IOL exchange, or piggyback IOL. The possible costs associated with the additional surgery should also be discussed with the patient.

■ CONCLUSION ■

The methodology for accurately calculating IOL power in eyes following corneal refractive surgery has improved dramatically in recent years. However, refractive surprises still occur. To effectively use the types of approaches described in this chapter, further progress is needed in the methods of measuring corneal power and in predicting ELP.

The "Holy Grail" in this field may be an adjustable IOL, which could facilitate correction, or at least reduction of residual spherical and astigmatic refractive errors, and residual higher-order aberrations. Ideally, such an IOL could be modified from time to time to adapt to the patient's changing visual needs and to compensate for aging changes of the cornea.[25] This and other future advances bode well for solving this challenging clinical problem.

References

[1] Koch DD, Liu JF, Hyde LL, Rock RL. Emery JM. Refractive complications of cataract surgery after radial keratotomy. Am J Ophthalmol 1989;108:676–682.

[2] Seitz B, Langenbucher A, Nguyen NX, Kus MM, Kuchle M. Underestimation of intraocular lens power for cataract surgery after myopic photorefractive keratectomy. Ophthalmology 1999;106:693–702.

[3] Hamed AM, Wang L, Misra M, Koch DD. A comparative analysis of five methods of determining corneal refractive power in eyes that have undergone myopic laser in situ keratomileusis. Ophthalmology 2002;109:651–658.

[4] Maldonado MJ, Nieto JC, Diez-Cuenca M, Pinero DP. Repeatability and reproducibility of posterior corneal curvature measurements by combined scanning-slit and placido-disc topography after LASIK. Ophthalmology 2006;113:1918–1926.

[5] Ciolino JB, Belin MW. Changes in the posterior cornea after laser in situ keratomileusis and photorefractive keratectomy. J Cataract Refract Surg 2006;32:1426–1431.

[6] Tang M, Li Y, Avila M, Huang D. Measuring total corneal power before and after laser in situ keratomileusis with high-speed optical coherence tomography. J Cataract Refract Surg 2006;32:1843–1850.

[7] Aramberri J. Intraocular lens power calculation after corneal refractive surgery: double-K method. J Cataract Refract Surg 2003;29:2063–2068.

[8] Wang L, Booth MA, Koch DD. Comparison of intraocular lens power calculation methods in eyes that have undergone LASIK. Ophthalmology 2004;111:1825–1831.

[9] Chan CC, Hodge C, Lawless M. Calculation of intraocular lens power after corneal refractive surgery. Clin Experiment Ophthalmol 2006;34:640–644.

[10] Koch DD, Wang L, Booth M. Intraocular lens calculations after LASIK. In: Probst L, editor. LASIK – advances, controversies and custom. Thorofare, NJ: Slack Inc; 2004. p. 259–267.

[11] Koch DD, Wang L. Calculating IOL power in eyes that have had refractive surgery. J Cataract Refract Surg 2003;29:2039–2042.

[12] Feiz V, Mannis MJ, Garcia-Ferrer F et al. Intraocular lens power calculation after laser in situ keratomileusis for myopia and hyperopia: a standardized approach. Cornea 2001;20:792–797.

[13] Randleman JB, Loupe DN, Song CD, Waring 3rd GO, Stulting RD. Intraocular lens power calculations after laser in situ keratomileusis. Cornea 2002;21:751–755.

[14] Walter KA, Gagnon MR, Hoopes Jr PC, Dickinson PJ. Accurate intraocular lens power calculation after myopic laser in situ keratomileusis, bypassing corneal power. J Cataract Refract Surg 2006;32:425–429.

[15] Wang L, Jackson DW, Koch DD. Methods of estimating corneal refractive power after hyperopic laser in situ keratomileusis. J Cataract Refract Surg 2002;28:954–961.

[16] Latkany RA, Chokshi AR, Speaker MG, Abramson J, Soloway BD, Yu G. Intraocular lens calculations after refractive surgery. J Cataract Refract Surg 2005;31:562–570.

[17] Masket S, Masket SE. Simple regression formula for intraocular lens power adjustment in eyes requiring cataract surgery after excimer laser photoablation. J Cataract Refract Surg 2006;32:430–434.

[18] Zeh WG, Koch DD. Comparison of contact lens overrefraction and standard keratometry for measuring corneal curvature in eyes with lenticular opacity. J Cataract Refract Surg 1999;25:898–903.

[19] Haigis W. Corneal power after refractive surgery for myopia: contact lens method. J Cataract Refract Surg 2003;29:1397–1411.

[20] Joslin CE, Koster J, Tu EY. Contact lens overrefraction variability in corneal power estimation after refractive surgery. J Cataract Refract Surg 2005;31:2287–2292.

[21] Gruenauer-Kloevekorn C, Fischer U, Kloevekorn-Norgall K, Duncker GI. Varieties of contact lens fittings after complicated hyperopic and myopic laser in situ keratomileusis. Eye Contact Lens 2006;32:233–239.

[22] Ianchulev T, Salz J, Hoffer K, Albini T, Hsu H, Labree L. Intraoperative optical refractive biometry for intraocular lens power estimation without axial length and keratometry measurements. J Cataract Refract Surg 2005;31:1530–1536.

[23] Mackool RJ, Ko W, Mackool R. Intraocular lens power calculation after laser in situ keratomileusis: aphakic refraction technique. J Cataract Refract Surg 2006;32:435–437.

[24] Borasio E, Stevens J, Smith GT. Estimation of true corneal power after keratorefractive surgery in eyes requiring cataract surgery: BESSt formula. J Cataract Refract Surg 2006;32:2004–2014.

[25] Wang L, Dai E, Koch DD, Nathoo A. Optical aberrations of the human anterior cornea. J Cataract Refract Surg 2003;29:1514–1521.

part ii

PREPARATION

Ophthalmic Viscosurgical Devices: Physical Characteristics, Clinical Applications, and Complications

Stephen S. Lane, MD and Richard L. Lindstrom, MD

CONTENTS

CHAPTER HIGHLIGHTS

>> Understanding viscosity, viscoelasticity, and pseudoplasticity

>> Physical and clinical correlation of dispersive and cohesive characteristics

>> Properties of commercial agents

>> Clinical applications of different ophthalmic viscosurgical devices

OPHTHALMIC VISCOSURGICAL DEVICES

PHYSICAL CHARACTERISTICS AND CLINICAL APPLICATIONS

The introduction of viscoelastic agents (now termed ophthalmic viscosurgical devices (OVD) by the International Standards Organization (ISO)) for uses in ophthalmic intraocular procedures has had a significant impact on the practice of ophthalmology. OVDs possess a unique set of properties, based on their chemical structure, that enable them to protect the corneal endothelium from mechanical trauma and to maintain an intraocular space, even in the face of an open incision. Viscosurgery,[1] a term used to designate the procedures and

manipulations performed with OVDs has been used in a broad spectrum of ophthalmic procedures. The use of OVDs has become commonplace in anterior segment surgery, and it is likely that the widespread use and availability of these materials facilitated and helped ease the transition in the conversion first from intracapsular to planned extracapsular surgery and then to phacoemulsification.

The physical properties of OVDs are the result of chain length, intrachain, and interchain molecular interactions. It is important to realize that the diverse rheologic properties of any given OVD have a direct impact on the clinical characteristics of that particular material. A thorough understanding of these properties will allow ophthalmic surgeons the opportunity to choose an OVD that is task specific. For example, a specific substance may be selected because of its space maintenance qualities, its corneal endothelial protection qualities, or its coating qualities.

RHEOLOGIC AND PHYSICAL PROPERTIES

The rheologic characteristics of OVDs that is most relevant when considering their usefulness in ophthalmic surgery are viscoelasticity, viscosity, pseudoplasticity, and surface tension (Tables 6-1 and 6-2).

Viscoelasticity

Elasticity refers to the ability of a solution to return to its original shape after being stressed. The rheologic property of viscoelasticity is the essence of the usefulness of these materials as surgical tools in ophthalmology. Elasticity allows the anterior chamber to reform after deformation by depression on the cornea when external forces are released. A non-elastic solution, such as balanced salt solution (BSS), will show no such reformation after release of forces.

The terms viscosity and viscoelasticity are not synonymous. Viscosity, viscoelasticity, and pseudoplasticity are, however, interrelated. The amount of elasticity of an elastic compound increases with increasing molecular weight and greater chain length of the molecules. Unfortunately, comparison of the different OVDs with regard to elasticity is not easily made because of the different ways and non-uniform expression of values by the various manufacturers.

Dr. Lane has no commercial or proprietary interest in the products discussed and will not receive any remuneration resulting from their use.

Table 6-1 Physical properties of viscoelastic substances

	Healon	Healon GV	Amvisc	Amvisc Plus	Chondroitin Sulfate	Viscoat	DisCoVisc
Resting viscosity (cps)*	> 200,000	2,000,000	100,000	140,000	17,000 at 50%	41,000	260,000
Dynamic viscosity (cps)†	40,000–64,000	80,000	40,000	55,000	30 at 20%	40,000	75,000
Color	Clear	Clear	Clear	Clear	Yellow	Clear	Clear
Pseudoplasticity	+++	++++	+++	+++	No	++	+++
Contact angle	60°	†¥	60°	†¥	†¥	52°	66.5°

	Ocucoat	Vitrax	ProVisc	Healon 5	Cellugel
Resting viscosity (cps)*	5,500	40,000	150,000	8.5 million	40,000
Dynamic viscosity (cps)†	4000	30,000	39,000	60,000–80,000	30,000
Color	Clear	Clear	Clear	Clear	Clear
Pseudoplasticity	+	+++	+++	++++	++
Contact angle	52°	†¥	60°	¥	48°

*At shear rate of zero.
+At shear rate of 1/s, 25°C.
¥†Not available.
Pseudoplasticity key: + = slight; ++ = fair; +++ = good; ++++ = excellent.
Modified from Liesegang TJ: Viscoelastic substances in ophthalmology, Surv Opththalmol.[38]

Viscosity

Viscosity (Table 6-1) reflects a solution's resistance to flow, which is in part a function of the molecular weight of the substance. Viscosity of viscoelastics is measured in centipoise (cPs) or centistokes (cSt), which are measures of the resistance to flow relative to a given shear force. Liquid solutions are generally considered to have viscosities of less than 10,000 cSt at rest, while solutions with resting viscosities greater than 100,000 cSt are gel-like. The higher the solution's molecular weight, the more it resists flow. Molecular weight, on the other hand, reflects the size of the solution's molecules. Viscosity is dependent on the degree of movement of a solution, which is also known as the shear rate, and varies inversely with temperature. The viscosity of a solution can be increased by increasing either the concentration or the molecular weight of the solution.

To facilitate optimal intraocular manipulation an OVD should maintain space and protect tissues (possess a high viscosity at low shear rates), allow movement of instruments, aid in IOL implantation (possess a moderate viscosity at medium shear rates), and allow easy introduction into the eye through a small cannula (possess a low viscosity at high shear rates).[2] At the present time, no OVD fulfills all of these requirements.

Pseudoplasticity

Pseudoplasticity refers to a solution's ability to transform when under pressure, from a gel-like substance to a more liquid substance. The more pseudoplastic a material is, the more rapidly it changes from being highly viscous at rest to a thin, watery solution at high shear rates. A change in molecular structure accompanies this pseudoplastic behavior. In clinical terms, a high-molecular-weight, high-viscosity OVD at rest (zero shear force) acts as an excellent lubricant, and coats tissues, and maintains space very well. When under the influence of stress (i.e., a high shear rate), however, the OVD will become an elastic molecular system behaving as an excellent shock absorbing gel. The highest shear rates occur when a solution is passed through a cannula, and viscosity becomes independent of molecular weight. When the molecules align themselves in the direction of flow, the viscosity is determined solely by the concentration. Pseudoplastic solutions, therefore, have a low viscosity at high shear rates and can be extruded easily through a small diameter cannula (27 or 30 gauge) (Figure 6-1). It is important to emphasize that the viscosity of a viscoelastic substance at rest (0 shear rate) is a function of concentration, molecular weight, and the size of the flexible molecular coils of the material (Figure 6-2A and B). At high shear rates, the viscosity is independent of molecular weight and is determined mainly by the concentration.[3]

Surface Tension

The coating ability of an OVD is determined not only by the surface tension of the material itself, but also by the surface tension of the contact tissue, surgical instrument, or IOL. By measuring the angle formed by a drop of the OVD on a flat surface (the contact angle), the coating ability of a substance can be estimated. Lower surface tension and lower contact angle indicate a better ability to coat. In this respect a solution of sodium hyaluronate (HA) has a significantly higher surface tension and contact angle than does a solution of chondroitin sulfate, sodium hyaluronate/chondroitin sulfate in combination, or HPMC, thus indicating these latter solutions provide superior coating.[4]

A comparison of the various physical properties of OVDs is summarized in Tables 6-1 and 6-2.

Table 6-2 Physical properties of various viscoelastic materials

	Healon 5	Healon GV	Healon	Vitrax	Amvisc	Amvisc Plus
Source	Rooster combs	Rooster combs	Rooster combs	Rooster combs	Rooster combs	Rooster combs
Manufacturer Molecular mass (daltons)	Advanced Medical Optics (AMO) 4×10^6	AMO 5×10^6	AMO 2.5–3.8×10^6	AMO 5×10^5	Bausch & Lomb 2×10^6	Bausch & Lomb 2×10^6
Content	2.3% sodium Hyaluronate	1.4% sodium hyaluronate	1% sodium hyaluronate	3% sodium hyaluronate	1% sodium hyaluronate	1.6% sodium hyaluronate
pH Buffer solvent	7.0–7.5 phosphate-buffered saline	7.0–7.5 phosphate-buffered saline	7.0–7.5 phosphate-buffered saline	7.0–7.5 physiological BSS	6.5–7.2 physiological saline	7.2 physiological saline
Osmalality (mOsm/kg H$_2$O)	320	302	309	310	318	340
Concentration (mg/mL)	23	14	10	30	10	16
Sizes	0.55 mL, 0.85 mL	0.55 mL, 0.85 mL	0.4 mL, 0.55 mL, 0.85 mL	0.65 mL	0.5 mL, 0.8 mL	0.5 mL, 0.8 mL

	Viscoat	Occucoat	DisCoVisc	ProVisc	Cellugel
Source	Bacterial fermentation (sodium hyaluronate): shark fin cartilage (sodium chondroitin sulfate)	Wood pulp	Bacterial fermentation (sodium hyaluronate): shark fin cartilage (sodium chondroitin sulfate)	Bacterial fermentation	Wood pulp
Manufacturer Molecular mass (daltons)	Alcon 500×10^3; 25×10^3	Bausch & Lomb 86×10^3	Alcon 1.7×10^6	Alcon 2.5×10^6	Alcon 3×10^5
Content	3% sodium hyaluronate; 4% sodium chondroitin sulfate	2% HPMC	1.6% sodium hyaluronate; 4% sodium chondroitin sulfate	1% sodium hyaluranate	2% HPMC
pH Buffer solvent	7.0–7.5 physiological phosphate buffer	7.2 BSS and variable buffers	6.8–7.6 physiological phosphate buffer	7.25 physiological sodium chloride phosphate buffer	N/A
Osmalality (mOsm/kg H$_2$O)	360	319	298	310	315
Concentration (mg/mL)	Sodium hyaluronate 30; Chondroitin sulfate 40	20	Sodium hyaluronate 17; Chondroitin sulfate 40	10	N/A
Sizes	0.5 mL, 0.75 mL	0.85 mL, 1.0 mL	1.0 mL	0.55 mL	1.0 mL

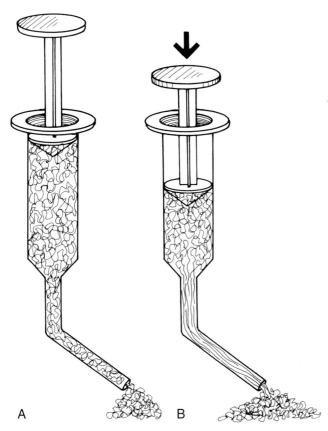

Figure 6-1 A, When shear is applied (flow through a cannula), the large, randomly entangled coils begin to uncoil, allowing flow. B, With increasing shear (more pressure on the syringe plunger), unfolding increases, entanglement drops, and the viscous solution flows easily through the cannula.

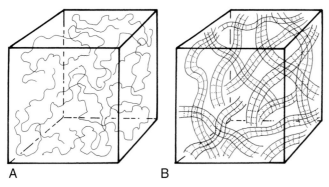

Figure 6-2 A, Sodium hyaluronate (NAHA) molecules in low concentration at rest (zero shear rate). In solution the NAHA chain folds on itself and forms a long, loose, randomly arranged coil. B, As the concentration of these large NAHA molecules is increased, the individual molecular coils start to overlap and become compressed. This crowding of the chains increased the chances for various noncovalent chain–chain interactions. This is turn increases the viscosity of the solution and also increases the elasticity of the solution.

COHESION AND DISPERSION

In an attempt to help us better understand the interaction between these various rheologic properties and their clinical usefulness, Arshinoff[5] has divided OVDs into two categories:

1. *ViscoCohesive* OVDs are characterized by high-viscosity materials, which adhere to themselves through intramolecular bonds, or intermolecular entanglement and resists breaking apart. In general, OVDs with long molecular chains will be more cohesive because the molecules become entangled. Cohesive OVDs possess a high molecular weight, a high degree of pseudoplasticity and high surface tension.

2. *ViscoDispersive* OVDs, exhibit opposite characteristics. They possess lower viscosity and adhere well to external surfaces, e.g., tissues and instruments. These materials tend to break apart easily compared to cohesive materials, exhibit lower molecular weight, lower surface tension and lower pseudoplasticity.

Although cohesiveness and dispersiveness are not measurable rheologic properties in themselves, they are useful constructs when considering the clinical behavior of OVDs as illustrated in Table 6-3.

OPHTHALMIC VISCOSURGICAL DEVICES CHARACTERISTICS

With the introduction of Healon 5™, a new descriptive term was introduced, "Viscoadaptive." This term refers to the ability of an OVD to adapt its behavior to the intended surgical task without the surgeon having to do anything except perform the task at hand. Unlike devices that fit one or the other of the above categories, the viscoadaptive agent ideally functions as both, *adapting* its behavior to a changing parameter in its environment. That changing parameter under most circumstances is the degree of turbulence present.

From a historical view, 1 million Daltons have been used as a convenient dividing line between a cohesive and a dispersive agent. With the introduction of DisCoVisc™ at 1.65 million Daltons, this older classification method would give the expectation of a cohesive product with little or no retention or protection.

However, while scientists understand that HA comes in a variety of molecular lengths and weights, this information is not well known, and is not intuitive to most clinicians. The combination of a medium weight and medium length HA molecule with chondroitin sulfate allows the product to have a triple negative charge resulting in an agent that has the dispersive (retentive) characteristics of chondroitin sulfate while maintaining space like a traditional cohesive product. As a result, previous classifications of OVDs would not accommodate DisCoVisc™ because they all assumed a high correlation between viscosity and cohesion. In 1998, Poyer et al.[4] described how the rate of removal of different OVDs varied when they were exposed to increasing vacuum forces. They found that the rate of removal was typical for a given

Table 6-3 OVD characteristics

Higher viscosity cohesive OVDs	Lower viscosity dispersive OVDs
Create and preserve spaces; displace and stabilize tissues	*Selectively* moves and isolates tissues
Low protection due to ease of aspiration	Very protective of corneal endothelium
Clear	Less clear visualization
Easy to remove	More difficult to remove

OVD and referred to this measurement as the cohesion-dispersion index (CDI) (Table 6-3). This index helped to establish an entirely new classification of OVDs as suggested by Arshinoff and Jafari[5] and as a consequence DisCoVisc™ became the first *"Viscous Dispersive OVD"* because of its unique attributes of cohesive and dispersive characteristics. This classification was recognized by the FDA in DisCoVisc's product insert and helps explain how one product can actually accomplish both dispersive and cohesive actions.

DESIRED PROPERTIES OF OPHTHALMIC VISCOSURGICAL DEVICES

It is apparent from the previous discussion that the interplay between the various rheologic properties is responsible for the clinical characteristics we desire in performing ophthalmic surgery. As a corollary, the degree to which we can maximize these desirable clinical characteristics is, for the most part, based upon our ability to optimize the unique rheologic and physical properties each OVD possesses. The desired properties of an ideal OVD are listed in Table 6-4.

■ VISCOELASTIC COMPOUNDS, THE BUILDING BLOCKS OF COMMERCIALLY AVAILABLE VISCOELASTIC MATERIALS ■

SODIUM HYALURONATE

Sodium hyaluronate (NaHa) is a biopolymer occurring in many connective tissues throughout the body, including both the aqueous and vitreous humors. Its basic structural unit is a disaccharide, joined by a beta one-4 glucosidic bond, which is linked in a repeating fashion with beta glucosidic bonds to form a long unbranched chain. This mucopolysaccharide chain subsequently forms a random coil when placed in a solution such as physiologic saline. As the concentration of large sodium hyaluronate molecules is increased (>0.5 mg/mL), individual molecular coils start to overlap and are compressed (Figure 6-2). This crowding of the chains increases the chances for various noncovalent chain–chain interactions. This, in turn, causes a considerable increase in the viscosity of the solution. For example, the kinematic viscosity of a 2 mg/mL concentration of sodium

Table 6-4 Desired properties of an ideal OVD

Ease of infusion
Retention under positive pressure in the eye
Retention during phacoemulsification
Easy removal/no removal required
Does not interfere with instruments or IOL placement
Protects the endothelium
Nontoxic
Does not obstruct aqueous outflow
Clear

hyaluronate in physiological buffer is only in the 100-cSt range: at 10 mg/mL, it is in the 100,000 cSt range. Therefore, a fivefold increase in the concentration causes a 1000-fold increase in the viscosity of the solution. With this increase in viscosity, the elastic properties of the solution also increase. This forms the rationalization of Amvisc Plus and Healon GV. The elastic behavior of a concentrated (>0.5 mg/mL) sodium hyaluronate solution is greatly dependent on the mechanical energy (shear force) applied to the solution. On a molecular level, this means that under the imposed strain, the polysaccharide coils slip between each other, and conformational and configurational rearrangements occur while the solution exhibits viscous flow (Figure 6-2). The hyaluronate acid fraction (NIF-NaHa)[7] used for ophthalmic procedures has a high molecular weight (2–5 million daltons (D)), a low protein content (<0.5%), and carries a single negative charge per disaccharide unit.

This fraction is highly purified and has been shown to be sterile, nontoxic, nonantigenic,[7] noninflammatory,[9] and pyrogen-free. In primate vitreous humors, sodium hyaluronate has a half-life of approximately 72 days.[10] In primate aqueous humors, the half-life is 2–7 days depending on the viscosity.[11] Clinical observations in humans have supported this result.

CHONDROITIN SULFATE

Chondroitin sulfate (CDS) is another viscoelastic biopolymer that is found as one of the three major mucopolysaccharides in the cornea. Its structure is similar to hyaluronic acid, consisting of the same repeating disaccharide unit. CDS is of medium molecular weight in the range of 50,000 D.

Chondroitin sulfate, like sodium hyaluronate, does not appear to be metabolized but is eliminated from the anterior chamber in approximately 24–30 h.

HYDROXYPROPYL METHYLCELLULOSE

Hydroxypropyl methylcellulose (HPMC) is yet another viscoelastic material used for intraocular procedures.[12] Unlike the previous two compounds, it does not occur naturally in animals but is distributed widely as a structural substance in plant fibers such as cotton and wood. It is a cellulose polymer composed of D-glucose molecules linked together by beta-glycosidic bonds.

Special care must be taken in the filtration of this material to ensure a highly purified preparation, as Rosen et al[14] noted the presence of vegetable fibers and other contaminates in samples they examined. Methylcellulose is a nonphysiologic compound and, as such, does not appear to be metabolized intraocularly but is eliminated from rabbit anterior chambers in approximately 3 days. It is also quite hydrophilic and hence can be irrigated from the eye.

■ COMMERCIAL OPHTHALMIC VISCOSURGICAL DEVICE PREPARATIONS ■

HEALON®, HEALON GV®, HEALON 5®

The first commercially available sodium hyaluronate, Healon, was developed by Balazs[15] who sold the rights to Pharmacia. In 1958, Balazs suggested the use of hyaluronic acid as a vitreous substitute and, subsequently, two different ophthalmic preparations were developed. Etamucaine (Laboratories Chibert, Clermount-Ferrand, France), a bovine hyaluronic acid preparation of low viscosity and concentration, was found to be well tolerated as a vitreous replacement despite a mild intravitreal inflammatory response.[16]

The second preparation, Healon, truly initiated the age of viscosurgery. This high viscosity, high-molecular-weight, sodium hyaluronate derived primarily from rooster combs was developed and purified by Balazs and associates to produce a specific non-inflammatory fraction.[9,10,15,17] In 1972, the first human intraocular injections of Healon into the vitreous and anterior chambers were reported, and its use in surgical procedures varying from vitreoretinal diseases to cataract extraction and keratoplasty was suggested. These suggestions have been pursued actively and, subsequently, OVDs have become an invaluable tool in a broad array of applications.

By increasing both the molecular weight and concentration, Pharmacia introduced Healon GV (greater viscosity) in 1992. With a resting viscosity of 2,000,000 cSt (at least ten times more viscous than most other viscoelastics), Healon GV provides superior viscosity for particularly demanding surgery.[18] Despite positive vitreous pressure, Healon GV is able to create and maintain a deep anterior chamber where other OVDs may fail (three times the resistance to pressure as Healon in the presence of high positive vitreous pressure). Procedures dealing with small pupils, pediatric cataract extraction, and capsulorhexis during positive vitreous pressure are facilitated with the use of Healon GV. However, because of its highly cohesive nature, Healon GV leaves the anterior chamber very quickly during irrigation/aspiration or phacoemulsification, leaving the corneal endothelium susceptible to compromise.

Pharmacia and Upjohn have developed a new OVD, which they believe possesses all of the best properties of Healon GV, and yet is retained in the anterior chamber throughout the phaco procedure. Healon 5 is the result of this effort and has been hailed as the first viscoadaptive OVD by the manufacturer. When exposed to low flow rates, it behaves as a super-viscous cohesive device like an enhanced Healon GV. However, as flow rates increase, Healon 5 begins to fracture into smaller pieces, making its behavior mimic some of the properties of dispersive OVDs. It was released for sale in the United States in early 2001. Recently, Pharmacia and Upjohn have sold Healon, Healon GV, and Healon 5 to Advanced Medical Optics (AMO) which now own sales and marketing rights to this family of OVDs.

AMVISC®, AMVISC PLUS®

Amvisc is another sodium hyaluronate product extracted from rooster combs. It was first distributed by Precision-Cosmet and now is distributed by Bausch and Lomb Surgical. Released in 1983, Amvisc is slightly less viscous than Healon. Amvisc Plus, a 1.6% sodium hyaluronate product with a higher viscosity than Amvisc, is also available. The viscosity of Amvisc Plus is 55,000 cps compared with Amvisc (40,000 cps). This higher viscosity obtained by increasing the total concentration (16 mg/mL) and using a sodium hyaluronate molecule of lower molecular weight, allows for improved space maintenance, tissue manipulation, and tissue immobilization when compared to Amvisc.[19]

AMOVITRAX®

AMOVitrax (Advanced Medical Optics) is a low-molecular-weight viscoelastic preparation of a highly purified, noninflammatory, fraction of sodium hyaluronate dissolved in BSS. Despite the relatively low molecular weight, AMOVitrax is highly concentrated, which provides for a significantly viscous material. Unlike other sodium hyaluronic compounds, AMOVitrax requires no refrigeration with a shelf life of 18 months. AMOVitrax (like Viscoat) possesses a lower viscosity than Healon at rest (0 shear) but maintains its viscosity under medium shear while Healon decreases sharply in a linear fashion.

PROVISC®

ProVisc (Alcon Surgical Inc.) is a sterile non-pyrogenic, high-molecular-weight, noninflammatory, highly-purified fraction of sodium hyaluronate dissolved in physiologic sodium chloride phosphate buffer. ProVisc material is obtained from microbial fermentation by a purified proprietary process. In this respect, it is similar to the process involved in the sodium hyaluronate fraction of Viscoat. Clinical testing demonstrates that ProVisc is equal to Healon in its efficacy for protecting the corneal endothelium and in its level of safety.[19] Like Viscoat, ProVisc requires refrigeration.[15]

VISCOAT®

Viscoat is a 1:3 mixture of 4% chondroitin sulfate and 3% sodium hyaluronate manufactured by Alcon Surgical Incorporated. The sodium hyaluronate fraction, like ProVisc, is produced by bacterial fermentation through genetic engineering techniques. The chondroitin sulfate is obtained from shark fin cartilage. This combination of the compounds combines the higher viscosity and chamber-maintaining properties of sodium hyaluronate with the coating and cell-protection properties of chondroitin sulfate. Koch, in a prospective randomized study, compared the endothelial protective effect of Healon and Viscoat during iris-plane phacoemulsification and posterior chamber phacoemulsification.[21] In the iris-plane phacoemulsification group, Viscoat provided greater corneal endothelial cell protection than Healon. In the posterior chamber phacoemulsification group, however, no significant differences in cell protection were noted with both materials exhibiting excellent endothelial cell protection.

DISCOVISC®

DisCoVisc (Alcon Surgical Inc.) is a sterile, nonpyrogenic, viscoelastic solution of highly purified, noninflammatory sodium chondroitin sulfate and sodium hyaluronate. DisCoVisc is specifically formulated to achieve an intermediate viscosity of $750,000 \pm 35,000$ Mpa.s (at shear rate $1\ s^{-1}$, $25°C$). Each mL of DisCoVisc OVD contains no more than 17 mg sodium hyaluronate, and 40 mg sodium chondroitin sulfate. Because it has an intermediate CDI, DisCoVisc is best described as the first viscous dispersive OVD, combining the key advantages of higher viscosity cohesives and lower viscosity dispersives in a single syringe. Its viscous character facilitates excellent space maintenance while its dispersive nature imparts exceptional tissue protection.

Petroll et al[13] demonstrated that residual OVD thickness following simulated phacoemulsification could be quantitatively measured using in vivo confocal microscopy and showed that DisCoVisc showed retention and adherence to the endothelium similar to Viscoat. Additionally, both DisCoVisc and Viscoat showed significantly better retention and adherence than any of the other agents tested.

OCUCOAT®

Ocucoat (Bausch and Lomb Surgical) is a highly purified synthetic, nonprotein, nontoxic preparation of 2% HPMC. Ocucoat has been marketed as a visco-adherent rather than a viscoelastic because of its significant coating ability and its relative lack of elastic properties. The reader must be aware that formulations produced by individual hospital pharmacies are not consistent proprietary products and can contain various solid particles, mainly vegetable matter remaining from the raw material.[14] Ocucoat is manufactured from the highest pharmaceutical grade HPMC and is subjected to a special dual-filtration process. A study presented in 1988 verified that Ocucoat is as free of particulate debris as Healon (Smith SG, European Intraocular Implant Council Meeting, 1988). Because of its poor elastic properties, a larger bore cannula, and increased infusion pressure are necessary for injection. Unlike other OVDs, Ocucoat can be sterilized by autoclaving and stored at room temperature. Because the raw materials are ubiquitous, there is potential for decreased cost. The complex biotechnical processes required to ensure purity, however, may limit this.

CELLUGEL®

Cellugel (Alcon Surgical Inc) is a sterile, nonpyrogenic, noninflammatory, single-use, ophthalmic viscosurgical device, of highly purified 2% HPMC supplied in a disposable syringe delivering 1 mL, packaged in a sterile peel pouch, and is terminally sterilized by autoclaving. Like Ocucoat, Cellugel can be stored at room temperature. Unlike Ocucoat, Cellugel has a 10-fold greater viscosity and fourfold higher molecular weight. As a result, the ability to maintain space is greater with Cellugel than with Ocucoat, despite both being 2% HPMC.

CLINICAL USES OF OPHTHALMIC VISCOSURGICAL DEVICES

Anterior segment surgery by its very nature induces corneal damage as has been documented by specular microscopy and pachymetry studies. Endothelial damage may occur at any stage, even in routine procedures, from the opening of the anterior chamber with manipulation of the cornea to insertion of an IOL after cataract extraction. The usefulness of OVDs in preventing mechanical injury to the corneal endothelium by inhibiting lens fragment collisions is well known. More recently it has also been shown that OVDs protect the corneal endothelium by reducing oxidative stress in the anterior chamber from free radicals produced during the ultrasonic phase of lens removal.[21A] Hence, the introduction of OVDs to anterior segment surgery can be easily appreciated from the perspective of corneal endothelial protection alone. Additional applications of these materials, however, have quickly become manifest, and the field of viscosurgery has broadened rapidly. Alpar[22] outlined some of the applications that

have been used in anterior segment surgery, many of which were developed specifically for cataract surgery. OVDs can be applied externally to provide corneal and conjunctival epithelial protection throughout the procedure without impairing visibility.[23] Both intraocularly and extraocularly, OVDs can be used to form a mechanical barrier to control hemorrhage. Maintenance of the anterior chamber while fashioning the surgical wound and during intraocular manipulations can be accomplished with the injection of an OVD through a small incision. The iris and other intraocular tissues can be manipulated with the "soft instrument" effect of OVDs even in the face of increased vitreous or orbital pressure, and they may contribute to greater surgical control in the case of an expulsive hemorrhage. Finally, the use of OVDs may help to decrease the incidence of postoperative cystoid macular edema by appropriate maintenance of intraocular pressure and alteration of the refraction of the operating microscope light (Table 6-5).

A review of each of the OVD's attributes should make it apparent that the use of a single agent during most ophthalmic intraocular procedures is accompanied by compromises in surgical suitability. In phacoemulsification for example, the ideal single OVD would offer a combination of cohesive and dispersive characteristics that would fulfill the range of needs through the course of the phacoemulsification procedure (Table 6-6).

Although a combination of agents can fulfill both cohesive and dispersive needs, the use of multiple agents may be cost prohibitive. Therefore, employing a needs-specific approach that takes into account the surgical needs (requirements), surgeons can more astutely match the agent with the task to improve the clinical outcome. Healon 5 viscoadaptive is an attempt to provide both cohesive and dispersive properties in a single agent. Continued experience with this agent will determine if this claim holds true.

COMPLICATIONS OF OPHTHALMIC VISCOSURGICAL DEVICE USE

Despite the many positive attributes of OVDs, their drawbacks and complications also must be given careful consideration. Most important is the elevation of intraocular pressure noted postoperatively after use in cataract surgery. First noted with the use of Healon,[25] the elevation is especially severe and prolonged if the material is not thoroughly removed at the conclusion of surgery,[25] giving rise to what has been termed, Healon-block glaucoma. This increase in intraocular pressure is dose-related and of a transient nature, occurring in the first 6–24 h and typically resolving spontaneously within 72 h postoperatively. It is presumed that this ocular hypertensive effect is the result of large molecules of the OVD creating mechanical resistance in the trabecular meshwork and hence decreasing outflow facility.

Table 6-5 Clinical uses of OVDs

Cataract surgery
Corneal surgery/penetrating keratoplasty
Glaucoma surgery
Anterior segment reconstruction as a result of trauma
Posterior segment surgery

Table 6-6 Viscoelastic requirements during phacoemulsification

Primary			
Surgical task	**Viscoelastic function**	**Required properties**	**Agent category**
Capsulorrhexis	Maintain deep anterior chamber	High viscosity at low shear rates; elasticity	Cohesive
Emulsify nucleus	Stay in eye to cushion and coat tissues, especially corneal endothelium	Low molecular weight; low surface tension; high viscosity at high shear rates	Dispersive
Remove cortex	Endothelial coating	Low surface tension	Dispersive
Open bag, insert IOL	Maintain deep anterior chamber and capsular bag	High viscosity at low shear rates; elasticity	Cohesive
Remove viscosurgical	Remove quickly and completely	High molecular weight; high surface tension	Cohesive

The clearance of an OVD through the trabecular meshwork is believed to be dependent upon a combination of the material's viscosity and molecular weight.[25] Theoretically, materials possessing lower viscosities and lower molecular weights clear the eye faster, thereby creating less intraocular pressure elevation.

Recently, our attention has been directed at the importance of early (1–8 h) postoperative intraocular pressure measurements when evaluating the effects of Healon[26] and other OVDs[24,27] on postoperative intraocular pressure. Significant intraocular pressure spikes can be missed if only 24-h postoperative measurements are taken.

Lane et al[28] compared the early postoperative intraocular pressures after the use of Healon, Viscoat, and Ocucoat in ECCE and IOL implantation. In this study, the Viscoat and Ocucoat groups were further randomized into subgroups in which the material was either retained at the conclusion of surgery or removed with irrigation/aspiration. The results of this study showed significant increases in intraocular pressure in all groups at the 4±1 h postoperative period. At 24 h all groups except for the Viscoat-removed group showed significant elevations in intraocular pressures from baseline values. More recently, Ranier et al[29] confirmed this, noting a significant IOP rise over baseline for both Healon 5 and Viscoat in the early postoperative period.

In an attempt to blunt the postoperative intraocular pressure rise, diluting, removing, and/or aspirating the OVD from the eyes at the conclusion of cataract surgery has been advocated by many.[16,24,30–34] It must be stressed, however, that this procedure has been shown only to shorten or reduce the incidence rather than eliminate the elevation of intraocular pressure.[32,33,35] Others recommend the use of pharmacologic prophylactic treatment in minimizing postoperative intraocular pressure rises. Acetazolamide,[36] intracameral miotics, beta blockers such as timolol[27,37] or levobunolol,[38] and/or pilocarpine 4% gel[39] have all been shown to be effective in reducing postoperative intraocular pressure.

It must be stressed, however, that all OVDs, as well as the surgical procedure alone, are capable of increasing the intraocular pressure in the early postoperative period. The removal of the viscoelastic substance and use of acetazolamide, as well as other glaucoma medications, blunt intraocular pressure elevations, but not in a predictable fashion. It is important to realize that the intraocular pressure response in any given individual after cataract surgery is only in part caused by which OVD is used.

Several other disadvantages of viscosurgery deserve brief mention. Because of the viscous nature and electrostatic charge of these materials, inflammatory and red blood cells may remain suspended in the anterior chamber after surgery, giving the appearance of a plastic anterior uveitis. Intraocular hemorrhage also may be trapped between the vitreous space and the OVD within the anterior chamber and hence mimic the appearance of a vitreous hemorrhage.[40]

Calcific band keratopathy has occurred as a complication peculiar to the initial formulation of chondroitin sulfate-containing OVDs. Several investigators noted that postoperative subepithelial corneal deposits identified histochemically as calcium phosphate precipitates were associated with the use of the intracameral Viscoat.[32,41–43] Since the re-formulation of Viscoat this complication has not recurred.

SUMMARY

OVDs have found applications within ophthalmology and have become indispensable tools in a variety of ophthalmic surgical procedures. The viscoelastic properties of these materials enable them to protect the corneal endothelium and epithelium effectively, maintain intraocular spaces, manipulate intraocular tissues, and control intraocular hemorrhage. Viscosurgery has helped to decrease the amount of corneal damage sustained during surgery and to facilitate difficult and delicate intraocular manipulations. At present, we have a choice of ten commercially available substances, seven sodium hyaluronate materials (Healon, Healon GV, Healon 5, Amvisc, Amvisc Plus, AMO Vitrax, and ProVisc), a combination of sodium hyaluronate and chondroitin sulfate (Viscoat), and two HPMC products (Ocucoat and Cellugel).

Widespread success in clinical situations has been achieved with the pure hyaluronate and combination hyaluronate sodium chondroitin sulfate material. Ocucoat and Cellugel possess the potential advantages of lower cost, no requirement of refrigeration, and a larger quantity of the material per unit (1 mL) while maintaining absolute purity because of the extensive refinement and filtration process. Because of the success of all of these products, a great deal of interest has been stimulated to develop other OVDs. We would expect that a number of new materials may become available in the coming years.

At the present time, no single OVD is ideal under all circumstances. For any particular surgical task, the surgeon should consider the multiple physiochemical characteristics of each OVD available, as well as their desirable and undesirable clinic effects, and then choose the most appropriate substance. With our current armamentarium of OVDs the ophthalmic surgeon can now optimize the surgical result by selecting the OVD most appropriate for the procedure. As new materials are developed and as our knowledge of the physical properties, clinical effects, and surgical indications are better defined, the selection process for choosing the best product should improve. Until then, as Arshinoff has stated "... OVDs remain peculiar fluids, occupying the physical boundary zone between fluids and solids, whose properties and use are limited only by our imagination and creativity."[5]

References

[1] Balazs EA, Miller D, Stegmann R. Viscosurgery and the use of Na hyaluronate in intraocular lens implantation. Presented at the International Congress and First Film Festival on Intraocular Implantation, Cannes, France; 1979.

[2] Bothner H, Wik O. Rheology of intraocular solutions. Viscoelastic Materials 1986;2:53–70.

[3] Bothner H, Wik O. Rheology of hyaluronate. Acta Otolaryngol (Stockh) 1987;442(Suppl.): 25–30.

[4] Poyer JF, Chan KY, Arshinoff SA. Quantitative method to determine the cohesion of viscoelastic agents by dynamic aspiration. J Cataract and Refract Surg 1998;24:1130–1135.

[5] Arshinoff SA, Jafari M. New classification of ophthalmic viscosurgical devices. J Cataract Refract Surg 2005;31:2167–2171.

[6] Arshinoff S. The safety and performance of ophthalmic viscoelastics in cataract surgery and its complications. In: Arshinoff S, editor. Proceedings of the Sixth Annual National Ophthalmic Speakers Program 1993. Montreal: Medicopea International; 1994. p. 21–28.

[7] Balazs EA. Sodium hyaluronate and viscosurgery. In: Miller D, Stegman R, editors. Healon – a guide to its use in ophthalmic surgery. New York: John Wiley; 1983. p. 5–28.

[8] Richter AW, Ryde EM, Zetterstrom EO. Non-immunogenicity of a purified sodium hyaluronate preparation in man. Int Arch Allergy Appl Immunol 1979;59:45–48.

[9] Denlinger JL, Eisner G, Balazs EA. Age-related changes in the vitreous and lens of rhesus monkeys (Macaca mulatta): I. Initial biomicroscopic and biochemical survey of free-ranging animals. Exp Eye Res 1980;31:67–69.

[10] Denlinger JL, Balazs EA. Replacement of the liquid vitreous with sodium hyaluronate in monkeys: I. Short-term evaluation. Exp Eye Res 1980;31:81–99.

[11] Schubert H, Denlinger JL, Galzs EA. Na-hyaluronate injected into the anterior chamber of the owl monkey: effect on IOP and range of disappearance. ARVO 1981;9(Abstr):118.

[12] Fechner PU, Rechner MU. Methylcellulose and lens implantation. Br J Ophthalmol 1983;67:259–263.

[13] Petroll WM, Jafari M, Lane S, Jester JV, Cavanagh HD. Quantitative assessment of ophthalmic viscosurgical device retention using in vivo confocal microscopy. J Cataract Refract Surg 2005;31:2363–2368.

[14] Rosen ES, Gregory RPF, Barnett F. Is 2% hydroxy propylmethylecellulose a safe solution for intraoperative clinical applications? J Cataract Refract Surg 1986;12:679–684.

[15] Balazs EA. Physiology of the vitreous body. In: Schepens CL, editor. Importance of the vitreous body in retina surgery with special emphasis on reoperations. St. Louis: Mosby; 1960. p. 29–48, 144–146.

[16] Girod P, Rouchy JP. L'acide hyaluronique dans la chirurgie du corps vitre: reflexions a propos de 24 cas. Annals Oculist 1970;203:25–40.

[17] Denlinger JL, El-Mofty AAM, Balazs EA. Replacement of the liquid vitreous with sodium hyaluronate in monkeys. II. Long-term evaluation. Exp Eye Res 1980;30:101–117.

[18] Hutz WW, Exkhardt B, Kohnen T. Comparison of viscoelastic substances used in phacoemulsification. J Cataract Refract Surg 1996;22:955–959.

[19] Probst L, Nichols B. Endothelial and intraocular pressure changes after phacoemulsification with AmVisc Plus and Viscoat. J Cataract Refract Surg 1993;19:725–730.

[20] Lehman R, Brint S, Stewart R, et al. Clinical comparison of ProVisc and Healon in cataract surgery. J Cataract Refract Surg 1995;21:543–547.

[21] Koch DD, Liu JF, Glasser DB, et al. A comparison of corneal endothelial changes after use of Healon or Viscoat during phacoemulsification. Am J Ophthalmol 1993;115:188–201.

[21A] Takahashi H, Suzuki S, Shiwa T, Sakamoto A. Alteration of free radical development by opthalmic viscosurgical devices in phacoemulsification. J Cataract Refract Surg 2006;32:1545–1548.

[22] Alpar JJ. Viscoelastic surgery. Ann Ophthalmol 1987;19:350–353.

[23] Norn MS. Preoperative protection of cornea and conjunctiva. Acta Ophthalmol 1981;59: 587–594.

[24] Barron BA, Busin M, Page C, et al. Comparison of the effects of Viscoat and Healon on postoperative intraocular pressure. Am J Ophthalmol 1985;100:377–384.

[25] Pape LG. Intracapsular and extracapsular technique of lens implantation with Healon. J Am Intraocul Implant Soc 1980;6:342–343.

[26] Henry JC, Olander K. Comparison of the effect of four viscoelastic agents on early postoperative intraocular pressure. J Cataract Refract Surg 1996;22:960–966.

[27] Cherfan GM, Rich WJ, Wright G. Raised intraocular pressure and other problems with sodium hyaluronate and cataract surgery. Transactions of the Ophthalmologic Society of the United Kingdom 1983;103:227–279.

[28] Lane SS, Naylor DW, Kullerstrand LJ, et al. Prospective comparison of the effects of Occucoat, Viscoat, and Healon on intraocular pressure and endothelial cell loss. J Cataract Refract Surg 1991;17:21–26.

[29] Rainer G, Menapace R, Findl O, et al. Intraocular pressure after small incision cataract surgery with Healon 5 and Viscoat. J Cataract Refrac Surg 2000;26:271–276.

[30] Choyce DP. Healon in anterior chamber lens implantation. J Am Intraocul Implant Soc 1981;7:138–139.

[31] Miller D, Stegmann R. The use of Healon in intraocular lens implantation. Int Ophthalmol Clin 1982;22:177.

[32] Nevyas AS, Raber IM, Eagle RC, et al. Acute band keratopathy following intracameral Viscoat. Arch Ophthalmol 1987;105:958–964.

[33] Olivius E, Thorburn W. Intraocular pressure after cataract surgery with Healon. J Am Intraocul Implant Soc 1985;11:480–482.

[34] Kohnen T, vonEhr M, Schutte E, Koch DD. Evaluation of intraocular pressure with Healon and Healon GV in sutureless cataract surgery with foldable lens implantation. J Cataract Refract Surg 1996;22:227–237.

[35] Glasser DB, Matsuda M, Edelhauser HF. A comparison of the efficacy and toxicity of and intraocular pressure response to viscous solutions in the anterior chamber. Arch Ophthalmol 1986;104:1819–1824.

[36] Lewen R, Insler MS. The effect of prophylactic acetazolamide on the intraocular pressure rise associated with Healon-aided intraocular lens surgery. Ann Ophthalmol 1985;17:315–318.

[37] Percival P. Complications from use of sodium hyaluronate (Healonid) in anterior segment surgery. Br J Ophthalmol 1982;66:714–716.

[38] Weidle EG, Lisch W, Thiel HJ. Excision of the posterior lens capsule without damaging the anterior vitreous face. Fortschr Ophthalmol 1985;82:256–258.

[39] Ruiz RS, Wilson CA, Musgrove KH. Management increased intraocular pressure after cataract extraction. Am J Ophthal 1987;103:487.

[40] Nirankari VS, Karesh J, Lakhanpal V. Pseudo vitreous hemorrhage: A new intraoperative complication of sodium hyaluronate. Ophthalmic Surg 1981;12:503–504.

[41] Binder PS, Deg JK, Kohl S. Calcific band keratopathy after intraocular chondroitin sulfate. Arch Ophthalmol 1987;105:1243–1247.

[42] Coffman MR, Mann PM. Corneal subepithelial deposits after use of sodium chondroitin. Am J Ophthalmol 1986;102:279–280.

[43] Ullman S, Lichtenstein SB, Heerlein K. Corneal opacities secondary to Viscoat. J Cataract Refract Surg 1986;12:489–492.

SUMMARY

The Phaco Machine: The Physical Principles Guiding its Operation

William J. Fishkind, MD, FACS, Thomas F. Neuhann, MD,
Roger F. Steinert, MD

7

CONTENTS

CHAPTER HIGHLIGHTS

>> Generation of ultrasonic energy

>> Mechanisms of lens disassembly

>> Control mechanisms of ultrasound power and fluidics

>> Anterior vitrectomy

>> Settings

Although the surgical techniques of phacoemulsification are often described, there is a tendency to overlook a basic aspect of this type of surgery: the physics of closed-system surgery and how it translates into clinical performance.

In addition, a basic knowledge of the principles of the physics and engineering of the machines, the power generators, and fluidics not only can assist in making a rational decision as to what kind of equipment to use but also can promote the performance of a surgical procedure that is more gentle and efficient, thus improving outcomes and minimizing complications.

All phaco machines consist of a computer to generate ultrasonic impulses and a transducer, usually piezoelectric crystals, to turn these electronic signals into mechanical energy. The energy thus created is harnessed, within the eye, to overcome the inertia of the lens and emulsify it. Once turned into emulsate, the fluidic systems remove the emulsate and replace it with balanced salt solution (BSS) in a closed, steady-state environment.

BASIC PRINCIPLES OF POWER GENERATION

The prerequisite for the removal of a cataract through a small incision is a technique to break up the hard nucleus into emulsate for aspiration. Inspired by the technique of dentistry to remove tarter with a metal tip that oscillates longitudinally at frequencies in the ultrasonic range, Kelman[1-3] adopted this principle, combining the oscillating tip and the evacuation tube into a hollow needle.[4] Titanium is the material of choice for such applications because it resists the fragmentation that occurs with more brittle metals. The mechanisms by which such an oscillating tip fragments the nucleus are examined in the following text.

TYPES OF TRANSDUCERS

Magnetostrictive Transducers

Magnetostrictive transducers are based on packs of ferromagnetic lamellae surrounded by an electric coil. The magnetic field induced by the high-frequency electric current flowing through the coil excites the oscillation.

The advantages of magnetostrictive transducers include contact-free excitation, thus avoiding deterioration at the junction of the current and the transducer. These transducers, coupling elements, and the entire handpiece are rugged. They can withstand mechanical injury and have a long life span. Their primary disadvantage is a relative low grade of efficiency. Only a small part of the energy input is transformed into mechanical action;

the majority becomes heat. Heating not only carries the risk of tissue burn but also makes the transducer lose efficiency with rising temperatures. Also, in the original design, the concentric aspiration line had to be brought out before the lamellar stack, necessitating two sharp bends that frequently clogged.

Recent improvements include considerably increased efficiency through sophisticated ferromagnetic metal alloys with rare earth elements and engineering modifications that allow both the irrigation and aspiration lines to be concentrically brought straight all the way through the tack to the tip. This not only avoids the clog-prone bends but also provides a double stream of constantly flowing cooling fluid through all the elements of the vibrating system, thus obviating the need for a separate cooling system, as was found to be necessary on the older handpiece.

PIEZOELECTRIC TRANSDUCERS

These transducers are based on the reversal of the piezoelectric phenomenon. Certain crystals, on compression, produce electric current. In reverse, electric current causes the crystal to contract. Applying current to a crystal at high frequency causes it to oscillate at that frequency.

The crystal is mounted on the "horn." This is a piece of tubing of narrowing diameter eventually ending with the attachment of the phaco needle. The decreasing diameter tube acts as an amplifier to generate adequate power for emulsification.

The advantages of piezoelectric crystals include a high grade of efficiency and, therefore, little inherent heat generation, with no need for extra cooling. Their low mass allows rapid movement and precise control. Newer machines use digital inputs to generate power. Digital control is more precise and instantaneous. Many new handpieces use multiple crystals (usually two to four sets) to maximize responsiveness and provide adequate power to emulsify the mature hard nucleus. Disadvantages include the connection points between crystal and electric current, the connections among the multiple layers of crystals that are necessary to provide adequate stroke amplitudes, and the structural brittleness of the crystal itself. These properties limit the longevity of such transducers. They are delicate and deteriorate both by accidental mechanical injury and by the oscillation they produce.

■ TUNING ■

Every material has an inherent frequency at which it vibrates naturally. This is called its resonant frequency. If excited to vibrate at this frequency, the transformation into mechanical amplitude will be optimal, and the creation of other forms of energy, principally heat, will be minimized. The creation of balanced crystals, their attachment to the horn, and the weight of the titanium phaco needle are, therefore, carefully controlled during manufacturing.

The phaco procedure itself is performed in a less rigidly controlled environment. In the course of phacoemulsification, the needle is passed through and inside material of inconsistent resistance. The aqueous humor is less resistant than a soft nucleus, and a soft nucleus less resistant than a mature one. Thus, for example, as the phaco needle travels through BSS into a hard nucleus, the resonant frequency must be adjusted, to prevent inefficient emulsification. The result of inefficient emulsification is

prolonged phaco time, higher powers, and ensuing increased heat generation.

Therefore, all modern phaco systems now have a built-in feedback loop constantly adjusting, or tuning, the oscillating frequency to an optimal resonance. This is a function of the central processing unit of the machine. It reads the change in resistance of the phaco needle and makes minute adjustments in the stroke length or frequency, dependent on which phaco machine is utilized, thus maximizing effectiveness. The rate of repetition with which the machine makes these adjustments is machine dependent. In the AMO Sovereign system, the tuning rate is 20 μs, in the Alcon Infiniti it is 100 times/s. It is intuitive, however, that the greater the frequency of these corrections, the more effective the emulsification.

■ POWER GENERATION ■

Power is created by the interaction of frequency and stroke length. Frequency is defined as the speed of the needle movement. It is determined by the manufacturer of the machine. Presently, most machines operate at a frequency of between 28,700 cycles per second (c/s; or hertz [Hz]) to 45,000 c/s (Table 7-1). This frequency range is the most efficient for nuclear emulsification. Lower frequencies appear to be less efficient, and higher frequencies create excess heat.[5]

Frequency is maintained constant by tuning circuitry designed into the machine computer. As noted earlier, tuning is vital because the phaco tip is required to operate in varied media. The computer recognizes the change in resistance by sensing a change in load. The appropriate response is then delivered to the phaco tip by a minute change of frequency or stroke length depending on the machine algorithm. The surgeon will subjectively appreciate good tuning circuitry by a sense of smoothness and power.

An innovative use of tuning circuitry software is found on the Alcon Infinit Machine. This modification is called "Smart Pulse" (Figure 7-1). When this proprietary programming is engaged, if the duration of the power stroke is less than 20 ms, a low power pulse, 1/2 of the programmed power (with a maximum of power of 10%) is generated prior to the application of the commanded power stroke. The low power pulse is used to sense the resistance of the nuclear fragment (load) and adjust the stroke length to provide the commanded power. This is important to allow maximum efficiency when ultrashort pulses of 5 ms are utilized. Without this modification, by the time the machine tuned the pulse would be over!

Stroke length is defined as the length of the needle movement (Figure 7-2). This length is generally 2–6 mil (thousandths of an inch). Most machines operate in the 2–4-mil range. Longer stroke lengths are prone to generate excess heat. Much like a hammer striking a nail through a greater distance, the longer the stroke length, the greater the physical impact on the nucleus and, in addition, the greater the generation of cavitational forces (Figure 7-3).

Stroke length is determined by foot pedal excursion in position three during linear control of phaco power. Although the frequency is unchanged, the amplitude of the sine wave is increased in direct proportion to the depression of the foot pedal (Figure 7-4).

Table 7-1 AMO sovereign settings for phaco chop*

Phaco 1 Hard chop	Phaco 2 Mod. chop	Phaco 3 Epinucleus unoccluded	Phaco 3 Epinucleus occluded	Phaco 4 Pre-occlusion
Vac. 315 Asp. 22 Power 30% Linear	Vac. 250 Asp.22 Power 25% Linear	Vac. 315 Asp. 22 Power 30% Thresh.150	Vac.150-315 Asp.22 Power 30%	Vac. 315 Asp. 22 Power 10%
0–25% CD 43%	0–25% BL 14%	0–25% BL 14%	4 long pulse (150 ms) BD 33%	0–100% CN 18%
26–50% CD 43%	26–50% CL 25%	26–50% CL 25%		
51–75% CB 60%	51–75% BD 33%	51–75% BD 33%		
76–100% DB 67%	76–100% CD 43%	76–100% CD 43%		
CD 6/8=14	BL 4/24=28	BL 4/24=28	BD 4/8=12	CN 6/28=34
CB 6/4=10	CL 6/24=30	CL 6/24=30		
DB 8/4=12	BD 4/8=12	BD 4/8=12		
	CD 6/8=14	CD 6/8=14		

*With 2.8 mm temporal clear corneal incision, 19-gauge 0° tip. Letter designations indicate duty cycles, i.e. DB is 8 ms on and 4 ms off in a 12 ms duty cycle.

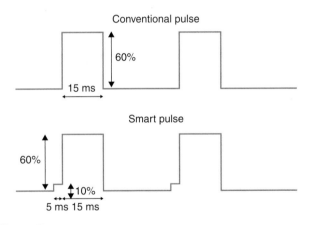

Figure 7-1 Smart pulse diagram.

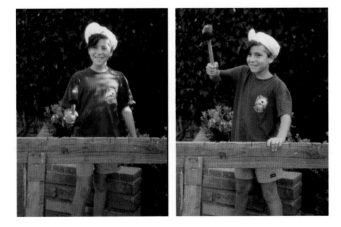

Figure 7-3 According to the formula F = MA (Force = Mass × Acceleration), as distance to the point of impact is increased, acceleration is increased, resulting in increased force.

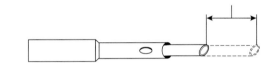

Figure 7-2 Stroke length.

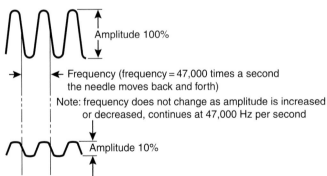

Figure 7-4 Frequency remains constant. The amplitude of the sine wave increases. This increases stroke length and resultant jackhammer and cavitational forces.

ENERGY AT THE PHACO TIP

The actual tangible forces, which emulsify the nucleus, are a blend of the "jackhammer" energy and cavitation energy.[1]

The jackhammer energy is the direct mechanical impact of the physical striking of the needle against the nucleus. The efficiency of this mechanism depends on two main prerequisites:

1. Rapid forward acceleration of the phaco tip. This overcomes the inertia of the nucleus penetrating it rather than driving it away.

77

2. Close mechanical contact between the tip and the nucleus. Engineers call this force coupling. It is accomplished by pressing the tip against the nucleus or by pressing the nucleus to the tip.

The jackhammer energy can be maximized or minimized depending on the tip selection as discussed in the text that follows.

The cavitation effect is more complex. The phaco needle, moving through the liquid medium of the aqueous humor at ultrasonic speeds, creates intense zones of high and low pressure. Low pressure, created with backward movement of the tip, literally pulls dissolved gases out of solution, thus giving rise to microbubbles (25.4^{-5} mm) in size. Forward tip movement creates an equally intense zone of high pressure. This produces compression of the microbubbles until they implode. At the moment of implosion, the bubbles create a temperature of 7204°C and a shock wave of 75,000 PSI. Of the microbubbles created, 75% implode, amassing to create a powerful shock wave radiating from the phaco tip in the direction of the bevel with annular spread. However, 25% of the bubbles are too large to implode. These microbubbles are swept up in the shock wave and radiate with it.

Utilizing high speed photography Dr. Teruki Miyoshi demonstated the development of cavitational energy in a video presented at ASCRS in 2005 (Figure 7-5).[1]

The cavitation energy thus created can be directed in any desired direction as the angle of the bevel of the phaco needle governs the direction of the generation of the shock wave and microbubbles.

An artificial but educational method of visualizing these forces, called enhanced cavitation, has been developed. Using this process, with a 45° tip, the cavitation wave is generated at 45° from the tip and comes to a focus 1 mm from it. Similarly a 30° tip generates cavitation at a 30° angle from the bevel, and a 15° tip, 15° from the bevel (Figure 7-6). A 0° tip creates the cavitation wave directly in front of the tip, and the focal point is 0.5 mm from the tip (Figure 7-7). The Kelman tip has a broad band of powerful cavitation, which radiates from the area of the angle in the shaft. A weak area of cavitation is developed from the bevel but is inconsequential (Figure 7-8).[8,9]

There is debate over the magnitude of the role of jackhammer and cavitation energy. Various investigators have found contrasting results on the subject of the power of cavitational energy.[2] Analysis of their data indicates that Jackhammer energy is the more

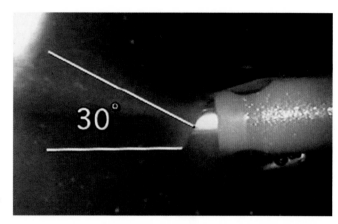

Figure 7-6 A 30° tip. Enhanced cavitation shows ultrasonic wave focused 1 mm from the tip, spreading at an angle of 30°.

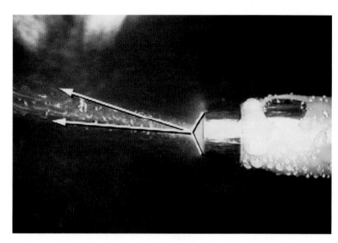

Figure 7-7 A 0° tip. Enhanced cavitation shows ultrasonic wave focused 0.5 mm in front of the tip, spreading directly in front of it.

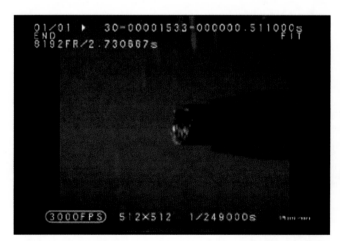

Figure 7-5 Miyoshi high-speed photograph of cavitation.

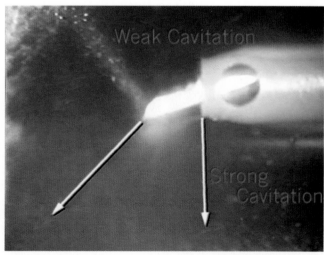

Figure 7-8 Kelman tip. Enhanced cavitation shows broad band of enhanced cavitation spreading inferiorly from the angle of the tip. A weak band of cavitation spreads from the tip.

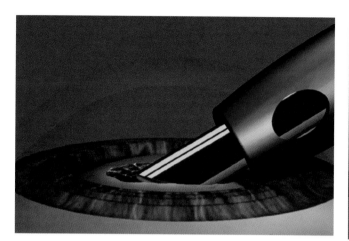

Figure 7-9 Turning the bevel of the phaco tip toward the nucleus focuses cavitation and jackhammer energy into the nucleus.

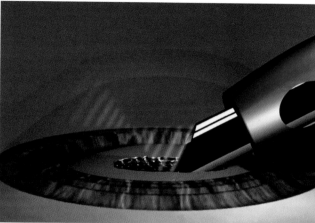

Figure 7-10 When the bevel is turned away from the nucleus ultrasonic energy is directed toward the iris and endothelium.

potent force in emulsification. Cavitation augments the emulsification when lens material is very close to, or within, the lumen of the phaco tip.

Taking into consideration analysis of enhanced cavitation, it can be concluded that emulsification is most efficient when both the jackhammer energy and cavitation energy are integrated. To accomplish this, utilize a 0° tip. When using an angled tip, the bevel of the needle should be turned toward the nucleus, or nuclear fragment. This simple maneuver causes the broad bevel of the needle to strike the nucleus. This enhances the physical force of the needle striking the nucleus. In addition, the cavitational force is concentrated into the nucleus rather than away from it (Figure 7-9). This causes the energy to emulsify the nucleus and be absorbed by it. When the bevel is turned away from the nucleus, the cavitational energy is directed up and away from the nucleus toward the iris and endothelium (Figure 7-10). Finally, in this configuration, the vacuum force (discussed later in this chapter) can be maximally exploited as occlusion is encouraged.

MODIFICATION OF PHACO POWER

Modification of phaco power must be accomplished to harness these powerful forces for a controlled phaco surgical procedure.

Application of the minimal amount of phaco power intensity necessary for emulsification of the nucleus is desirable. Unnecessary power intensity is a source of heat with subsequent wound damage. Moreover, excessive cavitational energy is a cause of endothelial cell damage and iris damage with resultant alteration of the blood–aqueous barrier. Phaco power intensity can be modified by altering phaco power amplitude, phaco power duration, and phaco power delivery.

ALTERATION OF PHACO POWER AMPLITUDE

Stroke length is determined by foot pedal excursion and, therefore, foot-pedal adjustment. When it is set for linear phaco, the depression of the foot pedal increases stroke length and, consequently, power.

Foot pedals, such as those found in the Allergan Sovereign and the Alcon Infiniti machines, permit surgeon adjustment of the throw length of the pedal in position 3. This can refine power application. The Bausch & Lomb (B&L) Millennium, and AMO Signature offer a dual linear foot pedal which permits the separation of the fluidic aspects of the foot pedal from the power elements, by adding a yaw movement to the foot pedal.

ALTERATION OF PHACO POWER DURATION-BURST, PULSE, MICRO-PULSE

The duration of application of phaco power has a dramatic effect on overall power delivered to the anterior segment. This is the use of power modulations. Power modulations include the use of burst, multiburst, and pulsed phaco. For example, if continuous power is employed for 1 min, the effective phaco time is 1 min. If the power is pulsed at 10 pulses per second, the effective phaco time is 30 seconds. The effective power delivered to the anterior segment is half of the continuous amount.

There are three different types of noncontinuous power modulations: burst, pulse, and hyperpulse, phaco.

In pulse phaco there is a fixed period of power with a fixed period of no power (aspiration only). The phaco power progressively increases as the foot pedal is depressed in position 3.

In burst phaco there is a fixed power with a reduced duration of the period of power on and power off (aspiration only) until there is continuous power.

Hyperpulse phaco has extremely short periods of power on and power off. Where a standard short pulse might be 50 ms a micropulse might by 5 ms.

Burst mode in the Allergan Sovereign (parameter is machine dependent) is characterized by 80 or 120 ms periods of power combined with variable short periods of aspiration only. Pulse mode uses fixed pulses of power of 50 or 150 ms with variable short periods of aspiration only. Phaco techniques such as phaco chop use minimal periods of power in pulse mode to reduce power delivery to the anterior chamber. In addition, the use of pulse mode, or hyperpulse mode, to remove the epinucleus provides an added margin of safety. When the epinucleus is emulsified, the posterior capsule is exposed to the phaco tip and may move forward toward it because of surge. Activation of pulse phaco mode creates a deeper anterior chamber to work within. This occurs because each period of phaco energy is followed by an interval of no phaco energy. During the interval of absence of energy the epinucleus is drawn toward the phaco tip, producing occlusion, interrupting outflow. This allows inflow to deepen the anterior chamber immediately before onset of another pulse of phaco energy. The surgeon will recognize the outcome as operating in a deeper, more stable anterior chamber.

Recent innovations by Alcon, AMO, B&L, and Staar have resulted in new forms of power modulation.

CAVITATIONAL MODIFICATIONS OF SOFTWARE

Abbott Medical Optics (AMO) introduced the WhiteStar System of hyperpulse phaco. In this modification, extremely short bursts of power are interspersed with similar, extremely short periods of aspiration. The relationship of these on/off periods are called a "duty cycle" (see Figure 7-13).

In a duty cycle pulse, the on time for ultrasonic energy is active for only a percentage of the total time of the pulse. For example, with a duty cycle of 50% the pulse on time/off time could be 4 ms on/8 ms off or 6 ms on/12 ms off. In the first example the pulse duration is 12 ms and in the second 18 ms. It can be seen with similar duty cycles the time of power on or off may be vastly different.

The duty cycle is selected by the surgeon. Using the AMO Sovereign there are many choices for on/off time and duty cycle (Table 7-2). The Alcon Infiniti system may generate up to 100 pps with programmable duty cycle between 5 and 95%. The B&L Millennium can generate up to 120 pps with duty cycles between 10 and 90%.

PULSE CONTOURING

The newest variation of phaco energy is the modification of the contour of the ultrasonic waveform. This is helpful in emulsification of cataract fragments. The traditional ultrasonic waveform is square (Figure 7-11). The B&L Millennium employs "rounded waveform" (Figure 7-11). This modulation changes the contour of the ultrasonic pulse so that within the duty cycle the pulse

Conventional	Advanced power modulation with CCS
Fixed duty cycle	Variable duty cycle (10–100%) – *To prevent continuous phaco energy even w/maximum pedal depression*
Fixed rise time	Variable rise time (waveform pulse) 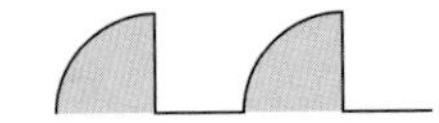 Unique to millennium technology – *less energy during nuclear removal* – *less heat build-up; less total energy*

Figure 7-11 The B&L Stellaris square waveform compared to the rounded waveform.

begins at low power and intensifies rapidly to the maximum preset power. The low power enhances the movement of the fragment toward the phaco tip enhancing occlusion. The higher power provides for the emulsification of the fragment.

The AMO Sovereign and Signature approach the problem of improved followability from a different perspective. They have engineered a pulse of ultrasonic power with a short burst of increased energy at the beginning of each ultrasonic waveform (Figure 7-12); this is named ICE (increased control and efficiency). The amplitude of this "kicker" can be programed up to 12% of the total power of the pulse. It can increase, decrease, or remain the same as the phaco power is increased. The concept is to drive the fragment a microscopic distance from the phaco tip as the tip is energized. The fragment is then available for emulsification without occlusion.

The change in phaco duty cycles leads to enhanced followability by altering the tendency for phaco power to repel cataractous material and modifying the fluidic characteristics of the pre-occlusion/post-occlusion cycle (discussed below). The end result is shorter phaco power on times, less delivery of total phaco energy to the anterior segment, and increased anterior chamber stability resulting is decreased incidence of ruptured posterior

Table 7-2 Alcon Infinity: torsional phaco*

	Sculpting	Quadrant removal	Epinucleus/cortex removal
Irrigation (cm H₂O)	95	95	95
Aspiration rate (cc/min)	24	38	33 linear
Vacuum limit (mm Hg)	120	360	300 linear
Torsional amplitude	100% linear	100% linear	100% linear

*20 gauge, 15° Kelman ABS Tip.

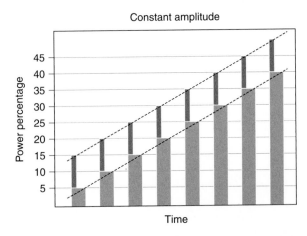

Constant amplitude

Figure 7-12 AMO ICE – a 1 ms "kicker" at the beginning of the pulse (not to scale).

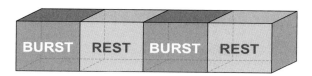

Figure 7-13 A duty cycle is the combined burst and rest time.

capsules and vitrectomy. In addition, the off time allows effective cooling of the phaco tip, minimizing the likelihood of wound burn, even during emulsification of a hard nucleus.

Wound Burn

The prevention of wound burn is an important feature of this software modification. Studies have shown that the wound will show the first signs of a wound burn at 45°C and frank signs of burn at 50°C. With WhiteStar, the maximal wound temperature at 100% power was measured at 28°C.[11] Therefore, the phaco tip can be placed though the wound without the cooling sleeve. Whenever there is decreased outflow through a phaco tip, especially when the wound is tight surrounding the tip compressing the sleeve or tip shaft, wound burn is possible. The greater the energy setting the greater the risk of wound burn. The surgeon must be vigilant to monitor bubbles around the tip wound interface or striae in the clear cornea over the phaco tip. Any suggestion of these phenomena mandates immediate cessation of phaco energy.

BIMANUAL MICROINCISIONAL PHACO

Micropulse phaco allows for the performance of a bimanual, microincisional, phacoemulsification procedure. The irrigation is provided by a 20-gauge irrigating chopping instrument through a 1.4 mm clear cornea incision. The 20-guage, 15° or 30° phaco tip *without the irrigation sleeve* is inserted through a 20-gauge clear cornea incision 90–100° away (21-gauge instrumentation with 1.1 mm incisions can also be utilized). The nucleus is emulsified by either a vertical or horizontal chopping procedure. The wound remains cool and the efficiency of the procedure is enhanced as the separate irrigation tends to wash fragments into the phaco tip.

Coaxial Microincisional PhacoMicropulse phaco also allows for another variation of microincisional phaco. This is coaxial phaco utilizing micro phaco tip of 20 gauge (Alcon Infiniti) and a thin-walled rigid infusion sleeve through a 2.4 mm. Torsional phaco (discussed below) is another excellent modality for coaxial microincisional phaco.

Employing similar modification to tip and sleeve the B&L Stellaris is capable of passing through a 1.8 mm incision for coaxial microincisional phaco.

ALTERATION OF PHACO POWER DELIVERY

The amplitude of phaco energy is modified by tip selection. Phaco tips can be modified to accentuate: (1) power intensity, (2) flow, or (3) a combination of both.

Power intensity is modified by altering bevel tip angle. As noted previously, the bevel of the phaco tip focuses power in the direction of the bevel. The 0° tip focuses both jackhammer and cavitational force directly in front of it. The 30° tip focuses

these forces at a 30° angle from the phaco tip (see Figures 7-6, 7-7, 7-9, and 7-10). The Kelman tip produces broad powerful cavitation directed away from the angle in the shaft (see Figure 7-8). This tip is excellent for the hardest of nuclei.

Power intensity and flow are modified by using a 0° tip. This tip focuses power directly ahead of the tip and enhances occlusion caused by the smaller surface area of its orifice.

Flare tips direct cavitation into the opening of the bevel of the tip. Thus random emission of phaco energy is minimized. The wide opening of the tip makes it easier to minipulate the fragment. The narrow "neck" of the tip functions as a flow restrictor by increasing the resistance to flow and reducing the tendency to create surge (Figure 7-14). Designer tips such as the "flathead" designed by Barry Seibel and power wedges designed by Douglas Mastel offer the ability to fine tune the focus of phaco energy as well as modify the aspiration flow dependent upon the configuration and diameter of the phaco tip. The rounded tip designed by Steven Dewey is interesting as it will maximize cavitational energy but is "capsular friendly." Thus, if the capsule should be aspirated by the phaco tip while energized, tearing the capsule is less likely.

Small-diameter tips, such as 21-gauge tips, change fluid flow rates. Although they do not in reality change the power intensity, they appear to have this effect, as the nucleus must be emulsified into smaller pieces for removal through the smaller diameter tip.

The Alcon aspiration bypass system (ABS) tip modification is available with many tip configurations. The tip type is a modification of power intensity, and the ABS is a flow modification. In the ABS system a 0.175 mm hole in the needle shaft permits a variable flow of fluid into the needle, even during occlusion (Figure 7-15). The amount of flow through the shaft hole is variable and depends on the vacuum level. The higher the vacuum level, the greater the flow. This flow adjustment serves to reduce postocclusion surge (discussed below).

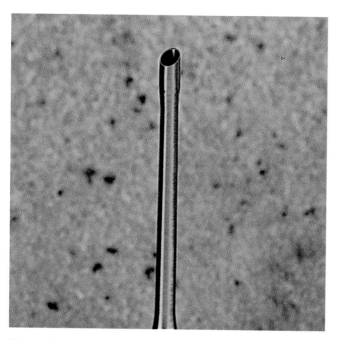

Figure 7-14 Flare tip focuses power at the tip secondary to the flare and acts as a flow restrictor secondary to the narrowing at the "neck." (Courtesy Micro Technology Inc.)

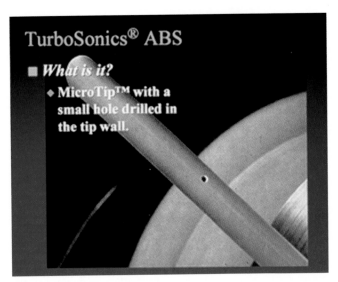

Figure 7-15 A 0.175 mm hole drilled in the shaft of the ABS tip provides an alternate path for fluid to flow into the needle when an occlusion occurs at the phaco tip.

ALTERATION OF PHACO POWER, DURATION AND CONFIGURATION – please see Pg 92 for an update to this section

Torsional Phaco

A new development in phaco is the harnessing of lateral or ocillatory movement of the phaco tips developed by Alcon in the Infiniti Machine. The OZiL torsional handpiece has both a longitudinal movement and torsional movement. The longitudinal movement, like a standard phaco needle is at 40 kHz. The torsional movement is at 32 kHz with 1° arc of motion (Figure 7-16). The torsional movement may be used alone or in combination with the longitudinal movement with many variations of timing. It requires an angled "kelman" tip of 15° or 30° to be effective. It appears to be most efficient when using a mix of longitudinal and torsional

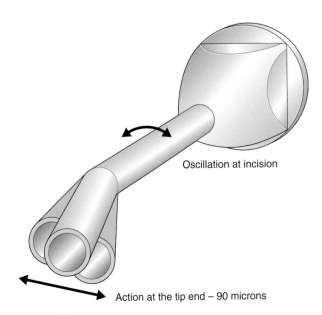

Oscillation at incision

Action at the tip end – 90 microns

Figure 7-16 Torsional needle.

movement. This modification, as well as needle configurations, is presently under modification. The final parameters for its use are yet to be determined. The torsional movement will emulsify with minimal chatter and improved followability. However, occasionally the low power phaco will cause chunks of nucleus to occlude the phaco needle lumen. Longitudinal movement is then used to emulsify the material present in the needle bore.

Torsional phaco is noteworthy for its efficient removal of nuclear material due to the propensity of torsional movement to favor pre-occlusion phaco (see below).

Phaco power intensity is the energy that emulsifies the lens nucleus. The phaco tip must operate in a cool environment and with adequate space to isolate its actions from delicate intraocular structures. This portion of the action of the machine is dependent on its fluidics.

◼ FLUIDICS ◼

The fluidics aspect of all machines is fundamentally a balance of fluid inflow and fluid outflow. The resultant balance of these two influences will be the maintenance of a constant intraocular volume and, therefore, a stable and deep anterior chamber. In addition, the intraocular pressure must be maintained within physiologically compatible limits.

INFUSION

Inflow (infusion) is the pressure gradient, which drives the infusion flow. In a gravity feed system, the bottle height above the eye of the patient creates an infusion pressure. When infusion pumps are employed, the amount of infusion pressure programmed into the pump will be responsible for the generation of infusion pressure. With temporal surgical approaches, the eye of the patient may be physically higher than in the past. This requires that the irrigation bottle be adequately elevated. In addition, when the machine flow rate is increased, increased fluid evacuation from the anterior chamber requires increased inflow to maintain the steady-state system. Therefore, when the machine flow rate is increased, the bottle height should also be increased. A shallow, unstable anterior chamber results otherwise.

Infusion tubing diameter and elasticity do not play a significant role in infusion volume control because high pressures and rapid pressure fluxes rarely occur on the irrigation bottle side of the system.

OUTFLOW

Control of outflow is notably more complex because many factors influence both volume and speed of fluid outflow during the phaco procedure. Among these variables are incision size, phaco tip diameter and sleeve diameter, pump type and settings, and tubing diameter and compliance. In addition, computer software design plays a significant role in regulating both outflow volume and speed.

Incision

The incision size is an important variable in the determination of fluid outflow. This is actually a controlled leak determined by the sleeve–incision relationship. The incision length selected should create a snug fit with the phaco tip and sleeve selected. This results in minimal controlled wound fluid outflow with resultant increased anterior chamber stability.

If the incision is too large for the selected phaco tip and sleeve combination, the excessive fluid outflow will necessitate increased fluid inflow to maintain a deep anterior chamber. The increased infusion volume not only is deleterious to the health of the endothelium but usually cannot sustain the sudden changes in volume that occur during the procedure. This leads to considerable chamber instability with increased risk of rupturing the posterior capsule.

If the incision is too small, crimping of the sleeve will lead to decreased inflow with resultant chamber shallowing. In addition, decreased inflow is the origin of decreased cooling and may produce wound burns.

Aspiration Settings

Aspiration rate, or flow, is defined as the flow of fluid, in cubic centimeters per minute (cc/min), through the aspiration tubing. With a peristaltic pump this rate is determined by the speed of the pump. Flow is the fluidic force that determines how well particulate material is attracted to the phaco tip. Flow adjustments act to speed up or slow down events in the anterior chamber. Therefore, if events appear to be occurring too rapidly, the flow rate is slowed. Alternatively, if events are occurring too slowly, the flow rate is increased.

Aspiration level, or vacuum, is a level and measured in millimeters of mercury (mm Hg). It is defined as the magnitude of negative pressure created within the tubing. Vacuum is the fluidic force determinant of how well, once occluded on the phaco tip, particulate material will be held to the tip.

Flow, therefore, is the setting that controls how well material is attracted to the phaco tip. Vacuum is the setting that determines how well material is held against the tip once occlusion occurs.

VACUUM SOURCES

The origin for the development of vacuum is the vacuum pump. The three categories of vacuum sources or pumps are: (1) flow pumps, (2) vacuum pumps,[3] and (3) hybrid pumps.

The prototype example of the flow pump is the peristaltic pump (Figure 7-17). This pump consists of a series of rotating rollers that successively compress the aspiration tubing, moving fluid within the tubing and creating vacuum. The speed of rotation of the pump head governs the flow rate. One important advantage of this class of pumps is the ability to allow independent control of both aspiration rate and aspiration level.

The primary example of the vacuum pump is the Venturi pump (Figure 7-18). In the Venturi pump, compressed gas is passed through a Venturi, which creates a vacuum. The Venturi is attached to a rigid reservoir that is attached to the aspiration tubing. The velocity of the compressed gas passage through the Venturi creates greater or lesser vacuum that is then transferred through the reservoir to the aspiration line. This results in varying amounts of vacuum.

Additional examples of this pump type are the rotary vane and diaphragmatic pumps.

Vacuum pumps allow direct control of only vacuum level. Flow control is dependent on the vacuum level setting. There is no independent setting of aspiration flow.

Modern modifications of the basic pump types have prompted the creation of a new pump category, the hybrid pump. These pumps are interesting in that they can act like either a vacuum or flow pump, independent of their original design, depending on their programming. They are the most recent supplement to pump types. They are universally controlled by digital inputs, producing extraordinary flexibility and responsiveness.

The primary example of the hybrid pump is the Allergan Sovereign peristaltic pump (Figure 7-19) or the B&L Concentrix pump (Figure 7-20).[12]

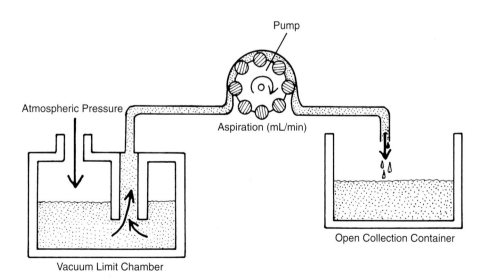

Figure 7-17 Peristaltic pump uses a rotating wheel with rollers to pinch off segments of the aspiration tubing, thereby moving separate columns of fluid through the tubing at a controlled rate of aspiration or flow. The vacuum limit is set separately and independently, limiting the maximal vacuum that is tolerated in the condition of complete occlusion of the aspiration line. The collection chamber, located after the vacuum limit chamber and the aspiration pump, is open to atmosphere.

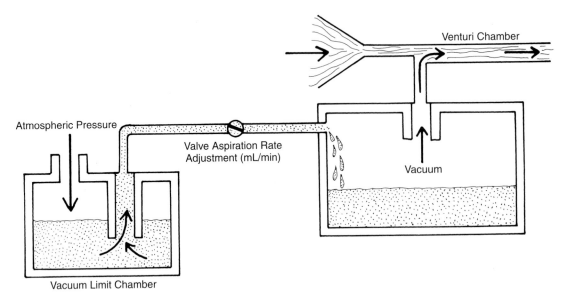

Figure 7-18 In a Venturi pump system, the flow of gas passed through tubing with increasing diameter creates a vacuum. The collection chamber is, therefore, a closed system. A separate valve can control the aspiration rate. A separate vacuum limit can be set, but a continuous internal vacuum is necessary to drive the aspiration of the fluid.

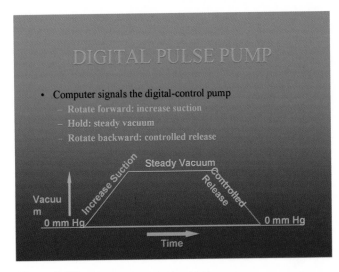

Figure 7-19 AMO Sovereign hybrid peristaltic pump.

Recognizing that surgeon preference over pump types may play a role in surgeon machine purchase, some new machines offer both types of pumps. The AMO Signature with Fusion Technology and the B&L Stellaris offer this option. The challenge to the surgeon is to balance the effect of phaco power intensity, which tends to push nuclear fragments away from the phaco tip, with the effect of flow, which attracts fragments toward the phaco tip, and vacuum, which holds the fragments on the phaco tip. Generally, low flow slows down intraocular events, and high flow or vacuum speeds them up. Low or zero vacuum is helpful during *sculpting* of a hard or a large nucleus. In this circumstance, the large, hard endonucleus may cause the surgeon to phacoemulsify near or under the iris, or anterior capsule, with a high-power intensity. With normal aspiration the phaco tip may aspirate the iris. The high power will cause immediate, severe damage to the iris. Therefore, zero (or very low) vacuum will prevent inadvertent aspiration of the iris or capsule, preventing significant morbidity.

SURGE

A principal limiting factor in the selection of high levels of vacuum or flow is the development of surge. When the phaco tip is occluded, flow is instantly interrupted, and vacuum rapidly builds to its preset maximum level (Figure 7-21). Emulsification of the occluding fragment then clears the occlusion. Flow instantaneously begins at the preset level in the presence of the high vacuum level. In addition, if the aspiration line tubing is not reinforced to prevent collapse (tubing compliance), the tubing will have constricted during the occlusion. It then expands on occlusion break. The expansion is an additional source of brisk vacuum production. These factors cause a rush of fluid from the anterior segment into the phaco tip (Figure 7-22). The fluid in the anterior chamber may not be replaced by infusion rapidly enough to prevent its shallowing. Therefore, subsequent, rapid anterior movement of the posterior capsule occurs. Often the cornea collapses. The violent snapping of the posterior capsule, or abrupt forceful stretching of the bag around nuclear fragments, may be a cause of capsular tears (Figure 7-23). In addition, the posterior capsule can be literally sucked into the phaco tip, tearing it. The magnitude of the surge is contingent on the presurge settings of flow and vacuum.

The phaco machine manufacturers help to decrease surge by providing noncompliant aspiration tubing. This does not constrict in the presence of high levels of vacuum.

Most manufacturers have created algorithms in their software that emulate the anterior chamber, moment to moment, during the phaco procedure. These algorithms can anticipate changes

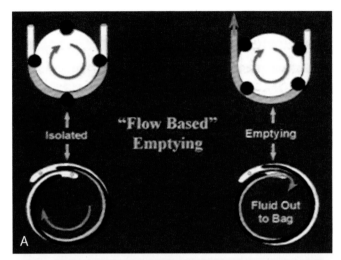

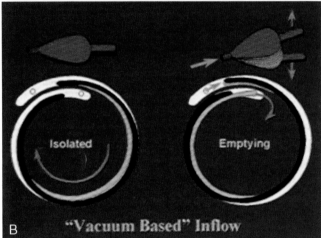

Figure 7-20 **A**, The scroll pumps' emptying phase is flow based, analogous to a peristaltic system. **B**, During the inflow phase, the male scroll opens like a bellows, creating vacuum response similar to a Venturi system.

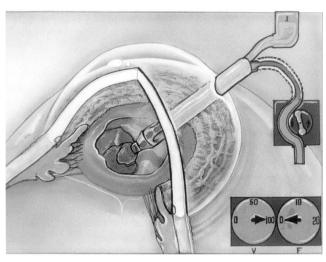

Figure 7-22 Early surge. Phaco power has partially emulsified the fragment. Flow is about to resume and instantaneously rise to the preset maximum. Vacuum, at maximum, is about to precipitously drop. The tubing is expanding. Outflow is exceeding inflow. The chamber is beginning to collapse. The posterior capsule is beginning to bulge around the remaining heminucleus. (Courtesy Thieme Publications, New York.)

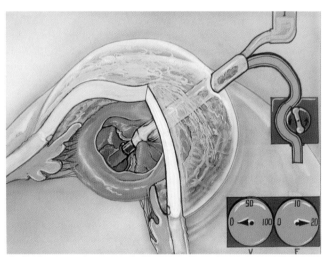

Figure 7-23 Midsurge. Flow is now at preset maximum. Vacuum is zero. The anterior chamber is markedly shallowed. The posterior capsule has snapped around the heminucleus, causing a tear. The cornea has collapsed. (Courtesy Thieme Publications, New York.)

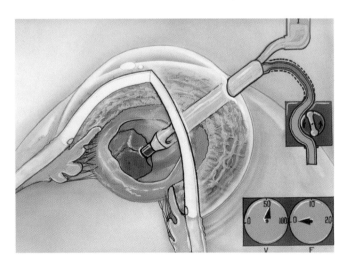

Figure 7-21 Immediate presurge. The nuclear fragment has occluded the phaco tip. Flow instantaneously drops to zero. Vacuum begins to rise toward the maximum preset. The aspiration tubing begins to collapse. The chamber is deep. (Courtesy Thieme Publications, New York.)

per microsecond in the real anterior chamber and make appropriate pump adjustments to minimize surge.

SURGE MODIFICATION

Surge is undoubtedly an unwanted event. The trampolining of the posterior capsule caused by surge has the effect of creating dismay among surgeons. In an effort to prevent capsular tears, they move the nucleus anteriorly, closer to iris and endothelium. To promote a more safe procedure and to spare the iris and endothelium unnecessary trauma, the astute surgeon will consider what changes in fluidics are necessary to prevent surge.

If the defining instant in the generation of surge is the occlusion break, the entire episode can be divided into: **preocclusive**, **occlusive**, and **postocclusive** segments.

Preocclusion

Historically, the only way to modify surge was to select lower levels of flow and vacuum. This category would be a modification in preocclusion (Figure 7-24). At present, many other methods exist to decrease surge. Another approach to surge management, in all phases of occlusion, is the use of an anterior chamber maintainer. The constant flow of this device acts to deepen the chamber in all phases of phacoemulsification. Constant infusion, when available, is another preocclusion modification, although its benefits are not significant.

The most powerful modification of fluidics to allow emulsification in the pre-occlusion phase is not a fluidic modification but a power modification. The development of micro pulse phaco (discussed earlier), a patented development of AMO, found originally in the Sovereign with Whitestar, and now available in all machines by all manufacturers, is an evolutionary change in creating a more stable anterior chamber during emulsification. The extremely short bursts of energy followed by a variable period of no energy and aspiration only, serves to hold a nuclear fragment very near, but not occluded on, the phaco tip. Therefore, the fragment is emulsified with a combination of jackhammer and cavitation energy without ever totally occluding the tip. If there is no occlusion, there cannot be surge. Therefore, the phaco is performed on the pre-occlusive side of the pattern.

Occlusion

Only a few modifications take place at the moment of occlusion. The first is the use of the ABS tip (Alcon). This tip, discussed earlier, has a 0.175 mm hole drilled in the shaft of the phaco needle (see Figure 7-15). When occlusion occurs at the tip, fluid flows into this hole. The amount of flow depends on the vacuum and flow settings. For example, the flow through this hole is 4 cc/min at a vacuum of 50 mm Hg and 11 cc/min at a vacuum of 400 mm Hg. Because some flow always exists, in reality there is never complete occlusion. This prevents the rise of high vacuum levels and thus diminishes postocclusion surge. This modification must be used with the high vacuum tubing or it does not function properly.

The second, as employed by AMO Sovereign/Signature, B&L Mellennium/Stellaris with the peristaltic pump (Advanced Fluidics System), and the Infinit (ALCON) with the dynamic rise time option, is a variable rise time. By slowing the pump speed during occlusion, the generation of high vacuum levels is decelerated, and surge is diminished.

A third method is demonstrated by the Signature (AMO), and Mellennium/Stellaris (B&L) with the dual linear foot pedal. Employing this device, by yawing the foot pedal, aspiration only can be selected. Utilizing linear vacuum the vacuum level can be increased to the exact amount to cause occlusion, but not higher, minimizing the post occlusion surge when phaco power is applied. This method of vacuum control changes both the occlusion and post occlusion function.

Postocclusion

Once occlusion has occurred, decreasing the vacuum or flow instantaneously to dramatically decrease flow into the phaco tip is a powerful method of diminishing surge.

The model for this type of surge modification is found in the AMO Sovereign unit. In this machine, microprocessors sample vacuum and flow parameters 50 times a second, creating a "virtual" anterior chamber model. At the moment of surge, the machine computer senses the increase in flow and instantaneously slows or reverses the pump to stop surge production. Pump management, rather than venting, is the mechanism to control surge.

In addition, this device has a programmable occlusion threshold setting. When the vacuum reaches this threshold, a new flow, as well as a new power modulation, can be programmed. Therefore, if a hard nucleus is being emulsified, when the vacuum reaches 80 mm Hg, for example, the flow, which might have been set at 350 mL/min, can now be automatically decreased to 100 mL/min. The result will be a noteworthy decrease in surge. Moreover, the pulse rate can be simultaneously slowed to further stabilize the anterior chamber.

Ever improving digital control is demonstrated in the Sovereign/Signature (AMO) with a fluidic modification they have named CASE (Chamber Stabilization Environment) technology. With this software the surgeon sets a vacuum threshold and time for an extremely fast, 26 ms, drop in vacuum to a pre-set new, lower vacuum. This drop occurs so fast that there is not enough time for vacuum to build and thus prevents the surge from occurring.

Another solution to this problem is demonstrated in the B&L Millennium/Stelaris machine. The dual linear foot pedal can be programmed to separate both the flow and vacuum from power. In this way, flow or vacuum can be lowered before beginning the emulsification of an occluding fragment. The emulsification, therefore, occurs in the presence of a lower vacuum or flow so that surge is minimized.

Finally, the Starr Wave machine solves this problem in another manner. The patented coiled aspiration tubing acts as a flow resistor. At low flow settings, up to 50 mL/min, the tubing acts like normal tubing. When flow exceeds this level, turbulence in the tubing inhibits further increases in flow. This dampens the fluid outflow, and subsequent vacuum rise. The result is decreased surge.

An add-on tubing restrictor, also manufactured by Starr, is called "cruise control." It is a dual sleeved tubing. The outer tubing creates the cartridge shell, and the inner tubing is fenestrated and is a filter (Figure 7-24A). The cartridge is inserted into the aspiration orifice of the handpiece and then connects to the aspiration tubing. Where it connects the cartridge narrows to 1 mm diameter. The inner cartridge filters emulsate particulates to prevent clogging at the flow restrictor, the 1 mm narrowing of the tubing. Thus a powerful flow restrictor decreases surge and stabilizes the anterior chamber insulating against fluid fluxes.

■ VENTING ■

Often during the performance of phacoemulsification, or irrigation and aspiration (I&A), undesirable material is aspirated on the phaco tip. This could be posterior capsule or a piece of

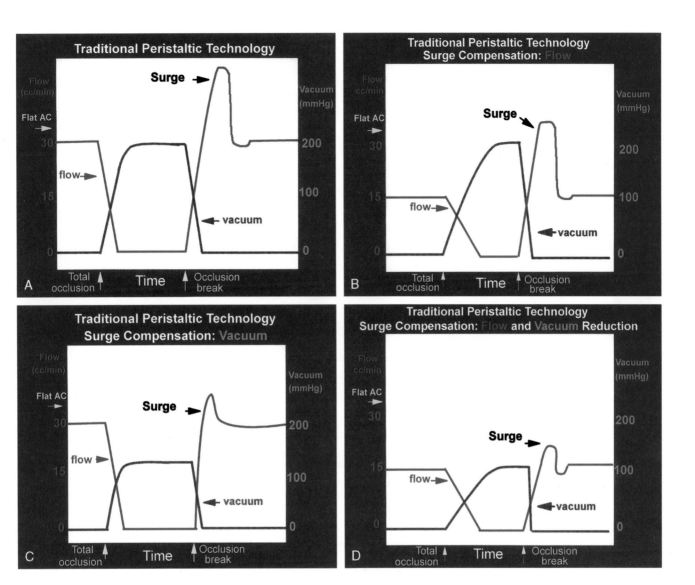

Figure 7-24 The dynamics of vacuum and flow, with particular emphasis on the phenomenon of surge. The values shown are illustrative and not necessarily those of any particular commercial system or surgical technique. **A,** In traditional peristaltic technology, flow ideally can be set at a relatively high rate just below that which would flatten the anterior chamber. In a nonoccluded system, the flow can be high, and the vacuum level at the phaco tip is nearly zero. When the tip is occluded, the aspiration rate rapidly falls to zero. The vacuum level rises correspondingly. The more rapid the flow rate, the more quickly the vacuum level rises. The vacuum level continues to build up to the preset limit, after which fluid is bled into the aspiration line, limiting the maximum vacuum. When occlusion is relieved, the vacuum then rapidly falls back to a near zero level at the tip. The stored potential energy in the aspiration line causes a momentary "surge" in the fluid flow before the flow stabilizes at the original level determined by the rotation of the peristaltic pump. If the potential energy causes a surge of fluid flow greater than the combined rate of irrigation fluid inflow and wound leak, flattening of the anterior chamber results. **B,** One mechanism for compensating for surge is to reduce flow. When flow or aspiration rate is reduced, two effects are seen. First, after occlusion is obtained, the rate at which the vacuum rises is slower. Ultimately, however, the vacuum still builds to the preset level. Second, after occlusion break, the height of the fluid surge is the same as in panel A. However, the surge is relative to the baseline level of nonoccluded flow. Because the flow has been reduced, the overall surge level may be at or below the level of a momentary flattening of the anterior chamber. **C,** An alternative compensation for surge is to reduce the vacuum level. Because the flow rate is unchanged, the speed at which the maximum vacuum is achieved is unchanged compared with the buildup of vacuum seen in panel A. After the occlusion is relieved, the amount of surge is reduced because the stored potential energy is reduced through the lower vacuum level. Because of the high flow rate, however, even this reduced amount of surge may exceed the level at which flattening of the anterior chamber is seen. **D,** In common clinical practice, both the flow and vacuum levels are reduced below the theoretical maximum to guard against surge. As illustrated, the reduction in flow rate and maximal vacuum level reduced the surge below the level at which the anterior chamber flattens. Through these compromises, safe phacoemulsification can be clinically performed. The dynamics of vacuum and flow are shown, with particular emphasis on the phenomenon of surge. The values shown are illustrative and not necessarily those of any particular commercial system or surgical technique.

(Continued)

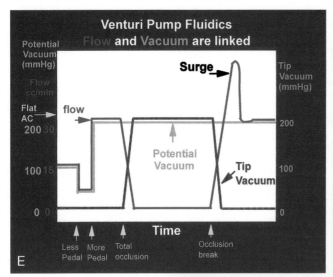

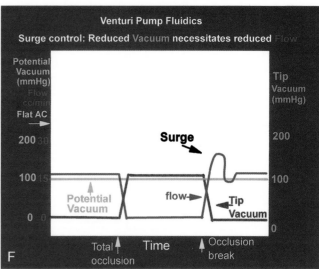

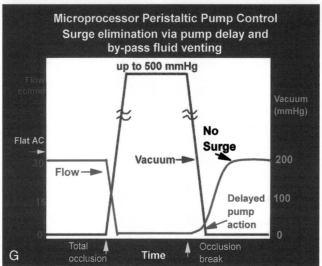

Figure 7-24, cont'd **E,** In a Venturi or diaphragm pump, flow and vacuum are intrinsically linked. The potential vacuum within the system caused by the Venturi and diaphragm pump is the principal determinant of the flow level. As illustrated in the left side of the figure, one attribute of the Venturi system is the rapid response time of the flow rate achieved by varying the potential vacuum within the system. After total occlusion occurs clinically, however, the performance at the phaco tip is similar to that of the peristaltic pump. The vacuum level at the tip rises to the preset level of the internal pump while the flow rate drops to zero. When occlusion is relieved, the vacuum at the tip once again drops to nearly zero. The stored potential energy in the system is translated into the clinical phenomenon of surge, just as in a peristaltic system. After the surge phenomenon, the flow rate stabilizes at the level determined by the internal vacuum of the Venturi pump. **F,** To compensate for surge and to maintain the anterior chamber, typically maximum potential vacuum and flow rate are reduced. Because of the intrinsic linkage of flow and vacuum in a Venturi or diaphragm pump system, reduction of the internal potential vacuum necessitates a reduced flow rate. By reducing both the flow and maximum vacuum, the surge level can be reduced below the level of flattening of the anterior chamber. **G,** New technology offers enhanced control over the surge phenomenon. As a result, phacoemulsification can be performed at vacuum levels that were previously highly unsafe. As illustrated, a microprocessor peristaltic pump control system may allow vacuum levels to build up to 500 mm Hg or more. After a break in the occlusion, the microprocessor delays the action of the pump by delaying its onset. In this manner, combined with other steps, such as reducing the compliance of the vacuum tubing, the phenomenon of surge is reduced to clinically tolerable levels, and high vacuum can be employed as a clinical tool without danger of collapse of the anterior chamber.

nucleus that is too large for efficient emulsification. Often the aspiration of these structures requires hasty release. Venting is the mechanism for this release by neutralizing vacuum in the aspiration line.

When the surgeon lifts the foot pedal from position 2 or 3, the venting mechanism is engaged. This allows air or fluid to flow into the aspiration line. Generally, venting to air has been abandoned by most manufacturers. When the aspiration line is vented to air, bubbles form in the aspiration tubing. When the foot pedal is again depressed, the development of vacuum is slowed because the air in the line must first be aspirated before vacuum can once more rise.

The preferred venting material is, therefore, fluid. Most machines use fluid from the infusion bottle for this purpose. The fluid flows into the aspiration tubing, neutralizing vacuum and permitting the release of unwanted material. Because no air has been introduced into the system, when the foot pedal is again engaged, there is brisk redevelopment of flow and vacuum. This technique produces a more responsive system.

In some machines, venting also occurs when the selected vacuum level is attained. Controlled venting stops further generation of vacuum and maintains the commanded vacuum level.

TUBING COMPLIANCE

The thickness and rigidity of the tubing, as well as the inner lumen diameter, contribute to the ability of the tubing to collapse and expand during the fluid fluxes which accompany phacoemulsification. The greater the tubing compliance, the less of a tendency it has to collapse when the phaco tip is occluded and vacuum rises. Generally, if the tubing collapses at high vacuum, it will expand when emulsification occurs, and vacuum suddenly drops to zero. This sudden expansion of the tubing is an additional factor in post-occlusion surge.

IRRIGATION AND ASPIRATION

Fluidic management techniques used in the phaco mode are now applied to the I&A segment. Therefore, surge management systems function to prevent surge when a large or "sticky" piece of cortex is aspirated.

Most I&A tips use a 0.3 mm orifice. They are now available in straight and angled configurations. Soft or hard metal sleeves are also offered to provide coaxial fluid inflow. Soft sleeves are now preferred to provide a tighter uniform seal within the surgical wound. This lessens superfluous outflow and leads to a more stable anterior chamber. Silicone I&A tips are also available and are, reportedly, less likely to tear the capsular bag.

BIMANUAL IRRIGATION AND ASPIRATION

Introduced in Europe by Dr. Peter Brauweiler, the use of separate cannulas for I&A has been widely accepted. In this technique, small paracentesis-like incisions are made for placement of the cannulas. The small incisions and smaller cannulas offer controlled inflow and outflow, which promotes anterior chamber stability. The ability to more easily reach recalcitrant cortex provides surgeons with a technique that simplifies I&A. The relative positions of the cannulas are simply exchanged to reach new areas of cortex.

Bimanual techniques are especially suited to removal of cortex in difficult situations. When the posterior capsule is torn, the additional control of aspiration cannula placement, as well as the decreased anterior chamber fluid fluctuations, minimizes the risk of rupturing the vitreous face with subsequent necessity for vitrectomy. In addition, in cases of zonular dehiscence, the added flexible placement and maneuverability of the aspiration cannula provide a margin of safety removing cortex without further disruption of zonules.

VITRECTOMY

All current machines have vitrectomy capability. Generally the same I&A tubing is used. They are attached to the vitrectomy handpiece. In the vitrectomy mode the foot pedal controls irrigation and aspiration and activates the vitrectomy handpiece cutter. If the cutter is actuated by compressed air, it must be connected with the dedicated compressed air tubing to the machine attachment port.

VITRECTOMY INSTRUMENTS

The three types of vitrectomy handpieces are rotary, oscillatory, and guillotine cutters.

Rotary cutters have a sharp blade, or blades, which rotate perpendicular to the long axis of the aspiration tube. They have the advantage of being self-sharpening and, therefore, perform excellent cutting when in proper working order. They are often actuated electrically. The potential problem with these cutters occurs when the blades are dull from extensive usage or are out of alignment. The rotary movement of the blades then has the capability of pulling the vitreous into the instrument without cutting it. The result is "spooling" of the vitreous, which is often the cause of postoperative vitreous traction with subsequent cystoid macular edema or retinal detachment.

Oscillatory cutters function similarly to rotary cutters, but rather than spinning in 360° circles, they rotate 180° and then reverse direction. They can be self-sharpening. They are electrically driven. Because they do not completely spin, they cannot spool the vitreous and are, therefore, safer to use. They require periodic maintenance because they are usually reusable.

Guillotine cutters are presently the most popular form of vitrectomy handpiece. The blade moves up and down in the long axis of the aspiration tube. These blades cannot be self-sharpening because of their design. Therefore, these instruments are usually disposable rather than reusable. This feature offers the benefit of well-lubricated, sharp blades each time they are used. They are actuated by compressed air. The higher the compression the more powerful the cutting downstroke. When compressed air flow stops, a spring forces the blade to open. These cutters remove vitreous cleanly, without spooling.

There have been recent improvements in vitrectomy instrumentation. First is the high speed vitreous cutter, cutting at 400–800 cuts/min. The second is the 23 ga and 25 ga vitrectomy instruments. These are available presently on the B&L Millennium, and the Alcon Infinity and Acuris machines. They will be available on the AMO Signature and B&L Solaris.

VITRECTOMY TECHNIQUE

When vitrectomy is necessary it can be performed from the limbus or pars plana. In either case a bimanual vitrectomy technique is preferred. If present the irrigation sleeve is removed from the vitrectomy handpiece and discarded. The main incision is closed. If not self-sealing, it should be sutured. The paracentesis incision is used for infusion. A 23-gauge cannula attached to the infusion bottle is inserted through the paracentesis. The infusion bottle is lowered to an adequate height to maintain the anterior chamber without excessive outflow. A new 2 mm paracentesis is created in a comfortable position. The vitrectomy handpiece, without the infusion sleeve, is placed through this incision. The machine is set to low vacuum (100–300 mm Hg). If a peristaltic pump is used, a flow of 20–30 mL/min will provide adequate generation of vacuum without excessive turbulence. The cutting speed should be high (400–800 cuts/min) so that the aspirated vitreous is cut before the vitreous strands are allowed to place traction on the vitreous base.

The tip of the cutter is placed into the anterior vitreous, and the vitrectomy is performed until vitreous is removed to the level of the posterior capsule (Figure 7-25). In this way the vitreous is literally shelled out of the posterior segment without disturbing the vitreous base at the pars plana or the vitreous connections to the macula or optic nerve. This approach minimizes the risk of postoperative cystoid macular edema and retinal detachment.

If performed from the pars plana, similar settings are used. The vitrectomy instrument is introduced through an incision created precisely 3.0–3.5 mm posterior to the limbus with a microvitreoretinal (MVR) blade. Under direct visualization the vitrector is placed into the anterior vitreous with the aspiration port up, and vitrectomy is performed as noted previously (Figure 7-26).[13]

Alternatively, a 25-gauge, self-sealing, transconjunctival approach can be used. A trocar-cannula system is used to enter the pars plana passing directly through the conjunctiva and sclera. After removing the trocar, the entry alignment cannula remains in place. The vitrector is placed through the cannula into the vitreous and the vitrectomy is performed carefully watching the vitrector tip. When the vitrectomy is judged to be adequate, the vitrector is removed and a plug is placed in the cannula. The cannula is removed when it is evident that no further vitrectomy is assumed. No sutures are necessary.

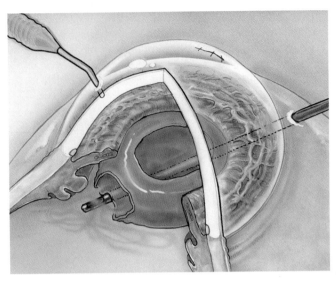

Figure 7-26 Vitrectomy through the pars plana. After an incision is made 3.5 mm posterior to the limbus with an MVR blade, the vitrectomy instrument is placed into the anterior vitreous under direct observation. (Courtesy Thieme Publications, New York.)

PHACO MACHINE SETTINGS

Currently, many new-generation sophisticated machines are available. Each of these controls the balance of power generation and fluidic features by different methods. In addition, surgeons now can tailor the machine parameters not only to their style of surgery, but also to each individual segment of the phaco procedure. Therefore, a listing of different settings for each procedure is beyond the scope of this chapter. However, a representative listing of different parameters for three surgeons using the same machine is illustrated in Tables 7-2–7-4. These tables show how power, flow, and vacuum vary from surgeon to surgeon and for each phase of phacoemulsification.

CONCLUSION

It has been said that the phaco procedure is blend of technology and technique. Awareness of the principles that influence phaco machine settings is required to perform a proficient and safe operation. In addition, often during the procedure, the initial parameters must be modified. A thorough understanding of fundamental principles will enhance the surgeon's capability to respond appropriately to this requirement.

It is a fundamental principle that through relentless evaluation of the interaction of the machine and the phaco technique, the skillful surgeon will find innovative methods to enhance technique. "The road to success is always under construction."

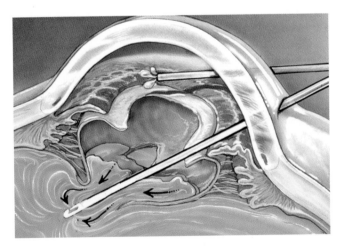

Figure 7-25 The vitrector, with the Charles Sleeve removed is placed through a paracentesis into the vitreous. Irrigation is provided by a 23-gauge cannula placed through another paracentesis. The vitreous is drawn back into the posterior segment and removed to the level of the posterior capsule. (Courtesy Thieme Publications, New York.)

Table 7-3 Alcon Infinity

Traditional phaco settings

Cataract density	1	2	3	4
Irrigation (cm H$_2$O)	110	110	110	110
Aspiration rate (cc/min)	40	40	40	40
Vacuum limit (mm Hg)	400	400	400	400
Dynamic rise	Off	2	2	2
Phaco power limit	15	30	50	70
On time (ms)	30	20	20	20

0.9 mm. Kelman ABS Tapered Needle.
Cataract grading system to limit repulsive forces and energy dissipation of traditional ultrasound.
Dynamic rise increases ability to hold tissue during energy activation.

Torsional phaco settings

	Initial Chop	Fragments	
Irrigation (cm H$_2$O)	110	110	
Aspiration rate (cc/min)	40	40	
Vacuum limit (mm Hg)	400	350	
Dynamic rise	2	Off	
Phaco power limit	Longitudinal 50 Torsional Off	Longitudinal 100 Torsional Amplitude 100	
On Time (ms)	20	5	100

0.9 mm. Kelman ABS Tapered Needle.
Initial chop using OZil Handpiece with traditional longitudinal burst.
Quadrant removal for all other segments use 5 ms linear traditional and 100 ms linear torsional burst for all cataract grades.
Dynamic rise is not utilized due to deceased repulsion.

Table 7-4 Bimanual Alcon Infinity

Ozil	0.9 microtip½ silver/1/2prpl (dewey-or-all purple, sharp: bent, no ABS)	Bimanual	Choose Grade 2

Grade 2
CHOP – Ozil Pulse

	Power			Torsional amplitude %		Irrig (bottle)	
limit	% on		pps	limit	% on	142	
40 (linear)	30		10	0	NA		
vac	320 (fixed)			asp rate	30 (fixed)		
			Dynamic rise 1				

QUAD – Ozil burst

	Power			Torsional amplitude %			Irrig (bottle)	
limit	% on			limit	msec on	msec off	142	
0				100% (linear)	35	50		
vac	350 (fixed)			asp rate	33 (fixed)			
			Dynamic rise 1					

(Continued)

Table 7-4 Bimanual Alcon Infinity—cont'd

EPI – Ozil continuous					
Power			**Torsional amplitude %**		**Irrig (bottle)**
limit	% on		limit	% on	142
0			25 (linear)	na	
vac	300 (fixed)		asp rate	32 (fixed)	
		Dynamic rise 0			
IA					
Cortex				**Irrig (bottle)**	
vac	600 (linear)	asp rate	50 (linear)	110	
Viscoat removal					
vac	650 (linear)	asp rate	50 (fixed)	110	
		Dynamic rise 0			
Vit cut I–A					
Cut rate	800	Vac (linear)	250	Asp	20 (linear)	Irrig (bottle)	60
		Dynamic rise 0			

References

[1] Kelman CD. Phaco-emulsification and aspiration. Am J Ophthalmol 1967;64:23–35.
[2] Kelman CD. History of emulsification and aspiration of senile cataracts. Trans Am Acad Ophthalmol Otolaryngol 1974;78:35–38.
[3] Kelman CD. Phacoemulsification in the anterior chamber. Ophthalmology 1979;86:1980–1982.
[4] Kratz RP, Colvard DM. Kelman phacoemulsification in the posterior chamber. Ophthalmology 1979;86:1983–1984.
[5] Cimino WW, Bond LJ. Physics of ultrasonic surgery using tissue fragmentation. II. Ultrasound Med Biol 1996;22:101–117.
[6] Miyoshi T. Ultra-high-speed images of the phaco tip under different power modes. ASCRS Film Festival Grand Prize Winner. Annual Meeting Spring; 2005.
[7] Fishkind WJ. Pop goes the microbubbles. Video Film Festival ASCRS 1998, Grand Prize winner ESCRS; 1998.
[8] Schafer M. Quantifying the impact of cavitation in phacoemulsification. Presentation ASCRS Annual Meeting, Best Paper of Session, Spring 2006.
[9] Zacharias J. Jackhammer or cavitation: the final answer. ASCRS Film Festival Grand Prize Winner. ASCRS Annual Meeting. Spring 2006.
[10] Serafano D. Upgrades to phaco system give surgeons more options. Ophthalmol Times 2001;26:16–17.
[11] Soscia W, Howard JG, Olson RJ. Microphacoemulsification with WhiteStar. A wound-temperature study. J Cataract Refract Surg 2002;28:1044–1046.
[12] Seibel BS. Section 1. In Phacodynamics, mastering the tools and techniques of phacoemulsification surgery. 3rd ed. Thoroughfare, NJ: Slack Inc; 1999.
[13] Nichamin LD. Prevention pearls. In: Fishkind WJ, editor. Complications in phacoemulsification. New York: Thieme; 2001. p. 260–270.

Bibliography

Chang DF. Phaco chop, mastering techniques, optimizing technology and avoiding complications. New Jersey: Slack Inc; 2004.
Fishkind WJ, editor. Complications in phacoemulsification, avoidance, recognition and management. New York: Thieme; 2001.
Garg A, Fine IH, Ali JL, et al. Mastering the phacodynamics. New Delhi, India: Jaypee Publishers; 2007.
Seibel BS. Phacodynamics, mastering the tools and techniques of phacoemulsification surgery. 3rd ed. Thoroughfare, NJ: Slack Inc; 2004.

NON-LONGITUDINAL PHACO: MODIFICATION OF FLUID CONTROL BY POWER MODULATIONS

Torsional Phaco (Alcon Infinity)

A new development in phaco is the harnessing of lateral or ocillatory movement of the phaco tips developed by Alcon in the Infiniti Machine. The OZiL Torsional Handpiece has both a longitudinal movement and torsional movement. The longitudinal movement, like a standard phaco needle is at 40 kHz. The torsional movement is at 32 kHz with 1 arc of motion (Figure 7-16). The torsional movement may be used alone or in combination with the longitudinal movement with many variations of timing. It requires an angled "Kelman" tip of 15° or 30° to be effective. It appears to be most efficient when using a mix of longitudinal and torsional movement. This modification, as well as needle configurations, is presently under modification. The final parameters for its use are yet to be determined. The torsional movement will emulsify with minimal chatter and improved follow-ability. However, occasionally the low power phaco will cause chunks of nucleus to occlude the phaco needle lumen. Longitudinal movement is then used to emulsify the material present in the needle bore.

Elliptical Phaco (AMO Signature)

In this system the longitudinal movement of the phaco tip at 38 kHz is combined with a transversal motion at 26 kHz. The resultant movement of the needle can be described as prolate-spheroid (shaped much like an egg cut in half). Elliptical power can be generated with any type of phaco tip.

While the longitudinal phaco cores the nuclear material, the non-longitudinal phaco shaves the nuclear material. Therefore this mode of needle movement is a noteworthy variation from other technology, since by its very movement, it generates partial occlusion phaco and therefore lessens the risk of surge.

Retrobulbar and Peribulbar Anesthesia for Cataract Surgery

8

Robert C. (Roy) Hamilton, MB, BCh, FRCPC

CONTENTS

- Desirable Prerequisites
- Anatomy and Applied Anatomy
- Ophthalmic Regional Block Anesthesia

CHAPTER HIGHLIGHTS

>> Relevant orbital anatomy

>> Principles of retrobulbar and peribulbar injection

>> Management of complications of anesthetic injection

Advances in surgical techniques, especially small-incision phacoemulsification, have lessened the universal demand for akinetic anesthesia using regional blocks. Other methods, including sub-Tenon's, subconjunctival, and solely topical corneoconjunctival anesthesia, have been introduced. However, solid regional block anesthesia including muscle akinesia is still the preferred choice of anesthesia for many cataract surgeons. Although peribulbar blocks were popularized in 1986, claiming to avoid serious complications of the retrobulbar method,[1] a recent survey of the annual American Society of Cataract and Refractive Surgeons with input from 1342 members indicates 30% using retrobulbar and 24% using peribulbar blocks.[2]

DESIRABLE PREREQUISITES

Knowledge of the basic science disciplines (pharmacology of ocular and local anesthetic drugs, physiology of the eye, anatomy of the orbit and its contents) is essential to safe practice of orbital regional anesthesia, including retrobulbar block.[3] Observation of and subsequent initial supervision by personnel with wide clinical experience and knowledge are recommended. The goal for each practitioner is to build up an experiential database from which increasingly good judgment can result.

Even when the blocking practitioner is an ophthalmologist, a strong argument can be made for the routine presence of an anesthesiologist.[4,5] Noninvasive blood pressure, electrocardiographic, and oxygen saturation monitoring should be routinely used before and during the induction of anesthesia and intraoperatively.

ANATOMY AND APPLIED ANATOMY

In this chapter the adjective, retrobulbar, refers to the conical compartment within the confines of the four rectus muscles and their intermuscular septa. Compared with the peripheral orbit where fat is more dense, the retrobulbar cone contains fat that is arranged in large globules, which permit free movement of the intraorbital portion of the optic nerve in the various duction positions of the globe. A matrix of connective tissues, which supports and allows dynamic function of the orbit contents, controls the spread of local anesthetic solutions.[6]

Motor nerves enter the muscle bellies of the four rectus muscles from their conal surface, 1–1.5 cm from the apex of the orbit. For conduction block of nerves and the resulting akinesia of their supplied muscles to occur, local anesthetics in blocking concentration have to reach and diffuse to the core of an exposed 5–10 mm segment of each of these motor nerves in the posterior retrobulbar space. Retained activity of the superior oblique muscle is often seen after retrobulbar local anesthetic injection because its motor nerve, the trochlear, runs outside the muscle cone. Total blockade of the smaller-diameter sensory and autonomic nerves, including the ciliary ganglion, on the other hand, is more easily achieved. Corneal and perilimbal conjunctival sensory innervation, along with the superior-nasal quadrant of the peripheral conjunctival sensation, are mediated through the nasociliary nerve, which lies within the retrobulbar space. The remainder of the peripheral conjunctival sensation, however, is supplied through the lacrimal, frontal, and infraorbital nerves coursing outside the muscle cone.[7] Because of this, intraoperative pain may be experienced in the peripheral orbit following a solely retrobulbar block.[8]

OPHTHALMIC REGIONAL BLOCK ANESTHESIA ■

TRADITIONAL RETROBULBAR BLOCK AND ITS INHERENT PROBLEMS

In 1934 Atkinson[9] described a technique that evolved into the traditional method of retrobulbar blockade. In his article:

> [With the patient's gaze directed] upward and inward, [a 35 mm needle entered percutaneously] a short distance below the inferior-temporal margin of the orbit... the skin is moved upward with the needle so that the point just clears the inferior orbital margin. The needle is then directed upward and inward, midway between the external and inferior recti muscles, and advanced toward the apex of the orbit for a distance of from 2.5 to 3.5 cm.

Although Atkinson did not use such a directive in his text (however, illustrations in his article may have led to the interpretation), traditional teaching regarding the inferior-temporal needle entry point has been to locate it at the junction of the medial two-thirds and lateral third of the inferior orbital rim. Generations of ophthalmology residents were trained in this way as a result; in fact, the technique continues to be reproduced in ophthalmology and anesthesiology texts even though "there is now no doubt that [it] is unsafe and there are medicolegal implications."[10] Unsöld, Stanley, and DeGroot[11] demonstrated conclusively in a cadaver model that the Atkinson "up-and-in" globe position places a stretched and taut optic nerve and the posterior pole of the globe in line for potential damage from the tip of the needle approaching from the inferior-temporal quadrant. In addition, tangential puncture of the optic nerve sheath can occur, leading to injection of anesthetic agent into the subarachnoid space resulting in brainstem anesthesia.[12] Pautler et al.[13] reported two cases of optic nerve trauma with resultant catastrophic loss of vision from long and sharp needles injected toward the orbital apex with the globe in the up-and-in position. Using information gained from the Unsöld paper, they recommended that for retrobulbar blocks patients should fixate in primary gaze and that needle length be reduced to 32 mm (1¼ inch) and directed toward an imaginary point behind the macula rather than aiming for the orbital apex. They reported that in the primary gaze globe position the optic nerve lies in a nontaut manner on the nasal side of the sagittal plane passing through the visual axis, in which location and state the risk of nerve damage is much reduced (Figure 8-1).

Katsev et al.[14] analyzed the dimensions of 120 orbits from 60 human skulls related to the length of needles used for retrobulbar anesthesia. The distance from the inferior orbital rim to the optic foramen ranged from a maximum of 58 mm to a minimum of 42 mm. Because a 38 mm (1½-inch) needle fully inserted toward the posterior orbit had the potential of damaging vital structures in fully one-fifth of the orbits examined (i.e., those of smaller dimension), they recommended that depth of needle penetration into the orbit be limited to a maximum of 31.5 mm (1¼ inch) from the inferior orbital rim. This would avoid damage to the tightly packed important structures (nerves, blood vessels, muscles) at the orbital apex.

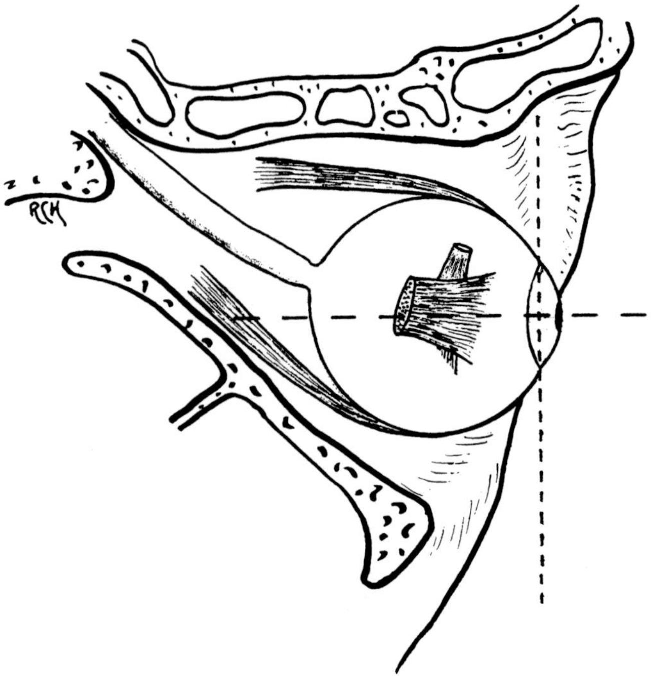

Figure 8-1 Plane of the iris and midsagittal plane of the globe in primary gaze; view from above. Fine dashed line indicates the plane of the iris (useful in gauging depth of needle advancement); coarse dashed line indicates the midsagittal plane of the eye and the visual axis through the center of the pupil. The optic nerve lies on the nasal side of the midsagittal plane of the eye. Note how the temporal orbital rim is set back from the rest of the orbital rim at or about the globe equator, making for easy needle access to the retrobulbar compartment. (Courtesy Gimbel Educational Services.)

Liu, Youl B, Moseley[10] repeated Unsöld's cadaver experiment in vivo using magnetic resonance imaging and confirmed the findings of a taut optic nerve in up-and-in position and of a sinuous loose nerve in the primary gaze position.

COMPLICATIONS OF OPHTHALMIC REGIONAL BLOCK ANESTHESIA

Optic Nerve Injury

Injection at the orbital apex, as was advocated in the distant past[15] and is now outmoded, has the potential of frank optic nerve injury. Katsev et al.[14] recommended that needle length introduced beyond the orbital rim for both intraconal and periconal injections should not exceed 31 mm (1¼ inch) to avoid damage to the optic nerve in all patients. In the execution of orbital blocks, it is possible for the needle tip to enter the optic nerve sheath and produce not only brainstem anesthesia, as described below, but also tamponade of the retinal vessels within the nerve and/or the small vessels supplying the nerve itself either by the volume of drug injected or by provoking intrasheath hemorrhage.[13,16–19]

Brainstem Anesthesia

Brainstem anesthesia is caused by direct spread of local anesthetic to the brain from the orbit along submeningeal pathways. It is the eyeblock complication most likely to warrant cardiopulmonary resuscitation. An essential prerequisite in all locations where regional ocular anesthesia is performed is the provision of oxygen saturation monitoring in the room where the block is done and in the operating room,[12] along with equipment to provide respiratory support and cardiopulmonary resuscitation.[5] The incidence has been reported as 1 in 350–500 retrobulbar injections.[12]

Globe Penetration and Perforation

The incidence range of globe penetration (solely entrance wound) and perforation (entrance and exit wounds) has been reported as low as 0 in a series of 2000 peribulbar blocks[1] to 1 in a series of 1000 retrobulbar blocks.[20] In myopic patients the incidence may be as high as 1 in 140 blocks.[21] The true incidence is not known because many cases are not reported;[22] more than 50% of cases go unrecognized at the time of their occurrence.[23] A rare and devastating complication, ocular explosion, has been reported several times;[24,25] it results from excessively high pressure being applied to the injecting syringe following unrecognized ocular penetration by the needle. Ultimate visual outcome is very poor.

Extraocular Muscle Malfunction

Because extraocular muscle malfunction can result from local anesthesia agent myotoxicity or needle trauma,[26,27] it is important to choose a block technique in which the needle placement avoids needle contact with muscle. The most common muscles affected, in order of frequency, are the inferior rectus muscle (Figure 8-2),[28–31] the inferior oblique muscle (including injury and trauma to its motor nerve) (Figure 8-3),[28] the superior rectus muscle (Figure 8-4),[32] and the medial rectus muscle (Figure 8-5).[33]

Hemorrhage

Retrobulbar hemorrhages vary in severity. Some are of venous origin and spread slowly. Signs of severe arterial hemorrhage are

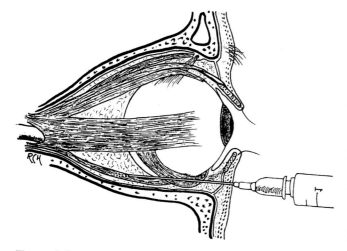

Figure 8-2 Inferior rectus muscle trauma, lateral view. A straight 31 mm (1¼-inch) needle being advanced from the inferior-temporal quadrant in an attempt to enter the retrobulbar compartment has failed to adequately rise from the orbit floor. The needle tip has entered the belly of the inferior rectus muscle. Hemorrhage into the muscle with subsequent fibrosis, or intramuscular injection of local anesthetic with subsequent myotoxicity, may result in prolonged or permanent imbalance between the superior and inferior rectus muscles and vertical diplopia.[31] (Courtesy Gimbel Educational Services.)

rapid and taut orbital swelling, marked proptosis with immobility of the globe, and massive blood staining of the lids and conjunctiva.[34] Serious impairment of the vascular supply to the globe may result.[35,36] By constant vigilance and keen observation of the signs immediately following needle withdrawal, bleeding may be minimized and confined by rapid application of digital pressure over a gauze pad placed on the closed lids. The incidence of serious retrobulbar bleeding was reported to be 1% to 3% in one paper[16] and as 0.44% in a series of 12,500 cases.[37] A strong argument can be made in favor of fine disposable needles over those of larger gauge,[8,13,38] on the grounds that if a vessel is perforated, less bleeding occurs through a small rent and the bleeding is less precipitous. Because the orbital apex contains the largest vessels entering and exiting the orbit, the depth to which needles are inserted should be strictly limited. When serious bleeding occurs in this area, there is the problem not only of general increase in orbital pressure, making surgery difficult, but also of the potential for obstruction to the blood supply to and from the globe.

The anterior orbit generally has smaller vessels than exist posteriorly. Two anterior orbital locations, which are relatively avascular and frequently used as sites for needle placement, are the inferior-temporal quadrant and the compartment directly on the nasal side of the medial rectus muscle. Needle placement into the superior nasal compartment should be avoided because the end vessels of the ophthalmic artery system are located there, as are some large veins and the complex trochlear mechanism of the superior oblique muscle.

In intraocular surgery it is considered advantageous if the intraocular pressure is low and pressure fluctuations are kept to a minimum.[39] The attainment of a "soft eye" in the avoidance of complications, particularly suprachoroidal hemorrhage,[40,41] was more important in a former era. Phacoemulsification techniques, which require a smaller surgical incision, are associated with smaller swings in intraocular pressure than the older intracapsular or extracapsular methods. At the completion of retrobulbar and peribulbar injections, mechanical orbital decompression devices[42–45] are commonly used to promote ocular hypotony and a reduction in vitreous volume,[46] especially when larger volumes of orbital injectate have been used (as in peribulbar blockade).

General Comment on Complications

The occurrence or avoidance of the complications mentioned previously is directly influenced by block technique. Elimination of known hazards (e.g., inappropriate globe position during block, inappropriate choice of needle path, inappropriate depth of needle placement) is the key to successfully avoiding complications.

COMPARISON OF RETROBULBAR WITH PERIBULBAR BLOCKADE

As discussed earlier, the peribulbar technique was introduced in 1986 as a less hazardous alternative to retrobulbar anesthesia in response to a concern about complications of the latter.[1] The rationale was that peribulbar technique, by avoiding needle placement within the rectus muscle cone, would avoid optic nerve damage and globe perforation. However, after initial enthusiasm, a significant number of globe perforations were reported.[47–49] Higher volumes of injectate were required to achieve akinesia, onset time of blockade was much slower than with retrobulbar,

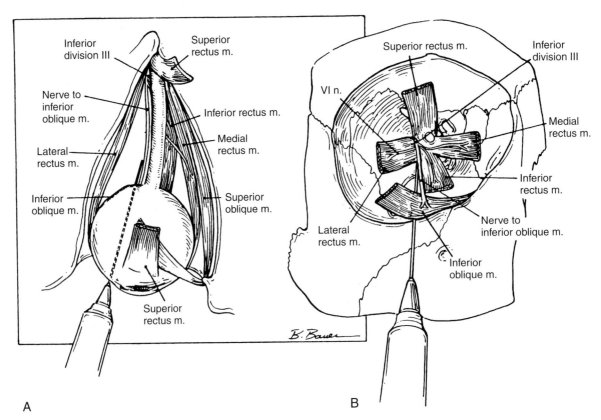

A   B

Figure 8-3 Risks of injection from the traditional entry point. Right orbit: **A**, view from above; **B**, view from in front with the globe removed. Observe the proximity of the needle path to the inferior oblique muscle belly, its motor nerve, and the lateral border of the inferior rectus muscle. One or more of these three structures can easily be damaged by a traditionally placed retrobulbar needle. (From Hunter DG, Lam GC, Guyton DL: Inferior oblique muscle injury from local anesthesia for cataract surgery, Ophthalmology 102:508, 1995. Copyright Elsevier 1995.)

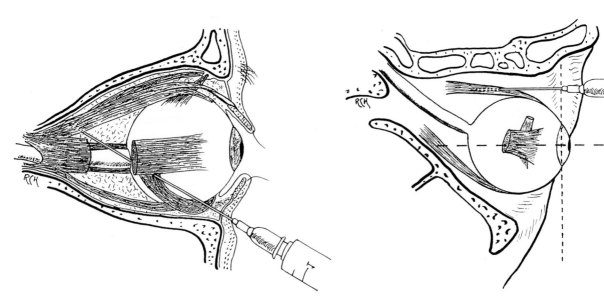

Figure 8-4 Superior rectus muscle trauma, lateral view. A straight 38 mm (1¹/₂-inch) needle being advanced from the inferior-temporal quadrant through the retrobulbar compartment too deeply has entered the belly of the superior rectus muscle. Hemorrhage into the muscle with subsequent fibrosis, or intramuscular injection of local anesthetic with subsequent myotoxicity, may result in prolonged or permanent imbalance between the superior and inferior rectus muscles and vertical diplopia.[32] (Courtesy of Gimbel Educational Services.)

Figure 8-5 Medial rectus muscle trauma, view from above. A straight needle being advanced in a sagittal plane from the extreme medial end of the palpebral fissure (on the nasal side of the caruncle) has traversed the medial compartment on the nasal side of the medial rectus muscle and entered into the belly of the medial rectus muscle. Hemorrhage into the muscle with subsequent fibrosis, or intramuscular injection of local anesthetic with subsequent myotoxicity, may result in prolonged or permanent malfunction of the medial rectus muscle. (Courtesy Gimbel Educational Services.)

and repeat injections (each with inherent risk of complication) were more frequently required. Although there are proponents of both retrobulbar and peribulbar techniques, safe anesthesia can be accomplished by both methods; likewise, serious complications can arise with both if carried out incorrectly. Two published large series preferred the more dependable outcome of retrobulbar needle placement.[8,50] Therefore, rather than condemn the retrobulbar technique outright, it merits revisitation and revision in the light of better understanding of the causes of various complications.[51]

REVISED RETROBULBAR BLOCK

Site and Depth of Injection

The inferior-temporal orbital quadrant is the preferred location for retrobulbar needle placement because it provides easy access to the retrobulbar cone compartment (see Figure 8-1). To avoid complications (hemorrhages, optic nerve trauma, brainstem anesthesia, muscle damage), needles must never be inserted deeply to the orbital apex.[14] Injectate placement in the anterior retrobulbar compartment is much safer; from there, posterior spread occurs to achieve motor nerve blocking concentration at the apex of the cone.[52]

Needle Type and Syringe Size

Traditional teaching favored dull-tipped, intermediate-gauge needles with the supposed advantages that blood vessels were pushed aside rather than traumatized and that tissue planes could be more accurately defined. Although a commonly held belief among ophthalmologists,[47] it is not true that it is more difficult to penetrate the globe, the optic nerve sheath, or blood vessels with a blunt needle.[3] Larger dull needles, compared with fine disposable ones, cause more serious damage if the globe is penetrated.[3] Because disposable cutting needles produce minimal tissue distortion, little or no pain results. Tactile discrimination is progressively reduced with increasing needle size.[38] The use of blunt-tipped, wider-gauge needles should be abandoned.[53] Special attention should be paid to the length of needle entering beyond the orbital rim; 31 mm as measured from the orbital rim should never be exceeded to rule out optic nerve impalement.[14] In regional block techniques (both retrobulbar and peribulbar), all needles should be orientated tangentially to the globe with the bevel opening faced toward the globe.[8] Because less force has to be exerted, a change in resistance to injectate flow is more easily detected by the injecting hand when using a needle mounted on a smaller syringe as compared with a larger size. This ability to more easily detect change in resistance to injection is important in avoiding complications, as is the regular use by all practitioners of standard sets of needles and syringes so that they become familiar with the normal flow resistance characteristics of their equipment. In addition, an "inject-as-you-advance" technique provides added safety.[54]

Advantage of Minimal or No Sedation

Fully conscious or minimally sedated patients on whom regional ophthalmic blocks are done painlessly can accurately report symptoms or demonstrate signs that may indicate onset of undesirable block complications. Thus, by being conscious they act as their own monitors. For example, the devastating complication of ocular explosion described previously[24,25] is not likely to occur in a conscious patient because the pain experienced by the patient would be so great. Elderly patients require less pharmacologic support for anxiety at the time of surgery than do young patients and take the discomforts of life more easily "in their stride." For a small percentage of elderly patients who benefit from preoperative sedation, fine judgment is required to select the correct drug dosage to produce a calm patient who remains alert and cooperative. The advantages of regional anesthesia can be negated rapidly with excessive use of sedation.[55] A recent multicenter study confirmed that intravenous anesthetic agents administered to reduce pain and anxiety are associated with an increased incidence of side effects and adverse medical events.[56] Incomplete regional anesthesia is best managed with block supplementation until complete; operating in the presence of obvious block failure subjects the patient to an unpleasant and stressful experience; and use of intravenous sedation to cover gross block inadequacy is hazardous and inappropriate.

Painless block techniques are achievable through the use of fine, sharp disposable needles and precision placement methods. The author strongly recommends a preblock transconjunctival injection of local anesthetic diluted 10 times with sterile balanced salt solution, which renders the percutaneous injection to follow totally painless (Figure 8-6).[57] This transconjunctival injection is carried out through conjunctiva previously rendered anesthetic with topical local anesthetic eye drops.

Preblock Assessment

A safe prerequisite to regional anesthesia of the orbit is to know the axial length measurement of the eye before the block to warn of the higher risk in longer-than-average eyes.[58] In cataract surgery a precise axial length measurement is usually available because it is required for intraocular lens diopter power calculation. In the presence of high myopia, peribulbar block or even general anesthesia, as opposed to retrobulbar block, may be more prudent. Similar caution would apply when a pre-existing scleral buckle exists from an earlier retinal operative procedure.

The axial length of the globe to be blocked is noted, as is the position of the globe in the orbit (enophthalmos versus exophthalmos), by observing the plane of the iris and the location of the globe equator relative to the temporal orbital rim.

Recommended Block Technique

The author, with an experience of 27,500 retrobulbar blocks and 5,700 peribulbar blocks over the past 18 years, has adopted a rational approach to safe retrobulbar blocking that stresses the importance of aiming the retrobulbar needle (27-gauge sharp disposable, 31 mm length) "midway between the inferior and lateral rectus muscles"[30] from an inferior-temporal entry point at the junction of the temporal and inferior orbital rims (Figure 8-7). This modified entry point allows easy and safe access to the retrobulbar space because the temporal orbital rim is set back from the rest of the orbital rim (see Figure 8-1).

The inferior-temporal rim of the orbit is palpated and the desired entry point chosen just inside the orbital rim at the 7:30 position

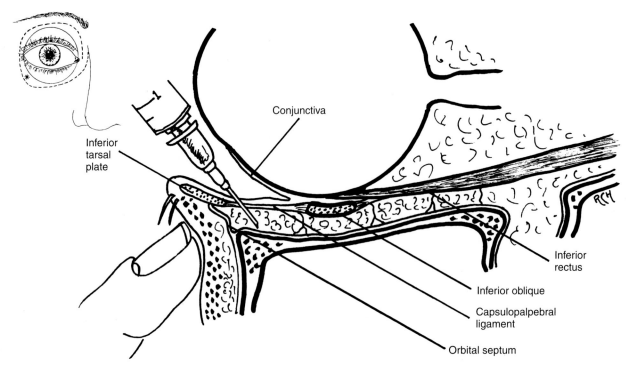

Figure 8-6 Injection of "painless local" in inferior-temporal quadrant, lateral view. After instillation of topical anesthesia drops in the inferior conjunctival fornix, the lower eyelid is gently retracted with a finger. A 30-gauge 12 mm needle enters transconjunctivally in the inferior-temporal area just posterior to the inferior tarsal plate with the shaft of the needle arranged tangentially to the globe. Following test aspiration, the initial injection is of 1 mL painless local* to a depth of 1 cm from the conjunctiva. The needle has easily and painlessly penetrated the conjunctiva, and deep to it the capsulopalpebral fascia. The needle entry point is at the lower end of the lateral orbital rim (small insert). After an interval of 3–4 min, the skin overlying the site of injection (lateral third of lower lid) will be anesthetic. (Courtesy Gimbel Educational Services.)
*Painless local made up from 1 part full-strength local anesthetic injectate and 10 parts balanced salt solution.[57]

for the right eye (Figure 8-8A) or the 4:30 position for the left eye. With the patient's eyes in primary gaze, the needle is advanced in a sagittal plane with a 10° upward inflection from the transverse plane, at first invaginating the skin while being directed safely between the globe and temporal orbit wall. It very soon penetrates the skin and can then be advanced to the depth of the globe equator before being redirected upward and inward toward an imaginary point behind the pupil, approaching but not passing the midsagittal plane (see Figures 8-1, 8-8, and 8-9). The globe is continuously observed during needle placement to detect globe rotation that would indicate engagement of the sclera by the needle tip. During this latter action the circumference of the globe can be "palpated" with the shaft of the needle as it passes around (Martin Livingston, MD, personal communication). The modified entry position provides safer access to the orbit because there is more physical space here compared with the traditional entry point (see Figure 8-7). In addition, the modified technique avoids possible needle damage to the inferior rectus and inferior oblique muscles and to the motor nerve supply to the inferior oblique (see Figure 8-3).[28] A percutaneous as opposed to a transconjunctival needle entry point is used because it avoids having to combat the orbicularis tone often present in the inferior eyelid or the problems created when there is a narrow palpebral fissure and wide lateral canthal fold. Slow needle advancement following first penetration of the skin is ideal, with injections of minidoses of anesthetic solution at multiple intervals. Having reached the desired final needle-tip location, and after

checking by aspiration for inadvertent intravascular placement, a slow injection of the desired volume of anesthetic solution is made. This interval method of needle advancement provides not only patient comfort but also constantly updated information about tissue resistances along the needle path. Should the needle tip penetrate the globe, the next minidose injection will announce itself loud and clear as severe pain (provided, of course, there has not been use of excessive sedation to render the patient beyond being able to act as his or her own monitor). A globe penetration picked up accurately and early in this fashion is far better than rapid needle placement to full depth in one swift motion with the possibility of globe perforation and its late diagnosis. Final depth of needle penetration of the orbit is gauged by observing the hub-shaft junction of the 31 mm needle in relation to the plane of the iris (Figures 8-1 and 8-8), instead of measuring from the inferior orbital rim as in the traditional technique; thus, in dealing with enophthalmic and exophthalmic globes, there is automatic correction for the anomaly. In dealing with a globe of average axial length (23.5 mm), when the midpoint of the 31 mm needle is at the plane of the iris, the point of the needle will already have passed the globe equator. In like manner, ovoid globes in myopic patients (greater axial length measurement) will require a longer section of the advancing needle to guarantee passage beyond the globe equator before redirection into the retrobulbar compartment. The final desired needle-tip position lies between the lateral rectus muscle and the optic nerve, as depicted in the cadaver dissection (see Figure 8-9).

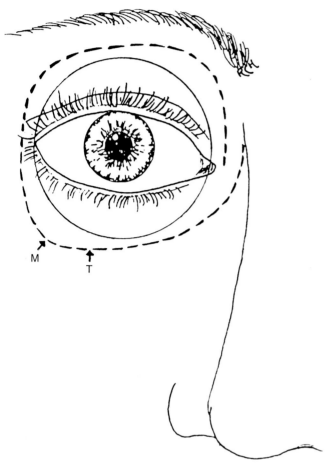

Figure 8-7 Traditional and modified needle entry positions. The outline of the globe is superimposed on a template of the orbital rim. Traditional inferior block injection site is just inside the orbital rim at T. The author's modified injection site is inferior-temporal, just inside the orbital rim at M. (Courtesy Gimbel Educational Services.)

Injectate Mixture and Volume

The selection of anesthetic agent with additives depends mainly on the desired duration of effect. Concentrations up to, but not exceeding, 2% lidocaine (or agent of equivalent potency) are appropriate. Admixture with epinephrine is commonly used to prolong block duration and to increase block solidity, but it may be contraindicated if orbital vascular pathology is present; a concentration of 1:200,000, given the volume of injectate used in ophthalmic regional anesthesia, is devoid of systemic effects.[59] Hyaluronidase, a highly purified bovine testicular enzyme that hydrolyzes extracellular hyaluronic acid,[60] is a desirable component for promotion of spread within the orbit and for hypotony.[61,62] Recently the product has been in short supply and, in fact, is no longer being produced.[60] Anecdotal reports have linked its absence from local anesthetic mixtures with a higher rate of complications, notably diplopias resulting from toxic levels of anesthetic in the extraocular muscles.[63] Having attained the desired safe depth of placement in the anterior retrobulbar compartment, and following a negative test aspiration for possible intravascular penetration, a volume of up to 4 mL of the chosen mixture is slowly injected. Younger adults present more of a challenge in achieving akinesia than the elderly because of more dense connective tissues, hindering the access of anesthetics to the motor nerves of the extraocular muscles.[64]

COMPLEMENTARY MEDIAL BLOCK

Because peripheral orbit sensation may be retained following retrobulbar block, as mentioned earlier (anatomy paragraph), a small-volume peribulbar local anesthetic injection provides an excellent complement. The site of choice is injection into the peribulbar fat compartment on the nasal side of the medial rectus muscle (Figure 8-10).[33] In addition to peripheral orbital anesthesia, this complemental injection provides effective blockade of the central fibers of orbicularis oculi, thus avoiding the need for van

OPHTHALMIC REGIONAL BLOCK ANESTHESIA

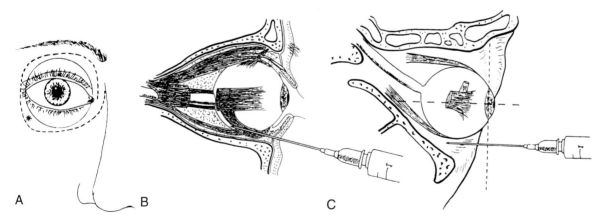

Figure 8-8 Revised inferior-temporal retrobulbar block. A and D, Frontal views; B and E, lateral views; C and F, views from above. The inferior-temporal rim of the orbit is palpated and the desired entry point (*) chosen just inside the orbital rim at the 7:30 position for the right *Eye* (A) or the 4:30 position for the left *Eye*. With the patient's *Eyes* in primary gaze, the 27-gauge 31 mm (1¼-inch) sharp disposable needle is advanced in a sagittal plane (C) with 10° upward inflection from the transverse plane (B), at first invaginating the skin while being directed safely between the globe and temporal orbit wall (C). It very soon penetrates the skin and can then be advanced to the depth of the globe equator (B and C). (If the needle were further advanced in the sagittal plane, contact with the lateral wall of the orbit would occur.)

(Continued)

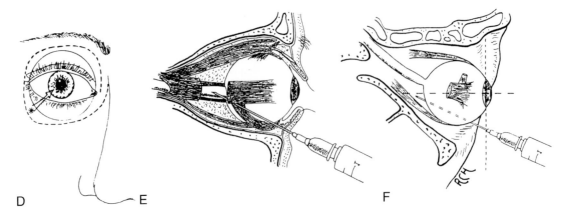

D   E   F

Figure 8-8, cont'd Revised inferior-temporal retrobulbar block. The needle is then redirected with medial and upward components (**D** and **E**) toward an imaginary point behind the pupil, approaching but not passing the midsagittal plane (**F**). The needle enters the retrobulbar space by passing through the intermuscular septum between the lateral and inferior rectus muscles (**E**). The globe is continuously observed during needle placement to detect globe rotation that would indicate engagement of the sclera by the needle tip. During needle placement, continuing observation of the relationship between the needle-hub junction and the plane of the iris establishes an appropriate depth of orbit insertion (**E** and **F**). In a globe with normal axial length as illustrated here, when the needle-hub junction has reached the plane of the iris, the tip of the needle lies 5–7 mm beyond the hind surface of the globe (**E** and **F**). Following test aspiration, up to 4 mL of anesthetic solution is slowly injected. (Courtesy Gimbel Educational Services.)

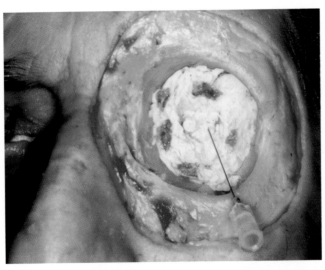

Figure 8-9 Cadaver dissection with final needle position in retrobulbar compartment; photograph of the left orbit. The anterior orbital contents have been removed as far back as 5 mm behind the posterior pole of the globe. Note the optic nerve stump and the amputated bellies of the four rectus muscles and the superior oblique muscle. The inferior oblique muscle has been removed along with the globe itself. A 27-gauge sharp disposable needle of 31 mm length has entered the retrobulbar compartment. It has passed between the lateral and inferior rectus muscles. Its tip lies between the lateral rectus muscle and the optic nerve. Note the medial and upward angling of the needle required for it to access its final desired location. (Courtesy Gimbel Educational Services.)

Lint or other type of facial nerve blockade. Injection into this compartment at a depth of 25 mm will contribute useful extraocular motor-nerve blockade, whereas more superficial placement (for which a 12 mm needle may be chosen) will provide excellent central orbicularis muscle blockade. The patient's eyes are directed in primary gaze. With the bevel facing the medial orbital wall, the needle is directed toward the interaural line and toward the midline of the skull at the occiput[65] and inserted to the desired depth. The volume injected can be within the range of 1–5 mL of local anesthetic solution, depending on the desired effect.

PERIBULBAR BLOCK

The adjective peribulbar refers to that location external to the confines of the four rectus muscles and their intermuscular septa. In the technique known as peribulbar block, local anesthetic agents or mixtures are deposited within the orbit but do not enter within the geometric confines of the cone of rectus muscles. The mechanism whereby it works was elucidated by Koornneef,[6] who demonstrated that the intermuscular septum between the rectus muscles was incomplete and permitted anesthetic deposited outside the cone of rectus muscles to spread centrally. Introduced as a safer method than intraconal blocking to avoid serious complications,[1] these nevertheless have been reported.[47–49] Knowledge of orbital anatomy is just as important as with the older method, and there are disadvantages to using periconal blocking. Davis and Mandel[1] in 1986 were first to publish a paper on the peribulbar block method. Calling their block technique posterior peribulbar, they used two intraorbital needle placements outside the muscle cone, one above and one below the cone, each to a depth of 3.5 cm with a total of up to 10 mL of solution injected.[1] Bloomberg[66] championed the cause of shorter needle peribulbar regional anesthesia and called his technique periocular block. In Bloomberg's method a 2.5-cm, or a 25- or 27-gauge needle entered the inferior-temporal orbital quadrant and was directed "deliberately toward the orbit floor" to a depth of 2 cm; a single 8- to 10-ml injection was given. He stated that only 5% of patients required supplemental blocking. Other authors report up to 50% failure to achieve akinesia with periconal blocking.[5,67] Onset of akinesia is considerably slower than with intraconal block,[5,68–70] volume requirement is greater,[71] postinjection orbital pressure is greater,[72] and the supplementation rate to achieve total akinesia is higher.[5,73,74] The incidence

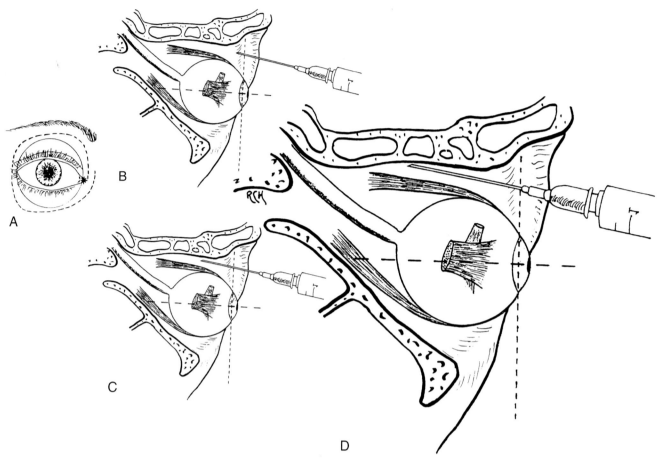

Figure 8-10 Complementary peribulbar block. Medial pericone block: needle entry point (*) is on the medial side of the caruncle at the extreme medial angle of the palpebral fissure (**A** and **B**). The patient's eyes are directed in primary gaze. With the bevel facing the medial orbit wall, the needle is directed toward the interaural line and toward the midline of the skull at the occiput;[65] that is at about 5° toward the medial orbit wall (**B** to **D**). Continuing observation of the relationship between the needle-hub junction and the plane of the iris controls appropriate depth of insertion (**D**). In a globe of normal axial length, the 25 mm needle tip will be at the depth of the hind surface of the eye. The eye in the drawing is 23.5 mm in diameter, and the needle is 25 mm long. Injection at a depth of 25 mm will contribute useful extraocular motor-nerve blockade, whereas more superficial placement will favor blockade of the central fibers of the orbicularis muscle. Volume injected can be within the range of 1–5 ml of local anesthetic solution, depending on the desired effect. (Courtesy Gimbel Educational Services.)

of periorbital ecchymoses[68] and conjunctival chemosis is also greater.[67,69,75] Of the many variations of the peribulbar technique, a common one is placement in two locations, one inferior-temporal and the other in the superior nasal orbit (a site that is vascular and, therefore, prone to hematoma formation). For those who wish to practice peribulbar blocking, the author suggests a two-needle technique: the first being an injection in the inferior-temporal quadrant, as described in Figure 8-11, and the second an injection into the medial fat compartment on the nasal side of the medial rectus muscle (complementary block as described in the previous section). Up to 5 mL of local anesthetic solution is injected at each site. Because there is insufficient space between the lateral rectus and inferior rectus muscles, and the lateral and inferior walls of the orbit, respectively, these areas cannot be used without risking extraocular muscle injury.

PARABULBAR (SUB-TENON'S) BLOCK

Anesthesia for cataract surgery produced by injection beneath Tenon's capsule of small volumes of local anesthetic was first described by Swan[52] in 1956. He indicated that the sub-Tenon's method produced better iris and anterior segment anesthesia than did subconjunctival injection. Since 1990 the sub-Tenon's injection technique has been extensively used.[76] This injection technique evolved into anesthesia produced by blunt cannula insertion[77] after surgical dissection into the sub-Tenon's space.[77–79] Onset of anesthesia is rapid;[81] the degree of abolition of extraocular muscle movement is proportional to the volume of injectate. Following placement of local anesthetic by cannula beneath Tenon's capsule, spread occurs into the anterior retrobulbar space.[82] Disadvantages of the method are an increased incidence of conjunctival chemosis and hemorrhage, and the potential of damaging one of the vortex veins.[77] Conjunctival hemorrhage is common if diathermy is not used.[82] Peripheral orbital anesthesia may be incomplete; supplemental local anesthetic injections may be necessary to achieve patient comfort.[83] Repeat sub-Tenon's injections can be performed simply in the presence of incomplete anesthesia.[53] Unlike topical corneoconjunctival anesthesia, sub-Tenon's, retrobulbar, and peribulbar techniques easily abolish iris and ciliary body sensation, and can be used to produce globe akinesia.[83]

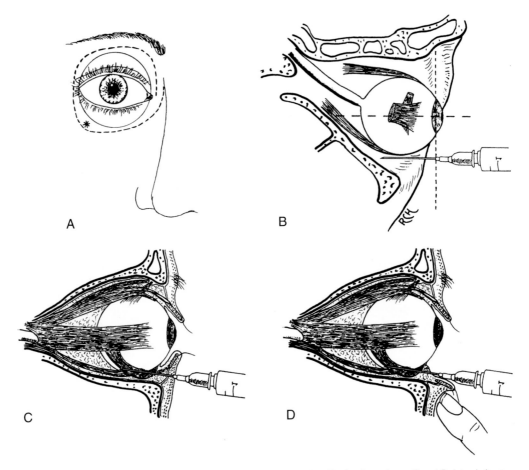

Figure 8-11 Peribulbar block, inferior-temporal injection. **A**, Frontal view; **B**, view from above; **C** and **D**, lateral views. The inferior-temporal rim of the orbit is palpated and the desired entry point (*) chosen just inside the orbital rim at the 7:30 position for the right eye (**A**) or the 4:30 position for the left eye. With the patient's eyes in primary gaze, the 27-gauge 25 mm sharp disposable needle is advanced in a sagittal plane (**B**) with 10° upward inflection from the transverse plane (**C** and **D**), and passes the globe equator to a depth controlled by observing the needle-hub junction reach the plane of the iris (**B**). Percutaneous needle entry is the preferred technique (**C**); however, the transconjunctival route is also possible (**D**). (Courtesy Gimbel Educational Services.)

References

[1] Davis DB, Mandel MR. Posterior peribulbar anesthesia: an alternative to retrobulbar anesthesia. J Cataract Refract Surg 1986;12:182–184.

[2] Leaming DV. Practice styles and preferences of ASCRS members: 1999 survey. J Cataract Refract Surg 2000;26:913–921.

[3] Grizzard WS, Kirk NM, Pavan PR et al. Perforating ocular injuries caused by anesthesia personnel. Ophthalmology 1991;98:1011–1016.

[4] Javitt JC, Addiego R, Friedberg HL et al. Brain stem anesthesia after retrobulbar block. Ophthalmology 1987;94:718–724.

[5] Morgan GE. Retrobulbar apnea syndrome: a case for the routine presence of an anesthesiologist. Reg Anesth 1990;15:106–107. [letter].

[6] Koornneef L. Orbital septa: anatomy and function. Ophthalmology 1979;86:876–880.

[7] Atkinson WS. Local anesthesia in ophthalmology. Am J Ophthalmol 1948;31:1607–1618.

[8] Hamilton RC, Gimbel HV, Strunin L. Regional anaesthesia for 12,000 cataract extraction and intraocular lens implantation procedures. Can J Anaesth 1988;35:615–623.

[9] Atkinson WS. Local anesthesia in ophthalmology. Trans Am Ophthalmol Soc 1934;32:399–451.

[10] Liu C, Youl B, Moseley I. Magnetic resonance imaging of the optic nerve in extremes of gaze: implications for the positioning of the globe for retrobulbar anaesthesia. Br J Ophthalmol 1992;76:728–733.

[11] Unsöld R, Stanley JA, DeGroot J. The CT-topography of retrobulbar anesthesia. Albrecht Von Graefes Arch Klin Exp Ophthalmol 1981;217:125–136.

[12] Hamilton RC. Brain-stem anesthesia as a complication of regional anesthesia for ophthalmic surgery. Can J Ophthalmol 1992;27:323–325.

[13] Pautler SE, Grizzard WS, Thompson LN et al. Blindness from retrobulbar injection into the optic nerve. Ophthalmic Surg 1986;17:334–337.

[14] Katsev DA, Drews RC, Rose BT. An anatomic study of retrobulbar needle path length. Ophthalmology 1989;96:1221–1224.

[15] Gifford H. Motor block of extraocular muscles by deep orbital injection. Arch Ophthalmol 1949;41:5–19.

[16] Morgan CM, Schatz H, Vine AK et al. Ocular complications associated with retrobulbar injections. Ophthalmology 1988;95:660–665.

[17] Brod RD. Transient central retinal occlusion and contralateral amaurosis after retrobulbar anesthetic injection. Ophthalmic Surg 1989;20:643–646.

[18] Giuffrè G, Vadala M, Manfrè L. Retrobulbar anesthesia complicated by combined central retinal vein and artery occlusion and massive vitreoretinal fibrosis. Retina 1995;15:439–441.

[19] Sullivan KL, Brown GC, Forman AR et al. Retrobulbar anesthesia and retinal vascular obstruction. Ophthalmology 1983;90:373–377.

[20] Cibis PA. Discussion. In: Schepens CL, Regan CDJ, editors. Controversial aspects of the management of retinal detachments. Boston: Little, Brown; 1965. p. 251.

[21] Duker JS, Belmont JB, Benson WE et al. Inadvertent globe perforation during retrobulbar and peribulbar anesthesia. Ophthalmology 1991;98:519–526.

[22] Schepens CL. A comparison of peribulbar and retrobulbar anesthesia for vitreoretinal surgical procedures. Arch Ophthalmol 1996;114:502. [letter].

[23] Ginsburg RN, Duker JS. Globe perforation associated with retrobulbar and peribulbar anesthesia. Semin Ophthalmol 1993;8:87–95.

[24] Magnante DO, Bullock JD, Green WR. Ocular explosion after peribulbar anesthesia. Ophthalmology 1997;104:608–615.

[25] Bullock JD, Warwar RE, Green WR. Ocular explosions from periocular anesthetic injections. Ophthalmology 1999;106:2341–2353.

[26] Carlson BM, Emerick S, Komorowski TE et al. Extraocular muscle regeneration in primates. Ophthalmology 1992;99:582–589.

[27] Rainin EA, Carlson BM. Postoperative diplopia and ptosis: a clinical hypothesis on the myotoxicity of local anesthetics. Arch Ophthalmol 1985;103:1337–1339.

[28] Hunter DG, Lam GC, Guyton DL. Inferior oblique muscle injury from local anesthesia for cataract surgery. Ophthalmology 1995;102:501–509.

[29] Ong-Tone L, Pearce WG. Inferior rectus muscle restriction after retrobulbar anesthesia for cataract extraction. Can J Ophthalmol 1989;24:162–165.

[30] Hamed LM. Strabismus presenting after cataract surgery. Ophthalmology 1991;98:247–252.

[31] Hamed LM, Mancuso A. Inferior rectus muscle contracture syndrome after retrobulbar anesthesia. Ophthalmology 1991;98:1506–1512.

[32] Capó H, Roth E, Johnson T et al. Vertical strabismus after cataract surgery. Ophthalmology 1996;103:918–921.

[33] Hustead RF, Hamilton RC, Loken RG. Periocular local anesthesia: medial orbital as an alternative to superior nasal injection. J Cataract Refract Surg 1994;20:197–201.

[34] Feibel RM. Current concepts in retrobulbar anesthesia. Surv Ophthalmol 1985;30:102–110.

[35] Goldsmith MO. Occlusion of the central retinal artery following retrobulbar hemorrhage. Ophthalmologica 1967;153:191–196.

[36] Kraushar MF, Seelenfreund MH, Freilich DB. Central retinal artery closure during orbital hemorrhage from retrobulbar injection. Trans Am Acad Ophthalmol Otolaryngol 1974;78:65–70.

[37] Edge KR, Nicoll JMV. Retrobulbar hemorrhage after 12,500 retrobulbar blocks. Anesth Analg 1993;76:1019–1022.

[38] Grizzard WS. Ophthalmic anesthesia. In: Reinecke RD, editor. Ophthalmology annual. New York: Raven Press; 1989. p. 265–294.

[39] Mackool RJ. Intraocular pressure fluctuations. J Cataract Refract Surg 1993;19:563–564. [letter, comment].

[40] Atkinson WS. Akinesia of the orbicularis. Am J Ophthalmol 1953;36:1255–1258.

[41] Atkinson WS. Observations on anesthesia for ocular surgery. Trans Am Acad Ophthalmol Otolaryngol 1956;60:376–380.

[42] Buys NS. Mercury balloon reducer for vitreous and orbital volume control. In: Emery J, editor. Current concepts in cataract surgery. St Louis: Mosby; 1980. p. 258.

[43] Davidson B, Kratz R, Mazzocco T et al. An evaluation of the Honan intraocular pressure reducer. J Am Intraocul Implant Soc 1979;5:237.

[44] Drews RC. The Nerf ball for preoperative reduction of intraocular pressure. Ophthalmic Surg 1982;13:761.

[45] Gills JP. Constant mild compression of the eye to produce hypotension. J Am Intraocul Implant Soc 1979;5:52–53.

[46] Palay DA, Stulting RD. The effect of external ocular compression on intraocular pressure following retrobulbar anesthesia. Ophthalmic Surg 1990;21:503–507.

[47] Kimble JA, Morris RE, Witherspoon CD et al. Globe perforation from peribulbar injection. Arch Ophthalmol 1987;105:749. [letter].

[48] Mount AM, Seward HC. Scleral perforations during peribulbar anaesthesia. Eye 1993;7:766–767.

[49] Gillow JT, Aggarwal RK, Kirby GR. A survey of ocular perforation during ophthalmic local anaesthesia in the United Kingdom. Eye 1996;10:537–538.

[50] Loots JH, Koorts AS, Venter JA. Peribulbar anesthesia: a prospective statistical analysis of the efficacy and predictability of bupivacaine and a lignocaine/bupivacaine mixture. J Cataract Refract Surg 1993;19:72–76.

[51] Hamilton RC. Retrobulbar block revisited and revised. J Cataract Refract Surg 1996;22:1147–1150.

[52] Swan KC. New drugs and techniques for ocular anesthesia. Trans Am Acad Ophthalmol Otolaryngol 1956;60:368–375.

[53] Gardner S, Ryall D. Local anaesthesia within the orbit. Curr Anaesth Crit Care 2000;11:299–305.

[54] Kuhn F, Mester V, Berta A. The continuous-injection technique to reduce complications during retrobulbar anesthesia. Ophthalmic Surg Lasers 1999;30:67–68.

[55] Smith DC, Crul JF. Oxygen desaturation following sedation for regional analgesia. Br J Anaesth 1989;62:206–209.

[56] Katz J, Feldman MA, Bass EB et al. Adverse intraoperative medical events and their association with anesthesia management strategies in cataract surgery. Ophthalmology 2001;108:1721–1726.

[57] Farley JS, Hustead RF, Becker KE. Diluting lidocaine and mepivacaine in balanced salt solution reduces the pain of intradermal injection. Reg Anesth 1994;19:48–51.

[58] Hamilton RC, Grizzard WS. Complications. In: Gills JP, Hustead RF, Sanders DR, editors. Ophthalmic anesthesia. Thorofare, NJ: Slack Inc; 1993. p. 187–202.

[59] Sarvela J, Nikki P, Paloheimo M. Orbicular muscle akinesia in regional ophthalmic anaesthesia with pH-adjusted bupivacaine: effects of hyaluronidase and epinephrine. Can J Anaesth 1993;40:1028–1033.

[60] American Academy of Ophthalmology Wydase Task Force Report. 2001.

[61] Nicoll JMV, Treuren B, Acharya PA et al. Retrobulbar anesthesia: the role of hyaluronidase. Anesth Analg 1986;65:1324–1328.

[62] Dempsey GA, Barrett PJ, Kirby IJ. Hyaluronidase and peribulbar block. Br J Anaesth 1997;78:671–674.

[63] Brown SM, Brooks SE, Mazow ML et al. Cluster of diplopia cases after periocular anesthesia without hyaluronidase. J Cataract Refract Surg 1999;25:1245–1249.

[64] Morsman CD, Holden R. The effects of adrenaline, hyaluronidase and age on peribulbar anaesthesia. Eye 1992;6:290–292.

[65] Sarvela J, Nikki P. Comparison of two needle lengths in regional ophthalmic anesthesia with etidocaine and hyaluronidase. Ophthalmic Surg 1992;23:742–745.

[66] Bloomberg LB. Anterior periocular anesthesia: five years experience. J Cataract Refract Surg 1991;17:508–511.

[67] Wang HS. Peribulbar anesthesia for ophthalmic procedures. J Cataract Refract Surg 1988;14:441–443.

[68] Drews RC, Malbran ES. Anesthesia, speculum free eye surgery, intraoperative fundus observation with the surgical microscope. In: Boyd BF, editor. Highlights of ophthalmology, vol. 1. Cali, Colombia: Carvajal; 1993. p. 1–26.

[69] Arora R, Verma L, Kumar A et al. Peribulbar anesthesia in retinal reattachment surgery. Ophthalmic Surg 1992;23:499–501.

[70] Khalil SN. Local anaesthesia for eye surgery. Anaesthesia 1991;46:232. [letter, comment].

[71] Straus JG. A new retrobulbar needle and injection technique. Ophthalmic Surg1988;19:134–139.

[72] Stevens J, Giubilei M, Lanigan L et al. Sub-Tenon, retrobulbar and peribulbar local anaesthesia: the effect upon intraocular pressure. Eur J Implant Ref Surg 1993;5:25–28.

[73] Ali-Melkkilä TM, Virkkilä M, Jyrkkiö H. Regional anesthesia for cataract surgery: comparison of retrobulbar and peribulbar techniques. Reg Anesth 1992;17:219–222.

[74] Lebuisson DA. Simplified and safer peribulbar anaesthesia. Eur J Implant Ref Surg 1990;2:123–124.

[75] Weiss JL, Deichman CB. A comparison of retrobulbar and periocular anesthesia for cataract surgery. Arch Ophthalmol 1989;107:96–98.

[76] Tsuneoka H, Ohki K, Taniuchi O et al. Tenon's capsule anaesthesia for cataract surgery with IOL implantation. Eur J Implant Ref Surg 1993;5:29–34.

[77] Stevens JD. A new local anaesthesia technique for cataract extraction by one quadrant sub-Tenon's infiltration. Br J Ophthalmol 1992;76:670–674.

[78] Mein CE, Woodcock MG. Local anesthesia for vitreoretinal surgery. Retina 1990;10:47–49.

[79] Greenbaum S. Parabulbar anesthesia. Am J Ophthalmol 1992;114:776.

[80] Greenbaum S. Anesthesia for cataract surgery. In: Greenbaum S, editor. Ocular anesthesia. Philadelphia: WB Saunders; 1997. p. 1–55.

[81] Markoff DD. Sub-Tenon's anesthesia. Operative Techniques Cataract Refractive Surg 2000;3:127–131.

[82] Stevens JD, Restori M. Ultrasound imaging of no-needle 1-quadrant sub-Tenon local anaesthesia for cataract surgery. Eur J Implant Ref Surg 1993;5:35–38.

[83] Simcock PR, Raymond GL, Lavin MJ. Peribulbar injection and direct infiltration for vitreoretinal surgery. Arch Ophthalmol 1992;110:1357–1358. [letter, comment].

OPHTHALMIC REGIONAL BLOCK ANESTHESIA

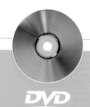

Topical Intracameral Anesthesia

Alan S. Crandall, MD

9

CONTENTS

CHAPTER HIGHLIGHTS

>> Techniques for topical anesthesia

>> Pupillary dilation through intracameral lidocaine

ANESTHESIA

Modern intraocular surgery involves many new technologies. These include, among many others:

- phacoemulsification
- foldable intraocular lenses
- clear corneal incisions
- capsular tension rings (and Cionni variations).

This infusion of new techniques has forced a reevaluation of the anesthetic needs for anterior segment surgery.

In the 1985 survey of members of the American Society of Cataract and Refractive Surgeons (ASCRS),[1] 76% of the responding ophthalmologists used a retrobulbar injection with a facial block; 4% used a periocular block, and 4% used general anesthesia. Thus, in 1985, 92% of the ophthalmologists who returned their survey used a retrobulbar anesthetic for cataract surgery. A similar survey conducted among members of the American Academy of Ophthalmology[2] showed that in 1992, 71% of those responding used retrobulbar anesthesia for cataract surgery, whereas 28% used a peribulbar technique. Subsequent ASCRS surveys showed a steady decline in the number of respondents using retrobulbar anesthesia.[3–11] By the 1998 survey, anesthesia preferences for cataract surgery had changed dramatically, with 32% of respondents using retrobulbar anesthesia; 27% using a periocular block; and 37% of respondents using topical anesthesia for cataract surgery, an anesthetic technique not even listed in the 1985 survey.

One might conclude from these data that topical anesthesia for cataract surgery is an entirely new notion. However, more correctly, one would say that topical anesthesia has been rediscovered. In 1884 Karl Koller first described the topical use of cocaine as an anesthetic agent for ocular surgery.[12] Later that same year, Knapp[13] described a method for enucleation using a retrobulbar injection of cocaine.[12] Widespread acceptance of injected cocaine anesthesia for cataract surgery was limited, however, by the toxicity of the drug. Thus, at the turn of the century, topical instillation of cocaine was the standard for cataract surgery. Topical cocaine, however, was not without local toxicity. Tetracaine later became available and was less locally toxic than cocaine; therefore, it was commonly substituted for cocaine as a topical agent for cataract surgery. Tetracaine, however, did not provide the same depth of anesthesia for intraocular structures as did cocaine. This fact, along with the more complicated surgical techniques developed in the 1920s and 1930s, pushed many ophthalmologists away from topical anesthesia to rely more on retrobulbar procaine injections to provide adequate surgical anesthesia for cataract surgery.[14] Infiltration of retrobulbar anesthetic was really the standard cataract surgery technique for decades thereafter. Ironically, it has been the complications associated with these infiltration anesthetic techniques that have led the ophthalmic community full circle, back to topical anesthesia for cataract surgery.

TOPICAL ANESTHESIA

Topical anesthesia is not new. In fact, it was considered an important discovery when Karl Koller observed that a solution of cocaine applied to the eye could prevent pain during eye surgery. (Koller likely also introduced Sigmund Freud[15] to cocaine.) With further advances in anesthesia and changes in ocular surgery, general anesthesia and injection techniques became the standard of care. The use of topical anesthesia was reintroduced by Fichman[16] in the early 1990s. This technique used topical 0.5% tetracaine. Soon other agents also became acceptable because other drops (such as 0.75% Marcaine (Sanofi Winthrop Pharmaceuticals, New York) and 1% to 2% lidocaine) were less toxic to the corneal epithelium.

Initially, some patients were not completely comfortable with the use of topical anesthesia alone, so some surgeons used intravenous sedation and analgesics to give further comfort. However, in 1995 Gills, Cherchio, and Raanan[17] introduced the use of nonpreserved lidocaine (1%) given intracamerally, which would provide further anesthesia. In an attempt to evaluate the new procedures, Patel et al.[18] randomized patients to receive a retrobulbar block versus topical anesthesia. A visual pain analogue scale was used to assess pain during surgery. They concluded that topical anesthesia can be used safely and that patient discomfort was only marginally higher postoperatively. Furthermore, the same group then randomly allocated patients to receive topical plus balanced salt solution, versus topical plus intracameral lidocaine, and found very slight differences between the two groups. They also found slightly better patient cooperation in the group that received the intracameral lidocaine.[19]

In routine small-incision cataract surgery, ocular anesthesia with topical anesthetics will usually suffice (Table 9-1). However, depending on the surgeon's experience[20] there may be contraindications (relative and absolute) to the use of topical anesthesia (Table 9-2).

Currently, this author uses topical anesthesia for cataract surgery, combined cataract and glaucoma surgery, trabeculectomy, viscocanalostomy, secondary lens implants, sutured posterior chamber intraocular lens, and sutured Cionni rings.

Table 9-1 Techniques of anesthesia for cataract surgery

General anesthesia
Retrobulbar
Peribulbar
Parabulbar
Topical

Table 9-2 Contraindications to topical anesthesia

Relative
Language barrier
Deafness
Uncooperative patients
Difficult surgery
Extended time for surgery
Nystagmus
Absolute
Allergy to the anesthetic
Coarse nystagmus

ADDITIONAL USES FOR INTRACAMERAL ANESTHESIA

USE OF INTRACAMERAL LIDOCAINE FOR PUPIL DILATION DURING CATARACT SURGERY

Cataract surgery papillary dilation is important; a standard regimen generally includes tropocaimide 1%, cyclogel 1% and neosynepherine 10%. Usually three sets of drops are applied over a 15–20 min time frame (sets every 5 min). Dilation with this combination is good but may last over many hours (patients are frequently still dilated on the day one visit). The multiple applications may also compromise the epithelial surface allowing abrasions to recur or reduce the clarity of the cornea making surgery more difficult.

Cionni et al[24] reported the use of unpreserved lidocaine intracamerally to paralyze the sphincter muscle which led to adequate pupil dilation within 90 s. They felt dilation was adequate and the pupil returned quickly to normal function.

To improve the speed of dilation we now use 1:1000 unpreserved epinephrine (Table 9-3); dilation is very rapid (Figure 9-1). The advantages of using intracameral techniques to dilate are:

1. the patients can be moved into the operating room quickly (not requiring three sets of drops separated by 5 min)

2. the corneas are subjected to fewer drops and are always pristine (especially valuable in diabetics or patients with anterior basement membrane disease)

3. the pupils return to normal function quickly

4. there is no risk for narrow angle closure.

Table 9-3 Formula for lidocaine/epinephrine

Lidocaine 1% preservative free 30 mL
Epinephrine 1:1000 mL amps (1cc)
Withdraw 0.3 mL Lidocaine 1% from vial, discard
Add back 0.3 mL Epinephrine to vial
Label: 24 h expires

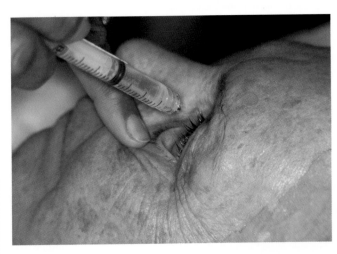

Figure 9-1 Bupivacaine 0.75% drops administered initially every 10 min three times.

Table 9-4 Epi-Shugarcaine

	pH
1:1000 Epinephrine (American Reagent)	3.133
4% non-preserved lidocaine (Abbott Labs)	6.333
BSS Plus (Alcon Labs)	7.197
Shugarcaine	6.97
3:1 Shugarcaine/epinephrine	6.899

Other regimens for intracameral dilation have proven helpful in patients with intraoperative floppy iris syndrome. Dr. Joel Shugar has found his intracameral solution[25] to rapidly dilate and help prevent iris problems in patient with IFIS (especially patients on Flomax (tamsulosin)). This combination is known as "epi-Shugarcaine" (Table 9-4).

PARABULBAR (SUB-TENON'S) ANESTHESIA

Tenon's capsule is, of course, an anterior extension of dura. It fuses with conjunctiva near the surgical limbus. Therefore, it can provide access to the retrobulbar space. Hansen, Mein, and Mazzoli[21] reported the use of sub-Tenon's surgery in 1990. Greenbaum[22] designed a specific flexible cannula to deliver the anesthesia. In this procedure, a dissection is made through conjunctiva and Tenon's capsule down to bare sclera; the Greenbaum cannula (or other blunt cannula) is used; and, by making the incision small enough, the fluid can be forced to dissect posteriorly, and, usually, only a few milliliters of anesthesia are required. The anesthesia is of rapid onset, but the globe akinesia takes a few minutes to occur. A similar technique was described by Stevens;[23] however, he used a blunt, curved, metal cannula and started his incision 5 mm posterior to the limbus.

TECHNIQUES FOR TOPICAL ANESTHESIA

1. In outpatients, drops with 0.5% proparacaine are initiated. Dilating drops and antibiotic plus Voltaren (Novartis Pharmaceutical Corp., East Hanover, NJ) are administered twice. Beginning with the third set and approximately 15 min before surgery, one more set of dilating drops and two sets of 0.75% bupivacaine drops are instilled (Figure 9-1). Next, two to three drops of half-strength Betadine (Purdue Frederick Co., Norwalk, Conn.) are instilled into the cul-de-sac (Figure 9-2).

2. Just before entering the operating room, viscous lidocaine is instilled into the cul-de-sac (Figure 9-3).

3. Once in the operating theater, one more drop is instilled and the patient has the sterile skin preparation administered. Another drop of anesthetic can be administered.

4. During draping, the patient's upper lid is held with a sterile 4 × 4 gauze bandage, and the patient is asked to look down. This usually allows application of the drape without difficulty (Figure 9-4). The patient can be told that there is an odd feeling during the process, especially when placing the lid speculum (Figure 9-5A and B). Most patients are quite

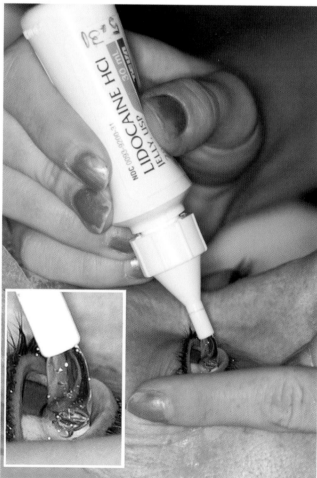

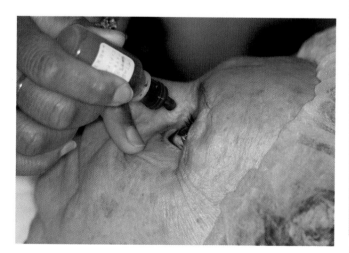

Figure 9-2 Betadine 5% drops administered before lidocaine gel.

Figure 9-3 Lidocaine 2% gel applied to ocular surface before preparation and draping of patient.

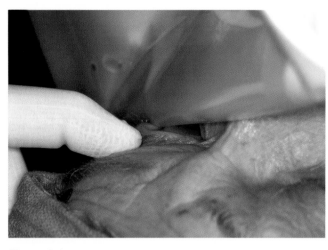

Figure 9-4 Drape applied after sterile prep as lids are retreated and patient looks down.

comfortable once the speculum is in place. It is important that the lashes are covered with the drape to reduce the stimulus. The light source is very low and slowly raised as the patient becomes comfortable.

5. A stab incision is made, and 0.3 mL of 1% unpreserved lidocaine is slowly injected. Patients can be warned that they may feel a slight sting, although most do not (Figures 9-6 and 9-7).

6. Versed (Roche Laboratories, Nutley, NJ), 0.5–1 mg, usually will be administered, although many patients require none.

Supported in part by a grant from Research to Prevent Blindness, Inc., New York, NY, to the Department of Ophthalmology and Visual Sciences, University of Utah.

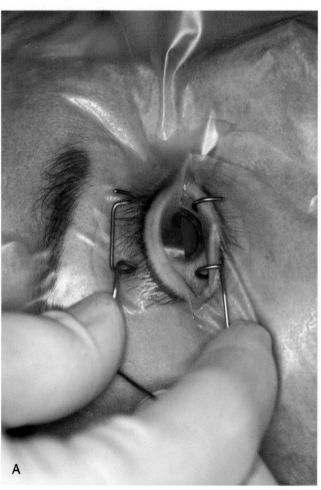

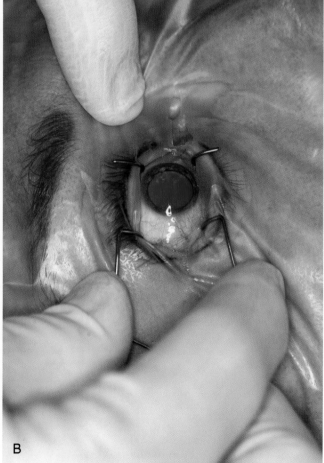

Figure 9-5 A and B, Lid speculum placed after incision of drape, ensuring adequate coverage of lid margin and lashes.

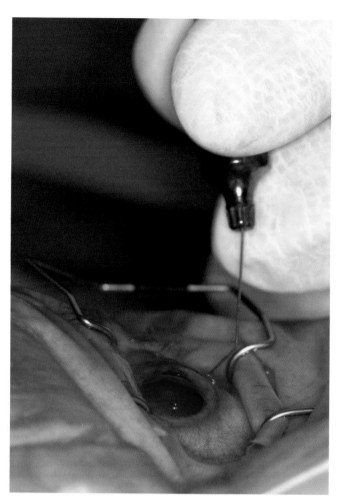

Figure 9-6 Nonpreserved lidocaine 1% injected into anterior chamber.

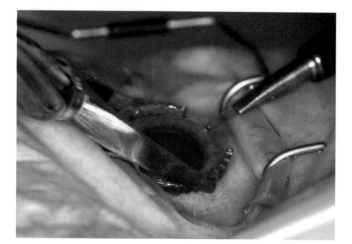

Figure 9-7 Thornton fixation ring used to stabilize globe for paracentesis.

References

[1] Leaming DV. Practice styles and preferences of ASCRS members – 1985 survey. J Cataract Refract Surg 1968;12:380–384.

[2] Schein OD, Bass EB, Sharkey P et al. Cataract surgical techniques: preferences and underlying beliefs. 1995;113:1108–1112.

[3] Leaming DV. Practice styles and preferences of ASCRS members – 1987 survey. J Cataract Refract Surg 1988;14:552–559.

[4] Leaming DV. Practice styles and preferences of ASCRS members – 1988 survey. J Cataract Refract Surg 1989;15:689–697.

[5] Leaming DV. Practice styles and preferences of ASCRS members – 1989 survey. J Cataract Refract Surg 1990;16:624–632.

[6] Leaming DV. Practice styles and preferences of ASCRS members – 1991 survey. J Cataract Refract Surg 1992;18:460–469.

[7] Leaming DV. Practice styles and preferences of ASCRS members – 1983 survey. J Cataract Refract Surg 1994;20:459–467.

[8] Leaming DV. Practice styles and preferences of ASCRS members – 1994 survey. J Cataract Refract Surg 1995;21:378–385.

[9] Leaming DV. Practice styles and preferences of ASCRS members – 1995 survey. J Cataract Refract Surg 1996;22:931–939.

[10] Leaming DV. Practice styles and preferences of ASCRS members – 1996 survey. J Cataract Refract Surg 1997;23:527–535.

[11] Leaming DV. Practice styles and preferences of ASCRS members – 1997 survey. J Cataract Refract Surg 1998;24:552–561.

[12] Altman AJ, Albert DM, Fournier GA. Cocaine's use in ophthalmology: our 100-year heritage. Surv Ophthalmol 1985;29:300–306.

[13] Knapp H. On cocaine and its use in ophthalmic and general surgery. Arch Ophthalmol 1884;13:402–448.

[14] Russell DA, Guyton JS. Retrobulbar injection of lidocaine (Xylocaine) for anesthesia and akinesia. Am J Ophthalmol 1954;38:78–84.

[15] Karch SB. Coca java and the Southeast Asia coca industry. In: Karch SB, editor. A brief history of cocaine. Boca Raton: CRC Press; 1997. p. 71–81.

[16] Fichman RA. Use of topical anesthesia alone in cataract surgery. J Cataract Refract Surg 1996;22:612–614.

[17] Gills JP, Cherchio M, Raanan M. Unpreserved lidocaine to control discomfort during cataract surgery using topical anesthesia. J Cataract Refract Surg 1997;23:545–550.

[18] Patel BCK, Burns TA, Crandall A et al. A comparison of topical and retrobulbar anesthesia for cataract surgery. Ophthalmology 1996;103:1196–1203.

[19] Crandall AS, Zabriskie NA, Patel BCK et al. A comparison of patient comfort during cataract surgery with topical anesthesia versus topical anesthesia and intracameral lidocaine. Ophthalmology 1999;1006:60–66.

[20] Patel BCK, Clinch TE, Burns TA et al. Prospective evaluation of topical versus retrobulbar anesthesia: a converting surgeon's experience. J Cataract Refract Surg 1998;24:853–860.

[21] Hansen EA, Mein CE, Mazzoli R. Ocular anesthesia for cataract surgery: a direct sub-Tenon's approach. Ophthalmic Surg 1990;21:696–699.

[22] Greenbaum S. Anesthesia in cataract surgery. In: Greenbaum S, editor. Ocular anesthesia. Philadelphia: WB Saunders; 1997. p. 1–55.

[23] Stevens JD. A new local anesthesia technique for cataract extraction by one quadrant sub-Tenon's infiltrations. Br J Ophthalmol 1992;76:670–674.

[24] Cionni RJ, Barros MG, Kaufman AH, Osher RH. Cataract surgery without preoperative eyedrops. J Cataract Refract Surg 2003;29:2281–2283.

[25] Shugar JK. Use of epinephrine for IFIS prophylaxis [letter]. J Cataract Refract Surg 2006;32:1074–1075.

part iii

EXTRACAPSULAR CATARACT EXTRACTION

Extracapsular Cataract Surgery: Indications and Techniques

10

Jared Emery, MD and Roger F. Steinert, MD

CONTENTS

CHAPTER HIGHLIGHTS

>> Standard technique for dense cataracts

>> Complication avoidance and management

>> Detailed illustrations of each surgical step

Extracapsular cataract surgery, strictly speaking, includes both phacoemulsification and planned extracapsular cataract extraction. By convention, the terms extracapsular and planned extracapsular refer to an operation in which the lens nucleus is delivered intact through a limbal incision of about 10 mm.

Since 1970, phacoemulsification and extracapsular cataract surgery have replaced intracapsular cataract extraction, except for rare instances, such as subluxated lenses or eyes in which a question of patient sensitivity to lens material exists. Phacoemulsification was used in about 15–20% of cataract cases in the United States from the mid-1970s through to 1987. Phacoemulsification then rapidly gained in popularity, becoming the procedure of choice for about 50% of surgeons by 1990, for 70% of surgeons by 1992,[1] and nearly 100% of responding surgeon members of the American Society of Cataract and Refractive Surgery in a survey in 2000.[2] However, the extracapsular cataract operation is still used by many surgeons in specific situations. In some cases, it is the procedure of choice. Every cataract surgeon should be skilled in extracapsular cataract surgery.

INDICATIONS

The extracapsular operation can be used successfully for almost any cataract. The method is not appropriate for luxated or subluxated lenses. Its main disadvantages compared with phacoemulsification include greater induced astigmatism,[3–7] less stability of the postoperative refraction,[3,8,9] more early postoperative inflammation,[10,11] and a higher rate of posterior capsular opacification.[12] Its main advantage is that in some cases it can provide a greater margin of safety. In cases in which the nucleus is very dense, the pupil dilates poorly, posterior synechiae are present, or zonular integrity is in question (as in pseudoexfoliation syndrome or after pars plana vitrectomy), some surgeons have a greater margin of safety with the extracapsular procedure.

The surgeon should use the procedure that is likely to give the most successful result. For example, if the surgeon perseveres with phacoemulsification made difficult by poor exposure, he or she might face a higher likelihood of capsular rupture with vitreous loss than might have been the case had the surgery been converted to large-incision extracapsular extraction. The careful surgeon judges each case in advance and chooses phacoemulsification or planned extracapsular surgery based on his or her expectation that this will produce the best result for the patient. In the majority of cases, this decision can be made before surgery. For some cases, however, one might choose during surgery to switch from phacoemulsification to a planned extracapsular technique. The extracapsular technique of Emery (discussion to follow) allows the surgeon to switch readily from phacoemulsification to large-incision planned extracapsular surgery at any stage of the operation.

TECHNIQUES

The best cataract surgical techniques give consistently reproducible results. The surgeon remains in control. The operation accomplishes removal of the nucleus with minimal stress on the zonules, secure placement of an intraocular lens (IOL) with an intact capsular bag, and closure with a watertight incision that gives minimal astigmatism. The procedure should be as simple as possible to promote success and should apply with minimal variations to all types of cases.

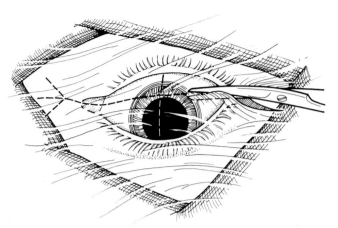

Figure 10-1 Technique for incision of plastic drape.

■ PREPARATION ■

After aseptic preparation of the operative site, dry the lid margins using cellulose sponges. Apply a large unperforated plastic drape (3M) to the open lids and incise (Figure 10-1).

Retract the upper and lower lids using the Jaffe wire lid speculum. Attach a rubber band to each speculum and use a hemostat to clip the rubber band to the drapes, applying the minimum amount of tension that will give adequate exposure of the globe. Place 4-0 black silk sutures beneath the insertions of the superior and inferior rectus muscles. Tuck in the flaps of the drape and attach the sutures to the rubber bands (Figure 10-2). Use only the necessary tension to produce adequate exposure above the superior limbus and maintain visibility of the inferior limbus.

■ CONJUNCTIVAL INCISION ■

Make a fornix-based flap to expose the limbus using a 7 mm peritomy with oblique relaxing incisions extending from the limbus about 3 mm posteriorly, as illustrated (Figure 10-3).

Apply light wet-field cautery to obliterate all visible surface vessels posterior to the intended incision site, which will be approximately 3 mm posterior to the anterior limbus (Figure 10-4). Clean the limbus with a Tooke knife to "squeeze" residual blood from vessels near the limbus. Avoid fraying the scleral surface with excessive scraping.

■ SCLERAL INCISION ■

Using calipers, measure a 10 mm chord length on the sclera, with the points positioned 3 mm posterior to the limbus (Figure 10-5). Make a 10 mm partially penetrating incision using a 30° disposable steel microsurgical blade. The incision groove will run parallel with the limbus and 3 mm posterior to the anterior limbal margin (Figure 10-6). The groove should be perpendicular to the scleral surface and to a depth of 50–75% of the scleral wall thickness.

Make a lamellar scleral dissection using a disposable crescent blade. Begin this dissection at the base of the preplaced groove. Dissect the flap anteriorly, beginning at the apex of the groove. Continue tangential to the globe for about 1 mm along the entire length of the groove. Then extend the tunnel in one direction, wherever access is easiest (Figure 10-7). Gradually come anterior, being careful to depress the heel of the crescent blade to avoid

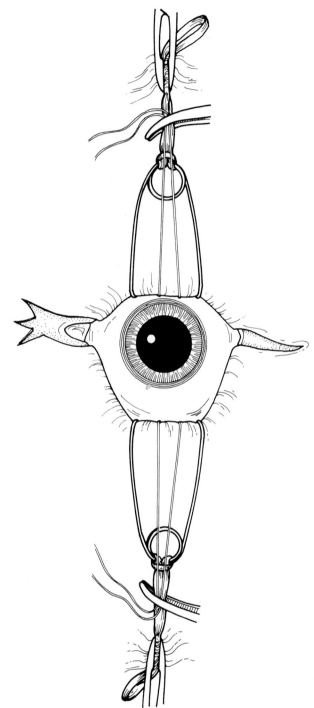

Figure 10-2 Surgeon's view of placement of Jaffe wire lid specula and rectus sutures. Note that good exposure of the operative site is achieved while still allowing visibility of the inferior limbus.

premature penetration at the site where the corneoscleral curvature steepens. Bring the incision anterior into clear cornea just beyond (central) to the limbal arcade (Figures 10-7 and 10-8). About 4 mm of scleral-corneal dissection should extend to the point of anterior chamber entry. Keeping the blade fully inserted, as in Figure 10-7, gently extend the plane of dissection right and left to the full 10 mm width; stabilize the globe by grasping the sclera posterior to the groove. Avoid grasping the scleral flap because it might tear. Judge the depth of the scleral-corneal

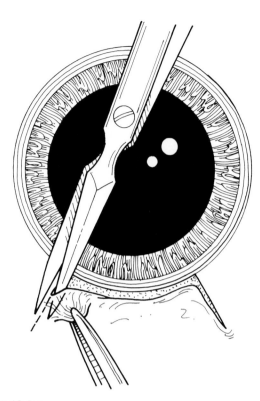

Figure 10-3 Expose the superior limbus with a 7 mm peritomy and oblique relaxing incisions.

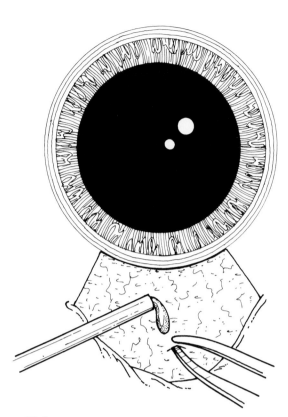

Figure 10-4 Cauterize surface vessels posterior to the incision site.

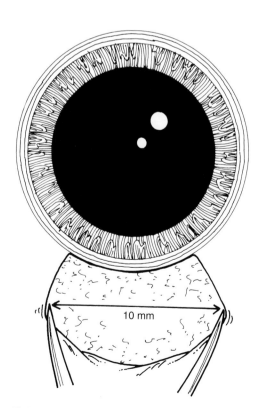

Figure 10-5 Incision site: a 10 mm chord length 3 mm posterior to the limbus.

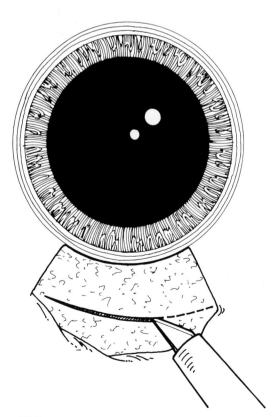

Figure 10-6 Place incision groove parallel with the limbus 3 mm posterior to the anterior limbal margin.

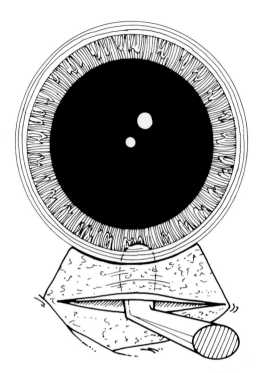

Figure 10-7 Dissection of scleral tunnel using crescent blade.

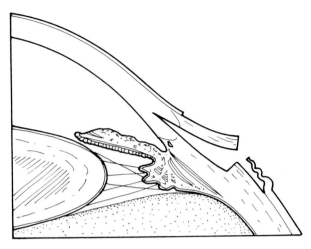

Figure 10-8 Cross-sectional view of cornea and sclera showing depth and extent of scleral tunnel.

dissection by viewing the blade through the translucent sclera. Keep the sclera moist to give greater visibility of the blade (see Figures 10-7 and 10-8).

Use a disposable phaco keratome to penetrate the anterior chamber, making an incision parallel to the iris plane. It helps to aim the point of the blade somewhat posteriorly until initial penetration is achieved to avoid sliding up along corneal lamellae and entering the anterior chamber more centrally than desired. After penetration of the blade point, level out the blade so that it remains parallel to the plane of the iris and then push in to make a 1.5 mm opening. You will extend this incision later after the anterior capsulectomy (Figure 10-9).

ANTERIOR CAPSULECTOMY

Fully inflate the anterior chamber with a viscoelastic such as sodium hyaluronate. Use a 27-gauge disposable needle with a small microhook at its tip to create a 6 or 7 mm circular anterior capsulectomy. Make very small bites directed parallel with the pupillary margin. Each bite after the first should begin on top of the anterior capsule about 1 mm from the adjacent capsular incision (Figure 10-10). A fluid movement of the microhook should first puncture the capsule with slight posterior pressure and then sweep parallel with the pupillary margin until the tear joins the adjacent incision.

The capsulectomy should be at least 6 mm in diameter. Smaller-diameter openings lead to rather large tears of the peripheral capsule that tend to destabilize the lens implant. An opening of 6–7 mm gives a reasonable margin of peripheral anterior capsule, while allowing the nucleus to prolapse with less pronounced radial tearing.

After completion of the circular anterior capsulectomy, reinsert the blade that was used to make the original entry into the anterior chamber and extend the entry site to about 3 mm. Inject additional viscoelastic before this step as needed. (The surgeon

may make the initial entry 3 mm wide to skip this step. The 1.5 mm initial entry was suggested to help retain the viscoelastic and to maintain the depth of the anterior chamber throughout the capsulectomy.) Remove the fragment of anterior capsule using toothless forceps. Insert the crescent blade and extend the third plane of the incision parallel to the iris plane to the full 10 mm width of the previous flap dissection (Figure 10-11). Use pushing strokes of the crescent blade to cut the third plane; this helps make a watertight valve incision.

REMOVAL OF THE NUCLEUS

Put three interrupted 8-0 Vicryl or 9-0 black silk sutures across the lips of the scleral groove, taking about a 1 mm bite on each side. Place them so that when they are tied they will be equally spaced across the wound, giving four 2.5 mm openings for passage of the irrigation–aspiration instrument (Figure 10-12). Loop the sutures around the margins of the groove, as shown in Figure 10-12.

Using the McIntyre 26-gauge cannula attached to an irrigating cystotome handpiece, prolapse the superior lens nucleus into the anterior chamber. Pass the McIntyre 26-gauge cannula into the anterior chamber at the 12 o'clock position. Move the tip over to the 2 o'clock position and slide it beneath the margin of the anterior capsular leaflet. Retract the leaflet toward the lens equator rather firmly to allow the cannula to pass beyond the equator. Then, press slightly posterior with the whole shaft (not just the tip) of the cannula while gently irrigating with gravity flow through the handpiece. Maintain posterior pressure against the scleral wound while holding the shaft of the instrument parallel to the plane of the iris to help bring the nucleus forward. The lens nucleus begins to cleave from the posterior capsule, allowing the tip of the cannula to pass beneath the equator of the nucleus. After cleavage begins and irrigation forms a space between the edge of the nucleus and the posterior capsule, lift slightly on the edge of the nucleus to enhance the cleavage, slide the cannula slightly to the right in the cleavage, lift on the edge of the nucleus again, depress slightly and slide into the cleavage to the right again, lift again on the nucleus, and so on, repeating this movement slowly to allow the nucleus to cleave and lift away from the posterior capsule. The movement should be slow and deliberate to give the

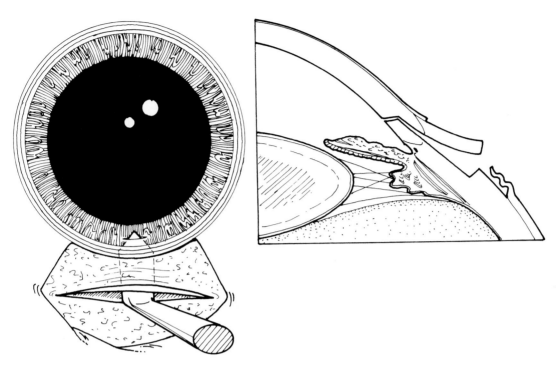

Figure 10-9 Plane three of the incision: penetration into the anterior chamber using a disposable phaco blade. Inset shows cross-sectional view of incisional planes.

nucleus time to separate gently from the posterior capsule. Continue this movement until the superior quarter to half of the nucleus emerges through the pupil into the anterior chamber (Figures 10-13 and 10-14).

Attach a Knolle-Pearce irrigating lens loop (Storz E0631) in the irrigating handpiece and adjust the bottle height to get a rapid drip of fluid. Pass the lens loop through the incision and then gently beneath the nucleus, allowing time for the fluid to dissect ample space between the nucleus and the posterior capsule. Lift slightly on the nucleus, slide into the cleavage plane, lift slightly again, slide further into the cleavage plane, and so on. Repeat this sequence until the nucleus floats up away from

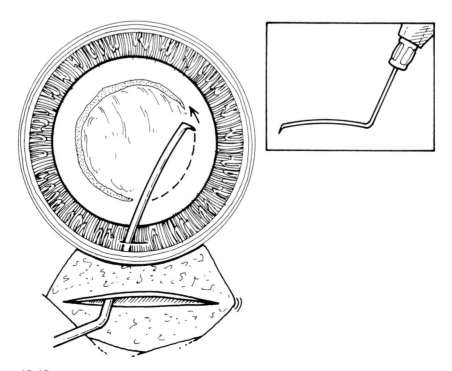

Figure 10-10 Anterior capsulectomy. For this, bend a 27-gauge disposable needle into the configuration shown in the inset. Attach the needle to a small syringe, which serves as a handle.

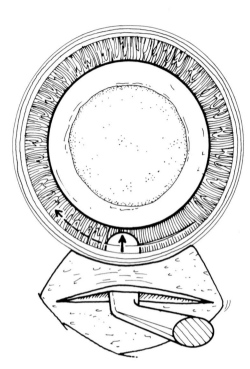

Figure 10-11 Extend plane three of the incision with the crescent blade.

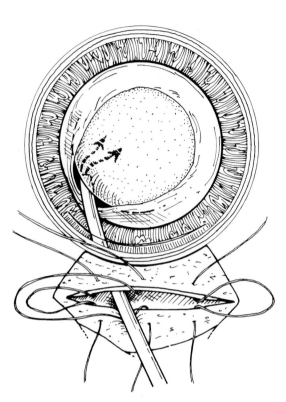

Figure 10-13 Technique for prolapse of superior nucleus into the anterior chamber using the McIntyre 26-gauge cannula with irrigation.

the posterior capsule and toward the wound. The lens loop should now be positioned beneath the central nucleus. Hesitate until fluid builds up and pushes the nucleus against the internal lip of the wound. Then withdraw the loop while applying slight posterior pressure at the same time, lift slightly on the anterior scleral lip with forceps held in the free hand. Most nuclei come readily through a 10 mm incision, but an occasional large hard compact nucleus comes out more readily after extending the scleral incision to a width of 11 mm (Figures 10-15 and 10-16).

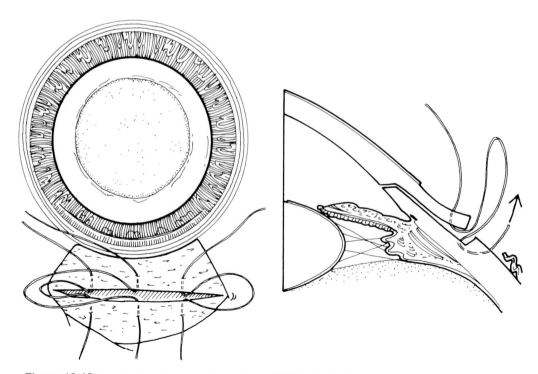

Figure 10-12 Technique for placement of three interrupted 9-0 black silk sutures.

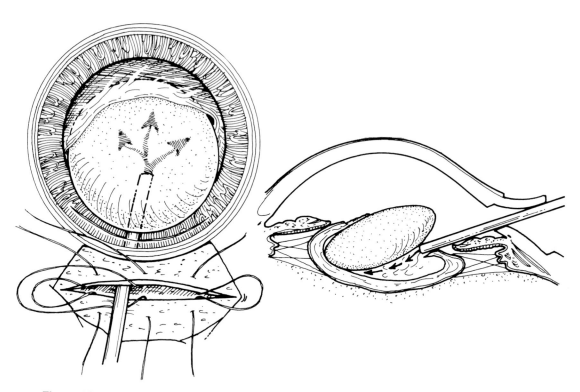

Figure 10-14 Prolapse of nucleus into anterior chamber is facilitated by infusion of balanced salt solution posterior to nucleus.

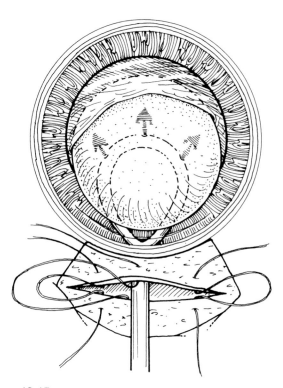

Figure 10-15 Extract the nucleus using a Knolle-Pearce irrigating lens loop.

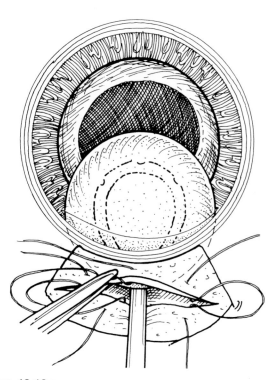

Figure 10-16 The lens loop draws the nucleus through the wound.

Commonly, a rumpled shell of epinuclear cortex strips away from the nucleus as it passes out of the eye and remains adjacent to the internal lip of the wound. Irrigate this loose cortex from the anterior chamber using a Randolph cannula attached to a squeeze bottle of balanced solution.

■ REMOVAL OF THE CORTEX ■

Tie the three preplaced sutures. Use either an automated irrigation-aspiration device, such as that found with equipment supplied for phacoemulsification or extracapsular surgery, or a manual irrigation–aspiration instrument. Insert the tip of the irrigation–aspiration device through any of the 2.5 mm wound segments between the sutures as needed for easy access. Insert the instrument with the aspiration hole aimed anteriorly.

Place the tip of the instrument gently into the capsular fornix while keeping close to the posterior capsule to avoid aspirating the free anterior capsular flap. This allows the cortex in the capsular fornix to occlude the opening as aspiration begins, helping prevent aspiration of the anterior capsular leaflet. About 1 s after initiating gentle aspiration, withdraw the tip of the aspiration device into the pupillary space to verify that cortex is attached to it. Once the surgeon confirms that the irrigation port is aspirating cortex and is free of other unwanted attachments, the aspiration vacuum can be increased to complete aspiration of the attached cortical fragment. Remove the cortex sequentially from adjacent sites until all has been removed. As each fragment is aspirated, slowly bring the tip of the instrument into the center

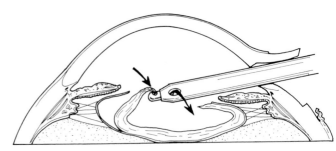

Figure 10-18 Cross-sectional view of cortical aspiration.

of the pupil to strip cortex away from the posterior capsule and simultaneously to aspirate it.

Begin aspirating cortex at the 6 o'clock position and then remove it gradually as illustrated until cortex remains only adjacent to the wound. Usually cortex adjacent to the wound can be removed by inserting the aspiration tip at the far right side of the incision to remove cortex next to the left part of the incision, and vice versa. If cortex near the wound is adherent, irrigate it using a curved Binkhorst aspiration cannula attached to a syringe. This usually loosens it so that it can be more easily removed by the aspiration tip (Figures 10-17 to 10-20). If these maneuvers do not remove the cortex, aspirate it carefully using a curved Binkhorst cannula attached to a syringe containing balanced salt solution after inflating the capsular bag with a viscoelastic agent.

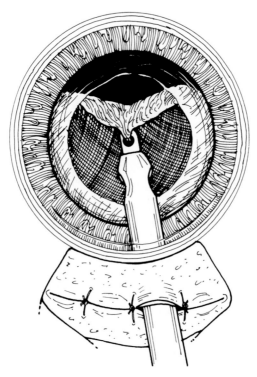

Figure 10-17 Remove residual cortex from posterior capsule using irrigation–aspiration instrument beginning at the 6 o'clock position (surgeon's view).

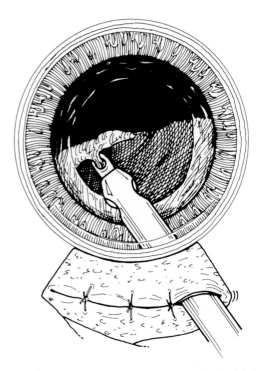

Figure 10-19 Cortex at 3 and 9 o'clock is removed after the inferior cortex.

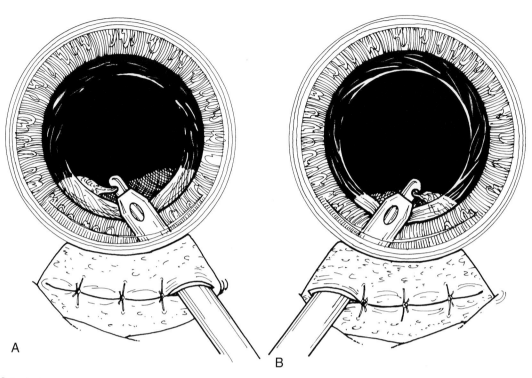

A

B

Figure 10-20 Aspiration of cortex at 12 o'clock position is made easier by inserting the irrigation–aspiration instrument through the far right side of the incision to remove cortex at the 12 to 1 o'clock position (**A**) and through the far left of the incision to remove cortex at the 11 to 12 o'clock position (**B**).

Polish the posterior capsule with a capsule polishing instrument (Figure 10-21). Any cortex that can be readily removed will be rubbed off the capsule. If residual fibrotic material does not readily come off, this may be left for later neodymium:yttrium-aluminum-garnet laser capsulotomy. With an appropriate aspiration device that includes a "capsule vacuuming" mode, residual cortical material can be vacuumed away from the posterior capsule with reasonable safety (Figure 10-22).

IMPLANTATION OF THE INTRAOCULAR LENS

With a viscoelastic agent, fill the central anterior chamber and place additional viscoelastic beneath the anterior capsular flaps to inflate the capsule for in-the-bag intraocular lens (IOL) insertion. If the surgeon desires to place the lens implant into the ciliary sulcus, such as in a situation when the posterior lens capsule has ruptured, use viscoelastic beneath the iris to flatten the residual anterior capsule flap against the posterior capsule to inflate the space of the ciliary sulcus rather than inflating the lens capsule as described previously.

Remove the 11 o'clock and 12 o'clock temporary sutures in preparation for the lens insertion. Holding the lens with lens-insertion forceps (such as Bechert forceps), slide it into the anterior chamber. As the optic passes through the wound, tilt it to position the haptic to pass into the capsular bag (or sulcus, if desired). The inferior haptic should slide close to the posterior capsule and into the bag (or sulcus) as the optic passes through the wound incision (Figure 10-23). As the right hand releases the optic, the left hand, holding the superior haptic, pushes it

in and to the left, thereby rotating the inferior haptic of the lens somewhat toward the 7 or 8 o'clock position.

After releasing the optic, grasp the superior haptic of the lens at its midpoint. In the left hand, use a blunt iris hook (Katena K3-5422) (Figure 10-24). Grasp the residual margin of the anterior

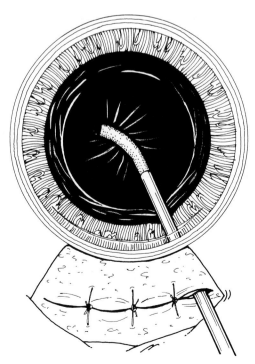

Figure 10-21 Polish the posterior capsule with a Kratz scratcher.

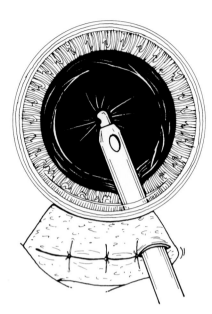

Figure 10-22 Aspiration of residual cortical material using irrigation–aspiration instrument and "capsule vacuuming" mode.

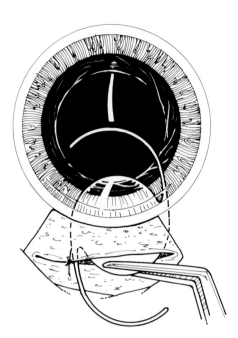

Figure 10-23 Technique for implantation of intraocular lens using viscoelastic.

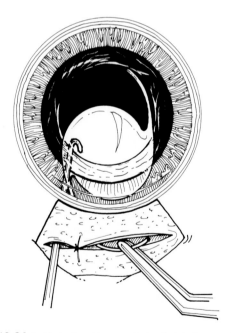

Figure 10-24 An iris hook guides superior haptic into the capsular bag.

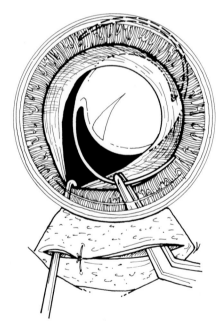

Figure 10-25 The iris hook can retract the anterior capsule and iris if necessary to allow accurate placement of the superior haptic into the capsular bag.

capsule along with the margin of the iris and retract slightly toward the wound, using the blunt iris hook in the left hand while passing the superior haptic into the anterior chamber and using the right hand with a vector of movement toward the position of the iris hook (Figure 10-25). This causes the lens to rotate into a horizontal position. The superior haptic is flexed sufficiently to clear the margin of the iris and the anterior capsule and to pass beneath the edge of the iris hook, which can, in effect, "shoe-horn" the superior haptic into the capsular bag by gliding the haptic beneath the hook. Once the superior haptic has been released into the capsule bag, a Sinskey hook may be used to rotate the lens slightly clockwise to settle it into a central position. Minimize manipulation of the lens to avoid dislocating a haptic from the bag into the ciliary sulcus.

■ WOUND CLOSURE ■

Place a corneal cover over the central cornea to block light from the microscope. Leave the temporary suture in place at the 1 o'clock position; close the incision to the right of that suture with a running 10-0 nylon suture placed in a shoelace fashion as illustrated. In Figure 10-26, the initial penetration point of each bite of the suture is labeled sequentially to demonstrate how the suture is placed. The first bite starts within the lips of the wound and passes through only the posterior lip; the final bite passes only through the anterior lip, thereby allowing the two suture ends to come together and to be tied within the wound. Begin each suture bite after the first, about 1mm from the anterior lip of the incision.

Pass the needle though the flap, then intralamellarly along the bed of the scleral dissection and finally through intact sclera. Exit 1 mm posterior to the scleral groove. Bury the knot within the lips of the wound next to the remaining temporary suture.

Aspirate residual viscoelastic material by passing the irrigation–aspiration instrument through the incision remaining open to the left of the temporary suture (Figure 10-27). Inject an intraocular miotic agent to constrict the pupil. Close the remainder of the wound with a 10-0 nylon suture using a modified shoelace configuration, as indicated (Figure 10-28). Close the conjunctival flap by applying wet-field coaptation forceps in the usual fashion along the oblique cuts nasally and temporally (Figure 10-29).

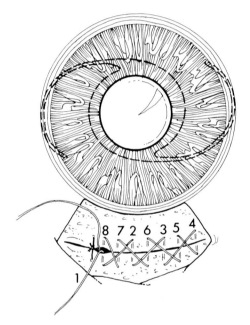

Figure 10-26 Technique for placement for shoelace suture – each bite is numbered in order. Suture is tied with knot in wound.

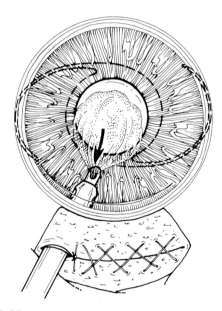

Figure 10-27 Removal of viscoelastic through remaining unsutured part of wound. Inject intraocular carbachol 0.01% to constrict pupil after removal of viscoelastic.

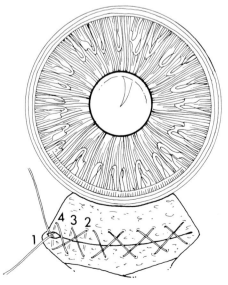

Figure 10-28 Remove remaining 9-0 silk suture and place 10-0 nylon shoelace suture as indicated, with each bite numbered in order of placement.

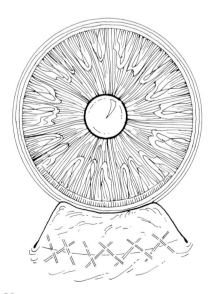

Figure 10-29 Appearance showing constricted pupil (carbachol) and conjunctival flap in place.

References

[1] Leaming DV. Practice styles and preferences of ASCRS members – 1992 survey. J Cataract Refract Surg 1993;19:603.

[2] Leaming DV. Practice styles and preferences of ASCRS members – 2000 survey. J Cataract Refract Surg 2001;27:948–955.

[3] Steinert RF, Brint SF, White SM et al. Astigmatism after small incision cataract surgery: a prospective, randomized, multicenter comparison of 4- and 6.5-mm incisions. Ophthalmology 1991;98:417–423.

[4] Hayashi K, Hayashi H, Nakao F et al. The correlation between incision size and corneal shape change in sutureless cataract surgery. Ophthalmology 1995;102:550–556.

[5] Kohnen T, Dick B, Jacobi KW. Comparison of induced astigmatism after temporal clear corneal tunnel incisions of different sizes. J Cataract Refract Surg 1995;21:417–424.

[6] Oshika T, Nagahara K, Yaguchi S et al. Three year prospective, randomized evaluation of intraocular lens implantation through 3.2 and 5.5 mm incisions. J Cataract Refract Surg 1998;24:509–514.

[7] Olson RJ, Crandall AS. Prospective randomized comparison of phacoemulsification cataract surgery with a 3.2-mm vs a 5.5-mm sutureless incision. Am J Ophthalmol 1990;125:612–620.

[8] Werblin TP. Astigmatism after cataract extraction: 6-year follow-up of 6.5- and 12-millimeter incisions. Refract Corneal Surg 1992;8:448.

[9] Watson A, Sunderraj P. Comparison of small-incision phacoemulsification with standard extracapsular cataract surgery: postoperative astigmatism and visual recovery. Eye 1992;6:626.

[10] Laurell CG, Zetterstrom C, Phillipson B et al. Randomized study of the blood–aqueous barrier reaction after phacoemulsification and extracapsular cataract extraction. Acta Ophthalmol Scand 1998;76:573–578.

[11] Pande MV, Spalton DJ, Kerr-Muir MG et al. Postoperative inflammatory response to phacoemulsification and extracapsular cataract surgery: aqueous flare and cells. J Cataract Refract Surg 1996;22:770–774.

[12] Minassian DC, Rosen P, Dart JK et al. Extracapsular cataract extraction compared with small incision surgery by phacoemulsification: a randomized trial. Br J Ophthalmol 2001;85:822–829.

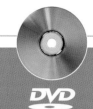

Small Incision Cataract Surgery in Underdeveloped Countries

Geoffrey Tabin, MA, MD

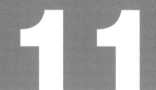

CONTENTS

CHAPTER HIGHLIGHTS

>> Special demands of cataract surgery in underdeveloped countries

>> Self-sealing large corneo-scleral incision

>> Triangular capsulotomy in advanced cataracts

>> Nuclear extraction

■ EVOLUTION OF THE OPTIMAL SURGICAL APPROACH TO CATARACTS IN THE DEVELOPING WORLD ■

Cataracts are currently the leading cause of blindness worldwide with the majority of cases in developing nations. Of the 38 million cases of blindness (visual acuity less than 20/400), an estimated 16 million are caused by age-related cataracts. In Nepal alone the percentage of curable blindness resulting from cataracts is more than 80%, and in India 3.8 million people develop cataract blindness yearly. As the world's population ages the incidence of cataract in developing nations will continue to rise and with no improvement in current practices, the World Health Organization estimates a doubling of blindness rates by 2020. Projections show that to eliminate the rapidly growing backlog within the next 25 years, the global number of cataracts operated on annually would have to increase from 7 to 32 million by the year 2020. There is clearly a pressing need for faster, less-expensive, and more effective delivery of high-quality cataract surgery.

New surgical techniques have minimized the use of expensive consumables and optimized efficiency, while preserving the highest level of quality in visual outcomes and minimizing complications.[1] Three steps have dramatically improved the speed and efficiency with which we are able to deliver high-quality sutureless, small-incision, cataract surgery (SICS). The first is a well-constructed scleral tunnel with a larger internal opening than the external scleral incision, which relies upon intraocular pressure to close the internal lip of the wound, thereby creating a self-sealing wound and eliminating postoperative suture-induced astigmatism. The second is a triangular capsulotomy technique, which eliminates the need for capsular staining with even the most mature cataracts. Finally, our lens-delivery technique relies on use of fluidics and eye positioning to irrigate the nucleus through our funnel-shaped wound and out of the eye. Finally, the once cost-prohibitive intraocular lenses (IOLs) and other consumables such as viscoelastic, have become affordable due to high-quality production in developing countries including Nepal and India. It has become increasingly clear that the modified version of extracapsular cataract extraction (ECCE) with posterior chamber (PC) IOL placement described in this chapter is the preferred approach to cataract surgery in the developing world.

PREOPERATIVE MANAGEMENT

Preoperative management begins with the surgeon examining patients who have been pre-screened for vision and relative afferent pupillary defects by ophthalmic assistants. As the majority of our patients have mature cataracts with no view to the posterior segment, the patients undergo B-scan ultrasound, when available, at the time of their biometry measurements.

The evening before surgery the patients' faces are vigorously washed and antibiotic drops and ointment are instilled at this time. Prior to surgery the eyelashes are closely cropped and fluoroquinolone eye drops are instilled at the time of dilation. The eye is then prepped with Betadine and a retrobulbar anesthetic is administered by an anesthetic technician, after which a Betadine soaked gauze is held over the eye. At the start of the case the surgeon performs a final Betadine prep with instillation of a small amount of 5% Betadine into the fornix of the eye. This preoperative cleaning and sterilization regimen leads to a low infection rate. The efficiency of patient turnover is maximized: as the surgeon is prepping and draping the eye, the scrub nurse is arranging a new instrument set, and surgery proceeds with a typical delay of less than 3 min between cases.

SURGICAL TECHNIQUE

Surgeon Positioning and Maximizing Surgical Field Exposure

We generally advocate that in the beginning surgeons learn SICS from a superior approach; however, many SICS surgeons operate from a temporal approach.

Temporal vs. Superior Surgical Approach

While a superior approach has long been the standard of care when performing ECCE, we routinely perform (98% of cases) ECCE using a temporal surgical approach as there is a significant difference between the amount of postoperative astigmatism induced by the two techniques. The mean induced astigmatic change is 1.75 diopters (D) following a superior surgical approach due to the effects of gravity and motion of the eyelids on the wound, while 0.75 D of astigmatism is induced following a temporal surgical approach.

A superior approach has remained the mainstream technique of choice given the following advantages: first, the upper eyelid covers the external wound following the operation when a superior approach is used, providing good wound protection. Second, surgeon positioning at the head of the operating table provides for a more streamlined flow of patients through the operating suite. Microscope heads, chair positions, and instrument tables need not be repositioned between cases.

Fortunately, most of these limitations have been overcome. The rate of postoperative infection is equivalent when using either a superior or a temporal approach; however, it is critical to close the conjunctiva over the external scleral wound with cauterization at the completion of the temporal approach surgery. We have also developed an operating table which facilitates patient flow when operating temporally. It allows the surgeon to be seated at one side; patients are then positioned with their feet perpendicular to the surgeon's line of sight, facing in either direction depending on the eye to be operated upon (Figure 11-1).

Access the Anterior Chamber by Creating a Sclerocorneal Tunnel

A superior rectus traction suture may be used if operating superiorly to enhance exposure. A fornix-based conjunctival peritomy to sclera is performed superiorly from 10 to 2 o'clock to bare sclera. Light cauterization is used to control bleeding and blanch episcleral vessels over the incision site. A straight to slightly frown-shaped incision centered at 12 o'clock is carried to 30–50% scleral depth tangential to the limbus for 6–7 mm and approximately 1.5–2 mm from the limbus. This incision can be made with a razor blade fragment or crescent blade, the former helping with cost containment. The crescent blade is then used to create a lamellar scleral corneal tunnel from the initial incision in a single plane approximately 1–1.5 mm into the clear cornea and parallel to the ocular surface. The dissected pocket should extend nasally and temporally to the limbus so that the transverse extent is much greater in the cornea than in the sclera (Figure 11-2).

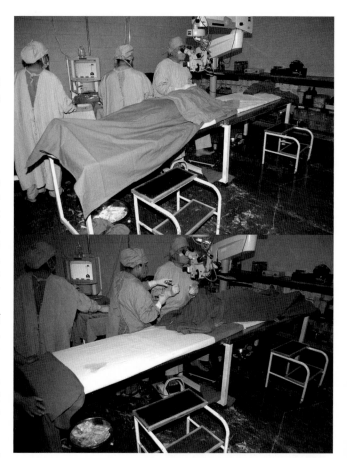

Figure 11-1 Operating table for cataract surgery from a temporal approach. The surgeon is seated at the side of the table and patients are positioned with their feet perpendicular to the surgeon's line of sight, facing one way or the other depending on the eye to be operated upon. *Upper image*, Operating on a patient's right eye. *Lower image*, Operating on a patient's left eye. A temporal surgical approach results in significantly less postoperative astigmatism compared to a superior surgical approach.

Triangular Capsulotomy vs. Continuous Curvilinear Capsulorrhexis

Triangular Capsulotomy

In the developing world mature, hypermature and Morgagnian cataracts are common; the anterior capsules associated with such dense cataracts are often tough and leathery, and there are frequently adhesions between the anterior capsule and the lens nucleus. Furthermore, poor surgical visibility is common due to corneal scars, pterygium, climatic keratopathy, and sub-optimal surgical microscopes. Under these circumstances, capsulorrhexis types of capsulotomies are difficult to complete and can lead to incomplete or inadequate capsular openings or tears in unexpected directions, increasing the risk of posterior capsular rupture.

Triangular capsulotomy has many advantages that make it a superb option in such sub-optimal surgical settings. First, it utilizes a straight needle, which facilitates entry into the AC and allows easy control of AC depth because the sclerocorneal tunnel has not yet been completed. Second, visibility is optimized as opaque lens material can be readily removed from the AC by aspiration or irrigation. Third, the capsulotomy is cut, not torn,

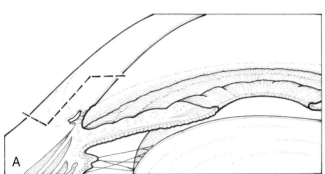 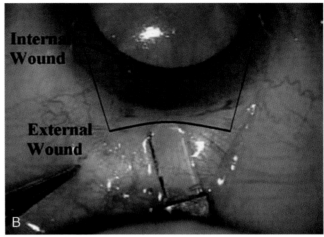

Figure 11-2 Sclerocorneal tunnel. A sclerocorneal tunnel whose external wound is in a different plane than the anterior chamber entrance wound facilitates sutureless, self-sealing wound closure. **A,** Cross section demonstrating the anatomical path of the sclerocorneal tunnel, which is demarcated by a black line. **B,** Intraoperative photograph of the sclerocorneal tunnel demarcated in black, illustrating that the internal opening of the tunnel into the anterior chamber is wider than the external opening. A razor blade fragment or crescent blade is used to create the sclerocorneal tunnel while forceps are used to stabilize the globe.

creating a reliably triangular shape, minimizing the number of capsular tags. Fourth, a triangular capsular flap provides clear visibility of the boundaries of the capsular bag, facilitating IOL placement.

Continuous Curvilinear Capsulorrhexis

We often employ a continuous curvilinear capsulorrhexis (CCC) for less advanced cataracts by using a 27-gauge needle introduced into the AC through a separate puncture site immediately adjacent to the external wound of the sclerocorneal tunnel. Viscoelastic is instilled prior to insertion of the needle into the anterior chamber. This capsular opening needs to be approximately 5–6mm in diameter, substantially larger than that utilized during phacoemulsification, as the entire lens must be expressed through this capsular window.

Triangular Capsulotomy

The triangular capsulotomy is performed before the sclerocorneal tunnel is completed so that the depth of the AC is maintained. A straight 26-gauge needle attached to a 1-mL syringe filled with balance saline solution is passed through the scleral tunnel with the entry point into the AC in sclera, not the more rigid corneal tissue. Using the beveled tip of the needle, the linear cut in the capsule is made from 4 o'clock to 12 o'clock and then from 8 o'clock to 12 o'clock so the two incisions meet at 12 o'clock. Thus, a triangular or V-shaped flap of anterior lens capsule still attached at its base is created (Figure 11-3). Each point of the triangular flap should be approximately 3mm from the center of the pupil. The apex of the capsulotomy is then lifted with the needle tip and peeled towards 6 o'clock to ensure the capsular cuts are complete. If the chamber shallows, a small amount of fluid may be irrigated through the needle to re-deepen the chamber.

Following capsulotomy, the sclerocorneal tunnel is then completed using a keratome blade to enter the anterior chamber. The sides of the blade are used to open the cornea from the temporal to the nasal aspects of the wound. The wound should be internally flared to encourage the nucleus to engage the tunnel at the time of expression. Viscoelastic may be placed in the AC to facilitate wound creation.

Nucleus Delivery into the Anterior Chamber

The lens nucleus is displaced from the capsular bag into the AC using both hydrostatic and gentle mechanical pressure. Irrigating under the displaced triangular anterior capsule flap, as well as under the temporal and nasal edges of the flap, with a flowing Simcoe cannula, will mobilize the lens nucleus and delaminate the lens components by hydrodissection. The nucleus is then gently directed inferiorly within the capsular bag while intermittently directing irrigation posterior to the nucleus, until the superior nuclear pole emerges from the capsular bag into the AC, forming a new cleavage plane between the nucleus and the iris. This newly formed cleavage between the nucleus and the iris is then accentuated by directing flow between the iris and the nucleus with the Simcoe cannula until the lens is entirely delivered into the AC. It is important not to force the nucleus in any one direction too strongly as this will strain and possibly compromise the zonules.

Extraction of the Nucleus from the Anterior Chamber

The lens nucleus is now removed from the eye. While several potential protocols are available for nucleus removal we recommend avoiding procedures that require sectioning or fragmentation of the nucleus, as these may traumatize the corneal endothelium. We recommend the following technique:

The vigorously flowing Simcoe cannula is passed posterior to the nucleus until the tip is fully visible beyond the distal pole of the nucleus. The eye is then gently rotated downward with toothed forceps held in the other hand. The accumulating irrigation fluid

Extracapsular Cataract Extraction

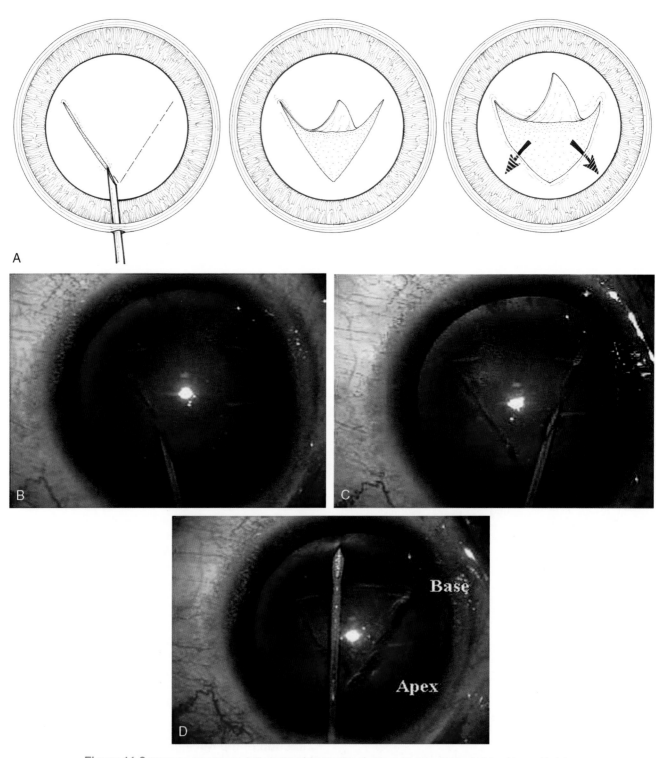

Figure 11-3 Triangular capsulotomy. **A,** Illustration of the creation of a triangular capsulotomy. *Left hand image*: First, two capsular incisions are made with a 27-gauge needle, demarcated by a dotted line, and joined to create a V-shaped window in the anterior lens capsule. *Center image*: The capsular window is then created by peeling the apex of the capsulotomy distally with the tip of the needle. *Right hand image*: The capsular bag is freed from the underlying lens cortex by injection of balanced saline solution. (Image courtesy of Brian Guercio.) Intraoperative photographs illustrating the first (**B**) and second (**C**) anterior lens capsular incisions created with a 27-gauge needle. **D,** Intraoperative photograph illustrating the creation of the capsular window by peeling the apex of the capsulotomy distally.

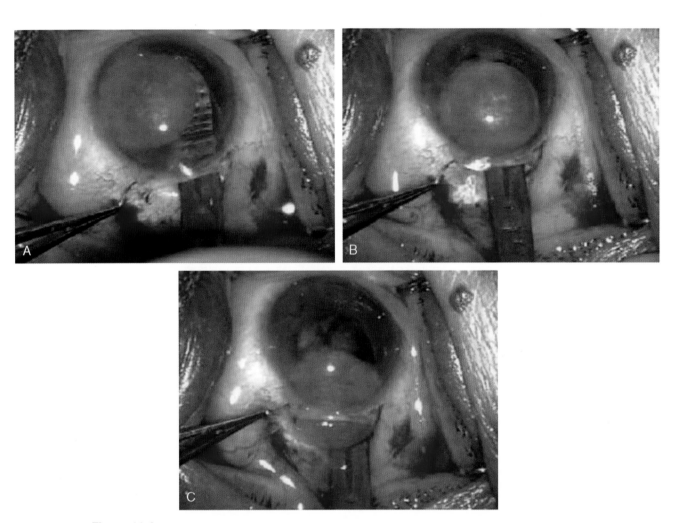

Figure 11-4 Extraction of the nucleus from the anterior chamber. Intraoperative photographs of a flowing Simcoe cannula aiding delivery of the lens nucleus from the anterior chamber. **A,** The tip of the cannula is passed posterior to the nucleus beyond the distal pole and the eye is gently rotated downward with toothed forceps. **B,** Accumulating irrigation fluid from the cannula beyond the distal pole of the nucleus engages the nucleus into the internal mouth of the sclerocorneal tunnel. **C,** Hydrostatic pressure plus gentle lifting and retraction with the tip of the cannula aides the nucleus into the tunnel and the nucleus is delivered through the external foramen of the tunnel with gentle downward pressure from the heel of the Simcoe cannula.

from the cannula will engage the nucleus into the internal mouth of the sclerocorneal tunnel. Hydrostatic pressure plus gentle lifting and retraction with the tip of the Simcoe cannula will force the nucleus further into the tunnel. Open the external foramen of the tunnel with gentle downward pressure using the heel of the Simcoe cannula and deliver the entire nucleus (Figure 11-4).

Posterior Chamber Intraocular Lens Placement

The Simcoe canula is then used in the standard fashion to remove all nuclear and cortical debris from the AC and capsular bag. Next, air is injected into the anterior chamber using the Rycroft cannula and a PMMA (polymethylmethacrylate) PC IOL is inserted into the capsular bag. Alternatively, the IOL can be inserted after filling the AC and expanding the capsular bag with viscoelastic. The apex of the V-shaped capsulotomy tear should also be folded backwards during this maneuver so that the flap lies on top of the anterior capsule. During insertion of the leading haptic, the anterior lip of the cornea is folded inward which protects the corneal endothelium during lens implantation. The

leading haptic is then passed into the capsular bag inferiorly, behind the base of the triangular capsulotomy (Figure 11-5). The folded anterior capsule flap at the base of the triangular capsulotomy serves as an easily identifiable landmark and facilitates correct PC IOL placement.

The trailing haptic is then passed into the capsular bag and correct placement of the PC IOL within the capsular bag is confirmed by observing the posterior capsule stretch lines that form perpendicular to the contacts between the IOL haptics and the capsule.

Capsulectomy

If a triangular capsulotomy was performed, the anterior capsular flap is removed to prevent any obscuring of the visual axis. A small incision is made in the anterior capsule at the edge of the base of the triangular flap with fine Vannas scissors while maintaining the AC depth with an irrigating Simcoe cannula. The capsular flap is engaged with aspiration using the Simcoe cannula (using low flow irrigation) and used to gently tear the flap entirely across its base which then should be removed from the AC (Figure 11-6).

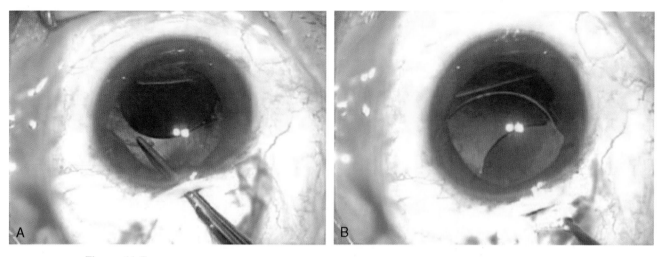

Figure 11-5 Posterior chamber intraocular lens (PCIOL) placement. Intraoperative photographs demonstrating insertion of a PCIOL into the capsular bag. **A,** The leading haptic of the PCIOL is passed into the capsular bag, posterior to the base of the triangular capsulotomy. **B,** The trailing haptic is then passed into the capsular bag.

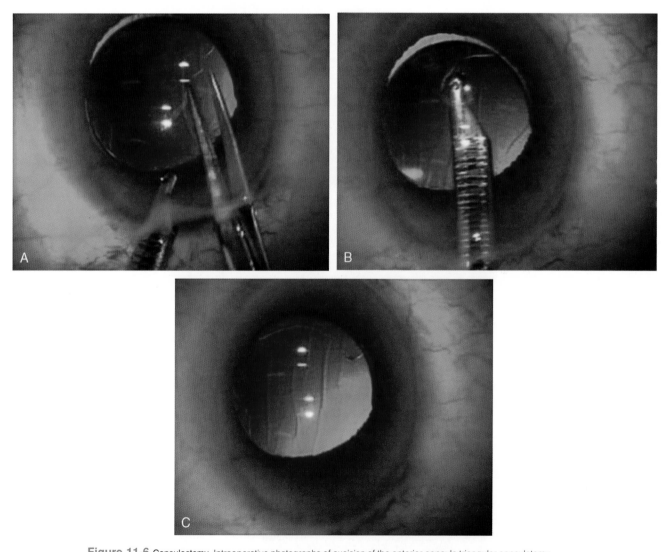

Figure 11-6 Capsulectomy. Intraoperative photographs of excision of the anterior capsule triangular capsulotomy. **A,** Vannas scissors are used to make a small incision in the anterior capsule at the base of the triangular flap while anterior chamber depth is maintained with an irrigating Simcoe cannula. **B,** The capsular flap is then engaged with the Simcoe cannula on aspiration, gently torn across its base and removed from the anterior chamber leaving an unobstructed visual axis (**C**).

Closure

The Simcoe cannula is used to irrigate and aspirate residual air or viscoelastic in the AC and intraocular pressure is restored. The 3-planed sclerocorneal tunnel will self-seal, which is confirmed by applying gentle pressure to the globe with an instrument and observing for wound leakage. Less than 1% of our wounds require suture placement for adequate closure. A subconjunctival injection of antibiotic and steroid is given just superior to the conjunctival wound, which balloons the conjunctiva and moves it over the limbus to cover the scleral wound. In the instance of a temporal surgical approach the conjunctiva is closed over the scleral wound with cauterization at the wound edges.

After removing the sterile drapes, antibiotic ointment is applied to the eye, which is then patched and shielded. Steroid and antibiotic drops are instilled every 2 h for the first postoperative day and then four times per day for 3 weeks.

SURGICAL OUTCOMES

Utilizing intraocular lenses manufactured in India or Nepal and local pharmaceuticals the cost per surgery is less than $20 per case. Moreover, experienced surgeons routinely perform more than 50 cases per day with an average operating time of 5 min per surgery.[2] The results of a prospective, randomized clinical trial in Nepal comparing our manual sutureless extracapsular surgical technique with phacoemulsification were published in the *American Journal of Ophthalmology*.[3] It was an "Expert Trial" with Professor David Chang operating with a phaco-chop (phaco) technique and Dr. Sanduk Ruit carrying out the temporal approach small incision ECCE (SICS). Both techniques achieved excellent and equivalent results. At 6 months 89% of the SICS patients had an uncorrected visual acuity (UCVA) of 20/60 or better and 98% had a best-corrected acuity (BCVA) of 20/60 or better; this outcome was equivalent to the visual acuity outcomes of the phaco patients (Figure 11-7). Furthermore, SICS is significantly faster, less expensive and less technology dependent than phacoemulsification and may be the more appropriate surgical procedure for the treatment of advanced cataracts in the developing world.

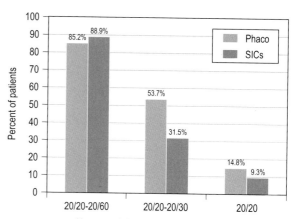

Figure 11-7 Visual acuity outcomes after small incision extracapsular cataract surgery is equivalent to those after phacoemulsification. Uncorrected visual acuity (UCVA) by functional level at 6 months after operation. Stratified into groups with visual acuity of 20/20, better than or equal to 20/30, and better than or equal to 20/60 in the phacoemulsification group (Phaco; black) vs. the manual sutureless small incision extracapsular cataract surgery (SICS; gray) group. (Image reproduced from Ruit S, Tabin G, Chang D: A prospective randomized clinical trial of phacoemulsification vs. manual sutureless small-incision extracapsular cataract surgery in Nepal, *Am J Ophthalmol* 143(1):32–38, 2007. With permission from Elsevier.)

References

[1] Ruit S, Paudyal G, Gurung R, Tabin G, Moran D, Brian G. An innovation in developing world cataract surgery: sutureless extracapsular cataract extraction with intraocular lens implantation. Clin Exper Ophthalmol 2000;28:274–279.

[2] Ruit S, Tabin GC, Nissman SA, Paudyal G, Gurung R. Low-cost high-volume extracapsular cataract extraction with posterior chamber intraocular lens implantation in Nepal. Ophthalmology 1999;106:1887–1892.

[3] Ruit S, Tabin G, Chang D. A prospective randomized clinical trial of phacoemulsification vs. manual sutureless small-incision extracapsular cataract surgery in Nepal. Am J Ophthalmol 2007;143 (1):32–38.

Bibliography

Brilliant GE, editor. The epidemiology of blindness in Nepal: report of the 1981 Nepal Blindness Survey. Chelsea, Michegan: Seva Foundation; 1988. p. 115–241.

Ruit S, Robin AL, Pokhrel RP, Sharma A, Defaller J, Maguire PT. Long-term results of extracapsular cataract extraction and posterior chamber intraocular lens insertion in Nepal. Tr Am Ophthalmol Soc 1991;LXXXIX:59–76.

part iv

PHACOEMULSIFICATION

Prophylactic Preoperative Preparation and Operative Measures for Control of Infection, Inflammation and Intraocular Pressure

Shaleen Belani, MD and Samuel Masket, MD

12

CONTENTS

CHAPTER HIGHLIGHTS

>> Differential diagnosis of postoperative inflammation

>> Preoperative prophylaxis of infection and inflammation

>> Issues in incision construction and sealing

INTRODUCTION

Clear corneal cataract surgery has been implicated as a causative factor in the rising rates of bacterial endophthalmitis. The accuracy of this implication regarding *cause* vs *correlation* as well as the *mechanism* of causation are not clear. The literature suggests that bacterial endopthalmitis following cataract surgery is more common with clear corneal incisions than with scleral tunnel incisions[1,2,3] and that this incidence is on the rise.[4,5] Regardless of mechanism, however, it is clear that measures to reduce infection rates are crucial to successful surgery. These measures include preoperative evaluation and treatment, operative measures to ensure sterility and close monitoring of the patient throughout the postoperative period.

If bacterial endophthalmitis is, indeed, on the rise, the main factor that is contributing to this is wound construction. Unstable wounds allow for bacterial contaminants from the tear film and ocular adnexa to enter into the anterior chamber.[6] Careful attention to wound construction is, therefore, imperative for clear corneal cataract surgery. It is important to be aware of other risk factors as well. For example, it is well known that diabetics have a higher incidence of endophthalmitis[7] and surgical complications, such as posterior capsule rupture, can at least quadruple that risk.[8]

However, as the incidence of infection is relatively low (currently 1 in 1000 in the United States) and there are a large number of variables in routine cataract surgery that might be implicated, it is unlikely that a large, multicentered, randomized controlled study could be completed to study all of the factors that are potentially related to the development of infection.[9] Therefore, measures to reduce infection, from the preoperative stage through the postoperative period, must be implemented routinely.

Postoperative inflammation is common after routine intraocular surgery and while it is usually self-limited, in rare cases it can result in permanent visual loss. An attempt should be made to minimize postoperative inflammation after routine cataract surgery. An increasingly reported problem in the past few years is an entity now well-described and known as toxic anterior segment syndrome (TASS). Believed to be caused by several factors including improper sterilization of instruments, ophthalmic ointments entering the eye, preservative-containing solution, and denatured viscoelastic agents, TASS must be recognized early and treated with high-dose topical steroids for the best prognosis.

Intraocular pressure (IOP) after cataract surgery and IOL implantation is readily controlled by the surgeon at the conclusion of the procedure in the presence of a well-constructed, hermetically sealed wound. Thorough removal of viscoelastic agents at the conclusion of the procedure is essential. However, in patients with pre-existing glaucoma, pharmacologic agents may be beneficial in providing additional IOP reduction.

PREOPERATIVE MEASURES TO REDUCE INFECTION

As bacterial flora implicated in bacterial endophthalmitis originate from fluid contaminated by the tear film, conjunctiva, lids and lashes, it is important to carefully examine these structures at the preoperative visit. One of the proposed mechanisms for infection is the ingress of fluid into the anterior chamber secondary to hypotony in the immediate postoperative period from physically unstable, potentially leaking wounds. This negative pressure gradient then allows periocular fluid with bacterial flora to enter into the anterior chamber.[10] Patients with blepharitis should be placed on a regimen to control their disease, including lid scrubs, warm compresses, antibiotics ointments or oral doxycycline in advanced or refractory cases. It may even be prudent to re-examine these patients once again before proceeding with surgery in order to ensure that the lashes are free of material that may be a source of contamination.

Although there is no good evidence to support a reduced risk of infection, preoperative antibiotic drops started 2–4 days prior to surgery have become common practice. This is based on studies which have shown a decrease in microbial flora in the tear film after a short course of antibiotics given topically.[10] To be effective in preventing endophthalmitis, a topical antibiotic must penetrate the eye with a significant concentration that well exceeds the MIC of the bacterial pathogens of concern, without causing significant toxicity to ocular structures. Studies involving fourth-generation fluoroquinolones have shown that they have good absorption into the aqueous humor[11] when applied topically, without causing toxicity to ocular structures. Moxifloxacin 0.5% may have better penetration compared to gatifloxacin 0.3% and the second-generation ciprofloxacin 0.3% when applied to the surface of the eye.[12,13] Although preoperative topical antibiotics are becoming the "standard of care," the downsides must be considered since these medications are expensive, can induce allergic reactions and widespread use may lead to bacterial resistance in the future. In addition, further studies are warranted to prove the efficacy of preoperative topical antibiotics with respect to infection prevention.

OPERATIVE MEASURES TO REDUCE INFECTION

The only proven method of prophylaxis against postoperative endophthalmitis is sterile ophthalmic preparation using povidone iodine solution on the skin (5–10%) and in the conjunctival sac (5%).[9,14,15] Povidone iodine is effective against a wide variety of pathogens including bacteria, fungi, spores, viruses and protozoa.[16] After the skin and ocular preparation with povidone iodine is completed, it is important to drape the patient so that the lashes and lid margin are isolated from the surgical field. After the drape is cut and lid speculum placed, it is helpful to push back or snip stray lashes before the procedure is begun. However, routine lash trimming prior to surgery has not been shown to be effective in reducing periocular bacterial flora and is not recommended.[17]

A 2005 survey of 800 ophthalmologists in UK teaching hospitals revealed that 99% of those surveyed used povidone iodine for skin preparation and 70% used povidone iodine 5% or 10% in the conjunctival sac. A large portion of surgeons surveyed also routinely use subconjunctival cefuroxime (66.4%) intraoperatively[18] and 18% of surgeons used intracameral antibiotics either directly into the eye or as part of the irrigation fluid. There is no definitive evidence to support the use of subconjunctival antibiotics at the conclusion of surgery or supplementation of the irrigating fluid with antibiotics. While studies involving antibiotic supplementation to the irrigation fluid have not yielded any conclusive benefit, recent studies involving intracameral antibiotics have shown promise. A large, multinational study conducted by the ESCRS Study group showed a significant benefit of intracameral cefuroxime in reducing rates of bacterial endophthalmitis

following routine cataract surgery. In this randomized controlled study, patients were given either intracameral cefuroxime or perioperative topical levofloxacin and a significantly reduced rate of endophthalmitis was reported in the cefuroxime group.[19] This result prompted the study to be halted early. However, while a fivefold reduction in infection was noted in the treatment group, the infection rate in the control group was higher than shown in other published data on post-cataract endophthalmitis and warrants further investigation. Regardless, the benefit of intracameral cefuroxime in reducing infection is apparent from this study. A recently published safety study of intracameral moxifloxacin 0.5%, instilled into the anterior chamber (0.1 mL) of 65 patients at the conclusion of surgery, demonstrated a lack of toxicity to ocular structures. Measures used to evaluate toxicity included endothelial cell counts, corneal pachymetry, anterior chamber reaction and visual recovery after phacoemulsification. While it appears to be safe for intraocular use, further studies are warranted to demonstrate the efficacy of intracameral moxifloxacin 0.5% for the prevention of infectious endophthalmitis.

The routine use of preoperative and/or operative antibiotics for infection prophylaxis must be carefully weighed against its risks, as bacterial resistance has become an increasing problem. Particularly, resistance to vancomycin has become a concern of the Centers for Disease Control who specifically recommend against the routine use of vancomycin for perioperative antibiotic prophylaxis.[20]

The most important step that the surgeon can make in controlling infection is to construct a wound with the proper surface architecture to allow for a hermetic seal and optimal stability. Several characteristics of wound construction are important, the most important being wound architecture. Ex vivo studies in cadaver eyes[21] have shown that square incisions are more stable than rectangular ones. The stability of square and nearly square clear corneal incisions has been confirmed by studies in human eyes.[22] There are several blades currently in use to create clear corneal wounds, many of which achieve similar results. More important than blade selection, however, is aiming for a square or nearly square incision to increase the probability of a stable, hermetically sealed wound. Other factors play a role such as size of incision, angle of insertion and shelving. Future standards for wound architecture and construction are warranted in order to determine the optimal surface architecture for wound stability with regards to reduced infection rates. (See Video 1 – Masket 2 min.)

Perhaps equally as important as wound construction is wound sealing, and confirmation of incisional sealing at the conclusion of surgery is mandatory. Manipulation of the clear corneal wound by surgical instrumentation can lead to wound stretch and threaten the stability of the wound.[23] It has been suggested that the use of unsleeved, rigid, round tubes, as in bimanual phacoemulsification, may compromise wound integrity.[24] If there is a suspicion of the potential for wound stretch because of surgical instrumentation during phacoemulsification or IOL placement, the Steinert-Deacon gauge can be used to confirm wound size (Figure 12-1). We recommend the use of intraoperative Seidel testing to demonstrate incisional sealing, however, other methods can be utilized as long as a hermetic seal is confirmed at the conclusion of the procedure. A fluorescein strip is applied to the wound after the wound has been hydrated and the wound is observed for leakage. If leakage is found, the wound is re-hydrated and/or a corneal suture is placed. In our view, hydration

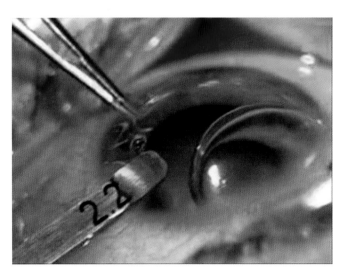

Figure 12-1 Steinert Deacon Gauge.

of the wound allows for apposition of the internal wound lips, thus facilitating wound seal. Although the efficacy of this technique has not been proven, it has become common practice. Attention should be given to hydration of the roof of the incision, as well as the sides, if stromal hydration is performed. There should be no hesitation in using a 10-0 suture to close the clear corneal incision in the presence of vitreous loss, iris prolapse, thermal burns or an unstable wound. Finally, a recheck of the intraocular pressure should be done, either with the use of a tonometer (Figure 12.2) or by digital palpation as hypotonous IOPs lead to unstable wounds.[25] It has been demonstrated that in the presence of a well-constructed, well-sealed wound, postoperative hypotony can be avoided.[22] (See Video 2 – Wound end.)

■ INFLAMMATION ■

Postoperative inflammation following cataract surgery is largely mediated by the arachidonic acid cascade (Figure 12.3). This results in the production of prostaglandins, which can ultimately lead to a breakdown of the blood–aqueous barrier. This inflammation results from surgical trauma and contributes to common postoperative complications including corneal edema, uveitis, and cystoid macular edema. Anti-inflammatory medications, such as corticosteroids and nonsteroidal anti-inflammatory drugs (NSAIDs), are commonly used to control the inflammatory response and reduce the frequency of the aforementioned complications. Whereas corticosteroids prevent the production of prostaglandins by inhibiting phospholipase A2, NSAIDs inhibit the cyclooxygenase enzyme later in the arachidonic acid cascade.[26]

Cystoid macular edema (CME) after cataract surgery was first described by Irvine in 1953 and results from the leakage of fluid from the perifoveal capillaries. CME can be categorized as either acute (less than 4 months after surgery) or chronic (persistence for more than 4 months after surgery). Several studies have examined the use of NSAIDs in the treatment of acute CME.[27,28] Although small, some of these studies have suggested that topical NSAIDs may have a therapeutic benefit in acute CME. In chronic CME, topical NSAIDs do appear to have a statistically significant benefit.[29] Newer NSAIDs, such as nepafenac, may prove to be more effective in controlling posterior segment inflammation because of their superior corneal penetration and bioactivation at target tissues.[30]

Because corticosteroids interfere with the arachidonic acid cycle at an earlier step, there is a higher incidence of adverse effects compared to that of NSAIDs. For example, in addition to their known anti-inflammatory properties, corticosteroids can be associated with elevations in intraocular pressure and impaired wound healing.[26] However, newer topical corticosteroids, such as loteprednol and rimexolone, have a lower risk of intraocular pressure changes.

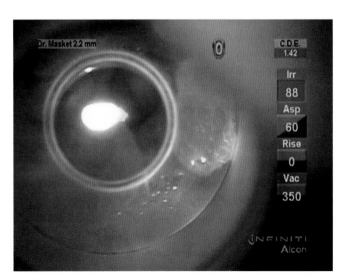

Figure 12-2 Barraquer Tonometer.

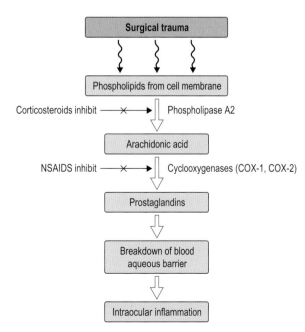

Figure 12-3 Arachidonic acid cascade.

PREOPERATIVE MEASURE TO REDUCE INFLAMMATION

NSAIDs

Since NSAIDs inhibit the production of prostaglandins, it is logical that they would be beneficial in preventing the inflammatory cascade before it begins. The use of preoperative NSAIDs has been shown to reduce postoperative inflammation, the incidence of cystoid macular edema, and patient discomfort.[31,32] It has become commonplace to use NSAIDs preoperatively and continue them postoperatively with topical steroids to reduce these complications.[33] The NSAID is started between 3 days and 1 h prior to surgery. Patients with diabetes mellitus are at increased risk of developing retinal edema, including CME, which has been confirmed by OCT.[34] While it has not been definitively shown that treating diabetics with topical NSAIDs preoperatively leads to reduced rates of postoperative CME, this should be considered in the preoperative evaluation, especially in patients with evidence of active retinopathy.

Patients with pre-existing inflammation prior to cataract extraction, such as those with chronic uveitis will likely require topical corticosteroids preoperatively and in some cases may also benefit from oral steroids in the immediate preoperative period. Active intraocular inflammation should be eliminated prior to scheduling surgery.

Prostaglandin analogs

Prostaglandin analogues may also lead to intraocular inflammation after routine cataract surgery and increase the chance of CME by disrupting the blood–aqueous barrier.[35] Hypotensive lipids such as latanoprost, travoprost, and bimatoprost, have been implicated in causing pseudophakic cystoid macular edema.[35–38] Is has been shown, however, that it is the preservative, benzalkonium chloride (BAK) in these medications that is responsible for inciting the inflammatory cascade; this is now termed *pseudophakic preservative maculopathy*.[39] A survey of UK ophthalmologists in 2003 revealed that 40.3% of ophthalmologists stopped prostaglandin analogs less than 1 week prior to surgery and resumed the medication 1–2 months after surgery.[40] Fortunately, in most instances, the induced CME is reversible upon discontinuation of the medication and administration of topical NSAIDs. A study to demonstrate a clear benefit to discontinuing the medication does not exist and most patients will probably not have a problem in uncomplicated surgery; however, consideration should be given to discontinuing the medication in selected patients who are at high risk of developing postoperative CME.

OPERATIVE MEASURES TO REDUCE INFLAMMATION

Factors which contribute to increased postoperative inflammation include prolonged surgery time, iris trauma, malpositioned IOLs, retained lens material and surgical complications including vitreous loss. Anterior chamber IOLs may be associated with postoperative inflammation if they are too large, too small, or positioned incorrectly. The introduction of immunogenic foreign material into the eye can incite a severe postoperative inflammatory reaction; this has been reported with increasing frequency in the past few years.

TASS is characterized by postoperative inflammation that usually begins in the first 24 h after cataract surgery and is believed to be due to toxic substances that enter the eye during surgery.[41] It was first described in 1992 by Monson et al. and is an inflammatory reaction, not an infectious process, that is limited to the anterior segment structures. Symptoms of TASS are similar to those of infectious endophthalmitis, which makes the diagnosis difficult to distinguish at times. However, the onset of TASS is often sooner than the typical 2–5 day onset of postoperative endophthalmitis. Clinical signs are also similar to patients with endophthalmitis with decreased vision, hypopyon formation and severe anterior segment inflammation. Mamalis et al.[41] describe other typical findings in TASS which include limbus-to-limbus corneal edema due to endothelial cell damage and pupillary abnormalities including a dilated, poorly reactive pupil. Severe intraocular inflammation in TASS can also lead to secondary glaucoma.

Implicated as causes for TASS are a wide variety of substances that are toxic to the eye including: intraocular anesthetics, detergents used to clean instruments, denatured viscoelastic agents, antibiotics, preservatives, ophthalmic ointments, and other contaminants that enter the eye during surgery. An increase in the number of TASS cases was noted in the early part of 2006 by the TASS Task Force, established by the ASCRS. In their published report,[42] a specific etiology responsible for this increase in cases was not identified; however, improper cleaning and sterilization of ophthalmic surgical instruments was believed to be a major factor contributing to the reported TASS cases. In this report, it was emphasized that any reused cannulated instruments, including phacoemulsification and I/A handpieces, be flushed thoroughly at the conclusion of surgery, and that single-use devices be discarded. These instruments may harbor residues of viscoelastic agents or lens material which may incite TASS. In addition, reused instruments that are cleaned with detergents or enzymes must be rinsed thoroughly with sterile, deionized/distilled water before use. They identified a potential contaminant in ultrasound water baths, as well as other water sources, which can harbor bacteria capable of producing heat-stable, unautoclavable endotoxins that can incite TASS. Preservative-containing medications or solutions containing sulfites or other toxic minerals should not be administered directly into the eye. This includes intracameral antibiotics/anesthetics or additives to irrigation solutions. In this report, no particular IOL was found to be more likely to contribute to TASS.

The initial approach to a patient suspected as having TASS is to rule out infection. Whereas infectious endophthalmitis involves the vitreous cavity, TASS related inflammation is typically confined to the anterior segment. However, in many cases, distinguishing the two conditions may be difficult and an aqueous tap may be required. Once the diagnosis of TASS is made, topical steroid should be administered with frequent dosing. The recommendation is to use prednisolone acetate 1% drops every 1–2 h. Intraocular pressure, which may be low initially due to ciliary body shutdown, may rise secondarily from damage to the trabecular meshwork. Gonioscopy as well as specular microscopy should be performed as soon as the cornea clears.

Prevention is the key to reducing the incidence of TASS. Particular attention should be placed on proper sterilization and cleaning of surgical instruments, and careful monitoring of all medications and solutions that enter the eye. When a new case of TASS is confirmed, a careful review of the operating room procedures and medications administered to the patient should be performed in order to promptly identify causative factors and modify them.

OPERATIVE MEASURES FOR CONTROL OF INTRAOCULAR PRESSURE ■

WOUND CONSTRUCTION

Previous work by Shingleton et al. has shown that postoperative hypotony may occur in as many as 20% of patients after clear corneal cataract extraction.[43] While hypotony is certainly a complication of any intraocular procedure, this risk can be reduced in the presence of a square or nearly square incision with meticulous control of incisional sealing. Postoperative IOP is, in fact, relatively stable compared to that set at the immediate conclusion of the procedure in the presence of a sealed wound.[22]

To allow for internal wound lip apposition, it is important that the IOP initially be set to a level higher than physiologic. However, it is not necessary to keep the pressure at this level at the conclusion of the procedure. The use of a Barraquer or Shiotz tonometer (see Figure 12-2) is useful in measuring intraoperative IOP. In our experience,[22] we use one of these devices to measure IOP after incisional sealing has been confirmed. The IOP can then be titrated to the desired level by removing small aliquots of fluid from the anterior chamber and, finally, rechecked using the tonometer.

USE OF INTRACAMERAL MIOTICS

The use of intracameral miotics has been studied to lower early postoperative IOP and may be useful when strict control of postoperative IOP is particularly important. The use of intracameral carbachol 0.01% (Miostat, Alcon) has been shown to result in lower IOPs in the first 24 h after clear corneal phacoemulsification with statistical significance.[44–48] However, the use of intracameral carbachol has also been demonstrated to result in increased postoperative inflammation, believed to be due to delayed restitution of the blood–aqueous barrier. Studies comparing carbachol to acetylcholine chloride (Miochol, Novartis Ophthalmics) have found a greater effectiveness of intracameral carbachol with respect to reduction of IOP after cataract extraction.[49,50]

CONCLUSION ■

As modern cataract surgery is accomplished with clear, corneal incisions, it is important that these wounds be constructed meticulously and consistently with the proper surface architecture. Creating a tightly sealed incision is perhaps the most important step that the surgeon can take in preventing, or at least reducing, the chances of a devastating infectious complication. Preoperative antibiotics have become routine practice and, in the near future, intracameral antibiotics may become the standard of care. However, it is important to weigh the benefits of antibiotic

prophylaxis with the risks of engendering bacterial resistance. With every substance and every instrument that is placed into the eye, care must taken to ensure that it is free of toxic contaminants, as TASS is becoming an increasingly recognized problem. Since prevention is always better than cure, preoperative and operatives measures to reduce infection, inflammation and IOP elevations are essential to optimize outcomes after cataract surgery.

References

[1] Cooper BA, Holekamp NM, Bohigian G, Thompson PA. Case-control study of endophthalmitis after cataract surgery comparing scleral tunnel and clear corneal wounds. Am J Ophthalmol 2003;136:300–305.

[2] Colleaux KM, Hamilton WK. Effect of prophylactic antibiotics and incision type on the incidence of endophthalmitis after cataract surgery. Can J Ophthalmol 2000;35:373–378.

[3] Nagaki Y, Hayasaka S, Kadoi C et al. Bacterial endophthalmitis after small-incision cataract surgery: effect of incision placement and intraocular lens type. J Cataract Refract Surg 2003;29:20–26.

[4] Taban M, Behrens A, Newcomb RL et al. Acute endophthalmitis following cataract surgery. Arch Ophthalmol 2005;123:613–620.

[5] West ES, Behrens A, McDonnell PJ et al. The incidence of endophthalmitis after cataract surgery among the U.S. Medicare population increased between 1994 and 2001. Ophthalmology 2005;112:1388–1394.

[6] Taban M, Sarayba MA, Ignacio TS, Behrens A, McDonnell PJ. Ingress of India ink into the anterior chamber through sutureless clear corneal cataract wounds. Arch Ophthalmol 2005;123: 643–648.

[7] Phillips 2nd WB, Tasman WS. Postoperative endophthalmitis in association with diabetes mellitus. Ophthalmology 1994;101:508–518.

[8] Norregaard JC, Thoning H, Bernth-Petersen P, Andersen TF, Javitt JC, Anderson GF. Risk of endophthalmitis after cataract extraction: results from the International Cataract Surgery Outcomes Study. Br J Ophthalmol 1997;81:102–106.

[9] Ciulla T, Starr M, Masket S. Bacterial endophthalmitis prophylaxis for cataract surgery: An evidence-based update. Ophthalmology 2002;109:13–24.

[10] Ta C, Egbert P, Singh K et al. Prospective randomized comparison of 3-day versus 1-hour preoperative ofloxacin prophylaxis for cataract surgery. Ophthalmology 2002;109:2036–2040.

[11] Katz HR, Masket S, Lane SS, Sall K, Orr SC, Faulkner RD, et al. Absorption of topical moxifloxacin ophthalmic solution into human aqueous humor. Cornea 2005;24:955–958.

[12] Kim DH, Stark WJ, O'Brien TP, Dick JD. Aqueous penetration and biological activity of moxifloxacin 0.5% ophthalmic solution and gatifloxacin 0.3% solution in cataract surgery patients. Ophthalmology 2005;112:1992–1996. [Epub 2005 Sep 23].

[13] Solomon R, Donnenfeld ED, Perry HD, Snyder RW, Nedrud C, Stein J, et al. Penetration of topically applied gatifloxacin 0.3%, moxifloxacin 0.5%, and ciprofloxacin 0.3% in the aqueous humor. Ophthalmology 2005;112:466–469.

[14] Trinavarat A, Atchaneeyasakul L, Nopmaneejumreslers C, Inson K. Reduction of endophthalmitis rate after cataract surgery with preoperative 5% povidone-iodine. Dermatology 2006;212 (Suppl. 1):35–40.

[15] Speaker MG, Menikoff. Prophylaxis of endophthalmitis with topical povidone-iodine. Ophthalmology 1991;98:1769–1775.

[16] Boes DA, Lindquist TD, Fritsche TR, Kalina RE. Effects of povidone-iodine chemical preparation and saline irrigation on the perilimbal flora. Ophthalmology 1992;99:1569–1574.

[17] Perry L, Skaggs C. Preoperative topical antibiotics and lash trimming in cataract surgery. Ophthalmic Surg 1977;8:44–48.

[18] Gordon-Bennett P, Karas A, Flanagan D, Stephenson C, Hingorani M. A survey of measures used for the prevention of postoperative endophthalmitis after cataract surgery in the United Kingdom. Eye 2008;22:620–627. [Epub 2006 Dec 15].

[19] Barry P, Seal DV, Gettinby G, Lees F, Peterson M, Revie CW. ESCRS Endophthalmitis Study Group: ESCRS study of prophylaxis of postoperative endophthalmitis after cataract surgery: preliminary report of principal results from a European multicenter study. J Cataract Refract Surg 2006;32:407–410.

[20] Centers for Diseases Control and Prevention. Recommendations for preventing the spread of vancomycin resistance. Recommendations of the Hospital Infection Control Practices Advisory Committee. MMWR Morb Mortal Wkly Rep 1995;44:1–13.

[21] Ernest PH, Lavery KT, Kiessling LA. Relative strength of scleral *Cornea* l and clear *Cornea* l incisions constructed in cadaver eyes. J Cataract Refract Surg 1994;20(6):626–629.

[22] Masket S, Belani S. Proper wound construction to prevent short-term ocular hypotony after clear corneal incision cataract surgery. J Cataract Refract Surg 2007;33:383–386.

[23] Nichamin L, Chang D, Johnson S, Mamalis N, Masket S, Packard R, et al. What is the association between clear cornea cataract incisions and postoperative endophthalmitis? ASCRS White Paper. J Cataract Refract Surg 2006;32(9):1556–1559.

[24] Masket S, editor. Consultation section; cataract surgical problem. J Cataract Refract Surg 2004;30:1613–1621.

[25] Taban M, Rao B, Reznik J et al. Dynamic morphology of sutureless cataract wounds – effect of incision angle and location. Surv Ophthalmol 2004;49(suppl 2):S62–S72.

[26] Simone JN, Whitacre MM. Effects of anti-inflammatory drugs following cataract extraction. Curr Opin Ophthalmol 2001;12:63–67.

[27] Flach AJ. The incidence, pathogenesis and treatment of cystoid macular edema following cataract surgery. Trans Am Ophthalmol Soc 1998;96:557–634.

[28] Heier JS, Topping TM, Baumann W, Dirks MS, Chern S. Ketorolac versus prednisolone verus combination therapy in the treatment of acute pseudophakic cystoid macular edema. Ophthalmology 2000;107(11):2034–2038.

[29] Sivaprasad S, Bunce C, Patel N. Non-steroidal anti-inflammatory agents for treating cystoid macular oedema following cataract surgery. Cochrane Database Syst Rev 2005;25(1):CD004239.

[30] Lindstrom R, Kim T. Ocular permeation and inhibition of retinal inflammation: an examination of data and expert opinion on the clinical utility of nepafenac. Curr Med Res Opin 2006;22 (2):397–404.

[31] Donnenfeld E, Perry H, Wittpenn J, Solomon R, Nattis A, Chou T. Preoperative ketorolac tromethamin 0.4% in phacoemulsification outcomes: pharmacokinetic–response curve. J Cataract Refract Surg 2006;32:1474–1482.

[32] Lane S, Modi S, Lehmann R, Holland E. Nepafenac ophthalmic suspension 0.1% for the prevention and treatment of ocular inflammation associated with cataract surgery. J Cataract Refract Surg 2007;33:53–58.

[33] Flach A. Topical nonsteroidal anti-inflammatory drugs in ophthalmology. Int Ophthalmol Clin 2002;42:1–11.

[34] Torron-Fernandex-Blanco C, Ruiz-Moreno O, Ferrer-Novella E, Sanchez-Cano A, Honrubia-Lopez FM. Pseudophakic cystoid macular edema. Assessment with optical coherence tomography. Arch Soc Esp Oftalmol 2006;81:147–153.

[35] Miyake K, Ota I, Maekuba K et al. Latanoprost accelerates disruption of the blood–aqueous barrier and the incidence of angiographic cystoid macular edema in early postoperative pseudophakias. Arch Ophthalmol 1999;117:34–40.

[36] Wand M, Gaudio AR, Shields MB. Latanoprost and cystoid macular edema in high-risk aphakic or pseudophakic eyes. J Cataract Refract Surg 2001;27:1397–1401.

[37] Kruse P, Rieck P, Sherif Z, Liekfeld A. Cystoid macular edema in a pseudophakic patient after several glaucoma procedures. Is local therapy with brimatoprost the reason? Klin Monatsbl Augenheilkd 2006;223(6):534–537.

[38] Arcieri ES, Santana A, Rocha FN, Guapo GL, Costa VP. Blood–aqueous barrier changes after the use of prostaglandin analogues in patients with pseudophakia and aphakia: a 6-month randomized trial. Arch Ophthalmol 2005;123(2):186–192.

[39] Miyake K, Ibaraki N, Goto Y et al. ESCRS Binkhorst Lecture 2002: pseudophakic preservative maculopathy.

[40] Ahad M, McKee H. Correspondence: stopping prostaglandin analogues in uneventful cataract surgery. J Cataract Refract Surg 2004;30(12):2644–2645.

[41] Mamalis N, Edelhauser H, Dawson D, Chew J, LeBoyer R, Werner L. Toxic anterior segment syndrome. J Cataract Refract Surg 2006;32:324–333.

[42] Mamalis N, Edelhauser H, Hellinger W, Kamae K. Toxic anterior segment syndrome (TASS) Outbreak Final Report. ASCRS Press Release 2006.

[43] Shingleton BJ, Wadhwani RA, O'Donoghue MW, Baylus S, Hoey H. Evaluation of intraocular pressure in the immediate period after phacoemulsification. J Cataract Refract Surg 2001;27:524–527.

[44] Cekic O, Batman C. Effect of intracameral carbachol on intraocular pressure following clear cornea phacoemulsification. Eye 1999;13(pt 2):209–211.

[45] Solomon KD, Stewart WC, Hunt HH, Stewar JA, Cate EA. Intraoperative intracameral carbachol in phacoemulsification and posterior chamber lens implantation. Am J Ophthalmol 1998;125(1):36–43.

[46] Kim JY, Sohn JH, Youn DH. Effects of intracameral carbachol and acetylcholing on early postoperative intraocular pressure after cataract extraction. Korean J Ophthalmol 1994;8:61–65.

[47] Wedrich A, Menapace R. Intraocular pressure following small-incision cataract surgery and poly-HEMA posterior chamber lens implantation. A comparison between acetylcholine and carbachol. J Cataract Refract Surg 1992;18:500–505.

[48] Wood. Effect of carbachol on postoperative intraocular pressure. J Cataract Refract Surg 1988;14:654–656.

[49] Hollands RH, Drance SM, House PH, Shulzer M. Control of intraocular pressure after cataract; extraction. Can J Ophthalmol 1990;25:128–132.

[50] Ruiz RS, Rhem MN, Prager TC. Effects of carbachol and acetylcholine on intraocular pressure after cataract extraction. Am J Ophthalmol 1989;107:7–10.

CONCLUSION

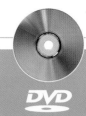

Incision Construction

I. Howard Fine, MD, Richard S. Hoffman, MD and Mark Packer, MD, FACS

13

CONTENTS

CHAPTER HIGHLIGHTS

>> Principles of self-sealing incisions

>> Development of clear corneal incisions

>> Techniques and profiles of clear corneal incisions

>> Controversies in self-sealing and sutured incision techniques

During the decade between the 1960s and the early 1970s, most cataract surgery in the United States and Europe was performed by the intracapsular cataract extraction technique using a limbal incision under a conjunctival flap. With few exceptions, there was little interest in reducing, minimizing, or altering surgically induced astigmatism.[1,2] The last 25 years have produced a rapid advancement in cataract surgery wound architecture. As the technology for removing cataracts has advanced, there has been a gradual trend towards smaller incisions, moving from the superior scleral to the temporal clear corneal location, in an attempt to reduce intraoperative complications and postoperative astigmatism.

EVOLUTION OF SMALL INCISIONS

With the advent of phacoemulsification, Kelman[3] predicted that incisions 3 mm wide would be astigmatism neutral because of their reduced size. However, within a very short time of the introduction of phacoemulsification, intraocular lens (IOL) implants became more commonplace. This situation necessitated the enlargement of the phacoemulsification incision to 6.5–7 mm for lens implantation.

Kratz is generally credited as the first surgeon to move from the limbus posteriorly to the sclera in order to increase appositional surfaces thus enhancing wound healing and reducing surgically induced astigmatism (Figure 13-1).[4,5] Girard and Hoffman[6] were first to call the posterior incision a *scleral tunnel incision* and were, along with Kratz, the first to make a point of actually entering the anterior chamber through the cornea creating a corneal shelf. This corneal shelf was designed to prevent iris prolapse. Maloney, who was a fellow of Kratz, advocated a corneal shelf to his incisions, which he described as strong and waterproof.[7]

With the availability of small-incision lenses that could be introduced through incisions of 4–mm or less, the stage was set for the development of techniques that resulted in the achievement of both relative astigmatism-neutral and self-sealing incisions. In 1989, Shepherd[8] introduced the *single horizontal suture*, which was actually a vertical mattress suture, for the closure of 4 mm scleral tunnel incisions in phacoemulsification and foldable lens implantation (Figure 13-2). The achievement of astigmatism neutrality was impressive. Others rapidly recognized that the compressive force of the single horizontal suture was tangential to the limbus and, therefore, exerted no force on the cornea, which would alter its curvature. As a result, variations of the Shepherd single stitch were soon developed for closure of incisions 5–7 mm wide, including the Fine infinity suture (Figure 13-3),[9] Masket's horizontal anchor suture (Figure 13-4),[10] and Fishkind's horizontal overlap suture (Figure 13-5).[11]

In 1989, McFarland[12] utilized the corneal shelf incision architecture and recognized that these incisions sized for foldable IOLs allowed for the phacoemulsification and implantation of lenses without the need for suturing. This involved lengthening the scleral tunnel and, in his early attempts, creating partial-thickness grooves in the floor of the scleral tunnel parallel to the long axis of the tunnel so that the incision could be reversibly stretched to admit a foldable lens.

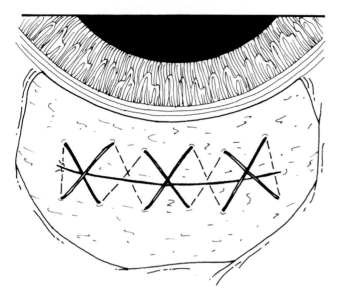

Figure 13-1 The scleral tunnel incision and running suture closure.

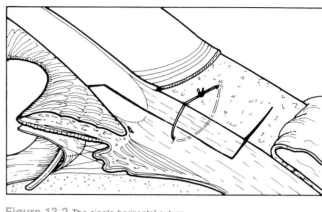

Figure 13-2 The single horizontal suture.

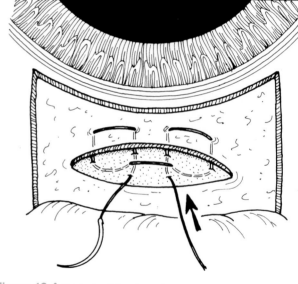

Figure 13-4 The horizontal anchor suture.

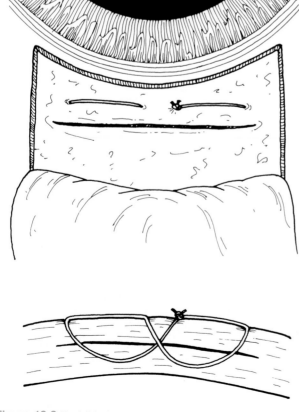

Figure 13-3 The infinity suture.

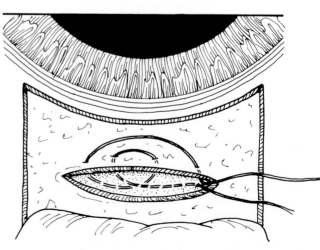

Figure 13-5 The horizontal overlap suture.

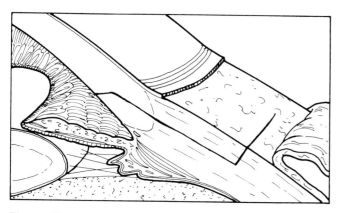

Figure 13-6 The self-sealing "corneal lip" scleral tunnel incision.

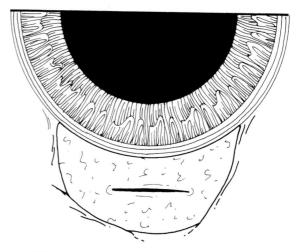

Figure 13-8 Scleral tunnel incision with straight groove.

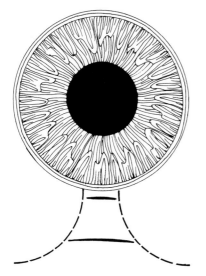

Figure 13-7 Incisional funnel with two possible incisions illustrated: both astigmatism neutral.

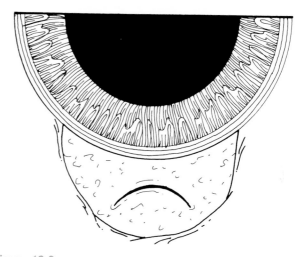

Figure 13-9 Frown incision.

SURGICAL TECHNIQUES FOR SCLERAL TUNNEL INCISIONS

Ernest[13] observed McFarland's surgery and recognized that McFarland's long scleral tunnel incision terminated in a decidedly corneal entrance and that the posterior lip of the incision, the so-called corneal lip, acted as a one-way valve imparting to this incision its self-sealing characteristics (Figure 13-6). Koch[14] described what he called the *incisional funnel* (Figure 13-7), indicating that there were certain characteristics of seal-sealing incisions with respect to length and configuration that imparted not only self-sealability, but also astigmatism neutrality to these incisions.

Self-sealing scleral tunnel incisions have varied with respect to width and the configuration of the groove (which represents the external or scleral incision as opposed to the internal or corneal portion of the incision). The groove has varied from circumlimbal to straight (Figure 13-8), frown (Figure 13-9) or chevron-shaped.[15–18]

■ SURGICAL TECHNIQUES FOR SCLERAL TUNNEL INCISIONS ■

In the following passage, we describe in detail the construction of a self-sealing scleral tunnel incision using a straight external scleral groove and a tunnel width of 4 mm, recognizing that the same tunnel can be made 7 mm wide with enlargement of the internal opening from 3 to 7 mm following completion of phacoemulsification and cortical cleanup, and just before lens implantation.

A conjunctival flap is made precisely by marking the width of the scleral tunnel at the limbus (Figure 13.10), and making vertical releasing incisions in the conjunctiva and Tenon's at exactly that width. These vertical releasing incisions extend back approximately 5 mm. The sub-tenon's space is bluntly dissected with a scissors (Figure 13.11) before a peritomy (Figure 13.12). After the peritomy, the conjunctiva-Tenon's flap is folded at its base upside down on top of the posterior conjunctiva. The peritomy leaves approximately a 0.5–1 mm lip of conjunctiva attached to the limbus. This acts as a buttress postoperatively to prevent anterior migration of the conjunctiva so that the flap never overhangs the limbus.

Mild cautery is performed near the limbus. Posteriorly, however, heavier cautery is used. The large vessels emanating from the rectus muscle and perforating the sclera between the muscle and the beginning of the tunnel are cauterized directly and adequately. (If these perforating vessels are cauterized before they enter the sclera, the tunnel should be dry during the entire

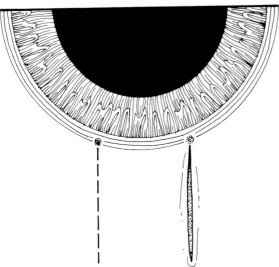

Figure 13-10 Caliper marks on conjunctiva to indicate position of vertical releasing incisions.

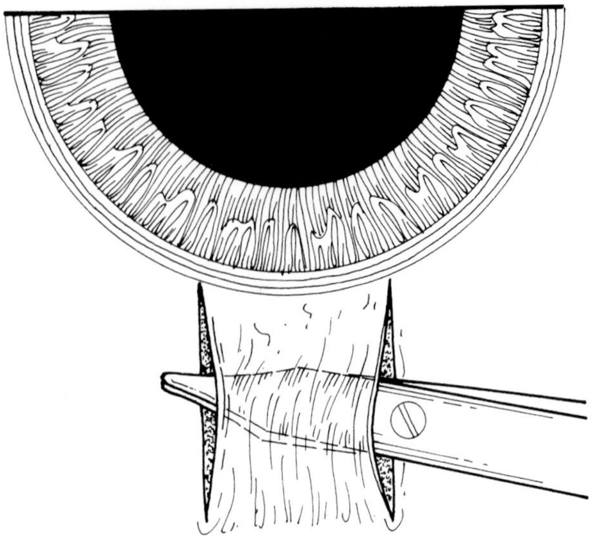

Figure 13-11 Blunt dissection of sub-Tenon's space with closed scissors.

procedure and there should be no bleeding either intraoperatively or postoperatively resulting in hyphema.)

Following cautery, a Fine millimeter marker (Rhein Medical No. 8-12106) is stamped in methylene blue and then pressed to the scleral bed, creating a 5 × 8 mm grid of dots 1 mm apart starting 1 mm posterior to the anterior edge of the corneal vascular arcade (Figure 13-13). This allows selection of an incision length, location and shape with great precision and reproducibility.[17] The globe is fixated with a twist grip (Weck No. 7640) posteriorly in the area of bared sclera and the sclera is cut perpendicularly to make a groove by incising the appropriate dots (Figure 13-14). The groove is sufficiently deep that the surgeon can look down the groove and pick the depth within the sclera at which he or she will dissect the scleral tunnel. A slight anterior edge is elevated with the No. 64 Beaver blade that is used to make the groove, and from that point on an Alcon

bevel-up crescent knife (Figure 13-15) (Alcon 8065-940002) is used to dissect the scleral tunnel. (It is important to keep the leading edge of the knife down, whether cutting anteriorly or to either side, as one moves the knife. This is a sharp knife that makes a very clean dissection in the scleral plane.) The dissection is carried forward to the Descemet's membrane at the anterior edge of the vascular arcade (Figure 13-16).

At this point, a side port is made with a trifacet freehand diamond knife (No. KOI KM218R). Viscoelastic is exchanged for aqueous humor through the side port by injecting the viscoelastic into the distal angle. As the expanding wave of viscoelastic moves towards the paracentesis, aqueous humor is expressed. This results in a very stiff and stable anterior chamber. A 3.5 mm keratome blade (Beaver No 5530) is lubricated with viscoelastic and brought into the tunnel. The blade is advanced so

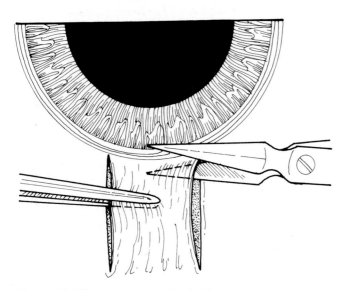

Figure 13-12 Peritomizing the conjunctival flap.

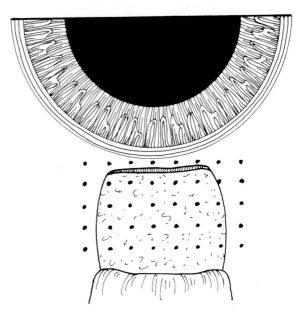

Figure 13-13 Millimeter grid on bare scleral bed.

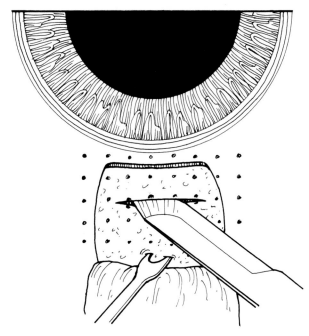

Figure 13-14 Initiation of the groove or external incision.

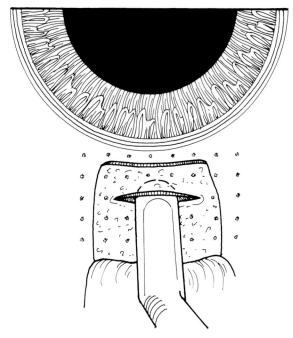

Figure 13-15 Initiation of the tunnel with a crescent knife.

that its point is just at the anterior edge of the vascular arcade. The point is tipped slightly posteriorly, resulting in a dimple on the anterior surface of the cornea, whose center is directly on the anterior edge of the arcade. The dimple is frequently outlined by a semicircular light reflex (Figure 13-17) with the tip of the keratome at the center. The keratome is then advanced horizontally, parallel to the iris, which results in a linear horizontal cut through Descemet's membrane into the anterior chamber, 0.5 mm anterior to the edge of the vascular arcade (Figure 13-18).

The surgeon must continuously guide the tip of the keratome as it is brought into the anterior chamber. If it is pointed too

posteriorly, the cut in Descemet's membrane will start to curve posteriorly at the ends in a "frown" configuration. On the other hand, if the tip of the keratome is elevated too much, the cut in Descemet's membrane will start to curve forward in a "smile" configuration rather than proceeding straight across and parallel to the groove. If the keratome is tilted to one side or the other, an "S-shaped" configuration may result. In all instances, observation of the cut as it proceeds in Descemet's membrane by advancing the keratome can allow for correction of the orientation of the keratome. A straight cut in Descemet's membrane is necessary for the correct architecture of the incision.

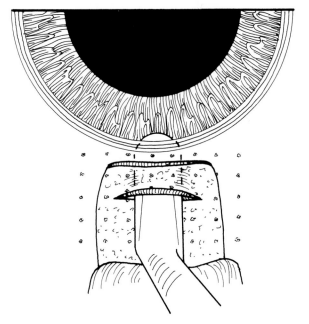

Figure 13-16 Dissection of the scleral tunnel into clear cornea.

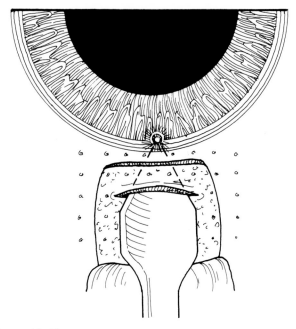

Figure 13-17 Dimpling of the cornea by depressing the point of the keratome.

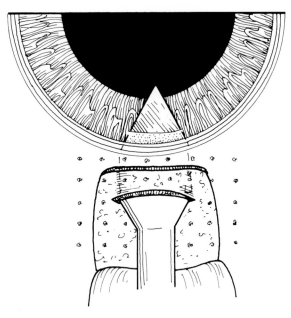

Figure 13-18 Straight-line incision in Descemet's membrane 0.5 mm anterior to the vascular arcade.

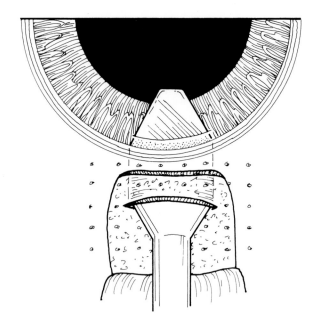

Figure 13-19 Enlargement of the 3.5 mm incision to 4.0 mm with a blunt tipped keratome.

The incision is complete when the parallel shoulders of the keratome enter the anterior chamber. The incision can be characterized by the presence of a short posterior lip of clear cornea that acts as a one-way valve.[19] Following the completion of the case, this valve is held closed by intraocular pressure which also acts to collapse the scleral tunnel.

If one goes more anteriorly into clear cornea before incising Descemet's membrane, the visualization during phacoemulsification is markedly impaired because of the striae that occur as the phaco tip is tilted down for endolenticular phacoemulsification.

It is important to avoid putting traction on the roof of the scleral tunnel with a forceps. A bridle suture is used during incision construction and the twist grip is placed posterior to the dot grid to stabilize the globe during construction of the scleral tunnel. The forceps is used to elevate the tunnel roof in placing the keratome inside the tunnel, but countertraction is placed on the posterior lip of the groove rather than the anterior lip during the cutting of Descemet's membrane with the keratome.

Phacoemulsification and later evacuation of viscoelastic take place with the bridle suture unattached to minimize stretching of the tunnel roof. After cortical cleanup and expansion of the bag with viscoelastic, the incision in Descemet's membrane is widened with a 4 mm blunt-tip keratome (Figure 13-19) (Beaver No. 374732) for folded silicone lenses. For 6 mm lenses, the initial keratome incision is enlarged with a super-sharp knife (15° Alcon ophthalmic knife No. 8065-921502) taking care to incise Descemet's membrane as a continuation of the straight-line cut made by the 3.5 mm keratome.

Following IOL implantation and evacuation of residual viscoelastic, the anterior chamber is fully repressurized with BSS through the side port. The lips of the wound are tested by applying pressure with a Weck cell sponge against the posterior lip of the wound (Figure 13-20) in an effort to make the incision leak.

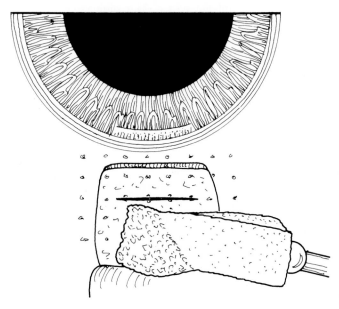

Figure 13-20 Testing the scleral incision for being watertight.

If it does leak, which happens less than 5% of the time, a single horizontal suture is placed (in the case of incisions 5 mm or larger, an infinity suture is placed). If no leakage is observed, the conjunctival flap is unfolded back over the incision and smoothed in place. Its corners are returned to the corners of the bed from which they were derived, up against the remaining lip of conjunctiva attached to the limbus (Figure 13-21). The flap is frequently adherent within 1 h, as observed in one-eyed patients who are not patched at the conclusion of surgery. A Maloney keratometer is used to estimate astigmatism at the conclusion of the surgery (Figure 13-22).[15]

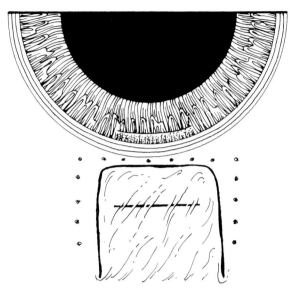

Figure 13-21 Conjunctival flap repositioned in its bed.

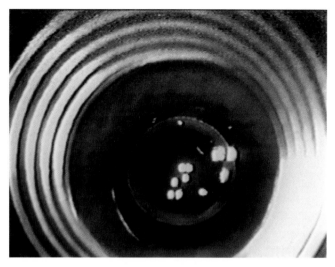

Figure 13-22 Estimation of corneal curvature using a Maloney intraoperative qualitative keratometer.

■ DEVELOPMENT OF CLEAR CORNEAL INCISIONS ■

There have been many surgeons who have favored corneal incisions for cataract surgery prior to their recent popularization. In 1968, Kelman[3] stated that the best approach for performing cataract surgery was with phacoemulsification through a clear corneal incision utilizing a triangular-tear capsulotomy and a grooving and cracking technique in the posterior chamber. Harms and Mackenson[20] in Germany published an intracapsular technique using a corneal incision in 1967 in an atlas called *Ocular Surgery Under the Microscope.* Troutman was an early advocate of controlling surgically induced astigmatism at the time of cataract surgery by means of the corneal-incision approach.[21] Arnott[22] in England used clear corneal incisions and a diamond keratome for phacoemulsification, although he had to enlarge the incision for introducing an IOL. Galand[23] in Belgium utilized clear corneal incisions for extracapsular

cataract extraction in his envelope technique and Stegmann of South Africa has a long history of having used the cornea as the site for incisions for extracapsular cataract extraction (Stegmann R. Personal communication, December 3, 1992). In April of 1992, Fine presented his self-sealing temporal clear corneal incision at the annual meeting of the American Society of Cataract and Refractive Surgery.[24] In May of 1992, at the Island Ophthalmology Seminar, Kellan demonstrated on video a technique that he referred to as the scleral-less incision. It was essentially a corneal limbal stab incision through conjunctiva and the limbus, entering the anterior chamber through clear cornea, leaving a corneal shelf or lip (Figure 13-23A and B). Finally, perhaps the leading proponent of clear corneal incisions for modern era phacoemulsification was Kimiya Shimizu of Japan.[25]

Fine's personal experience with corneal incisions began in 1979 when the temporal clear cornea was used as the site for secondary anterior chamber IOL implantation. The temporal

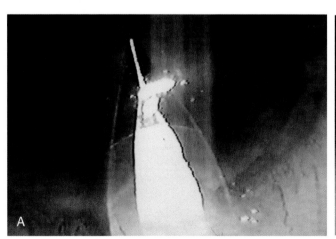

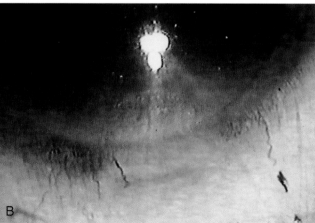

Figure 13-23 **A,** Kellan's corneal limbal stab incision through conjunctiva and the limbus. **B,** Corneal limbal incision following removal of the steel keratome.

approach was preferred because of the unpredictable nature of the disturbed anatomy present at the superior limbus in eyes that had previous intracapsular cataract extraction. As soon as foldable lenses were available, in 1986, he used sutured clear corneal incisions for phacoemulsification and foldable IOL implantation in patients who had pre-existing filtering blebs. After these procedures, a marked reduction in surgically induced astigmatism was noted despite the fact that these incisions were corneal rather than scleral. In 1992, Fine began routinely utilizing clear corneal cataract incisions for phacoemulsification and foldable IOL implantation with incision closure using a tangential suture modeled after John Shepherd's technique.[8] Within a very short period, the suture was abandoned in favor of self-sealing corneal incisions.[26]

INDICATIONS FOR CLEAR CORNEAL INCISIONS

Initially, the utilization of clear corneal incisions were limited to those patients with pre-existing filtering blebs, patients taking anti-coagulants or with blood dyscrasias, or patients with cicatrizing disease such as ocular cicatricial pemphigoid or Stevens–Johnson syndrome. Subsequently, because of the natural fit of clear corneal cataract incisions with topical anesthesia, the indications for clear corneal cataract surgery expanded. With the ability to avoid any injections into the orbit and utilization of intravenous medications, those patients who had cardiovascular, pulmonary, and other systemic diseases that might have contraindicated cataract surgery became surgical candidates. Subsequently, through the safety and increasing utilization of these incisions by some pioneers in the United States, including Williamson, Shepherd, Martin, and Grabow,[27] these incisions became increasingly popular and utilized on an international basis.

Studies by Rosen[28] using topographical analyses of these incisions demonstrated that clear corneal incisions sized 3 mm in width or less were topographically astigmatism-neutral. This led to an increasing interest in these incisions because of an increasing utilization of techniques including T-cuts, arcuate cuts, and limbal relaxing incisions for managing pre-existing astigmatism at the time of cataract surgery. Without astigmatism neutrality in the cataract incision, the predictability of adjunctive astigmatism-reducing procedures would be decreased, making it more difficult to achieve the desired result. In the initial studies and ultimate utilization of multifocal IOLs, the need for astigmatism neutrality was again a factor for stimulating interest in clear corneal incisions. Finally, the availability of phakic IOLs and the need for control of astigmatism at the time of implantation of these lenses has driven many surgeons to consider clear corneal incisions as the route for phakic IOL implantation.

Other advantages of the temporal clear corneal incision include:

- better preservation of pre-existing filtering blebs[29]
- preservation of options for future filtering surgery
- increased stability in the refractive results because of the neutralization of the forces from lid blink and gravity
- the ease of approach to the incision site
- the lack of need for bridle sutures and resultant iatrogenic ptosis
- the location of the lateral canthal angle under the incision which facilitates drainage.

CLASSIFICATION OF CLEAR CORNEAL INCISIONS

Early on there was criticism surrounding the use of self-sealing clear corneal incisions because of the fear of a possible increase in the incidence of endophthalmitis secondary to poor wound healing and sealability. This potential controversy stimulated many studies into the strength and safety of clear corneal incisions compared to limbal and scleral tunnel incisions. Unfortunately, because of a lack of standardization in the definition of what constitutes a limbal versus clear corneal incision, considerable confusion has been generated in this area making it difficult for surgeons to communicate and compare the relative claims of their individual techniques. Based on Hogan's *Histology of the Human Eye*: "The conjunctival vessels are seen with the slit lamp as fine arcades that extend into clear cornea for about 0.5 mm beyond the limbal edge",[30] and topographical studies of incisions done by Menapace[31] in Vienna, Fine has categorized these incisions using the parameters of location and architecture.[32] An incision is termed *clear corneal* when the external edge is anterior to the conjunctival insertion, *limbal corneal* when the external edge is through conjunctiva and limbus, and *scleral corneal* when it is posterior to the limbus (Figure 13-24). In addition to the anatomic designation of the external incision, these incisions are also classified by their architecture as being *single plane* when there is no groove at the external edge of the incision, *shallow groove* when the initial groove is less than 400 μ, and *deeply grooved* when it is deeper than 400 μ (Figures 13-25 and 13-26). To reduce the confusion and facilitate communication regarding these incisions, we believe they should be classified as clear corneal, limbal corneal, or scleral corneal incisions and as single planed, shallow grooved, or deep grooved.

PREOPERATIVE EVALUATION

Certain studies that may be of value as part of a preoperative work-up include endothelial cell counts in patients with endothelial dystrophies, and perhaps computerized corneal topography when refractive surgical procedures are going to be combined with cataract surgery in the management of pre-existing astigmatism. This is especially true when refractive and keratometric measurements do not coincide. There has been a recent trend

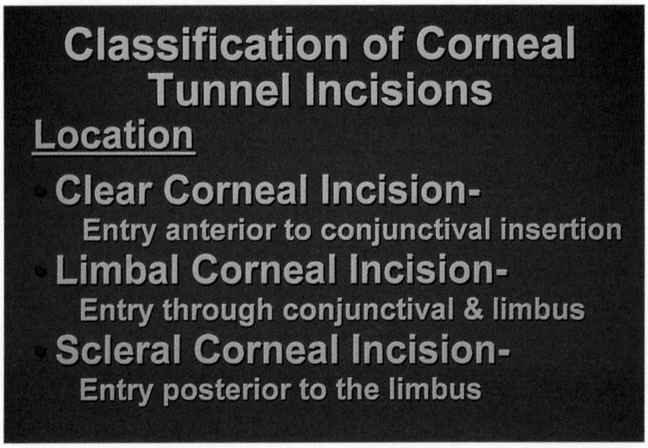

Classification of Corneal Tunnel Incisions

Location
- **Clear Corneal Incision-** Entry anterior to conjunctival insertion
- **Limbal Corneal Incision-** Entry through conjunctival & limbus
- **Scleral Corneal Incision-** Entry posterior to the limbus

Figure 13-24 Classification of corneal tunnel incisions by external incision location.

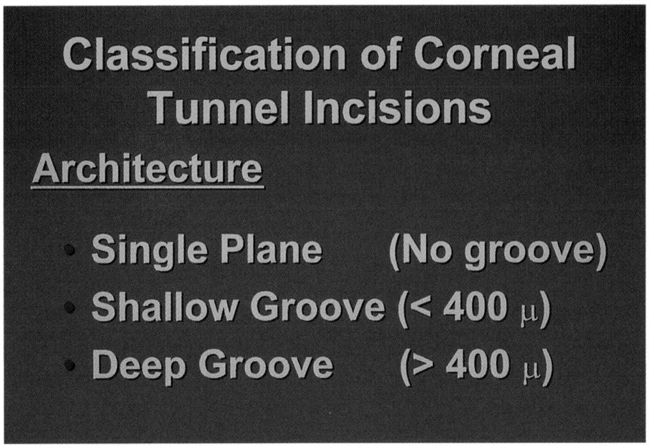

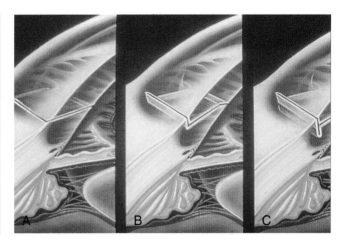

Classification of Corneal Tunnel Incisions

Architecture

- **Single Plane   (No groove)**
- **Shallow Groove (< 400 μ)**
- **Deep Groove   (> 400 μ)**

Figure 13-25 Classification of corneal tunnel incisions by wound architecture.

Figure 13-26 Cross-sectional view of single plane (**A**), shallow groove (**B**), and deep groove (hinged) clear corneal incisions (**C**).

for surgeons to use fourth-generation fluoroquinalone drops four times per day for 3 days prior to the day of surgery.

■ TECHNIQUES ■

Single plane incisions, as first described by Fine,[33] utilized a 3 mm diamond knife.

A Fine-Thornton 13 mm fixation ring (Mastel Instruments, Rapid City, SD) (Figure 13-27) stabilizes the globe and allows

manipulation without creating conjunctival tears, subconjunctival hemorrhages, or corneal abrasions (Figure 13-28). Aqueous humor is replaced by viscoelastic material through the side-port incision (Figure 13-29). After pressurization of the eye with viscoelastic, a 300 micron groove may be placed at the anterior edge of the vascular arcade (Figure 13-30), however, this is optional. If the groove has been placed, an incision is made by depressing the posterior edge of the groove with the diamond blade, flattening the blade against the surface of the eye. The knife is moved in

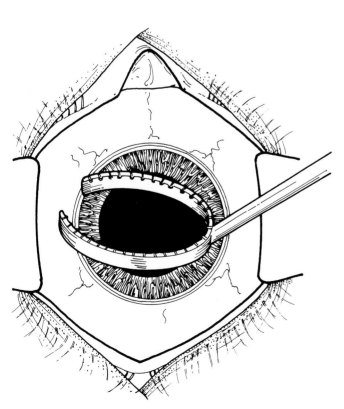

Figure 13-27 The Fine Thornton ring, shown in partial profile. Temporal limbus is seen inferiorly.

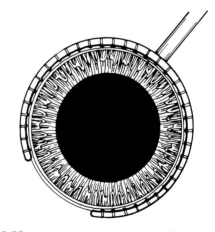

Figure 13-28 Purchase of the globe by the Fine-Thornton ring.

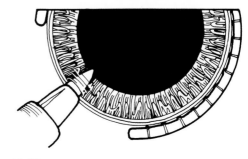

Figure 13-29 Paracentesis being made.

149

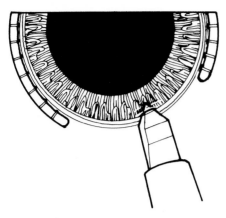

Figure 13-30 Grooving of the peripheral cornea.

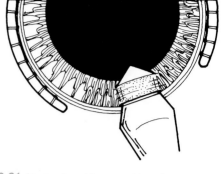

Figure 13-31 Construction of the corneal tunnel.

the plane of the cornea until the shoulders, which are 2 mm posterior to the point of the knife, touch the external edge of the incision and then a dimple down technique is used to initiate the cut through Descemet's membrane. After the tip enters the anterior chamber, the initial plane of the knife is re-established to cut through Descemet's in a straight-line configuration (Figure 13-31). Following phacoemulsification, lens implantation, and removal of residual viscoelastic, stromal hydration of the clear corneal incision can be performed in order to help seal the incision.[26] This is performed by placing the tip of a 26- or 27-gauge cannula in the side walls of the incision and gently irrigating balanced salt solution into the stroma (Figure 13-32). This is performed at both edges of the incision in order to help appose the roof and floor of the incision. Once apposition takes place, the hydrostatic forces of the endothelial pump will help seal the incision. In those rare instances of questionable wound integrity, a single radial 10-0 nylon suture is placed to ensure a tight seal.

Williamson[34] was the first to utilize a shallow 300–400 micron grooved clear corneal incision. The rationale for the Williamson incision was that it led to a thicker external edge to the roof of the tunnel and less likelihood of tearing. Langerman[35] later described the single hinge incision in which requirements for the initial groove were 90% of the depth of the cornea anterior to the edge of the conjunctiva. Initially he utilized a depth of

600 μ and subsequently made the tunnel itself superficially in that groove, believing that this led to enhanced resistance of the incision to external deformation. Minimal differences in surgically induced astigmatism have been demonstrated between beveled and hinged clear corneal incisions.[36]

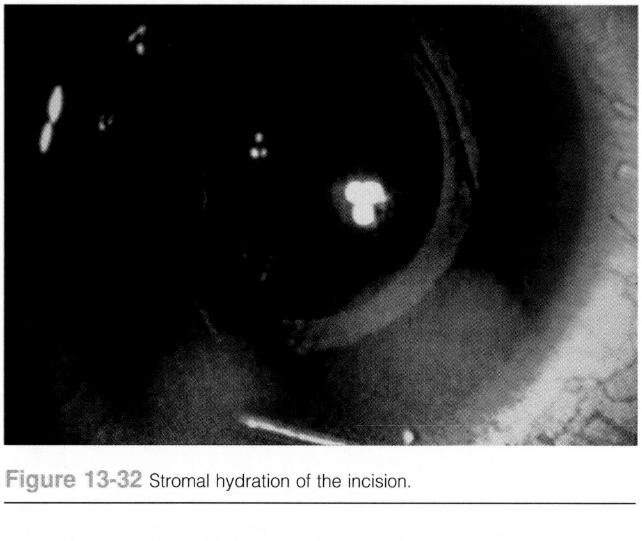

Adjunctive techniques were utilized to combine refractive surgery incisions with clear corneal cataract incisions. Until recently, Fine used the temporal location for the cataract incisions and added one or two T-cuts made by the Feaster Knife (Rhein Medical No. 05-8200) with a 7 mm ocular zone for the management of pre-existing astigmatism. Others, including Lindstrom and Rosen, rotated the location of the incision to the steep axis in order to achieve some increased flattening at the steepest axis to address pre-existing astigmatism. Kershner[37] utilized the corneal incision in the temporal half of the eye by starting with a nearly full-thickness T-cut through, which he then made his corneal tunnel incision. For large amounts of astigmatism he used a paired T-cut in the opposite side of the same meridian. Finally, the popularization of limbal relaxing incisions by Gills[38] and Nichamin[39] added an additional means of reducing pre-existing astigmatism by using the groove for the limbal relaxing incision as the site of entry for the clear corneal cataract incision. This has been found to be a simple and practical approach for reducing pre-existing astigmatism at the time of cataract surgery.[40] At this time, Fine places all of his incisions at the temporal periphery and addresses pre-existing astigmatism with limbal relaxing incisions at the steep axis and/or toric IOLs.

New technology blades have been developed which have helped perfect incision architecture. The Fine Triamond Knife (Mastel No. 0851913191) was developed in conjunction with Mastel Precision Instruments (Rapid City, SD) so that the incision could be made with an extremely sharp, thin and narrow knife without a necessity for dimpling down, which resulted in some tendency for there to be tearing of tissue or scrolling of Descemet's membrane. Subsequently, in conjunction with Rhein Medical (Tampa, FL), the 3-D blade (No. 05-5083) was developed, which had differential slope angles to the bevels on the anterior versus the posterior surface (Figures 13-33A, B, C) resulting in an ability to just touch the eye at the site of the external incision location and advance the blade in the plane of the cornea. The differential slopes on the anterior versus posterior aspects of the blade allowed the forces of tissue resistance to create an incision that

Figure 13-32 Stromal hydration of the incision.

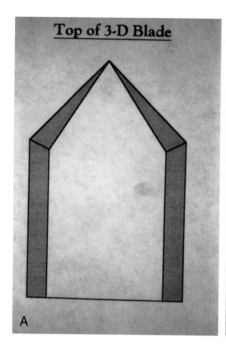

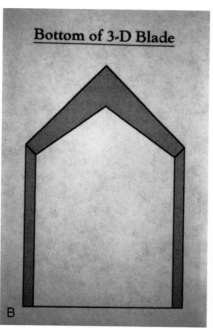

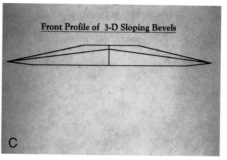

A B C

Figure 13-33 Schematic representation of top view (**A**) and bottom view (**B**) of the 3 mm Rhein 3-D diamond keratome. The front profile of the keratome (**C**) demonstrates the differential slopes on the anterior versus posterior aspects of the blade which allow the forces of tissue resistance to create the proper incision architecture.

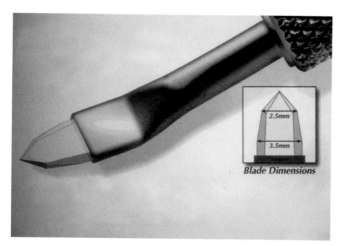

Figure 13-34 The Rhein 3-D Trapezoidal Blade with 2.5–3.5 mm blade dimensions.

was characterized by a linear external incision, a 2 mm tunnel, and a linear internal incision without the need to dimple down or distort tissues to create the proper incision architecture.[41] The trapezoidal 3-D blade (Rhein No. 05-5086) also allows enlargement of the incision to 3.5 mm for IOL insertion without altering incision architecture (Figure 13-34). Histologic studies of clear corneal incisions performed with steel keratomes and diamond keratomes have shown more disruption of corneal stromal tissue with steel keratomes and more likelihood of severe stromal damage after insertion of foldable IOLs, suggesting that diamond keratomes may have a beneficial effect on incision healing.[42,43]

Many companies, in addition to Rhein Medical, are designing diamond knives for clear corneal incisions. Mastel Precision Surgical Instruments have designed a sleek trapezoidal blade that

they have named the Superstealth (Figure 13-35). The Stealth blade is an ultra-thin diamond with asymmetric facets that result in a self-directing bevel similar to the Rhein 3-D blade. ASICO (American Surgical Instruments Company, Westmont, Illinois) has designed two new diamond knives for clear corneal incisions: the Pathfinder (Figure 13-36) and the Clearpath (Figure 13-37). Both blades contain a shelf on the surface of the blade that creates an inner corneal valve of consistent length by forcing the leading

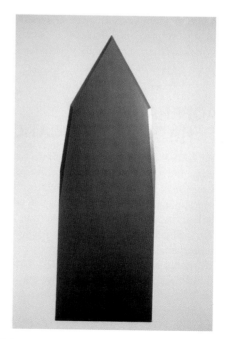

Figure 13-35 Mastel Trapezoidal Diamond Stealth Blade.

151

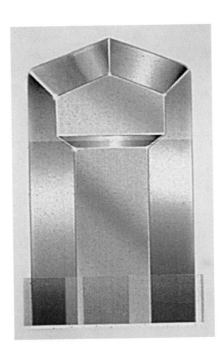

Figure 13-36 ASICO Pathfinder Blade.

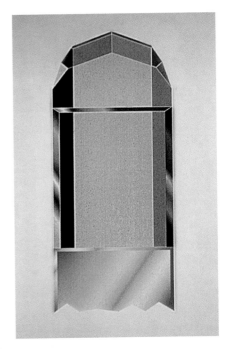

Figure 13-37 ASICO Clearpath Blade.

edge of the blade into the anterior chamber when the shelf reaches the external incision. Stromal hydration of the wound is claimed to be unnecessary with the Clearpath blade due to the facet design.

A recent study by Mamalis[44] has revealed small predictable enlargements of clear corneal incisions after insertion of foldable IOLs with both forceps and injectors. The degree of wound enlargement increased with higher IOL powers when lenses were inserted with forceps but did not increase with increasing IOL powers when injectors were used. In general, injectors were associated with a smaller percentage increase in wound stretching than forceps, making them a preferable choice for foldable lens insertion through clear corneal incisions.

■ INTRAOPERATIVE AND POSTOPERATIVE COMPLICATIONS ■

Although clear corneal and scleral incision cataract surgery share many of the same intraoperative and postoperative complications, clear corneal incisions, by nature of their architecture and location, have some unique complications associated with them. If one accidentally incises the conjunctiva at the time of the clear corneal incision, ballooning of the conjunctiva can develop, which may compromise visualization of anterior structures. When this develops, the use of a suction catheter is usually required by the assistant to aid in visualization. Early entry into the cornea might result in an incision of insufficient length to be self sealing, and thus a single suture may be required in order to ensure a secure wound at the conclusion of the procedure. A late entry may result in a corneal tunnel incision sufficiently long that the phacoemulsification tip would create striae in the cornea and compromise

visualization of the anterior chamber. In addition, incisions that are too short or improperly constructed can result in an increased tendency for iris prolapse.

Manipulation of the phacoemulsification handpiece intraoperatively may result in tearing of the roof of the tunnel, especially at the edges, potentially compromising the ability for the incision to self seal. Tearing of the internal lip can also occur, resulting in compromised self-sealability or, in rare instances, small detachments or scrolling of Descemet's membrane in the anterior edge of the incision. Of greater concern has been the potential for incisional burns.[45,46] When incisional burns develop in clear corneal incisions, there may be a loss of self-sealability, corneal edema, and severe induced astigmatism.[47] In addition, manipulation of the incision can result in an epithelial abrasion which can compromise self-sealability because of the lack of a fluid barrier by an intact epithelium. Without an intact epithelial layer, the corneal endothelium does not have the ability to help appose the roof and floor of the incision through hydrostatic forces.

Postoperatively, hypotony might result in some compromised ability for these incisions to seal. Wound leaks and iris prolapse have been very infrequent postoperative complications[48] and are usually present in incisions greater than 3.5 mm in width. In a large survey performed for the American Society of Cataract and Refractive Surgery by Masket and Tennen,[49] there was a slightly increased incidence of endophthalmitis in clear corneal cataract surgery compared to scleral tunnel surgery. However, the survey failed to note the incision sizes in those cases where endophthalmitis in clear corneal incisions had occurred, and thus it is possible that any increase in the incidence of endophthalmitis is associated with unsutured clear corneal incisions greater than 4 mm in width.

POSTOPERATIVE CLINICAL COURSE AND OUTCOMES ■

The usual postoperative regime involves examination on the first postoperative day and a second examination at 10 to 14 days at which time spectacle correction is prescribed. Use of drops postoperatively includes instillation two to three times a day of a fluoroquinalone, prednisolone acetate and a topical non-steroidal anti-inflammatory drug (NSAID). The antibiotic and steroid are discontinued at 10 to 14 days and the NSAID is continued for an additional 10 days.[50]

Numerous studies have been performed documenting the safety and low magnitudes of astigmatism induced by these incisions depending on their size. Masket and Tennen[51] have documented by vector analysis 0.50 diopter (D) of induced cylinder and less than 0.25 D of cylinder change in the surgical meridian using 3.0 × 2.5 mm self-sealing temporal clear corneal incisions. They were also able to demonstrate the refractive stability of these incisions 2 weeks following surgery. Kohnen, Dick, and Jacobi[52] compared the surgically induced astigmatism of 3.5, 4, and 5 mm grooved temporal clear corneal incisions and found a mean induced astigmatism of 0.37 D, 0.56 D, and 0.70 D respectively after 6 months. A similar study by Pfleger et al.[53] revealed even smaller amounts of induced astigmatism from 3.2, 4, and 5.2 mm temporal clear corneal incisions with the 3.2 mm incision demonstrating astigmatic neutrality with only 0.09 D of induced cylinder.

In addition to comparing the effects of different-sized temporal clear corneal incisions on induced astigmatism, numerous studies have evaluated the relative astigmatic effects of incision location in regard to clear corneal incisions versus corneoscleral incisions, and of the temporal versus superior meridian. Nielsen[54] evaluated surgically induced astigmatism from 3.5 mm and 5.2 mm temporal and superior clear corneal incisions, and compared them with 3.5 mm and 5.2 mm corneoscleral incisions at the superior location. The 3.5 mm clear corneal incisions induced roughly 0.5 D of with-the-rule or against-the-rule drift, depending on temporal or superior location. Larger amounts of astigmatism were induced with the larger clear corneal incisions. He found that the refractive effect of clear corneal incisions was stable between postoperative day 1 and postoperative week 6, making their astigmatic keratotomy effect more useful and predictable if one wished to consider preoperative cylinder when selecting incision type or location.

Cillino et al.[55] compared the astigmatic effects of unsutured 5.2 mm temporal clear corneal incisions with 5.2 mm superior corneoscleral incisions and found comparable amounts of induced astigmatism. Rainer et al.,[56] however, has found a small but significant amount of surgically induced astigmatism continuing up to 5 years postoperatively with 5 mm superior scleral incisions. Although the use of unsutured 5.2 mm clear corneal incisions is considered unsafe because of a possible increase in rates of wound complications and endophthalmitis, Holweger and Marefat[57] have demonstrated that absorbable sutured 5-clear corneal incisions were topographically comparable to 3.5 mm sutureless clear corneal incisions, 6–8 months postoperatively, making this incision and closure technique a viable option for surgeons.

When temporal clear corneal incisions of 3.2 mm or less have been compared with superiorly placed scleral tunnel incisions of the same size, similarly low numbers of induced astigmatism have been documented for the two incision locations.[58,59] In contrast, similarly sized incisions when compared in regard to temporal versus superior clear corneal location have demonstrated more meridional flattening in the superior axis than the temporal axis.[60–62] This has also been demonstrated in the oblique superolateral clear corneal incision compared with a temporal incision, confirming the bias for the temporal location for clear cornea incisions when astigmatic neutrality is desired.[63]

Although small clear corneal incisions appear to have similar astigmatic effects as superior corneoscleral incisions, recent concern has surrounded the possibility of increased endothelial cell loss with these incisions. Grabow[64] reported an increased incidence of endothelial cell loss for superior clear corneal incisions, which increased linearly with increasing ultrasound times. Amon et al.[65] discovered a significant increase in endothelial cell loss in 3.5 mm temporal clear corneal incisions when compared to 3.5 mm superior scleral tunnel incisions. However, a recent study by Dick et al.[66] found that the total endothelial cell loss at 1 year with clear corneal incisions compared favorably with endothelial cell loss rates of other cataract extraction techniques. As ultrasound times decrease in the future with advancing technologies and techniques, such as lens chopping and the use of power modulations,[67] endothelial cell loss rates should become insignificant.

Dick et al.[68] have also recently demonstrated that cataract extraction through a clear corneal incision results in less inflammation in the immediate postoperative period when compared to surgery through a sclerocorneal incision. This may ultimately have a beneficial effect in reducing posterior capsule opacification, cystoid macular edema, and keratopathy.

PROFILES OF CLEAR CORNEAL INCISIONS ■

Clear corneal incisions involving an incision in the plane of the cornea with a length equal to 2 mm are still being constructed in the same manner today. In 1992, the incisions were as wide as 4 mm, but have more recently been reduced to a maximum width of 3.5 mm, if not sutured. Figure 13-26 shows an artist's view of what the profile of clear corneal incisions were thought to look like. Part A shows the single plane incision and its apparent inherent lack of stability as one surface can easily slide over another. Charles Williamson, MD, from Baton Rouge, innovated an alteration of that incision which involves a shallow, perpendicular groove prior to incising the cornea into the anterior chamber (Part B). David Langerman, MD, deepened the perpendicular groove with the belief that it led to greater stability (Part C). These grooved incisions have been abandoned by the authors in favor of a paracentesis-style incision due to the difficulties associated with a persistent foreign body sensation in the grooved incisions and the pooling of mucus and debris in the gaping groove. More importantly, the grooved incisions represent a disruption in the fluid barrier that intact epithelium create, which allows for a vacuum seal as a result of endothelial pumping.

Initial incision construction technique began with a blade applanated to the surface of the eyeball with the point at the edge of the clear cornea, which advanced for 2 mm into the plane of the cornea before incising Descemet's membrane (Figure 13-38). These early incisions were made with knives with straight sides; however, these knives were subsequently replaced by trapezoidal-

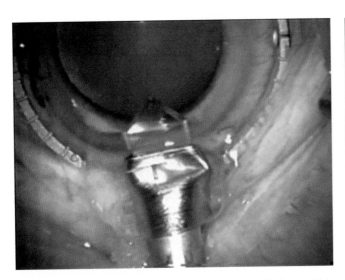

Figure 13-38 Clear corneal incision construction with the blade completely inserted.

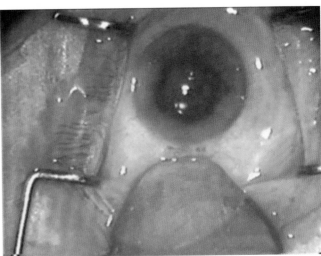

Figure 13-39 Testing the seal of the incision with a Seidel test using fluorescein and tactile pressure.

shaped knives in order to allow the enlargement of the incision without violating the architecture by cutting sideways. From the onset of the use of clear corneal incisions, stromal hydration of the incisions, which thickens the cornea, forcing the roof of the incision onto the floor of the incision and facilitating endothelial pumping to the upper reaches of the cornea, was strongly advocated. Testing the seal of the incision with a Seidel test using fluorescein (Figure 13-39) was also strongly advocated. These practices have not changed since 1992, except that we now infrequently depress the posterior lip of the incision.

To obtain a better understanding of the architecture of clear corneal incisions, the authors conducted a study of the profiles of clear corneal incisions using the Zeiss Visante Optical Coherence Tomography (OCT) Anterior Segment Imaging System (Figure 13-40). This technology has allowed the first view of the clear corneal incision in the living eye in the early postoperative period. All previous views were in autopsy eyes sectioned

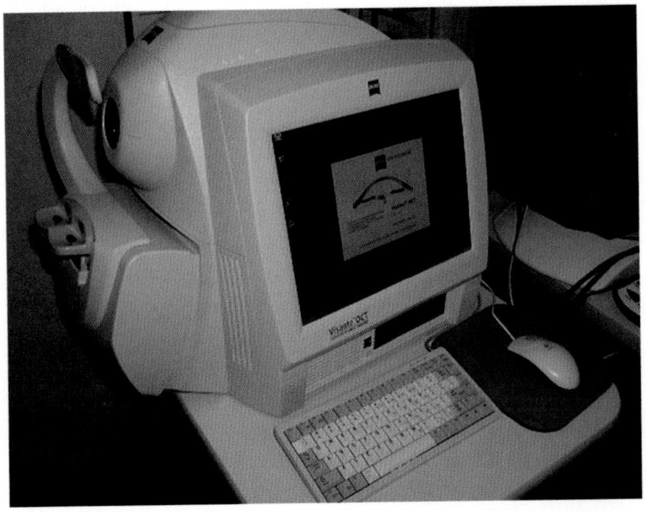

through the incision, which introduces artifacts. Figure 13-41 shows an example of the corneal periphery in a control eye which includes the anterior chamber angle. The regularity of the corneal epithelium blending in the conjunctiva and the clear corneal stroma blending into sclera can be clearly seen.

A variety of knives were used to create the clear corneal incisions during cataract surgery. All clear corneal incisions were made by one surgeon (IHF). OCT images of each operative eye were taken on the first postoperative day, within 24 h of cataract surgery and are representative of multiple images from multiple patients.

As seen in Figure 13-42, which was taken on the first day postoperatively, the clear corneal incision is actually curvilinear, not a straight line, as seen in the artist's depiction of clear corneal incisions (Figure 13-26). It is an arcuate incision which is considerably longer than the chord length originally estimated for the length of the incision. It is very important to note that the architecture of the incision allows for a fit not unlike tongue and groove paneling, which adds a measure of stability to these incisions and makes sliding of one surface over the other considerably less likely. Figure 13-43 shows an incision that was made with a 300 micron groove at the external edge of the incision prior to incision construction. The incision itself still has a similar curved or arcuate configuration, but the gaping of the external groove, which is noted on the first day postoperatively, is accompanied by a similar offset of the internal lips of the incision, which appears to be somewhat less stable than a paracentesis-style incision.

These images also demonstrate the persistence of stromal swelling from stromal hydration on the first postoperative day, which many critics of clear corneal incisions believed disappeared within 1 or 2 h.

Figure 13-44 shows a clear corneal incision made with the Rhein Medical (Tampa, FL), the Rhein 3D Trapezoidal blade, 2–2.5 mm (#05-5088), for incision construction using single-piece acrylic lenses with a Royale injector (ASICO, LLC, Westmont, IL, #AE-9045). Once again, the very advantageous architecture of the incision is observed. It is interesting to note that the arc length is considerably longer than the chord length and is probably a hypersquare incision in that it is only 2 mm wide. As Figures 13-45–48

Figure 13-40 The Zeiss Visante Optical Coherence Tomography Anterior Segment Imaging System.

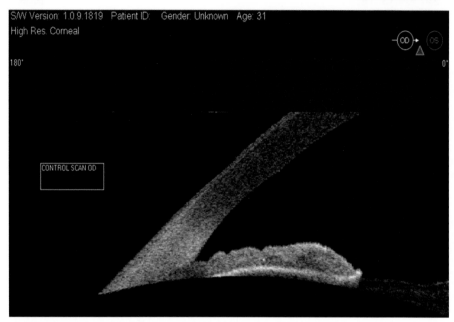

PROFILES OF CLEAR CORNEAL INCISIONS

Figure 13-41 OCT image of a control eye showing the corneal periphery including the anterior chamber angle.

Figure 13-42 OCT image of a clear corneal incision made with the Rhein 3D Trapezoidal 2.5–3.5 mm Blade. Image of the blade is inset.

demonstrate, all clear corneal incisions made with a variety of blades demonstrated a similar, arcuate architecture.

The BD Kojo Slit (BD Medical-Ophthalmic Systems, Franklin Lakes, NJ, #372032) is a blade that is curved in the direction of the width of the incision. This creates an arcuate incision paralleling the curvature of the peripheral cornea with a chord length whose width is considerably smaller than the incision itself, which may add a greater degree of stability. The first few times that this blade is used, its unusual configuration makes it somewhat more difficult to create an incision in the plane of the cornea and the

incision can end up considerably shorter than anticipated (see Figures 13-49 and 13-50). However, as one learns how to use this blade, the desired architecture is much easier to achieve (Figure 13-51).

One of the surprising findings was that proper incision construction resulted in a longer incision than the chord length that was measured and in greater stability (like tongue in groove paneling) of the incision. Another surprising finding was that stromal swelling does, indeed, last for at least 24 h. These findings demonstrate those characteristics that have contributed to

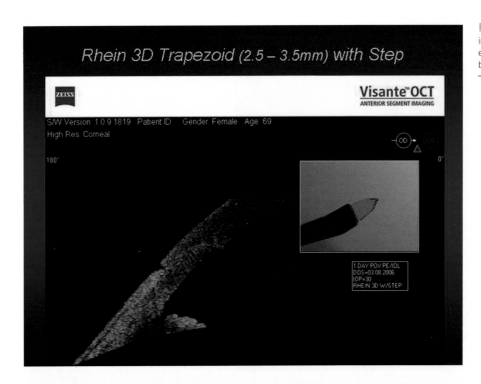

Figure 13-43 OCT image of a clear corneal incision with a 300 micron groove at the external edge of the incision. Image of the Rhein 3D blade is inset.

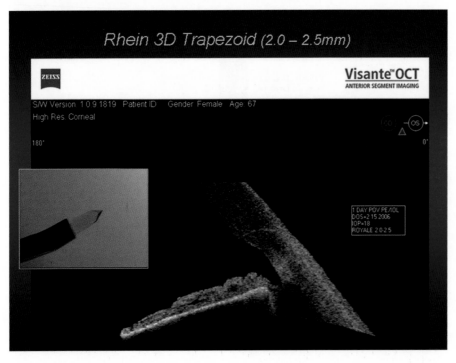

Figure 13-44 OCT image of a clear corneal incision made with the Rhein 3D Trapezoidal 2–2.5 mm Blade. Image of the blade is inset.

an added measure of safety in clear corneal incisions that can result in the absence of endophthalmitis.

CONTROVERSIES SURROUNDING CLEAR CORNEAL INCISIONS

One of the most controversial criticisms of clear corneal incisions has been their relative strength compared to limbal or scleral incisions. Ernest et al.[69,70] demonstrated that rectangular clear corneal incisions in cadaver eye models were less resistant to external deformation utilizing pinpoint pressure than were square limbal or scleral tunnel incisions. Subsequently, Mackool and Russell[71] demonstrated that once the incision width was ≤3.5 mm and the length ≥2 mm, there was an equal resistance to external deformation in clear cornea incisions as compared to scleral tunnel incisions. In Ernest's work as well, as incision sizes became increasingly small, the force required to cause failure of these incisions became very similar for limbal and clear corneal incisions, and thus this could be used to further document the safety of incisions sized 3 mm or less.

A major criticism of these cadaver studies is that there is a lack of functioning endothelium contributing to wound sealing. Others

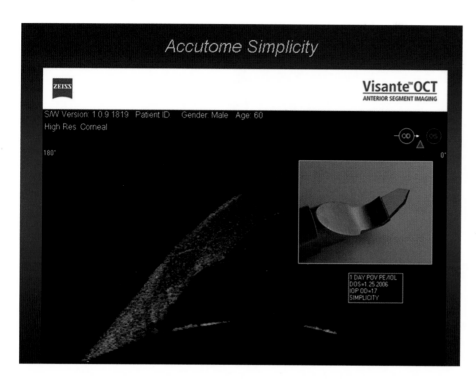

Figure 13-45 OCT image of a clear corneal incision made with the Accutome Simplicity Blade. Image of the blade is inset.

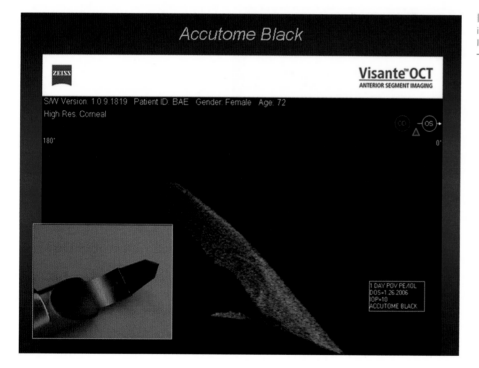

Figure 13-46 OCT image of a clear corneal incision made with the Accutome Black Blade. Image of the blade is inset.

have also indicated that cadaver eye incision strength cannot be compared to incisions in vivo.[28] Ernest and Neuhann[72] have compared in vivo posterior limbal incisions with clear corneal incisions and found that deep-grooved incisions performed better than shallow-grooved or single-plane incisions, in addition to finding that posterior limbal incisions performed better than clear corneal incisions when challenged by pinpoint pressure.

Many surgeons have called into question the validity of pinpoint pressure as a clinically relevant test for cataract wound strength because the probability that anyone would challenge their own incision by pressing on it with something as fine as the instruments utilized to apply pinpoint pressure in these studies is highly unlikely. Regardless of whether more posteriorly placed incisions demonstrate increased strength compared to clear corneal incisions, the real question is whether that added strength is clinically significant or relevant. Fine[73] and others have demonstrated the stability of clear corneal incisions when a knuckle or a finger tip, the most likely way patients would challenge these incisions, was used. In addition, it is a well-known fact that a 1 mm "hypersquare" paracentesis will leak the day after surgery if pinpoint pressure is applied to its posterior lip; however, the likelihood

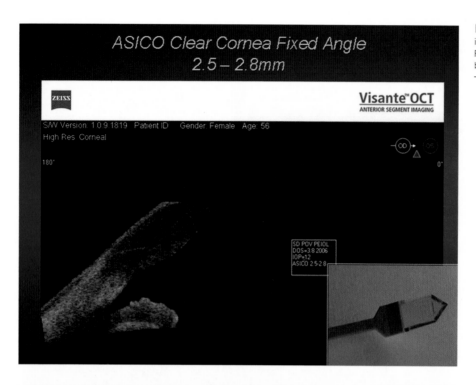

Figure 13-47 OCT image of a clear corneal incision made with the ASICO Clear Cornea Fixed Angle 2.8–2.8 mm Blade. Image of the blade is inset.

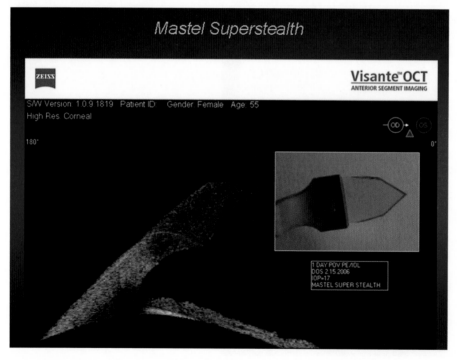

Figure 13-48 OCT image of a clear corneal incision made with the Mastel Superstealth Blade. Image of the blade is inset.

of any paracentesis incision leaking spontaneously or with blunt pressure the day following surgery is extremely low.

Another point of controversy is in regard to the studies in cat eyes performed by Ernest et al.[74] These studies revealed a fibrovascular response in incisions placed in the limbus with extensive wound healing in 7 days compared to a lack of fibrovascular healing in clear corneal incisions. This study has been used to propose an increased safety for limbal incisions as compared to clear corneal incisions. Unfortunately, the real issue for these various incisions is not healing but sealing. We believe that as long as an incision is sealed at the conclusion of surgery, and it remains sealed thereafter, the time before complete healing of the incision is accomplished is almost irrelevant, especially since there is still a 7-day period in which limbal incisions are not truly "healed." An analogy can be drawn to the sealing which takes place during laser-assisted in-situ keratomileusis (LASIK) in which there is no fibrovascular healing of the clear corneal interface, which has little effect on the strength, effectiveness or safety of the wound and, in fact, is an advantage by limiting scarring and an inflammatory healing response.

One of the clear disadvantages of limbal corneal incisions is the greater likelihood of ballooning of conjunctiva, which can make visualization of anterior chamber structures during the surgical

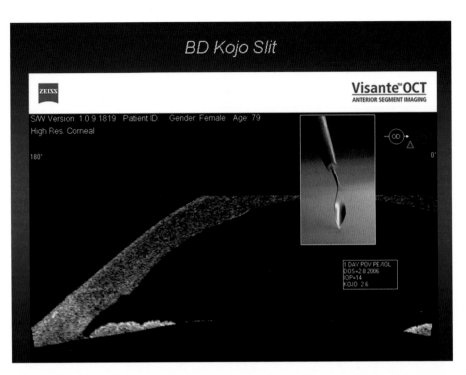

Figure 13-49 OCT image of a clear corneal incision made with the BD Kojo Slit Blade during the learning curve. Image of the blade is inset.

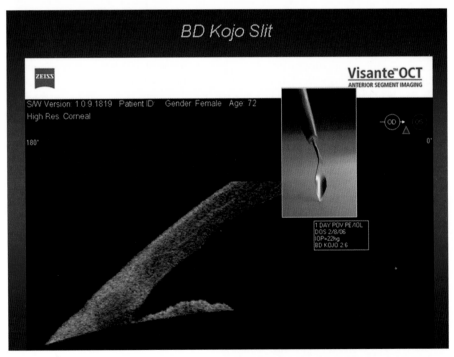

Figure 13-50 OCT image of a clear corneal incision made with the BD Kojo Slit Blade during the learning curve. Image of the blade is inset.

procedure more difficult. In addition, studies by Park et al.[29] demonstrated that violation of the conjunctiva threatens the integrity not only of pre-existing filtering blebs but of the conjunctiva which would participate in filtering surgery at some future date. Finally, the presence of subconjunctival hemorrhage, although not important with respect to the ultimate function of the eye, may be of importance from a cosmetic perspective to the patient as well as to the survival of filtering blebs.

Contraindications for clear corneal incisions include the presence of radial keratotomy incisions that extend to the limbus that might be challenged by clear corneal incisions,[75] marginal degenerations associated with thinning of the peripheral cornea and, perhaps, advanced corneal endothelial dystrophy.

■ ENDOPHTHALMITIS: IS THERE AN INCREASED RISK? ■

Endophthalmitis prophylaxis involves a large number of factors including:

* a proper preoperative antibiotic regime
* preparation of the surgical field, including Betadine and draping

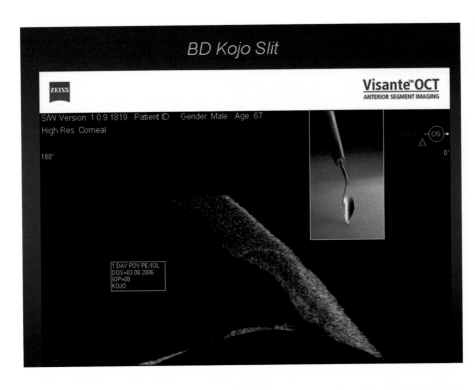

- incision construction
- surgical technique, including atraumatic surgery
- power modulations to avoid heating the incision
- avoiding grasp of the roof of the incision with a toothed forceps, which would abrade the epithelium and disrupt the fluid barrier for endothelial pumping
- incision closure
- testing for leakage
- postoperative antibiotics.

The authors have practiced for longer than 10 years, on over 9000 cases without a single case of infectious endophthalmitis.

The role of unsutured clear corneal incisions for cataract surgery and the apparent increased incidence of postoperative endophthalmitis in many reports are under rather intense scrutiny.[76–86] The role of changing antibiotic sensitivity has been an issue (Figure 13-52). In Sweden, there has been a decreased incidence of endophthalmitis associated with an increased use of clear corneal incisions.[87,88] The recent ESCRS study of endophthalmitis showed an 80% reduction with the use of intracameral

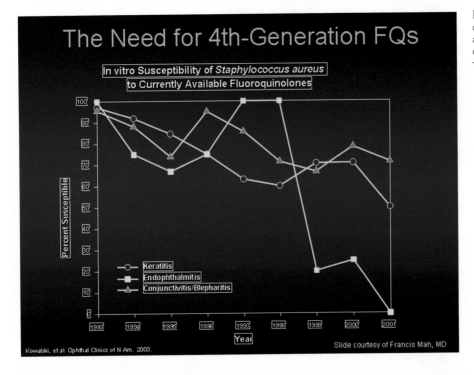

cefuroxime.[89] There are other reports of no increased incidence of endophthalmitis with the use of clear corneal incisions.[76,90–92]

Attention to all of the details for endophthalmitis prophylaxis is of primary importance. Incision construction leading to proper architecture is of primary importance among all of the variables that are part of endophthalmitis prophylaxis, and certainly not all clear corneal incisions are the same. An incision in the plane of the cornea with a chord length of at least 2 mm appears to give uniquely advantageous architecture for adequate self-sealability.

CONCLUSION

Clear corneal cataract incisions are becoming a more popular option for cataract extraction and IOL implantation throughout the world. Through the use of clear corneal incisions and topical and intracameral anesthesia, we have achieved surgery that is the least invasive of any time in the history of cataract surgery, with visual rehabilitation that is almost immediate. Just 25 years ago, inpatient intracapsular cataract surgery, often performed under general anesthesia, followed by aphakic spectacles, was the standard of care. It is striking to realize how far we have come in such a short time.

References

[1] Paton D, Troutman R, Ryan S. Present trends in incision and closure of the cataract wound. Highlights Ophthalmol 1973;14(3):176.
[2] Jaffe NS, Clayman HM. The pathophysiology of corneal astigmatism after cataract extraction. Trans Am Acad Ophthalmol Otolaryngol 1975;79:OP615–630.
[3] Kelman CD. Phacoemulsification and aspiration: a new technique of cataract removal: a preliminary report. Am J Ophth 1967;64:23.
[4] Colvard DM, Kratz RP, Mazzocco TR, Davidson B. Clinical evaluation of the Terry surgical keratometer. Am Intraocular Implant Soc J 1980;6:249–251.
[5] Masket S. Origin of scleral tunnel methods. J Cataract Refract Surg 1993;19:812–813. [letter to the editor].
[6] Girard LJ, Hoffman RF. Scleral tunnel to prevent induced astigmatism. Am J Ophthalmol 1984;97:450–456.
[7] Maloney WF, Grindle L. Textbook of phacoemulsification. Fallbrook, CA: Lasenda Publishers; 1988.
[8] Shephard JR. Induced astigmatism in small incision cataract surgery. J Cataract Refract Surg 1989;15:85–88.
[9] Fine IH. Infinity suture: modified horizontal suture for 6.5 mm incisions. In: Gills JP, Sanders DR, editors. Small-incision cataract surgery: foldable lenses, one-stitch surgery, sutureless surgery, astigmatic keratotomy. Thorofare, NJ: Slack, Inc; 1990. p. 191–196.
[10] Masket S. Horizontal anchor suture closure method for small incision cataract surgery. J Cataract Refract Surg 1991;17(Suppl.):689–695.
[11] Fishkind WJ. Horizontal overlap suture: a new astigmatism-free closure, focus on phaco. Ocular Surgery News 1990;8.
[12] McFarland MS. Surgeon undertakes phaco, foldable IOL series sans sutures. Ocular Surgery News 1990;8.
[13] Ernest PH. Presentation at the Department of Ophthalmology. Detroit, MI: Wayne State University School of Medicine; Feb 28, 1990.
[14] Koch PS. Structural analysis of cataract incision construction. J Cataract Refract Surg 1991;17 (Suppl.):661–667.
[15] Kershner RM. Sutureless one-handed intercapsular phacoemulsification: the keyhole technique. J Cataract Refract Surg 1991;17(Suppl.):719–725.
[16] Fine IH. Architecture and construction of a self-sealing incision for cataract surgery. J Cataract Refract Surg 1991;17:672–676.
[17] Singer JA. Frown incision for minimizing induced astigmatism after small incision cataract surgery with rigid optic intraocular lens implantation. J Cataract Refract Surg 1991;17(Suppl.):677–688.
[18] Pallin SL. Chevron sutureless closure: a preliminary report. J Cataract Refract Surg 1991;17 (Suppl.):706–709.
[19] Ernest PH. Introduction to sutureless surgery. In: Gills JP, Sanders DR, editors. Small incision cataract surgery: foldable lenses, one-stitch surgery, sutureless surgery, astigmatic keratotomy. Thorofare, NJ: Slack, Inc; 1990. p. 103–105.
[20] Harms H, Mackensen G. Intracapsular extraction with a corneal incision using the Graefe knife. In: Ocular surgery under the microscope. Stuttgart, Germany: Georg Thieme Verlag; 1967. p. 144–153.
[21] Paton D, Troutman R, Ryan S. Present trends in incision and closure of the cataract wound. Highlights of Ophthalmology 1973;14(3):176.
[22] Arnott EJ. Intraocular implants. Tran Ophthalmol Soc UK 1981;101:58–60.
[23] Galand A. La technique de l'enveloppe. Liege, Belgium: Pierre Mardaga publisher; 1988.
[24] Brown DC, Fine IH, Gills JP et al. The future of foldables. Panel discussion held at the 1992 annual meeting of the American Society of Cataract and Refractive Surgery. Ocular Surgery News 1992;(Suppl.).
[25] Shimizu K. Pure corneal incision. Phaco & Foldables 1992;5:5–8.
[26] Fine IH. Corneal tunnel incision with a temporal approach. In: Fine IH, Fichman RA, Grabow HB, editors. Clear-corneal cataract surgery & topical anesthesia. Thorofare, NJ: Slack, Inc; 1993. p. 5–26.
[27] Fine IH, Fichman RA, Grabow HB. Clear-corneal cataract surgery & topical anesthesia. Thorofare, NJ: Slack, Inc; 1993.
[28] Rosen ES. Clear corneal incisions: a good option for cataract patients. A roundtable discussion. Ocular Surgery News 1998.
[29] Park HJ, Kwon YH, Weitzman M, Caprioli J. Temporal corneal phacoemulsification in patients with filtered glaucoma. Arch Ophthalmol 1997;115:1375–1380.
[30] Hogan MJ, Alvarado JA, Weddell JE, editors. Histology of the human eye: an atlas and textbook. Philadelphia: W.B. Saunders Company; 1971.
[31] Menapace RM. Preferred incisions for current foldable lenses and their impact on corneal topography. Abstract. Luxor-Aswan, Egypt: Cataract Workshop on the Nile; November 20, 1996.
[32] Fine IH. Descriptions can improve communication. Ophthalmology Times 1996;21:30.
[33] Fine IH. Self-sealing corneal tunnel incision for small-incision cataract surgery. Ocular Surgery News 1992.
[34] Williamson CH. Cataract keratotomy surgery. In: Fine IH, Fichman RA, Grabow HB, editors. Clear-corneal cataract surgery & topical anesthesia. Thorofare, NJ: Slack, Inc; 1993. p. 87–93.
[35] Langerman DW. Architectural design of a self-sealing corneal tunnel, single-hinge incision. J Cataract Refract Surg 1994;20:84–88.
[36] Vass C, Menapace R, Rainer G et al. Comparative study of corneal topographic changes after 3.0 mm beveled and hinged clear corneal incisions. J Cataract Refract Surg 1998;24:1498–1504.
[37] Kershner RM. Clear corneal cataract surgery and the correction of myopia, hyperopia, and astigmatism. Ophthalmology 1997;104:381–389.
[38] Gills JP, Gayton JL. Reducing pre-existing astigmatism. In: Gills JP, editor. Cataract surgery: the state of the art. Thorofare, NJ: Slack, Inc; 1998. p. 53–66.
[39] Nichamin L. Refining astigmatic keratotomy during cataract surgery. Ocular Surgery News 1993.
[40] Budak K, Friedman NJ, Koch DD. Limbal relaxing incisions with cataract surgery. J Cataract Refract Surg 1998;24:503–508.
[41] Fine IH. Techniques spotlight: new blade enhances cataract surgery. Ophthalmology Times 1996.
[42] Jacobi FK, Dick B, Bohle R. Histological and ultrastructural study of corneal tunnel incisions using diamond and steel keratomes. J Cataract Refract Surg 1998;24:498–502.
[43] Radner W, Menapace R, Zehetmayer M, Mallinger R. Ultrastructure of clear corneal incisions. Part I: Effect of keratomes and incision width on corneal trauma after lens implantation. J Cataract Refract Surg 1998;24:487–492.
[44] Mamalis N. Incision width after phacoemulsification with foldable intraocular lens implantation. J Cataract Refract Surg 2000;26:237–241.
[45] Fine IH. Special Report to ASCRS Members: Phacoemulsification Incision Burns. Letter to American Society of Cataract and Refractive Surgery members, 1997.
[46] Majid MA, Sharma MK, Harding SP. Corneoscleral burn during phacoemulsification surgery. J Cataract Refract Surg 1998;24:1413–1415.
[47] Sugar A, Schertzer RM. Clinical course of phacoemulsification wound burns. J Cataract Refract Surg 1999;25:688–692.
[48] Menapace R. Delayed iris prolapse with unsutured 5.1 mm clear corneal incisions. J Cataract Refract Surg 1995;21:353–357.
[49] Endophthalmitis: State of the prophylactic art. Eyeworld News 1997;42–43.
[50] Nishi O, Nishi K, Fujiwara T, Shirasawa E. Effects of diclofenac sodium and indomethacin on proliferation and collagen synthesis of lens epithelial cells in vitro. J Cataract Refract Surg 1995;21:461–465.
[51] Masket S, Tennen DG. Astigmatic stabilization of 3.0 mm temporal clear corneal cataract incisions. J Cataract Refract Surg 1996;22:1451–1455.
[52] Kohnen T, Dick B, Jacobi KW. Comparison of the induced astigmatism after temporal clear corneal tunnel incisions of different sizes. J Cataract Refract Surg 1995;21:417–424.
[53] Pfleger T, Skorpik C, Menapace R, Scholz U, Weghaupt H, Zehetmayer M. Long-term course of induced astigmatism after clear corneal incision cataract surgery. J Cataract Refract Surg 1996;22:72–77.
[54] Nielsen PJ. Prospective evaluation of surgically induced astigmatism and astigmatic keratotomy effects of various self-sealing small incisions. J Cataract Refract Surg 1995;21:43–48.
[55] Cillino S, Morreale D, Mauceri A et al. Temporal versus superior approach phacoemulsification: short-term postoperative astigmatism. J Cataract Refract Surg 1997;23:267–271.
[56] Rainer G, Vass C, Menapace R et al. Long-term course of surgically induced astigmatism after 5.0 mm sclerocorneal valve incision. J Cataract Refract Surg 1998;24:1642–1646.
[57] Holweger R, Marefat B. Corneal changes after cataract surgery with 5.0 mm sutured and 3.5 mm sutureless clear corneal incisions. J Cataract Refract Surg 1997;23:342–346.
[58] Oshima Y, Tsujikawa K, Oh A, Harino S. Comparative study of intraocular lens implantation through 3.0 mm temporal clear corneal and superior scleral tunnel self-sealing incisions. J Cataract Refract Surg 1997;23:347–353.
[59] Poort-van Nouhuijs HM, Hendrickx KHM, van Marle WF et al. Corneal astigmatism after clear corneal and corneoscleral incisions for cataract surgery. J Cataract Refract Surg 1997;23: 758–760.
[60] Long DA, Monica ML. A prospective evaluation of corneal curvature changes with 3.0 to 3.5 mm corneal tunnel phacoemulsification. Ophthalmology 1996;103:226–232.
[61] Simsek S, Yasar T, Demirok A et al. Effect of superior and temporal clear corneal incisions on astigmatism after sutureless phacoemulsification. J Cataract Refract Surg 1998;24:515–518.
[62] Roman SJ, Auclin F, Chong-Sit DA, Ullern M. Surgically induced astigmatism with superior and temporal incisions in cases of with-the-rule preoperative astigmatism. J Cataract Refract Surg 1998;24:1636–1641.
[63] Rainer G, Menapace R, Vass C et al. Corneal shape changes after temporal and superolateral 3.0 mm clear corneal incisions. J Cataract Refract Surg 1999;25:1121–1126.
[64] Grabow HB. The clear-corneal incision. In: Fine IH, Fichman RA, Grabow HB, editors. Clear-corneal cataract surgery & topical anesthesia. Thorofare, NJ: Slack Inc; 1993. p. 29–62.
[65] Amon M, Menapace R, Vass C, Radax U. Endothelial cell loss after 3.5 mm temporal clear corneal incision and 3.5 mm superior scleral tunnel incision. Eur J Implant Refract Surg 1995;7:229–232.
[66] Dick HB, Kohnen T, Jacobi FK, Jacobi KW. Long-term endothelial cell loss following phacoemulsification through a temporal clear corneal incision. J Cataract Refract Surg 1996;22:63–71.
[67] Fine IH. Ongoing research in uses of power modulations to achieve low-energy phacoemulsification of cataracts. Presentation at the ASCRS Innovators' Session; Seattle, April 12, 1999.
[68] Dick HB, Schwenn O, Krummenauer F et al. Inflammation after sclerocorneal versus clear corneal tunnel phacoemulsification. Ophthalmology 2000;107:241–247.
[69] Ernest PH, Lavery KT, Kiessling LA. Relative strength of scleral corneal and clear corneal incisions constructed in cadaver eyes. J Cataract Refract Surg 1994;20:626–629.
[70] Ernest PH, Fenzl R, Lavery KT, Sensoli A. Relative stability of clear corneal incisions in a cadaver eye model. J Cataract Refract Surg 1995;21:39–42.
[71] Mackool RJ, Russell RS. Strength of clear corneal incisions in cadaver eyes. J Cataract Refract Surg 1996;22:721–725.
[72] Ernest PH, Neuhann T. Posterior limbal incision. J Cataract Refract Surg 1996;22:78–84.

[73] Fine IH. New thoughts on self-sealing clear corneal cataract incisions. Presented at Hawaii '96; Maui, Hawaii, January 22, 1996.

[74] Ernest P, Tipperman R, Eagle R et al. Is there a difference in incision healing based on location? J Cataract Refract Surg 1998;24:482–486.

[75] Budak K, Friedman NJ, Koch DD. Dehiscence of a radial keratotomy incision during clear corneal cataract surgery. J Cataract Refract Surg 1998;24:278–280.

[76] Eifrig CW, Flynn HW, Scott IU, Newton J. Acute-onset postoperative endophthalmitis: review of incidence and visual outcomes (1995–2001). Ophthalmic Surg Lasers 2002;33:373–378.

[77] Miller JJ, Scott IU, Flynn HW, Smiddy WE, Newton J, Miller D. Acute-onset endophthalmitis after cataract surgery (2000–2004): incidence, clinical settings, and visual acuity outcomes after treatment. Am J Ophthalmol 2005;139:983–987.

[78] Cooper BA, Holekamp NM, Bohigian G, Thompson PA. Case-control study of endophthalmitis after cataract surgery comparing scleral tunnel and clear corneal wounds. Am J Ophthalmol 2003;136:300–305.

[79] Colleaux KM, Hamilton WK. Effect of prophylactic antibiotics and incision type on the incidence of endophthalmitis after cataract surgery. Can J Ophthalmol 2000;35:373–378.

[80] Nagaki Y, Hayasaka S, Kadoi C et al. Bacterial endophthalmitis after small-incision cataract surgery: effect of incision placement and intraocular lens type. J Cataract Refract Surg 2003;29:20–26.

[81] Taban M, Behrens A, Newcomb RL, Nobe MY, Saedi G, Sweet PM, et al. Acute endophthalmitis following cataract surgery. Arch Ophthalmol 2005;123:613–620.

[82] West ES, Behrens A, McDonnell PJ, Tielsch JM, Schein OD. The incidence of endophthalmitis after cataract surgery among U.S. Medicare population increased between 1994 and 2001. Ophthalmology 2005;112:1338–1394.

[83] McDonnell PJ, Taban M, Sarayba MA et al. Dynamic morphology of clear corneal cataract incisions. Ophthalmology 2003;110:2342–2348.

[84] Taban M, Rao B, Reznik J et al. Dynamic morphology of sutureless cataract wounds – effects of incision angle and location. Surv Ophthalmol 2004;46:S62–S72.

[85] Sarayba MA, Taban M, Almeda TI et al. Inflow of ocular surface fluid through clear corneal cataract incisions: a laboratory model. Am J Ophthalmol 2004;138:206–210.

[86] Wallin T, Parker J, Jin Y, Kefalopolous G, Olson RJ. Cohort study of 27 cases of endophthalmitis at a single institution. J Cataract Refract Surg 2005;31:735–741.

[87] Montan PG, Wejde G, Seterquist H et al. Prophylactic intracameral cefuroxime; evaluation of safety and kinetics in cataract surgery. J Cataract Refract Surg 2002;28:982–987.

[88] Montan PG, Wejde G, Koranyi G, Rylander M. Prophylactic intracameral cefuroxime: efficacy in preventing endophthalmitis after cataract surgery. J Cataract Refract Surg 2002;28:977–981.

[89] Barry P, Seal DV, Gettinby DP, Lees F, Peterson M, Crawford WR. ESCRS study of prophylaxis of postoperative endophthalmitis after cataract surgery: preliminary report of principle results from a European multicenter study. J Cataract Refract Surg 2006;32:407–410.

[90] Monica ML, Long DA. Nine-year safety with self-sealing corneal tunnel incision in clear cornea cataract surgery. Ophthalmology 2005;112(6):985–986.

[91] Masket S. Is there a relationship between clear corneal cataract incisions and endophthalmitis? J Cataract Refract Surg 2005;31(4):735–741.

[92] Oshika T. Update on cataract surgery in Japan: annual survey of the Japanese Society of Cataract and Refractive Surgery. *Presentation at the annual meeting of the Japanese Society of Cataract and Refractive Surgery*, Joint Symposium with the American Society of Cataract and Refractive Surgery, June 16, 2006.

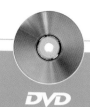

Capsulorrhexis

Thomas F. Neuhann, MD and Roger F. Steinert, MD

14

CONTENTS

- History
- Development of Capsulorrhexis
- Terminology
- Principles and Advantages of Capsulorrhexis
- Current Standard Techniques of Capsulorrhexis
- Difficult Situations
- Special Surgical Techniques
- Complications and Pitfalls

CHAPTER HIGHLIGHTS

>> Technical tips
>> Several techniques illustrated
>> Management of complicated capsulotomy

■ HISTORY ■

The rebirth of extracapsular cataract extraction in its modern, refined, microsurgical version has brought with it the need for an adequate technique for anterior capsulectomy. Vogt's technique, using toothed forceps to grasp and rip out a part of the anterior capsule, was definitely thought to be too traumatic to both the endothelium and the zonular apparatus, as well as too uncontrollable. Kelman's "Christmas tree" technique was a considerable improvement in terms of both better control and less trauma. Soon, however, interconnected perforations of the anterior capsule with a cystotome in a circular pattern, the "can-opener" technique, became the most popular and almost universally used approach worldwide. It allowed relatively precise control of the diameter and shape of the excised anterior capsular flap and, by using a cannula infusion cystotome, allowed the anterior chamber to be maintained throughout the procedure. Later, in an attempt to use the anterior capsule for additional endothelial protection during the surgical procedure, the "letterbox" technique was developed and gained considerable popularity, especially among surgeons preferring planned extracapsular cataract extraction. This two-stage technique also offered

considerable advantages for controlled lens implantation into the capsular bag because the anterior capsular window was not completed until after implantation of the intraocular lens (IOL).

Although these techniques and their modifications adequately fulfilled the aim of removing the central part of the anterior capsule, they proved to have one major disadvantage. The necessary manipulations during either phacoemulsification or extraction of the entire nucleus were almost invariably associated with the creation of one or more tears of the remaining peripheral anterior capsular rim, extending at least into the capsular equator. This has a number of undesirable side effects. Not infrequently, the tears extended beyond the capsular equator and into the posterior capsule, accompanied by the associated complications of vitreous loss and loss of the nucleus into the vitreous, especially when occurring early in the course of the operation. In addition, these tears divided the peripheral anterior capsule into a number of separate flaps, which could then interfere with the surgical procedure, especially the aspiration of peripheral cortical remnants. Finally, accumulating clinical evidence led an increasing number of surgeons to prefer IOL implantation into the capsular bag over sulcus implantation; however, it became evident after a while that at least 50% of the IOLs thought to be securely implanted with both loops in the capsular bag had, in reality, only one fixation loop in the bag or none at all. Anterior capsule tears were frequently the source of IOL loops escaping from the capsular bag.

■ DEVELOPMENT OF CAPSULORRHEXIS ■

From what may later be called a general surgical "instinct" (which was later fully substantiated by the clinical experience), a number of surgeons had realized for some time that the ideal anterior capsulectomy would be one with a smooth, continuous, ideally circular, margin, but the technique to achieve this ideal remained elusive. In 1984, Howard Gimbel in Calgary, Alberta, Canada, and Thomas Neuhann in Munich independently, but simultaneously, developed a technique that essentially consisted of tearing rather than cutting out a central anterior capsular window. What was so decisively new about this technique was not the tearing itself in fact, it had been used for part of the anterior capsulotomy before. The difference was that the tear was brought around the entire circumference, resulting in a circular opening with no beginning or end, nor an outward-pointing edge from which a radial tear could originate. Gimbel and Neuhann used different technical approaches, yet with the same underlying basic principle, benefiting from the specific tearing properties of the lens capsule. Much like cellophane, the lens capsule splits easily from a sharp-edged point of departure, whereas it is extremely resistant to tears into a smooth margin. Both surgeons showed their first video film in 1985 – Gimbel at the annual meeting of the American Society of Cataract and Refractive Surgery in Boston and Neuhann at the meeting of the German Ophthalmological Society in Heidelberg. In his film, Neuhann also proposed the term capsulorrhexis. The first formal publication in a scientific journal appeared in 1987;[1] in 1990 Gimbel and Neuhann published a joint article in the Journal of Cataract and Refractive Surgery.[2]

Both Gimbel and Neuhann have always regarded capsulorrhexis as having been developed by them equally, though independently, respectfully acknowledging the work of others on which the technique is based.[3]

■ TERMINOLOGY ■

The term *kapsulorhexis* was proposed by Neuhann to make it clear that it was a truly new surgical technique, a new surgical principle (namely tearing instead of cutting) and not just another modification of previous techniques. Gimbel originally called his technique "continuous tear capsulotomy." Bringing both their terms together yielded "continuous curvilinear (more general than circular) capsulorrhexis" (CCC).

■ PRINCIPLES AND ADVANTAGES OF CAPSULORRHEXIS ■

Capsulorrhexis leaves a capsular bag with mechanical and structural integrity, despite there being an opening large enough to deliver the lens through. This is due to the lens capsule's shearing property, which resembles cellophane. Although the capsule tears easily when departing from a sharply pointed defect in an edge, requiring a minimal amount of force, much greater force is required to rupture a straight, smooth margin.[4–6] This property is commonly experienced when opening the cellophane wrapper of a package. Tearing open a cellophane-wrapped package is greatly facilitated when the manufacturer provides a linear break in the wrapper and an arrow to that point with the instructions "Start here." If an opening in the lens capsule has a continuous smooth margin, the remaining capsule stays on stretch like a trampoline, as if no hole were present. The obvious advantages of this are as follows:

1. No tags or flaps of anterior capsule remnants interfere with surgery, especially the aspiration of the peripheral cortex.

2. The mechanical forces exerted onto the capsule, and thereby onto the zonules, are minimized.

3. The capsular bag is deeply open during surgery with a closed-system approach: the posterior capsule is ballooned posteriorly and thus held on stretch, reducing the danger of it getting caught and broken, while the anterior capsule remains on stretch horizontally, maintaining intracapsular space for surgical maneuvers.

4. With an intact capsulorrhexis, manipulations within the capsular bag (which are always in some way associated with

distention), such as tilting or cracking the nucleus or implanting an IOL, no longer entail the risk of extending radial tears in the anterior capsule into the posterior capsule.

5. Capsulorrhexis is the prerequisite for a reproducibly secure, verifiable, and permanent capsular bag fixation of IOL implant haptics.[7]

6. Even in the case of a posterior capsule defect, regardless of its size, an intact anterior capsulorrhexis provides the possibility of implanting an IOL safely into the ciliary sulcus. If the capsulorrhexis opening is well centered and smaller than the optic, it may be used additionally to fixate the implant by capturing the optic ("rhexis fixation") posteriorly while the haptics remain anterior in the ciliary sulcus.

7. It can be learned "by doing" without exposing the patient or the physician to any risk.

8. Capsulorrhexis is the prerequisite for all attempts to minimize or control posterior capsule opacification after cataract formation by the principle of a sharp posterior edge of the IOL.

■ CURRENT STANDARD TECHNIQUES OF CAPSULORRHEXIS ■

There are three basic choices that a surgeon must make for establishing his or her standard technique:

1. The instrument: a cystotome or a forceps

2. The access: via the main incision or via a side-port paracentesis

3. The medium: irrigation with fluid or viscoelastic.

Although all three options may theoretically be freely combined, in practice there are two main options:

1. A bent needle or cystotome through a side-port paracentesis under fluid irrigation (or viscoelastic)

2. A forceps through the main incision (or a side-port paracentesis) under viscoelastic.

For the needle technique, a 23-gauge needle is bent to about a one-quarter circle and with the tip 45° away from the bevel. The needle is mounted on an infusion handpiece, connected to the gravity-fed infusion at maximum height. With the infusion continuously running, the anterior chamber is entered through the side port, the size of which should just be large enough to permit passage of the needle. The chamber will thus be formed as deep as possible. The anterior capsule is perforated near the center with the needle tip and then slitted in a curvilinear manner with the cutting side edge of the needle in such a way that the desired radius of the capsulorrhexis is reached in a blend-in manner (Figure 14-1). When about to reach the desired circumference, the capsule is lifted from underneath, close to the leading tear edge, and pushed upward and forward to propagate the tear. Soon, enough of a flap will be created to permit flipping it over and engaging it from its backside, its epithelial side, now facing up toward the cornea. The needle engages the flap by exerting just enough pressure to create the friction necessary for engagement, but not enough pressure for the needle tip to perforate. Having the capsular flap thus engaged, it is torn in a circular fashion (Figure 14-2A) by appropriately influencing the tear vectors. The more distant the point of engagement is from the leading

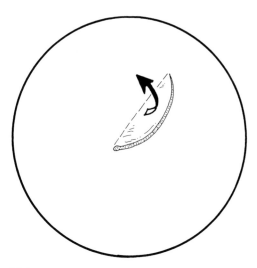

Figure 14-1 In the standard technique for capsulorrhexis, a central puncture with a cystotome followed by an arched curve creates a slit. The capsular flap is pulled and lifted at its edge.

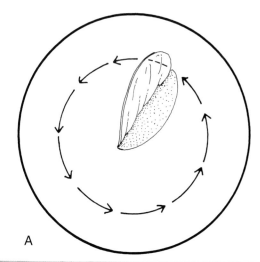

edge of the tear, the more centripetally one must tear; the closer the point of engagement is to the leading edge, the more directly the tear will follow the direction of traction. It is, therefore, most advisable to refixate the tear with the cystotome point frequently, close to the leading edge – a basic principle that governs the entire technique and its variations. When brought around full circle, the tear is blended into itself, automatically coming from outside in, which is a basic prerequisite to avoid a discontinuity.

The same technique can also be performed with the anterior chamber filled with a viscoelastic substance. In this instance one would basically follow the same guidelines, with the exception of the continuously running infusion.

The forceps technique makes the use of a viscoelastic substance mandatory to maintain the anterior chamber. When using a Utrata-type forceps, access through the main incision, which for that purpose must be fully widened to at least 3 mm, must

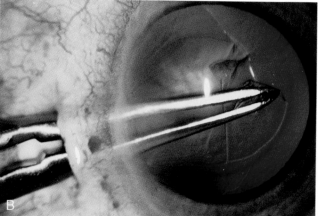

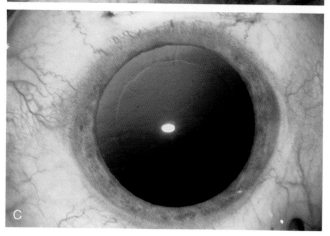

TECHNICAL TIPS

Starting the tear somewhere in the center in the capsule has the advantage of virtually eliminating the possibility of creating a discontinuity that would be caused by finishing the tear from inside out; this becomes especially valuable in cases with reduced visibility (e.g., small pupils, no red reflex). The tear must be performed over the full 360° in the direction in which it was started.

Puncturing the capsule within the contour of the capsulorrhexis has the disadvantage that it may cause a stellate burst (with extensions to the capsular periphery) if the needle is not perfectly sharp. If such a burst goes unnoticed (e.g., for visibility reasons) or if its extensions reach too far peripherally to be recovered, a peripheral tear will result at this location (Figure 14-3). In addition, with this technique the risk of inadvertently completing the capsulorrhexis from inside out is slightly higher. On the other hand, by beginning with a puncture, the surgeon has two options as to where to proceed with the tear, developing it and bringing both ends together at the point of maximal control (Figures 14-2C and 14-4). Today, most surgeons probably start somewhere in the capsular center.

Figure 14-2 A, Flap is inverted, and the underside of the capsule edge, now anterior, is engaged with the needle tip or forceps and pulled circularly. **B,** Circular tear capsulorrhexis is illustrated using a capsulorrhexis forceps. **C,** Perfect large circular capsulorrhexis is seen on red reflex through the operating microscope.

be chosen. When using a coaxial forceps of a pars plana-type construction, such as the Koch forceps, a paracentesis opening of appropriate size is sufficient. Otherwise, the forceps technique follows the same principles and guidelines as outlined earlier for the needle technique (see Figure 14-2B).

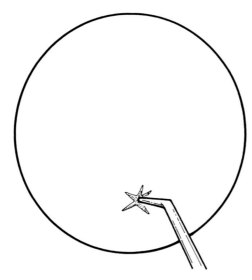

Figure 14-3 Use of a blunt needle to puncture the capsule in the periphery may create a stellate burst with outward pointing edges from which peripheral tears may originate.

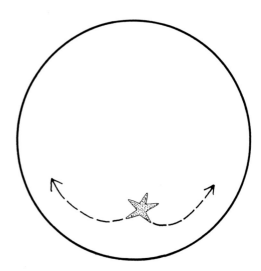

Figure 14-4 After a stellate opening, a continuous curve capsulorrhexis can be achieved by tearing in both directions from the most peripheral edges of the stellate opening.

TECHNICAL TIPS

With irrigation, the capsular flap floats freely in the anterior chamber, improving visualization, maneuverability, and control. Conversely, the incision must be tight, necessitating a very accurate and meticulous fulcrum technique. A viscoelastic substance is more forgiving with a leaking incision. However, visualization, especially of the leading tear edge, may be impaired as the torn-out portion of the capsule gets larger, crimps, and is "frozen" in the viscoelastic, possibly mixed with anterior cortex, and may lead to loss of control over the flap. Therefore, the flap should always be well spread out over the undersurface.

TECHNICAL TIPS

A drawback of the forceps technique is that it necessitates a larger incision and, therefore, can be safely performed only with a viscoelastic agent. Conversely, grasping with a forceps is somewhat more secure than grasping with a needle and is independent of the solidity of the underlying cortical material (which, with the needle technique, really constitutes the "second hand"). This latter aspect also makes it the technique of choice in some special situations (see later).

Two additional aspects regarding capsulorrhexis techniques merit discussion: firstly, the question of the ideal size of the anterior capsule opening. Ideally, the size should be:

- as large as possible. The larger the opening, the easier the manipulation of the nucleus
- small enough to allow the anterior capsular margin to just cover the optical part of the IOL, completely sealing it into the capsular bag. This "sealing-in" effect appears to be a prerequisite for the inhibitory effect of sharp IOL edges on the formation of secondary cataract.

Secondly, the limitations in obtaining the ideal size, which include the following:

- The size of the pupil
- The central insertion of the zonular fibers.

The surgeon must recognize that corneal magnification will make the initial capsulorrhexis appear larger than its true size; once the IOL is inserted, the capsulorrhexis will appear to have shrunken in comparison with the IOL optic.[8]

An asymmetric opening, that is, partly covering and partly not covering the optic margin, is to be avoided because of its potential for causing IOL optic decentration.

LEARNING CAPSULORRHEXIS

One of the major advantages of capsulorrhexis is that it can be learned "by doing," without exposing the patient to any additional risk. Coming from whatever prior technique of anterior capsulotomy, the surgeon may begin along the given guidelines. If the tear starts moving into an unwanted direction, the surgeon can revert to the previous technique.

TECHNICAL TIPS

When using Utrata-type forceps through the main incision, insidious loss of viscoelastic is very likely to occur. This leads to a flattening of the anterior chamber and, consequently, a forward movement of the lens. This, in turn, leads to an increase of the outward vector forces inherent in the lens capsule, making it increasingly more difficult to keep the tear from running outward. Knowing the danger means banning it: refilling the chamber with viscoelastic patiently as losses occur can prevent this most frequent source of losing control over the capsular tear. Instruments that open only at the tip (coaxial vitrectomy type) introduced through a paracentesis reduce viscoelastic loss. Use of a low-molecular-weight, retentive viscoelastic agent also reduces the amount of viscoelastic lost through the main incision.

To practice, good surrogates for the lens capsule are cellophane, as used in shrink-wrap packages, or tomato skin. Pigs' eyes, with thicker and more elastic anterior capsules, can serve as excellent models for learning to master the difficulties in infantile and juvenile capsules.

■ DIFFICULT SITUATIONS ■

Capsulorrhexis is best learned under ideal conditions: good-to-adequate pupillary dilation, good red reflex, deep anterior chamber, and no positive pressure.

The following four basic types of difficulties present challenges for capsulorrhexis:

1. No red reflex
2. Small pupil
3. Positive back pressure
4. Extreme elasticity: the infantile/juvenile capsule.

Although they often occur in various combinations, each of these situations is discussed separately to clarify the basic principles of management.

NO RED REFLEX

When there is no adequate reflex from the fundus to retroilluminate the surgical site for visualization, other clues must be used to "detect" the capsular margin in order to control the tear at every moment. The introduction of capsular dyeing, usually with trypan blue, is certainly the most notable progress in solving problems of visualization of the anterior capsule (for details, see Chapter 27, The Intumescent Cataract). Additional help can be contributed by other technical details; for instance, inclining the eye slightly with regard to the observation and illumination paths can sometimes produce enough of a red reflex to safely proceed. Also, side illumination, in addition to, or instead of, coaxial illumination, can be helpful. Often, one can benefit from the orange-skin-like specular reflex of the coaxial light source on the capsule. Constant manipulation of the eye position in such a way that the progressing tear edge remains in that reflex zone outlines the tear very clearly. Also, one should always choose as high a magnification as possible that does not interfere with the necessary overview. Finally, proceeding slowly in small steps and with frequent regrasping will help the surgeon not to lose control of the flap.

THE SMALL PUPIL

In addition to precluding visualization of the capsular area where one wishes to place the tear, the small pupil, in most instances, also causes reduction of the red reflex. Therefore, all of the previous measures are advisable as needed. (For an extensive discussion of small-pupil techniques, see Chapter 21.) When the pupil is smaller than the desired capsulorrhexis diameter, one may combine different principles. With experience, the surgeon will be able to tear a capsular flap "blindly," larger than the pupil diameter. Starting from the capsular center within the visible pupillary

area will ensure completion from "outside in." If one chooses to start the capsulorrhexis from the peripheral circumference, the needle may be used to retract the pupillary margin to the desired eccentricity, sliding along it while creating the initial slit and developing the flap away from the site of entry. Previous dyeing of the capsule with trypan blue can be helpful in judging the flap diameter. Measures to increase the pupillary diameter may include injection of atropine and/or epinephrine into the anterior chamber; filling the chamber with viscoelastic; peeling off the fibrous lining of the posterior aspect of the pupil, which so often limits its dilation; dilation of the pupil with self-retaining hooks or dilators (e.g. Malyugin ring) or only local dilation of the pupil with a second instrument through a second paracentesis, sliding along the pupillary edge with the progression of the tear. Multiple snip-sphincterotomies or sphincter stretching has been advocated. When in doubt, I prefer a keyhole iridotomy, which is later resutured, because it restores the iris diaphragm and thereby helps prevent later broad adhesions between an atonic, flaccid iris and the anterior capsule, or even the posterior capsule from migrating behind the implant. Finally, another possibility is performing phacoemulsification through an initially smaller capsulorrhexis and enlarging it later in a two-step technique.

POSITIVE PRESSURE

Positive pressure tends to force the tear outward. Therefore, these cases require an intentionally small diameter to begin with – which can be widened as soon as the pressure is relieved – and continuous, pronounced centripetal traction in small steps, regrasping frequently close to the tear edge. Also, exerting counterpressure by pushing the lens back with viscoelastic is very helpful.

INFANTILE/JUVENILE CAPSULE

The special challenge in infantile and juvenile capsulotomy is the increased elasticity of the lens capsule. When placing tension on an anterior capsule flap, it will first distend considerably before propagating the tear; once the tear starts, it has a great propensity to get lost outward because of the tractional "preload" and the elasticity, creating a pronounced outward pulling vector force. It is, therefore, advisable to aim for a tear that is smaller than one really wishes it to be because it will become wider by itself. The capsulorrhexis tear should progress slowly, in small steps, and with frequent regrasping and directing the tearing more centripetally than for a typical adult cataract. The disadvantage of the extreme elasticity, however, has a positive side also. Should a discontinuity in the capsulorrhexis margin occur, it is, for the same reason, less likely to progress peripherally when due caution during surgery is maintained.

The only situation in which capsulorrhexis is impossible in principle is the totally fibrosed capsule. Cases of heavy fibrosis or fibrous plaques extending so far peripherally that one cannot tear around them without hitting zonules mandate the use of scissors to cut through the fibrosis. The scissor cut should end just barely at the margin of the fibrosis, and from there on into regular capsule the opening should be continued as a tear.

The intumescent lens combines the difficulties of positive pressure with those of a lack of red reflex. Filling the anterior chamber with a thick viscoelastic is advisable to block opaque liquefied cortex from leaking into the aqueous humor and compromising visibility. Usually a forceps technique is preferable because the cortex is liquefied and, therefore, presents no resistance to a needle tip. The second major problem is the increased pressure within the capsule as a result of the swollen lens, which increases the risk of uncontrollable extension of the partially completed capsular opening to the periphery. The surgeon must try to counteract this tendency by filling the anterior chamber with a high-viscosity viscoelastic, to the extent of indenting the anterior lens pole. Sometimes one can decompress the lens by making a small puncture in the central anterior lens and aspirating some of the liquid content through the puncturing needle.

SPECIAL SURGICAL TECHNIQUES

Applying the same basic principles as described earlier has led to the development of maneuvers that may prove helpful in certain situations.

BIMANUAL FORCEPS

In certain situations, it may become difficult to grasp and manipulate the capsular flap using just the needle tip. The surgeon may, in these situations, prefer to change to a forceps technique. However, when removing the irrigating cystotome, the lens diaphragm may come forward, causing the tear to divert outward. To avoid this, a bifurcated spatula of the Bechert type (or similar modification) is introduced into the chamber through an opposite paracentesis. The capsular flap is pinched between the needle tip and spatula tip. The capsule flap can then be manipulated as with a forceps.

An alternative is to introduce viscoelastic through the second paracentesis before withdrawing an irrigating cystotome needle. The anterior chamber will remain formed while the surgeon changes to a forceps.

BIMANUAL/BI-INSTRUMENTAL CAPSULORRHEXIS

When the zonules are very weak, pulling centripetally on the flap may risk disinsertion of the capsule. Holding the flap with capsular forceps with one hand and gently pushing the peripheral margin outward (centrifugally) with a blunt instrument can propagate the tear with less stress on the zonules. The surgeon should strongly consider placing a capsule tension ring as soon as the capsulorrhexis is completed in these very tenuous cases.

POSTERIOR CAPSULORRHEXIS

Leaving the posterior capsule intact is one of the major objectives of extracapsular surgery. Nevertheless, this goal cannot always be attained. Examples are a dense, nonremovable posterior capsular opacification that will doubtlessly interfere significantly with vision; an infantile cataract in which rapid opacification of the osterior capsule is inevitable and neodymium:yttrium-aluminum-garnet (Nd:YAG) laser capsulotomy is impractical (see Chapter 26, Surgical Management of Pediatric Cataracts and Aphakia); or, most frequently, accidental posterior capsular rupture. In all of these cases, the opening in the posterior capsule should have the same quality, if possible, as that of the anterior capsulorrhexis, namely being not further extendable because of a continuous smooth margin. This can be obtained by applying the same technique of capsulorrhexis as that of the posterior capsule. In cases of intentional posterior capsule opening, the posterior capsule should be nicked centrally with a needle tip, viscoelastic is injected through the first tiny triangular defect to separate and posteriorly displace the anterior vitreous face, and the posterior capsular triangle is grasped by capsular forceps and torn out as a curvilinear posterior capsulorrhexis.

When an unintended capsular defect occurs, extension can be limited by the same technique, as long as the original posterior capsule rent is limited enough to permit this. This technique will then preserve a capsular bag into which an IOL can be implanted securely, maintaining all the advantages of intracapsular implantation.

"RHEXIS-FIXATION"

In the case of a posterior capsular rupture that cannot be limited by posterior capsulorrhexis, another maneuver may maintain most of the advantages of capsular implant fixation. If the anterior capsulorrhexis margin is intact and smaller than the IOL optic, the IOL can be implanted into the ciliary sulcus and the optic captured, that is, "buttoned in" backward through the capsulorrhexis in the technique first described by Tobias Neuhann. This provides secure mechanical fixation of the lens by the capsule and centration in relation to the capsular opening, with the lens haptics only acting as secondary support. The IOL in this position will have the same optical power as though intracapsularly implanted.

COMPLICATIONS AND PITFALLS

The following are three classic intraoperative complications that can occur with capsulorrhexis:

1. Discontinuity of the anterior capsular margin
2. Tear into the zonules
3. Diameter being too small.

The following are two classic postoperative complications:

1. Purse-string contraction
2. Incarceration of viscoelastic.

DISCONTINUITY OF THE ANTERIOR CAPSULAR MARGIN

The major causative factors in this instance are: completing the capsulorrhexis "from inside outward" (Figure 14-5), nicking an originally intact margin with the second instrument during lens extraction, or breaking the rim with the activated phaco tip. A discontinuity in an otherwise intact CCC margin will, in most cases, extend into a radial tear into the capsular fornix; it will do so very readily because the distensive forces will concentrate

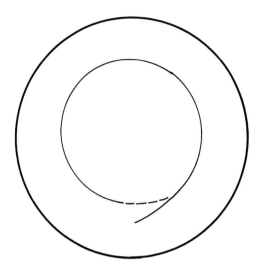

Figure 14-5 Illustration of a capsulorrhexis that is progressively enlarging so that it finishes from the inside toward the outside.

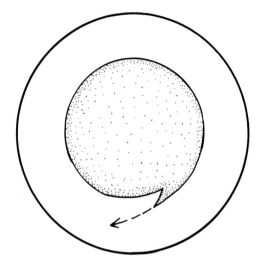

Figure 14-6 Discontinuity in the capsule is created by an inside-to-outside finish. From that point, a peripheral tear may originate. The same situation results when a previously intact capsulorrhexis margin is cut with an instrument or with the phacoemulsification tip.

on this single point of weakness (Figure 14-6). The risk of this radial tear extending around the capsular fornix into the posterior capsule increases with sparse and friable zonules and with all maneuvers that distend the anterior capsular opening, such as hydrodissection, expression of the nucleus, nuclear fracturing techniques that rely on pushing the nuclear sections widely apart, and IOL implantation maneuvers.

TECHNICAL TIPS

The most important rule is to always close the circle from outside inward. This will automatically occur when starting the tear somewhere in the center of the capsule, as described earlier (Figure 14-7). If the flap breaks off during the course of the tear, the surgeon must be sure to grasp the remaining flap and continue the outward pointing tear edge. When a discontinuity happens, timely recognition is of key importance. Its edge must instantly be grasped with forceps and blunted off by blending into the main contour (Figure 14-8). When a tear has occurred into the capsular fornix, utmost caution is warranted not to extend the tear further by avoiding the previous risk factors. A relaxing counterincision opposite the first tear may be considered. A radial tear does not preclude capsular bag implantation if manipulations are appropriately gentle. The lens haptics should be placed at 90° from the radial tear. Such a tear is a relative contraindication for implantation of plate haptic IOLs.

TEAR INTO THE ZONULES

If the tear encounters zonular fibers, either because it is too peripheral or because zonules are inserted abnormally centrally, it cannot readily be continued. Further tearing will risk deviation of the tear to the periphery, like tearing paper alongside a ruler (Figure 14-9). With the help of high microscope magnification, an optimized red reflex or specular reflex, and optimal focusing, the responsible zonules can be identified and their insertions removed from the capsule with the needle or forceps tip. Then the surgeon brings the tear more centrally and continues.

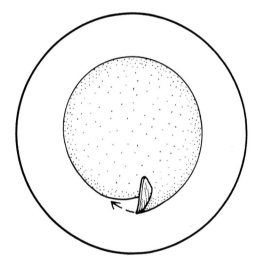

Figure 14-7 When an inside-outside discontinuity occurs, it can be repaired by picking up the resulting triangle, inverting it, and tearing centripetally to bring the tear edge back toward the capsulorrhexis margin, ultimately blending it in.

Sometimes this situation can also be managed by grasping the flap close to its edge and briskly pulling it centrally. This maneuver, however, carries a higher risk and is only advised when the more controlled approach does not seem possible.

Healon 5 (Pharmacia), with its exceptionally high density, can also help redirect an extending capsulorrhexis tear. A relatively small amount of Healon 5 is injected into the angle, with the expanding bolus reaching the edge of the tear. The dense Healon 5 will help redirect the tear back centrally.

CAPSULORRHEXIS WITH TOO SMALL A DIAMETER

If the surgeon realizes that the diameter of the CCC is becoming smaller than desired, he or she may just continue the tear in a spiral manner until the desired diameter is reached (Figure 14-10).

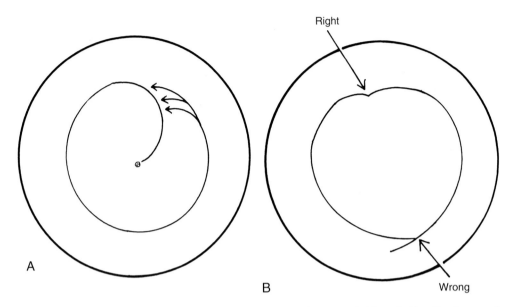

Figure 14-8 **A,** Starting the capsulorrhexis from the center makes it virtually impossible to end in an inside-out fashion. Creating a continuous margin is much more likely. **B,** When a capsulorrhexis is completed correctly, a small centrally pointing tag is created. When the capsulorrhexis is incorrectly finished, a discontinuity occurs.

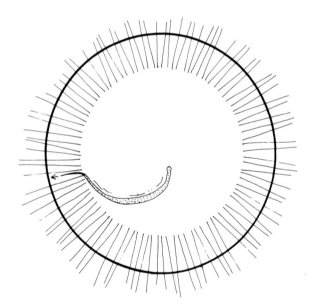

Figure 14-9 When a capsular tear encounters a zonular fiber, the resulting zonular forces direct the tear peripherally toward the equator.

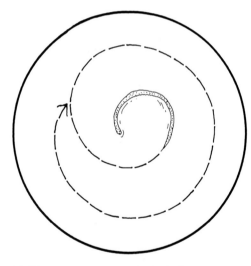

Figure 14-10 In performing the capsulorrhexis, the surgeon may realize that the original arc is too small. The capsulorrhexis can be expanded by "spiraling" outward to the desired diameter and then "closing the circle."

When a large and hard nucleus coincides with a very small diameter of the anterior capsular opening, hydrodissection may lead to a pressure-induced rupture of the posterior capsule. The nucleus blocks the capsular opening, and the injected fluid has only one way to escape: posteriorly. An initial bulging forward of the lens followed by a sudden, snaplike drop backward indicates the occurrence. In such an event, conversion to planned extracapsular cataract extraction is indicated. A lens loop behind the nucleus is necessary. Consideration should be given to "posterior assisted levitation" with either an instrument or injection of viscoelastic through a pars plana sclerotomy to support the nucleus from behind.[9]

PURSE-STRING CONTRACTION

The remaining lens epithelial cells on the back surface of the anterior capsule postoperatively undergo fibrous metaplasia. The contraction of this fibrous layer is normally counteracted by the centrifugal forces of the zonular apparatus. However, when either the zonules are weak (e.g., in pseudoexfoliation, trauma, and retinitis pigmentosa) or the fibrosis is excessive (e.g., after increased postoperative inflammation, with some silicone lenses and other factors) or in combinations of both, the anterior capsular opening may contract ("capsular phimosis") (Figure 14-11). The contracture may block the visual axis or exert excessive contracture on the ciliary body, leading to hypotony.[10]

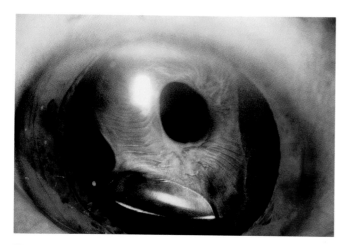

Figure 14-11 Postoperative photograph illustrating contracture of the capsulorrhexis. This situation is more common when the original capsulorrhexis is 4 mm or smaller.

TECHNICAL TIPS

In cases identified at risk for excessive contraction, the surgeon should aim for a relatively large opening, implant lenses with stiff haptics with an overall diameter of about 13 mm, consider implantation of a capsular tension ring (or even two), and perhaps avoid silicone as a lens material. Postoperatively, these cases should be monitored closely. At the first sign of contraction, the anterior capsular margin should be incised with an Nd:YAG laser at three or four equidistant locations. Extension of these discontinuities need not be feared at this stage, owing to the fibrous lining itself and the already secure sealing in of the IOL.

INCARCERATION OF VISCOELASTIC ("CAPSULAR BLOCK SYNDROME")

Residual viscoelastic may be trapped behind an implant when the IOL optic margin is completely covered by the capsulorrhexis. The retained viscoelastic attracts water osmotically and swells. The implant acts as a valve, permitting the influx of aqueous behind the lens, but not the efflux of the thick viscoelastic–aqueous mixture. This phenomenon is more pronounced with plate haptic lenses but may happen with all types of implants. The consequence may be gross inflation of the capsular bag with posterior ballooning of the posterior capsule and anterior displacement of the IOL, heralded by a shallow anterior chamber and a myopic shift in the refraction.[11]

This complication can best be avoided by complete removal of the viscoelastic material, actively aspirating it from behind the lens. Once capsular block has occurred, the retained material can be released into the anterior chamber by puncturing the anterior capsule beyond the optical margin with Nd:YAG laser pulses. If the pupil cannot be dilated adequately to expose the anterior capsule peripheral to the IOL optic, a laser peripheral iridectomy can be made, followed by further laser pulses deeper through the iridectomy to open the anterior capsule. If this cannot be achieved, the posterior capsule must be punctured, releasing the material into the vitreous. Prophylactic treatment with topical steroids, nonsteroidal anti-inflammatory agents, and glaucoma medications is given because of expected transient inflammation and elevated intraocular pressure from the abruptly released viscoelastic agent.

References

[1] Neuhann T. Theorie und operationstechnik der kapsulorhexis. Klin Monatsbl Augenheilkd 1987;190:542–545.

[2] Gimbel HV, Neuhann T. Development, advantages, and methods of the continuous curvilinear capsulorrhexis. J Cataract Refract Surg 1991;17:110–111.

[3] Assia EI, Apple DJ, Barden A et al. An experimental study comparing various anterior capsulectomy techniques. Arch Ophthalmol 1991;109:642–647.

[4] Thim K, Krag S, Corydon L. Stretching capacity of capsulorrhexis and nucleus delivery. J Cataract Refract Surg 1991;17:27–31.

[5] Krag S, Thim K, Corydon L. Stretching capacity of capsulorrhexis: an experimental study on animal cadaver eyes. Eur J Implant Refract Surg 1990;2:43–45.

[6] Assia EI, Apple DJ, Tsai JC et al. The elastic properties of the lens capsule in capsulorrhexis. Am J Ophthalmol 1991;111:628–632.

[7] Colvard DM, Dunn SA. Intraocular lens centration with continuous tear capsulotomy. J Cataract Refract Surg 1990;16:312–304.

[8] Waltz KL, Rubin ML. Capsulorrhexis and corneal magnification. Arch Ophthalmol 1992;110:170. [letter].

[9] Harris DJ, Specht CS. Intracapsular lens delivery during attempted extracapsular cataract extraction: association with capsulorrhexis. Ophthalmology 1991;98:623–627.

[10] Fritsch E, Bopp S, Lucke K et al. Pars-plana-kapselresektion zur therapie des okulären hypotoniesyndroms durch kapselschrumpfung mit ziliarkörpertraktion. Fortschr Ophthalmol 1991;88:802–805.

[11] Davison JA. Capsular bag distension after endophacoemulsification and posterior chamber intraocular lens implantation. J Cataract Refract Surg 1990;16:99–108.

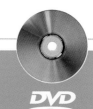

Hydrodissection and Hydrodelineation

**I. Howard Fine, MD, Richard S. Hoffman, MD and
Mark Packer, MD, FACS**

15

CONTENTS

- Hydrodissection
- Technique
- Hydrodelineation
- Completion of the Procedure
- Conclusions

CHAPTER HIGHLIGHTS

>> Hydrodissection techniques
>> Hydrodelineation techniques
>> Cortical cleaving hydrodissection

■ HYDRODISSECTION ■

Hydrodissection of the nucleus in cataract surgery has traditionally been perceived as the injection of fluid into the cortical layer of the lens under the lens capsule to separate the lens nucleus from the cortex and capsule.[1] With increased use of continuous curvilinear capsulorrhexis[2,3] and phacoemulsification in cataract surgery, hydrodissection became a very important step to mobilize the nucleus within the capsule for disassembly and removal.[4-8] Following nuclear removal, cortical cleanup proceeded as a separate step, using irrigation and aspiration handpieces.

Fine[9] has previously described cortical cleaving hydrodissection, which is a hydrodissection technique designed to cleave the cortex from the lens capsule and thus leave the cortex attached to the epinucleus. Cortical cleaving hydrodissection usually eliminates the need for cortical cleanup as a separate step in cataract surgery by phacoemulsification, thereby eliminating the associated risk of capsular rupture.

■ TECHNIQUE ■

A small capsulorrhexis, 5–5.5 mm, optimizes the procedure. The large anterior capsular flap makes this type of hydrodissection easier to perform. The anterior capsular flap is elevated away from

the cortical material with a 26-gauge blunt cannula (e.g., Katena Instruments No. K7-5150) before hydrodissection (Figures 15-1–15-3). The cannula maintains the anterior capsule in a tented-up position at the injection site near the lens equator. Irrigation before elevation of the anterior capsule should be avoided because it will result in transmission of a fluid wave circumferentially within the cortical layer, hydrating the cortex and creating a path of least resistance that will disallow later cortical cleaving hydrodissection (Figure 15-4). Once the cannula is properly placed and the anterior capsule is elevated, gentle, continuous irrigation results in a fluid wave that passes circumferentially in the zone just under the capsule, cleaving the cortex from the posterior capsule in most locations. When the fluid wave has passed around the posterior aspect of the lens, the entire lens bulges forward because the fluid is trapped by the firm equatorial cortical-capsular connections (Figures 15-5 and 15-6). The procedure creates, in effect, a temporary intraoperative version of capsular block syndrome as seen by the enlargement of the diameter of the capsulorrhexis. At this point, if fluid injection is continued, a portion of the lens prolapses through the capsulorrhexis. However, if the capsule is decompressed before prolapse by depressing the central portion of the lens with the side of the cannula in a way that forces fluid to come around the lens equator from behind (Figures 15-7 and 15-8), the cortical-capsular connections in the capsular fornix and under the anterior capsular flap are cleaved. The cleavage of cortex from the capsule equatorially and anteriorly allows fluid to exit from the capsular bag via the capsulorrhexis, which constricts to its original size, and mobilizes the lens in such a way that it can spin freely within the capsular bag. Repeating the hydrodissection and capsular decompression starting in the opposite distal quadrant may be helpful. Adequate hydrodissection at this point can be demonstrated by the ease with which the nuclear–cortical complex can be rotated by the cannula.

■ HYDRODELINEATION ■

Hydrodelineation is a term first used by Anis[10] to describe the act of separating an outer epinuclear shell or multiple shells from the central compact mass of inner nuclear material, the endonucleus, by the forceful irrigation of fluids (balanced salt solution) into the mass of the nucleus.

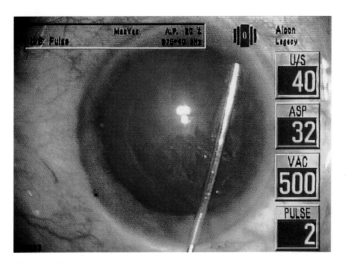

Figure 15-1 Placement of the cannula under the anterior capsulorrhexis in one of quadrants, elevating the capsule.

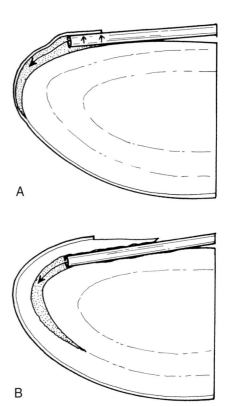

Figure 15-3 A, In cortical cleaving hydrodissection, the fluid wave passes between the capsule and cortex. **B,** In conventional hydrodissection, the natural fluid cleavage plane is between the cortex and epinucleus.

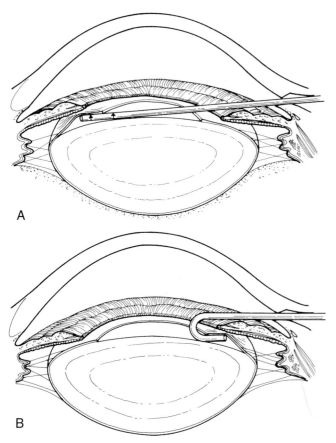

Figure 15-2 Cortical cleaving hydrodissection. **A,** In the original technique, the cannula is passed inferiorly, with tenting up of the anterior capsule before injection of fluid. **B,** The alternative technique described by Steinert uses a 180° Binkhorst cannula to direct the initial fluid wave superiorly. The cannula is rotated to elevate the anterior capsule and to direct the fluid wave between the capsule and the cortex.

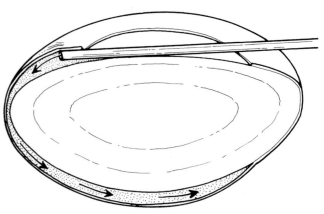

Figure 15-4 As the fluid is injected, a posterior fluid wave is created.

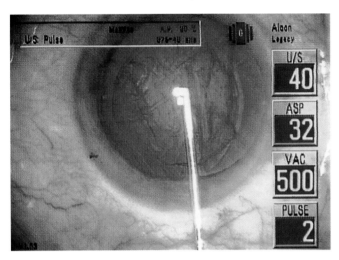

Figure 15-5 Enlargement of capsulorrhexis as seen following second cortical-cleaving hydrodissection, fluid wave placed in the opposite distal quadrant just before decompression of the capsular bag.

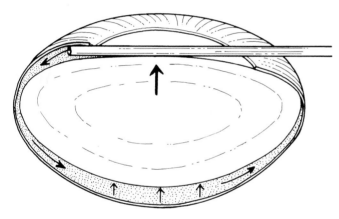

Figure 15-6 As cortical-cleaving hydrodissection proceeds, fluid is trapped posteriorly, with anterior displacement of the lens in the capsular bag.

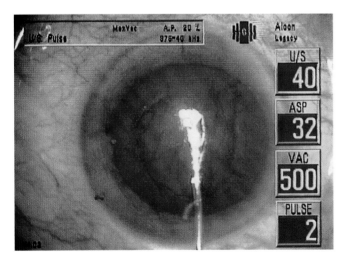

Figure 15-7 Return of capsulorrhexis to its original size following decompression of the bag.

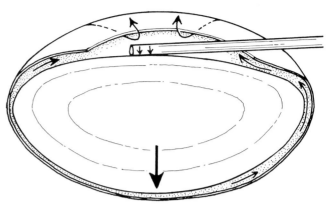

Figure 15-8 Posteriorly loculated fluid is decompressed by downward pressure on the lens with the cannula. Trapped fluid then advances around the equator, releasing equatorial cortical-capsular adhesions.

Our technique uses the same hydrodissection cannula as previously described. The cannula is placed in the nucleus, off center to either side, and directed at an angle downward and forward towards the central plane of the nucleus. When the nucleus starts to move, the endonucleus has been reached; it is not penetrated by the cannula. At this point, the cannula is directed tangentially to the endonucleus, and a to-and-fro movement of the cannula is used to create a tract within the nucleus. The cannula is backed out of the tract approximately halfway (Figure 15-9), and a gentle but steady pressure on the syringe allows fluid to enter the "empty" distal tract without resistance. Driven by the hydraulic force of the syringe, the fluid will find the path of least resistance, which is the junction between the endonucleus and the epinucleus, and flow circumferentially in this contour (Figure 15-10). Most often, a circumferential golden ring will be seen outlining the cleavage between the epinucleus and the endonucleus. Sometimes the ring will appear as a dark circle rather than a golden ring.

Occasionally, an arc will result and surround approximately one quadrant of the endonucleus. In this instance, creating another tract the same depth as the first but ending at one end of the arc, and injecting into the middle of the second tract, will extend that arc (usually another full quadrant). This can be repeated until a golden or dark ring verifies circumferential division of the nucleus.

For very soft nuclei, the placement of the cannula allows creation of an epinuclear shell of variable thickness. The cannula may pass through the entire nucleus if it is soft enough, so the placement of the tract and the location of the injection allow an epinuclear shell to be fashioned as desired. In very firm nuclei, one appears to be injecting into the cortex on the anterior surface of the nucleus, and the golden ring will not be seen. However, a thin, hard epinuclear shell is achieved even in the most brunescent nuclei. That shell will offer the same protection as a thicker epinucleus in a softer cataract.

Hydrodelineation circumferentially divides the nucleus and has many advantages. Circumferential division reduces the volume of the central portion of nucleus removed by phacoemulsification by up to 50%. This allows less deep and less peripheral grooving and smaller, more easily mobilized quadrants after cracking or chopping. The epinucleus acts as a protective cushion within which all of the chopping, cracking and phacoemulsification forces can be confined. In addition, the epinucleus keeps the bag on stretch throughout the procedure, making it unlikely that a knuckle of capsule will come forward, occlude the phaco tip, and rupture.

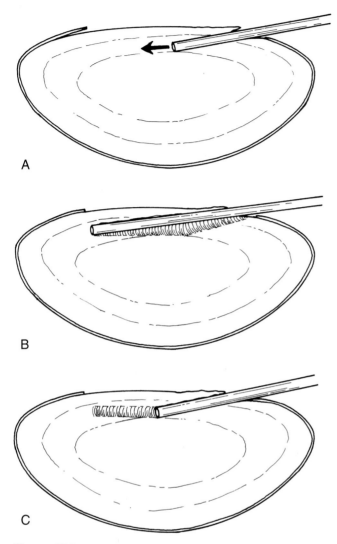

A

B

C

Figure 15-9 Hydrodelineation is performed by determining the natural cleavage plane between the nucleus and epinucleus. **A,** Blunt-tipped cannula is advanced as deeply as possible, thereby riding across the tops of the firm nucleus. **B,** Cannula is advanced inferiorly. **C,** Cannula is then partially withdrawn within the tract. Sufficient cannula length is embedded in the lens material to trap fluid to be injected, but the open tract created allows the fluid pressure to seek out the natural cleavage plane between the inner nucleus and the middle epinuclear layer.

More recently, Vasavada has described a technique for hydrodelineation in very hard cataract called "inside-out hydrodelineation."[11] The nucleus is bowled out and then fluid is injected from inside the bowl outward. This then allows endonuclear rotation and chopping of the peripheral endonucleus bowl and removal of the epinucleus in the usual manner.

■ COMPLETION OF THE PROCEDURE ■

After evacuation of all endonuclear material, the epinuclear rim is trimmed in each of the three quadrants (Figure 15-11), mobilizing cortex as well in the following way. As each quadrant of the epinuclear rim is rotated to the distal position in the capsule and trimmed, the cortex in the adjacent capsular fornix flows over the floor of the epinucleus and into the phaco tip (Figure 15-12).

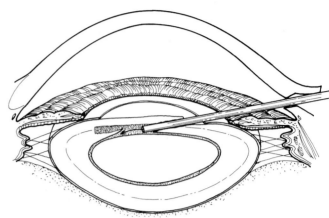

Figure 15-10 Complete hydrodelineation is obtained. If the pupil is widely dilated relative to the size of the nucleus, a "golden ring" is seen because of the microscope light reflex.

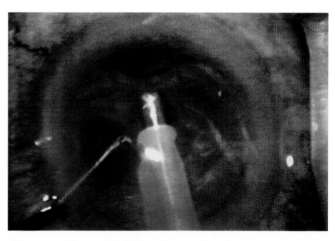

Figure 15-11 Purchase of the epinuclear rim and roof in foot position 2, being pulled central to the capsulorrhexis. The cortical layer is seen superior to the rim and roof of the epinuclear shell.

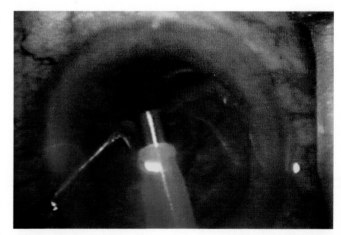

Figure 15-12 Following trimming of the initial purchase of the rim and roof in foot position 3, one can see the cortex flow over the floor and into the tip, removing it from that same quadrant.

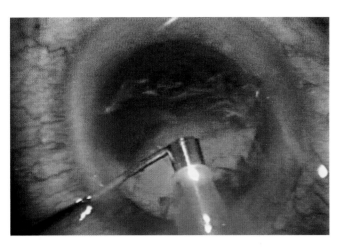

Figure 15-13 Repositioning the floor of the epinucleus after rim and roof of the epinuclear shell have been trimmed and the cortex has been evacuated from the third epinuclear quadrant.

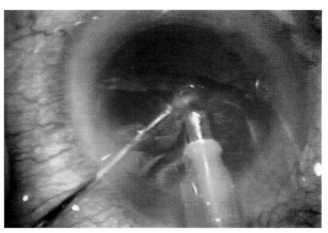

Figure 15-14 Initiating the flipping maneuver of the residual epinucleus using the fourth quadrant of epinuclear rim and shell.

Then the floor is pushed back to keep the bag on stretch until three of the four quadrants of the epinuclear rim and forniceal cortex have been evacuated (Figure 15-13). It is important not to allow the epinucleus to flip too early, thus avoiding a large amount of residual cortex remaining after evacuation of the epinucleus.

The epinuclear rim of the fourth quadrant is then used as a handle to flip the epinucleus (Figures 15-14 and 15-15). As the remaining portion of the epinuclear floor and rim is evacuated from the eye, 70% of the time the entire cortex is evacuated with it (Figure 15-16).[12] Downsized phaco tips with their increased resistance to flow are less capable of mobilizing the cortex because of the decreased minisurge accompanying the clearance of the tip when going from foot position 2 to foot position 3 in trimming of the epinucleus. After the intraocular lens is inserted, these strands and any residual viscoelastic material are removed using the irrigation–aspiration tip, leaving a clean capsular bag.

If there is cortex still remaining following removal of all the nucleus and epinucleus, there are three options:

1. The phacoemulsification handpiece can be left high in the anterior chamber while the second handpiece strokes the cortex-filled capsular fornices. Often, this results in floating up of the cortical shell as a single piece and its exit through the phacoemulsification tip (in foot position 2) because cortical cleaving hydrodissection has cleaved most of the cortical capsular adhesions.

2. If the surgeon wishes to complete cortical cleanup with the irrigation–aspiration handpiece before lens implantation, the residual cortex can almost always be mobilized as a separate and discrete shell (reminiscent of the epinucleus) and removed without ever turning the aspiration port down to face the posterior capsule (see Figure 15-15).

3. The final option is to viscodissect the residual cortex by injecting the viscoelastic through the posterior cortex onto the

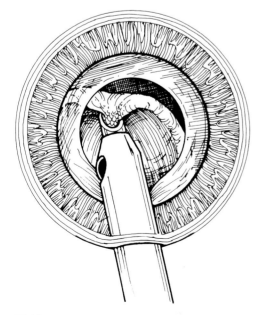

Figure 15-15 Aspiration of residual epinuclear and cortical envelope.

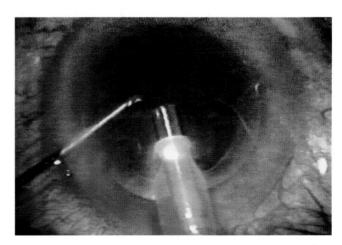

Figure 15-16 Capsular bag is clear of cortex, except for a single strand to the right following flipping and evacuation of the residual epinucleus.

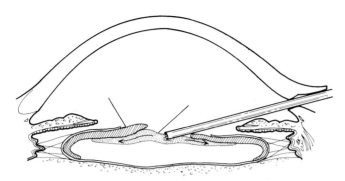

Figure 15-17 Residual cortex can be aspirated after intraocular lens insertion. The first step is to carefully instill a viscoelastic agent under the residual cortex.

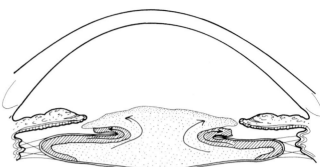

Figure 15-18 As the viscoelastic agent fills the capsular bag, tags of remaining cortex are brought anteriorly, draping over the anterior capsule.

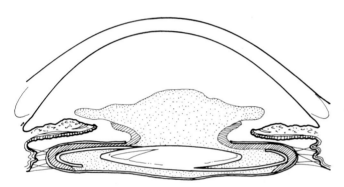

Figure 15-19 After the intraocular lens (IOL) is placed in the capsular bag, residual cortex is then anterior to the IOL optic.

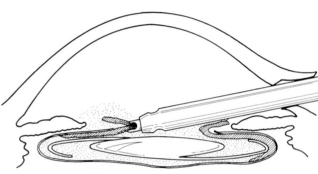

Figure 15-20 Irrigation–aspiration tip can now access the remaining cortex and successfully aspirate the cortex while the intraocular lens remains within the capsular bag.

posterior capsule. We prefer the dispersive viscoelastic device chondroitin sulfate-hyaluronate [Viscoat]. The viscoelastic material spreads horizontally, elevating the posterior cortex and draping it over the anterior capsular flap (Figure 15-17). At the same time the peripheral cortex is forced into the capsular fornix (Figure 15-18). The posterior capsule is then deepened with a cohesive viscoelastic device [e.g., Provisc] and the IOL is implanted through the capsulorrhexis, leaving the anterior extension of the residual cortex anterior to the IOL (Figure 15-19).

Removal of residual viscoelastic material accompanies mobilization and aspiration of residual cortex anterior to the IOL (Figure 15-20), which protects the posterior capsule, leaving a clean capsular bag.

■ CONCLUSIONS ■

In summary, the lens can be divided into an epinuclear zone with most of the cortex attached and a more compact central nuclear mass. The central portion of the cataract can be removed by any endolenticular technique, after which the protective epinucleus is removed with all or most of the cortex attached. In most cases, irrigation and aspiration of the cortex as a separate step are not required, thereby eliminating that portion of the surgical procedure and its attendant risk of capsular disruption. Residual cortical cleanup may be accomplished in the presence of a posterior chamber IOL, which protects the posterior capsule by holding it remote from the aspiration port.

References

[1] Faust KJ. Hydrodissection of soft nuclei. Am Intraocular Implant Soc J 1984;10:75–77.
[2] Neuhann T. Theorie und operationstechnik der kapsulorhexis. Klin Monatsbl Augenheilkd 1987;190:542–545.
[3] Gimbel HV, Heuhann T. Development, advantages, and methods of the continuous circular capsulorrhexis technique. J Cataract Refract Surg 1990;16:31–37.
[4] Davison JA. Bimodal capsular bag phacoemulsification: a serial cutting and suction ultrasonic nuclear dissection technique. J Cataract Refract Surg 1989;15:272–282.
[5] Sheperd JR. In situ fracture. J Cataract Refract Surg 1990;16:436–440.
[6] Gimbel HV. Divide and conquer nucleofractis phacoemulsification: development and variations. J Cataract Refract Surg 1991;17:281–291.
[7] Fine IH. The chip and flip phacoemulsification technique. J Cataract Refract Surg 1991;17:366–371.
[8] Fine IH, Maloney WF, Dillman DM. Crack and flip phacoemulsification. J Cataract Refract Surg 1993;19:797–802.
[9] Fine IH. Cortical cleaving hydrodissection. J Cataract Refract Surg 1992;18:508–512.
[10] Anis A. Understanding hydrodelineation: the term and related procedures. Ocular Surg News 1991;9:134–137.
[11] Vasavada AR, Raj SM. Inside-out delineation. J Cataract Refract Surg 2004;30:1167–1169.
[12] Fine IH. The choo-choo chop and flip phacoemulsification technique. Op Tech Cataract Refract Surg 1998;1:61–65.

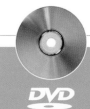

Principles of Nuclear Phacoemulsification

Howard V. Gimbel, MD, MPH

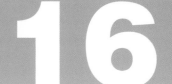

16

CONTENTS

CHAPTER HIGHLIGHTS

>> Evolution of nuclear phacoemulsification

>> Nuclear fracturing techniques

>> Special clinical presentations

>> Avoidance of complications during phaco

■ PHACOEMULSIFICATION TODAY ■

Cataract surgery using phacoemulsification techniques and instrumentation offers a number of attractive benefits to both the surgeon and patient. The principal advantage is a smaller incision size, which decreases the amount of tissue injury, reduces the amount of postoperative pain and inflammation, and provides a more rapid refractive stabilization[1,2] with less astigmatism induced by the procedure.[1–4] The smaller incision also allows minimal restrictions on the patient's physical activities, even in the early postoperative period.

Although early phacoemulsification techniques performed in the anterior chamber were associated with a high loss of endothelial cells,[5–12] the corneal problems have been significantly minimized by the advent of in situ, or what has become known as posterior chamber, phacoemulsification[13–18] and the protective properties of viscoelastic substances.[19–26] These have in turn enhanced intraoperative safety and surgeon control, while minimizing iris trauma,[27] capsule tears, and the possibility of intra-operative suprachoroidal hemorrhage by maintaining a pressurized surgical environment.

Other advantages of phacoemulsification that are difficult to quantify include a more efficient use of operating room time by the surgeon and staff, highly satisfied patients, and a quicker return to personal independence and to the workforce by many patients, which has tremendous potential economic repercussions.

These benefits and favorable outcomes continue to drive a growing interest in, and an acceptance and application of phacoemulsification. In the Leaming studies,[28] phacoemulsification as the surgical procedure of choice increased from 12% in 1985 to 79% in 1992, and to 97% in 2000. It is worth noting, that this survey only reflects the opinion of a portion of the American Society of Cataract and Refractive Surgery membership and may not precisely indicate the trend among American cataract surgeons in general.[29,30] Nonetheless, the upswing in usage of the technique is undeniable. In other countries, such as Australia,[31] the United Kingdom,[32] and Canada, the conversion has probably not been as remarkable, but the momentum for change seems to be building. Similar trends have also been reported in Asia[33–36] and in other parts of Europe.[32,37–40]

The acceptance of phacoemulsification in most countries can be directly correlated with the introduction of continuous curvilinear capsulorrhexis (CCC) in 1985.[41–43] In concert with the vast majority of today's in situ phacoemulsification techniques, CCC preserves the anterior capsule rim and helps to ensure in-the-bag placement and long-lasting centration of an intraocular lens.[44]

■ THE EVOLUTION OF PHACOEMULSIFICATION ■

The origins of phacoemulsification can be traced to the pioneering efforts of Kelman. In 1967, Kelman described a single-instrument technique for cataract extraction using ultrasound vibration to remove lens material through a 3 mm corneoscleral incision.[45] To minimize posterior capsule tears and dropped nuclei, the nucleus was prolapsed into the anterior chamber and subsequently emulsified. Over the course of the next several years, Kelman shared his experiences of the technique;[46–50] this included the publication of results using this new procedure that compared favorably with the results of intracapsular cataract extraction,[51,52] the method of cataract extraction most commonly used at that time. Kelman's enthusiasm for a procedure that reduced astigmatism and provided early rehabilitation was shared by a number of surgeons. Between 1973 and 1979, the results of thousands of Kelman phacoemulsification cases performed by numerous surgeons were reported.[53–75] However, several factors limited the universal application of Kelman phacoemulsification as the procedure of choice for cataract extraction.

First, a number of reports were published citing damage to the corneal endothelium using the technique. Second was the realization that the very dense, brunescent nucleus resisted ultrasonic fragmentation, making many cases difficult, dangerous, or impossible to accomplish with the techniques and instruments then available. Finally, the shape of intraocular implants of the day required an incision substantially larger than 3 mm, potentially discounting any advantage of a smaller wound to remove the cataract. Nonetheless, Kelman had set the stage for further refinement of his ingenious invention.

In the early 1970s, Sinskey, because of the difficulty of delivering softer nuclei into the anterior chamber, used a 15° phacoemulsification tip to sculpt the central nucleus down almost to the posterior capsule before removing the peripheral nuclear shell.[76] By performing the phacoemulsification posteriorly in the capsular bag, and thus deep in the anterior chamber, damage to the corneal endothelial cells was significantly reduced.

During this same period, Little[77] and Kratz[78–80] popularized two-handed emulsification of the nucleus using a spatula as a second instrument. Little passed the spatula into the anterior chamber directly alongside the ultrasound tip through the 12 o'clock incision. He sculpted the anterior nucleus centrally with a 45° tip, then tilted and prolapsed the remaining nucleus out of the superior equator of the capsular bag for further emulsification. Kratz chose to use a side-port second incision at 3 o'clock for this purpose. The goal of his iris plane-tilt technique was to increase the efficiency of Sinskey's method, especially for lenses with a hard epinucleus as well as a hard nucleus, while reducing contact with the endothelium and still protecting the posterior capsule. Maloney adopted this technique and taught it to many surgeons.[81]

The author was originally trained as an intracapsular surgeon but attended Kelman's New York phacoemulsification course in January 1974. With modifications learned from Kratz, Sinskey, and Little, combined with the author's own experience and innovation, a technique soon evolved from a one-handed anterior chamber technique to a two-handed posterior chamber technique for soft nuclei with Kratz's tipping technique for hard lenses. The author developed the CCC technique in 1984, and by 1985 had developed the "divide and conquer nucleofractis" method of in situ phacoemulsification.[82,83] This approach evolved because hard, large nuclei could not be tipped out of a 5–6 mm CCC and could not be safely emulsified in situ. It was found to be necessary to emulsify these lenses by systematically dividing and fragmenting the dense nuclear rim after sculpting all that could be safely sculpted. The fracturing technique was then applied to less dense cataracts before extensive sculpting was done. The maneuver of fracturing the nucleus, which the author termed "nucleofractis,"[83] can be used in many different ways. It has added efficiency and safety during the emulsification of moderately dense lenses and has allowed all but rock-hard cataracts to be easily conquered by phacoemulsification. The techniques make use of several aspects of lens anatomy.

■ THE PRINCIPLE OF NUCLEOFRACTIS ■

CLINICAL ANATOMY OF THE LENS

The cataractous lens consists primarily of three structures: the capsule, the cortex, and the nucleus (Figure 16-1). The lens capsule is the outermost layer of the lens and consists of the anterior capsule transitioning to the posterior capsule at the equator of the lens.[84–86] Surrounding the central nucleus and epinucleus is the lens cortex. The germinal epithelium of the lens is the source of the lens fibers.[87,88] The nucleus is the central core of the lens and varies in hardness from the center to the periphery in most cataracts, depending on the progression of the cataract. As the typical age-related cataract progresses, the central and then the peripheral nucleus tend to become more brunescent, changing from clear to yellow to dark brown.

A number of lamellar zones are present in the lens, starting with the fetal nucleus, which becomes the hard central nucleus as new fibers are laid down through life.[89,90] These fibers join in a Y-shaped suture anteriorly and posteriorly. The lens thus develops in layers, but orientation of the lens fibers creates radial cleavage planes through which cracks can be made (Figure 16-2). It is the author's clinical observation that, although the Y sutures are the zones most susceptible to fracturing, "fault lines" that may be utilized for cracking are present to a lesser degree throughout the lens. In a very soft lens, such as in a younger person, it may be difficult to identify these fault lines because of decreased fiber density within the nucleus and because interdigitating portions of the lens fibers still hold the nucleus together.

The radial and lamellar zones are analogous to those seen in a tree. If a cross-section of a tree is examined, just inside the outer bark, an actively replicating living tissue lays down concentric lamellae of tree fiber. The existence of these lamellae is confirmed by the annular rings of the cut tree trunk. These are less densely packed in the periphery and much more dense and closer together in the center of the tree core. The cataract's outer capsule simulates the tree bark. Just inside the capsule are lens epithelial cells, which lay down concentric lamellae of nuclear tissue that are

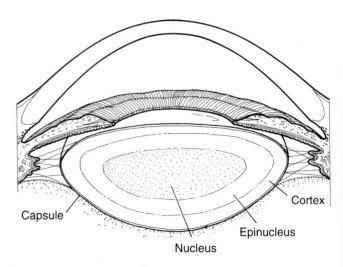

Figure 16-1 Cross-sectional view of the crystalline lens.

Capsule

Cortex

Epinucleus

Nucleus

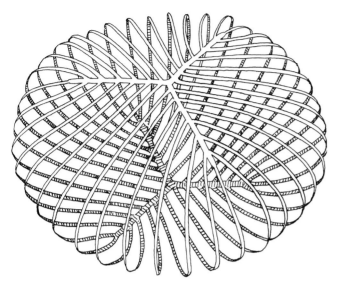

Figure 16-2 Artist's conception of radial and lamellar zones.

looser in the periphery and much denser in the center. A log for use in a fireplace has lamellar separations of bark and annular rings corresponding to the cortex being separated by lamellar hydrodissection. However, for efficient burning, the core of the log is also split with radial fractures, many of which are seen as natural cleavage planes as the wood dries. Another analogy is the watermelon, which has radial as well as circumferential cleavage planes. When sculpting down through the nucleus of the cataract, one can often see the natural radial cleavage planes in the nucleus of the lens corresponding to the aforementioned Y sutures seen on slit-lamp examination. Although the radial fractures often follow these primary cleavage planes, the instruments can easily create other radial cleavage planes.

Drews has used neodymium:yttrium-aluminum-garnet (Nd: YAG) laser energy to demonstrate the position of the core of the lens nucleus, to confirm the existence of these radial fracture lines within the nuclear core, and to provide an anatomical basis for the formation of grooves across the nucleus during phacoemulsification.[91,92] Hydrodissection of the epinuclear layers from the nuclear core occasionally fractures the nucleus radially, demonstrating the existence of these anatomical divisions. Mechanical fracturing of the nucleus can make very effective use of these anatomical features to achieve safer and more efficient phacoemulsification.

ORIGINS OF NUCLEOFRACTIS

The concept of fracturing or cracking the nucleus is not new. As far back as 1967, Kelman used Ringberg forceps to crack the nucleus (Kelman C, Personal communication, 1985). For safety reasons, this technique was abandoned in favor of the nuclear prolapse method. The author's introduction of a bimanual nucleofractis technique resulted from a combination of a number of factors. In the late 1970s the author used the spatula instrument for rotation of the lens, thereby facilitating sculpting. The spatula was also used as needed during phacoemulsification to stabilize and position the nucleus. By 1984, that author was using

a technique to subdivide chunks of the nucleus before breaking them up and suctioning them out, and, in 1985, found that rotation of the lens could result in an inadvertent fracture of the nucleus. This discovery led to the development of a technique to purposefully fracture the nuclear rim.

In 1986 the author applied the term *divide and conquer* to this in situ phacoemulsification technique, which is derived from the Latin *divide et impera*. The divide and conquer technique was first introduced by way of a videotape at the 1987 European Intraocular Implantlens Council (now called the European Society of Cataract and Refractive Surgery) meeting in Jerusalem. The technique was subsequently presented at numerous courses and was demonstrated by live surgery at the 1988 Canadian Rockies Symposium on Cataract and Refractive Surgery in Calgary, Alberta, Canada.

The fracturing maneuver of divide and conquer can be accomplished once the instruments can be positioned sufficiently deep in the lens, which is achieved after the sculpting of a trough, trench, groove, or crater in the lens nucleus. The goal is then to split the nucleus where it is intact posteriorly and equatorially by a rim of peripheral nucleus. The ideal place to apply the splitting force is at the bottom of the groove first and then at the rim. The reverse can also be used and is the order when chopping techniques are used.

In the author's experience, this is best accomplished using a bimanual, direct, or at times a cross-fracturing technique, in which the phaco probe is moved to the opposite side of the rim and the second instrument is moved to the other. Although, in the author's opinion, the use of a Haefliger phaco cleaver (Moria, Paris, France) for these purposes is preferable, a number of customized instruments, including chopping instruments, have been designed to facilitate this maneuver.[93–95] The nucleus is thus bisected with a minimum of instrument and nuclear movement, so the force is effectively applied at the parallel faces of the groove, splitting the rim directly apart (Figure 16-3). If the instruments are placed too anteriorly in the trench, the bottom of the rim is not split, because the inappropriate placement of the instruments has created a torque in this area rather than a splitting force (Figure 16-4).[96] The capsule may redirect the horizontal vector forces and actually compress the deeper nuclear layers.

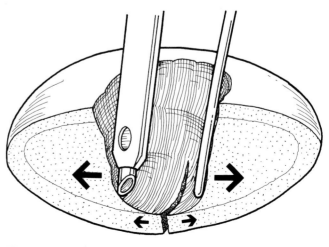

Figure 16-3 Posterior placement of the two instruments for bidirectional fracturing or nucleofractis.

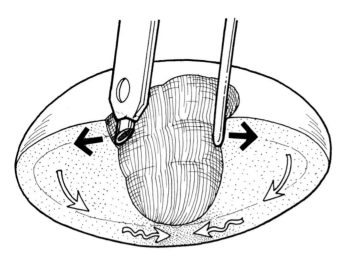

Figure 16-4 Inappropriate anterior placement of the instruments, resulting in misapplication of vector forces and ineffective fracturing.

In addition to the direct and cross-action fracturing techniques, several other methods of cracking are available. Parallel cracking[97] is accomplished by lining up the groove with the point midway between the main incision and the side-port opening. The second instrument is laid deep within the trench while the phaco handpiece rests on top of it. The instruments are then moved away from each other in a parallel position, resulting in the easy cracking. The nucleus can then be rotated to make additional grooves and then each groove can be aligned and cracked in exactly the same manner.

Nonrotational cracking is parallel, direct, or cross-handed, and takes place within the nucleus without rotation. Learning this technique is advantageous, as it may facilitate nuclear fracturing in the presence of a rent in the CCC opening with less risk of extending the tear. This can usually be safely accomplished by cracking 90° away from the rent to minimize stress to this area. Chopping rather than splitting is the safest method of nucleus disassembly in the presence of an anterior or posterior capsule tear.

Divide and conquer nucleofractis demands a slight stretch or distortion of the lens capsule, and subsequent tears are resisted only by the strong tear-resistant border of the CCC. Conversely, the integrity of the capsule border cannot always be preserved in planned extracapsular extraction or in anterior chamber phacoemulsification, particularly when attempted in large, dense, brunescent nuclei. Hence, a clear interdependence has been recognized between the two techniques. Thus, the technique of in situ phacoemulsification is uniquely suited to the technique of CCC. The demand for the coexistence of the two techniques is furthered by the great resilience and strength of the smooth-edged border of the CCC, which has been demonstrated experimentally[98–100] and by protection of the corneal endothelium by a larger rim of anterior capsule during in situ or in-the-bag phacoemulsification.[101]

Because of the mechanics and complexities of nucleofractis, the advent of divide and conquer rendered sculpting no longer a random process, but a defined means of achieving nuclear cracking. In fact, two broad variations of divide and conquer nucleofractis[83,102–104] have been developed to deal with different types of cataracts:

1. The trench technique, for soft to moderately hard nuclei
2. The crater technique for moderately hard to very hard and even dense, brunescent nuclei.

DIVIDE AND CONQUER

Following CCC, hydrodissection is utilized to facilitate divide and conquer nucleofractis phacoemulsification. Both phacoemulsification techniques incorporate four basic steps: (1) deep sculpting until a fracture is possible, (2) nucleofractis of the nuclear rim and posterior plate of the nucleus, (3) fracturing again and breaking away a wedge-shaped section of nuclear material for emulsification, and (4) rotation or repositioning of the nucleus for further fracturing and emulsification.

Crater Divide and Conquer

The deep sculpting of the nucleus was part of the author's first divide and conquer technique back in 1985. At that time, the technique involved sculpting out to the nuclear rim and removing as much of the right side of the lens as could be safely done. The left side of the lens continued to be stabilized with the spatula and then, rather than just being sculpted, sections were broken away with radial fractures and emulsified.

As this technique was applied to very hard lenses, the author began using the fracturing technique for brunescent lenses after deep central sculpting. This technique became the *crater divide and conquer* (CDC) technique because of the large crater sculpted, leaving a dense peripheral rim to fracture into multiple sections (Figure 16-5). This required considerable patience as the nucleus was shaved progressively deeper. It also became apparent that the entire rim could be fractured into sections and then these sections brought into the center in a manner similar to the way that sections were broken away in the earlier technique. A trench, trough, or groove is not used in these cases in which a dense, brunescent lens is present, because it does not weaken the entire lens nucleus enough to easily fracture, and the resulting segments are too large to manage safely.

Before hydrodissection was introduced, the nucleus was mechanically broken away from the cortex by rocking clockwise and counterclockwise using two instruments, until the lens could be rotated within the cortical shell. As mentioned previously, complete hydrodissection is now routinely utilized because nuclear shifting or rotation is required for the nucleofractis

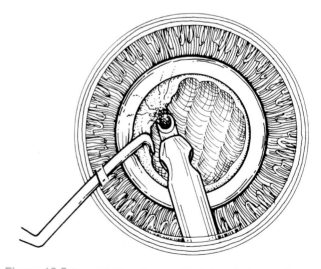

Figure 16-5 Crater "divide and conquer" technique. In dense and brunescent cataracts, nucleofractis is facilitated by emulsification of a deep and wide central crater of nucleus.

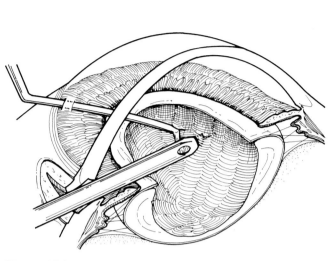

Figure 16-6 Cross-sectional view of sculpted crater.

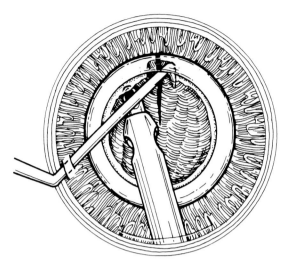

Figure 16-7 Using the cyclodialysis spatula and the phaco tip, the resultant peripheral nuclear rim is fractured.

technique. Hydrodissection has made this easier and safer by reducing stress on the zonular ligaments during rotation.

Some experience is required to enable the surgeon to judge how deeply the central coring may safely proceed without rupturing the posterior capsule. A safety mechanism built into the CDC technique is the maintenance of a peripheral nuclear rim after creation of the crater, which maintains distention of the capsular bag, keeping the posterior capsule deep and stretched during sculpting and nucleofractis. Once central coring is complete (Figure 16-6), the nuclear rim is fractured using the bimanual method, whereby the spatula and phaco tip create a counter-pressure (Figure 16-7). The lens is rotated, and a second crack is made, isolating a pie-shaped section (Figure 16-8). The nuclear rim is then rotated clockwise for right-handed surgeons, facilitating systematic piece-by-piece nucleofractis. The harder the nuclear rim, the smaller the wedge-shaped sections should be to allow manageability of the individual pieces and to reduce the possibility of tearing the posterior capsule.

TECHNICAL TIPS

The phaco tip itself may be more efficient for cutting through tissue in dense nuclei than the resistance of the phaco sleeve allows. That is why in very dense, brunescent lenses, deep burrowing is facilitated by retracting the sleeve to expose more of the tip. The extra amount exposed is conditional upon the size of the pupil to minimize the potential for touching the edge of the iris with the metal part of the tip in small pupils. Usually, however, increasing the amount of tip exposed from the standard distance of 1.5–2 mm is advantageous in the denser lenses.

When the CDC technique is used, and especially in very dense and brunescent cataracts, rather than immediately emulsifying each wedge-shaped section, the nuclear sections are generally left in place for capsular bag distention (Figure 16-9). Once the fracturing is complete, each pie-shaped wedge of the nuclear rim

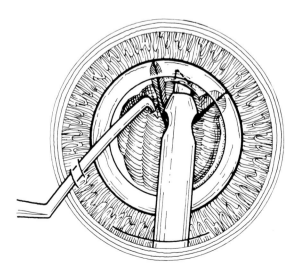

Figure 16-8 Nucleus is rotated, and a second fracture is made. The section is left in place, ensuring stabilization of the nucleus and capsule.

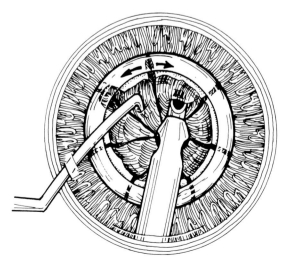

Figure 16-9 Remaining "donut" of nucleus is systematically fractured using the bimanual technique.

THE PRINCIPLE OF NUCLEOFRACTIS

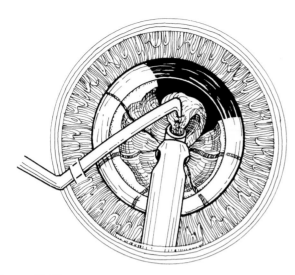

Figure 16-10 Individual sections are brought into the center for emulsification.

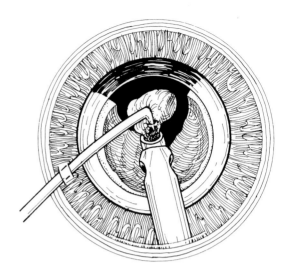

Figure 16-11 Alternatively, the first section may be isolated and emulsified to allow space for subsequent fracturing.

is brought to the center of the capsule, where phacoemulsification is safely accomplished (Figure 16-10). High flow, high vacuum, and low ultrasound power using a 15° or 30° tip keeps these segments fastened to the tip, reducing the chance of the segments tumbling into the chamber. The spatula is used to control what is coming to the tip and remains under the last segments being emulsified to protect the posterior capsule. The ultrasonic turbulence is contained within the lens bag and absorbed by the lens and capsule for all but the last one or two small nuclear fragments.

As an alternative during CDC, the first sector may be removed prior to performing additional space for tissue separation (Figure 16-11). This technique is best performed in firm, but easily fractured lenses such as in mature, white cataracts. Each section may be emulsified as it is broken away (Figure 16-12). This is analogous to the choice one has when serving pieces of birthday cake. One can either cut the entire cake into pieces before serving any or cut a single piece, serve it, and then cut another and so forth.

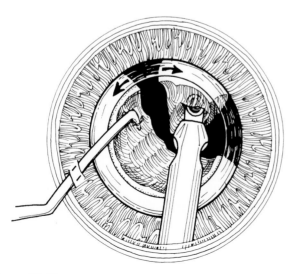

Figure 16-12 Remaining nuclear rim is individually fractured and emulsified.

Trench Divide and Conquer

Realizing the efficiency of the fracturing maneuvers during CDC, the author made the decision to stop sculpting the right side of soft lenses after making the central trench and instead make a central fracture. Then not only was the left side divided by fracturing, but also the right side. These variations were named the *trench divide and conquer* (TDC) technique. For the purposes of these descriptions, a superior orientation of the incision with a subincisional area in the 12 o'clock position is assumed.

Trench Divide and Conquer with "Down Slope" Sculpting

The author appreciated a slight variation from the traditional sculpting method being employed with the nucleofractis techniques. By nudging the lens inferiorly with the second instrument, the upper central part of the nucleus can be sculpted very deeply, to the point of sculpting directly parallel and close to the posterior capsule. This allows the tip to remove more of the upper part of the nucleus during sculpting and to reach the posterior pole of the lens very early for effective fracturing. With the lens nucleus nudged toward the 6 o'clock position, the surgeon can sculpt very deeply down the slope of the posterior curvature of the upper part of the capsule. The author termed this method TDC with "down slope" sculpting.[104,105]

First using this nudging maneuver in small pupil cases out of necessity, because of the limitations of the size of the pupil and capsule opening, the author then began extending its applicability to almost all cases. This has been found to greatly enhance the speed and efficiency of the nucleofractis techniques and has increased the safety, because the sculpting is parallel rather than somewhat perpendicular to the posterior capsule, as occurs when traditionally sculpting the inferior part of the lens.

Using a 30° or 45° tip, the TDC technique begins with a shallow trench or trough sculpted slightly to the right of the center of the lens surface (Figures 16-13 and 16-14). The lens is stabilized with the spatula or chopper through the paracentesis. Then, nudging the loosened lens nucleus inferiorly with the second

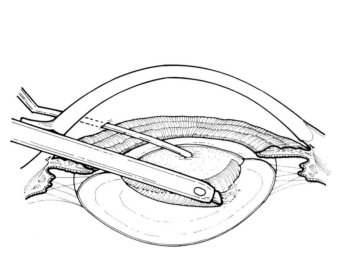

Figure 16-13 Cross-sectional view of initial sculpting of a trench or trough.

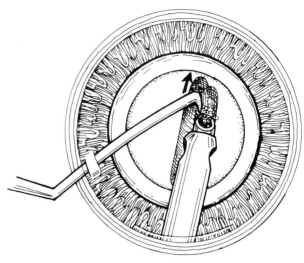

Figure 16-14 After nudging the lens inferiorly with the second instrument, the down slope technique starts with a trench or trough sculpted to just past the center of the lens surface.

instrument, down slope sculpting is accomplished, sculpting very deeply to the posterior pole of the lens (Figure 16-15). Hydrodissection is essential to achieve down slope sculpting because then the nucleus is not attached to the peripheral cortex and capsule, and the nucleus can easily be displaced in the capsular bag.

Placing the instrument tips deep in the center of the lens, fracturing is accomplished by pushing toward the right with the phaco tip as the cyclodialysis spatula or chopper is pushed to the left (Figure 16-16). This is accomplished in foot position 2 (irrigation/aspiration only and no ultrasound power). The lens usually splits from the center to the superior and inferior rim of the nucleus if the instruments are held deep in the center. If the split does not readily extend to the equator inferiorly or superiorly, moving the instruments away from the center can produce the mechanical advantage necessary to extend the fracture through the nuclear rim.

After this first crack has been obtained, the depth of the sculpted groove in the lens can be determined, and thus the surgeon can gauge how much deeper sculpting should be continued to facilitate further fracturing. In all but brunescent nuclei, usually three to five sculpting passes allow one to get deep enough into the lens to start fracturing.

Either before the first fracture or immediately afterward, the down slope technique may be used to sculpt the majority of the upper part of the lens. Keeping the probe deep in the tissue and close to the posterior cortex, the surgeon then burrows deeply into the left hemisection and creates a second crack that intersects with the first, isolating a pie-shaped section of nucleus. In soft nuclei, this is usually performed about 60° from the first fracture, but in hard nuclei, the crack is shortened to about 30° away (Figures 16-17 and 16-18).

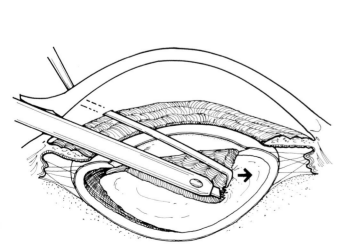

Figure 16-15 Cross-sectional view of nudging maneuver and down slope sculpting.

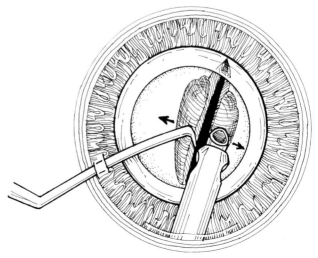

Figure 16-16 With the instrument tips deep in the center of the lens, a fracture can be obtained easily and early.

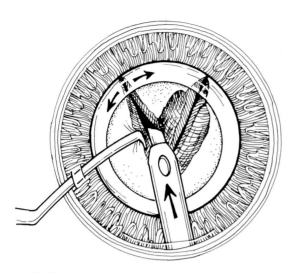

Figure 16-17 Using the bimanual technique again, a second crack is made and either emulsified or left in place for further fracturing.

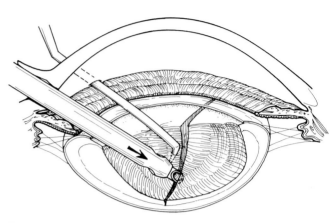

Figure 16-18 Cross-sectional view of second fracture.

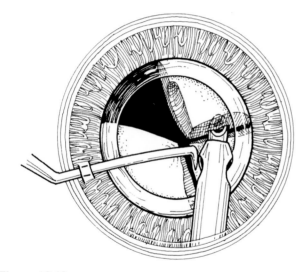

Figure 16-19 Right section is maneuvered into midpupillary zone for further nucleofractis.

The isolated pie-shaped section can then either be emulsified or left in place as the next crack is made in a similar fashion. The remaining right section of nucleus is then maneuvered with the second instrument and brought to the midpupillary zone (Figure 16-19). A final split is made after impaling the tip with a short burst of ultrasound, pushing with the phaco tip toward the 6 o'clock position while stabilizing the upper portion. The piece can then be fractured into halves or thirds and emulsified as they are fractured. Alternatively, the right hemisection may be rotated to the left side and fractured in a way similar to the first hemisection (Figure 16-20).

The down slope method can also be used to remove a large portion of the upper part of the lens, creating a horizontal anterior to posterior wall in the nucleus. The phaco tip is then used to stabilize the upper portion, while the second instrument pushes inferiorly against this wall creating a horizontal fracture (Figure 16-21). The inferior hemisection is then divided into three or more sections by burrowing into the right side and breaking away a section for emulsification while stabilizing the

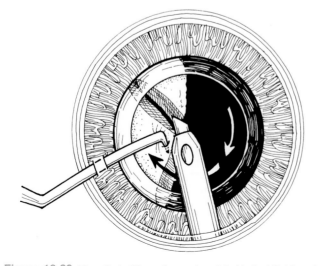

Figure 16-20 Alternatively, this section can be rotated to the left side and fractured.

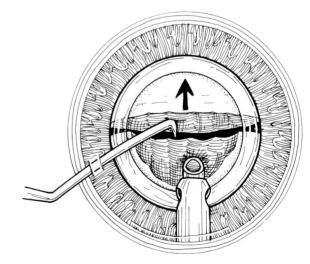

Figure 16-21 Using down slope sculpting and nucleofractis, a horizontal split can be created.

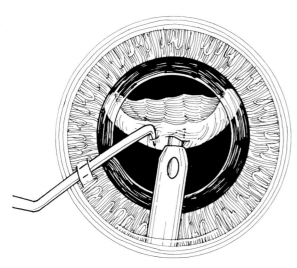

Figure 16-22 Inferior hemisection brought to center for division and emulsification.

left piece with the spatula. The thin upper hemisection is then brought to the center and divided similarly (Figure 16-22).

With traditional sculpting techniques, the deepest part of the sculpting inevitably ends up inferior to the center of the lens. If the surgeon rotates the lens 90° after sculpting each quadrant, then the nuclear material deep in the center or posterior pole of the nucleus may still impede complete fracturing to the center and the sections will tend to hang together in the middle of the lens (Figure 16-23). However, with down slope sculpting, complete and efficient fracturing and subsequent emulsification can be accomplished by sculpting deeply and fracturing through the entire posterior plate of the nucleus. Rather than utilizing grooves to start the fractures, the surgeon simply needs to get the instruments deep into the center of the lens to fracture through the naturally occurring radial fault lines of the lens. Except in brunescent nuclei, where notches are sculpted in the nuclear rim so that the spatula has a wall to push against, the principal advantage of the technique is that pregrooving the nucleus for subsequent fracturing is completely unnecessary and may be accomplished successfully without a chopper.

Down slope sculpting in the upper pole of the lens to just past the center reduces the chance of posterior capsule rupture with the phaco port. If the lens is nudged inferiorly by the second instrument and deep sculpting is done from just inside the continuous curvilinear capsulorrhexis to the center of the lens, then the tip travel will be parallel to the concave slope of the posterior aspect of the nucleus and the posterior capsule. Although the surgeon cannot visualize the tip when going "down slope," the depth of the sculpting is determined by visualizing the depth of the groove and translucency of the remaining tissue.

With traditional techniques, if the nucleus is broken through unexpectedly when sculpting a deep, long trench toward 6 o'clock, the tip is more perpendicular to the inferior portion of the posterior capsule because of its concavity and is directly perpendicular to the equatorial capsule (Figure 16-24). With down slope sculpting, considerable

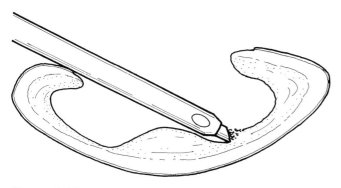

Figure 16-23 With traditional sculpting techniques, excessive central nuclear material may impede fracturing.

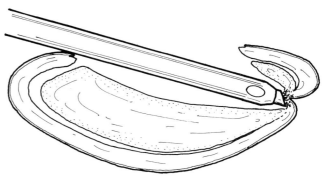

Figure 16-24 In addition, traditional shallow sculpting can create potential for direct contact with the posterior capsule.

nuclear material remains ahead of the tip at the end of each sculpting pass. Therefore, breaking though is unlikely with this "cushion" present. The risk of engaging the capsule is thus minimized.

The surgeon must be cautious when the CCC is small to avoid tearing the edge of the anterior capsule superiorly with the tip or the sleeve of the phaco instrument. In my experience, this is most likely to occur in cases with poor visualization, such as when hypermature, white cataracts are present. Ordinarily, the risk is low because one is not sculpting much past the center when first beginning the trench.

Care must also be exercised in displacing the nucleus within the capsular bag so that the whole bag is not displaced and the upper zonular ligaments are not unduly stretched and broken. Also, when tipping the handle of the phaco handpiece up to sculpt down toward the posterior pole, the surgeon must not push the tip posteriorly faster than the tip is chiseling its way through the lens material. The zonular ligaments may also be torn in such a manner. These risks are greatest in lenses with hard epinucleus and where the zonula are already weakened.

Limiting sculpting to the superior part of the nucleus adds safety because of the reduced risk of contacting the posterior capsule, and it adds efficiency because of the rapidity with which the posterior pole of the nucleus is reached with the phaco tip. With instruments this deep in the nucleus, the fracturing can be effectively initiated and safely completed.

SPECIAL SITUATIONS

Modifications to these general techniques may be necessary when a surgeon is confronted with any of a number of special, challenging situations. In *soft lenses*, Sinskey's technique of phacoemulsification[106] should be applied using basic sculpting without fracturing and without lifting the nucleus out of the bag. It is important to achieve hydrodissection in these lenses, but it may be difficult to achieve without prolapsing the nucleus out of the capsule. Therefore, hydrodissection should be attempted with caution, and perhaps even only partial hydrodissection should be the goal. Hydrodissecting a small amount in a number of quadrants or using the technique of hydrofree dissection[104,107,108] may be applicable here. Additionally, hydrodelineation can facilitate removing these softer lenses by achieving separation between nucleus and epinucleus. The epinucleus is often large and thick but also very soft. It folds and flips more readily if the central nucleus has been completely removed first.

In cases in which a history of *trauma* exists, a fibrotic anterior capsule may be present, or zonules may be missing in one quadrant or more, and the lens may be partially subluxated. Additionally, an old perforating or penetrating capsule injury may be present and the capsule resealed. It is important to look for iridodonesis to confirm whether the zonules are weak, anticipating that intracapsular surgery may be required. If zonules are absent or very weak in one quadrant or hemisection, they may be strong in the other sections and allow standard techniques. It is important to recognize that traumatic cataracts may develop very quickly, necessitating surgery within days or weeks of the injury. If the zonules are weakened but no capsule puncture has occurred, complete hydrodissection and hydrodelineation are essential. If the capsule has been injured or damaged during pars plana vitrectomy, hydrodissection should not be attempted. Tedious, delicate sculpting, as described by Fine[109-111] and Koch,[112-114] should be used.

PHACOEMULSIFICATION AND REVERSE PUPILLARY BLOCK

Upon entering the anterior chamber with the phaco tip, particularly with high-infusion sleeves and high bottles, reverse pupillary block or iris concavity may occur, resulting in patient discomfort, especially in eyes under topical anesthesia. Although it is more common in the highly myopic or pediatric eye, iris concavity may occur without notice. Reverse pupillary block is the stretching or extension of the iris posteriorly causing iris concavity and contact with the anterior lens capsule. This block can be immediately released by lifting the iris off from the top of the capsule with a spatula or any second instrument.

To prevent reverse pupillary block and avoid discomfort it is preferable to have an instrument between the iris and capsule as the irrigation is turned on. This will allow fluid to circulate in behind the iris, thus preventing pupillary block. Another technique to help prevent reverse pupillary block is to control the irrigation using short staccato-like taps on the foot switch. If reverse pupillary block should occur, with this technique one may interrupt the development of iris concavity before excessive deepening of the anterior chamber and minimize discomfort to the patient.

With *highly myopic cases*, the principal concern is the potential for lack of vitreous support. The lens iris diaphragm may be quite unstable and may fluctuate widely during on and off irrigation, and even when shifting between foot positions one and two. Machines with an adjustable flow rate are more advantageous in these cases and should be used to ensure more stable hydrodynamics.

Cases with a *shallow chamber* can be challenging even with the use of viscoelastics, because it is difficult to achieve an average chamber depth in cases with high hyperopia; very old, thick cataracts; and/or loose zonules. The most important consideration under these circumstances is to use a tunnel incision with a corneal entry, performed more anterior in location than usual. This helps to prevent iris prolapse through the wound during phacoemulsification. Even during the capsulotomy, the viscoelastic can potentially extrude from the eye, although the use of dispersive or noncohesive, low-molecular-weight, hyaluronate viscoelastic may minimize this problem. Maintaining the chamber for capsulorrhexis is important because iris prolapse at this stage can lead to iris trauma when inserting the phaco probe. Iris trauma may occur just from the friction of the phaco sleeve passing over the iris.

TECHNICAL TIPS
A lower bottle position is advocated to allow the lens iris diaphragm not to be pushed far posteriorly as soon as irrigation is started. If the anterior-chamber depth does fluctuate widely, the pupil is usually more dilated when the lens iris diaphragm is posterior and tends to be more constricted when the lens iris diaphragm is in a normal or anterior position (chamber collapse). Repeated episodes of chamber collapse can lead to a constricted pupil. Additionally, a deep chamber should be avoided, so that the phaco tip does not have to tip so far posteriorly. Simply stated, keeping the bottle low keeps the chamber a normal depth and more stable.

TECHNICAL TIPS

It is also important to ensure proper wound size in these cases. Avoiding too large an incision is critical. Unless using a standard keratome, erring on the conservative side is recommended. In addition, the bottle may need to be raised for extra pressure to deepen the anterior chamber during phacoemulsification. As soon as possible, the phaco tip should be used to develop a trench rather than shaving more of the superficial anterior surface where turbulence can reach the cornea. By achieving depth into the lens early, the turbulence is dissipated.

Loose zonules can typically be detected on the first puncture of the capsule for capsulorrhexis. The integrity of the zonules can be tested with the instrument being used to puncture the capsule: bent needle, cystotome, or forceps. If the lens is quite mobile and the zonules are very loose, an intracapsular tension ring may need to be used. To manage cases with lost or weak zonules in cataract surgery and to lower the incidence of postoperative capsular contraction, it is essential to maintain the circular contour of the capsular bag both intraoperatively and postoperatively. IOLs with loop shapes that conformed to that of the capsular bag, or a loopless IOL that would exactly fit the capsular bag were initially used to achieve this goal. However, the large size of these IOLs required larger incisions resulting in longer healing times and the increased likelihood of significant postoperative astigmatism.

Clinically, the capsular tension ring (CTR) has been used in the management of patients with moderate loss of zonular support in cataract surgery. However, for cases with a significant loss of zonular support (more than a quadrant) the capsular tension ring and remaining zonules may be unable to provide enough support to stabilize the capsular bag. For these cases Cionni, in 1998, modified the conventional capsular tension ring by adding a PMMA hook on the loop. At the free end of the hook is an eyelet for manipulation and suture placement. When the ring is implanted in the capsular bag, a suture can be secured to this eyelet to allow scleral fixation without violating the integrity of the capsular bag. Clinical outcomes have shown that this ring provides excellent support and centration of the capsular bag and IOL both intraoperatively and postoperatively.

Another set of conditions such as coloboma, complete aniridia, or eye trauma which may result in loss of iris tissue or sphincter function, may be managed with an aniridia ring that creates an artificial iris diaphragm. Several types are commercially available.

Capsular tension rings are indicated during any cataract surgery in which the stability of the capsular bag is compromised. An unstable capsular bag can result from previous trauma, pseudoexfoliation syndrome, floppy capsule syndrome, or in various developmental or congenital syndromes. Instability of the capsular bag increases the risk of complications during or after cataract extraction and IOL implantation as discussed earlier. Capsular tension rings can significantly reduce this risk.

In many situations, inadequate capsular support is apparent prior to surgery. Placement of a capsular tension ring in these situations should be planned prior to surgery. There is debate as to weather or not to place a capsular tension ring in all eyes with pseudoexfoliation syndrome. Although this is not presently recommended in all cases, its use should be planned in all cases. In other situations, the need for a capsular tension ring may not be apparent until after the crystalline lens has been removed. For example, in the case of floppy capsule syndrome, the capsular bag is slowly stretched by a large crystalline lens. It is not until the lens is removed and the bag is released from this stretch that the floppy nature is apparent. In these cases a capsular tension ring may be placed at this time to prevent postoperative folds or wrinkles in the posterior capsule, which may transsect in the visual axis. In other cases, there is no preoperative history, or slit-lamp biomicroscopic findings to suggest inadequate capsular support. It is in these cases where the attention to detail during surgery is paramount. If the surgeon performs a round continuous curvilinear capsulorrhexis, then removes the crystalline lens and implants an IOL, the CCC should still be round if the capsular support is adequate. If the CCC becomes oval, it indicates inadequate capsular support in the meridian in which there is no IOL haptic support. In this situation a capsular tension ring may be placed and the surgeon will note that the CCC is round once again. This should reduce the risk of late capsular bag subluxation. Late capsular bag subluxation may also be prevented by using capsular tension rings in cases of suspiciously unstable capsular bags after IOL implantation, especially in pseudoexfoliation syndrome.

In cases of zonular dehiscence involving one quadrant, i.e., less than 90°, a capsular tension ring, or a capsular edge ring is indicated. If two or less quadrants are involved, i.e., 90° to 180°, a single hook Cionni ring is indicated. A double hook Cionni ring is indicated if the zonular dehiscence is greater than 180°.

Capsular tension rings stabilize the capsular bag by exerting outward force on the bag; therefore, it is mandatory that the bag be able to withstand this force for the tension ring to be safe and effective. A capsular tension ring, therefore, cannot be placed into an eye that does not have a good-quality CCC. If the CCC is torn, very eccentric, or very large, a tension ring may extend the tear and dislocate from its position within the bag.

If the posterior capsule is torn prior to inserting a tension ring, the ring can only be inserted if the surgeon is able to convert the torn posterior capsule into a posterior CCC. If this is accomplished then a ring may be inserted safely. If the posterior capsule is torn after a ring has already been placed, it is not always necessary to remove the ring. All efforts should be made to convert the tear into a posterior CCC, but if this cannot be accomplished and the ring cannot be easily removed (i.e., via a safety suture) the ring may be left in place. There may, however, be a higher likelihood of extension of the posterior capsule tear with resultant posterior dislocation of the ring and the IOL.

The lens nucleus and epinucleus act as an endoskeleton to the capsular bag. For this reason, if there is any suspicion of zonular dialysis, or if the bag starts collapsing during surgery, a capsular tension ring should be inserted into the bag before or during phacoemulsification to act as an alternate endoskeleton to the bag before removing its own natural endoskeleton. In cases of severe zonular dehiscence and capsular dialysis, and when vitreous has prolapsed around the dehisced area, requiring anterior vitrectomy, the vitrectomy should be postponed until the ring is in place. The ring will exert an outward pressure on the capsular bag thus preventing vitreous from further prolapsing anteriorly from around the edges of the dehisced capsular bag during the vitrectomy. Thus, causing further collapse of the capsular bag and further tearing of its zonular attachments, leading to a vicious circle of vitreous prolapse and zonular dehiscence.

TECHNICAL TIPS

When performing capsulorrhexis, the lens can be inadvertently nudged to one side by the instrument. Centration of the CCC can be deceiving, but releasing the instrument from the anterior capsule as one is tearing it allows the lens to assume its natural position. Reinspecting is then crucial to ascertain where the edge of the tear is progressing. The same recommendation applies in pediatric cases, in which very elastic zonules and a somewhat elastic capsule typically are present. During phacoemulsification, the two-handed technique is crucial for stabilizing the nucleus in cases with loose zonules.

TECHNICAL TIPS

Hydrodissection is helpful to atraumatically loosen the nucleus but must be limited to avoid overhydrating the vitreous and expanding its volume. Low flow and vacuum reduce fluctuations in chamber depth and minimize lens movements that might further damage zonules.

A *subluxated lens* is usually diagnosed prior to surgery by observation of iridodonesis, displaced Y sutures, and chamber angle abnormalities. As mentioned previously, however, pre-existing zonular damage may first be detected during attempts to puncture the anterior capsule. Assuming the instrument is sharp, failure to puncture – with noticeable wrinkling of the capsule and movement of the lens – should suggest a loosened zonula.

Cataract surgery in patients with *pseudoexfoliation syndrome* carries a significantly higher risk of intraoperative postoperative complications.[115] Zonular dialysis, capsular rupture, vitreous loss, and late intraocular lens dislocation have been reported to occur more frequently in the presence of pseudoexfoliation.[116–118] Also, fragile lens zonules, abnormal ciliary body interface, and poor papillary dilation have been implicated as a basis for more frequent complications.[119,120]

Pharmacological agents should be used to maintain maximal pupil dilation through the surgery. All contact with the iris must be strictly avoided during phacoemulsification to prevent additional constriction of the pupil. The bimanual in situ nucleofractis techniques with minimal zonular stress are ideally suited for safe phacoemulsification in cases with pseudoexfoliation, and their safety has been confirmed in a multicenter study.[121]

VARIATIONS

Since divide and conquer's inception, a number of popular variations have emerged. Shepherd was one of the early advocates of fracturing and soon developed his in situ fracture technique,[122,123] which also relies heavily on nuclear rotation. Using either a 30° tip or a 45° tip, a groove two tip widths wide is sculpted from the 12 to 6 o'clock positions (Figure 16-25). The nucleus is then rotated by placing the phaco tip in the proximal and the spatula in the distal end of the groove and turning clockwise (Figure 16-26). Shepherd believes that this is most easily accomplished if no fracture has taken place. A second groove is carved, crosshatched across the first and then carried slightly deeper (Figure 16-27). The phaco tip is pushed against the left wall of the distal groove, the spatula is placed cross-action against the right wall, and the nuclear rim is gently separated (Figure 16-28). The nucleus is then rotated one-quarter turn, and the fracturing procedure is repeated until all four grooves are broken (Figure 16-29). Shepherd uses a "tumble" rather than "follow" method for removing the segments. To initiate tumbling, a spatula is used to push down on the apex of an inferior fragment until the fragment flips over, and the piece is rotated centrally with the apex trailing (Figures 16-30 and 16-31). This quadrant can then be emulsified (Figure 16-32). Each quadrant is similarly manipulated into the central area and removed (Figure 16-33). Davison has also developed a similar technique, in which the nuclear segments are managed using increased vacuum level settings.[124–127]

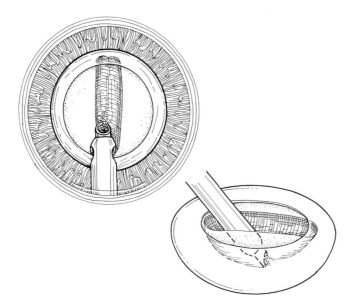

Figure 16-25 Shepherd's technique begins with a groove sculpted from 12 to 6 o'clock.

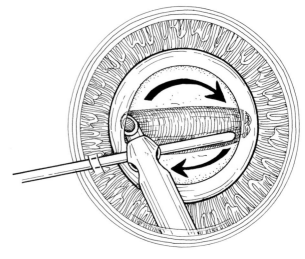

Figure 16-26 Clockwise pressure is exerted by both instruments to rotate the groove 90°.

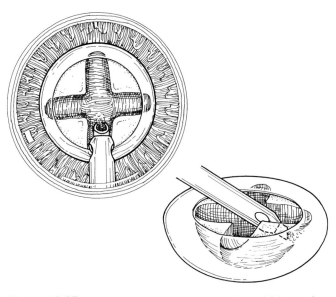

Figure 16-27 Original groove is then crossed with the establishment of a second groove.

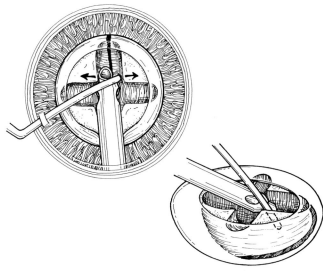

Figure 16-28 Spatula and phaco tip are pushed apart, fracturing the nucleus.

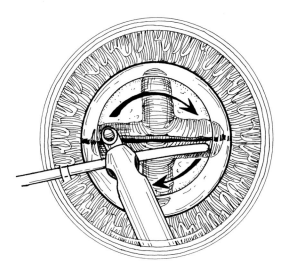

Figure 16-29 Following nuclear rotation, another groove is cracked, resulting in four quadrants of nucleus.

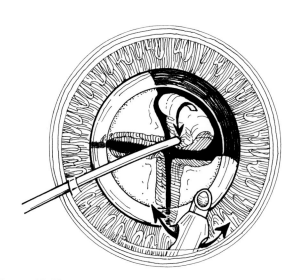

Figure 16-30 Spatula is used to depress the apex of a wedge and to tumble it into an upside-down position.

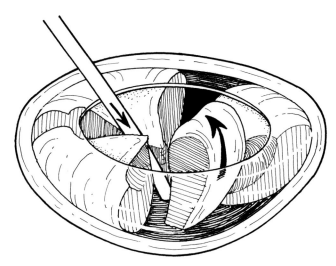

Figure 16-31 Base of the tumbled wedge ends up in a central position.

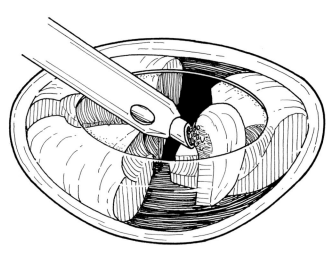

Figure 16-32 First wedge is emulsified.

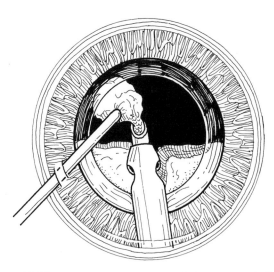

Figure 16-33 Remaining wedges are then similarly maneuvered within the bag and emulsified.

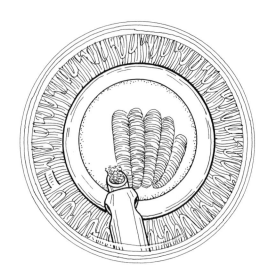

Figure 16-34 Fine's "chip and flip" technique begins with central sculpting of the nucleus.

One criticism of Shepherd's technique is that the tumbling maneuver may cause the central portion of the nuclear segments to point down toward the posterior capsule and possibly cause a tear.[128] In the author's opinion, this risk may be exaggerated. The base soon leaves the capsule and is displaced anteriorly, reducing pressure on the posterior capsule by the tip. Some surgeons have advocated engaging the apex and lifting it up to facilitate removal. A more practical and efficient method to avoid this situation would be to create more and smaller pieces that turn sideways upon removal. Even if the segment starts to tumble, the top can be shaved off in one or two passes to reduce the thicker, equatorial portion of the lens. If the sculpting has been sufficiently wide and deep centrally, these apexes are thin, soft, and nonthreatening, because one has reached the epinucleus during sculpting.

In an effort to enhance the safety and control of quadrant management, Fine attempted to create a central nuclear component and an outer epinuclear component and to perform phacoemulsification using the two zones. This became his "chip and flip" technique.[108–110] Following hydrodelineation to create the zones, the chip and flip technique is initiated by performing central sculpting using a 30° tip (Figure 16-34). A Bechert nucleus rotator or cyclodialysis spatula is introduced, and the nucleus is pushed toward 12 o'clock (Figure 16-35). The rim of the inner nuclear bowl is removed at 5 to 6 o'clock, and the nucleus is rotated clockwise to sequentially facilitate each hour of rim being removed from the 5 to 6 o'clock region (Figure 16-36). Once the rim of the inner nuclear bowl is removed, the second handpiece is brought into the cleavage plane between the inner nuclear chip and the outer nuclear bowl and swept under the chip, elevating

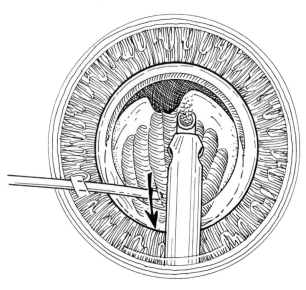

Figure 16-35 At the 5 to 6 o'clock position, the inner nuclear rim is removed.

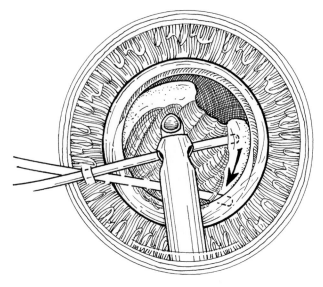

Figure 16-36 Second instrument is used below the phaco probe to rotate the nucleus and further facilitate removal in this region.

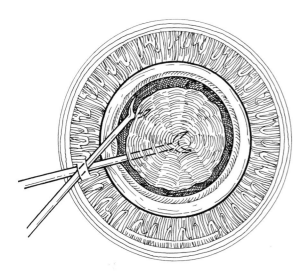

Figure 16-37 Bechert rotator is used to sweep under the nuclear chip and elevate it into the center of the bag.

it into the center of the bag (Figure 16-37). By using the second handpiece to control the nuclear chip, the chip can then be quickly and safely removed (Figure 16-38).

In the late 1980s and early 1990s, Fine described two endolenticular phacoemulsification techniques: chip and flip,[109] and chop and flip.[97,109–111] The techniques used the pulse mode to remove nuclear material which decreased chattering and increased

holding power of the nuclear material. Many modulations in the delivery of power are now available. With these modulations, significantly less total ultrasound is delivered into the eye. The Alcon 20,000 Legacy has a bimodal option that allows the surgeon to use linear aspiration flow rate or vacuum in foot position 2. Fine takes maximum advantage of the new technologies available with this system as described in his choo-choo chop and flip phacoemulsification technique.[129,130] This uses the burst mode and bevel down technique with high vacuum and US power settings for enhanced efficiency.

The soft outer nuclear bowl, which has cushioned all previous phacoemulsification, is now displaced from the capsular fornix at 5 to 6 o'clock (Figure 16-39). The nuclear bowl is mobilized by pulling the rim at 5 to 6 o'clock toward 12 o'clock and pushing with the second handpiece in the bottom of the nuclear bowl toward 5 to 6 o'clock to tumble or flip the soft outer nuclear bowl (Figure 16-40). By flipping the bowl away from the capsule it can be removed safely, either with aspiration or with low-powered emulsification without jeopardizing the capsule (Figure 16-41).

A number of similar techniques for soft-to-moderate lenses have been published in the literature.[129,131–134] By necessity, these techniques are limited to lenses whose consistency is sufficiently soft to permit the creation of a cleavage plane within the nucleus by hydrodelineation.

Dillman and Maloney recognized the benefits of cracking and teamed with Fine to develop the "crack and flip" technique,[97] which is essentially a hybrid of Shepherd's in situ fracture, Fine's

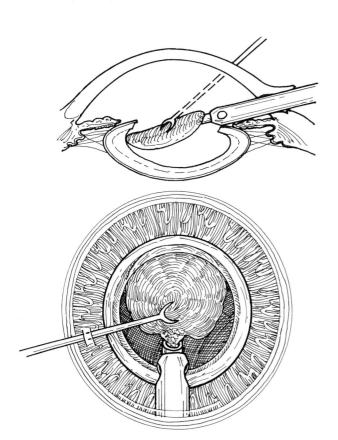

Figure 16-38 Remaining central nucleus is controlled and subsequently emulsified using a two-handed technique.

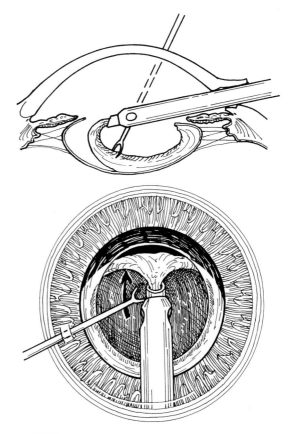

Figure 16-39 In the 5 to 6 o'clock position, the phaco tip engages the rim with aspiration only as the second instrument pushes the bottom of the bowl.

THE PRINCIPLE OF NUCLEOFRACTIS

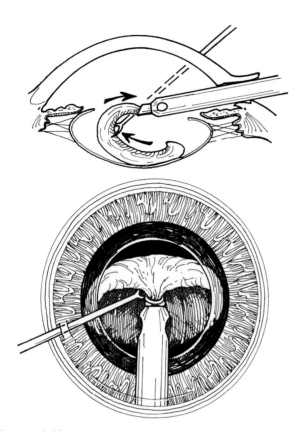

Figure 16-40 Nuclear bowl should begin to flip away from the posterior capsule.

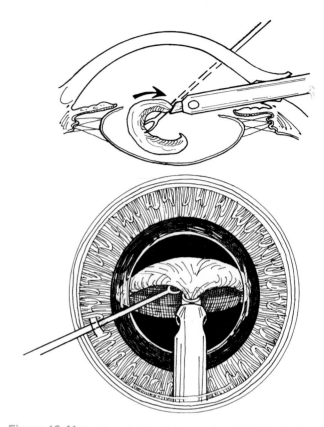

Figure 16-41 Bowl is worked out of the capsule and folded on itself.

chip and flip, and Maloney and Dillman's fractional 2:4 phaco-emulsification techniques.[135-137] With crack and flip, the sculpting starts centrally, and the first groove is made toward 6 o'clock (Figure 16-42). The sculpting takes place entirely within the central compact mass, and every effort is made to avoid actually reaching the golden hydrodelineation ring during sculpting. At the same time as one groove is completed, the nucleus is rotated clockwise 90° and the next groove is started (Figure 16-43).

After four grooves have been placed cracking is accomplished, which divides the nucleus into quadrants (Figure 16-44). If

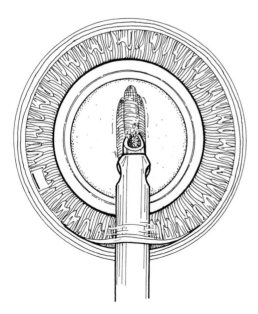

Figure 16-42 "Crack and flip" technique begins with a central groove toward 6 o'clock.

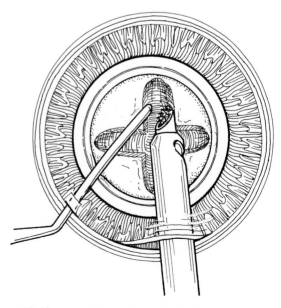

Figure 16-43 Nucleus is rotated 90°, and a similar groove is created.

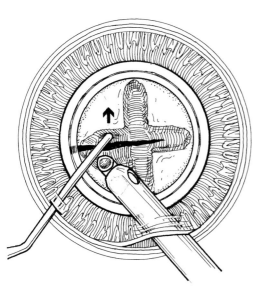

Figure 16-44 Following the formation of four grooves, the nucleus is split into quadrants.

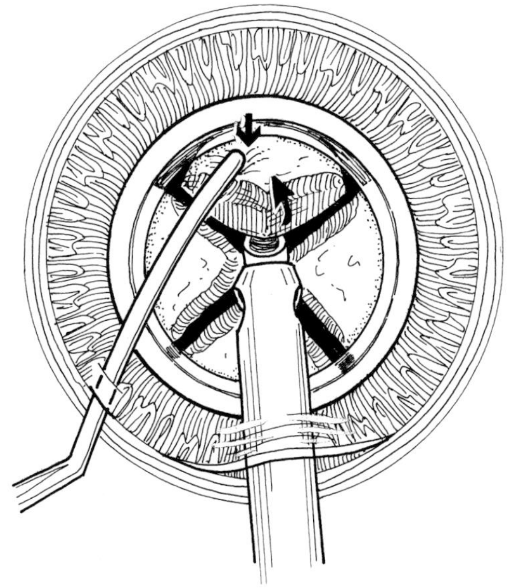

Figure 16-45 Second instrument is used to rotate the blunt periphery downward and to lift the sharp apex safely upward.

grooving has taken place in such a way that it was contained centrally and did not reach the epinuclear shell, then the cracking process itself will extend only to the hydrodelineation circle and will leave the epinucleus entirely intact. Pressure by the second handpiece is brought against the upper aspect of the base of the quadrant to rotate the blunt periphery of the quadrant downward and to elevate the sharp apex (Figure 16-45). Elevating the apex minimizes the threat of a sharp edge tearing the posterior capsule. Once the apex is elevated, it is engaged deeply within the epinuclear shell by the phaco tip, and the second handpiece is brought under the quadrant to support it until occlusion occurs (Figure 16-46). As occlusion occurs, the quadrant is brought toward the middle of the epinuclear

shell, and the second handpiece can be utilized to either hold the quadrant down, to mash it toward the phaco tip, or to crack it into eighths. Once the quadrant is emulsified by the phaco tip, the second handpiece holds the remaining fragments deep within the epinucleus until they are sequentially removed by the phaco tip from within the epinuclear shell.

The remaining quadrants are rotated to bring another quadrant to the distal position for removal in the same manner. Each quadrant is sequentially removed in this way, working in the central portion of the epinucleus. Every attempt is made to keep a quadrant or any of its fragments from coming up into the anterior chamber. After removal of the quadrants, an empty but intact epinuclear shell remains.

Clearly, two schools of thought have emerged regarding hydrodelineation. Some surgeons believe that hydrodelineation detracts from the effectiveness and efficiency of the operation and prefer not to perform it. Others, including Dillman, Maloney, and Fine, use hydrodelineation to maintain the peripheral protective cushion of the outer nucleus. For the author's own technique, hydrodelineation is performed on a regular basis; however, under certain circumstances, as with a very dense lens, the option of fracturing right out to the periphery is preferential.

The goal of the *endocapsular* phacoemulsification surgeon is to maximize the amount of anterior capsule in place during phacoemulsification. The anterior capsule is seen to serve as a physical barrier to protect the corneal endothelium during phacoemulsification and to limit the turbulence within the confines of the capsular bag. A number of endocapsular phacoemulsification techniques have been proposed in the literature, but have not been integrated into current practice.[138–148]

Both Solomon and Michelson described what Michelson has termed a minicapsulorrhexis.[149–151] The minicapsulorrhexis is small enough to maximize this barrier effect of the anterior capsule while being adequately large to allow lateral excursion of the phaco tip without creating undue stress on the margins of the capsulotomy (Figures 16-47 and 16-48). The technique

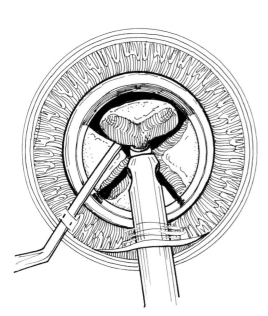

Figure 16-46 Once elevated, the apex is engaged and occluded using the second instrument as a maintenance tool.

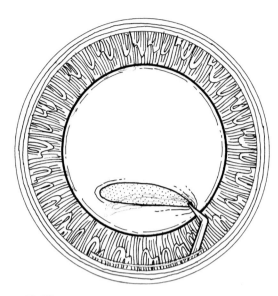

Figure 16-47 "Minicapsulorrhexis" of endocapsular phacoemulsification is initiated with a puncture near the superior iris border in a well-dilated pupil.

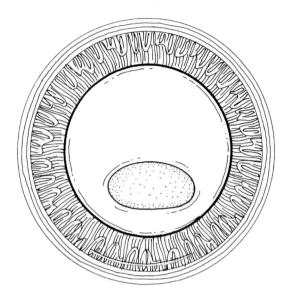

Figure 16-48 "Minicap" should be large enough to accommodate the phaco tip and sleeve while allowing easy access to the nucleus.

facilitates near total compartmentalization of the emulsification process within the lens capsule, thereby providing significant protection to the iris and corneal endothelium. The minicap is typically 0.5 by 4 mm in size, made near the superior iris border. Reported advantages of this location include an enhanced barrier effect for the anterior chamber and better access to the 12 o'clock position. It is important to note that when emulsifying below the anterior capsule, visibility becomes extremely important, and the space-maintaining properties of viscoelastic materials should be used to their fullest potential.

Before commencing sculpting, working space may be created with several short bursts of low-power linear phacoemulsification under the leading edge of the anterior capsule. Solomon recommends passing the handpiece through the anterior chamber in a "bevel down" position to prevent stripping the Descemet membrane and then rotating the tip to the "bevel up" position.[149] The initial sculpting maneuver should be limited to half the nucleus, leaving the epinuclear rim intact. The depth of the sculpting should proceed to include at least two-thirds to three-fourths of the central nuclear thickness (Figure 16-49). The dislocation and rotation maneuver is accomplished by first impaling the phaco tip into the base of the superior ledge of the unsculpted rim of the nucleus. Gentle force is applied with the phaco tip to rotate the nucleus 90°. The unsculpted nucleus is now inferiorly located (Figure 16-50). This remaining central material is thus sculpted, completing the nuclear bowl. The epinuclear rim may be emulsified under low phacoemulsification power (Figure 16-51). The residual nuclear plate is emulsified after it has been dislocated off the posterior capsule and floated anteriorly toward the iris plane (Figures 16-52–16-54).

Using this technique, Michelson claimed to observe no endothelial cell loss in between 40% and 65% of his cases, and minimal cell loss (4% or less) in the remaining cases. Similar low cell loss levels have been reported by a number of surgeons using an endocapsular phacoemulsification method.[98,139,152,153]

Nishi has also reported good results using a buttonhole capsulotomy opening, wherein a 3.5–4 mm horizontal capsulotomy is made in the superior portion of the capsule (Figure 16-55).[154,155] The ends of the capsulotomy are then rounded off, using forceps or a microcapsulopunch (Figure 16-56). Nishi reported that the buttonhole configuration reduces stress concentrations so that the capsulotomy does not easily tear.

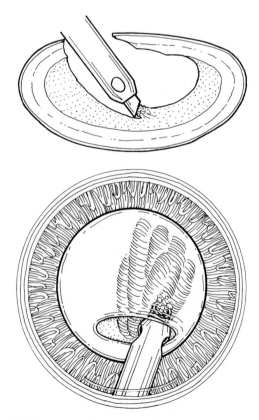

Figure 16-49 Initial sculpting includes at least two-thirds to three-fourths of the central nuclear thickness in depth. The epinuclear rim is left intact.

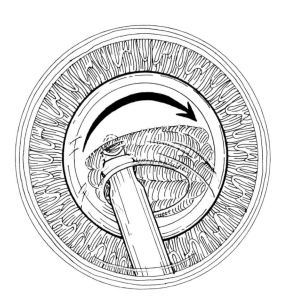

Figure 16-50 Phaco tip is used to rotate the nucleus 90°, rendering the unsculpted portion in the easily accessible inferior position.

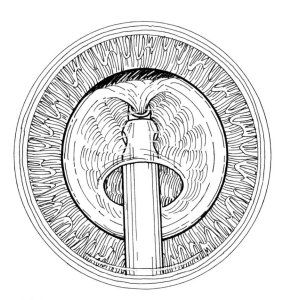

Figure 16-51 Following removal of the nuclear bowl, the epinuclear rim can be emulsified under low power.

Having a superiorly placed minicapsulotomy mandates a one-handed technique, because the capsulotomy is not sufficiently large to introduce a second instrument. However, two-port endocapsular phacoemulsification has been proposed by Pop.[156] Under viscoelastic, a very small capsulorrhexis for entrance of a spatula is created at the 2 o'clock position; a second capsulorrhexis, about 3 mm in diameter, is made at about 11 o'clock for the phaco tip (Figure 16-57). The side port is created only after the initial capsulorrhexis is performed to allow the incision line to be on the same plane as the port. The surgeon can then proceed with a bimanual phacoemulsification technique in up to 3+ density nuclei or more. Following phacoemulsification, the bridge between the two CCCs is incised (Figure 16-58). Once

the IOL is implanted, a very small snip is made in the margin of the 3 mm CCC, and one large opening from the original two is made (Figures 16-59–16-60). Pop reports that the procedure does not take much time and provides excellent protection to the corneal endothelium and anterior chamber. However, he concedes that the technique is not for beginners and requires excellent visualization.

In addition to the corneal protection afforded by the endocapsular phacoemulsification, many advocates of the technique report less stress on the zonules and assurance of a maintained anterior capsule for IOL placement in the sulcus in the presence of a torn posterior capsule.[157,158] Furthermore, during anterior vitrectomy after a posterior capsule tear when prolonged

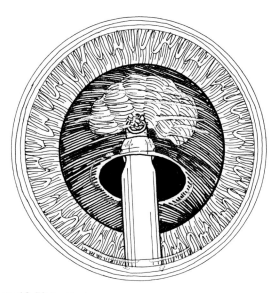

Figure 16-52 Residual nuclear plate is then dislocated off the posterior capsule, floated anteriorly toward the iris plane, and emulsified.

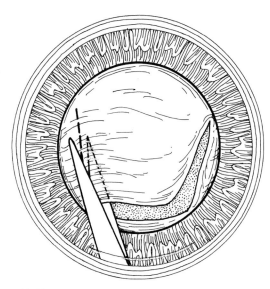

Figure 16-53 Following emulsification and before intraocular lens implantation, capsule scissors are used to initiate a second-stage capsulorrhexis.

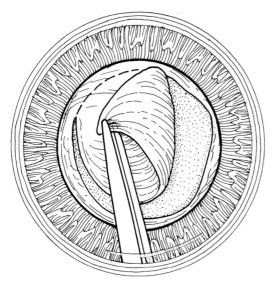

Figure 16-54 Capsule forceps are used to complete the second-stage capsulorrhexis.

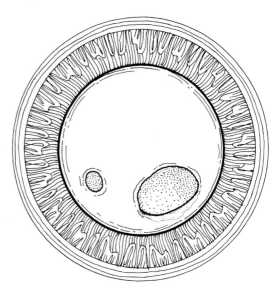

Figure 16-57 Respective locations of Pop's two capsule ports.

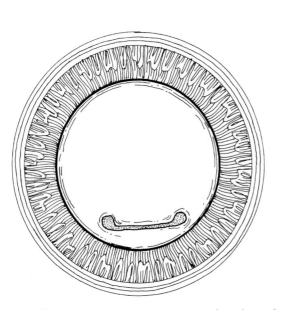

Figure 16-55 Nishi's buttonhole anterior capsulotomy for endocapsular phacoemulsification.

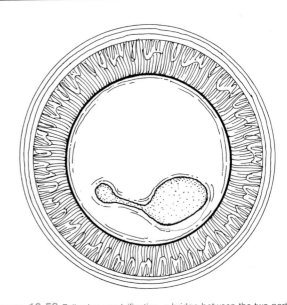

Figure 16-58 Following emulsification, a bridge between the two ports is created.

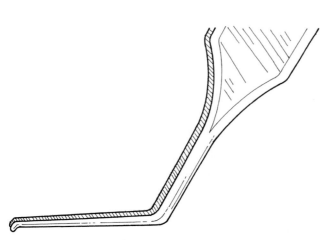

Figure 16-56 Angulated 60° Nishi-Utrata capsulorrhexis forceps.

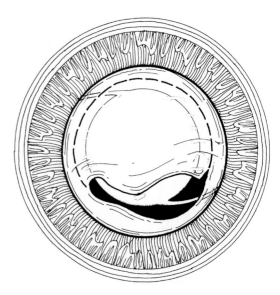

Figure 16-59 Following implantation of the lens, a complete capsulorrhexis is performed.

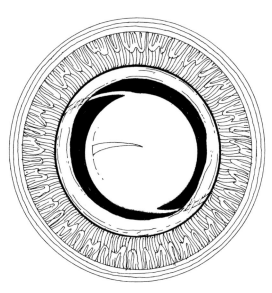

Figure 16-60 Appearance after completion of the capsulorrhexis.

infusion may occur, the anterior capsule provides a protective barrier against endothelial damage.

Certainly, the endocapsular technique provides less opportunity for fragments to come up against the corneal endothelium, but one must balance this against the increased potential for posterior capsule tears. A posterior capsule tear occurring during emulsification is more frequently associated with loss of nuclear material into the vitreous when a large part of anterior capsule is present. Anterior capsule tears may occur during manipulation of the instruments within the small CCC. Should the zonules be stretched or separated during emulsification, the zonular dehiscence may be worsened during the subsequent two-staged capsulotomy, resulting in a disinserted capsular bag.[102,104,159,160] The range of movement of the emulsification tip may be diminished or hindered by the limited nature of anterior capsule opening. This

can challenge the surgeon's dexterity and create the possibility of extending an anterior capsular tear around the equator to the posterior capsule. Endolenticular phacoemulsification, with adequate experience, is a safe procedure and minimizes endothelial cell loss. In addition, any concerns regarding cell loss, for example in patients with low endothelial cell counts preoperatively, can be alleviated to a great degree by using a more adhesive or viscous viscoelastic.

Endocapsular phacoemulsification is a technique that may provide the surgeon with an entry point into the future of ophthalmology and cataract surgery, given the research now taking place in the fields of injectable IOLs and endocapsular balloons, and in many other developing technologies.[141,142,146,161–163]

ONE-HANDED VS. TWO-HANDED PHACOEMULSIFICATION

Many surgeons have reported good results using a one-handed technique to perform central sculpting and removal of the nuclear rim and nuclear plate.[106,164–168] Pacifico has developed a one-handed variation of the author's divide and conquer technique.[169] Instead of bimanual cracking, the lens sections are cut, rotated, cut, and removed in sequence. The normal anatomical structures of the eye are used in a sense to act as a second instrument. Alternatively, sculpting can be performed with a one-handed technique, a viscoelastic injected, and a cracking device can be inserted and used for nucleofractis. Then emulsification is completed with the tip alone.

Typically, one-handed phacoemulsification is accomplished by sculpting a bowl and removing the bulk of the nuclear top, center, and rim (Figure 16-61). Pointing the phaco tip toward 9 o'clock and pushing counterclockwise toward 6 o'clock dislocates the nucleus to allow the equator to be aspirated into the tip (Figure 16-62). Pointing the tip toward 3 o'clock and pushing clockwise sometimes works better than using the 9 o'clock maneuver. The softer the nucleus, the harder this rotation maneuver is to

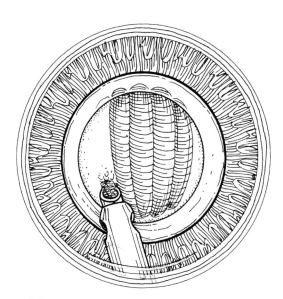

Figure 16-61 One-handed phacoemulsification. Very deep sculpting through the nucleus and into the soft transitional material.

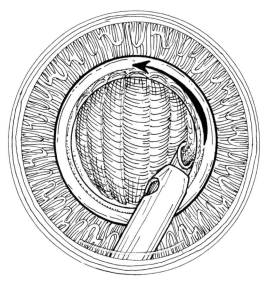

Figure 16-62 After maximum sculpting has been accomplished, the tip engages the nucleus at 9 o'clock and rotates that point to the 6 o'clock position.

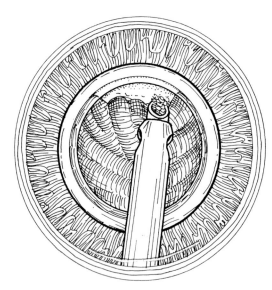

Figure 16-63 After a number of similar rotations, the entire nucleus has been sculpted in the 6 o'clock position.

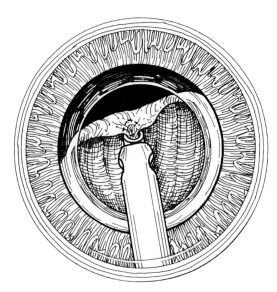

Figure 16-64 Phaco tip is used to engage and split the thin nuclear rim away from the capsule.

accomplish; however, softer nuclei are easier to aspirate into the tip. For a hard nucleus, low power occludes the tip and emulsifies the nucleus more effectively than if power is simply increased. Once the tip is occluded, moving the tip toward 12 o'clock allows the nucleus to follow (Figure 16-63). The remaining posterior nuclear plate is sufficiently small to be freely attracted to the phaco tip for safe central emulsification in a circumferential manner in the posterior chamber (Figure 16-64). Again here, deep central sculpting to debulk the nucleus determines the ease with which the resultant nuclear plate can be removed.

One-handed techniques can be quite stressful to the lens capsule and zonules when the phaco handpiece is used as both manipulator and emulsifier. Movements against the lens capsule may be much more pronounced with one-handed techniques. In the author's experience, these techniques are not as efficient or safe as the bimanual methods. Nonetheless, for surgeons who feel more confident with a one-handed technique, these techniques are reasonably safe and can provide excellent results.

MACHINE PARAMETERS

One commonly overlooked step in the mastery of phacoemulsification is a clear understanding of the equipment. A number of articles have been published that provide for an elementary understanding of the basic dynamics of phacoemulsification energy and fluidics within the eye.[170–178] A familiarity with these principles should allow surgeons to better manage the mechanical energy and heat present.[179]

When the ultrasound tip impacts the nucleus, it mechanically slices, cuts, and emulsifies it. Additionally, a physical effect known as cavitation occurs. With cavitation, a physical process creates microbubbles that implode as the sound waves expand and compress.[180] During the compression cycle, a positive pressure is exerted on the liquid, which pushes the molecules together; during the expansion cycle, negative pressure pulls them

apart. If the reaction is sufficiently intense, a cavity is formed, thus dissolving the nucleus in front of the phaco needle.

Variable surgeon control of phacoemulsification power or stroke has provided a great advantage to the cataract surgeon. Increasing the phacoemulsification power or stroke means that the to-and-fro thrust distance of each cycle of the phaco tip is increased, whereas decreased phacoemulsification power or stroke results in a decrease in the distance that the phaco tip moves. Average phacoemulsification power is calculated by dividing cumulative delivered energy by total ultrasound time and multiplying it by 100.

Typically, four phaco cutting tip angles are available: 15°, 30°, 45°, and 60°.[181] The key to selecting a good tip angle is achieving a balance between occludability and burrowing effect, both of which are influenced by the lens type. With a standard lens that fractures quite easily and allows nuclear fragments to be emulsified as they are fractured, the 45° tip is probably more efficient. These sharper, more acutely angled tips are more useful in mobilizing the nucleus, cut more effectively at the same power level, and are much easier to observe when sculpting very deep in the nucleus. After cracking is complete, however, the emphasis changes to use more aspiration and less cutting. It can be difficult to completely occlude the broad 45° tip because of the larger elliptical area. To counter this, some surgeons change to a 30° tip, which more easily occludes and, therefore, builds vacuum on a peristaltic pump. In a dense, brunescent lens where a more delicate touch can be required to retrieve firmer epinuclear material out of the equatorial area, a smaller angle, such as the 15° or 30° tip, may be more advantageous. It is clear that one particular tip angle is not best for every surgeon on every case.

A number of specialized tips have been designed. The mini-cobra tip is reported to allow the surgeon to emulsify cataracts with less ultrasound energy than conventional tips and to have the ability to be inserted through a 2.5 mm incision.[182] Smaller port sizes are available as well, and this wider range certainly provides benefits to the surgeon.[183]

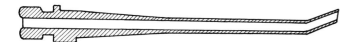

Figure 16-65 Cross-sectional schematic of the modified Kelman phaco tip.

Soft nuclei can be better served by a smaller port, which assists with the sculpting portion. However, the smaller ports do not work as efficiently in very hard nuclei. Currently the author uses a modified 30° Kelman tip, which has a bend close to its distal end (Figure 16-65), which creates shear stresses on the lower edge and performs like a serrated knife. With this hook end, gripping and pulling are quite easily accomplished for fracturing purposes. This fingerlike effect additionally allows turning of the tip to work on either the left or right side of a central trench. Additionally, the tip permits very effective and efficient down slope sculpting in the superior portion of the lens, allowing prompt access to the posterior pole for fracturing.

The cataract surgeon should choose the equipment that best responds to his or her needs and technique. For instance, two ways to move nuclear quadrants into the center of the lens exist. The first is to go to the periphery with the phaco tip, impale the nuclear quadrant, and physically tow it into the center. This technique is safest when used with low settings and a peristaltic pump. If the nucleus is not staying on the tip, a faster aspiration flow rate and higher vacuum are needed to achieve more grabbing and holding power. Alternatively, venturi or diaphragm pumps can increase the pulling power by increasing immediate vacuum levels and, therefore, the strength of fluid flow toward the phaco tip. An analogy has been made to a mountain stream. If the stream flows at a leisurely pace, it is unable to carry with it anything but the smallest pieces. However, if the stream is moving rapidly, the increased flow can carry larger objects.

For the past several years, the author has used phaco machines with a peristaltic pump system that allows aspiration flow rates to be preset, i.e., the rate in cc per minute at which the ultrasound needle aspirates fluid and lens material. The faster the flow, the more rapid the vacuum build-up is once the tip is occluded. This ability is preferable when adjusting the rise time of vacuum build-up, as this dictates the safety margin or how fast materials come to the port. This can be invaluable in challenging cases such as those involving small pupils or in the presence of a loose capsule. The establishment of a different aspiration flow rate in foot positions 2 and 3 allows the surgeon to engage material with a safer vacuum level at foot position 2 and then change to position 3 for emulsification. This change of position can be monitored by the audio feedback that results from altering pump speeds.

A number of good articles are available in the literature surveying the available machines, and a number of ophthalmic newspapers usually run an annual feature highlighting the latest innovations in the phacoemulsification machine marketplace.[184–195] It is because most units have their own unique advantages and disadvantages, that manufacturers have been attempting to marry the best features of each system. By testing each type of pump, the surgeon can determine which one best suits his or her technique and needs. It may be that in the future the surgeon will be able to switch between peristaltic and venturi systems within the same unit. With this in mind, the consumer should consider the manufacturer's policy on future upgrades prior to purchase.

THE LEARNING CURVE

It is because of the need for reduced costs and increased efficiency, that some surgeons in countries with a developing economy are very skilled at sutureless extracapsular surgery. Some of these experienced extracapsular cataract surgeons may delay converting to the phacoemulsification technique because of a perceived formidable "learning curve."[196,197] However, both prospective and retrospective studies of surgeons converting from extracapsular cataract extraction (ECCE) to phacoemulsification have demonstrated excellent results with no significant increase in the complication rate.[198,199] Pederson, in a study of his first 125 unselected cases of phacoemulsification, found no significant increase in the complication rates and attained a visual acuity of 20/40 or better in 98.4% of the patients.[200]

Ophthalmology training programs are now routinely teaching phacoemulsification to residents, under immediate supervision, with excellent results. A number of papers have established that residents can learn to perform phacoemulsification safely with acceptable results when appropriately trained and supervised, and a good method for this type of teaching has been suggested by one particular author.[201–205] A number of surgical training systems have been developed to assist with the learning process.[206–207] The particular technique being taught may be an important factor to consider as well. In two concurrent studies teaching phacoemulsification to residents, Allison initially reported a 14.7% vitreous loss compared with previous studies that cited a 2.4–9% loss using ECCE.[206–211] In the follow-up study, in which a nuclear fracturing technique was taught, the complication rate dropped to 1.6%.[212]

PHYSICAL AND MENTAL PREPAREDNESS

Both the experienced and inexperienced among us can form a number of habits that will maximize our surgical abilities before we ever enter the operating room. The physical preparedness of the surgeon is comparable to that of the athlete. The literature on the benefits of a healthy personal lifestyle is voluminous, so this section is intended only as a brief overview.

In the area of nutrition, a number of studies indicate that eating too much food or choosing high-fat foods can produce sluggish thinking.[213] The practice of eating balanced meals and having regular eating habits is seen as important to keep the level of glucose at a consistent, optimal level for critical thinking. Proper hydration is a must for peak performance. Pitts, at the Harvard University School of Health has established that an athlete's stamina is directly proportional to his or her level of hydration.[214] Aside from the general health benefits, temperance or abstinence from stimulants or depressants is extremely important. It has been demonstrated that nicotine interferes with muscle coordination and control, at least partly because of its ability to upset the acetylcholine balance in the nerve junctions. It has also been reported that caffeine causes a worsening of fine motor coordination because of increases in hand and arm tremors.[215] On the author's first course with Kelman, it was advised that if the participants wanted to carry out this type of surgery using an instrument that vibrated at 40,000 cycles per second, neither coffee nor alcohol should be drunk for 24 to 48 hours beforehand. This advice confirmed the author's convictions on that subject.

Horne has suggested that the loss of a night's sleep undermines creative thinking and the ability to deal with unfamiliar situations.[216] We can all appreciate that a stable personal and professional life allows one optimal concentration, happiness, and a positive outlook. The importance of regular exercise is attested to by the research of Rauhala and colleagues in Finland.[217] A lack of exercise allows some persistence of muscle activity at rest. The authors have established that regular exercise helps a person to relax muscles more completely, which seemingly would result in a steadier hand and, indeed, a steadier body. A study by Nieman has established that exercise increases the size of mitochondria by up to 40% and the number by up to 120%, which gives one the capacity to produce much more energy.[218] Additionally, Neiman reports that decreased anxiety, improved short-term cognition, decreased incidences of depression and even an elevation of mood are all benefits of exercise.[219] A final benefit that people often mention as being a result of regular exercise is an increased feeling of self-confidence.

A healthy professional environment is also beneficial. By ensuring that one has proper equipment, systems, and staff with a cooperative "team" spirit, then maximum attention can be allotted to surgery itself.

■ CONCLUSIONS ■

AVOIDING "FORMULA" PHACOEMULSIFICATION

Keeping abreast of the rapid advances in our field is a challenge in and of itself. With every new technique, instrument, or application of technology, we are forced to modify our approach and adjust to changes in our routine. Perhaps more than ever before, we must develop problem-solving skills, as opposed to memorizing an established body of knowledge.

This chapter provides a summary of what has been accomplished in the past 30 years, a look at where we are today, and, perhaps, a preview of where we may be heading in the future. Certainly, each case should be approached with a strategy in mind, but an ability to adjust, interpret, modify, and improvise should be close at hand. It is the author's sincerest hope that this text has assisted in stimulating this type of thinking and in nurturing these abilities.

References

[1] Heslin KB, Guerriero PN. Clinical retrospective study comparing planned extracapsular cataract extraction and phacoemulsification with and without lens implantation. Ann Ophthalmol 1984;16:956–962.

[2] Watson A, Sunderraj P. Comparison of small incision phacoemulsification with standard extracapsular cataract surgery: post-operative astigmatism and visual recovery. Eye 1992;6:626–629.

[3] Kraff MC, Sanders DR. Planned extracapsular extraction versus phacoemulsification with IOL implantation: A comparison of concurrent series. J Am Intraocular Implant Soc 1982;8:38–41.

[4] Neumann AC, McCarty GR, Sanders DR, et al. Small incisions to control astigmatism during cataract surgery. J Cataract Refract Surg 1989;15:78–84.

[5] Polack FM, Sugar A. The phacoemulsification procedure II: corneal endothelial changes. Invest Ophthalmol 1976;15:458–469.

[6] Arentsen JJ, Rodriques MM, Laibson PR. Corneal opacification occurring after phacoemulsification and phacofragmentation. Am J Ophthalmol 1977;83:794–804.

[7] Binder PS, Sternberg H, Wickham MG, et al. Corneal endothelial damage associated with phacoemulsification. Am J Ophthalmol 1976;82:48–54.

[8] Polack FM, Sugar A. The phacoemulsification procedure III: corneal complications. Invest Ophthalmol 1977;16:39–46.

[9] Sugar J, Mitchelson J, Kraff M. The effect of corneal endothelial cell density. Arch Ophthalmol 1978;96:446–448.

[10] Waltman SR, Cozean CH. The effect of phacoemulsification on the corneal endothelium. Ophthalmic Surg 1979;10:31–33.

[11] Abbott RL, Forster RK. Clinical specular microscopy and intraocular surgery. Arch Ophthalmol 1979;97:1476–1479.

[12] Yang HK, Kline Jr OR. Specular microscopy with intraocular implantations. Am Intraocular Implant Soc J 1981;7:31–35.

[13] Irvin AR, Kratz RP, O'Donnell JJ. Endothelial damage with phacoemulsification and intraocular lens implantation. Arch Ophthalmol 1978;96:1023–1026.

[14] Kraff MC, Sanders DR, Lieberman HL. Specular; microscopy in cataract and intraocular lens patients. Arch Ophthalmol 1980;98:1782–1784.

[15] Colvard DM, Kratz RP, Mazzoco TR, et al. Endothelial cell loss following phacoemulsification in the pupillary plane. Am Intraocular Implant Soc J 1981;7:334–336.

[16] Graether JM, Harris GW, Davison JA, et al. A comparison of the effects of phacoemulsification and nucleus expression on endothelial cell density. Am Intraocular Implant Soc J 1983;9:420–423.

[17] Gwin RM, Warrant JK, Samuelson DA, et al. Effects of phacoemulsification and extracapsular lens removal on corneal thickness and endothelial cell density in the dog. Invest Ophthalmol Vis Sci 1983;24:227–236.

[18] Davison JA. Endothelial cell loss during the transition from nucleus expression to posterior chamber-iris plane phacoemulsification. Am Intraocular Implant Soc J 1984;10:10–13.

[19] Hoffer KJ. Effects of extracapsular implant techniques on endothelial density. Arch Ophthalmol 1982;100:791–792.

[20] Holmberg AS, Philipson BT. Sodium hyaluronate in cataract surgery II: report on the use of Healon in extracapsular cataract surgery using phacoemulsification. Ophthalmology 1984;91:53–57.

[21] Bourne WM, Liesegang TJ, Waller RR, et al. The effect of phacoemulsification on corneal endothelial cell density. Am J Ophthalmol 1984;98:759–762.

[22] Bleckman H, Vogt R. Experimental endothelial lesions by means of an ultrasound phacoemulsifier. Graefes Arch Clin Exp Ophthalmol 1986;224:457–462.

[23] Glasser DB, Katz HR, Boyd JE. Protective effects of viscous solutions in phacoemulsification and traumatic lens subluxation. Arch Ophthalmol 1989;107:1047–1051.

[24] Craig MT, Olson RJ, Mamalis N, et al. Air bubble endothelial damage during phacoemulsification in human eye bank eyes: the protective effects of Healon and Viscoat. J Cataract Refract Surg 1990;16:597–601.

[25] Glasser DB, Osborn DC, Nordeen JF, et al. Endothelial protection and viscoelastic retention during phacoemulsification and intraocular lens implantation. Arch Ophthalmol 1991;109:1438–1440.

[26] Lane SS, Naylor DW, Kullerstarnd LJ, et al. Prospective comparison of the effects of Occucoat, Viscoat, and Healon on intraocular pressure and endothelial cell loss. J Cataract Refract Surg 1991;17:21–26.

[27] Sheets JH. A step beyond ECCE. CLAO J 1987;13:67–70.

[28] Leaming DV. Practice styles and preferences of ASCRS members – 2003 survey. J Cataract Refract Surg 2004;30(4):892–900.

[29] Hattenhauer JM. To 'phaco' or notfi Arch Ophthalmol 1991;109:315 [letter].

[30] Prince RB, Tax RL, Miller DH. Conversion to small-incision phacoemulsification: experience with the first 50 eyes. J Cataract Refract Surg 1993;19:246–250.

[31] Landers JAG. Phacoemulsification in cataract surgery. Med J Aust 1990;153:742 [letter].

[32] Hodgkins PR, Luff AJ, Morrell AJ, et al. Current practice of cataract extraction and anaesthesia. Br J Ophthalmol 1992;76:323–326.

[33] Miyajima H. Phacoemulsification surges forward in Japan. Ocular Surg News 1992;10(16):38–39.

[34] Oshika T, Amano S, Araie M, Majima Y, Leaming DV. Current trends in cataract and refractive surgery in Japan: 1998 survey. Jpn J Ophthalmol 2000;44(3):268–276.

[35] Dada VK, Sindhu N. Management of cataract – a revolutionary change that occurred during last two decades [Review]. J Indian Med Assoc 1999;97(8):313–317.

[36] Lee SY, Tan D. Changing trends in cataract surgery in Singapore. Singapore Med J 1999;40(4):256–259.

[37] Weiser M. Et voila! Phaco in France on the rise. Ocular Surg News 1992;10(14):54.

[38] Krootila K. Practice styles and preferences of Finnish cataract surgeons – 1998 survey. Acta Ophthalmol Scand 1999;77(5):544–547.

[39] Masek P. Cataract surgery in the Czech Republic 1988–1997. Cesk Slov Oftalmol 1999;55(3):117–122.

[40] Ehrich C, Pham DT, Haberle H, Wollensak J. Cataract surgery of ther Berlin Virchow clinic. Overview of the last 16 years. Ophthalmologe 1998;95(6):427–431.

[41] Gimbel HV, Neuhann T. Development, advantages and methods of the continuous circular capsulorhexis technique. J Cataract Refract Surg 1990;16:31–37.

[42] Neuhann T. Theorie und Operationstechnik der Kapsulorhexis. Klin Monatsbl Augenheilkd 1987;190:542–545.

[43] Gimbel HV, Neuhann T. Continuous curvilinear capsulorhexis. J Cataract Refract Surg 1991;17:110 [letter].

[44] Apple DJ, Park SB, Merkley KH, et al. Posterior chamber intraocular lens implantation in a series of 75 autopsy eyes. Parts I–III. J Cataract Refract Surg 1986;12:358–371.

[45] Kelman CD. Phacoemulsification and aspiration – a new technique of cataract removal. A Preliminary report. Am J Ophthalmol 1967;64:23–35.

[46] Kelman CD. Phacoemulsification and aspiration: a progress report. Am J Ophthalmol 1969;67:464.

[47] Kelman CD. Cataract emulsification and aspiration. Trans Ophthalmol Soc UK 1970;90:13.

[48] Kelman CD. Personal interview on phacoemulsification. Highlights Ophthalmol 1971;1970–13:40–61.

[49] Kelman CD. Summary of personal experience. Trans Am Acad Ophthalmol Otolaryngol 1974;78:35–38.

[50] Kelman CD. Phacoemulsification and aspiration. the Kelman technique of cataract removal. Birmingham: Aesculapius Publishing Co; 1975.

[51] Kelman CD. Phacoemulsification and aspiration: a report of 500 consecutive cases. Am J Ophthalmol 1973;75:764–768.

[52] Kelman CD. Phacoemulsification and aspiration of senile cataracts. A comparative study with intracapsular extraction. Can J Ophthalmol 1973;8:24.

[53] Shock JP. Phacofragmentation and irrigation of cataracts: a preliminary report. Am J Ophthalmol 1972;74:187.

[54] Paton D. Phacoemulsification: trials and tribulations. Invest Ophthalmol 1973;12:318.

[55] Hiles DA, Hurite FG. Results of the first year's experience with phacoemulsification. Am J Ophthalmol 1973;75:473–477.

[56] Hurite FG, Kennerdel JS. Experiences with phacoemulsification. Trans Pa Acad Ophthalmol Otolaryngol 1973;26:126–130.

[57] Kratz RP. Difficulties, complications, and management. Symposium on phacoemulsification. Trans Am Acad Ophthalmol Otolaryngol 1974;78:18.

[58] Shock JP. Alternative techniques: phacofragmentation, phacocryolysis and irrigation of cataracts. Trans Am Acad Ophthalmol Otolaryngol 1974;78:22.

[59] Troutman RC. Preliminary report of the committee on phacoemulsification. Trans Am Acad Ophthalmol Otolaryngol 1974;75:41–42.

[60] Hurite FG. The contraindications to phacoemulsification and summary of personal experience. Trans Am Acad Ophthalmol Otolaryngol 1974;78:14–17.

[61] Emery JM, Paton D. Phacoemulsification: a survey of 2875 cases. Trans Am Acad Ophthalmol Otolaryngol 1974;78:OP31–34.
[62] Cleasaby GW, Fung WE, Webster RG. The lens fragmentation and aspiration procedure (phacoemulsification). Am J Ophthalmol 1974;77:384–387.
[63] Cleasby GW. The advantages and disadvantages of Kelman phacoemulsification (KPE). Ophthalmology 1974;81:1973–1974.
[64] Benolken RM, Emergy JM, Landis DJ. Temperature profiles in the anterior chamber during phacoemulsification. Invest Ophthalmol 1974;13:71–74.
[65] Dayton GO, Hulquist CR. Complications of phacoemulsification. Can J Ophthalmol 1975;10:61–68.
[66] Troutman RC, Clahane AC, Emery JM, et al. Cataract survey of the cataract-phacoemulsification committee. Trans Am Acad Ophthalmol Otolaryngol 1975;79:178–185.
[67] Kline OR. Phacoemulsification visual results and complications: report of 800 cases. Ophthalmic Surg 1976;8:94–97.
[68] Fung WE. Phacoemulsification. Ophthalmology 1978;85:46–51.
[69] Emery JM. Phacoemulsification – cataract surgery of the future. Int Ophthalmol Clin 1978;18:155–170.
[70] Emery JM, Wilhelmus KA, Rosenburg S. Complications of phacoemulsification. Ophthalmology 1978;85:141–150.
[71] Kratz RP. Intracapsular versus extracapsular cataract extraction for intraocular lens implantation. Int Ophthalmol Clin 1979;19:179–194.
[72] Ewing C. Phacoemulsification. Can J Ophthalmol 1979;14:1–2.
[73] Kraff MC, Sanders DR, Lieberman HL. Total cataract extraction through a 3 mm incision. A report of 650 cases. Ophthalmic Surg 1979;10:46–54.
[74] Emery JM, Little JH. Phacoemulsification and aspiration of cataracts: surgical techniques, complications, and results. St. Louis: Mosby; 1979.
[75] Knolle GE, Justice J, Spears WD. Discussion of presentation by Dr. Gilbert W. Cleasby. Ophthalmology 1979;86:1975–1979.
[76] Sinskey RM, Cain W. The posterior capsule and phacoemulsification. Am Intraocular Implant Soc J 1978;4:206–207.
[77] Little JH. Outline of phacoemulsification for the ophthalmic surgeon. 2nd ed. Oklahoma City: Samco Color Press; 1975.
[78] Kratz RP. Teaching phacoemulsification in California and 200 cases of phacoemulsification. In: Emery JM, Paton D, editors. Current concepts in cataract surgery: selected proceedings of the fourth biennial cataract surgical congress. St. Louis: Mosby; 1976. p. 196–200.
[79] Kratz RP, Colvard DM. Kelman phacoemulsification in the posterior chamber. Ophthalmology 1979;86:1983–1984.
[80] Kratz RP, Mazzocco TR, Davidson B, et al. The shearing intraocular lens: a report of 1,000 cases. Am Intraocular Implant Soc J 1981;7:55–57.
[81] Maloney WF, Grindle L. Textbook of phacoemulsification. Fallbrook, CA: Lasenda Publishers; 1990.
[82] Gimbel HV. Divide and conquer [video]. Presented at the European Intraocular Implantlens Council meeting. 1987.
[83] Gimbel HV. Divide and conquer nucleofractis phacoemulsification: development and variations. J Cataract Refract Surg 1991;17:281–291.
[84] Worgul BV. Lens. In: Duane TD, Jaeger EA, editors. Biomedical foundations of ophthalmology. Philadelphia: Harper and Row; 1983.
[85] Marshall J, Beaconsfield M, Rothery S. The anatomy and development of the human lens and zonules. Trans Ophthalmol Soc UK 1982;102:423–440.
[86] Drews RC. The lens capsule: a lens implant surgeon's understanding. The Mary Louise Prentice Lecture. Trans Ophthalmol Soc UK 1986;105:265–272.
[87] Worst J. A morphological description of human cataractous lenses by SEM. Doc Ophthalmol 1987;67:197–207.
[88] Worst J. Some aspects of cataract morphology: a SEM study. Doc Ophthalmol 1988;70:155–163.
[89] Duke-Elder S. Anatomy of the visual system. In: System of ophthalmology, Vol II. St. Louis: Mosby; 1961. p. 320–323.
[90] Bron A, Smith G, Smith R, et al. Changes in light scatter and width measurements from the human lens cortex with age. Eye 1992;6:55–59.
[91] Drews RC. YAG laser demonstration of the anatomy of the lens nucleus. Ophthalmic Surg 1992;23:811–824.
[92] Drews RC. Phacoemulsification without ultrasound. Eur J Implant Refract Surg 1993;5:80–81.
[93] Pisacano AM, Levy JH, Anello RD. New spatula to facilitate bimanual phacoemulsification. J Cataract Refract Surg 1990;16:259–261.
[94] Levy JH, Pisacano AM, Anello RD. A new endocapsular nucleus controller to facilitate nuclear splitting during bimanual endocapsular phacoemulsification. Eur J Implant Refract Surg 1992;4:121–122.
[95] Brauweiler P. Bimanual irrigation/aspiration. J Cataract Refract Surg 1996;22:1013–1016.
[96] Seibel BS. Phacodynamics: mastering the tools and techniques of phacoemulsification. Thorofare, NJ: Slack, Inc; 1993.
[97] Fine IH, Maloney WF, Dillman DM. Crack and flip phacoemulsification technique. J Cataract Refract Surg 1993;19:797–802.
[98] Patel J, Apple D. Protective effect of the anterior lens capsule during extracapsular cataract extraction. Ophthalmology 1989;96:598–602.
[99] Krag S, Thim K, Corydon L. The stretching capacity of capsulorhexis – an experimental study on animal cadaver eyes. Eur J Implant Refract Surg 1990;2:43–45.
[100] Thim K, Krag S, Corydon L. Stretching capacity of capsulorhexis and nucleus delivery. J Cataract Refract Surg 1991;17:31.
[101] Ohrloff C, Oldendorp J, Puck A. Minimal endothelial cell loss following phacoemulsification and posterior chamber lens implantation. Klin Monatsble Augentreilkd 1985;186:302–306.
[102] Gimbel HV. Continuous curvilinear capsulorhexis and nucleus fracturing. Evolution, technique and complications. Ophthalmology Clin N Am 1991;4:235–249.
[103] Gimbel HV. Trough and crater divide and conquer nucleofractis techniques. Eur J Implant Refract Surg 1991;3:123–126.
[104] Gimbel HV. Evolving techniques of cataract surgery: continuous curvilinear capsulorhexis, down-slope sculpting and nucleofractis. Semin Ophthalmol 1992;7:193–207.
[105] Gimbel HV. Down-slope sculpting. J Cataract Refract Surg 1992;18:614–618.
[106] Sinskey RM, Patel JV. Manual of cataract surgery. New York: Churchill Livingstone; 1987.
[107] Gimbel HV. Hydro-free dissection [video]. Presented at the ASCRS film festival, San Diego. 1992.
[108] Gimbel HV. Hydro dissection/hydrodelineation. Int Ophthalmol Clin 1994;34:73–90.
[109] Fine IH. The chip and flip phacoemulsification technique. J Cataract Refract Surg 1991;17:366–371.
[110] Fine IH. Two-handed phacoemulsification through a small circular capsulorhexis. In: Koch P, Davison J, editors. Phacoemulsification techniques. Thorofare, NJ: Slack Inc; 1991. p. 191–205.
[111] Fine IH. The chip and flip phacoemulsification technique. In: Yalon M, editor. Techniques of phacoemulsification surgery and IOL implantation. Thorofare, NJ: Slack Inc; 1992. p. 3–23.
[112] Koch PS. Converting to phacoemulsification: a manual for the surgeon in transition. Thorofare, NJ: Slack, Inc; 1988.
[113] Koch PS. Spring surgery. In: Koch P, Davison J, editors. Phacoemulsification techniques. Thorofare, NJ: Slack Inc; 1991. p. 207–238.
[114] Koch PS. A strategic approach to phacoemulsification based on nuclear density. Semin Ophthalmol 1992;7:234–244.
[115] Raitta C, Setala K. Intraocular lens implantation in exfoliation syndrome and capsular glaucoma. Acta Ophthalmol (Copenh) 1986;64:130–133.
[116] Guzek JP, Holm M, Cameron JA, et al. Risk factors for intraoperative complications in 1000 extracapsular cataract cases. Ophthalmology 1987;97:461–466.
[117] Skuta G, Parrish RK, Hodapp E, et al. Zonular dialysis during extracapsular cataract extraction in pseudoexfoliation syndrome. Arch Ophthalmol 1987;105:532–534.
[118] Dark A. Cataract extraction complicated by capsular glaucoma. Br J Ophthalmol 1979;63:465–468.
[119] Ghosh M, Speakman J. The ciliary body in senile exfoliation of the lens. Can J Ophthalmol 1973;8:394–403.
[120] Tarkkanen AHA. Exfoliation syndrome. Trans Ophthalmol Soc UK 1986;105:233–236.
[121] Osher RH, Cionni RJ, Gimbel HV, et al. Cataract surgery in patients with pseudoexfoliation syndrome. Eur J Implant Refract Surg 1993;5:46–50.
[122] Shepherd JR. In situ fracture. J Cataract Refract Surg 1990;16:436–440.
[123] Shepherd JR. Shepherd phaco fracture. In: Devine TM, Banko W, editors. Phacoemulsification surgery. Toronto: Pergamon Press Canada Ltd; 1991. p. 67–72.
[124] Davison JA. Minimal lift-multiple rotation technique for capsular bag phacoemulsification and intraocular lens fixation. J Cataract Refract Surg 1988;14:25–34.
[125] Fine IH, Packer M, Hoffman RS. Use of power modulations in phacoemulsification. Choo-choo chop and flip phacoemulsification. J Cataract Refract Surg 2001;27(2):188–197.
[126] Davison JA. No-lift capsular bag phacoemulsification and dialing technique for no-hole intraocular lens optics. J Cataract Refract Surg 1988;14:346–349 [letter].
[127] Davison JA. Bimodal capsular bag phacoemulsification: a serial cutting and suction ultrasonic nuclear dissection technique. J Cataract Refract Surg 1989;15:272–282.
[128] Davison JA. Hybrid nuclear dissection technique for capsular bag phacoemulsification. J Cataract Refract Surg 1990;16:441–450.
[129] Johnson SH. Split and lift: nuclear quadrant management for phacoemulsification. J Cataract Refract Surg 1993;19:420–424.
[130] Fine IH. The choo-choo chop and flip phacoemulsification technique. Operative Tech Cataract Refract Surg 1998;1:61–65.
[131] Faust KJ. Hydrodissection of soft nuclei. J Am Intraocul Implant Soc 1984;10(1):75–77.
[132] Krasnov MM, Makarov IA. Said Naim Iussef: Densitometric analysis of crystalline lens nucleus in the choice of strategy of surgical treatment of cataracts. Vestn Oftalmol 2000;116(4):6–8.
[133] Walkow T, Anders N, Klebe S. Endothelial cell loss after phacoemulsification: relation to preoperative and intraoperative parameters. J Cataract Refract Surg 2000;26(5):727–732.
[134] Corydon L, Krag S, Thim K. One-handed phacoemulsification with low settings. J Cataract Refract Surg 1997;23(8):1143–1148.
[135] Maloney WF. Tutorial in phacoemulsification. Eur J Implant Refract Surg 1990;2:125–133.
[136] Maloney WF, Dillman D. Fractional 2:4 phaco. In: Koch P, Davison J, editors. Phacoemulsification techniques. Thorofare, NJ: Slack Inc; 1991. p. 241–255.
[137] Maloney WF, Dillman D. A comprehensive approach to phacoemulsification from beginning to advanced techniques. Ophthalmol Clin N Am 1991;4:221–234.
[138] Sakka Y. Phacoemulsification without anterior capsulectomy. Folia Ophthalmol Jpn 1982;33:233–235.
[139] Hara T, Hara T. Subcapsular phacoemulsification and aspiration. Am Intraocular Implant Soc J 1984;10:333–337.
[140] Gindi JJ, Wan WL, Schanzlin DJ. Endocapsular cataract surgery – I. Surgical technique. Cataract 1985;2:6–10.
[141] Hara T, Hara T. Recent advance in intracapsular phacoemulsification and complete in-the-bag intraocular lens implantation. Am Intraocular Implant Soc J 1985;11:488–490.
[142] Parel JM, Gelender H, Trafers WF, et al. Phacoersatz: cataract surgery designed to preserve accommodation. Graefes Arch Clin Exp Ophthalmol 1986;224:165–173.
[143] Hara T, Hara T. Fate of the capsular bag in endocapsular phacoemulsification and complete in-the-bag intraocular lens fixation. J Cataract Refract Surg 1986;12:408–412.
[144] Hara T, Hara T. Clinical results of endocapsular phacoemulsification and complete in-the- bag intraocular lens fixation. J Cataract Refract Surg 1987;13:279–286.
[145] Hara T, Hara T. Endocapsular phacoemulsification and aspiration (ECPEA) – recent surgical technique and clinical results. Ophthalmic Surg 1987;20:469–475.
[146] Haeflinger E, Parel JM, Fantes F, et al. Accommodation of an endocapsular silicone lens (phacoersatz) in the nonhuman primate. Ophthalmology 1987;94:471–477.
[147] Hara T, Hara T. Roundel phacoemulsification technique for in-the-bag intraocular lens fixation. J Cataract Refract Surg 1987;13:441–446.
[148] Hara T, Azuma N, Chiba K, et al. Anterior capsular opacification after endocapsular cataract surgery. Ophthalmic Surg 1992;23:94–98.
[149] Solomon LD. Endocapsular phacoemulsification. In: Solomon LD, editor. Practical phacoemulsification: proceedings of the 2nd annual workshop [Supplement to Ophthalmic Practice]. 1990. p. 10–13.
[150] Solomon LD. Endocapsular (intercapsular) phacoemulsification. In: Solomon LD, editor. Practical phacoemulsification. Proceedings of the 3rd Annual Workshop [Supplement to Ophthalmic Practice]. 1991. p. 29–39.
[151] Michelson MA. Endocapsular phacoemulsification with mini-capsulorhexis. In: Koch P, Davison J, editors. Phacoemulsification techniques. Thorofare, NJ: Slack Inc; 1991. p. 275–309.
[152] Wan WL, Gindi JJ, Schanzlin DJ. Endocapsular cataract surgery – II. Effects on the corneal endothelium. Cataract 1985;2:11–14.
[153] Solomon KD, Gwin TD, O'Morchoe DJC, et al. Protective effect of the anterior lens capsule during extracapsular cataract extraction. Part I: experimental animal study. Ophthalmology 1989;96:591–597.
[154] Nishi O, Nishi K. Endocapsular phacoemulsification following buttonhole anterior capsulotomy: a preliminary report. J Cataract Refract Surg 1990;16:575–762.
[155] Nishi O. Endo-Intercapsular cataract surgery following buttonhole anterior capsulotomy. In: Yalon M, editor. Techniques of phacoemulsification and surgery and IOL implantation. Thorofare, NJ: Slack Inc; 1992. p. 249–266.
[156] Pop M. Two-port endocap phaco: safe and quick. Ocular Surg News 1991;9:1–40.
[157] Stark WJ, Streeten B. The anterior capsulotomy of extracapsular cataract extraction. Ophthalmic Surg 1984;15:911–917.
[158] Apple DJ, Kincaid MC, Mamalis N, et al. Intraocular lenses: evolution, designs, complications and pathology. Baltimore: Williams & Wilkins; 1989. p. 141–143.
[159] Gimbel HV. Two-stage capsulorhexis for endocapsular phacoemulsification. J Cataract Refract Surg 1990;16:246–249.

[160] Gimbel HV. Continuous circular, two-stage and posterior continuous circular capsulorhexis: description and analysis. Ophthalmic Practice 1990;8:81–85.

[161] Nishi O. Refilling the lens of the rabbit eye after intracapsular cataract surgery using an endocapsular balloon and an anterior capsule suturing technique. J Cataract Refract Surg 1989;15:450–454.

[162] Nishi O, Hara T, Hara T, et al. Further development of experimental techniques for refilling the lens of animal eyes with a balloon. J Cataract Refract Surg 1989;15:584–588.

[163] Teichmann KD. Endocapsular closed chamber technique for disc lens implantation. J Cataract Refract Surg 1989;16:253–256.

[164] Arnold PN. One-handed method of posterior chamber phacoemulsification. J Cataract Refract Surg 1990;16:646–648.

[165] Fishkind WJ. In situ phacoemulsification. In: Koch P, Davison J, editors. Phacoemulsification techniques. Thorofare, NJ: Slack Inc; 1991. p. 143–152.

[166] Arnold PN. Nuclear flip technique in small pupil phacoemulsification. J Cataract Refract Surg 1991;17:225–227.

[167] Kershner RM. Sutureless one-handed intercapsular phacoemulsification. The keyhole technique. J Cataract Refract Surg 1991;17:719–725.

[168] Klemen UM. V-style phacoemulsification. J Cataract Refract Surg 1993;19:548–550.

[169] Pacifico RL. Divide and conquer phacoemulsification: one-handed variant. J Cataract Refract Surg 1992;18:513–517.

[170] Krey HF. Ultrasonic turbulences at the phacoemulsification tip. J Cataract Refract Surg 1989;15:343–344.

[171] Scleral and corneal burns during phacoemulsification with viscoelastic materials. Health Devices 1988;17:377–379.

[172] Shimmura S, Tsubota K, Oguchi Y, et al. Oxiradical-dependent photoemission induced by phacoemulsification probe. Invest Ophthalmol Vis Sci 1992;33:2904–2907.

[173] Davis PL. Phaco transducers: Basic principles and corneal thermal injury. Eur J Implant Refract Surg 1993;5:109–112.

[174] Wilbrandt HR, Wilbrandt TH. Evaluation of intraocular pressure fluctuations with differing phacoemulsification approaches. J Cataract Refract Surg 1993;19:223–231.

[175] Zetterstrom C, Laurell CG. Comparison of endothelial cell loss and phacoemulsification energy during endocapsular phacoemulsification surgery. J Cataract Refract Surg 1995;21(1):55–58.

[176] Hayashi K, Nakao F, Hayashi F. Corneal endothelial cell loss following phacoemulsification using the small-port phaco. Ophthalmic Surg 1994;25(8):510–513.

[177] Pacifico RL. Ultrasonic energy in phacoemulsification: mechanical cutting and cavitation. J Cataract Refract Surg 1994;20(3):338–341.

[178] Probst LE, Nichols BD. Corneal endothelial and intraocular pressure changes after phacoemulsification with Amvisc Plus and Viscoat. J Cataract Refract Surg 1993;19(6):725–730.

[179] Strobel J, Jacobi KW. Phaco-emulsification and planned ECCE: intraoperative differences in intraocular heating. Eur J Implant Refract Surg 1991;3:135–138.

[180] Hunkeler JD. Peristaltic-based pump maximizes control. Ocular Surg News 1993;11(16):22, 23.

[181] Weiss IS. Aspiration pressure of phacoemulsification tips. J Cataract Refract Surg 1986;12:173.

[182] Singer JA. Funnel shaped tip controls ultrasound energy during phaco. Ocular Surg News 1992;10(13):48.

[183] Zelman J. Small-port phacoemulsification. In: Solomon LD, editor. Practical phacoemulsification: proceedings of the 3rd annual workshop [Supplement to Ophthalmic Practice]. 1991. p. 40–42.

[184] Heslin KB. Phacoemulsification with the Heslin/Mackool ocusystem: results of a retrospective study. Am Intraocular Implant Soc J 1983;9:445–449.

[185] Heslin KB, Guerriero PN. Phacoemulsification with the Heslin/Mackool ocusystem. A follow-up report. Ann Ophthalmol 1985;17:601–603.

[186] Neumann AC, Molyet E, Teal C, et al. Phacoemulsification devices. A consumer's update. J Cataract Refract Surg 1978;13:669–677.

[187] Neumann AC, Molyet E, Teal C, et al. Phacoemulsification devices: a consumer's report. J Cataract Refract Surg 1987;13:70–75.

[188] Davison JA. Personal correction of a phacoemulsification machine problem. J Cataract Refract Surg 1988;14:456–458 [letter].

[189] Eggleston RJ. One consumer's experience with a phacoemulsification device. J Cataract Refract Surg 1988;14:232–233.

[190] Phacoemulsification systems. Health Devices 1989;18:377–404.

[191] Ohneck JA. Comparative efficiency of current phacoemulsification units. Ophthalmic Practice 1990;8:73–75.

[192] Javier JA, Devine TM. Thermal comparison of the Bausch & Lomb Millennium, Alcon AdvanTec Legacy, and the AMO Sovereign WhiteStar phacoemulsification Systems. J Cataract Refract Surg 2006;32(11):1896–1897.

[193] Adams W, Brinton J, Floyd M, Olson RJ. Phacodynamics: an aspiration flow vx vacuum comparison. Am J Ophthalmol 2006;142:320–322.

[194] Rose AD, Kanade V. Thermal imaging study comparing phacoemulsification with the Sovereign with WhiteStar system to the Legacy with AdvanTec and NeoSoniX system. Am J Ophthalmol 2006;141(2):322–326.

[195] Fine IH, Packer M, Hoffman RS. Power modulations in new phacoemulsification technology: improved outcomes. J Cataract Refract Surg 2004;30:1014–1019.

[196] Olson RJ. Is the phacoemulsification learning curve too steep? Arch Ophthalmol 1991;109:1510 [letter].

[197] Cotlier E. Phacoemulsification by residents. Ophthalmology 1992;99:1481 [letter].

[198] Hagan JC. A prospective study of the transition to phacoemulsification and small incision cataract surgery. Mo Med 1992;89:663–667.

[199] Prince RB, Tax RL, Miller DH. Conversion to small-incision phacoemulsification: experience with the first 50 eyes. J Cataract Refract Surg 1993;19:246–250.

[200] Pedersen O. Phacoemulsification and intraocular lens implantation in patients with cataract. Acta Ophthalmol 1990;68:59–64.

[201] Cotlier E, Rose M. Cataract extraction by the intracapsular methods and by phacoemulsification: the results of surgeons in training. Trans Am Acad Ophthalmol Otolaryngol 1976;81:163–182.

[202] Csordas JE. The surgeon's transition to phacoemulsification. In Solomon LD, editors. Practical phacoemulsification: proceedings of the 2nd annual workshop [Supplement to ophthalmic practice]. 1990. p. 5–9.

[203] Cruz OA, Wallace GW, Gay CA, et al. Visual results and complications of phacoemulsification with intraocular lens implantation performed by ophthalmology residents. Ophthalmology 1992;99:448–452.

[204] Kreisler KR, Mortenson SW, Mamalis N. Endothelial cell loss following "modern" phacoemulsification by a senior resident. Ophthalmic Surg 1992;23:158–160.

[205] Goetz JS. Teaching phacoemulsification to residents. Ophthalmic Practice 1992;10:219–222.

[206] Maloney WF, Hall D, Parkinson DB. Synthetic cataract teaching system for phacoemulsification. J Cataract Refract Surg 1988;14:218–221.

[207] Zirm ME, Rosen ES. The high communication wetlab: a unique innovation in teaching ophthalmic surgery. Eur J Implant Refract Surg 1992;4:145–148.

[208] Allinson RW, Metrikin DC, Fante RG. Incidence of vitreous loss among third-year residents performing phacoemulsification. Ophthalmology 1992;99:726–730.

[209] Browning DJ, Cobo LM. Early experience in extracapsular cataract surgery by residents. Ophthalmology 1985;92:1647–1653.

[210] Pearson PA, Owen DG, Van Meter WS, et al. Vitreous loss rates in extracapsular surgery by residents. Ophthalmology 1989;96:1225–1227.

[211] Sappenfield DL, Driebe Jr WT. Resident extracapsular surgery: results and a comparison of automated and manual technique. Ophthalmic Surg 1989;20:619–624.

[212] Allinson RW, Palmer ML, Fante R, et al. Vitreous loss during phacoemulsification by residents. Ophthalmology 1993;100:1181 [letter].

[213] Spring B. Effects of food and nutrients on the behavior of normal individuals. In: Wurtman RJ, Wurtman JJ, editors. Nutrition and the brain. New York: Raven Press; 1986. p. 1–41.

[214] Pitts GL, Johnson RE, Consolzio FC. Work in the heat as affected by intake of water, salt and glucose. Am J Physiol 1944;142:253–259.

[215] Craig WJ. Nutrition for the nineties. Eau Claire, WI: Golden Harvest Books; 1992. p. 283.

[216] Home JA. Human sleep, sleep loss and behaviour implications for the prenatal cortex and psychiatric disorders. Br J Psychiatry 1993;162:413–419.

[217] Rauhala E. Relaxation training combined with increased physical activity lowers the psychophysiological activation in community-home boys. Int J Psychophysiol 1990;10:63–68.

[218] Neiman DC. Fitness and sports medicine. Palo Alto: Bull Publishing Co; 1990. 167.

[219] Neiman DC. Fitness and sports medicine. Palo Alto: Bull Publishing Co; 1990. 389–392.

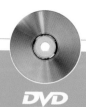
DVD

Phaco Chop

Roger F. Steinert, MD

17

CONTENTS

CHAPTER HIGHLIGHTS

>> Understanding the mechanics of the phaco chop maneuver

>> Technique for horizontal and vertical phaco chop

>> Special circumstances:

>> Weak zonules

>> Dense nuclei

>> Small pupils

>> Complication avoidance

In 1993, Kunihiro Nagahara introduced the concept of a new technique for nuclear disassembly during phacoemulsification. His insight was that natural cleavage planes existed in the nucleus that had not been used previously (Figure 17-1A). By impaling the nucleus with the phacoemulsification tip, and thereby stabilizing it, the second "chopping" instrument could be pulled from the equatorial side of the outer nucleus toward the center. The nucleus was split readily by the chopping instrument, taking advantage of these natural cleavage planes. Nagahara made an analogy to the technique of chopping or, more accurately, splitting a log of wood with a wedge, taking advantage of the wood's grain, or cleavage planes (Figure 17-1B).

■ EVOLUTION OF PHACO CHOP ■

STOP AND CHOP

Several surgeons were stimulated by Nagahara's method and evolved techniques in an effort to improve on the reliability and repeatability of phaco chop. Paul Koch found that the initial chop, intended to bisect the nucleus, was the most difficult. He reverted to creating an initial deep trough with the phaco tip and then cracking the trough with lateral pressure from the phaco tip and a second instrument, identical to the beginning of the quadrant cracking technique. At this point, however, Koch stopped the quadrant cracking approach and then began chopping the remaining pieces of nucleus; he labeled this technique as "stop and chop."[1] This technique (Figure 17-2) remains popular with many surgeons, and it is an important transition for almost anyone learning phaco chop because it eliminates the most difficult chopping step: the initial chop.

CHOP AND DEBULK

To maximize the safety of the corneal endothelium and be able to continue to perform phacoemulsification in the posterior chamber and iris plane, the surgeon should create some central space to allow the chopping technique to be used in disassembling the nucleus posterior to the iris. Similar to a multipiece jigsaw puzzle, taking pieces apart becomes easier once the initial piece is removed. In addition, the majority of ultrasound power is used to phacoemulsify the central hard nucleus, not the periphery. Steinert[2] described a technique that began identically to Nagahara's with an initial phaco chop to bisect the nucleus. Although perhaps more difficult to master, this initial chop is a more efficient maneuver than the creation of a trough and then splitting it, as in the stop and chop technique. After the initial chop, however, the central hard nucleus is emulsified along the fault line of the initial crack before proceeding to chopping further pieces of nuclei. In softer nuclei, very little central material is removed at this step. In harder, larger nuclei, more central nucleus can be removed at this step; in very advanced cataracts, the center is bowled out to the midperiphery before beginning to chop further (Figure 17-3).

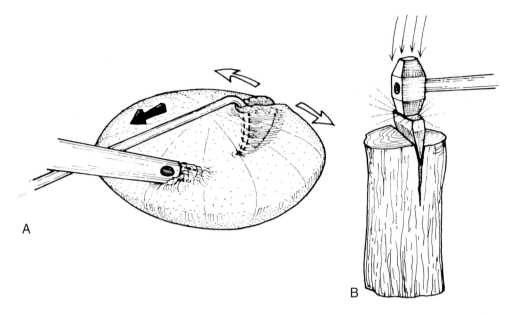

Figure 17-1 A, Nagahara's insight was to split the nucleus along its natural cleavage planes. B, The principle of chopping is the same as using a wedge to split a log along its natural planes.

CIRCUMFERENTIAL SEQUENTIAL DISASSEMBLY

Both Koch and Steinert found that the chop technique was better applied as a method of the progressive chopping of small wedges in a circumferential direction, rather than the chopping of four full quadrants as originally described by Nagahara. The reason for this is that the progressive circumferential chopping of small wedges results in only one small piece being removed at any given time. Because of the bulk, the large nuclear pieces remain stable within the posterior capsular sac. Therefore, control of the phacoemulsification process is enhanced.

Howard Gimbel[3] earlier described several techniques of nuclear fracture whose principles have been incorporated in phaco chop as it has evolved. Gimbel pointed out the importance of debulking the central nucleus, forming a narrow trough for softer nuclei and a larger crater for hard nuclei. In addition, he demonstrated the ability to break off pieces of the peripheral nucleus with lateral separation movements after engaging them with the phacoemulsification tip, proceeding in a circumferential direction. Gimbel called this technique "nucleofractis." In essence, a phaco chop is the nucleofractis technique, greatly facilitated by the second "chopping" instrument instead of relying on forceful lateral movements of the phacoemulsification tip.

HIGH-VACUUM PHACO CHOP

In addition to his incorporation of central debulking techniques and use of progressive circumferential chopping steps, Steinert recognized that using high vacuum during chopping further improves nuclear control and reduces the total ultrasound energy required. High vacuum allows the surgeon to grasp and hold the

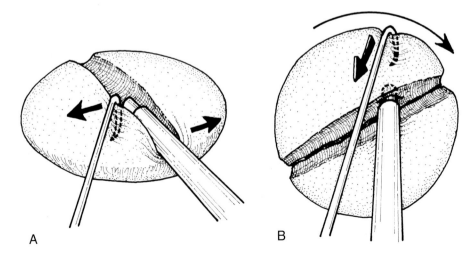

Figure 17-2 A, Paul Koch's "stop and chop" technique begins with a groove and cracking of the nucleus into two halves, identical to the start of "divide and conquer" nuclear fracture. B, Nucleus is rotated 1 to 2 clock hours, and the surgeon stops the "divide and conquer" technique and begins to "chop."

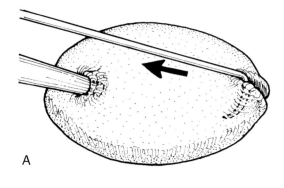

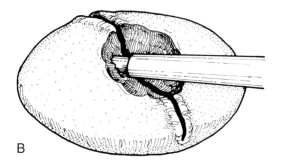

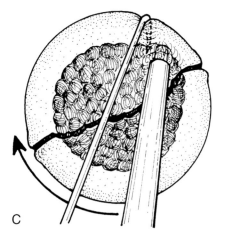

Figure 17-3 A, Full phaco chop approach uses the chopper to split the nucleus into two halves. B, Space is created, and the hardest central portion of the nucleus is removed, leaving enough peripheral nucleus to gain purchase by the phaco tip with a small amount of ultrasound and high vacuum. C, nucleus is rotated clockwise (for a right-handed surgeon; a left-handed surgeon rotates counterclockwise and performs mirror-image maneuvers), and pie-shaped wedges are split off and removed with short bursts of ultrasound.

nuclear wedges and draw them toward the central zone of safety before completing the emulsification. Moreover, the manual energy input from the phaco chop, combined with the energy input from the high vacuum, reduces the total amount of ultrasonic energy required. Overall, the technique appears to be safer and more controlled. Because of its efficiency, the nuclear disassembly step of phacoemulsification cataract surgery is generally substantially faster than alternative techniques such as quadrant cracking.[4-6]

PHACO QUICK CHOP ("VERTICAL PHACO CHOP")

Vladimir Pfeifer of Slovenia is generally credited for originating the fundamental concept of vertical forces that also fragment the nucleus. This technique has been developed and taught by David Dillman and Louis Nichamin as "phaco quick chop." Nagahara's fundamental concept is to stabilize the nucleus with the phaco tip and then pull the chopping instrument in the horizontal plane from the equator toward the center. Vertical chop differs by embedding the phaco tip deeply into the nucleus and then impaling a sharp-tipped chopping instrument into the anterior nucleus in front and adjacent to the phaco tip. The chopper pushes downward sharply while the phaco tip lifts upward (Figure 17-4A). Each instrument moves about one-half of the total amount of vertical separation needed to generate a fissure. As soon as the vertical (anteroposterior) split begins to develop, the two instruments also spread horizontally slightly to complete the cleavage of the two sections (Figure 17-4B). Vertical chop is then continued to break off smaller sections of nucleus for emulsification, progressing circumferentially, as in the technique described earlier (Figures 17-4C and D).

The principal advantage of vertical chopping is the elimination of the need to pass the chopper under the anterior capsule out to the equator of the nucleus. Because neither the anterior capsule edge nor the equator can always be seen, some surgeons dislike the necessity of relying on tactile feedback and judgment of distances under the iris. On the other hand, vertical chopping works best in moderate-density nuclei. It often fails in softer nuclei, where the phaco tip and chopper pull through the nucleus, or in hard nuclei, where so much force is required that, when cleavage does occur, the abrupt movement threatens the integrity of the posterior capsule and/or zonules.

The "complete" phaco surgeon should be comfortable with both horizontal and vertical chopping maneuvers, as each has its place.

■ DETAILED TECHNIQUE OF PHACO CHOP ■

The basic concept of horizontal phaco chop, as it is usually practiced, is illustrated in Figure 17-5. The nucleus is stabilized with the phacoemulsification tip, which is impaled with moderate vacuum (typically 50–80 mm Hg) and low ultrasonic power, in a position near the center, but off-center by about 1 mm towards the incision. The irrigation sleeve should be retracted more than is customary for divide and conquer nuclear fracture, in order to permit the phaco tip to advance to the depth of midnucleus (1.5–2 mm). While impaling the nucleus, the phaco handpiece is markedly tipped in the vertical direction, as if aiming for the optic disc. The chopping instrument is passed through a paracentesis that is about 1½ clock hours away from the incision. The chopper can assist the proper location of the impaling of the

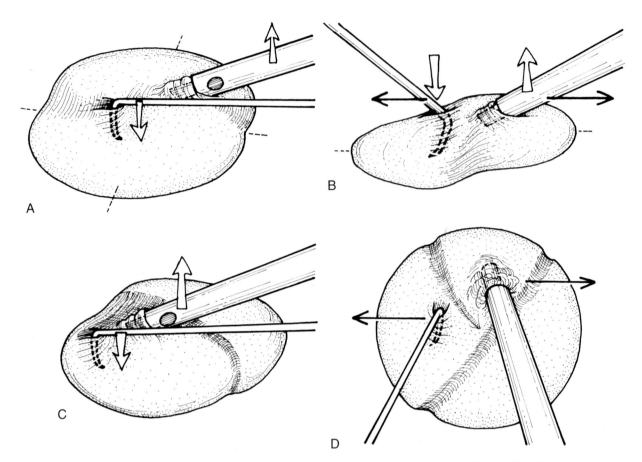

Figure 17-4 **A,** In vertical phaco chop ("phaco quick chop"), the deeply buried phaco tip is lifted up while a sharp-tipped chopper presses downward. **B,** Once the endonucleus starts to split, the instruments are separated slightly laterally as well to enhance full cleavage of the two sections of nucleus. **C,** and **D,** Nucleus is rotated, and the vertical chop maneuver is repeated to create smaller nuclear fragments that can be removed with ultrasound and aspiration. (**C,** Side view; **D,** surgeon's view.)

phaco tip by pressing lightly on the nuclear surface and shifting the nucleus gently (about 1 mm) away from the incision.

The chopper is advanced under the anterior capsule until it can pass around the equator of the nucleus at the nucleus–epinucleus border, about 180° opposite the paracentesis. If the nuclear equatorial border can be visualized as either a "golden ring" (smaller nucleus) or a dark ring (larger nucleus) as a result of effective hydrodelineation, the chopper can be placed into this ring under direct visualization (see Figures 17-5A and B). If the nucleus is very large or the pupil does not adequately dilate, the surgeon will nevertheless be able to feel the abrupt change as the chopper tip passes from the hard nucleus to the relatively soft epinucleus. The chopping instrument will shift posteriorly by at least 1 mm when this border is encountered (see Figure 17-5C).

The chopping instrument is then drawn across the center of the nucleus, moving from opposite the paracentesis in the direction of the paracentesis (see Figure 17-5D). Once the center of the nucleus is approached or fully transected, the nucleus fractures readily. To successfully split the nucleus, the chopper tip should be at least at half depth in the nucleus anteroposteriorly, as well as chopping across half of the nucleus radially. The impaled phaco tip will also have weakened the central nucleus and contributes to a successful chopping hemisection of the nucleus. This basic chop maneuver works well in nuclei ranging from low to high density.

The next step is to debulk the center of the nucleus. If the lens has mild-to-moderate density, the debulking is restricted to a zone no larger than a conventional trough. In that manner, the peripheral nuclear pieces retain enough integrity for the circumferential peripheral chopping maneuvers. On the other hand, if the lens is firmer, a crater or bowl is phacoemulsified to further debulk the center (see Figure 17-5E). In all cases, it is important to leave sufficient firm peripheral nuclear material to allow the nucleus to be safely engaged and held by the phaco tip during the progressive circumferential chopping.

Circumferential peripheral nuclear chopping then proceeds. For a right-handed surgeon, the heminucleus being chopped should be located to the surgeon's left, and the nucleus rotated in a clockwise direction. The phacoemulsification tip engages the leading edge of the heminucleus, and then the chopper transects the peripheral wedge, leaving the wedge engaged in the phacoemulsification tip (see Figure 17-5F). For a left-handed surgeon, the maneuvers are performed in a mirror-image fashion, with the direction of the nuclear rotation counterclockwise.

The size of the pie-shaped wedges of nucleus to be chopped depends on the density of the nucleus. The harder the nucleus, the smaller the fragment should be. The pie-shaped pieces can be created in virtually any size. For 2+ nuclear density, only three wedges should be created in each heminucleus; for a very dense

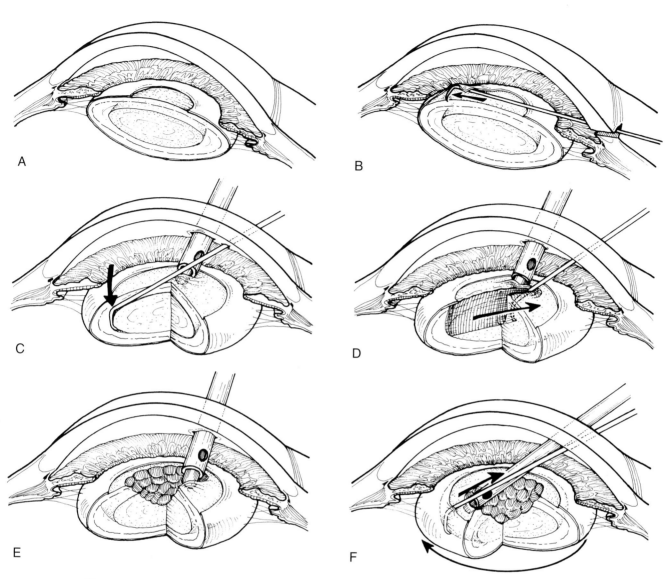

Figure 17-5 **A,** With a widely dilated pupil and small-to-moderate-sized endonucleus, hydrodelineation will create a separation of the endonucleus from the epinucleus, seen as a golden ring or a black ring, depending on the illumination and red reflex. **B,** The surgeon directs the chopper under the anterior capsule and down into the ring. **C,** If the pupillary dilation is smaller than the size of the endonucleus, the surgeon must advance the tip of the chopper without being able to see the equator. The surgeon, with experience, will have a good sense of how much the chopper must be advanced to reach the zone of the ring and will be able to feel when the chopper tip reaches this point and is able to drop. **D,** The phaco tip impales the nucleus and is advanced to the depth of the midnucleus. The chopper pulls toward the phaco tip, splitting the nucleus in half. **E,** The central, hardest portion of the nucleus is removed. The harder the nucleus, the larger the area sculpted. Enough nuclear material must remain that the phaco tip can engage and become occluded on the periphery, while the chopper breaks off pie-shaped wedges for removal (**F**).

4+ nucleus, six to eight wedges should be created. If a piece is chopped and appears to be too large, it can be chopped once again. The goal is to create "bite-sized" pieces that are appropriate for the phacoemulsification tip.

■ CHOPPING INSTRUMENTS ■

A large number of chopping instruments have been developed. Although this can perplex a novice, the variety of chopping instruments gives the surgeon many options with which to solve technical problems. Once the surgeon becomes proficient with a specific design, however, there is little value in further change.

Original chopping instruments were fashioned out of Sinskey hooks, with the tip rebent to a length of approximately 1.5 mm. This type of instrument is generally inadvisable, however. The very-fine-gauge wire of a Sinskey hook can cut through a nucleus, but the absence of any bulk in the wire prevents the full realization of the potential of phaco chop. Recall that Nagahara's fundamental principle was that the chopping instrument should act like a wedge. Most models of chopping instruments have a thicker gauge than the Sinskey hook, often with sharp internal cutting surfaces, thus obtaining the desired wedge-splitting effect.

Sharp cutting surfaces in chopping instruments may be on only one surface, generally directed along the shaft of the chopper, or

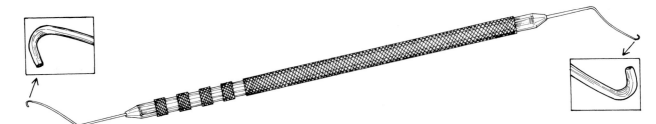

Figure 17-6 Steinert double-ended claw chopper. One end is 1.5 mm in length, for chopping most nuclei; the other end is 1.75 mm length, for chopping large, hard nuclei. (Courtesy Rhein Medical.)

two or three surfaces may be sharpened, allowing more successful "lateral chopping" maneuvers. The shaft may also be angled for right- or left-hand approaches.

Steinert designed a curved chopping instrument (Figure 17-6; Rhein Medical, Tampa, Fla.) to incorporate all of these principles and also to facilitate keeping the chopper engaged in the center of the nucleus. The curved distal element acts in the same manner as a cat's claw or a farmer's hoe. The chopper naturally engages the curved equator of the nucleus, which can be felt by the surgeon. The claw configuration then keeps the chopper engaged deeply into the nucleus, avoiding the tendency for straight choppers to rise up and out of the nucleus as they pass toward the center.

■ THE PHACOEMULSIFICATION NEEDLE ■

For many years, phacoemulsification instrument manufacturers progressively increased the angle of the phacoemulsification tip to gain increased "cutting power." The phaco chop technique has reversed that trend, however. The greater the angle of the phacoemulsification tip, the larger the cross-sectional area of the phaco tip port. With a greater tip angle, more of the tip must be buried into the nuclear fragment to obtain occlusion, which is necessary for stabilizing the nucleus before the initial phaco chop and for engaging and controlling the peripheral circumferential wedges. In fact, Nagahara returned to a true 0° phacoemulsification tip. The 0° tip greatly facilitates obtaining occlusion of the circumferential nuclear fragments and their manipulation.

WHY DOES THIS NOT REDUCE ULTRASOUND POWER UNACCEPTABLY?

Phacoemulsification handpieces have greatly increased in power over recent years. More importantly, however, better understanding of ultrasonics had led to manipulations in the configuration of the phacoemulsification tip to improve the efficiency of ultrasonification of the nucleus through the creation of cavitation. For example, Nagahara's 0° tip has an internal bevel that vastly improves ultrasound power through internal cavitation, as well as reducing the cross-sectional area of the phacoemulsification needle tip.

Some surgeons use a bent needle phaco tip, a design originally introduced by the late Charles Kelman. The bent tip is necessary

for the action of torsional phaco. However, obtaining occlusion at the tip in order to build high vacuum levels and then manipulate a wedge of nucleus becomes more difficult.

■ TRANSITION TO PHACO CHOP ■

The surgeon should first become proficient in anterior capsulorrhexis, hydrodissection, and hydrodelineation; the nucleus must be freely mobile to allow easy rotation once chopping begins. An intact and well-defined circular-tear anterior capsulotomy provides a clear landmark for the surgeon, as well as the capsular strength for extra manipulation.[7] Hydrodelineation frees the nucleus from the epinucleus, which is necessary for chopped fragments to be removed, as well as disclosing the location of the nuclear equator.

The surgeon wishing to learn phaco chop should begin by chopping the second half of the nucleus in a case where the first half of the nucleus is removed with a conventional divide and conquer quadrant technique (Figure 17-7A). The second half of the nucleus is usually quite mobile at that point, and the basic technique and tactile feel of phaco chop can be appreciated within several cases by chopping the second half of the heminucleus (Figure 17-7B).

Once the surgeon feels comfortable with chopping the second heminucleus, the next step is to perform the stop and chop technique for both halves of the heminucleus, while still retaining the initial trough and split hemisection of the traditional divide and conquer technique (see Figure 17-2).

The last step in the progress to full phaco chop is to bisect the nucleus with the phaco chopper (see Figures 17-3A and 17-5D). Although some surgeons have found this to be the most challenging step in the technique, it also is the most rewarding. Full phaco chop markedly improves the efficiency of the disassembly of the nucleus, particularly because of the elimination of the multiple steps of rotation and trough creation in the standard quadrant cracking techniques.

CHALLENGES IN PHACO CHOP

Small Pupils

A novice will be insecure about the inability to visualize the periphery during chopping maneuvers. Small pupil cases should only be undertaken with phaco chop after the surgeon has gained reasonable comfort in more straightforward cases with large pupils and moderate-density nuclei. However, once this basic

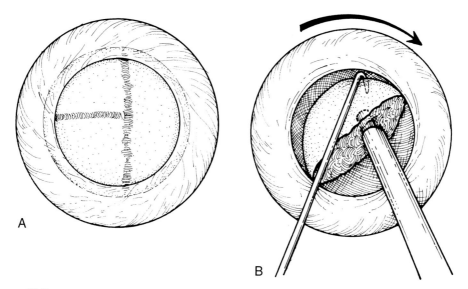

Figure 17-7 A, To begin learning phaco chop, the first half of the nucleus is removed using standard divide and conquer technique; the second heminucleus remains undivided. **B,** The second half of the nucleus can now be chopped with good direct visualization.

skill is achieved, chopping is preferred over the quadrant cracking or the divide and conquer techniques because chopping does not require peripheral passes with the ultrasound tip, and it is not dependent on a good red reflex.[8–10]

THE 4+ NUCLEUS

Chopping a 4+ hard nucleus can be particularly difficult, both because a hard nucleus is also a thick nucleus and because of the physical properties of a hard brunescent nucleus.[10] Nevertheless, chopping offers distinct advantages in the phacoemulsification of very advanced cataracts.[11] Because the nucleus is thick, a standard 1.5 mm phaco chopper will not have adequate length to pass through the center of a nucleus (Figure 17-8A). As a result, a superficial vertical split will occur, but the deeper layer of the nucleus will tend to split in a more lateral fashion, creating a posterior plate (Figure 17-8B). If this occurs, the surgeon must identify which half of the heminucleus is above the plate and which half is attached to the plate. The half of the nucleus that is above the plate should be removed first, which allows the larger fragment to be mobilized and chopped. Several chopping instruments are now available with longer tips, in the order of 1.75–2 mm, which greatly facilitates successful chopping of these thicker nuclei. These choppers, although longer, are still well short of endangering the posterior capsule, considering that a brunescent nucleus is at least 3.5 mm thick (Figure 17-8C).

A very hard brunescent nucleus also tends to have a posterior "leathery" quality. Chopped fragments have posterior bridging strands that keep nuclear fragments attached to each other. These posterior strands represent posterior epinucleus that has partially hardened, with strong adhesion to the posterior nucleus and with a tough, strandlike quality. When these strands occur, they are seen against the red reflex as they bridge between two chopped nuclear fragments (see Figure 17-8D). The surgeon can rotate the phaco chopper 90° in his or her fingers, then carefully pass the chopper posterior to the nuclear fragment and transect the

bridging fibers (see Figure 17-8E). This maneuver has led to variations of phaco chop generally known as "posterior cracking." Techniques for phacoemulsification of the dense brunescent cataract are discussed in detail in Chapter 28.

ZONULAR ABNORMALITIES

Once experience is gained with phaco chop, it is the preferred technique in the presence of weak or missing zonules. This situation occurs most commonly in pseudoexfoliation syndrome or after trauma.[12–15] It is because horizontal chopping creates opposing forces between the two instruments that it minimizes forces on the zonules.[16]

■ COMPLICATIONS OF PHACO CHOP ■

MULTIPLE INCOMPLETE CHOPS

A surgeon inexperienced at phaco chop often tends to "scratch" the nucleus without accomplishing front-to-back cleavage. This usually occurs for two reasons. The first is because the chopper is not passed far enough into the periphery in order to allow the chopper to "hook" and engage the equator. The surgeon can test whether the chopper is around the equator by gently pulling on the chopper and verifying that the nucleus moves with it. The second is because the chopper is allowed to ride up and out of the nucleus. The claw-shaped chopper was designed by Steinert to resist this tendency. For all chopper styles, the surgeon must learn to maintain appropriate posterior pressure on the chopping instrument.

When fragmented and incomplete chops do occur, the most important step is for the surgeon to remain patient. He or she should continue rotating and attempt to chop a new area, concentrating on proper technique. In addition, the chopper can

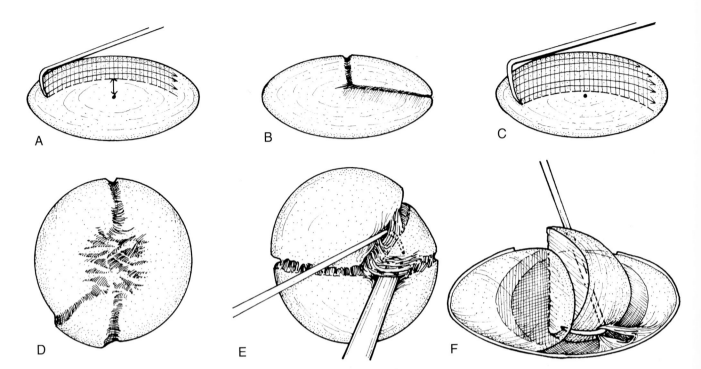

Figure 17-8 A, Thick, advanced nuclear cataract will not chop well with a standard chopping instrument because the length of the tip is inadequate to split the center of the nucleus. **B,** If the thick nucleus splits at all, a short-tip chopper will tend to split the upper portion of the nucleus, but the fracture line will lateralize, leaving a posterior nuclear plate attached to one portion of the two pieces of nucleus. **C,** A longer length chopper will have a better likelihood of cleanly splitting the nucleus. The extra length of the chopper tip is far from the posterior capsule. **D,** In advanced nuclear sclerosis, "leathery" posterior nuclear strands will bridge across a chopped wedge and interfere with its removal, particularly at the posterior apex. **E,** Chopper can be rotated 90°, parallel to the posterior capsule, and used to snap across these strands and free the nuclear wedge.

act as a "finger" to hook around the equator of a fragment and help bring it toward the phaco tip in the central zone. This maneuver is particularly helpful when the vacuum is inadequate or complete occlusion cannot be achieved, and the nuclear fragment keeps "falling back," away from the phaco tip.

POSTERIOR CAPSULE RUPTURE

The most feared complication for novice surgeons with phaco chop is the rupture of the posterior capsule with the chopper. In fact, this is rare and should not occur at all with adherence to the principles of phaco chop. The phaco chop instrument is typically only 1.5 mm long and, even with phaco chop instruments that have been elongated for dealing with a 4+ nucleus, the length never exceeds 2 mm (see Figure 17-8A and C). The conventional lens is thicker than this in the periphery and increases to between 3 mm and 4 mm centrally (and sometimes even thicker). As a result, the phaco chopping instrument is well away from the posterior capsule. Many of the phaco chopping instruments have a blunted tip, which is also less likely to engage the posterior capsule.

ANTERIOR CAPSULE/ZONULAR RUPTURE

A more common complication is misjudging the location of the anterior capsule, such that the phaco chopper is anterior to the peripheral anterior capsule rather than within the capsular bag (Figure 17-9A). This mistake can be avoided by placing the phaco chopping instrument against the nucleus centrally within the capsulorrhexis, and keeping a small amount of posterior pressure against the nucleus as the chopper is passed peripherally. In a very hard nucleus with almost no anterior cortex, little space is present between the anterior capsule and the nucleus. In this case, the surgeon should rotate the phaco chopping instrument 90° within the surgeon's fingers so that it can slip under the anterior capsule in a "flat" position (Figure 17-9B). As the chopper passes out to the edge of the endonucleus, it is rotated back 90° to the vertical chopping position (Figure 17-9C).

■ CONCLUSION ■

With careful attention to detail in following the progressive learning technique that was suggested earlier, any two-handed phacoemulsification surgeon should be able to master the maneuvers of phaco chop. Phaco chop is faster, and, as a result, ultrasound time is reduced, with a reduction in corneal endothelial damage and the potential for rupture of the posterior capsule.

Moreover, because phaco chop is a technique that involves stabilizing the nucleus with a phaco instrument centrally and then applying centripetal forces with the phaco chopper against the ultrasound tip, there is much less zonular stress than in

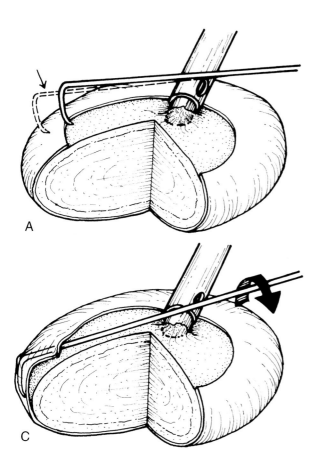

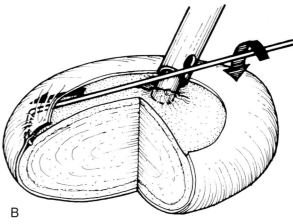

Figure 17-9 A, The surgeon must be careful to avoid passing the chopper over the anterior capsule instead of under it. This error is more likely in a large, dense cataract where little anterior cortex remains to separate the anterior capsule from the anterior nucleus. **B,** By rotating the chopper 90°, in a horizontal position parallel to the iris plane, the tip can pass easily between the anterior capsule and the nucleus. **C,** As the chopper tip is advanced out to the level of the equator of the nucleus, the tip is then rotated back 90°, from horizontal back to vertical, where it will pass around the nuclear equator and be positioned for chopping.

standard cracking techniques. After phaco chop is mastered, it becomes a central element in the phacoemulsification surgeon's technique.

References

[1] Koch PS, Katzen LE. Stop and chop phacoemulsification. J Cataract Refract Surg 1994;20: 566–570.

[2] Steinert RF. Phaco chop. In: Steinert RF, editor. Cataract surgery: technique, complications, and management. Philadelphia: WB Saunders; 1995.

[3] Gimbel HV. Divide and conquer nucleofractis phacoemulsification: development and variations. J Cataract Refract Surg 1991;17:281–291.

[4] Pirazzoli G, D'Eliseo D, Ziosi M, et al. Effects of phacoemulsification time on the corneal endothelium using phacofracture and phaco chop techniques. J Cataract Refract Surg 1996;22:967–969.

[5] DeBry P, Olson RJ, Crandall AS. Comparison of energy required for phaco-chop and divide and conquer phacoemulsification. J Cataract Refract Surg 1998;24:689–692.

[6] Ram J, Wesendahl TA, Auffarth GU, et al. Evaluation of in situ fracture versus phaco chop techniques. J Cataract Refract Surg 1998;24:1464–1468.

[7] Gimbel HV, Neuhann T. Development, advantages, and methods of the continuous circular capsulotomy technique. J Cataract Refract Surg 1990;16:31–37.

[8] Lumme P, Laatikainen LT. Risk factors for intraoperative and early postoperative complications in extracapsular surgery. Eur J Ophthalmol 1994;4:151–158.

[9] Joseph J, Wang HS. Phacoemulsification with poorly dilated pupils. J Cataract Refract Surg 1993;19:551–556.

[10] Hayashi K, Nakao F, Hayashi F. Corneal endothelial cell loss after phacoemulsification using nuclear cracking procedures. J Cataract Refract Surg 1994;20:44–47.

[11] Vasavada A, Singh R. Step-by-step chop in situ and separation of very dense cataracts. J Cataract Refract Surg 1998;24:156–159.

[12] Lunne P, Laatikainen L. Exfoliation syndrome and cataract extraction. Am J Ophthalmol 1993;116:51–55.

[13] Osher RH, Cionni RJ, Gimbel HV, et al. Cataract surgery in patients with pseudoexfoliation syndrome. Eur J Implant Refract Surg 1993;5:45–50.

[14] Fine IH, Hoffman RS. Phacoemulsification in the presence of pseudoexfoliation: challenges and options. J Cataract Refract Surg 1997;23:160–165.

[15] Moreno J, Duch S, Lajara J. Pseudoexfoliation syndrome: clinical factors related to capsular rupture in cataract surgery. Acta Ophthalmol 1993;71:181–184.

[16] Masket S, editor. Consultation section. J Cataract Refract Surg 1998;24:1289–1298.

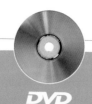

Tilt and Tumble Phacoemulsification: Coaxial and Bimanual

Elizabeth A. Davis, MD, FACS, Dennis C. Lu, MD, David R. Hardten, MD, FACS and Richard L. Lindstrom, MD

18

CONTENTS

- Indications
- Preoperative Preparation
- Operative Procedure
- Bimanual Technique
- Postoperative Care
- Conclusion

CHAPTER HIGHLIGHTS

>> Prolapsing the nucleus equator for ouside-in phaco

>> Hydrodissection method

>> Capsulorrhexis requirements

>> Coaxial and bimanual technique comparison

The technique of tilt and tumble is a modified form of supracapsular phacoemulsification. It uses a technique to tilt one pole of the nucleus above the anterior capsule. Phacoemulsification is then performed while supporting the lens in the iris plane with a nucleus rotator.

In the following paragraphs this procedure will be described and illustrated with both a coaxial and a bimanual technique.

INDICATIONS

The indications for the tilt and tumble phacoemulsification technique are quite broad. It can be utilized in either a large or small pupil situation. Some surgeons favor the technique with small pupils where the nucleus can be tilted up such that the equator is resting in the center of the pupil and is then carefully emulsified. It does require a larger continuous-tear, anterior capsulectomy of at least 5 mm. If a small anterior capsulectomy is created, the hydrodissection step of tilting the nucleus can be dangerous, and it is possible to rupture the posterior capsule during the hydrodissection step. If, inadvertently, a small anterior

capsulectomy is created, it is probably safest to convert to an endocapsular phacoemulsification technique or enlarge the capsulorrhexis. If it is not possible to tilt the nucleus with either hydrodissection or a manual technique, the surgeon should also convert to an endocapsular approach. Occasionally, the entire nucleus will subluxate into the anterior chamber. In this setting if the cornea is healthy, the anterior chamber deep, and the nucleus soft, then the phacoemulsification can be completed in the anterior chamber supporting the nucleus away from the corneal endothelium. The nucleus can also be pushed back inferiorly over the capsular bag to allow the iris plane tilt and tumble technique to be completed.

In patients with severely compromised endothelium, such as Fuchs' dystrophy or previous keratoplasty patients with a low endothelial cell count, endocapsular phacoemulsification is preferred to reduce endothelial cell loss. In a normal eye, corneal clarity on the first day postoperatively is excellent. Nevertheless, the tilting and tumbling maneuvers do increase the chance of endothelial cell contact of lens material compared to an endocapsular phacoemulsification. Therefore, the endocapsular technique should not be employed in eyes with borderline corneas or shallow anterior chambers.

PREOPERATIVE PREPARATION

The patient enters the anesthesia induction or preoperative area and Tetracaine drops are put in both eyes. The administration of these drops increases the patient's comfort during the placement of the multiple dilating and preoperative medications, decreases blepharospasm and also increases the corneal penetration of the drops to follow.

The eye is dilated with 2.5% neosynephrine and 1% cyclopentolate every 5 min for three doses. Additionally, preoperative topical antibiotic and anti-inflammatory drops are administered at the same time as the dilating drops. The authors favor the combination of a preoperative topical antibiotic, topical steroid and topical nonsteroidal. The rationale for this is to pre-load the eye with antibiotic and non-steroidal prior to surgery. The pharmacology of these drugs and the pathophysiology of postoperative infection and inflammation support this approach. An eye that is pre-loaded with anti-inflammatories prior to the surgical insult is likely to have a much reduced postoperative inflammatory response. Both topical steroids and non-steroidals have been found to be synergistic in the reduction of postoperative inflammation. In addition, the use of perioperative antibiotics is supported in the literature as reducing the small chance of postoperative endophthalmitis. Since the patient will be sent home on the same drops utilized preoperatively, there is no additional cost.

Our usual anesthesia is topical tetracaine reinforced with intraoperative intracameral 1% non-preserved (methylparaben free) xylocaine. For patients with blepharospasm a "miniblock" O'Brien facial nerve anesthesia, utilizing 2% xylocaine with 150 units of hyaluronidase per 5 cc of xylocaine, can be quite helpful in reducing squeezing. This block lasts 30–45 min and makes surgery easier for the patient and the surgeon. Patients are sedated prior to the block to eliminate any memory of discomfort. One way to determine when this facial nerve block might be useful is to ask the technicians to make a note in the chart when they have difficulty performing applanation pressures or A-scan because of blepharospasm. In these patients a mini facial nerve block can be quite helpful.

In younger anxious patients and in those with difficulty cooperating, the authors perform a peribulbar block. Naturally, general anesthesia is used for very uncooperative patients and children. While this is controversial, in some patients where general anesthesia is chosen and a significant bilateral cataract is present, the authors will perform consecutive bilateral surgery completely re-prepping and starting with fresh instruments for the second eye. Again, this is a clinical decision weighing the risk-to-benefit ratio of operating both eyes on the same day versus the risk of two general anesthetics.

Upon entering the surgical suite the patient table is centered on pre-placed marks so that it is appropriately placed for microscope, surgeon, scrub nurse and anesthetist access. The authors favor a wrist rest, and the patient's head is adjusted such that a ruler placed on the forehead and cheek will be parallel to the floor. The patient's head is stabilized with tape to the head board to reduce unexpected movements, particularly if the patient falls asleep during the procedure and suddenly awakens. A second drop of tetracaine is placed in each eye. If the tetracaine is placed in each eye, blepharospasm is reduced. A periocular prep with 5% povidone-iodine solution is completed. The ocular surface and fornices are not irrigated with povidone-iodine. Under topical anesthesia the authors have found that the patients note a significant burning. If a few drops leak into the eye this is certainly acceptable.

An aperture drape is helpful for topical anesthesia to increase comfort. It has been noted by the authors that when the drape is tucked under the lids this often irritates the patient's eye and also reduces the malleability of the lids, decreasing exposure. Since it is important to isolate the meibomian glands and lashes, a Tegaderm adhesive cut in half for the upper and lower lids may be used.

Balanced salt solution is used in all cases. For the short duration of a phacoemulsification case, BSS plus does not provide any clinically meaningful benefit. The authors place 0.5 cc of the intracardiac non-preserved (sodium bisulfate free) epinephrine in the bottle for assistance in dilation and perhaps hemostasis. Heparin sulfate 1 mL (1000 units) is also added to reduce

the possibility of postoperative fibrin. This is also a good anti-inflammatory and coating agent. At this dose there is no risk of enhancing bleeding or reducing hemostasis.

The lids are separated with a Lindstrom/Chu aspirating speculum (Rhein Medical). A final drop of tetracaine is placed in the operative eye or the surface is irrigated with the non-preserved xylocaine. The authors do not like to utilize more than three drops of tetracaine or other topical anesthetic, as excess softening of the epithelium can occur, resulting in punctate epithelial keratitis, corneal erosion and delayed postoperative rehabilitation.

■ OPERATIVE PROCEDURE ■

The patient is asked to look down. The globe is supported with a dry Merocel sponge, and a counter puncture is performed superiorly at 12 o'clock with a diamond stab knife (Osher/Storz). The incision is about 1 mm in length (Figure 18-1). Approximately 0.25 mL of 1% non-preserved methylparaben free xylocaine is injected into the eye (Figure 18-2). The patient is advised that they will feel a "tingling" or "burning" for a second, and then "the eye will go numb." This provides a psychological support for the patient that they will now have a totally anesthetized eye and should not anticipate any discomfort. The patient is told that while they will feel some touch and fluid on the eye, they will not feel anything sharp, and if they do, the anesthesia can be supplemented. This injection also firms up the eye for the clear corneal incision. The authors do not find it necessary to inject viscoelastic prior to constructing the corneal wound.

A temporal or nasal anterior limbal or posterior clear corneal incision is performed. Care is taken not to incise the conjunctiva, as this can result in ballooning during phacoemulsification and irrigation aspiration. Some surgeons define this as being a posterior clear corneal incision and others as an anterior limbal incision.

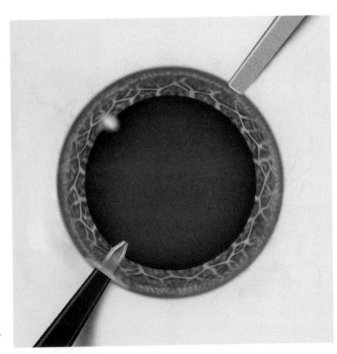

Figure 18-1 Counterpuncture site of 1 mm is made with a diamond stab knife.

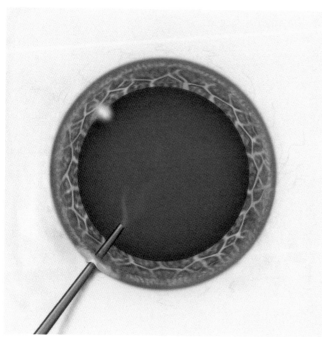

Figure 18-2 Preservative-free xylocaine is injected intracamerally.

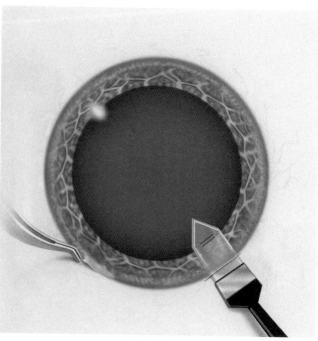

Figure 18-3 A clear corneal incision is made temporally in right eyes and nasally in left eyes.

The anatomical landmark is the perilimbal capillary plexus and the insertion of the conjunctiva. Since the incision is into a vascular area, long-term wound healing can be expected to be stronger than it is with a true clear corneal incision. True clear corneal incisions, such as performed in radial keratotomy, clearly do not have the wound-healing capabilities that a limbal incision demonstrates where there are functioning blood vessels present.

The anterior chamber is then entered parallel to the iris at a depth of approximately 300 μ. This creates a hinge type of incision (Figure 18-3).

In right eyes the incision is temporal, and in left eyes, nasal. This allows the surgeon to sit in the same position for right and left eyes. The nasal cornea is thicker, has a higher endothelial cell count and allows very good access for phacoemulsification. The nasal limbus is approximately 0.3 mm closer to the center of the cornea than the temporal limbus, and this can, in some cases where there is excess edema, reduce first-day postoperative vision more than one might anticipate with a temporal incision. There also can, in some patients, be pooling of irrigating fluid. For this reason, an aspirating speculum is useful. It is also helpful to tip the head slightly to the left side. Nonetheless, in left eyes a nasal clear corneal approach is an excellent option, particularly for surgeons who find the left temporal position uncomfortable.

In some patients it may be safest to create a corneal scleral incision. Examples of these include patients who have had a previous radial keratotomy or demonstrate findings of peripheral corneal ulcerative keratitis, in some patients with very low endothelial cell counts, and any case where there is any significant peripheral pathology or thinning. The anterior limbal or posterior corneal incision described above can be made temporally, nasally, in the oblique meridian or even superiorly without induction of significant corneal edema or endothelial cell loss.

The incision, if it is 3 mm in length, tends to cause an induction of 0.25 ± 0.25 diopters (D) of astigmatism. If the incision is placed on the steeper meridian, the astigmatism can, therefore, be expected to be reduced to somewhere between 0 and 0.50 D. An incision in the 3 mm range will almost always be self-sealing. With modern injector systems most foldable intraocular lenses can be implanted through a 3 mm anterior limbal incision.

In select patients an intraoperative astigmatic keratotomy can be performed at the 7–8 mm optical zone. This can be done at the beginning of the operation. The patient's astigmatism axis is marked carefully using an intraoperative surgical keratometer which allows one to delineate the steeper and flatter meridian and not be concerned about globe rotation. One 2 mm incision at a 7–8 mm optical zone will correct 1 D of astigmatism and two 2 mm incisions will correct 2 D of astigmatism in a cataract-age patient. One 3 mm incision will correct 2 D, and two 3 mm incisions 4 D. One can combine a 3 mm and a 2 mm incision to correct 3 D. Larger amounts of astigmatism can also be corrected utilizing the Arc-T nomogram. Depending on the age of the patient one can correct up to 8 D of astigmatism with two 90° arcs. Many surgeons have moved to a more peripheral corneal limbal arcuate incision, but the authors favor the 7–8 mm optical zone because of years of experience with this approach. There certainly is a variation in response, but there have not been any significant, induced complications with this approach. The outcome goal is 1 D or less of astigmatism in the preoperative axis. It is preferable to under-correct rather than over-correct. The key in astigmatism surgery is "axis, axis, axis." *If one is not careful in preoperative planning and the incision is placed more than 15° off axis, one is better avoiding this approach.*

The anterior chamber is constituted with a viscoelastic. Studies carried out by the authors have not found any significant difference between one viscoelastic or another in regards to postoperative

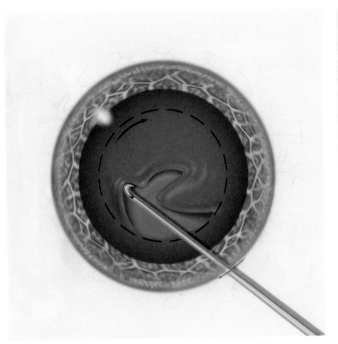

Figure 18-4 A continuous curvilinear capsulotomy is made with a cystatome.

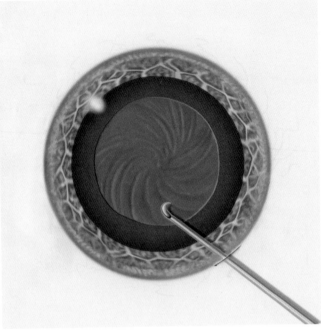

Figure 18-5 The capsulotomy is optimally 5–6 mm in diameter.

endothelial cell counts. Amvisc Plus works well and 0.8 cc can be obtained at a very fair price.

Next a relatively large diameter continuous tear anterior capsulectomy is fashioned (Figures 18-4 and 18-5). This can be made with a cystatome or forceps. The optimal size is 5–6 mm in diameter and inside the insertion of the zonules (usually at 7 mm). Larger is better than smaller, as there is less subcapsular epithelium and thus lower risk of capsular opacification. Additionally, a larger capsulorrhexis makes for an easier cataract operation. With this technique there has not been any change in the incidence of intraocular lens decentration. With some intraocular lenses the capsule will seal down to the posterior capsule around the loops rather than be symmetrically placed over the anterior surface of the intraocular lens. These eyes do extremely well and this might be preferable to having the capsule anterior to the optic. This is also certainly a controversial position.

Hydrodissection is then performed utilizing a Pearce hydrodissection cannula on a 3 cc syringe filled with BSS. Slow continuous hydrodissection is performed gently lifting the anterior capsular rim until a fluid wave is seen. At this point irrigation is continued until the nucleus tilts on one side, up and out of the capsular bag (Figure 18-6). If one retracts the capsule at approximately the 7:30 o'clock position with the hydrodissection cannula, usually the nucleus will tilt superiorly. If it tilts in another position, it is simply rotated until it is facing the incision (Figure 18-7).

Once the nucleus it tilted some additional viscoelastic can be injected under the nucleus pushing the iris and capsule back. Also, additional viscoelastic can be placed over the nuclear edge to protect the endothelium. The nucleus is emulsified from outside–in while supporting the nucleus in the iris plane with a second instrument, such as a Rhein Medical, Storz Lindstrom Star or Lindstrom Trident nucleus rotator (Figure 18-8). Once half the nucleus is

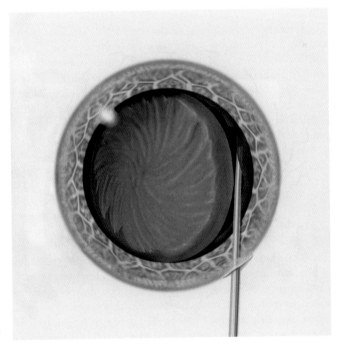

Figure 18-6 Continuous slow hydrodissection leads to tilting of the nucleus out of the bag.

removed, the remaining one half is tumbled upside-down and approached from the opposite pole (Figure 18-9). Again, it is supported in the iris plane until the emulsification is completed (Figure 18-10). Alternatively, the nucleus can be rotated and emulsified from the outside edge in a carousel or cartwheel type of technique. Finally, in some cases, the nucleus can be continuously emulsified in the iris plane if there is good followability until the entire nucleus is gone.

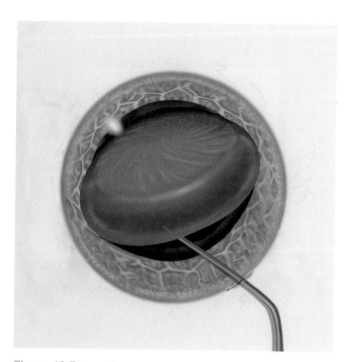

Figure 18-7 The nucleus is rotated to face the incision.

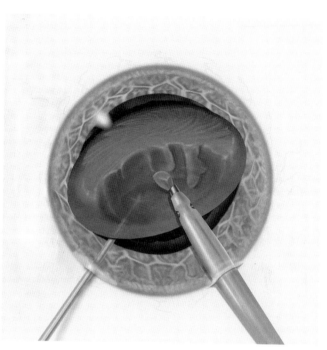

Figure 18-8 The nucleus is supported during phacoemulsification with a second instrument.

This is a very fast and very safe technique and, as mentioned before, it is a modification of the iris plane technique taught by Richard Kratz in the late 1970s and 1980s. It is basically "back to Kratz" with help from Brown and Maloney in the modern phacoemulsification, capsulorrhexis, hydrodissection and viscoelastic era. Surgery times now range between 4 and 7 min with this approach rather than 10–15 min for endocapsular phacoemulsification.

In addition, the capsular tear rate has now gone under 1%. Therefore, the authors find this technique to be easier, faster and safer. It is true that in this technique the phacoemulsification tip is closer to the iris margin and also somewhat closer to the corneal endothelium. There is, however, a significantly greater margin of error in regards to the posterior capsule. Care needs to be taken to position the nucleus away from the corneal

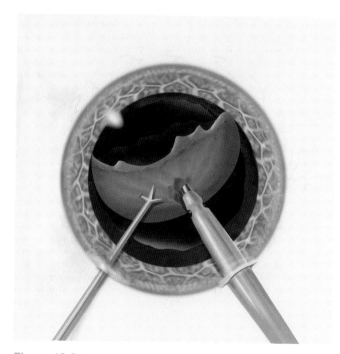

Figure 18-9 The second half of the nucleus is tumbled upside down.

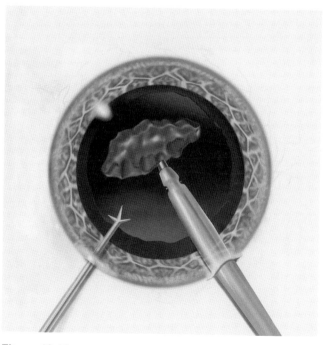

Figure 18-10 Emulsification is completed in the iris plane.

endothelium and away from the iris margin when utilizing this approach.

If the nucleus does not tilt with simple hydrodissection, it can be tilted with viscoelastic or a second instrument such as a nuclear rotator, Graether collar button or hydrodissection cannula.

The dual function Bausch & Lomb Millennium™ is excellent for all cataract techniques including "tilt and tumble." The vacuum is set with a range of 325–400 mm Hg and the ultrasound power set in a pulse mode from 10% to 30%. The foot pedal is arranged such that there is surgeon control over ultrasound on the vertical or pitch motion of the foot pedal, and then on the yaw or right motion foot pedal, there will be vacuum control. This allows very efficient emulsification, and the Millennium™ is currently the authors' preferred machine. The microflow plus needle with a 30° angle tip works well with the Millenium.

Following completion of nuclear removal, the cortex is removed with the irrigation aspiration hand piece. The authors prefer a 0.3 mm tip and utilize the universal hand piece with interchangeable tips. A curvilinear tip is used for most cortex removal. Sub-incisional cortex can be aspirated with a Lindstrom right angle sand blasted tip currently manufactured by Rhein and Storz (Figure 18-11). If there is significant debris or plaque on the posterior capsule, one can attempt some polishing and vacuum cleaning but not so aggressively as to risk capsular tears.

The anterior chamber is reconstituted with viscoelastic and the intraocular lens is inserted utilizing an injector system (Figures 18-12 and 18-13).

Excess viscoelastic is removed with irrigation aspiration. Pushing back on the intraocular lens and slowly turning the irrigation aspiration to the right and left two or three times allows a fairly complete removal of viscoelastic under the intraocular lens.

The authors favor injection of a miotic and tend to prefer carbachol over miochol at this time, as it is more effective in reducing postoperative intraocular tension spikes and has a longer

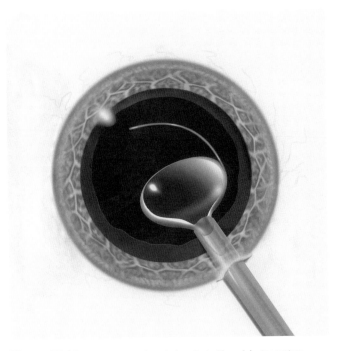

Figure 18-12 The intraocular lens is inserted with an injector system.

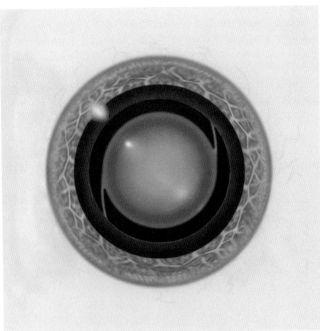

Figure 18-13 The lens is centered in the capsular bag.

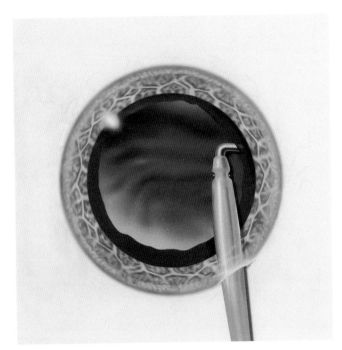

Figure 18-11 Subincisional cortex is removed with a right angled tip.

duration of action. It is best to dilute the carbachol 5:1, or one can obtain an excessively small pupil which results in dark vision for the patient at night for 1–2 days. The anterior chamber is then refilled through the counter-puncture and the incision is inspected. If the chamber remains well constituted and there is no spontaneous leak from the incision, wound hydration is not necessary. If there is some shallowing in the anterior chamber and a spontaneous leak, wound hydration is performed by injecting BSS peripherally into the incision and hydrating it to push the edges together. We suspect that within a few minutes these clear corneal or posterior limbal incisions seal, much as a LASIK flap will stick down, through the negative swelling pressure of the cornea and capillary action. It is important to leave the eye slightly firm at 20 mm Hg or so to reduce the side effects of hypotony and also help the internal valve incision appropriately seal.

At completion of the procedure another drop of antibiotic, steroid and non-steroidal is placed on the eye. Additionally, one drop of an anti-hypertensive such as Betagan or Alphagan is applied to reduce postoperative intraocular tension spikes.

■ BIMANUAL TECHNIQUE ■

Recently, the concept of bimanual sleeveless phacoemulsification, which has been promoted by Amar Agarwal, has led to the development of sub-1 mm incision phacoemulsification.[1] New skills must be learned and several alterations in the technique must be made when incorporating the technique (tilt and tumble or any other) to bimanual sleeveless microphacoemulsification:

1. Three 1 mm stab incisions are made to allow for the sleeveless phaco probe, the irrigating second instrument, and the anterior chamber maintainer.

2. It is because the smaller incision cannot accommodate current capsulorrhexis forceps, that the authors prefer the use of a cystotome to perform the capsulorrhexis. New designs for microincision capsulorrhexis forceps have recently been developed, but typically require a steeper learning curve.

3. The instruments will behave as if they are "oar-locked" by the small incisions and, thus, the surgeon must adapt to the reduced mobility of the instrument.[2]

4. Probably the skill that is most foreign to ophthalmologists is learning how to use the irrigating second instrument and learning how to use irrigation itself as a tool.[3] It is because the irrigation is no longer coaxial with the phaco probe, that it may be used to drive material towards the phaco tip rather than away from the tip as in coaxial irrigation sleeves. Other novel uses of the irrigating second instrument include using the irrigation to flip the epinucleus, as Fine has described.[3] In addition, the irrigation may be used to drive the iris away from the phaco tip as in pseudoexfoliation cases with small pupils.

5. Microphacoemulsification is a truly bimanual procedure where the instruments may be interchanged between any of the incisions. For example, removal of subincisional cortex may be accomplished by interchanging the irrigating and aspirating handpieces in order to obtain better access to the cortical material. Similarly, interchanging the phaco probe and the irrigating second instrument may be necessary in certain situations, such as in the cases of zonular dialysis where traction may be relieved doing this maneuver. Consequently, right-handed surgeons must learn how to phaco with the left hand and left-handed surgeons must learn how to phaco with the right hand.

OPERATIVE PROCEDURE

The preoperative preparation is no different when adapting the tilt and tumble technique to a bimanual sleeveless microphacoemulsification technique. A counterpuncture is performed superiorly at

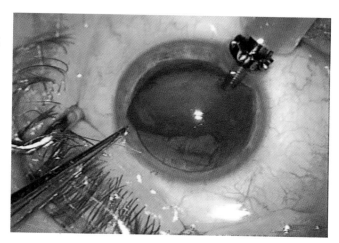

Figure 18-14 Three port microemulsification. The nucleus is supported during phacoemulsification with a second instrument.

12 o'clock with a diamond stab knife. Preservative-free lidocaine is injected into the eye. Two additional stab incisions of approximately 1 mm in width are created in clear cornea for insertion of the phaco probe and the anterior chamber maintainer (Figure 18-14). The stab incision for the anterior chamber maintainer is placed inferiorly at 6 o'clock. For the phaco probe, we perform a temporal (2 o'clock) or nasal (10 o'clock) anterior limbal or posterior clear corneal incision in a direction that is paralleled to the iris plane. The direction of this incision prevents an excessively long tunnel and thereby minimizes "oar-locking," but is shelved enough to be self-sealing.[3] Incision size is critical in bimanual phacoemulsification, as a too large incision compromises anterior chamber stability while a too small incision causes oar-locking of the instruments. Care must be taken not to incise the conjunctiva as this can result in ballooning during the procedure. Some surgeons define this as being a posterior clear corneal incision and others as an anterior limbal incision. The anatomical landmark is the perilimbal capillary plexus and the insertion of the conjunctiva. When the incision is made, there will be a small amount of capillary bleeding. Since the incision is into a vascular area, long-term wound healing can be expected to be stronger than it is with a true clear corneal incision. The anterior chamber is then constituted with viscoelastic. A dispersive viscoelastic may provide protection to the endothelium. Ocucoat (Bausch & Lomb, Miami, FL) has proved to be an excellent viscoelastic and can also be utilized to coat the epithelial surface during surgery. This eliminates the need for continuous irrigation with BSS. It gives a very clear view. It is also economically a good choice in most settings. Amvisc Plus also works well.

As in coaxial tilt and tumble, a relatively large-diameter, continuous-tear, anterior capsulectomy is fashioned. It is because the 1 mm incision cannot accommodate comfortably traditional capsulorrhexis forceps, that the capsulorrhexis may be completed with a cystotome or a bent needle.[3] Alternatively, the surgeon may learn how to use the newer forceps specifically designed for microincision phacoemulsification.

Hydrodissection is then performed as described above in the coaxial technique. During the hydrodissection, the posterior lip of the wound is depressed in order to prevent the anterior chamber from becoming too deep, which may cause excessive stress on the zonules or disrupt the posterior capsule. However, with the small incisions of microphacoemulsification, depression of the posterior lip may not be as easy.

The anterior chamber maintainer is then inserted through the inferior paracentesis. The authors prefer to use an anterior chamber maintainer designed with screw-type threads on the infusion tip in order to secure the device within the paracentesis.

A deep anterior chamber is paramount in the tilt and tumble technique. Thus, it is preferable to use an anterior chamber maintainer inserted through a third port, as it provides superior chamber stability over two port techniques that rely solely on the irrigation from current 20-gauge irrigating second instruments. The nucleus is then emulsified from outside–in while supporting the nucleus in the iris plane with an irrigating second instrument, such as a nucleus rotator.

When utilizing a peristaltic machine, a high flow rate is used, which enhances followability. It is best to set the bottle high in order to maintain a deep anterior chamber, particularly if one chooses to undertake bimanual sleeveless phacoemulsification without an anterior chamber maintainer.

The Storz Millennium™, which features Concentrix™ that provides both flow (as in peristaltic pumps) and vacuum (as with a venture pump) response, has the dual linear system that is excellent for all cataract techniques including "tilt and tumble," as it permits simultaneous linear control of ultrasound and vacuum or flow. The authors set the maximum vacuum in the range of 250–300 mm Hg, with the bottle height between 120 cm and 130 cm, which facilitates maintenance of a deep anterior chamber. The maximum ultrasound power is typically set at 60%, with average use of 11–15%, depending upon the density of the cataract. As with standard phaco, performing the microphacoemulsification technique (sleeveless phaco tip), we take care to avoid the use of excessive ultrasound power in order to prevent wound burn. In addition, caution must be exercised with higher vacuum levels as it is possible to core through the nucleus and aspirate the iris margin if very high vacuums are utilized.

Following completion of nuclear removal, the cortex is removed with bimanual irrigation and aspiration. In the absence of an anterior chamber maintainer, the irrigating second instrument may provide irrigation through the paracentesis port while the aspiration device is inserted through the main incision. However, in the presence of an anterior chamber maintainer, irrigation from the second instrument is not necessary (Figure 18-15). Cortical and epinuclear removal is then performed in the usual manner. For subincisional cortical material, the irrigation and aspirating devices may be interchanged through their respective incisions in order to gain better access. If there is significant debris or plaque on the posterior capsule, one can attempt some polishing and vacuum cleaning but not so aggressively as to risk capsular tears. Often there is an unexpected small burr of sharp defect on the irrigation–aspiration tip, which results in a capsular tear following a surgery that otherwise went well.

Although intraocular lenses (IOLs) that can be inserted through small incisions are under development, current IOLs cannot take advantage of microincision surgery. Thus, one of the stab incisions must be enlarged to allow for insertion of the IOL. Alternatively, a new incision may be created, which ensures a well-constructed, self-sealing incision that has not been previously stretched by oar-locked instruments.[1] After the capsular bag is reconstituted with viscoelastic, the intraocular lens is

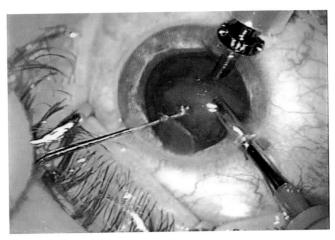

Figure 18-15 Subincisional cortex is removed with the aspiration hand piece. Irrigation is provided by the anterior chamber maintainer.

inserted utilizing an injector system. The remainder of the surgery is completed as above for the coaxial technique.

■ POSTOPERATIVE CARE ■

No patch is routinely utilized for the topical and intracameral approach. If a mini-block of the lids has been performed, this will wear off in 30–45 min, and there is usually adequate lid function for a normal blink at the completion of the procedure. Patients are advised that they will have some erythropsia, meaning they will see a pink after-image for the rest of the day, but usually this will resolve by the next morning. They are also told that their vision may be a little dark at night from the miotic, and not to be concerned if they wake up at night and their vision seems dimmer.

The patient is seen on the first day postoperative and then at approximately 2–3 weeks postoperatively. At this time a refraction, slit lamp, and funduscopic examination is performed. If there is no inflammation, patients are seen again 1 year postoperatively. If at 3 weeks there is still persistent inflammation, additional postoperative anti-inflammatory medications are recommended, and the patient is asked to return again in 2–3 months.

Topical antibiotic, steroid and non-steroidal, are utilized twice a day, usually requiring a 5 cc bottle and 3–4 weeks of therapy. Occasionally a second bottle of steroid and non-steroidal antibiotic is necessary if flare and cell persist at the 3-week examination. There are minimal restrictions, including a request that there be no swimming and no very heavy lifting for 2 weeks. The authors consider the ideal postoperative refractive spherical equivalent for a monofocal lens to be -0.62 D with less than 0.50 D of astigmatism in the same axis as existed preoperatively. Most patients can see 20/30+ and J3+ with this type of correction. Monovision can be utilized in the appropriate settings. Good results can also be obtained with an accommodating or multifocal IOL.

The second eye is done at ≥2 weeks postoperatively, except in rare situations. Any YAG lasers are deferred for 90 days in order to allow the blood–aqueous barrier to become intact and capsular fixation to be firm.

■ CONCLUSION ■

The authors hope that other surgeons will find this approach to cataract surgery useful. These techniques must be personalized, and every surgeon will find that slight variations in the technique are required to achieve the optimum results for their own patients in their own environment. Continuous efforts at incremental improvement result in meaningful advances in the surgeon's ability to help the cataract patient obtain rapid, safe, visual recovery following surgery.

References

[1] Agarwal A, Agarwal S, Narang P, Narang S. Phakonit: phacoemulsification through a 0.9 mm corneal incision. J Cataract Refract Surg 2001;27:1548–1552.
[2] Ronge L. Step-by-step guide to micro phaco. EyeNet 2004;8:23–26.
[3] Ifft D. Bimanual microincision phaco. Ophthalmology Management November 2003;45–56.

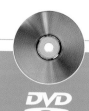

Biaxial Phacoemulsification

H. Burkhard Dick, MD, PhD

19

CHAPTER HIGHLIGHTS

>> Incision length classification and clinical importance

>> Instrumentation for biaxial phaco

>> Surgical technique

>> Avoiding and managing complications

INTRODUCTION

When one considers that biaxial phacoemulsification was first described in 1985 and, therefore, has been one of the options available to cataract surgeons, it remains interesting that the approach can be viewed with some suspicion. Each time a particular surgeon has advocated the approach, interest was raised and then seemed to drift away. This was due, in part, to a lack of equipment and instrumentation to facilitate the technique. In fact, it has only been in the past 3 years that improvements in instrumentation and phacoemulsification equipment have enabled cataract surgeons to fully explore a biaxial approach and sub-2 mm incisions. Today, a growing number of cataract surgeons are becoming converts to the biaxial technique for phacoemulsification. This chapter will explore the evolution of biaxial microsurgical phacoemulsification, as well as the current technique, instrumentation and software available.

TERMINOLOGY

The term *bimanual* phacoemulsification does not appropriately describe noncoaxial phacoemulsification. Arshinoff recently observed that even with coaxial phacoemulsification, because most surgeons have been operating for many years with both hands, the standard coaxial procedure has been bimanual (Figure 19-1).[1]

Since the new technique of unsleeved phacoemulsification has been introduced, it has been referred to by various names by various surgeons, including *cold phacoemulsification*. The new non-sleeved phacoemulsification procedure has enabled surgeons to perform phacoemulsification through a smaller incision. If phacoemulsification and aspiration are considered as one axis and the now-separated irrigation a second axis, then *biaxial* (as proposed by Arshinoff) is an appropriate term for the procedure. Biaxial is simply what is different from coaxial in biaxial phacoemulsification (Figure 19-2). The naming should be "biaxial" phacoemulsification, because it clearly refers to the fundamental difference in the procedure separating it from coaxial phacoemulsification. Biaxial makes no specific reference to incision size, although this may change over time.

To emphasize the smaller incision (1.5 mm as opposed to 2.8 mm), the new procedure could appropriately be called *microincision phacoemulsification* (or MICS – microincision cataract surgery). When discussing incision length, Grabow recently suggested distinguishing the various lengths by the following terms:

- *Long incision* for extracapsular cataract extraction/intracapsular cataract extraction (10 mm incision)
- *Small* incision for phacoemulsification with a poly(methyl methacrylate) intraocular lens (6 mm incision)
- *Mini*-incision for phacoemulsification with a foldable intraocular lens (IOL) (3 mm incision)
- *Microincision* for phacoemulsification with a foldable IOL (≤1.5 mm incision).[2]

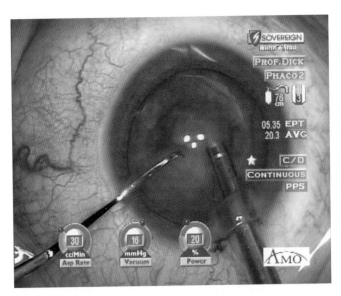

Figure 19-1 Bimanual, coaxial phacoemulsification using a sleeved phaco tip and a chopper in the second hand.

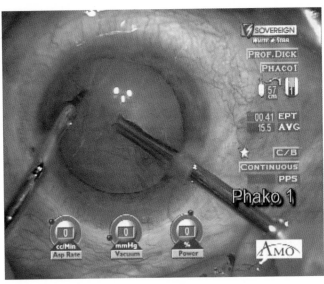

Figure 19-2 Bimanual non-sleeved phacoemulsification: aspiration is considered as one axis and the separated irrigation (chopper) as a second axis. With this configuration, *biaxial* phacoemulsification is the appropriate term for the procedure.

As the procedure is still in evolution, some cases are performed using nonsleeved phacoemulsification through two 1.5 mm incisions with IOL implantation through an enlarged (or separate) incision. In this case, one could describe the procedure as biaxial phacoemulsification or microincision phacoemulsification, but could not truly call the whole procedure microincision, as only the phacoemulsification portion would have been performed through a microincision. Only when both phacoemulsification *and* IOL implantation are performed through 1.5 mm incisions can we truly call the entire procedure microincision. But even this might be questionable to some extent, as previously pointed out by Osher. If two 1.5 mm incisions (totalling 3 mm of incision length) are used, is it still microincision surgery?[3]

If one incision is enlarged to 2.8 mm and the other is left at 1.5 mm (totaling 4.3 mm), it would be mini-incision surgery. Surgery using a 1.7 mm (mini-incision) sleeved coaxial phacoemulsification with IOL implantation through a 1.8 mm incision would be called coaxial mini-incision surgery. It seems to be appropriate to describe our procedures using both, the phacoemulsification technique (coaxial or biaxial) and the incision size, such as coaxial miniincision or biaxial microincision.

■ BENEFITS OF BIAXIAL ■

The outcomes achieved with standard phacoemulsification techniques are quite good, making it a procedure that is difficult to improve upon. Still, there are some quantifiable benefits to using a biaxial approach:

- Greater anterior chamber stability – owing to microincisions limiting wound leakage and collateral fluid egress
- Closed environment – reduced risk of infection
- Corneal endothelial cell protection – due to less flow volume
- Safer procedure in challenging cases – such as in eyes with compromised zonules and post-vitrectomy cataract removal
- Minimal induced astigmatism.

Biaxial phacoemulsification separates irrigation and phacoemulsification for cataract removal, through micro incisions that range from 1.2 mm to 1.5 mm in size, although it is possible to perform through incisions of less than 1 mm. Irrigation is typically accomplished with an irrigating chopper, while the cataract is emulsified and aspirated using a sleeveless phaco needle.[4] The biaxial approach provides surgeons better visualization and maneuverability due to smaller instrumentations and can be a safer procedure in complicated cases. Further, various clinical studies have shown that biaxial phacoemulsification can be used on any grade of cataract.[5–17] Although there was a large degree of skepticism about the safety of removing cataracts through a microincision with a sleeveless phaco tip, a variety of advancements in phacoemulsification power modulation along with improved understanding of fluid dynamics have removed many of the perceived barriers to biaxial phacoemulsification.

Compared with coaxial phacoemulsification, biaxial phacoemulsification can lower mean phacoemulsification time, mean total phacoemulsification time and surgically induced astigmatism.[18] A number of studies also show that the two techniques are, substantially, equivalent in terms of endothelial cell loss and visual outcomes.[7,19–21]

■ HISTORICAL PERSPECTIVE ■

Introduced by Kelman in 1967, phacoemulsification has evolved to become safe and highly successful.[22] As mentioned, the first attempts of biaxial phacoemulsification through a 1 mm incision were described in 1985 by Shearing.[23] However, attempts to separate aspiration and irrigation from ultrasound were first described in the 1970s by Girard.[24] He made a number of attempts at ultrasound and aspiration infusion separation but was unsuccessful, abandoning his efforts because of extensive thermal corneal damage.[24–26] Shearing and his colleagues continued where Girard left off and succeeded in performing biaxial phacoemulsification through two 1 mm incisions, concluding that the technique was feasible.[23,27]

The biaxial approach has since evolved to become safer and more successful, with a published report of the advantages specifically related to the biaxial technique in 1997 by Colvard, which states the benefits of the two-needle technique for irrigation–aspiration (I–A) in comparison to the aspiration of subincisional cortical material with a standard I–A handpiece.[27] In Japan, Tsuneoka et al. successfully performed cataract surgery through an incision of 1.4 mm with a 20-gauge sleeveless ultrasound tip, avoiding thermal burns at the incision site by maintaining a level of leakage through the incision for cooling purposes.[28]

One of the critical components in the success of the biaxial approach is incision creation, with a number of surgeons advancing their level of knowledge of the optimal incision for this microsurgery. Ernest, developer of the sutureless technique, performed studies of wound geometry on cadaver eyes to conclude that wound leakage could be avoided, despite any internal or external pressure, through a square wound and an internal corneal lip of at least 1.5 mm.[29,30] Fine introduced temporal self-sealing clear corneal incisions, which significantly lessened surgical time, reduced the risk of induced astigmatism and promoted quicker postoperative recovery.[31,32] Fine also developed several phacoemulsification techniques, including the crack and flip, chip and flip, and the choo-choo chop and flip techniques. Agarwal introduced the concept of Phakonit (Phako with Needle Incision Technology) in 1998 where the lens was emulsified through a clear corneal incision of 0.9 mm, using a bare phaco needle and an irrigating chopper.[10]

In terms of instrumentation development, the goal was to create instruments capable of maximum efficiency through these microincisions. An infrared laser device for cataract removal was developed by Dodick in the early 1990s, evolving to become the Dodick photolysis system, which claimed safe operation within the capsular bag, reduced heat release and intraocular energy and clear corneal incisions of under 1.5 mm.[33–35] Agarwal developed instrumentation for his Phakonit technique, including the irrigation chopper and the Phakonit knife, and Fine developed numerous instruments and implants including lens insertion forceps, bimanual handpiece sets and irrigating choppers.[16,36,37] The 'tilt and tumble' phacoemulsification technique was developed by Lindstrom, which was a variant of supracapsular phacoemulsification where a beveled phaco tip was used with the superior pole of the nucleus tilted above the capsule.[38]

The drawbacks to the biaxial phacoemulsification technique revolve mainly around the risk of thermal damage to the cornea and wound leakage, which can potentially lead to anterior chamber collapse. As is commonly known, in biaxial phacoemulsification, there is no sleeve surrounding the phaco tip. This sleeve serves three purposes: (1) it helps deliver irrigation fluid into the eye; (2) it keeps the phaco tip cool; and (3) protects the cornea from direct contact with the phaco tip.[4]

Part of the solution to reducing the risk of biaxial phacoemulsification has been to reduce the amount of ultrasonic energy that is delivered into the eye. The main phacoemulsification equipment manufacturers, including Advanced Medical Optics (AMO, Santa Ana, CA), Alcon Laboratories (Ft. Worth, TX) and Bausch & Lomb (Rochester, NY), all began to introduce software changes to their systems that would enable biaxial

surgeons to better control ultrasound energy during the procedure. The AMO offering, Sovereign with WhiteStar technology, enabled 'ultrapulse' modulation, making it possible to adjust the duty cycle and pulse duration.[39] Studies by Donnenfeld, Soscia and Olson, et al, and Packard reported the results of using a 21-gauge irrigating chopper and a 21-gauge bare phaco needle and using WhiteStar micro-pulse power modulation with the Sovereign phacoemulsification machine. Soscia, et al, also reported in a study of cadaver eyes that thermal injury did not occur during the procedure, even with 100% power and aspiration completely occluded.[7,40] Packard noted that the Sovereign system did not produce wound burns and provided adequate surgical efficiency through sub-2 mm incisions.[41]

Braga-Mele studied biaxial microincision surgery using the Bausch & Lomb Millennium Microsurgical System with burst mode and moderate incisional outflow, which allowed frequency, energy and pulse width control, promoting cooling and preventing wound burn and contracture. The linear footpedal interval control and constant percent power enabled minimal ultrasonic energy and, subsequently, heat release.[42]

Alcon, with its Infiniti Vision System, introduced sonic oscillatory motion with longitudinal ultrasonic vibration, as well as modifiable pulse and burst modes, which were designed for minimal occlusion and reduced energy use.[4] The Infiniti system also features Aqualase using saline pulses rather than ultrasound to further reduce thermal corneal damage risk.[43]

To avoid fluid instability and subsequent anterior chamber collapse, fluid infusion is required to be greater than the vitreous pressure and the atmospheric pressure, but its measurement is dependent on specific variables. Choppers and cannulae have been developed especially for this procedure to ensure that a safe amount of fluid reaches the eye regardless of forced or passive infusion. Agarwal attempted to solve the problem of fluidic instability by developing a three-port Phakonit technique that utilizes a separate anterior chamber maintainer. Agarwal and Agarwal also introduced the concept of pressurized infusion by injecting air into the infusion bottle, allowing the use of 20- and 21-gauge irrigating choppers during phacoemulsification. Agarwal also resolved the issue of fluid spraying over the cornea during phakonit by ensuring that the hub of the infusion sleeve was only present at the base of the needle.[17,44]

INSTRUMENTATION

The advent of biaxial phacoemulsification has resulted in the development of numerous instruments designed to improve the efficiency of this procedure. These endeavors have primarily focused on sleeveless phaco needles and irrigating choppers, but also include microkeratomes for the incisions and microincision capsulorrhexis forceps for the creation of the capsulorrhexis. Typically, 19- or 20-gauge instrumentation is used in biaxial phacoemulsification:

- *Keratomes*. Diamond, sapphire or metal keratomes can be used to create the 1.2–1.4 mm clear-corneal trapezoidal incisions for the irrigation chopper and the phaco needle.

- *Needle or microforceps for capsulorrhexis*. The instrument used for creation of the capsulorrhexis really is a matter of personal preference. If using a needle, a 24- or 27-gauge bent needle

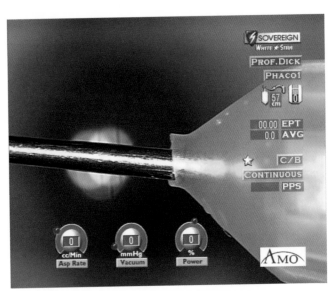

Figure 19-3 A phaco needle with a cut sleeve for biaxial phacoemulsification.

works best.[21] If forceps are the preferred method, a number of instrument companies have created microincision 23-gauge capsulorrhexis forceps for the task.[45]

- *Phaco needle.* The optimum needle for biaxial phacoemulsification is a 21- or 20-gauge needle (Figure 19-3) with a 0–30° beveled tip.[46]

- *Irrigating choppers.* There are two types of irrigating choppers: side irrigating and forward irrigating. Once again, numerous instrument manufacturers have developed irrigating choppers for biaxial phacoemulsification. The authors' preference is to use a 19-gauge chopper with two irrigation ports to the side (Figure 19-4) or one at the end of the tip (G-32059, Geuder, Heidelberg, Germany).[21]

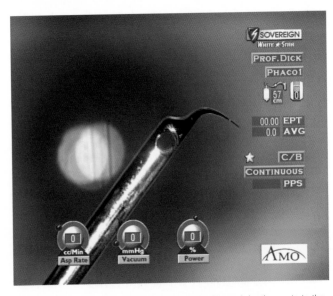

Figure 19-4 A 19-gauge chopper (1.1 mm) with two irrigation ports to the side (2 x 0.75 mm) for biaxial phacoemulsification. This chopper is also available in an oval diameter with a terminal opening.

- *Bimanual irrigation and aspiration.* As with the phaco needle and irrigating chopper, for cortical clean-up the recommended gauge size for these tips is 20-gauge. Most instrument companies now also offer disposable I–A tips that can be easily switched around to facilitate the removal of subincisional cortex.[4]

PHACO MACHINES, PUMPS AND SOFTWARE

With the increased use of biaxial phacoemulsification, most equipment manufacturers have worked with cataract surgeons to develop modifications and improvements to their systems that enable surgeons to better control ultrasound power. The overall goal is to use minimal ultrasound power to emulsify the cataract, avoiding or reducing corneal tissue trauma – this technique has come to be known as "cold phaco:"

- *Advanced Medical Optics (AMO):* AMO's offering for biaxial phacoemulsification, its WhiteStar Technology, utilizes what the company calls "ultrapulse" modulation of the ultrasound energy. This software is used on either the Sovereign and Sovereign Compact systems. WhiteStar has been clinically proven to result in clearer corneas on the first postoperative day.[47] The patented microburst technology is designed to increase cutting power vs. continuous ultrasound in many situations, and there is no need to switch handpieces or modes during lens removal to adjust for lens density. It also reduces the energy directed into the eye to minimize thermal damage and improve outcomes. WhiteStar Biaxial microphacoemulsification can be used for removal of all lens types through incisions as small as 1.4 mm using little or no ultrasound. The software allows the surgeon to adjust both the duty cycle and pulse duration.[48] A 10-patient study to evaluate WhiteStar in biaxial phacoemulsification by Donnenfeld et al. showed that there was a decreased thermal effect with the software, with corneal wound temperatures well below those that can cause corneal shrinkage.[7] An in-vitro study by Soscia et al. using human cadaver eyes showed similar results when using settings well beyond the norm of those found in cataract surgery.[41]

- *Alcon:* Alcon's offering for biaxial phacoemulsification with its Infiniti Vision System includes adjustable pulse and burst modes, as well as the ability to customize fluidic parameters based on the surgeon's preferred surgical technique and patient pathology. The Infiniti's Custom Fluidics Software monitors and adjusts fluidic parameters, providing increased fluidic versatility and control. It also allows customized lens removal while minimizing fluidic flow and turbulence. The system's custom power modulations offer precise energy delivery with an improved thermal safety profile and reduced repulsion of the cataract. A new feature of the Alcon system is the OZil Torsional Handpiece that uses an ultrasonic, oscillating, side-to-side movement to break up the lens. It is designed to help improve followability and reduce cavitation.[48] Another feature on the Infiniti system is the AquaLase Liquefaction Device. Aqualase utilizes 4 µL pulses of heated balanced salt solution to liquefy the cataract and appears to be most successful in mild-to-moderate nuclear sclerosis.[48] It is intended to reduce the risk of thermal damage to the cornea, however, there have been no published studies to confirm this.

- *Bausch & Lomb*: The Millennium Microsurgical System gives biaxial surgeons a number of options for controlling phacoemulsification power during surgery, including, conventional pulse mode, fixed-burst mode and multiple-burst mode with its Custom Control Software (CCS). In addition, the Millennium system operates at a lower ultrasound frequency (28.5 kHz), which is thought to reduce friction and cause less tissue damage. However, the Millennium has a longer stroke length, which means the same amount of heat is likely produced during emulsification.[48] The Millennium System also offers cataract surgeons a choice of pumps systems – either a peristaltic pump (Advanced Flow System [AFS]) or a venturi pump. The AFS pump is designed to provide improved intraoperative stability, efficiency and control, while the direct-response venturi vacuum system provides simultaneous, dual-linear foot pedal control of flow, aspiration and ultrasound power.

An in-vitro study looking at wound temperatures using the CCS software on the Millennium by Braga-Mele found that the microburst and hyperpulse settings in the software reduced wound temperatures during biaxial phacoemulsification. In the pig-eye study, temperatures were lower in all power settings below 80% and never exceeded 45°C.[5]

- *Geuder*: The Megatron S3 VIP, for cataract and vitreoretinal surgery, features a Venturi Inclusive Peristaltic (VIP) dual pump system, CFM Phaco Matrix with numerous ultrasound settings including Geuder's new Cool Flash Mode for biaxial phacoemulsification technique and SOS – minimized ultrasound energy through Safe Occlusion System. The Realtime Vac Sensor (RVS) in combination with innovative software is intended to provide superior anterior chamber stability.

AIR PUMP AND INTERNAL INFUSION

One of the greater challenges in biaxial phacoemulsification is proper fluidics and maintenance of a stable anterior chamber. Because the instruments used are smaller in gauge, the amount of fluid into the eye is reduced. There are a number of options available for addressing this issue, including using large-bore irrigating choppers, raising the infusion bottle, reducing the rate of vacuum/aspiration or forcing infusion with an external mechanism such as an air pump. A number of equipment manufacturers have also introduced innovations that help answer the fluid issue:

- *Air pump*. An air pump is attached to the infusion bottle and is used to inject air into the bottle in order to increase the flow rate. As described by Agarwal in his book, the benefits to this approach are increased infusion through the irrigating chopper, as well as helping to maintain a stable anterior chamber.[49] With the availability of new instruments and phacoemulsification systems for biaxial phacoemulsification the use of an air pump is not necessary.

- *Thin-walled tubing*. Along with raising the height of the infusion bottle, thin-walled tubing will help to increase inflow and keep the chamber stable.[46]

- *Intellesis Sensor Accuracy*. This offering by AMO is said to monitor the pressure variations at the phaco tip, providing vacuum control over the tubing, and reducing the potential for surge and a loss of chamber stability.[50]

- *Innovative Stable Chamber System.* Offered by Bausch & Lomb on its Millennium Microsurgical System, this system is also said to reduce post-occlusion surge and improve chamber stability. It is available as part of the Millennium Micro Incision Vacuum Pack.[51]

- *Cruise Control.* Staar Surgical offers low compliance (thin-walled) tubing and post-occlusion surge control (Cruise Control) for its phacoemulsification system.

■ SURGICAL TECHNIQUE FOR BIAXIAL PHACOEMULSIFICATION ■

Our preferred technique for biaxial phacoemulsification begins with a 1.3 mm trapezoidal corneal incision with a tunnel that is 1.3 mm in length. This is made at 11 o'clock and is parallel to the limbus. Prior to creation of the biaxial incisions, the pupil is dilated with tropicamide 0.5% and phenylephrine 0.5%, followed by 1 drop of diclofenac. Anesthesia was accomplished with an injection of bupivicaine 0.5% with lidocaine 2% into the eyelid and tetracaine 1% onto the conjunctiva.

To create the trapezoidal incision (Figure 19-5), we use a trapezoidal steel microkeratome that is designed specifically for biaxial cataract surgery (Nanoedge, Geuder, Heidelberg, Germany). The second incision for the irrigating chopper is made at 2 o'clock and is 1 mm in width. After filling the anterior chamber with ophthalmic viscosurgical device (OVD), we perform a capsulorrhexis with a 24-gauge bent needle and then do hydrodissection and hydrodelineation. According to Hoffman, free rotation of the entire epinucleus helps to make lens removal easier during biaxial phacoemulsification. As a result, he recommends performing hydrodissection, then rotation of the lens before performing hydrodelineation. Hoffman also recommends applying external pressure on the posterior lip of the microincision during this step in order to avoid excessive pressure in the anterior chamber.[45]

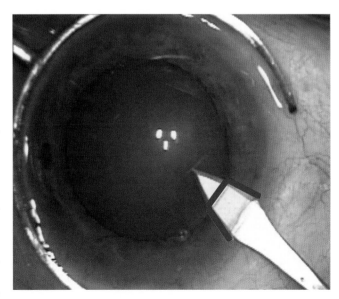

Figure 19-5 Creation of the trapezoidal clear corneal incision using a trapezoidal steel microkeratome designed specifically for biaxial cataract surgery (Nanoedge, Geuder, Heidelberg, Germany).

After completion of hydrodissection and hydrodelineation, the next step is to insert a 20-gauge phacoemulsification needle through the 11 o'clock incision and a 19-gauge irrigating chopper, with two irrigation ports, through the 2 o'clock incision. Our preferred method for cataract removal is to use a stop-and-chop technique using the Sovereign machine with WhiteStar Software (v. 6). The normal settings are:

- Maximum phacoemulsification power: 55%
- Bottle height: 57 cm
- Aspiration rate: 29 cm^3/min
- Maximum vacuum: 50 mm Hg.

For the emulsification and aspiration of the nucleus, the following settings are typically used:

- Maximum phacoemulsification power: 40%
- Bottle height: 76 cm
- Aspiration rate: 30 cm^3/min
- Maximum vacuum: 300 mm Hg.

The phacoemulsification energy was done in pulses with a duty cycle of 33%, which means that phacoemulsification energy was on for 33% of every 1 s.[21] The WhiteStar Software enables the surgeon to make two critical changes to the manner in which ultrasound energy is used. First, the surgeon can shorten the duration of the phacoemulsification pulse to as little as 6 ms. Second, the surgeon can change the duty cycle to prolong and vary the amount of time the ultrasound cycles off. Chang reports that there are three benefits to these features: (1) a lower duty cycle means less ultrasound energy into the capsular bag; (2) in combination with the interrupted ultrasound, more frequently delivery means the build-up of less heat; and (3), the two features means less repelling forces at the tip of the phaco needle.[49]

There is another aspect about the effect this software has on ultrasound power. Baudouin describes this pulsing as a "microburst"

effect that helps to sustain transient cavitation – the effect that occurs at the beginning of ultrasound power and leads to the breakdown of tissue.[52] By using microbursts to sustain transient cavitation, the use of ultrasound is expected to be more efficient, requiring less heat and energy introduced into the eye. The vast majority of biaxial surgeons agree that a chopping technique works best for this procedure, except in cases with extremely soft nuclei or in refractive lens exchange when biaxial I–A is typically all that is necessary.[5–17,45]

The maintenance of a stable anterior chamber during biaxial phacoemulsification is down to using appropriately sized incisions, proper bottle height, as well as an ophthalmic viscosurgical device (OVD) to help keep the eye pressurized.[51] Although much has been made about unstable anterior chambers during biaxial phacoemulsification, the reality is that the chamber should actually be more stable, because there should be very little outflow from the eye.[18]

In a study conducted at the authors' university comparing the biaxial technique with coaxial phacoemulsification, the effective phacoemulsification time (EPT) was <3 s in the majority of the biaxial cases (66%). This compared to an EPT of 32% in the coaxial eyes.[21] This study found that a shorter EPT was associated with more rapid visual recovery in the biaxial eyes.

To perform biaxial I–A, the bottle height is raised, and irrigation and aspiration tips are inserted through the nasal and temporal incisions to remove the residual cortex and polish the posterior capsule. We then inject additional OVD into the eye and enlarge the incision. The amount of enlargement is currently determined by the IOL to be implanted (Figure 19-6). In almost all cases of biaxial surgery, it is necessary to enlarge the incision in order to insert IOL. A few surgeons opt to create a third incision in order to insert the IOL, placed between the nasal and temporal incisions.[48] In case of a trapezoidal corneal incision this additional incision is not necessary. Precise measurement of the small incision (starting with 1 mm size) can be performed using a titanium microincision caliper (Figure 19-7, Duckworth & Kent, 9-646).

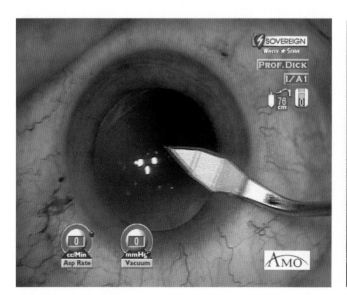

Figure 19-6 Enlargement of the incision for subsequent intraocular lens implantation.

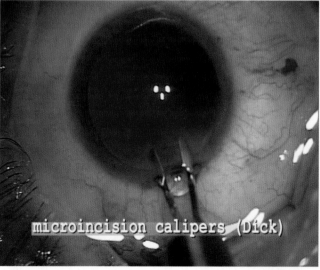

Figure 19-7 The titanium microincision caliper accurately measures very small incisions as used in biaxial phacoemulsification. (Duckworth & Kent, 9-646.)

After IOL implantation and removal of the OVD, both incisions were checked to ensure that they were watertight and left sutureless.

BIAXIAL ADVANTAGES

As was shown in our study, the results between biaxial phacoemulsification and coaxial phacoemulsification are relatively similar – both patient groups had no complications and very good clinical results. So, why bother with biaxial cataract surgery? There are a number of very sound reasons for using this approach. Consider that in this particular study, the biaxial group showed an earlier improvement in best-corrected visual acuity (BCVA) compared to the coaxial group.[21] Similar results have been reported by Agarwal and Olson.[7,10]

There are additional advantages outlined by Paul and Braga-Mele:[4]

- Smaller incisions should lead, theoretically, to a more stable anterior chamber due to a closed operating environment with less leakage of balanced salt solution and OVD.

- These microincisions should heal more quickly and further reduce postoperative astigmatism. They should also be associated with a lessened risk of postoperative endophthalmitis.

- By separating the irrigation from the phaco needle, removal of the nucleus fragments should be simplified because irrigation from the needle no longer pushes the pieces away.

- As the microincision sizes are similar, the I–A handpiece ports can be interchanged to better manage subincisional cortex or nuclear fragments.

- The micro-instrumentation used in biaxial phacoemulsification makes visualization of the operating field much better, which improves the safety of the procedure.

More importantly, are these advantages:

- *Reduced phacoemulsification energy.* As evidenced by our prospective randomized study, as well as those by Alio, Donnenfeld, Chang and others, there is a statistically significant reduction in the amount of phacoemulsification energy that is used in biaxial phacoemulsification when compared to coaxial phacoemulsification surgery.[7,18,49] As Chang notes there does not really exist an apples to apples method of comparing the effective phacoemulsification times, because all equipment manufacturers have different ways of measuring EPT. However, there is little doubt that less ultrasound energy is better for the eye and the corneal incision.[49] In Alio's study, he found that total surgical time was less in biaxial surgery than in the coaxial cases and that by decreasing the surgical time it reduced the ultrasound energy introduced into the eye, making it the superior procedure.[18]

The key is the use of pulsed ultrasound energy. With software like WhiteStar available, cataract surgeons can very precisely control the delivery of energy into the eye, making it possible to break down the nucleus without a sleeve. Without the need for a phaco sleeve, incisions can be downsized even further without risking thermal damage.[21] Not only that, these microincisions mean less corneal stromal damage and less surgically induced astigmatism.

- *Improved control and chamber stability.* As a result of the separation of ultrasound power and irrigation, in biaxial phacoemulsification, surgeons actually have a much greater degree of control over what is happening within the capsular bag. With traditional phacoemulsification, the irrigation from the phaco needle has a tendency to push the lens fragments away from the tip. This necessitates the need to "chase" after fragments and guide them back to the phaco tip. In biaxial phacoemulsification, the irrigating chopper can be used to direct fragments to the tip making it quicker to emulsify and remove the nucleus. There is also less "acoustical streaming" from the phaco tip to push lens fragments away, according to Baudouin, due to the reduction and modulation of ultrasound energy.[52]

Management of the chamber is a frequently cited drawback of biaxial phacoemulsification. However, in the authors' experience, as well as the experience of others, these chambers tend to be more stable than in coaxial surgery. Fishkind notes that because fluid volumes are decreased in biaxial phacoemulsification and, owing to the fact that there is less uncontrolled fluid egress because of tight-fitting incisions, the chamber is more stable. This experience is shared by Fine and Hoffman, who have hypothesized that there may actually be a lower risk of surgically induced posterior vitreous detachment and cystoid macular edema in eyes where a biaxial approach is used. This would be due to less movement of the lens, iris and vitreous, because there are not extreme changes in chamber pressure.[46]

- *Enhanced safety and efficacy.* The authors' clinical study, as well as those conducted by Alio, Donnenfeld and others, point to the improved safety and efficacy of biaxial phacoemulsification when compared to coaxial and other standard techniques.[7,18,53–55] There is a trend toward quicker visual recovery in these eyes, as well as reduced induced astigmatism. Studies have also shown that there is no difference in corneal endothelial cell loss or endothelial morphology when biaxial phacoemulsification is used.[19,56]

CHALLENGES OF BIAXIAL PHACOEMULSIFICATION

Realistically, there are some challenges to successfully performing biaxial phacoemulsification. Chief among these is the learning curve, particularly for cataract surgeons who have not adopted a chopping technique for cataract removal. The smaller incisions used in biaxial phacoemulsification can also limit movement of the instruments that is necessary in order to avoid tissue trauma. Fluid leakage can be a problem if there is not a perfect fit between instruments and incisions, leading to chamber instability.[48] This is illustrated by a case report of leakage from an irrigation port incision.[57]

There is also the lack of an IOL that can go through an unenlarged microincision. In almost all cases, it is necessary to enlarge the incision in order to implant the IOL. A number of biaxial critics, therefore, see this need for enlargement as defeating the purpose of creating the tiny incisions initially.[4] Next, is the concern that the bare phaco needle will overheat and cause corneal tissue damage and wound burns. Granted this is a risk, but as studies by

Agarwal, Donnenfeld, Olsen and Braga-Mele have demonstrated by using new software that enables to minimize and control ultrasound energy, the risk of wound burn during biaxial phacoemulsification is actually extremely low.[7,10,43,51,58]

Finally, biaxial cataract procedures can take more overall surgical time, particularly in eyes with a greater than +4 cataract. This is due to the downsizing of the instruments, as well as the tighter fit around the phaco needle and irrigating chopper. When starting out with biaxial phacoemulsification, it is important to choose your first cases with care in order to learn to understand and manage these challenges.

CURRENT CLINICAL FINDINGS

Results on biaxial cataract surgery published over the past 18 months certainly confirm the positive view we have of this procedure. In a study of the thermal effect of microburst and hyperpulse settings during sleeveless biaxial phacoemulsification with advanced power modulations, Braga-Mele concluded that this technique reduced wound temperatures during the phacoemulsification procedure, enhancing safety and efficiency. With power varying from 20% to 80% in 10% increments, pulse modes were set with and without aspiration-line occlusion, and wound temperatures were measured three times per second. The results verified that wound temperature did not exceed 39°C using 80% power during 3 min of occlusion, and 29°C with fixed microbursts of 4 ms on, 4 ms off.[5]

As discussed earlier in this chapter, the clinical outcomes of biaxial microincision were compared to those of coaxial small-incision clear cornea cataract surgery in the authors' prospective series. In this study, phacoemulsification using pulsed ultrasound energy with variable duty cycles was used, followed by mini-incision IOL implantation. The outcomes of BCVA, astigmatism, laser flare photometry value, effective phacoemulsification time (EPT), and endothelial cell count were assessed, revealing that BCVA improved more rapidly and EPT was shorter in the biaxial group. The median BCVA was 20/20 in the biaxial group and 20/25 in the coaxial group, and 68% of coaxial procedures had an EPT of over 3 s compared to only 34% of biaxial procedures.[21]

Another study of biaxial microincision phacoemulsification through two 1.4 mm incisions for posterior polar cataract extraction found that adequate anterior chamber stability was provided by the low-infusion and low-vacuum system, and lens fragments were removed without hydrodissection or nucleus rotation. The study concluded that the biaxial technique enhanced safety by reducing risks of complication.[59]

In an assessment of the feasibility of biaxial microincisional phacoemulsification in hard cataracts of N3+ using the AMO Sovereign with WhiteStar technology, the ultrasound power was set at 30–25% according to nuclei hardness, with a duty cycle of 33%. The results showed no cases of thermal burn, and the amount of infusion solution used was less than that used in conventional coaxial phacoemulsification, placing this technique at an advantage over coaxial phacoemulsification.[12]

Prakash et al. assessed the efficiency of biaxial microincision phacoemulsification followed by the implantation of an injectable ThinOptX IOL in the capsular bag. The results verified that ThinOptX IOLs could be safely inserted through 1.7 mm incisions used for biaxial phacoemulsification, with adequate distance

and near visual acuity. Although the results suggested there was no notable change in keratometric astigmatism, the posterior capsular opacification rate was substantially higher with the ThinOptX IOL.[60]

Khng et al. looked at the changes in intraocular pressure (IOP) during standard coaxial and biaxial microincision phacoemulsification using a pressure transducer positioned in the vitreous cavity, which recorded IPO at 100 readings per second. The results revealed that biaxial microincision phacoemulsification was safer. The findings showed that IOP was lower for at least one of the biaxial phacoemulsification eyes than for the standard coaxial phacoemulsification eye in four of the eight stages of the procedure: hydrodissection and delineation, nuclear disassembly, irrigation–aspiration and anterior chamber reformation.[20]

Fine et al. also recently published a technique for refractive lens exchange using biaxial microincision phacoemulsification. Their study involved removal of the crystalline lens through two 1.2 mm incisions, with capsulorrhexis formation, cortical cleaving hydrodissection, lens extraction in the iris plane and residual cortex removal all performed through the microincisions. The study found that this technique offered more surgical control during the procedure, in addition to the safety of a constant pressurization of the eye during the removal of the lens far from the posterior capsule.[61] Fine noted that this technique was safe and the least invasive, as the irrigating cannula was held above the lens to eliminate the risk of corneal damage. Hydrolineation was also avoided due to the use of a sleeveless phacoemulsification needle with the bevel turned towards the lens equator, which was carouselled in the plane of the capsulorrhexis without ultrasound energy and with high vacuum. Visual acuity results showed that 43% of the patients achieved both 20/25 and J2 or better.[62]

RISK MANAGEMENT

Certainly, there is a greater risk of complications when a surgeon first begins biaxial phacoemulsification. What follows is a listing of some of the most common problems and how to manage them effectively, where appropriate:

- *Wound construction.* There may be differences in removal techniques in biaxial phacoemulsification surgery, but all biaxial surgeons agree on one point: the need for a well-constructed incision. A poorly constructed incision will lead to wound leakage, chamber instability, corneal trauma and astigmatism.[49]

- *Phaco tip occlusion.* This can occur when a highly viscous OVD is used. This type of OVD can also be difficult to remove at the end of biaxial cases, leading to IOP spikes and occlusion of the anterior chamber. In routine cases, it is best to use a regular medium viscous OVD such as Healon (AMO, Santa Ana, CA).[21]

- *Irrigation flow rate.* Particularly when high vacuum is in use or following occlusion, the irrigation rate from the smaller gauge choppers used in biaxial surgery may not be able to maintain a stable anterior chamber. The surgeon must take these factors into account and adjust the infusion rate, aspiration rate and vacuum accordingly.[21] When exiting the eye the phaco tip has to be taken out first followed by the irrigating chopper to prevent anterior chamber collapse (Figure 19-8).

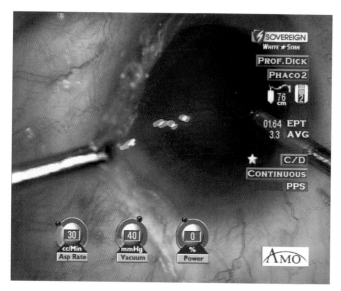

Figure 19-8 Anterior chamber collapse due to removal of the irrigating chopper prior to the removal of the phaco tip.

COMPLICATED AND SPECIAL CASES ▪

As a result of the microincisions required for biaxial cataract surgery, as well as the almost completely closed environment, the procedure actually lends itself very well to some of the more complicated cataract cases (Figure 19-9).

Among them are advanced and hypermature cataracts with a tense capsule. Under a grant from the Research to Prevent Blindness, Olson looked at which complicated cases would benefit from the biaxial approach. In hypermature cataracts with a tense capsule, a biaxial approach enables the cataract surgeon to

perform an incision, inject a highly OVD material and create a capsulorrhexis without the risk of the capsulorrhexis going out of control, or for visualization to become obscured due to the milky cortex.[63] The same approach can also work in cases where iris prolapse is a concern due to a flat anterior chamber. In eyes with zonular dialysis, the biaxial approach allows the surgeon to place the two incisions away from the area of risk and, thus, operate with reduced risk.

Another complication that can benefit from biaxial cataract surgery is in the management of floppy iris syndrome. Douglas Koch combines a highly viscous OVD with a biaxial phacoemulsification technique in these cases using a modified stop-and-chop technique to keep the iris under control.[64]

A final potential use for biaxial cataract surgery is in pediatric and young cataract cases. Although there are no published reports establishing the use of biaxial surgery in these young eyes, the need for a completely closed environment would seem to lend itself to the procedure.[65]

▪ FUTURE TRENDS ▪

Based on studies published in the past 2 years, as well as on anecdotal reports, there is an upsurge in the number of surgeons who now make biaxial cataract surgery a part of their surgical armamentarium. This situation has been helped by equipment manufacturers developing software that helps facilitate sleeveless, microincision cataract surgery, as well as by surgeons and instrument manufacturers working together to develop tools that can effectively work through these minute incisions.

The next piece of the puzzle is an IOL that can be delivered easily and safely through an un-enlarged microincision. At the present time, there are a number of IOLs that can be inserted through incisions of between 1.7 and 2.2 mm. In the authors' series, an aspheric acrylic mini-incision IOL (Figure 19-10, Acri.Smart 36A, Acritec, Hennigsdorf, Germany) was injected

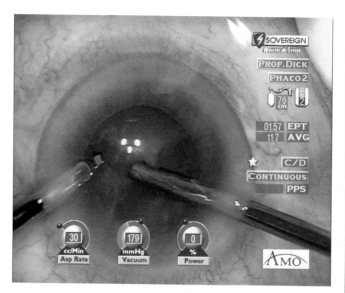

Figure 19-9 The biaxial approach facilitates phacoemulsification in an eye with a hard nucleus, reduced pupil size and loose zonules (pseudoexfoliation syndrome): e.g., non-sleeved (improved approach into the nucleus) phacoemulsification to the intended zonular direction (interchangeable).

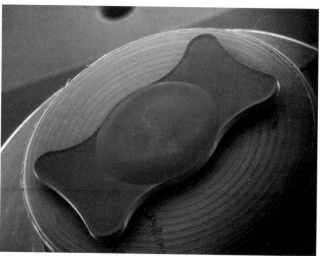

Figure 19-10 Scanning electron microscopy overview of the aspheric acrylic Acri.Smart 36A intraocular lens for mini-incisional implantation. (Acri.Smart 36A, Acritec, Hennigsdorf, Germany)

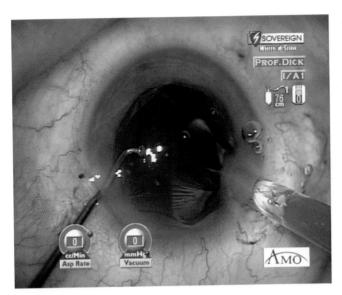

Figure 19-11 Implantation of an aspheric acrylic microincision intraocular lens (IOL) (Acri.Smart 36A) after uncomplicated biaxial phacoemulsification using a second instrument (iris manipulator) to ensure one-step direct IOL implantation into the capsular bag.

through a 1.7 mm incision (Figure 19-11). This company also manufactures the Acry.Lyc acrylic IOL that is capable of being inserted through a 1.5 mm incision when the injector is placed just inside the incision. ThinOptX (Abingdon, VA) developed a hydrophilic acrylic IOL that is rolled and placed into a special injector for insertion into the capsular bag. Published reports indicate that this lens was injected through a 1.5 mm incision.[4,16] Insufficient capsular bag performance and high posterior capsule

opacification rates with this IOL were reported.[64] Finally, Bausch & Lomb (Rochester, NY) recently introduced an aspheric (aberration-free), hydrophilic acrylic one-piece IOL called MI60 (26% water content) with 10° average angulation that can be injected through a 1.8 mm incision using the wound-assisted technique. The 4-point fixation design is proven to offer good stability with its parent design, Akreos Adapt (Figure 19-12). Moreover, three overall diameters are available to better fit capsular bag sizes. The 360° barrier and square edge design in the Akreos MI60 incorporates the 360° posterior ridge as its Akreos predecessors in resisting posterior capsular opacification. Its 10° angulation is a further improvement, reinforcing the lens contact with the posterior capsule.

When phacoemulsification came into the mainstream, the IOLs being implanted were between 5.5 and 6 mm and required enlargement of the incision. The need for incisional enlargement is not a new phenomenon. However, the argument in favor of biaxial phacoemulsification will certainly become an easier one when there are IOLs widely available that can go through a <1.5 mm incision.

The authors have become convinced that biaxial cataract surgery is the way forward. With the equipment, software and instrumentation now available, the surgery is safe, efficient and minimally invasive. Patients have better visual recovery in the immediate postoperative period with very low complication rates. The arguments used for many years against the biaxial approach really no longer stand. In fact, this technique may actually show a benefit in complicated cases and in hard cataracts. It is entirely possible that longer-term follow-up will show that there are fewer cases of cystoid macular edema and retinal detachment in these eyes due to the almost completely closed environment in which the cataract surgery is performed.

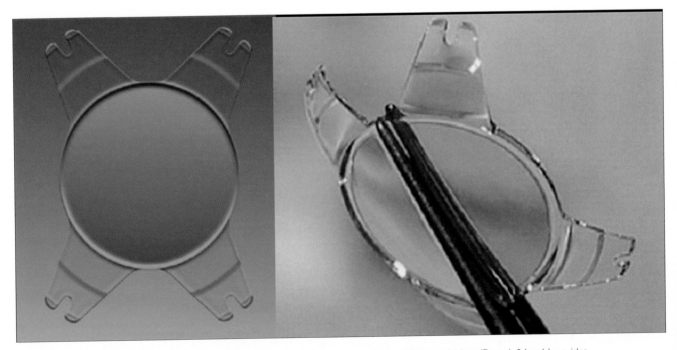

Figure 19-12 Aspheric (aberration-free), hydrophilic acrylic one-piece MI 60 intraocular lens (Bausch & Lomb) provides a 4-point fixation design for good stability and a 360° square edge barrier for posterior capsular opacification prevention.

References

[1] Arshinoff SA. Biaxial phacoemulsification. J Cataract Refract Surg 2005;31:646–647. [letter].

[2] Grabow HB. Letter. J Cataract Refract Surg 2006;32:547–548.

[3] Osher RH. Microcoxial phacoemulsification. Part 2: clinical study. J Cataract Refract Surg 2007;33:408–412.

[4] Paul, T, Braga-Mele, R. Bimanual microincisional phacoemulsification: the future of cataract surgery? Current Opin Ophthalmol 2005;16:2–7.

[5] Braga-Mele R. Thermal effect of microburst and hyperpulse settings during sleeveless bimanual phacoemulsification with advanced power modulations. J Cataract Refract Surg 2006;32:639–642.

[6] Spencer MH. Direct puncture capsulorrhexis. J Cataract Refract Surg 2005;31:1490–1492.

[7] Donnenfeld ED, Olson RJ, Solomon R, et al. Efficacy and wound-temperature gradient of Whitestar phacoemulsification through a 1.2 mm incision. J Cataract Refract Surg 2003; 29:1097–1100.

[8] Tsuneoka H, Hayama A, Takahama M. Ultrasmall-incision bimanual phacoemulsification and AcrySof SA30AL implantation through a 2.2 mm incision. J Cataract Refract Surg 2003; 29:1070–1076.

[9] Tsuneoka H, Shiba T, Takahashi Y. Ultrasonic phacoemulsification using a 1.4 mm incision: clinical results. J Cataract Refract Surg 2002;28:81–86.

[10] Agarwal A, Agarwal A, Agarwal S, Narang P, Narang S. Phakonit: phacoemulsification through a 0.9 mm corneal incision. J Cataract Refract Surg 2001;27:1548–1552.

[11] Colvard DM. Bimanual technique to manage subincisional cortical material. J Cataract Refract Surg 1997;23:707–709.

[12] Assaf A, El-Moatassem AM. Feasibility of bimanual microincision phacoemulsification in hard cataracts. Eye 2007;21:807–811. [Epub 2006 May 5].

[13] Sethi HS, Dada T, Rai HK, Seth P. Closed chamber globe stabilization and needle capsulorhexis using irrigation hand piece of bimanual irrigation and aspiration system. BMC Ophthalmol 2005;5:21.

[14] Yaylali V, Yildirim C, Tatlipinar S, Demirlenk I, Arik S, Ozden S. Subjective visual experience and pain level during phacoemulsification and intraocular lens implantation under topical anesthesia. Ophthalmologica 2003;217:413–416.

[15] Brazitikos PD, Androudi S, Alexandridis A, Ekonomidis P, Papadopoulos NT. Up-irrigation of dropped nuclear fragments during phacoemulsification with the bimanual irrigation–aspiration system. Acta Ophthalmol Scand 2003;81:76–77.

[16] Agarwal A. The evolution of phakonit. Cataract & Refractive Surgery Today 2004;September: 39–41.

[17] Packard R. Techniques and instrumentation for bimanual microincisional cataract surgery. Cataract & Refractive Surgery Today 2004;September:50–54.

[18] Alio J, Rodriguez-Prats JL, Galal A, Ramzy M. Outcomes of microincision cataract surgery versus coaxial phacoemulsification. Ophthalmology 2005;112:1997–2003.

[19] Mencucci, R, Ponchietti, C, Virgili, G, Giansanti, F, Menchini, U. Corneal endothelial damage after cataract surgery: microincision versus standard technique. J Cataract Refract Surg 2006;32:1351–1354.

[20] Khng C, Packer M, Fine IH, Hoffman RS, Moreira FB. Intraocular pressure during phacoemulsification. J Cataract Refract Surg 2006;32:301–308.

[21] Kurz S, Krummenauer F, Gabriel P, Pfeiffer N, Dick HB. Biaxial microincision versus coaxial small-incision clear cornea cataract surgery. Ophthalmology 2006;113:1818–1826.

[22] Maloney WF. Architect of our future: Charles D. Kelman, MD. Ocular Surgery News Europe/ Asia-Pacific Edition. August 2004.

[23] Shearing SP, Relyea RL, Loaiza A, Shearing RL. Routine phacoemulsification through a one-millimeter non-sutured incision. Cataract 1985;2:6–10.

[24] Girard LJ. Ultrasonic fragmentation for cataract extraction and cataract complications. Adv Ophthalmol 1978;37:127–135.

[25] Packer M. Bimanual microincision cataract surgery is the wave of the future. Ophthalmology Times 2004;March 15.

[26] Girard LJ. Pars plana lensectomy by ultrasonic fragmentation 1984, part II: operative and postoperative complications, avoidance or management. Ophthalmic Surg 1984;15:217–220.

[27] Colvard DM. Bimanual technique to manage subincisional cortical material. J Cataract Refract Surg 1997;23:707–708.

[28] Tsuneoka H, Shiba T, Takahashi Y. Feasibility of ultrasound cataract surgery with a 1.4 mm incision. J Cataract Refract Surg 2001;27:934–940.

[29] Ernest PH, Kiessling LA, Lavery KT. Relative strength of cataract incisions in cadaver eyes. J Cataract Refract Surg 1991;17(Suppl.):668–671.

[30] Ernest PH, Fenzl R, Lavery KT, Sensoli A. Relative stability of clear corneal incisions in a cadaver eye mode. J Cataract Refract Surg 21(1):39–42. Jan.

[31] Bhairavi V, Kharod TK. Clear corneal incisions in cataract surgery. Ophthalmology Management December 2006.

[32] Fine IH. Architecture and construction of a self-sealing incision for cataract surgery. J Cataract Refract Surg 1991;17(Suppl.):672–676.

[33] Sperber LT, Dodick JM. Laser therapy in cataract surgery. Curr Opin Ophthalmol 1994;5: 105–109.

[34] Dodick JM, Lally JM, Sperber LT. Lasers in cataract surgery. Curr Opin Ophthalmol 1993;4:107–109.

[35] Kanellopoulos AJ, Dodick JM, Brauweiler P, Alzner E. Dodick photolysis for cataract surgery: early experience with the Q-switched neodymium: YAG laser in 100 consecutive patients. Ophthalmology 1999;106:2197–2202.

[36] www.finemd.com

[37] Fine HI, Packer M, Hoffman RS. Use of power modulations in phacoemulsification: Choo-choo chop and flip. J Cataract Refract Surg 2001;27:188–197.

[38] Davis EA, Lindstrom RL. Tilt and tumble phacoemulsification. Dev Ophthalmol 2002;34:44–58.

[39] Hoffman RS, Fine IH, Packer M. New phacoemulsification technology. Curr Opin Ophthalmol 2005;16:38–43.

[40] Soscia W, Howard JG, Olson RJ. Microphacoemulsification with WhiteStar. A wound-temperature study. J Cataract Refract Surg 2002;28:1044–1046.

[41] Packard R. Evaluation of a new approach to phacoemulsification: bimanual phaco with the Sovereign system rapid pulse software. XIII Congress of the European Society of Ophthalmology Istanbul, June 2001.

[42] Braga-Mele R, Liu E. Feasibility of sleeveless bimanual phacoemulsification with the millennium microsurgical system. J Cataract Refract Surg 2003;29:2199–2203.

[43] Mackool RJ, Brint SF. AquaLase: a new technology for cataract extraction. Curr Opin Ophthalmol 2004;15:40–43.

[44] Agarwal A, Agarwal AT, et al. Antichamber collapser. J Cataract Refract Surg 2002;28: 1085–1086.

[45] Hoffman RS. 10 tips reflect shift toward bimanual phaco. Ophthalmology Times 2005; November 15.

[46] Ifft D. Bimanual microincision phaco. Ophthalmology Management November 2003.

[47] Advanced Medical Optics (AMO). Santa Ana, CA. Data on file, 2007.

[48] Weikert MP. Update on bimanual microincisional cataract surgery. Current Opin Ophthal 2006;17:62–67.

[49] Agarwal A. Bimanual phaco: mastering the phakonit/mics technique. Thorofare, NJ: Slack Inc; 2005.

[50] Advanced Medical Optics (AMO). Santa Ana, CA. Data on file, 2007.

[51] Bausch & Lomb. Rochester, NY. Data on file, 2007.

[52] Advanced Medical Optics. Santa Ana, CA. Data on file, 2007.

[53] Milla E, Verges C, Cipres M. Corneal endothelium evaluation after phacoemulsification with continuous anterior chamber infusion, Cornea 2005;24:278–282.

[54] Wong VW, Lai TY, Lee GK, Lam PT, Lam DS. Safety and efficacy of microincisional cataract surgery with bimanual phacoemulsification for white mature cataract. Ophthalmologica 2007; 221:24–28.

[55] Nawrocki J, Michalewski J, Michalewska Z, Cisiecki S. Cool phaco – new option in cataract surgery. Klin Oczna 2005;107:36–38.

[56] Wilczynski M, Drobniewski I, Synder A, Omulecki W. Evaluation of early corneal endothelial cell loss in bimanual microincision cataract surgery (MICS) in comparison with standard phacoemulsification. Eur J Ophthalmol 2006;16:798–803.

[57] Stratas BA. Clear corneal paracentesis: a case of chronic wound leakage in a patient having bimanual phacoemulsification. J Cataract Refract Surg 2005;31:1075.

[58] Soscia W, Howard JG, Olson RJ. Bimanual phacoemulsification through 2 stab incisions. A wound-temperature study. J Cataract Refract Surg 2002;28:1039–1043.

[59] Haripriya A, Aravind S, Vadi K, Natchiar G. Bimanual microphaco for posterior polar cataracts. J Cataract Refract Surg 2006;32:914–917.

[60] Prakash, P, Kasaby, HE, Aggarwal, RK, Humfrey, S. Microincision bimanual phacoemulsification and Thinoptx((R)) implantation through a 1.70 mm incision. Eye 2007;21:177–182.

[61] Fine, IH, Hoffman, RS, Packer, M. Optimizing refractive lens exchange with bimanual microincision phacoemulsification. J Cataract Refract Surg 2004;30:550–554.

[62] Fine IH. Bimanual MICS has much to offer over coaxial. EuroTimes March 2006.

[63] Olson RJ. Bimanual phacoemulsification for complicated cases. Cataract & Refractive Surgery Today September 2004.

[64] Koch DD. Managing intraoperative floppy iris syndrome. Cataract & Refractive Surgery Today November/December 2005.

[65] Vasavada AR, Nihalani BR. Pediatric cataract surgery. Curr Opin Ophthalmol 2006;17:54–61.

FUTURE TRENDS

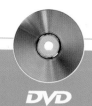

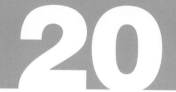

Microcoaxial Phacoemulsification with Torsional Ultrasound

Robert H. Osher, MD

20

CHAPTER HIGHLIGHTS

>> Microcoaxial technology
>> Validation in laboratory studies
>> Clinical technique
>> The role of torsional ultrasound

Cataract surgery has evolved into a very safe outpatient procedure with unprecedented visual outcomes. Yet new technologies continue to emerge that allow the operation to be performed through smaller, less-invasive incisions with more efficient delivery of energy. One method, sleeveless bimanual microphacoemulsification, relies on the separation of irrigation through one port while ultrasound and aspiration functions are utilized through a second incision. Microcoaxial phacoemulsification is another approach in which all functions can be performed through a smaller incision simply by reducing the size of the sleeve. Coupled with surge-reducing fluidic technologies and a new ultrasonic energy delivery modality utilizing an oscillating needle creating torsional side-to-side movement, a highly efficient and extremely safe technology has been achieved. It is the purpose of this chapter to provide the reader with an overview of microcoaxial phacoemulsification and to describe the benefits of torsional ultrasound.

TECHNOLOGICAL INNOVATIONS

The INFINITI Vision System (Alcon Surgical Ft. Worth, Texas) introduced the MicroSmooth Ultra Sleeve designed to facilitate coaxial phacoemulsification and implantation of an intraocular lens with a 6 mm optic through an unenlarged 2.2 mm incision. The thin-walled silicone sleeve (Figure 20-1) with large irrigating ports maximizes irrigation inflow which is necessary for maintaining optimal chamber stability. The sleeve itself provides insulation within the incision, separating the vibrating needle from the surrounding tissue. Its coaxial design also allows the use of aspiration bypass, a thermo-protective safety feature only possible with a coaxial set-up. The same sleeve is used during cortical removal, vacuuming of the capsule, and removal of the ophthalmic viscosurgical device (OVD) at the conclusion of the procedure.

LABORATORY EVALUATION

Rigorous laboratory investigations were undertaken comparing micro-coaxial performance to that of sleeveless bimanual micro-phacoemulsification.[1] Fluidic testing demonstrated that the smaller sleeve reduced the infusion to 75% of that available with a normal sleeve. However, the irrigation flow was considerably higher than the volume available using 19-, 20-, and 21-gauge irrigating choppers, as much as 60% more than the 20-gauge (Figure 20-2). In addition, there was less leakage due to the sealing of the sleeve. These results suggested a fluidic advantage that could provide a deeper chamber with less fluctuation when challenged by either a higher aspiration rate or occlusion break. When this experiment was performed in a test chamber, the results demonstrated greater chamber stability with less surges when using the micro-coaxial system at five different vacuum levels (Table 20-1).

As incisions get smaller and smaller, temperature within the incision must remain at a safe level in order to avoid thermal

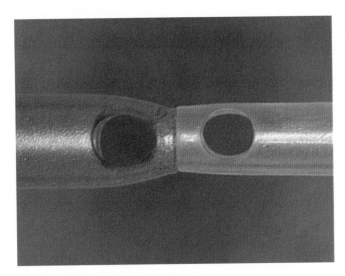

Figure 20-1 Comparative size of traditional coaxial phaco sleeve to MicroSmooth Ultra Sleeve.

injury.[2] Micro-coaxial phaco has the advantage of an insulating sleeve between the metal of the vibrating needle and the surrounding tissue as well as having the aspiration bypass system. The temperature was measured inside multiple incisions constructed in cadaver eyes. Using a Flir Systems Therma P60 infrared camera (Figure 20-3), a very safe temperature profile was identified. An even greater margin of safety was confirmed by utilizing power modulation with a duty cycle. Moreover, laboratory testing demonstrated an additional temperature reduction with torsional ultrasound.

Incisional competency was also studied since the author had first-hand clinical experience with occasional wound leak using sleeveless bimanual microphacoemulsification. Several histopathologic studies have disclosed collagen damage with the use of a bare phaco tip.[3,4,5] All laboratory testing of incisional sealing in cadaver eyes showed better incision competency with micro-coaxial phacoemulsification (Figure 20-4).

■ INTRAOCULAR LENS IMPLANTATION ■

A final laboratory study was designed to discover a safe and reproducible method of implanting a single-piece AcrySof acrylic intraocular lens (IOL) (Alcon Laboratories) with a 6 mm optic through an unenlarged 2.2 mm incision. We arrived independently at a very similar technique to that developed by Takayuki Akahoshi, MD, the Japanese surgeon who pioneered this procedure using a sub-2 mm incision with NANO Sleeve (Alcon Laboratories). A new injector was designed by Duckworth & Kent (DK 7797) to allow the insertion of the lens using one hand while the second hand introduced an instrument through the stab incision to provide counter-traction. After loading the IOL into the cartridge and folding the lens, using the method shown in the diagram, the chamber and capsular bag were filled with a retentive OVD. The incision was entered with the bevel-down tip of the Monarch C cartridge and counter-traction was applied with an Osher nucleus manipulator (Duckworth & Kent 6-472-2) through a 1 mm side-port incision. The cartridge was advanced into the lip of the incision as far as possible without excessive force but not into the chamber. While maintaining

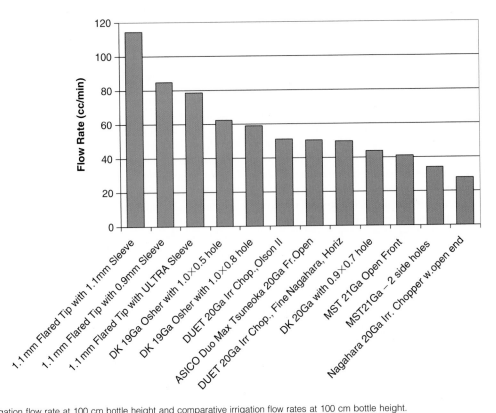

Figure 20-2 Irrigation flow rate at 100 cm bottle height and comparative irrigation flow rates at 100 cm bottle height.

Table 20-1 Coaxial set-up produces more stable occlusion break response. Comparison of surge: occlusion-break response.

Occlusion Break from Specified Vacuum Level (mm Hg) & 78 cm Btl. Height	Surgical outcome			
	Microcoaxial (Infiniti with ULTRA Sleeve and 1.1 mm Flared ABS)	Bimanual with 21Ga MST Open Front irrig. chopper through 1.2 mm	Bimanual with 20 Ga. Fine/Nagahara. irrig. Chopper through 1.2 mm	Bimanual with 19Ga D&K Osher 1.0x0.8 irrig. Chopper through 1.3 mm
100	trace	trace	mild	trace
200	trace/mild	mild	mild	trace
300	mild/moderate	significant	moderate	trace/mild
400	moderate	significant	significant	significant
500	significant	significant	significant	significant

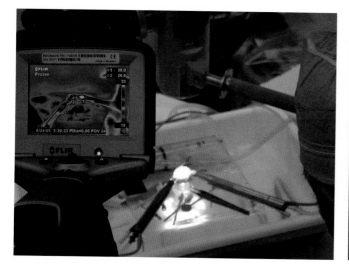

Figure 20-3 Comparative thermal testing with simultaneous temperature recordings.

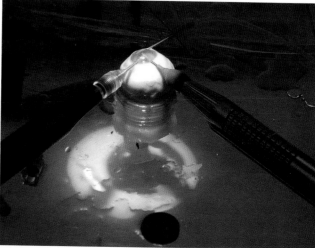

Figure 20-4 Incisional competency test setup.

counter-traction, the spring-loaded plunger was advanced steadily without hesitation and the leading edge of the lens was delivered into the OVD-filled capsular bag (Figure 20-5). The nucleus manipulator was used to depress the trailing edge of the optic–haptic junction and was then withdrawn from the side-port incision. An Osher dull-fingered Y-hook (Duckworth & Kent MP205) was used to rotate the trailing haptic of the unfolding lens into the capsular bag.

■ CLINICAL EVALUATION ■

The author designed a prospective clinical study to evaluate microcoaxial phacoemulsification in which 100 consecutive patients undergoing routine cataract surgery were enrolled.[6] All eyes were demonstrated to have consistent chamber stability and incisional competency. All phacoemulsifications were uncomplicated with no special instrumentation required, except for a 2.2 mm diamond keratome. The only machine parameter that required modification was the bottle height, which was increased from 45 cm to 70 cm. Otherwise, the phacoemulsification was

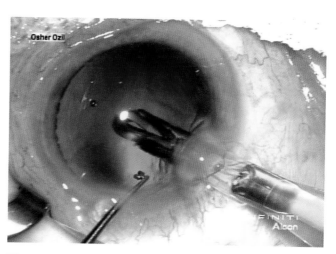

Figure 20-5 Counter-traction technique for inserting intraocular lens through a 2.2 mm incision.

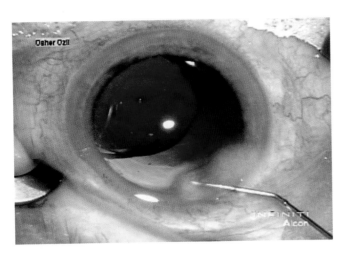

Figure 20-6 Stromal hydration is performed before removal of ophthalmic viscosurgical device.

identical to the author's preferred slow-motion divide and chop technique. The IOL was injected using the one-handed counter-traction technique. In contrast to the phacoemulsification, the IOL insertion was initially challenging until the counter-traction method was mastered then all difficulties vanished. The closure was sutureless in all but the very last patient, whose incision was the only one that leaked until a 10-0 nylon suture was passed. The surgeon found that stromal hydration was more effective when performed before the OVD was removed (Figure 20-6).

Intraoperative and postoperative complications were absent and the patients consistently experienced excellent uncorrected vision on the first postoperative day. The details of the laboratory and clinical studies have been published in the 2007 *Journal of Cataract and Refractive Surgery*.[1,6]

■ TORSIONAL ULTRASOUND AND MICROCOAXIAL PHACOEMULSIFICATION ■

Traditional longitudinal phacoemulsification developed by Charles Kelman, MD, utilizing a forward and back "jackhammer" effect has remained relatively unchanged for more than 3 decades. Improved handpieces, instrumentation, and surgical techniques have certainly been introduced, along with other machine innovations, such as continuous irrigation, surgeon control of parameters, and power modulation, using the concept of duty cycle to enhance efficiency while reducing temperature within the incision. Yet, the basic principle of emulsifying the nucleus with longitudinal ultrasound has never been modified. As the nucleus is removed, there is some degree of repulsion and thermal friction within the incision followed by retraction of the tip that creates cavitational energy and free radicals.

In early 2006, Alcon introduced a new concept, OZIL; an option of torsional ultrasound on the Infiniti Vision System. A dedicated handpiece which utilized an angled or curved tip would ultrasonically oscillate from side-to-side creating a more efficient emulsification with less friction-generated heat within the incision (Figure 20-7). The oscillatory motion of the hub occurred at a frequency of 32,000 Hz creating an equivalent stroke at the tip of approximately 90 μ at 100% power, similar to traditional phacoemulsification. However, unlike longitudinal stroke, the torsional stroke decreases away from the tip so there is significantly less movement within the incision (e.g. 30 μ at 100%).

The effect of this modification of ultrasound is quite profound. First, cutting efficiency is greatly increased. Traditional ultrasound is only 50% effective because the backwards motion of the stroke does not contact lens material. Rather than cutting only 50% of the time when the tip is moving forward, nuclear material is being emulsified or sheared constantly with torsional ultrasound, as the tip is moving in both directions.

Comparison of Stroke Movement

Traditional Ultrasound

Torsional Ultrasound

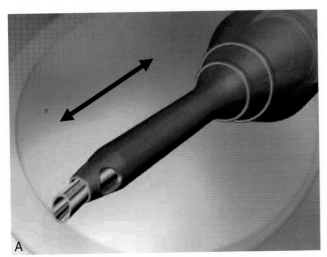
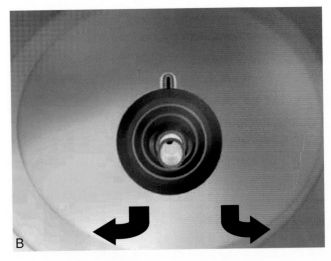

Figure 20-7 Torsional ultrasound creates side-to-side oscillation of tip rather than traditional "back and forth" longitudinal motion.

Second, the behavior of the nuclear material is quite different because there is no repulsion and chasing after pieces is unnecessary. There is visibly less chatter and dispersion of lens material versus traditional longitudinal ultrasound. The ability to maintain nuclear material at the tip is increased and turbulence is reduced.

Third, there is an improved thermal safety profile. The primary source of heat is friction and, because there is less movement in the incision, the heat that would normally be produced from traditional phaco is reduced by approximately two-thirds given the same power level.[7] Operating at the lower frequency of 32 KHz versus 40 KHz also has a thermal benefit and an energy saving of 20%. Power modulation can also be used with various duty cycles further improving the thermal safety profile. Coupled with the insulation of the silicone sleeve and the presence of aspiration bypass, there is even more thermal protection with the reduced incision size.

It should be emphasized that the surgeon may individualize the torsional settings. Torsional ultrasound can be combined with longitudinal ultrasound (sequential not simultaneous) in different ratios selected by the surgeon, which is a very effective approach to the harder nucleus (Figure 20-8). The ability to program the traditional duty cycle into the energy delivery equation also has been an important development. As a result, surgeons trying this new technology have found that the emulsification requires less cumulative energy and machine fluidic parameters can be reduced. In a laboratory study using small silicone beads suspended in balanced salt solution in cadaver eyes, torsional ultrasound resulted in better fluidics with much less repulsion.[8] It was possible to achieve the same efficiency with lower fluidic parameters. In a randomized comparative clinical study involving 525 eyes undergoing phacoemulsification with either conventional or torsional ultrasound, results showed that the torsional mode produced more effective lens removal and a smaller amount of phaco time and energy.[9]

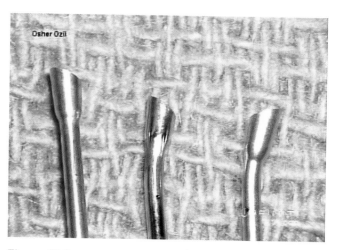

Figure 20-9 Straight tip, Kelman tip, and new blended tip designed independently by Dr. Akahoshi and Dr. Osher.

One challenge that is being addressed is the requirement to use the curved Kelman-style tip in order to reap the benefits of this new technology. While it is possible to emulsify the nucleus using torsional ultrasound with a straight tip, intermittent bursts of longitudinal ultrasound are necessary to prevent "apple coring" of the nucleus. Since it has been estimated that 80% of the world's phaco surgeons use a straight tip, there is a need for a less curved design that would be easier to use than the traditional 30° curve of the Kelman tip (Figure 20-9). Dr. Akahoshi in Japan and Dr. Osher in the United States have independently arrived at a blended tip with a curve of approximately 12°, which shares similar efficiency and thermal benefits as the more angled Kelman tip. While Dr. Akahoshi prefers a square configuration on his tip and Dr. Osher prefers a 30° round tip, a variety of tip options and innovations are likely to appear in the future.

■ CONCLUSION ■

Favorable results strongly suggest that these new technologies will be explored and expanded upon by many ophthalmologists.[1,5,6] In the author's personal opinion, microcoaxial phacoemulsification with torsional ultrasound is a lovely marriage that should endure the test of time.

References

[1] Osher RH, Injev VP. Microcoaxial phacoemulsification Part 1: Laboratory studies. J Cataract Refract Surg 2007;33(3):401–407.

[2] Osher RH, Injev VP. Thermal study of bare tips with various system parameters and incision sizes. J Cataract Refract Surg 2006;32:867–872.

[3] Vasavada AR. Phaco tips and corneal tissue: histomorphology and immunohistochemistry reveal the effects of sleeveless and sleeved tips. Cataract & Refractive Surgery Today 2005;June (Suppl.):9–10.

[4] Weikert MP, Koch DD. Phaco wound study: alterations in corneal wound architecture with bimanual microincisional phacoemulsification. Cataract & Refractive Surgery Today 2005;June (suppl):11–13.

[5] Berdahl JP, DeStafeno JJ, Kim T. Corneal wound architecture and integrity after phacoemulsification. Evaluation of coaxial micro incision and micro incision bimanual technique. J Cataract Refract Surg 2007;33:510–515.

[6] Osher RH. Microcoaxial phacoemulsification Part 2: Clinical study. J Cataract Refract Surg 2007;33:408–412.

[7] Boukhny M. Laboratory performance comparison between torsional and conventional longitudinal phacoemulsification. Presented at ASCRS, Session 1-G. 2006.

[8] Solomon K. Alcon CME Program. American Academy of Ophthalmology. 2006.

[9] Liu Y, Zeng M, Liu X, Luo L, Yuan Z, Xia Y, et-al. Torsional mode versus conventional ultrasound mode phacoemulsification: Randomized comparative clinical study. J Cataract Refract Surg 2007;33:287–292.

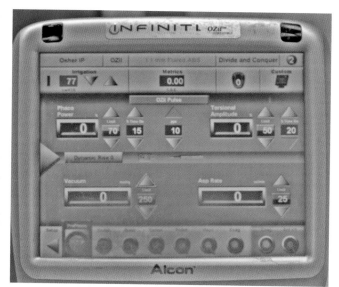

Figure 20-8 Ratio of torsional and longitudinal power can be programmed in addition to duty cycle.

part V

SPECIAL TECHNIQUES FOR CATARACT EXTRACTION

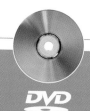
DVD

Phacoemulsification in the Presence of a Small Pupil

I. Howard Fine, MD, Mark Packer, MD, FACS and Richard S. Hoffman, MD

21

TECHNIQUES FOR MANIPULATION OF THE PUPIL

CONTENTS

CHAPTER HIGHLIGHTS

>> Instrumenting a small pupil
>> Use of viscoadaptive devices
>> Iris hooks and expansion rings
>> Intraoperative floppy iris syndrome management

During cataract surgery, the pupil that dilates poorly, is fibrosed or is hyalinized frequently is associated with complications, and can be, therefore, the determining factor in the decision not to proceed with phacoemulsification.

With newer endolenticular techniques, especially with nucleo-fractis procedures and chop techniques,[1–4] pupils do not have to be as large as previously required. This is because much of the procedure takes place in the endolenticular space, within the center of the capsulorrhexis, rather than at the equator of the lens, as in anterior chamber phacoemulsification[5] and nuclear tilt pupillary plane phacoemulsification techniques.[6] However, there still are numerous instances in which the pupil is inadequate to allow the surgeon to proceed, and some form of manipulation or surgery is required.

■ TECHNIQUES FOR MANIPULATION OF THE PUPIL ■

PHARMACEUTICALS

The surgeon may tailor the initial pharmacological intervention for pupillary mydriasis in cataract surgery in order to achieve greater dilation. The use of phenylephrine 10% and cyclopentolate 2% will sometimes produce more effective mydriasis than lower concentrations of these or other agents, especially when administered in multiple doses over 1 h. The use of preoperative nonsteroidal anti-inflammatory agents (NSAIDs), such as flurbiprofen sodium 0.03% (Ocufen, Allergan) or suprofen 1.0% (Profenal, Alcon) mitigates any intraoperative pupillary constriction. Additionally, preservative-free epinephrine 1:10,000 may increase the diameter of the pupil when injected into the anterior chamber at the start of surgery.

VISCOADAPTIVE AGENTS

A viscoelastic device, particularly a high-molecular-weight product, can increase mydriasis by the application of direct mechanical pressure on the pupillary margin during instillation. In particular, we have found Healon 5 (Advanced Medical Optics) to produce stable mydriasis during phacoemulsification. When poor mydriasis is caused by the presence of posterior synechiae and there is adequate zonular support, the surgeon may introduce the viscoelastic cannula between the anterior capsule and the pupillary margin and then inject viscoelastic in order to disrupt the iridocapsular adhesions. The cannula is angled in a tangential fashion to create a wave of viscoelastic, which will dissect the synechiae. Multiple injection sites may be utilized to fully free the pupil. Following dissection of the synechiae, additional dispersive viscoelastic may be injected in the center of the pupil to achieve even greater dilation of the pupillary margin.

INSTRUMENTATION

Often, the pupil can be manipulated with the phacoemulsification handpiece. The surgeon can retract the proximal portion of the pupil through the incision with the sleeve on the phacoemulsification handpiece and effectively enlarge its size (Figure 21-1). This technique requires a great deal of skill and may result in thermal injury with chafing of the pupil and focal depigmentation of the iris. An additional advantage can be obtained by using the second handpiece in such a way as to stretch the pupil in advance of the phacoemulsification tip, once again enlarging the pupil for adequate visualization of structures just under the margin of the pupil (Figure 21-2).

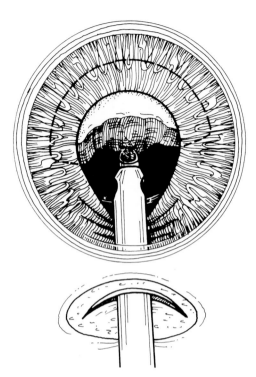

Figure 21-1 Retraction of the proximal pupil with the silicone sleeve of the phaco handpiece.

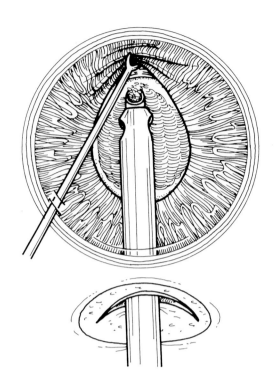

Figure 21-2 Stretching the distal pupil with an instrument through the side-port incision.

In other circumstances, a portion of the lens may be manipulated through the pupil to maintain the pupil in a semi-dilated state. The protruding portion of the nucleus can then be consumed by the phacoemulsification handpiece before repositioning the nucleus within the pupil (Figure 21-3). The surgeon may accomplish mechanical stretching of the pupil with a variety of instruments. Frye[7] has taught a technique that he attributes to Keener of Indianapolis, Indiana. Two hooks are used to engage the pupillary margin at opposite points and steady, gentle pressure is applied across the full extent of the anterior chamber to produce a pupillary diameter of 5–6 mm. A second stretch placed orthogonal to the first increases the diameter further. Viscoelastic protects the anterior lens capsule during this maneuver.

Alternatively, the Beehler pupil dilator (Moria #19009) is uniformly applicable in the presence of small pupils. Inserted through a 2.5 mm single-plane clear corneal incision, it usually stretches the pupil to 6–7 mm while creating tiny microsphincterotomies circumferentially around the pupil (Figure 21-4). The pupil can then be mechanically reduced at the end of the procedure with a Lester hook supplemented with an intraocular miotic agent. Pupils enlarged in this manner maintain a good cosmetic appearance and an ability to react to light, but may require a miotic agent for some time after cataract surgery to prevent the formation of iridocapsular synechiae.

PUPIL DILATING HOOKS AND EXPANSION RINGS

Recently, we have seen a renewed interest in the use of iris hooks as described by McReynolds.[8] Mackool[9] has designed self-retaining titanium hooks that can be placed through paracenteses

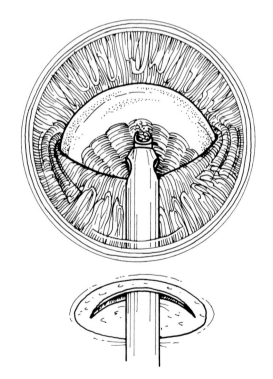

Figure 21-3 Expanding the pupil with nuclear material.

so that the pupil can be positioned and held widely dilated in a triangular or square shape, thus allowing the surgeon to adequately perform phacoemulsification regardless of the initial size of the pupil (Figures 21-5 and 21-6). Although this procedure is somewhat time consuming and results in considerable fluid loss

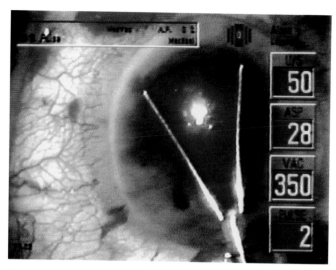

Figure 21-4 The Beehler pupil dilator effectively stretches the pupil to a diameter of 6–7 mm by creating tiny minisphincterotomies.

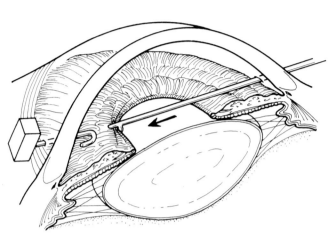

Figure 21-5 Stretching the pupil with an iris repositor in the process of engaging the pupil by the iris hook.

from the eye, as a result of leakage through the paracenteses during phacoemulsification, it is an effective method of pupillary dilation and visualization of the structures for phacoemulsification. De Juan has designed disposable nylon hooks with an adjustable silicone retaining sleeve that can be used through smaller paracentesis (Figures 21-7 and 21-8). Although more costly per case, they may offer some additional advantages as reported by Nichamin,[10] particularly facilitation of removal of the hooks through the paracentesis incisions. More recently, many surgeons have favored a diamond configuration of the pupil by hooks, with one hook under the clear corneal phaco incision.

Pupil expander rings represent another option in the surgical armamentarium for small pupil cases. The Hydroview Iris Protector Ring (Grieshaber) forms a compressed oval in its dehydrated state (Figure 21-9). It can then be placed in the anterior chamber through a 3 mm incision and inserted into the small pupil. This hydrogel device expands with hydration (Figure 21-10), and captures the pupillary margin by means of flanges (Figure 21-11). The ring can be manipulated to expand the pupil as it hydrates. The device then remains in place for the entire surgical procedure, including implantation of the intraocular lens (Figure 21-12), and can then be removed through the same small incision (Figure 21-13). The Morcher Pupil Expander Ring Type 5S is a solid polymethylmethacrylate (PMMA) ring that is placed at the pupillary margin and

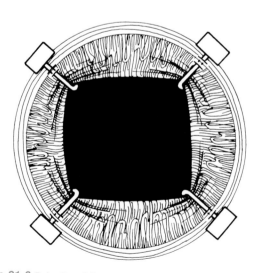

Figure 21-6 Refraction of the pupil by self-retaining titanium iris hooks.

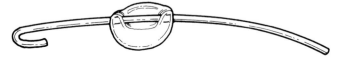

Figure 21-7 Disposable nylon hook with adjustable silicone retaining sleeve.

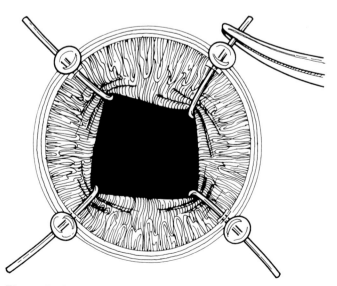

Figure 21-8 Tightening the sleeve on the retractor to adjust the pupillary aperture.

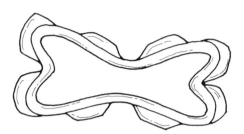

Figure 21-9 Dehydrated iris protector ring.

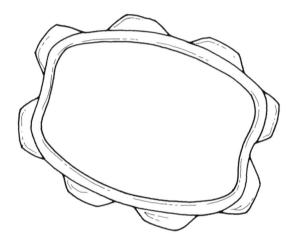

Figure 21-10 Iris protector ring expanding as it hydrates.

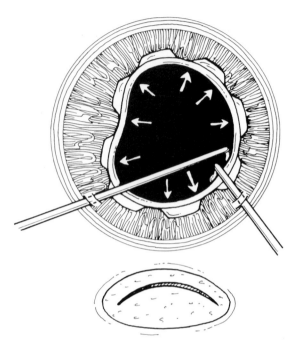

Figure 21-11 Manipulation of the ring into position and dilation of the pupil as the ring expands.

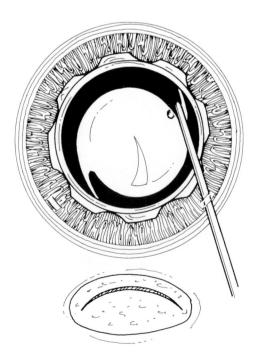

Figure 21-12 Implantation of intraocular lens through iris protector ring.

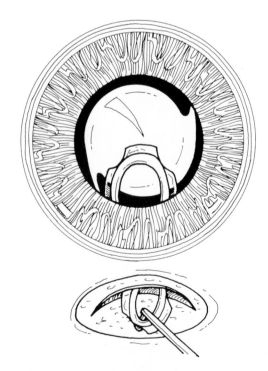

Figure 21-13 Removal of the iris protector ring.

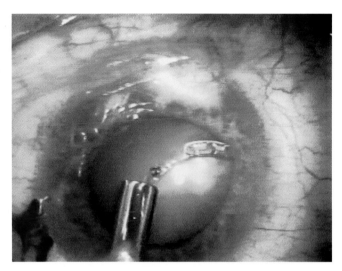

Figure 21-14 The Morcher pupil dilator may be injected via a device available from Geuder, as seen in this case of floppy iris.

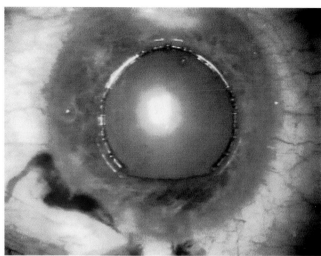

Figure 21-15 The Morcher pupil dilator in place, permitting capsulorrhexis and completion of the surgery.

expands the pupil through 300° of even tension, thus reducing the likelihood of iris sphincter tears and postoperative pupillary deformity. The ring may be introduced into the anterior chamber with forceps and then placed within the pupillary margin with a small hook. The central segment of the ring is manipulated into position, first in apposition to the distal pupillary margin, and then the ends of the ring are placed with the aid of eyelets on the ring. Following implantation of the intraocular lens, the ring is removed by first freeing the ends from their point of apposition with the pupil by means of the small hook, again placed in each eyelet. The ring may then be withdrawn from the anterior chamber with forceps. An injection device is also available for the ring from Geuder (Figures 21-14 and 21-15) (see section on Intraoperative Floppy Iris Syndrome).

The Perfect Pupil (Becton-Dickinson) represents a new and effective option for both maintaining mydriasis and protecting the pupillary margin during surgery. This polyurethane device features a 7 mm internal diameter and an available injection device.

Another helpful and easy-to-use expansion ring is the Malyugin ring (Microsurgical Technology (MST)). This ring is supplied with a disposible injector that compresses the ring to allow its insertion and then its controlled expansion within the eye.

■ IRIS SURGERY ■

A variety of techniques using iris surgery enable enlargement of the pupil. A proximal sphincterotomy can be performed by grasping the superior sphincter and pulling it out of the incision. A small segment of the sphincter can be excised, after which the iris is repositioned (Figure 21-16).[11] Although this procedure results in a permanently enlarged pupil that may be somewhat oval (Figure 21-17), it does

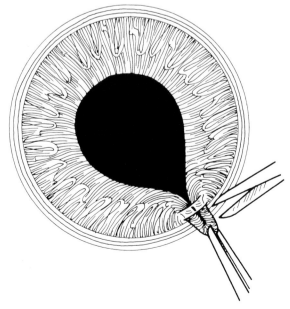

Figure 21-16 Excising a portion of the proximal iris sphincter.

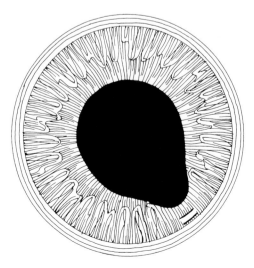

Figure 21-17 Enlargement of the pupil following partial sphincterotomy.

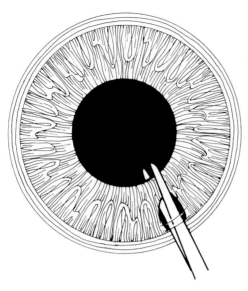

Figure 21-18 Midiris iridectomy.

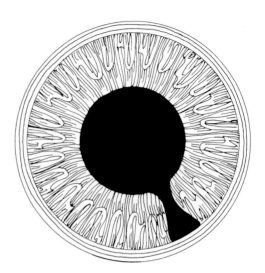

Figure 21-19 Appearance of sector iridectomy following sphincterotomy through midiris iridotomy.

frequently achieve adequate dilation for completion of the surgery. This has been found especially useful in glaucoma patients undergoing cataract surgery and may be combined with a small inferior sphincterotomy.

Performing a superior sector iridectomy is frequently used for pupillary enlargement. However, this technique subjects the patient to glare and other undesirable retinal images postoperatively because of the permanently enlarged pupil and the potential for edge effects from lenses and haptics uncovered by the prominently enlarged pupils.

A modification of the superior sector iridectomy, which tends to give adequate dilation for surgery and yet is less of a problem postoperatively, is the superior midiris iridectomy followed by sphincterotomy. This allows the pillars of the iris to come together more closely following completion of the surgery than does a sector iridectomy (Figures 21-18 and 21-19).

Many surgeons use a suture to close the sphincterotomy at the completion of surgery, hoping to avoid potential sources of glare and trying to achieve a more cosmetically acceptable appearance postoperatively. These sutures may be preplaced through the clear cornea. The posterior loop is drawn out of the peripheral iridectomy with a hook before sphincterotomy (Figures 21-20–21-23). Alternatively, the suture may be placed through clear cornea at the end of the surgical procedure. The ends are drawn out of

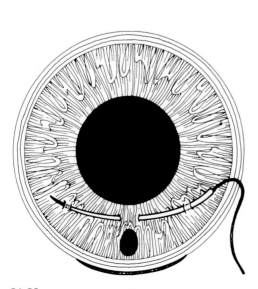

Figure 21-20 Needle is passed through clear cornea through each of the iris pillars and back out through cornea on the other side.

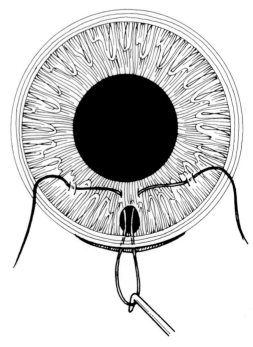

Figure 21-21 Central loop pulled through the peripheral iridotomy out of the incision before sphincterotomy.

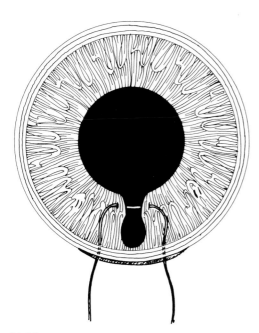

Figure 21-22 Suture is cut from the needle, and both ends are brought out of the incision for tying after lens implantation.

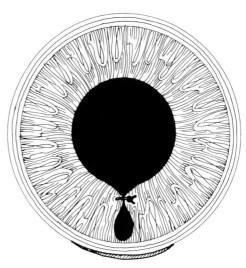

Figure 21-23 Appearance of the iris following tying of the suture to close the sphincterotomy.

the cataract incision and tied in the same way as originally described by Worst and reported by Drews.[12]

Masket[13] has described a technique for using a preplaced suture in the inferior or distal portion of the iris (Figure 21-24), drawing a loop of the central segment of the suture out of the incision (Figure 21-25) and then performing a sphincterotomy inferiorly or distally (Figure 21-26). After implantation of the intraocular lens, the ends of the suture are drawn out of an inferior or distal limbal self-sealing paracentesis and tied (Figure 21-27). This can

dramatically increase exposure to the area in which most of the phacoemulsification takes place. Exposure is increased specifically at the distal portion of the capsulorrhexis and the capsular bag just under the distal capsular flap (Figure 21-28). This suture can restore an acceptable cosmetic appearance to the pupil postoperatively and remove the potential for unwanted glare (Figure 21-29). An additional iris surgical procedure for pupillary enlargement is the pupilloplasty technique of Fine.[14] After lysing synechiae, partial-thickness sphincterotomies are made using

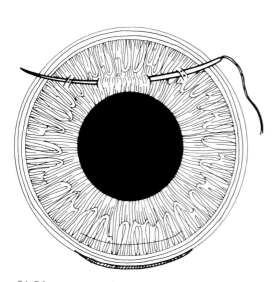

Figure 21-24 Preplacement through clear cornea of iris suture distally.

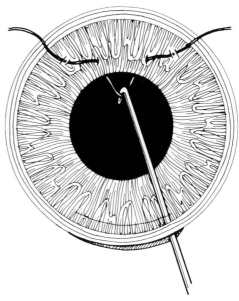

Figure 21-25 Retrieval of central loop of suture from under the iris and through the incision.

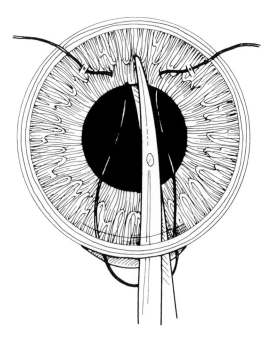

Figure 21-26 Inferior sphincterotomy.

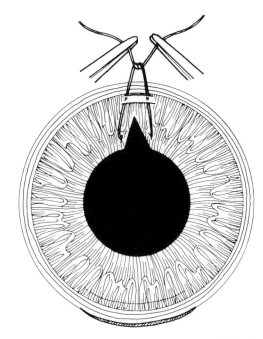

Figure 21-27 Closure of distal iris sphincter after lens implantation.

Rappazzo scissors (Storz Instruments, E-1961-A) through the paracentesis or through the cataract incision (Figures 21-30 and 21-31). The sphincterotomies cut full thickness through approximately half the width of the musculus sphincter pupillae (Figure 21-32) at each of eight sites (Figure 21-33). Following sphincterotomies, each of the sites is stretched to the root of the iris. We believe that this results in the fracturing of the hyalinized fibrotic portions of the pupil but only stretching of the residual circular muscle in the pupil that was not transected. This technique usually achieves 6–7 mm pupil diameters, regardless of the initial size of the pupil (Figure 21-34). At the completion of the phacoemulsification and implantation procedure, a Lester-type hook is used to mechanically return the pupil to as small a configuration as possible (Figures 21-35 and 21-36). The patient uses miotic drops and ointments postoperatively to keep the pupil small and to avoid synechiae from the sphincterotomy sites to the anterior edge of the capsulorrhexis. This technique tends to achieve an excellent cosmetic appearance postoperatively (Figures 21-37 and 21-38) and also allows more normal and physiologic behavior of the pupil.

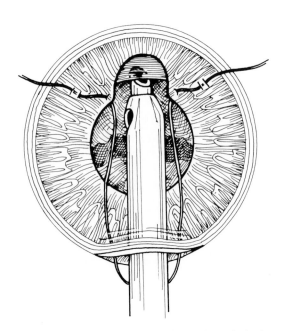

Figure 21-28 Maximum exposure under the distal capsulorrhexis.

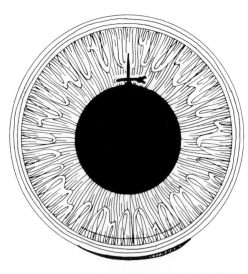

Figure 21-29 Undilated view of the patient postoperatively.

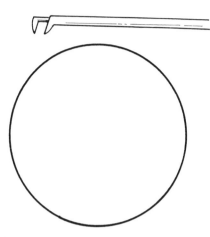

Figure 21-30 Rappazzo scissors relative to size of a US government dime.

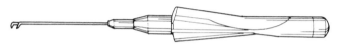

Figure 21-31 Rappazzo scissors showing squeeze-action handles that cause opposing blades to shear.

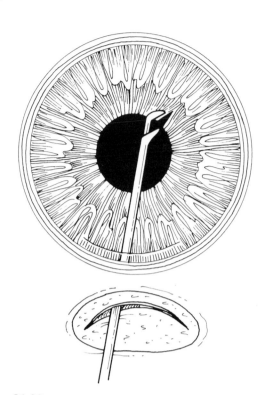

Figure 21-32 Half-width sphincterotomy.

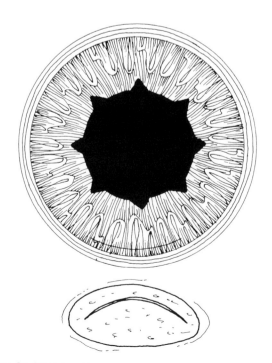

Figure 21-33 Eight sphincterotomies.

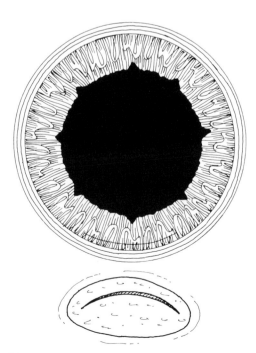

Figure 21-34 Appearance of pupil after stretching.

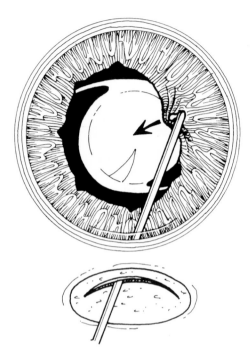

Figure 21-35 Mechanical reduction of pupil size using Lester hook.

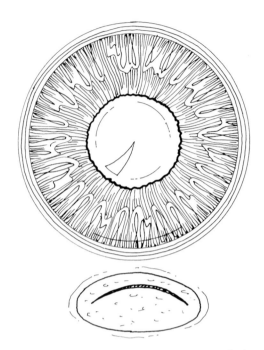

Figure 21-36 Appearance of pupil immediately postoperatively.

Osher[15] has described pupillary membrane dissection as a technique to allow dilation of the pupil to an adequate diameter. This procedure involves meticulous dissection with a bent needle or microforceps to free and remove a fibrotic pupillary membrane (Figures 21-39 and 21-40). This technique is time consuming and may produce some bleeding, but it has proved a valuable aid in the management of some cases of small pupil.

■ INTRAOPERATIVE FLOPPY IRIS SYNDROME ■

Intraoperative floppy iris syndrome (IFIS) has presented new challenges to cataract surgeons.[16] Over a short period of time,

we have learned a variety of new tricks for managing this challenge.

As advised by Sam Masket, MD,[17] we do not discontinue Flomax, but have the patients instill 1% atropine drops qid for 1 week preoperatively. At the time of surgery, we never stretch the pupil, because that seems to exacerbate the tendency for the iris to be floppy and to prolapse.

BIMANUAL TECHNIQUE

Bimanual microincision phacoemulsification in the case of soft or moderate nuclear densities is quite advantageous, because the small size of the incisions makes it less likely that the iris will actually prolapse if it comes to the incision. Cortical cleaving hydrodissection and hydrodelineation are performed and then

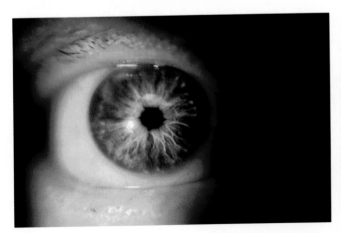

Figure 21-37 Late postoperative appearance of sphincterotomized and stretched light brown pupil.

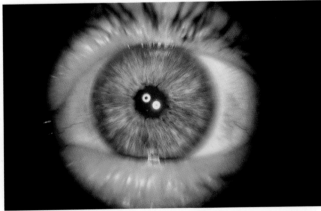

Figure 21-38 Late postoperative appearance of sphincterotomized and stretched blue pupil.

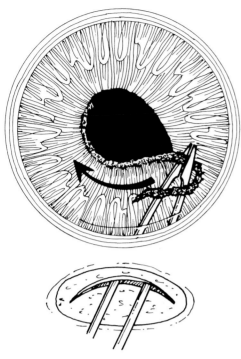

Figure 21-39 Dissection of pupillary membrane.

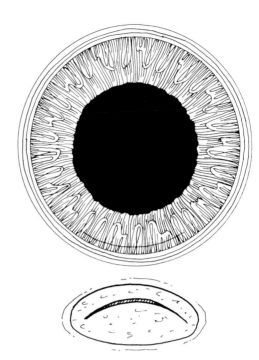

Figure 21-40 Dilation of pupil after dissection and peeling of pupillary membrane.

the lens is hydroexpressed into the plane of the iris. The unsleeved phaco needle in the right-hand incision with the bevel turned toward the cataract, and the irrigator in the left hand, sitting high in the anterior chamber above the lens are used. The lens itself keeps the iris back and the fact that the irrigation is anterior to the iris tends to keep the iris taught and prevents it from billowing. Using very little ultrasound energy and high vacuum, the endonucleus is removed while carouselling the nuclear complex in the plane of the iris. At the completion of the removal of the endonucleus, one can see how the iris was held back by the remaining epinuclear shell (Figure 21-41). That is then removed by the phacoemulsification needle while the anteriorly positioned irrigator keeps the iris taut and posteriorly located so that it cannot billow with a constriction of the pupil.

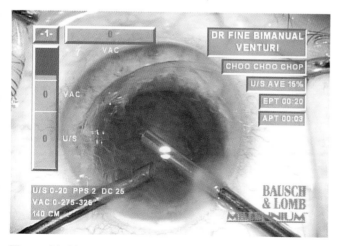

Figure 21-41 The epinuclear shell holds the iris back, keeping it in an adequately dilated state.

THE USE OF HEALON 5 WITH BIMANUAL PHACO AND INTRAOPERATIVE FLOPPY IRIS SYNDROME

The use of Healon 5 is very advantageous for bimanual phaco-emulsification of harder nuclei. The pupil is manually dilated with the Healon 5 and a slightly larger capsulorrhexis is performed. We do one endolenticular horizontal chop, and then we keep the irrigating chopper high in the anterior chamber throughout the remainder of the phacoemulsification procedure, mobilizing nuclear material from the endolenticular space and bringing it up the chopper for further disassembly. We try to keep the phaco tip occluded as much as possible, and if there is a clearance of occlusion, we try to go directly to foot position 1 rather than 2 to avoid evacuating Healon 5 from the eye. The irrigating chopper high in the anterior chamber allows fluid from it to press against the iris and keep it retroplaced disallowing billowing or floppiness of the iris and helping to maintain pupillary dilation. It is very easy to mobilize nuclear material with a bevel-down tip from the endolenticular space. We then will evacuate the epinucleus in the usual form and throughout the procedure we do lose some Healon 5 and as a result the pupil will come down some, but the iris will never be allowed to billow or become floppy.

Following the completion of phacoemulsification, we will once again maximally dilate the pupil with Healon 5. To avoid mobilizing Healon 5 during cortical cleanup, the aspirator is used in a circumferential pattern along the capsulorrhexis evacuating cortical material from the capsular fornices without allowing a clearance of occlusion. Once again, the anterior position of the irrigator was advantageous for maintaining a retroplaced iris and disallowing billowing or floppiness of the iris with concomitant constriction. We end up with a very good-looking iris, free from any trauma.

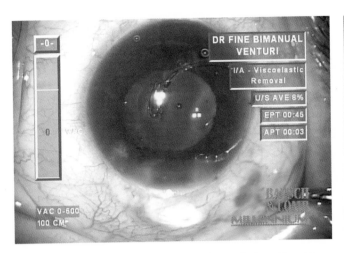

Figure 21-42 The Morcher Pupil Expander Ring perfectly positioned for retrieval out of the eye with the injector.

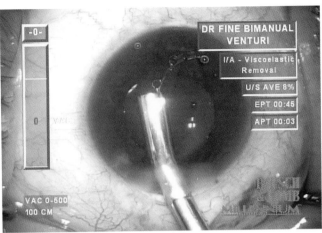

Figure 21-43 The Morcher Pupil Expander Ring is removed from the eye with the injector.

THE USE OF PUPIL EXPANDER RINGS IN INTRAOPERATIVE FLOPPY IRIS SYNDROME

The use of the Morcher Pupil Expander Ring (Type 5S, FCI Ophthalmics, Marshfield Hills, MA) is extremely advantageous in conjunction with coaxial phacoemulsification. The ring can be inserted through a 2.5 mm incision with an injection system (Geuder Pupil Dilator Injector, #G-32970, FCI Ophthalmics, Marshfield Hills, MA) so that the flanges engage the pupil as it is being introduced. The ring is introduced following incision construction and filling of the anterior chamber with a dispersive viscoelastic. The position of the pupil can actually be adjusted by adjusting the position of the ring. With the ring in place, capsulorrhexis, the hydrosteps, phacoemulsification, cortical clean-up, and intraocular lens implantation are performed. Prior to removing the viscoelastic, the ring is disengaged from the pupil and moved to the extreme right side of the anterior chamber with the leading edge of the open portion of the ring directly confronting the incision (Figure 21-42). The injection instrument can then be placed back into the incision and the hook in the injection system can engage the leading eyelet and draw the ring back into the injector by the spring-loaded plunger (Figure 21-43). If the ring enters the injector at an angle, a piece of the leading positioning hole will snap off leaving the surgeon with a disadvantageous circumstance of a transparent intraocular foreign body, so it is very important to properly position the ring prior to removing it with the injector. However, the use of the injector for the removal of the ring dramatically reduces the potential for any injury to intraocular contents or to the incision itself.

CHALLENGING CASES

In the disadvantageous set of circumstances in which one is confronted with a small pupil from Flomax, pseudoexfoliation, and extremely shallow anterior chamber, we have found it preferable to do a pars plana, transcleral, 25-gauge vitrectomy (25 Gauge High Speed Vitrectomy cutter tip, Bausch & Lomb, San Dimas, CA, #CX 5825) as an initial step in the operation (Figure 21-44).

This deepens the chamber, facilitates retroplacement of the iris, and creates adequate room for further manipulations. One has to maintain tactile feedback with regards to the softness of the eye, as this high-speed vitrector can overly soften the eye, which can retroplace the lens enough to challenge further the already weakened zonular apparatus. Following the completion of the transcleral vitrectomy, the conjunctival and scleral incisions do not need to be sutured. The anterior chamber is then filled with viscoelastic, the pupil expander ring is injected, and capsulorrhexis is performed. Gentle cortical cleaving hydrodissection is performed to facilitate later cortical clean-up. A capsular tension ring is then injected into the capsular fornix to stabilize the lens during the extraction procedure and to provide some additional long-term centration of the intraocular lens (IOL). Horizontal chopping is preferred because it avoids downward pressure on the lens which could challenge the weakened zonules.[18]

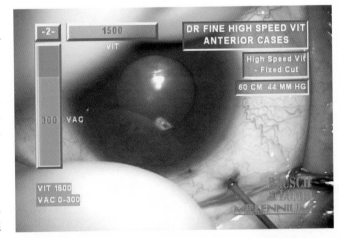

Figure 21-44 Pars plana transcleral 25-gauge vitrectomy prior to commencing cataract surgery in a patient with pseudoexfoliation, floppy iris syndrome and a very shallow anterior chamber. Tactile feedback of the softening of the eye is evidenced by the fingers shown in the illustration.

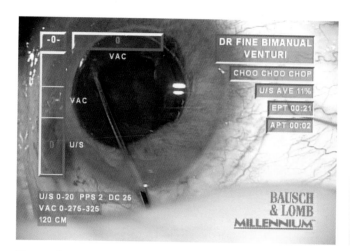

Figure 21-45 Inside-out hydrodelineation following bowling-out of the central portion of the endonucleus in a case in which no hydrodissection or hydrodelineation had previously been performed.

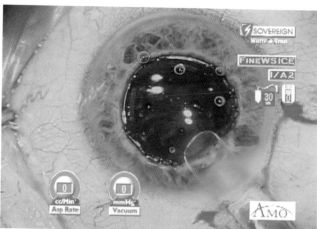

Figure 21-46 Subincisional cortex is removed with a microincision aspirator while the iris is held back with coaxial irrigator.

It is very important that one be aggressive during cortical clean-up in the presence of a capsular tension ring because there can be substantial amounts of cortex hidden from view. Going behind the iris with an aspirator and stripping cortex circumferentially, rather than centrally, vastly facilitates the removal of the cortex from around the ring, rather than trapping the capsular tension ring by engaging the anterior and posterior leaf of the cortex and stripping centrally. The use of cortical cleaving hydrodissection just prior to the introduction to the capsular tension ring is very beneficial for later removal of the cortex.

HYDROSTEPS

In IFIS, hydrodissection and hydrodelineation are difficult because of the tendency for the iris to prolapse out of the eye. In cases in which there is inadequate hydrodissection and hydrodelineation, rotation of the cataract may not be possible. We can do vertical chopping to create very thin, small pie-shaped segments distally. With the removal of three or four distal pie-shaped segments, enough room within the capsular bag has been created so that rotation can then be done. This allows chopping circumferentially, after which the epinucleus can be flipped and mobilized.

In cases in which there is no opportunity to perform hydrodissection or hydrodelineation because of the tendency of the iris to prolapse, one can bowl out a small portion of the central endonucleus and then do hydrodelineation from inside-out (Figure 21-45) as first described by Abhay Vasavada, MD, for hard cataracts.[19] This will result in an ability to then rotate the endonucleus and then chop the residual endonuclear bowl in the usual manner. One can then flip the epinucleus in the usual manner.

COAXIAL PHACOEMULSIFICATION

On occasion, with coaxial phacoemulsification it can be very advantageous to remove subincisional cortex by using a small 1.1 mm paracentesis from the side of the eye opposite the incision for microincision aspirator while utilizing the coaxial handpiece as the irrigator to hold the iris back in the subincisional area (Figure 21-46). This has been a useful trick for us in a variety of cases.

INTRAOCULAR LENS IMPLANTATION

It is important in floppy irises that the cartridge of the injection system for IOL implantation be turned bevel-up as it is introduced into the incision in order to prevent prolapse of iris into the cartridge. The cartridge is turned bevel-down to deliver the lens as usual, but after the lens is in the bag, it is turned bevel-up again so that it acts as a shoe-horn as it exits the eye and doesn't allow the iris to prolapse either into the cartridge or out of the eye (Figure 21-47).

These maneuvers are easily performed by all phaco surgeons. They reduce the challenges and the complications[16] of operating on Flomax patients.

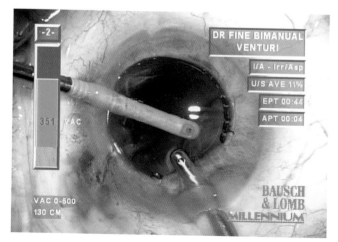

Figure 21-47 Bevel-up withdrawal of the cartridge following injecting of an intraocular lens into the capsular bag.

■ CONCLUSION ■

In conclusion, phacoemulsification in the presence of a small pupil continues to pose a challenge to the surgeon. However, the diverse techniques for management of these pupils present us with options for reducing complication rates to the standard low level.

References

[1] Gimbel HV. Divide and conquer nucleofractis phacoemulsification: development and variations. J Cataract Refract Surg 1991;17:281–291.

[2] Shepherd JF. In situ fracture. J Cataract Refract Surg 1990;16:436–440.

[3] Fine IH, Maloney WF, Dillman DM. Crack and flip phacoemulsification technique. J Cataract Refract Surg 1993;19:797–802.

[4] Fine IH. The choo-choo chop and flip phacoemulsification technique. Operative Techniques in Cataract and Refractive Surgery 1:61–65.

[5] Kelman CD. Phacoemulsification in the anterior chamber. Ophthalmology 1979;86:1980–1982.

[6] Kratz RP, Colvard DM. Kelman phacoemulsification in the posterior chamber. Ophthalmology 1979;86:1983–1984.

[7] Frye LL. Pupil stretch maneuver. Course No. 454 (Modern Phaco/ECCE Implant Surgery: XII, Wed. Nov 11, 1992). Dallas, TX: American Academy of Ophthalmology.

[8] McReynolds WU. Pupil dilator for phacoemulsification. In: Emery JM, Paton D, editors. Current concepts in cataract surgery. Selected Proceedings of the First Biennial Cataract Surgery Congress. St. Louis: CV Mosby Co; 1976.

[9] Mackool RJ. Small pupil enlargement during cataract extraction: a new method. J Cataract Refract Surg 1992;18:523–526.

[10] Nichamin LD. Enlarging the pupil for cataract extractions using flexible nylon iris retractors. J Cataract Refract Surg 1993;19:795–796.

[11] Fishkind WA, Koch PS. Managing the small pupil. In: Koch PS, Davison JA, editors. Textbook of advanced phacoemulsification techniques. Thorofare, NJ: Slack, Inc; 1991. p. 79–90.

[12] Drews RC. Straight needle technique. In: Emery JM, Jacobson AC, editors. Current concepts in cataract surgery. Selected Proceedings of the Eight Biennial Cataract Surgical Congress. Norwalk, CT: Appleton-Century-Crofts; 1984.

[13] Masket S. Preplaced inferior iris suture method for small pupil phacoemulsification. J Cataract Refract Surg 1992;18:518–522.

[14] Fine IH. Pupilloplasty for small pupil phacoemulsification. J Cataract Refract Surg 1994;20: 192–196.

[15] Osher RH. Pupillary membranectomy [Videotape]. Audiovisual J Cataract implant Surg 1991;7.

[16] Chang DF, Campbell JR. Intraoperative floppy iris syndrome associated with tamsulosin. J Cataract Refract Surg 2005;31:664–673.

[17] Personal communication with Samuel Masket, MD.

[18] Fine IH, Hoffman RS. Phacoemulsification in the presence of pseudoexfoliation: challenges and options. J Cataract Refract Surg 1997;23:160–165.

[19] Vasavada AR, Raj SM. Inside-out delineation. J Cataract Refract Surg 2004;30:1167–1169.

Combined Cataract Implant and Filtering Surgery

Anup K. Khatana, MD, John S. Cohen, MD and
Robert H. Osher, MD

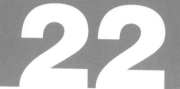

CONTENTS

CHAPTER HIGHLIGHTS

>> Indications for combined surgery
>> Step-by-step surgical technique
>> Management of complications

HISTORY

The indications for combined surgery have evolved full circle during the past several decades. In the 1970s and early 1980s, cataract surgery alone was thought to have a beneficial effect on long-term glaucoma control.[1-3] Although the precise mechanism for this is not known, large incisions and large sutures often resulted in unintentional filtering blebs in some eyes and probable subclinical filtration in others, which had beneficial effects on intraocular pressure (IOP) in glaucoma eyes. Combined surgery at that time was technically more complex than present techniques and was associated with greater risks and limited success. To avoid the increased risks of this more complex surgery, patients often underwent staged surgery with performance of one procedure and then the other, resulting in a longer total period of rehabilitation.

In the 1980s, with newer techniques of extracapsular surgery and safer intraocular lenses (IOLs), cataract surgery was performed earlier with improved visual results. In the late 1980s and 1990s, more secure closure of surgical incisions and concern about the risks of postoperative IOP elevations prompted greater interest in combined cataract and glaucoma surgery.[4-8] Enthusiasm, however, was dampened with clinicians' belief that the more extensive combined procedure resulted in less filtration than trabeculectomy surgery when performed alone. With the ability to increase filtration after combined surgery by modifying wound healing with antimetabolite therapy, the indications became more liberal. Expectations increased that short- and long-term IOP control would be improved, many patients would be able to discontinue glaucoma medications altogether, and both cataract and glaucoma would be effectively managed with one surgical procedure. Several studies showed the benefits of this approach with minimal complications.[9-11] In time, however, it became evident that antimetabolite use was associated with a small but troubling incidence of complications such as leaking blebs, hypotony, "blebitis," and endophthalmitis, which represented a significant contrast to the infrequent incidence of complications of cataract surgery alone. In addition, with the development of small-incision surgery, clear corneal incisions, foldable IOLs placed in the capsular bag, and improvements in techniques of anesthesia and virtually same-day rehabilitation, cataract surgery alone became much more desirable if it could be performed without risk of glaucoma damage from perioperative IOP elevation.

With the realization that IOP elevations were uncommon (although still possible) following the present minimally traumatic technique of phacoemulsification and IOL implantation, cataract surgery alone is becoming the procedure of choice in many patients with diagnoses of ocular hypertension, glaucoma suspect, and early-to-moderate glaucoma. Combined surgery may rarely be considered in eyes with diagnoses of ocular hypertension and glaucoma suspect when IOP is significantly elevated despite the use of multiple medications. (This may also be a situation in which cataract surgery combined with nonpenetrating deep sclerectomy/viscocanalostomy or other still unproven newer options such as endocyclophotocoagulation (ECP), Schlemm's canal surgery, etc., can be considered.) Combined surgery is usually advisable when glaucoma is uncontrolled with maximum medical therapy, glaucoma control requires more than two medications (or fewer if unused medications are contraindicated), and damage is advanced with visual field loss threatening or involving fixation even if the IOP is controlled.

■ SURGICAL OPTIONS IN PATIENTS WITH CATARACT AND GLAUCOMA ■

Before any surgical procedure is performed, advantages and disadvantages must be considered, taking into account the severity of the disease, condition of the fellow eye, availability and affordability of medications, compliance with medication schedules, and compliance with follow-up visits. Patient compliance with long-term follow-up is important to provide continued monitoring of the IOP, discs, visual fields and bleb appearance. As with most surgical procedures, the precise indications for combined surgery vary among surgeons depending on the level of comfort, experience, and skill. The surgeon and patient must balance the benefits and risks of performing combined cataract and glaucoma surgery with those of performing either procedure alone.

CATARACT SURGERY ALONE (PHACOEMULSIFICATION)

Cataract surgery alone can be performed efficiently with rapid, if not immediate, visual recovery in most cases. Postoperative elevation of IOP is a risk in all eyes. Its occurrence must be considered when choosing a surgical procedure in eyes with ocular hypertension, pigment dispersion syndrome, pseudoexfoliation, primary open-angle glaucoma, postoperative pressure spike in the fellow eye, and a family history of glaucoma. One study measured IOP after phacoemulsification performed with clear corneal and sclerocorneal incisions in eyes without glaucoma. Peak elevations were higher for sclerocorneal than clear corneal incisions, measuring 43 and 37 mm Hg 6 h postoperatively for each group, respectively, and 30 mm Hg for both groups 24 h postoperatively. At 15 months, peak IOP measured 19 mm Hg in both groups. Eyes with glaucoma would be expected to be at greater risk of IOP elevation.[6,12–14]

Although no formal surveys have polled surgeons regarding approaches to coexisting cataract and glaucoma, as a general rule of thumb, cataract surgery alone will be considered if the glaucoma is adequately controlled with two or fewer medications (with no contraindications or allergy to the remaining available medications) and visual field loss does not involve fixation (Table 22-1). The surgeon must anticipate the possibility of an acute and/or chronic postoperative elevation of IOP that could require an increase in medical therapy. Perioperative beta-blocker and carbonic anhydrase inhibitor therapy should be considered to reduce this risk. Postoperative IOP elevation may be more likely in the presence of coexisting uveitis, when iris manipulation or posterior synechialysis is required, if peripheral anterior synechiae are present, when cortex or viscoelastic agents are incompletely removed, and so on. In addition, there may be a relative contraindication to the use of prostaglandin analogues and miotics postoperatively because of the potential increased risk of inflammation and cystoid macular edema. If visual field loss involves or threatens fixation, delay in lowering a postoperative IOP spike could result in progression of glaucoma damage with increased visual disability. These risks warrant consideration of combined surgery. The authors favor a conservative approach and, when in doubt, consider combined surgery.

Table 22-1 Indications for single or combined surgery

Phacoemulsification
Indications
Presence of a cataract that impairs visual function or prevents adequate view of the optic nerve, with:

- IOP controlled with fewer than two medications
- ability to use remaining available medications
- mild-to-moderate visual field loss that does not involve or threaten fixation

Trabeculectomy
Indications
Cataract does not decrease visual function or impair view of optic nerve, and cataract progression that would require surgery is not anticipated (surgeon's judgment), with:

- uncontrolled IOP with maximum tolerated medical therapy
- extreme IOP elevation (e.g., with corneal edema, even if significant cataract is present) unless glaucoma is lens induced

Combined surgery
Indications
Cataract decreases visual function or prevents view of optic nerve or is likely to do so if trabeculectomy alone were performed (surgeon's judgment), and:

- uncontrolled IOP with two or more medications
- uncontrolled IOP with less than two medications with others ineffective or contraindicated
- unable to use medications because of cost, compliance, physical limitations, and so on
- pupil stretch or extensive posterior synechialysis required (with resulting debris potentially blocking trabecular outflow and increasing IOP postoperatively)
- extensive peripheral anterior synechia (increasing potential for postoperative IOP elevation)
- visual field loss is moderate to advanced or involves fixation

Cataract surgery employing techniques other than small-incision clear corneal phacoemulsification (such as extracapsular cataract extraction, which usually requires a larger incision and may be associated with more extensive inflammation) may have a greater risk of postoperative IOP elevation and glaucoma damage. Larger incisions and the use of superior incisions, especially ones that involve conjunctiva and sclera, can make future trabeculectomy surgery technically more difficult. This is another reason that temporal "near clear" or clear corneal incisions are preferred, particularly in glaucoma patients.

TRABECULECTOMY SURGERY

Trabeculectomy surgery alone may be considered when the IOP is uncontrolled despite maximum medical therapy and the cataract does not decrease visual function. Even with uneventful trabeculectomy surgery, however, a cataract can progress. If cataract surgery is necessary in the near future, even a clear corneal approach may result in scarring of the filtering bleb with elevation of IOP, requiring additional medical therapy or glaucoma surgery.[15,16] The surgeon's judgment must be used in determining the best procedure for these patients (see Table 22-1).

In cases of marked IOP elevation (e.g., with corneal edema, neovascular glaucoma, traumatic glaucoma) with coexisting cataract, a staged approach with either trabeculectomy with mitomycin C (MMC) or tube implant surgery may be the safest and best choice, deferring consideration of the cataract to a future time when conditions are more controlled. On the other hand, if lens-induced glaucoma is suspected, combined surgery may be the best approach.

COMBINED CATARACT AND TRABECULECTOMY SURGERY

Combined surgery attempts to manage both cataract and glaucoma using one surgical procedure. The choice of this procedure should be determined on an individual basis for each patient (see Table 22-1). Although combined surgery has been considered controversial in the past, it is now accepted as an indicated procedure in selected eyes with coexisting cataract and glaucoma. (For this discussion, combined surgery is defined as phacoemulsification with posterior chamber IOL implantation and trabeculectomy.)[7]

Glaucomatous eyes have compromised trabecular meshwork and reduced aqueous outflow. There is a greater risk of postoperative IOP elevation that may further increase when posterior synechialysis or pupil manipulation is required. Although visual recovery after combined surgery may be delayed compared with cataract surgery alone, it is more rapid than when the glaucoma and cataract are managed separately in a two-stage approach. Combined surgery facilitates the management of postoperative IOP elevations versus cataract surgery alone.[17] However, early postoperative elevations of IOP can occur when combined surgery is performed.[8,18] Use of releasable sutures with combined surgery permits secure wound closure, minimizing risk of a flat or shallow anterior chamber, and permits suture removal to increase aqueous flow and lower IOP postoperatively when the eye is stable.[9] (Laser suture lysis of simple interrupted sutures can be used in place of releasable sutures.)[19]

Although most filtering blebs function successfully, those that fail are more likely to do so within 6 months, with the rest failing years later.[20] Although the use of antimetabolites decreases the incidence of bleb failure, it is important to preserve conjunctiva for possible future filtering surgery. Conjunctival dissection in combined surgery should be restricted to a single superior quadrant (the superotemporal quadrant provides the greatest exposure), leaving the remaining superior quadrant for future glaucoma surgery if needed.

Combined surgery with MMC has been reported to reduce IOP from 13.4% to 34% with 1.2 to 1.4 fewer glaucoma medications. These results were statistically better than both combined surgery with 5-fluorouracil (5-FU) and with no antimetabolite use, which were the same.[9,11] Lack of efficacy of MMC in an additional study may have been due to surgical technique or the risk factors in the patient population studied.[21] It has been suggested that more intensive follow-up and postoperative manipulations were required in the non-MMC group to achieve results statistically similar to the MMC group.

Combined phacoemulsification, IOL implantation, and trabeculectomy surgery with MMC is most applicable in eyes that

have uncontrolled glaucoma with maximum medical therapy and a cataract that impairs vision. Eyes requiring more than two glaucoma medications, eyes controlled on fewer than two medications with others contraindicated or ineffective, and eyes with visual field damage that is advanced or involves fixation may also be good candidates for combined surgery with MMC to minimize the possibility of potentially damaging postoperative IOP elevation. Combined surgery will permit better management of postoperative IOP elevation and provide a high probability of improved short-term and long-term IOP control with fewer medications. In these eyes, it is safer to perform one combined procedure than two separate procedures. Although trabeculectomy with MMC performed alone may have the potential for greater reduction of IOP and glaucoma medications than combined surgery with MMC, the success of combined surgery with MMC more than justifies its use in appropriate patients. In addition, the techniques presently employed in combined surgery do not increase risk more than performing the procedures separately and may even reduce the risk with only one trip to the operating room.

If the glaucoma is controlled with fewer than two medications, with the ability to add others, and visual field loss is mild in an eye with a visually disabling cataract, combined surgery with MMC may not be required. Phacoemulsification with IOL alone may be performed to avoid some of the potential complications of combined surgery, such as bleb dysesthesia, bleb infection, endophthalmitis, etc. Although unlikely, significant IOP elevation can occur. One study showed that one of 17 eyes with stable open-angle glaucoma requiring one or two medications for control had an IOP elevation to 30 mm Hg 1 day following clear corneal phacoemulsification surgery.[22] If postoperative elevation of IOP does occur, significant glaucoma progression is unlikely.

Eyes with a functioning filtering bleb and controlled IOP also require special decision making when planning cataract removal. Present techniques of clear corneal phacoemulsification have a decreased risk of early postoperative elevations of IOP. In 69 eyes undergoing small-incision clear corneal phacoemulsification with a functioning filtering bleb, two eyes required subsequent additional glaucoma surgery. Sixteen eyes required more glaucoma medications postoperatively than preoperatively. If preoperative IOP was less than 15 mm Hg, the chance of needing more medications was 27.6%, and if greater than 15 mm Hg, the chance of needing more was 41.7%. Thus, the surgeon must be aware that, even in this situation, dangerous elevations of IOP could occur with cataract surgery alone and that there is a risk that increased glaucoma therapy will be required.[15,16] If a previously filtered eye has a questionably functioning filtering bleb with a significant cataract and IOP is uncontrolled or controlled with multiple medications in the presence of advanced glaucoma damage, combined surgery may be a good option. Internal or external revision of the existing trabeculectomy combined with phacoemulsification could also be considered.

■ ANTIMETABOLITES ■

Daily postoperative subconjunctival 5-FU injections enhanced filtration success when trabeculectomy was performed alone.[23–25] Although in an early report 5-FU mildly improved filtration success in combined surgery, other studies found no benefit.[26–29]

Chen's pioneering work with MMC,[30] a stronger antimetabolite than 5-FU that could be applied topically at the time of filtering surgery, offered the potential of improved filtration success with combined surgery. The initial report of combined surgery with MMC showed improved IOP control with fewer glaucoma medications at 1-year follow-up. Subsequent investigations have supported these results.[9,30–32]

Although MMC improves the success of filtration in combined surgery, it also may increase the risk of complications such as hypotony maculopathy, bleb leaks, bleb infection, and endophthalmitis. As a result, the concentration of MMC and duration of application have decreased since its initial use. Although MMC appears to have a fairly flat dose–response curve, reduced exposure seems to decrease the incidence of complications.[26,27,33,34]

Many variables are associated with MMC use. Surgeons using similar concentrations and exposure times of MMC may get different results, and surgeons using different concentrations and exposure times may get similar results. The choice of sponge material may be one of these variables. Different cellulose spears, instrument wipes, and corneal caps may each absorb different amounts of MMC and, when placed in contact with tissue, result in different antimetabolite effect. Surgeons may choose materials that will not tear or fragment during application, cut variable-sized pieces of the material to be placed in contact with the tissue, place pressure on the material containing MMC through the overlying conjunctiva to squeeze MMC into the tissues, or use a cellulose spear to absorb any MMC containing liquid that seeps out from beneath the conjunctival flap and threatens to contact the edges of the conjunctival incision. In addition, many surgeons wipe the subconjunctival space lateral and posterior (the space posterior to the conjunctival incision in limbus-based flaps) to the bleb area for about 15–20 s with the hope that a more diffuse, lower-profile filtering bleb will form. This may result in a less localized and cystic bleb with less potential to develop a late leak through a thinned wall.

Each surgeon should develop his or her own technique, starting with conservative MMC exposure times to minimize the risk of complications. The surgeon should consider the risk/benefit ratio of MMC use and err on the side of less rather than more antimetabolite exposure to avoid complications, realizing that additional glaucoma surgery could be required. When the surgeon is comfortable with the technique and the results, the exposure times can be modified and individualized depending on the severity of glaucoma, risk factors for failure, ability to perform additional glaucoma surgery in the future, and so on. (See Application of Mitomycin for specific parameters of one technique of MMC use.)

APPLICATION OF MITOMYCIN BEFORE OR AFTER ENTERING THE ANTERIOR CHAMBER

When MMC was first used in combined surgery, many surgeons applied the antifibrotic agent near the end of the procedure, after watertight closure of the scleral flap. The area was irrigated with balanced salt solution (BSS), and the conjunctiva was closed. No clinically evident adverse effects were noted. Concern subsequently developed over the possibility of toxicity to corneal endothelial cells and the ciliary body epithelium. Experiments in rabbits showed that MMC penetrated the sclera and resulted in detectable aqueous levels. A reversible decrease in aqueous production followed application of MMC to the scleral surface in monkey eyes. However, the dose of MMC used in these studies was larger than that used clinically in humans.[35–38]

MMC can be applied before entering the anterior chamber or after removing the cataract and securely closing the wound to prevent MMC entry into the eye. Cohen[26] provided evidence that topical application of MMC at the end of the procedure after secure closure of the scleral incision does not cause loss of corneal endothelial cells. This method permits the surgeon to abort the use of MMC if a defect occurred in the conjunctiva or in the scleral wound that would contraindicate its use and, therefore, might be safer for the surgeon who is less experienced with combined surgery. When the surgeon is comfortable with the surgical technique, if desired, MMC can be applied before entering the anterior chamber. (See Application of Mitomycin.) Because of the variability of response to MMC seen in the conjunctiva of individual eyes, some surgeons have recently advocated a subconjunctival injection of a standard dose of MMC that is usually performed at the beginning of the operation.

SUBCONJUNCTIVAL OR SUB-TENON'S INJECTION OF ANTIMETABOLITE POSTOPERATIVELY

Based on the work by Gressel, Parrish, and Folberg,[23] which initially showed that daily postoperative subconjunctival injections of 5-FU improve success of trabeculectomy surgery, many surgeons will augment intraoperative antimetabolite therapy with postoperative 5-FU if bleb failure is threatened (increased bleb vascularization, decreased filtration, etc.). Kapetansky has very recently shown a beneficial effect with the use of (usually a single) postoperative subconjunctival injection of the vascular endothelial growth factor (VEGF) inhibitor, bevacizumab, in trabeculectomy eyes at high risk of failure in the first 1–2 months postoperatively (personal communication).

■ RESULTS FOLLOWING COMBINED SURGERY ■

Several prospective and retrospective studies, using varying techniques of MMC application in varying concentrations, found significantly lower IOP with fewer glaucoma medications. Mean IOP decreased 5 mm Hg in the MMC group versus 3 mm Hg in the placebo group. The mean number of medications required for IOP control decreased 0.5 to 2.7 in the MMC groups versus 0.7 to 0.9 in the placebo groups. Fifty percent to 100% of eyes in the MMC groups versus 10% to 67% in the placebo groups were controlled without medications.[9–11,39]

■ COMPLICATIONS FOLLOWING COMBINED SURGERY ■

Complications and their frequency were listed in several prospective and retrospective studies and included vitreous loss (2–7%), wound leak (1–30%), iris incarceration in sclerostomy (2%), shallow anterior chamber (7–14%), serous choroidal detachment (14–27%), hypotony (6–18%), and fibrin formation in the anterior chamber (7–19%). With improved surgical techniques and modified methods and durations of MMC application, complications have been significantly reduced. (The management of complications is discussed under Postoperative Management and Complications.)

■ COMBINED SURGERY METHOD ■

PREOPERATIVE PREPARATIONS

Medications

As with operative technique, the preoperative regimen varies by surgeon. Topical corticosteroid eyedrops are used every 2 h starting the day before surgery. Topical antibiotic eyedrops are used every 2 h starting the evening before surgery. A combination antibiotic-steroid ointment is applied to the eyelashes at bedtime the evening before surgery. A nonsteroidal anti-inflammatory eyedrop is applied twice the morning of surgery. Cyclopentolate 1%, phenylephrine 2.5%, and homatropine 2% eyedrops are applied every 5–10 min for four applications before surgery. One drop of betaxolol (Betoptic) is applied 30 min before surgery. One drop of 5% povidone-iodine (Betadine) solution is administered immediately before the facial prep.[40]

Topical antiglaucoma therapy has been shown to have an adverse effect on the conjunctival inflammatory cellular profile and on filtering surgery success. The use of steroid drops has been shown to have a beneficial effect on both of these parameters. This is why corticosteroid eyedrops are started preoperatively.[41] Consideration should be given to discontinuing IOP-lowering agents that compromise the blood–aqueous barrier, increase the risk of iritis, and make pupillary dilation difficult (such as miotics) several days to a week before surgery. This should not be done if other glaucoma medications cannot be substituted to blunt possible IOP elevation in eyes with advanced glaucoma.

Anesthesia

Although topical anesthesia is used by many surgeons for combined surgery, the authors usually use either a short- or long-acting retrobulbar block. The short-acting block is performed with 3–4 mL of 2% lidocaine (xylocaine) with 150 units of hyaluronidase. The long-acting retrobulbar block is performed with 3–4 mL of 4% lidocaine (xylocaine) and 0.75% bupivacaine (marcaine) in a 1:1 mixture, with 150 units of hyaluronidase combined with a Van Lint block using the same anesthetic mixture and requiring a patch postoperatively. Preoperative discussion with the patient of anesthetic options may be helpful. A postoperative eye patch is not used with short-acting blocks.

The long-acting block may be helpful in more difficult cases when pupil stretch or posterior synechialysis is required and phacoemulsification and cortex removal will be done through a small pupil and capsulorrhexis.

OPERATIVE TECHNIQUE

Conjunctival Flap

One author (JC) prefers a limbus-based flap, while another (AK) prefers a fornix-based flap. Although a limbus-based flap requires more manipulation and is technically more cumbersome than a fornix-based flap, it provides greater certainty of watertight closure and avoidance of postoperative incision leak. In contrast, the fornix-based flap provides easier and better surgical exposure but has a greater risk of postoperative wound leak. Although there is evidence that limbus- and fornix-based flaps result in

the same long-term IOP results, an incision leak is counterproductive to bleb formation.[18,42] When antimetabolites are used with the surgery, leaks may heal more slowly and be more difficult to repair with a fornix-based flap.[9,23] However, the authors will usually perform a fornix-based flap if significant subconjunctival scar tissue exists from previous surgery. The morphology of the blebs that form with limbus-based vs. fornix-based flaps is different. Although both techniques can create broad and diffuse blebs, the bleb may be more elevated, increasing the risk of dysesthesia, with limbus-based flaps. The modified fornix-based technique of creating the conjunctival incision approximately 1.5 mm posterior to the conjunctival insertion at the limbus can create a bleb that is fairly flat anteriorly. This may decrease the risk of dysesthesia and increase the possibility of being able to resume contact lens wear after the incision has healed.

Limbus-based conjunctival flap

Dissection is performed in the superotemporal quadrant to minimize anatomic restrictions from the brow and the superior orbital rim. The initial incision should be made 8–9 mm posterior to the limbus and penetrate the conjunctiva and Tenon's capsule to expose the sclera, using sharp scissors and toothed forceps. Blunt scissors and nontoothed forceps (e.g., Pierse forceps, instrument #2-136, Duckworth & Kent, St. Louis, Mo.) extend the incision parallel to the limbus and laterally in both directions to permit adequate exposure. The incision width usually approximates 12 mm (Figure 22-1). The incision should remain about 8–9 mm from the limbus along the entire length to minimize the limitation of filtration from the incision scar and to avoid the thinner and more delicate conjunctiva that is sometimes present closer to the limbus. Tenon's tissue is bluntly pushed anteriorly with a dry cellulose sponge or curved edge of a blade to expose the limbus. (Sometimes the insertion of Tenon's tissue must be cut to provide adequate exposure. If at all possible, Tenon's capsule insertion should be left intact to provide extra integrity to the bleb.) Blunt dissection is also performed beneath the edge of the conjunctival incision posteriorly with scissors.

Fornix-based conjunctival flap

Either directly superiorly or in the superotemporal quadrant, nontoothed tissue forceps and sharp scissors are used to create a limbal conjunctival incision approximately 7 mm wide. The authors prefer making the conjunctival incision approximately 1.5 mm posterior to the conjunctival insertion in contrast to the standard fornix-based technique of incising the conjunctiva at its insertion to the cornea. Blunt scissors are used to extensively bluntly dissect posteriorly to provide adequate exposure for the scleral incision and a larger potential space for filtration (Figure 22-2).

Scleral Incision and Paracentesis

A three-stage tunnel incision is made with the initial vertical incision approximately 2 mm posterior to the limbus. The first-stage vertical incision is performed at about one-half scleral depth and the necessary width for insertion of the desired IOL (the authors use a 0.37 mm preset diamond blade) (Figure 22-3A). The second stage of the incision is made horizontally, parallel to Descemet's membrane (the authors use a crescent steel blade), and

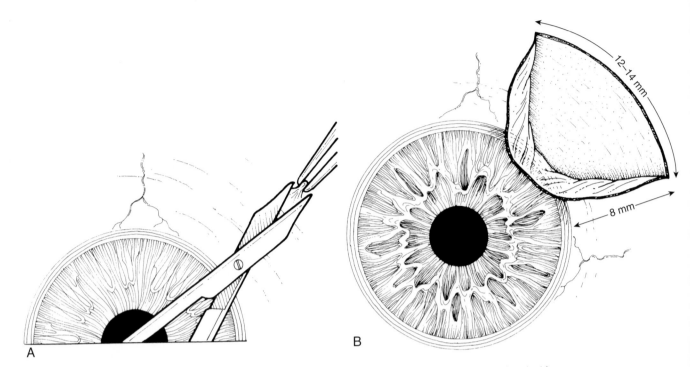

Figure 22-1 A, Initial incision for limbus-based conjunctival flap is made with sharp scissors and toothed forceps, 8–9 mm posterior to the limbus, exposing sclera. B, Limbus-based flap should be about 12 mm wide to provide adequate exposure.

extends approximately 1–2 mm anterior to the limbus. MMC is now used. (See Application of Mitomycin later in text.) If the initial scleral incision inadvertently is made full thickness (as in eyes with thin sclera), the flap can still be dissected anteriorly using only half the scleral thickness. However, it is important to tightly suture the deeper full-thickness area of the incision separately from the rest of the superficial flap prior to MMC application to prevent the development of postoperative hypotony from ciliary body toxicity or a second pathway for aqueous outflow. A keratome blade (appropriate for the size of the phacoemulsification tip) makes the vertical third stage of the incision and enters the anterior chamber (see Figure 22-3B). A narrow, sharp-pointed blade is then used to make a small peripheral paracentesis opening in the cornea, at a position 3 clock hours to the left of the scleral incision (right-handed surgeon) for insertion of a manipulating instrument. A viscoelastic agent is then injected to fill and maintain the anterior chamber.

Alternatively, some surgeons prefer creating the same type of scleral flap they usually create for a straight trabeculectomy – whether triangular, trapezoidal, rectangular or square. This can help to create consistency in management and results between straight trabeculectomies and combined phaco-trabeculectomies.

Application of Mitomycin

Two small pieces of a cellulose spear (the authors use i-Spear ophthalmic sponge, Alcon, Fort Worth, Tex.), each the approximate size of the scleral flap, are soaked in MMC (0.4 mg/mL). These two pieces are then placed on the scleral surface, overlying and extending beyond the scleral tunnel on both sides

(Figure 22-4A). This will spread the MMC effect beyond the area overlying the scleral tunnel and hopefully extend the area of filtration laterally in both directions. The conjunctiva is brought down over the sponges (see Figure 22-4B). The edges of the conjunctival incision should not touch the sponges or any liquid containing MMC. A cellulose sponge should be used to absorb any excess liquid that flows out from under the conjunctival flap. After 1 min of tissue exposure, one of the sponges is removed, and the remaining sponge is positioned centrally on the scleral flap. After an additional minute, the second sponge is removed, and the conjunctival and corneal surfaces, the tissues beneath the edges of the conjunctiva laterally, and the scleral tunnel are irrigated with 15 mL of BSS. An intact piece of cellulose sponge, about 2×3 mm in size, is securely grasped by toothed forceps and wiped beneath the previously dissected posterior subconjunctival space (limbus-based flap) for 15–30 s (see Figure 22-4C). This area is also irrigated with 15 ml of BSS. (When a fornix-based flap is used, a similar maneuver can be performed deeper than the area previously exposed.)

A total of 1 ¾ min of MMC exposure time beneath the limbus-based conjunctival flap is used for most eyes. The duration of exposure may be decreased by 15–30 s if the need for IOP reduction is less because of less severe glaucoma, a reduced tendency for healing related to older age, systemic use of corticosteroids or other immunocompromising drugs, and so on. The duration may be increased by 15–30 s if there are risk factors for failure, such as thicker tissue, younger age, previous surgery, African-American race, or history of inflammation. Evidence has shown that the dose–response curve of MMC is fairly flat but that longer exposure times may have an increased incidence of complications.[33]

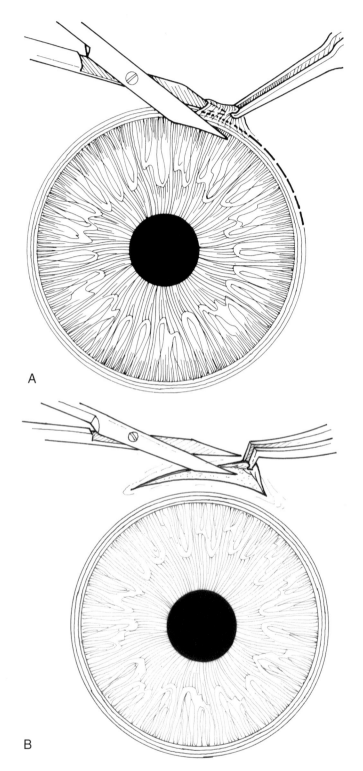

A

B

Figure 22-2 A, Limbal conjunctival incision is made to create a standard fornix-based conjunctival flap. B, Alternate technique for fornix-based conjunctival flap, with the conjunctival incision performed 1.5 mm from the conjunctival insertion.

With fornix-based flaps, two round methylcellulose corneal shields are cut in half. The corneal shield material has excellent integrity, eliminating any concerns over pieces of the sponge material falling apart or being left behind. It also keeps a fairly low profile even after being soaked, allowing a greater surface area of contact with the sclera and Tenon's capsule. The first two pieces are wiped around and then placed in the superonasal and superotemporal subconjunctival space. The third piece is placed over the superior rectus insertion, and the fourth piece is wiped around anteriorly, both nasally and temporally, and then

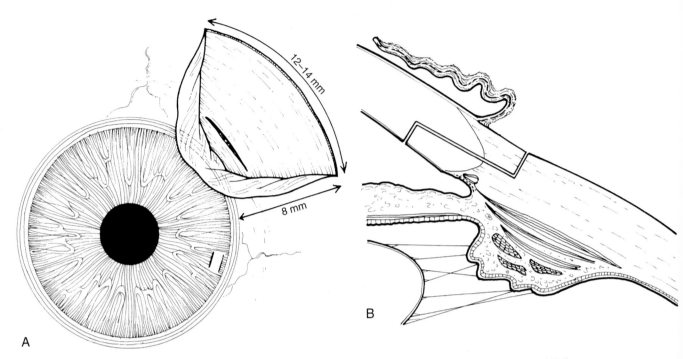

Figure 22-3 **A,** First-stage vertical incision is performed at about one-half scleral depth and the necessary width for insertion of the desired intraocular lens. **B,** Three-stage scleral incision is made into the anterior chamber.

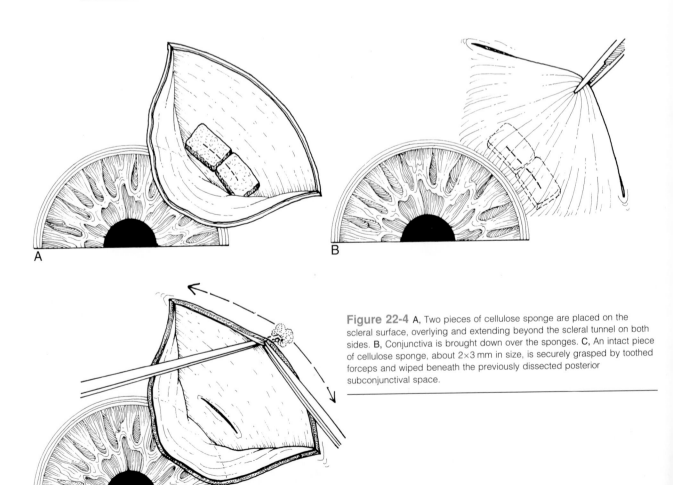

Figure 22-4 **A,** Two pieces of cellulose sponge are placed on the scleral surface, overlying and extending beyond the scleral tunnel on both sides. **B,** Conjunctiva is brought down over the sponges. **C,** An intact piece of cellulose sponge, about 2×3 mm in size, is securely grasped by toothed forceps and wiped beneath the previously dissected posterior subconjunctival space.

placed anteriorly near the area where the posterior edge of the scleral flap will be created. This creates a wedge-shaped area of MMC exposure with the greatest exposure applied posteriorly. While the sponges are in place, the anterior edge of the conjunctival flap is pressed down onto the sclera at the incision site with a cyclodialysis spatula to prevent any external leakage of MMC. The incision surface is then briefly irrigated with BSS to remove any MMC that may have oozed out while the sponges were being inserted. Exposure time varies from a total of 1.5 to 2.5 min for combined surgery, depending on the multiple factors listed in the previous paragraph.

Management of the Small Pupil and Posterior Synechia

Long-term use of glaucoma (especially miotic) eyedrops may limit the effectiveness of pupillary dilation in preparation for phacoemulsification. If the patient is using miotic eyedrops and the IOP and stage of glaucoma permit, discontinuation of the miotics and, if possible, substitution of other glaucoma drops may enhance the mydriasis. The minimum acceptable and comfortable pupil size may vary depending on the specific type and severity of the cataract. A "soft" cataract may not require surgical enlargement of the pupil even if dilation is poor. A brunescent cataract, however, may require surgical enlargement of the pupil even if it dilates moderately. Although manipulation of the pupil may result in decreased sphincter function, patients rarely complain of any problems and are far better off avoiding more serious events such as a capsule defect or vitreous loss. Each surgeon must determine what pupil size is adequate.

The dilated preoperative examination helps predict whether pupil manipulation will be necessary. Stripping a pupillary membrane or lysis of posterior synechia may significantly enhance pupil size. "Viscodilation" with a cohesive viscoelastic may be all that is required to enlarge the pupil to a comfortable size for capsulorrhexis. If further enlargement is required, the authors have found pupil stretch to be successful virtually 100% of the time. Although iris hooks, pupil ring expanders, and minisphincterotomies will enhance pupil size, they are rarely required because of the success of pupil stretch, improved techniques of phacoemulsification, and newer viscoelastics. (See Chapter 21, Phacoemulsification in the Presence of a Small Pupil.)

If pupil enlargement is required, the authors employ a bimanual stretch maneuver. Two instruments designed for iris manipulation are used (Osher Y-hook, E0577, Storz, Claremont, Calif.; Kuglen Iris Hook and IOL Manipulator, 6-400 and 6-402, Duckworth & Kent, St. Louis, Mo.). One instrument is placed in the anterior chamber through the paracentesis opening while the other enters through the phacoemulsification incision, and the pupil is stretched by simultaneously pushing and pulling the pupillary edge of the iris in opposite directions in the same meridian (6 clock hours apart) (Figure 22-5A).[43–45] For additional enlargement, a second stretch maneuver can be performed in a meridian about 90° from the first (see Figure 22-5B), or the two stretch instruments can be placed less than 6 clock hours apart before stretching. A slow and gradual stretch will minimize the risk of an atonic pupil. Self-limited bleeding may occur from the tears in the pupillary margin of the iris. Elevation of the IOP

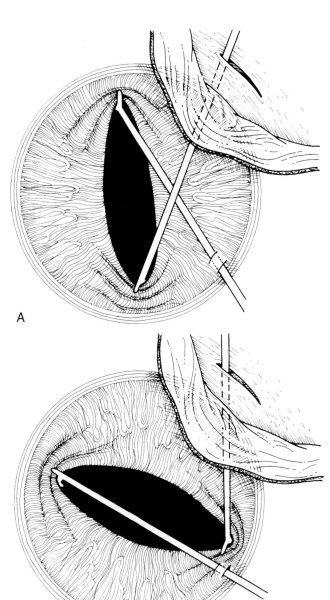

A

B

Figure 22-5 A, Pupil is stretched by simultaneously pushing and pulling the pupillary edge of the iris in opposite directions in the same meridian (6 clock hours apart). B, Additional enlargement can be achieved by performing a second stretch maneuver 90° away from the first.

by filling the anterior chamber with BSS or viscoelastic can help tamponade the bleeding.

In the rare cases when bimanual stretch inadequately dilates the pupil, iris retraction hooks can be helpful. Pupil stretching usually does not have any long-term effect on postoperative vision, IOP or inflammation.[72,73]

Capsulorrhexis

Continuous circular capsulorrhexis is performed using a 22-gauge needle with a right-angle bend made about 1 mm from the tip. An alternate method using capsule forceps is preferred by many surgeons. The size of the capsulorrhexis is often limited by sub-optimal pupillary dilation and may require enlargement later in the procedure when the chamber has been deepened by a viscoelastic agent. (See earlier section, Management of the Small Pupil and Posterior Synechia.) Too small a capsulorrhexis may compromise phacoemulsification and cortical aspiration, increase the risk of a radial extension of the capsulorrhexis, and result in intraoperative and postoperative complications. (Also see Chapter 14, Capsulorrhexis.)

Hydrodissection, Hydrodelineation, and Viscodissection

The nuclear and cortical lens layers are hydrodissected from the lens capsule by gently injecting BSS just beneath the edge of the capsulorrhexis with a blunt 27-gauge cannula, using moderate infusion pressure. The pupil is observed for passage of a fluid wave across the red reflex. When dense cataracts preclude observation of the fluid wave, slight anterior movement of the nucleus confirms hydrodissection. Injection of fluid into the cataractous lens can achieve hydrodelineation by separating the nuclear, epinuclear, and cortical layers. (A 27-gauge J-shaped cannula can direct the hydrodissection to the cortex beneath the scleral incision and achieve better mobilization of the more difficult-to-remove cortex in this area.) Successful hydrodissection is crucial in poorly dilated pupils. It is helpful to test for adequate hydrodissection by rotating the nucleus (with viscoelastic in the anterior chamber) using one or two manipulating instruments. The injection of a viscoelastic may also be used to dissect cortex or nucleus away from the lens capsule when normal irrigation–aspiration techniques may be dangerous (e.g., with a small pupil or capsulorrhexis, capsule defect). (Also see Chapter 15, Hydrodissection and Hydrodelineation.)

Phacoemulsification and Cortical Aspiration

Phacoemulsification is performed using the preferred technique of the surgeon. The authors usually create a central groove greater than two-thirds of the depth of the lens and use a second instrument to help crack the nucleus into two halves. Each half is then rotated and chopped into smaller pieces, which permit easier and safer phacoemulsification in the posterior chamber.

Aspiration of the cortex is performed in the usual manner. This can be more challenging in the presence of a small pupil and capsulorrhexis. An iris manipulating hook should be used to push the iris peripherally and expose the peripheral capsular bag, when it is inadequately seen, to ensure removal of hidden cortex. Use of a separate aspiration cannula (Surgical Design Corporation, Long Island City, NY; Oasis Medical Inc., Glendora, Calif.) that is small enough to be passed through the paracentesis opening or the use of a 90° angled irrigation–aspiration tip can be extremely helpful in removing cortex from the capsular bag opposite the paracentesis and beneath the area of the scleral incision (Figure 22-6A). A J-shaped cannula on a syringe containing BSS can also be used to remove the subincisional cortex after having inflated the bag and anterior chamber with viscoelastic (see Figure 22-6B). (Also see Chapter 16, Principles of Nuclear Phacoemulsification, and Chapter 17, Phaco Chop.)

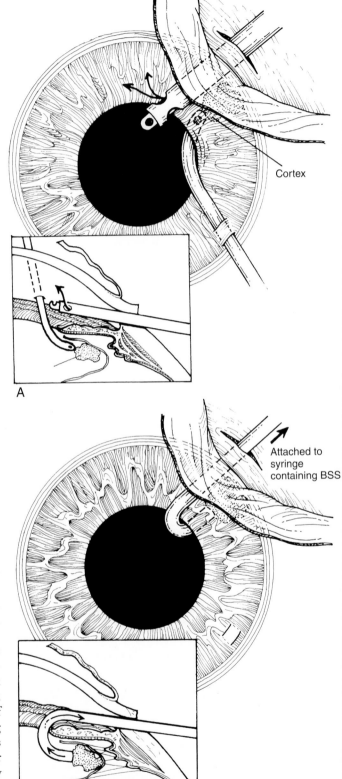

Cortex

Attached to syringe containing BSS

A

B

Figure 22-6 **A,** Separate aspiration canula, small enough to be passed through the paracentesis opening, can be extremely helpful in removing cortex from beneath the area of the scleral incision. **B,** J-shaped cannula on a syringe containing balanced salt solution can also be used to remove the subincisional cortex after inflating the capsular bag with viscoelastic.

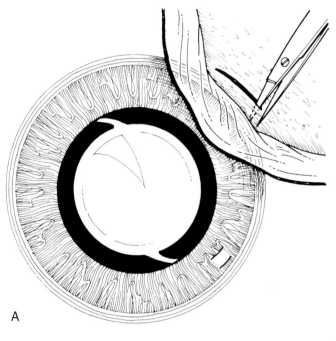

A

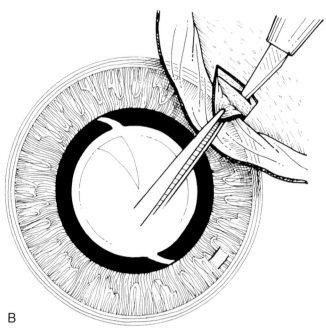

B

Figure 22-7 A, Left side of the scleral tunnel is cut anteriorly to permit elevation of the corner and exposure of the tunnel floor. **B,** Sharp blade is used to make an incision in the scleral floor of the tunnel, parallel to the limbus, about 0.5–1 mm anterior to the posterior edge of the tunnel. **C,** Kelly punch is used to create a sclerectomy on the left side of the tunnel.

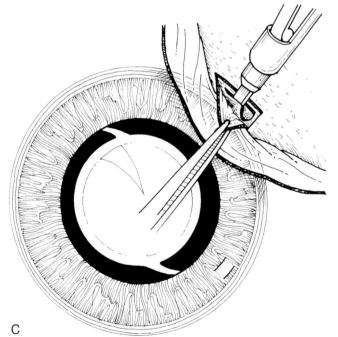

C

Intraocular Lens Implantation

The tunnel incision is enlarged to the required size for IOL implantation. Use of IOL injectors may require little or no enlargement, depending on the specific IOL, cartridge and injector used. (Also see Part VI, Intraocular Lenses.)

Trabeculectomy or Sclerectomy

The left side of the scleral tunnel is cut anteriorly to permit elevation of the corner and exposure of the tunnel floor (Figure 22-7A). This creates an "L" shaped flap. A pair of nontoothed forceps is used to

elevate the roof of the scleral tunnel to perform the trabeculectomy or sclerectomy.

A sharp blade is used to make an incision in the scleral floor of the tunnel, parallel to the limbus, about 0.5–1 mm anterior to the posterior edge of the tunnel (see Figure 22-7B). A Kelly punch (instrument #E-2798, Storz, Claremont, Calif.) is used to create a 1×2 mm opening into the anterior chamber on the left side of the tunnel (Figures 22-7C and 22-8A). Trabecular meshwork or peripheral cornea anterior to the trabeculum is removed. (Alternatively, the punch can be passed into the phacoemulsification incision and punch posteriorly; see

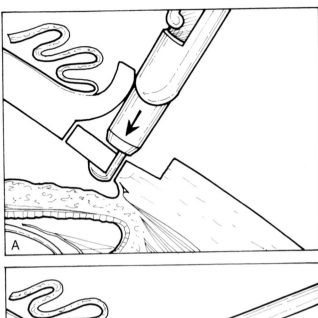

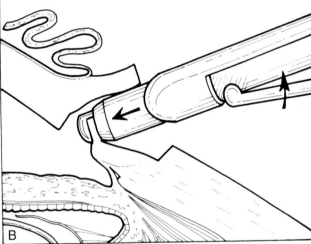

Figure 22-8 A, Kelly punch creates a sclerectomy (side view of Figure 22-7C). B, Alternatively, the punch can be passed into the phacoemulsification incision and punch posteriorly.

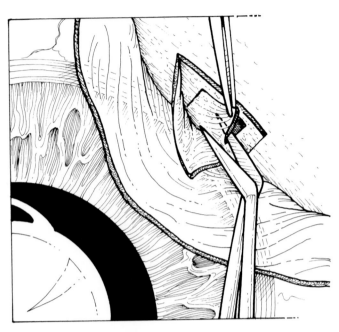

Figure 22-9 Sclerectomy can be created freehand with scissors and forceps.

Figure 22-8B.) If preferred, a freehand dissection is performed by making the same incision in the tunnel floor. Radial incisions are made anteriorly with a fine scissors (e.g., Vannas, instrument #E3389, Storz, Claremont, Calif.) on both sides of this incision. While the deep scleral tissue is grasped with toothed forceps, the scissors are used to cut the anterior edge, excising the tissue and creating a 1–2 mm filtration opening (Figure 22-9). An assistant can elevate the roof of the tunnel with nontoothed forceps or a cellulose sponge, or the surgeon can use the edge of the Vannas scissors to elevate the scleral flap during this dissection.

It is important to avoid extending the sclerectomy to the posterior edge of the tunnel floor to prevent simulation of a "full-thickness filtering procedure" with free access of aqueous flow through the incision to the scleral surface. Leaving a portion (0.5–1 mm) of the scleral floor intact forces the aqueous humor to percolate from the trabeculectomy or sclerectomy opening, across a short portion of the scleral floor, and through the incision to the scleral surface, resulting in slight resistance to flow. If the

trabeculectomy or sclerectomy opening is inadvertently created over the ciliary body and uvea, the dissection should be extended anteriorly over the iris. If required, a fine-needle-tip cautery can be used at low power to control bleeding.

Peripheral Iridectomy

Although some surgeons have suggested that an iridectomy is not necessary, it is safest to perform one.[74] Without an iridectomy, a shallow anterior chamber or application of digital pressure could result in occlusion of the trabeculectomy or sclerectomy opening from iris prolapse.

The iridectomy is performed by carefully grasping the peripheral iris as posteriorly as possible through the trabeculectomy or sclerectomy opening with a fine-toothed forceps. The peripheral iris is elevated with a slight side-to-side pulling motion, and Vannas scissors create the iridectomy opening (Figure 22-10A). The size of the iridectomy should approximate the size of the trabeculectomy or sclerectomy opening. Prolapsed iris tissue should be irrigated or gently massaged into the anterior chamber by bluntly rubbing in a peripheral to central motion on the corneal surface over the iridectomy with the elbow of the 19-gauge irrigation cannula. Aqueous humor will pass through the sclerectomy opening and the scleral incision into the subconjunctival space (Figure 22-10B). A fine-needle-tip cautery can be used at low power to control bleeding from the iridectomy edge. Great caution must be taken while cauterizing in this area. If the cautery disrupts the zonules in the area, vitreous can prolapse through the iridectomy and sclerostomy even in a phakic eye. Vitreous prolapse from any cause must be meticulously managed to prevent the vitreous from occluding the internal sclerostomy and causing failure of the trabeculectomy.

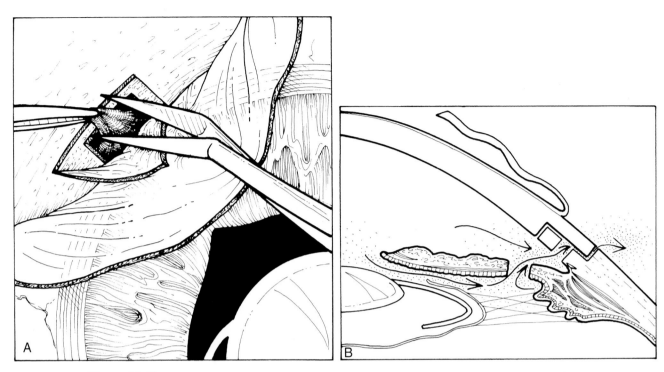

Figure 22-10 A, Peripheral iris is elevated with a slight side-to-side pulling motion, and Vannas scissors are used to create the iridectomy opening. **B,** Aqueous passes through the sclerectomy opening and the scleral incision into the subconjunctival space.

Scleral Flap Closure with Releasable Sutures

The scleral flap is closed with releasable sutures.[46] These will secure the wound and provide nearly watertight closure, preventing early postoperative hypotony, flat anterior chamber, and associated complications. Three or four releasable sutures are usually used, placing one at the corner and two along the scleral incision. A fourth suture can be placed in the side scleral incision. When the anterior chamber has stabilized and bleb healing has produced some resistance to aqueous flow, the sutures can be released to increase aqueous flow and help reach the target IOP. The number of sutures placed varies significantly among surgeons. However, the greater the number of sutures placed, the greater control one can have in reaching the goal IOP by reducing the effect of each suture as it is released or lysed.

The releasable sutures are placed in three steps. Using a narrow cutting needle on a 9-0 nylon suture (#7760, Ethicon, Sommerville, NJ) the first bite is placed through partial-thickness cornea, about 2 mm central and parallel to the limbus (Figures 22-11A and B). The second bite is placed radial to the limbus (approximately 90° to the first bite), passing through partial-thickness cornea beneath the conjunctival insertion at the limbus and exiting on the scleral side of the limbus (see Figures 22-11C and D). (In the early postoperative period, epithelial cells grow over the suture lying on the corneal surface between the first and second bites.) The third bite is placed across the scleral flap incision (see Figures 22-11E and F). After placing the first suture, the second and third sutures are also placed (see Figure 22-11G). Before tying the releasable sutures, the viscoelastic is aspirated from behind and in front of the IOL.

The releasable sutures are tied by grasping the suture exiting the sclera from the third bite and passing three throws around a tying forceps (see Figure 22-11H). The tying forceps then are used to grasp the suture on the scleral flap surface between the second bite and the third bite (see Figure 22-11I), and the three throws are brought down over the grasped suture, creating a loop knot that secures the scleral incision (see Figure 22-11J). The suture is trimmed long enough so that it lies flat on the scleral surface (see Figure 22-11K). The suture lying on the corneal surface is trimmed where it entered the cornea for the first bite (see Figure 22-11L). Forceps are used to pull gently on the suture, and scissors are used to push gently on the cornea so that when the suture is cut at the corneal surface, it retracts into the corneal tissue.

After placement of the releasable sutures, acetylcholine (Miochol-E) is injected through the paracentesis tract to deepen the anterior chamber and to constrict the pupil. Scleral flap closure should be secure enough to prevent aqueous leak from pressure elsewhere on the globe, but to permit slight aqueous leak when blunt pressure is applied to the posterior lip. An elevated IOP on the first postoperative day is preferable to hypotony, particularly if MMC has been used. It is easier to manage the former. (Management of IOP and release of sutures are discussed later in this chapter.)[46–48]

The technique of laser suture lysis of standard simple interrupted sutures is described later in this chapter. Three other releasable suture techniques have been described by Hoskins and Migliazzo,[49] Savage et al.,[50] McAllister and Wilson,[51] Shin,[52] and Johnstone[53] and can be researched if desired.

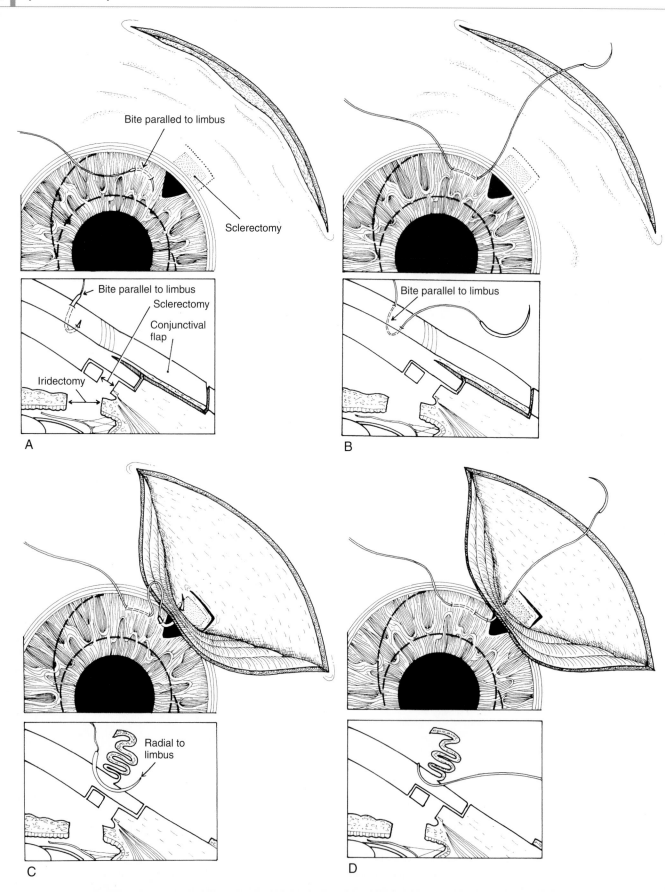

Figure 22-11 A and **B,** First bite is passed through partial-thickness cornea, about 2 mm central and parallel to the limbus. **C** and **D,** Second bite is placed radial to the limbus (approximately 90° to the first bite), passing through partial-thickness cornea beneath the conjunctival insertion at the limbus and exiting on the scleral side of the limbus.

(Continued)

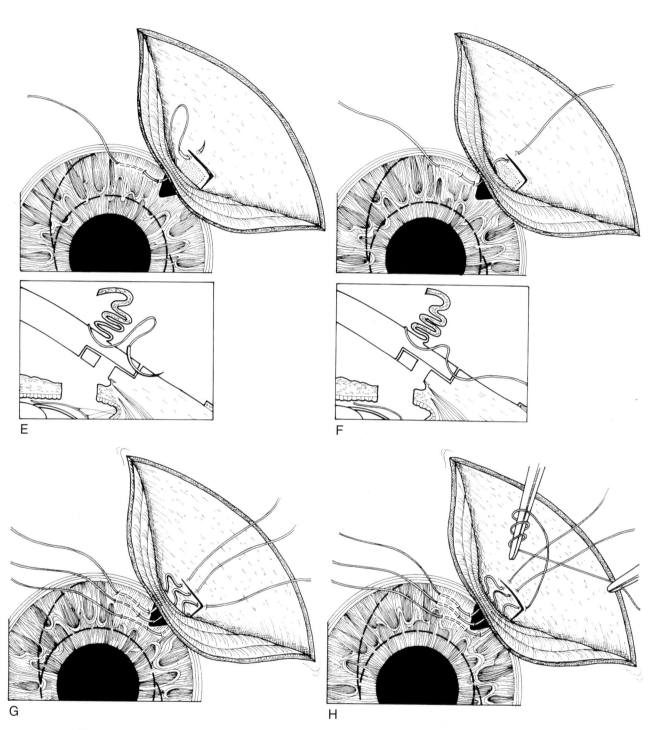

Figure 22-11, cont'd E and F, Third bite is placed across the scleral flap incision. G, After placing the first suture, the second and third sutures are also placed. H, Releasable sutures are tied by grasping the suture exiting the sclera from the third bite and passing three throws around a tying forceps.

(Continued)

Conjunctival Flap Closure

The limbus-based conjunctival flap is closed with a 9-0 absorbable monofilament suture on a tapered vascular (noncutting) needle. Using a running suture technique, the deeper Tenon's layer is closed with locking stitches, and the superficial conjunctival layer is closed with a nonlocking stitch. Widely spaced stitches are used in the deeper Tenon's layer, and stitches 0.5–1 mm from the incision edge and separated by 1–2 mm are used in the conjunctival layer (Figure 22-12A).

On the other hand, if the standard fornix-based flap incision was created by disinserting the conjunctiva at the limbus, it can be closed by securing one side of the conjunctival flap to the

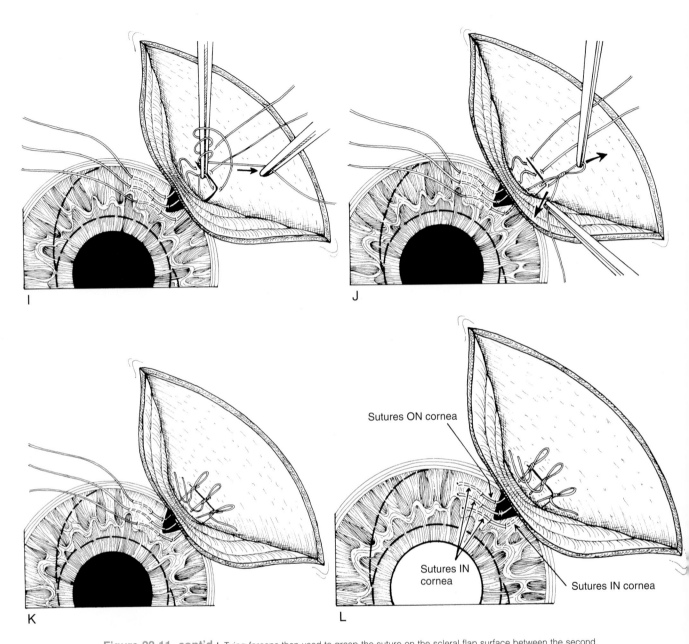

Figure 22-11, cont'd I, Tying forceps then used to grasp the suture on the scleral flap surface between the second bite and the third bite. J, Three throws are brought down over the grasped suture, creating a loop knot that secures the scleral incision. K, Suture is trimmed long enough so that it lies flat on the scleral surface. L, Suture lying on corneal surface is trimmed where it entered the cornea for the first bite.

peripheral cornea with a mattress suture. The other side of the conjunctival flap incision is then pulled, stretching the conjunctival edge against the peripheral cornea, and another mattress suture is placed. The limbal edge of conjunctiva is inspected, and additional mattress sutures are placed as necessary for secure closure. The surgeon must be sure that the exposed "elbow" of the releasable suture, between the first and second bites (the place where the suture is grasped when removed postoperatively), is not covered by the conjunctival flap. A running (noncutting needle on 9-0 or 10-0 absorbable) suture closes the conjunctiva laterally (see Figure 22-12B). It is helpful to start this closure with a bite of episclera at the limbus. An overlapping running suture, using

9-0 nylon (Ethicon 2890) can also be used to close the conjunctiva at the limbus (see Figure 22-12C).

An alternative closure of a standard fornix-based conjunctival flap has been reported by Wise,[54] using a 9-0 nylon suture on a VAS-100 needle (Ethicon 2890, Ethicon, Inc., Somerville, NJ). The VAS-100 needle is a very useful needle in glaucoma surgery. It is finer than a standard spatulated needle, thus creating a smaller hole (particularly useful in thin conjunctiva), yet it is stronger than a standard tapered vascular needle and can be passed through cornea and sclera without bending easily. The VAS-100 needle is also available on a monofilament 9-0 Vicryl suture by special order.

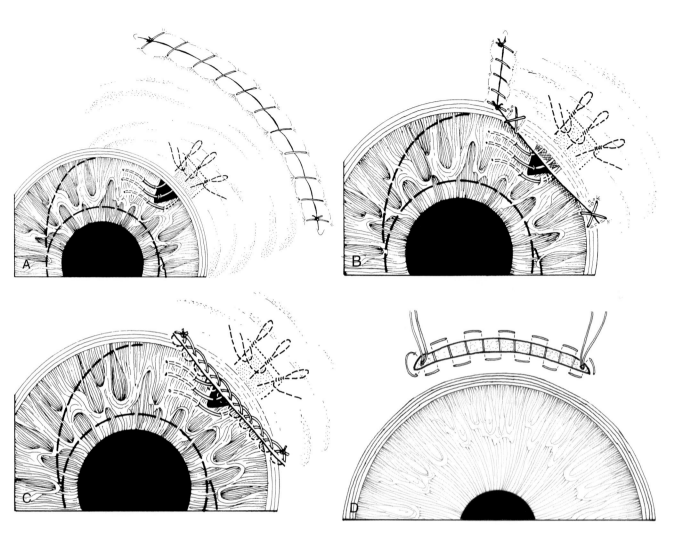

Figure 22-12 **A,** Using a running suture technique, the deeper Tenon's layer is closed with locking stitches, and the superficial conjunctival layer is closed with a nonlocking stitch. **B,** Mattress and a lateral running (noncutting needle on 9-0 or 10-0 Vicryl) suture closes the conjunctiva laterally. **C,** Overlapping running suture, using 9-0 nylon (Ethicon 2890) can also be used to close the conjunctiva at the limbus. **D,** Running horizontal mattress suture conjunctiva to conjunctiva closure with 9-0 monofilament Vicryl on a tapered vascular needle (Ethicon V402G) for alternate fornix-based technique (from Figure 22-2B).

The alternative technique fornix based conjunctival flap (with the conjunctival incision 1.5 mm posterior to the limbus) is closed with a running horizontal mattress technique using a monofilament 9-0 Vicryl on a tapered vascular needle (Ethicon V402G, Sommerville, NJ) suturing conjunctiva to conjunctiva. The narrow anterior lip of conjunctiva is often quite thin near the limbus and requires gentle care. The suture is pulled down toward through the cornea after each pass out through the anterior edge of the incision, to cinch the incision edges together (Figure 22-12D).

Phacoemulsification and Trabeculectomy at Separate Sites

Combined surgery with separate-site temporal clear corneal phacoemulsification and superonasal trabeculectomy has been advocated by some surgeons. This approach requires the surgeon to change positions and move the microscope when switching from one surgical site to the other. For younger surgeons who have trained in the era of temporal corneal phacoemulsification, they

may feel more comfortable using this same approach instead of a scleral tunnel technique used with one-site surgery. If a two-site approach is used, it is important to make sure that the incision is completely corneal to avoid any disruption of the temporal conjunctiva that could create a leak in the bleb. Although one study suggested slight benefit in IOP control, another study did not confirm this finding.[55,56] The authors generally use this approach when superotemporal scarring requires superonasal filtration, when the presence of extremely thin conjunctiva increases the risk of a defect from the added manipulation, or in very deep set eyes.

INTRAOPERATIVE MEDICATIONS

At the completion of the procedure aqueous betamethasone (Celestone) is injected subconjunctivally. An antibiotic preparation may also be injected subconjunctivally at the surgeon's discretion. In addition, one drop of 5% povidone-iodine solution (Betadine) is placed in the fornix at the conclusion of the procedure. If the anesthetic block requires postoperative patching, antibiotic-steroid ointment is also applied.

BASIC POSTOPERATIVE MANAGEMENT

Frequency of Examinations

The early postoperative period is critical to the success of combined surgery. This is when elevated IOP is most likely to occur and when it can most effectively be managed. Examinations should be performed 1 day after surgery and at least weekly during the first postoperative month.

Postoperative Medications

Topical prednisolone acetate 1% corticosteroid eyedrops are used every 2 h while awake for the first few weeks following surgery, and are then gradually tapered and discontinued around the end of the third postoperative month. There has been some very recent debate about the potential benefits/risks of long-term, low-dose maintenance anti-inflammatory therapy to reduce the risk of wound remodeling and late fibrosis causing bleb failure. However, there have not been any randomized, peer-reviewed studies that have critically evaluated these claims. Topical antibiotic eyedrops (the authors use a quinolone eyedrop) are used four times a day during the first 7–10 days and then discontinued. If releasable suture removal is anticipated, the antibiotic drops are continued. Topical nonsteroidal antiinflammatory eyedrops are used three times a day for about 3 weeks. Postoperative subconjunctival injections of 5-FU may be administered for augmentation of intraoperative antifibrosis effect.

POSTOPERATIVE MANAGEMENT AND COMPLICATIONS

Postoperative Elevated Intraocular Pressure

Determining the cause of elevated intraocular pressure

Elevation of IOP often occurs in the early postoperative period. It is important to proceed through a stepwise logical evaluation of potential causes along the path of aqueous filtration from the anterior chamber to the subconjunctival space. Careful examination of the anterior chamber may reveal the presence of noncirculating cells, indicating retained viscoelastic material that interferes with flow at the trabeculectomy or sclerectomy opening. Gonioscopy should be performed to rule out obstruction of the internal sclerostomy opening by vitreous, iris, fibrin, or a blood clot or incompletely removed Descemet's membrane, sclera, or cornea. Because of the risk of prolapsed vitreous occluding the internal sclerostomy, it is very important that a capsular tear and vitreous prolapse is managed with an adequate anterior vitrectomy. Examination of the filtering bleb may reveal a shallow or flat bleb from tight wound closure and inadequate filtration, an encysted filtering bleb, a subconjunctival hemorrhage, or blood clot blocking filtration through the scleral flap. Hemorrhage in the filtering bleb may occur intraoperatively from bleeding associated with tissue dissection; from anesthetic, antibiotic, or steroid injection; or postoperatively from suture release or laser lysis. Rarely,

postoperative subconjunctival hemorrhage can occur from relaxation of a vessel in spasm or from clot lysis before a vessel has healed.

Late postoperative elevation of IOP is almost always due to episcleral scarring in the filtering bleb. This may occur gradually over time or may be precipitated by episodes of inflammation from uveitis, subsequent eye surgery, and so on. However, gonioscopy should still also be performed in these cases to rule out internal obstruction.

Treatment of Early Postoperative Elevation of Intraocular Pressure

Blockage of internal filtration opening

If the internal sclerectomy is blocked by a blood clot or fibrin, injection of tissue plasminogen activator into the anterior chamber may correct the obstruction.[57] If the iris, vitreous, Descemet's membrane, or lens capsule is preventing aqueous outflow, Nd:YAG or argon laser treatment may open the obstruction, but surgical intervention and wound revision will probably be required. Some cases of iris incarceration can be successfully managed with the use of a miotic such as pilocarpine. However, even if successful, the risk of recurrence is high and should be managed by some maneuver to prevent recurrence. Long-term miotic use in these cases is not ideal. Argon laser iridoplasty can be used to shrink and stretch the iris around the iridectomy to reduce its laxity and prevent recurrent incarceration.

Tight wound closure and technique of removal of releasable sutures

If the elevated IOP is due to inadequate filtration from tight scleral flap closure, removing releasable sutures can loosen the scleral flap and increase filtration. (Similar principles also apply to laser lysis of conventional sutures.) Before considering suture release or lysis, digital or instrument pressure is critical to determine the current resistance to outflow. If the IOP drops and a significant bleb rises with light pressure, then suture release will carry a high risk of inducing hypotony. On the other hand, if the IOP does not drop and a bleb can not be raised even with firm pressure, then the risk of inducing hypotony is usually low. In general, the authors try to avoid resuming anti-glaucoma drops, if possible, because of their potential of increasing conjunctival inflammation. At the same time, this must also be weighed with the IOP level and the severity of glaucoma damage. If the current IOP is at a level deemed to be dangerously high even for a few weeks, then consideration must be given to temporarily restarting at least some IOP lowering medical therapy. The surgeon, however, must use a reasoned and rational approach (Table 22-2). If the sutures are released before adequate healing has occurred, hypotony and overfiltration can result. If suture release is delayed too long and too much healing has occurred, increased filtration and lowered IOP will not be achieved. Virtually all combined procedures are now performed with adjunctive antimetabolite therapy. In most patients, this will slow wound healing and delay suture release compared with when antimetabolite therapy is not used.

The vascularity of the filtering bleb serves as a helpful indication of the extent of underlying wound healing. Highly vascularized filtering blebs indicate a high probability of more rapid

Table 22-2 Removal of releasable sutures*

A. Surgery performed with antimetabolites

1. Elevated IOP first postoperative week

   a. Try to avoid suture removal because of risk of:

      • Hypotony and flat anterior chamber

      • Wound leak (and potential bleb failure) in fornix-based conjunctival flap

   b. Lower IOP by:

      • IOP-lowering medications (beta-blocker or CAI preferred to avoid hyperemia)

      • Mild digital or instrument pressure on edge of incision in limbus-based conjunctival flap

      • Decompression through paracentesis

      • Recheck IOP after 20 min

2. Elevated IOP after first postoperative week

   a. Trial of digital or instrument pressure

      • Recheck IOP after 20 minutes

   b. Remove one releasable suture if needed

      • If no IOP decrease, augment with instrument or digital pressure

      • Remove only one suture on any day (usually)

      • Depending on IOP, recheck in 1 day

3. Effect of bleb appearance on decision to remove suture

   a. Can remove suture earlier if bleb is vascular

   b. Delay removal if bleb is avascular

   c. If bleb is avascular with low IOP

      • Permit healing (2 or 3 months)

      • Consider tapering steroids more rapidly

      • Then trim suture at the corneal surface

B. Surgery performed without antimetabolites

1. Healing is more rapid

2. Effort is made to avoid removal during first week

3. Removal after second week usually has minimal or no effect

*These principles also apply to laser suture lysis.

---

healing and should prompt consideration of earlier suture removal. Avascular or relatively avascular filtering blebs suggest slower healing and should prompt consideration of delayed suture removal. (It is advisable to consider discussing with the patient the pros and cons of suture removal or laser suture lysis so that they are aware of the possible complications.) Rather than using a "cookbook" approach to the steroid drop regimen, the regimen is based on the vascularity and appearance of the bleb. If significant conjunctival injection develops and persists, the authors will not hesitate to increase the steroid drops to hourly for as long as necessary. In the end, once the eye has completely healed, the ideal bleb is minimally ischemic. Significant residual vascularity of the bleb even beyond 3 months postoperatively still indicates a greater risk of long-term bleb failure.

During the first postoperative week, every effort should be made to avoid suture removal because of the increased risk of overfiltration, hypotony, chamber flattening, and associated complications. An IOP in the 20s for a short period will usually not cause progression of glaucoma damage. If a limbus-based conjunctival flap was used, digital, cotton swab, or instrument pressure can be applied while observing the bleb for enlargement.[53,58] If a fornix-based conjunctival flap was used, digital pressure or instrument pressure could cause a bleb leak and may need to be avoided during this period, depending on the closure technique used. However, with the technique of closing the fornix-based conjunctival flap with a running horizontal mattress suture, wound leaks are quite rare, even with the application of pressure on the first postoperative day. Topical and, if needed, oral therapy (including acetazolamide and hyperosmotic) can be administered, and, if necessary, paracentesis can be performed at the slit lamp examination (preceded by a drop of topical anesthetic, topical antibiotic, and 5% povidone-iodine solution [Betadine]). However, it is important to keep in mind that complete turnover of aqueous volume occurs in approximately 100 min, limiting the duration of effect of a therapeutic paracentesis. This also applies to digital pressure and massage. The IOP should be monitored for 30–60 min and then rechecked the following day to ensure stability.

During the second postoperative week, healing has progressed and removal of releasable sutures is safer. It is preferable to first apply gentle and then stronger digital pressure to stimulate filtration. Sometimes this maneuver will dislodge a fibrin clot or disrupt initial wound healing and result in lasting IOP control. IOP should be rechecked in 20–30 min to determine if the effect is lasting. If the IOP has returned to an undesirable level, and depending on the stage of glaucoma damage and the risk factors for failure (previous surgery, race, type of glaucoma, etc.), suture release can be performed. The surgeon should realize that complications of suture release can still occur.

During the third postoperative week, suture removal is usually safe. If suture removal is performed, the principles of adjunctive digital pressure, reevaluation of IOP in 30 min and avoidance of multiple suture removal in 1 day, should be followed. As healing progresses, the effect of suture release decreases, depending on the duration and concentration of MMC, surgical technique, individual patient variables, etc.

The technique of suture release involves elevation of the upper eyelid (an assistant may be helpful but is not required) and use of a fine forceps to grasp the suture where it changes direction at the elbow between the first (intracorneal) and the second (sublimbal) bites of the releasable suture. If necessary, the superficial layers of the corneal epithelium (which have grown over this portion of suture that was on the epithelial surface at the time of surgery) are penetrated to grasp the suture. The intracorneal segment of suture is teased out of the tissue and then pulled with constant gentle traction to release the loop knot and remove the suture (Figure 22-13A and B). In the rare cases where whilst trying to remove a releasable suture it breaks, the scleral portion of the suture can still by lysed with an argon laser as described below. The bleb is observed for enlargement during suture removal, and the IOP is measured. If the IOP is unchanged, gentle digital pressure can be applied to initiate or promote filtration. If IOP decreased, it may be checked again in about 20 min to determine if the effect is lasting. Follow-up can be planned for the next day or in 1 week, depending on the surgeon's preference. As a general rule, only

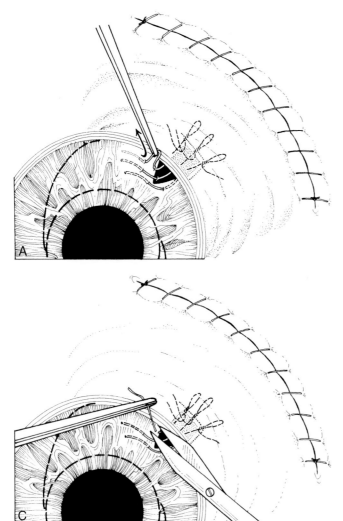

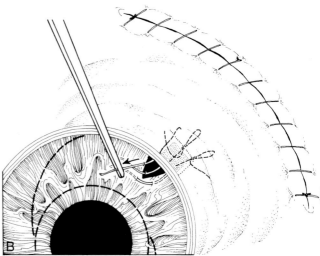

Figure 22-13 A, Intracorneal segment of suture is teased out of the tissue. **B,** Suture is pulled to release the loop knot and remove the suture. **C,** If suture removal is not needed, the sutures can be trimmed by teasing the intracorneal portion out of the tissue, pulling slightly with forceps and depressing the cornea with scissors so that the cut end will retract into the tissue.

one suture should be released on any day, and the sutures are removed from left to right, with the corner suture removed last.

If the surgeon decides that suture removal will not be necessary, the sutures can remain (the 9-0 nylon will dissolve over the next 2–3 years) or can be trimmed by teasing the intracorneal portion (the first of the three bites) out of the tissue, pulling it slightly with forceps while depressing the cornea with scissors so that the cut end will retract into the tissue (see Figure 22-13C).

Laser suture lysis

Argon laser suture lysis can be very useful in the postoperative management of trabeculectomy surgery. The timing of suture lysis is similar to the removal of releasable sutures. If available, the Hoskins or the Ritch lens (Ocular Instruments, Bellevue, Wash.) can compress the overlying conjunctiva (and its blood vessels) and aid in visualization of the scleral flap sutures. If these lenses are not available, the corner of a four-mirror Posner goniolens (Ocular Instruments, Bellevue, Wash.) can serve the same purpose. If visualization is difficult because of thick or boggy overlying tissue or engorged blood vessels, topical phenylephrine may be helpful.

In eyes with residual subconjunctival blood overlying the scleral flap sutures, use of the argon or green wavelength risks absorption of the laser energy by the blood and the overlying conjunctiva.

This could result in a full-thickness conjunctival defect that may not heal. Laser suture lysis with a krypton or red wavelength laser permits selective treatment of the suture and minimizes risk to the conjunctiva. The diode infrared wavelength can also be used for laser suture lysis, but is less effective.

Laser suture lysis settings are 50 μ spot size, 70–100 ms burn duration, and 260–400 mW of power (Table 22-3). Ideally, one should attempt to cut the suture at both ends to ensure that the long episcleral piece of suture lays flat and does not perforate the conjunctiva.

Management of Subconjunctival Hemorrhage

Subconjunctival hemorrhage in the filtering bleb may increase the risk of bleb failure. More aggressive use of topical corticosteroid eyedrops is usually adequate to preserve the filtering bleb. Earlier

Table 22-3 Laser suture lysis settings

Spot size: 50 μm
Burn duration: 70 to 100 ms
Power: 260 to 400 (average 300) mW

suture release, subconjunctival injection of corticosteroids adjacent to the filtering bleb, and subconjunctival 5-FU injections may be considered.

Encysted Filtering Bleb

An encysted filtering bleb is characterized by a localized highly elevated bleb associated with a high IOP. It is usually evident within the first postoperative month and may develop as early as several weeks following surgery. Conservative management with addition of IOP-lowering agents is usually successful in controlling IOP. Needling the filtering bleb at the slit lamp examination (preceded by topical anesthetic, broad-spectrum topical antibiotic, and 5% povidone-iodine solution [Betadine]) or in the operating room may restore diffuse filtration and lower IOP. However, the success of needling revisions tends to be lower in eyes with true encapsulated blebs. The conjunctiva is slightly elevated by a subconjunctival injection of sterile BSS or anesthetic such as 1% lidocaine (xylocaine) with epinephrine for vasoconstriction, administered about 1 cm from the bleb. A cotton-tipped applicator is used to push the BSS toward the bleb. A needle knife is passed into the subconjunctival space through the same entry point used for the BSS injection. The knife is passed beneath the elevated conjunctiva to the bleb where the wall is punctured and cut. If the nature of the bleb permits, the knife can also be passed across the bleb to cut the opposite wall. This procedure can be augmented with daily subconjunctival injections of 5-FU or a pre-needling injection of mitomycin C to prevent healing. Hypotony can result from this procedure. A recent case report showed a beneficial effect of adjunctive bevacizumab on the outcome of a needling revision of an encapsulated bleb that had previously failed an earlier needling with adjunctive mitomycin C.[71]

Treatment of Late Postoperative Intraocular Pressure Elevation

Scarring of the filtering bleb, the most common cause of late IOP elevation, may be managed by needling the bleb and scleral flap. This technique is best performed when the scleral flap edges can be seen through the conjunctiva by slit-lamp examination. (IOP reduction first may be attempted by the addition of eyedrops to avoid the risks of subconjunctival hemorrhage and hypotony.) Although some surgeons prefer to perform this at the slit lamp, others may prefer the operating room.

Late scleral flap needling (and injection of antimetabolite)

The eye is prepared by several applications of a topical anesthetic eyedrop and a drop of 5% povidone-iodine solution (Betadine). A subconjunctival injection of BSS separates scar tissue and creates a plane for safer passage of the needle. A 27-gauge or 30-gauge needle or needle knife is inserted into the subconjunctival space at least 1 cm from the scleral flap and is passed beneath the conjunctiva to the scarred filtering bleb or the scleral flap incision. A back-and-forth motion is used to disrupt the scar tissue, elevate the scleral flap, and, if necessary, penetrate the sclerostomy. Restoration of aqueous flow is indicated by elevation of the filtering bleb. After removal of the needle, the entry point is observed

for aqueous leakage. If necessary, careful light cautery can be applied to shrink the conjunctiva surrounding the leak to achieve closure. The leaking area is first dehydrated with a sterile cotton tip applicator. A low-temp disposable cautery unit is then brought very close to the conjunctiva, without actually touching the conjunctiva, and a brief light treatment of cautery applied. Direct contact with the conjunctiva can sometimes have the opposite effect and enlarge the defect. Suture closure is rarely necessary.

Antimetabolite can be injected before needling. A mixture of bupivacaine 0.75% with epinephrine (marcaine) or lidocaine 1% with epinephrine (xylocaine), and MMC 0.4 mg/mL is prepared for injection by aspirating 0.01 mL of the MMC into a 30-gauge needle on a 1 mL syringe, followed by 0.02 mL of bupivacaine (or lidocaine). This small volume only partially fills the hub of the needle. The needle is inserted into the subconjunctival space 1 cm from the bleb, and the mixture is injected near the site of revision, elevating the tissue. A sterile cotton swab is used to spread the mixture in the subconjunctival space. After 15 or 20 min, a second needle (or "Angled Stiletto" knife, Becton-Dickinson), passed through the same entry point as the first, is used to revise the bleb, scleral flap, and, if necessary, the sclerostomy.[59] Great care must be taken to avoid any risk of the antimetabolite entering the central portion of the bleb cavity and potentially entering the anterior chamber which could lead to corneal decompensation.

A similar technique has been reported, employing a needle revision of the filtering bleb with postoperative injections of 5-FU.[60]

Other Causes of Intraocular Pressure Elevation

Rare causes of postoperative elevation of IOP may include aqueous misdirection (malignant glaucoma, ciliary block glaucoma), suprachoroidal hemorrhage, choroidal effusion, and so on. Management of these entities is complex. Publications and texts should be consulted to develop appropriate strategies of treatment.

Postoperative hypotony mechanisms

Hypotony may result from excessive outflow or inadequate production of aqueous. In the early postoperative period, excessive outflow from a wound leak or bleb leak is more common than overfiltration with a large bleb, aqueous flow through a cyclodialysis cleft or aqueous underproduction from iridocyclitis, choroidal detachment, or, rarely, from a previous cyclodestructive procedure. (Hyposecretion of aqueous from iridocyclitis may be clinically diagnosed by noting stagnant or slowly moving cells in the anterior chamber after residual viscoelastic has been ruled out.)

An aqueous leak can usually be identified by applying fluorescein solution and patiently observing the bleb surface under blue light for an interruption in the fluorescein pattern. Painting the area of interest with a fluorescein strip will sometimes reveal aqueous leaks that may be difficult to identify with liquid fluorescein. Sometimes hypotonous eyes will only demonstrate a leak with application of gentle digital pressure to the globe.

The need for intervention becomes more urgent if secondary complications from hypotony are present, such as flat anterior chamber, significant choroidal effusions, macular choroidal folds sometimes associated with disc edema or congestion (hypotony maculopathy), and, of course, choroidal hemorrhage.

Overfiltration with leak: early

A wound leak or conjunctival button hole is counter-productive to the development of a bleb and should be closed as soon as possible. However, some incision leaks may close spontaneously, particularly at the limbus. The management options for a wound leak depend on the leak location and appearance, and include: bandage contact lens for tamponade; application of cyanoacrylate or tissue glue to seal the leak and use of a large bandage contact lens to prevent discomfort;[61,62] reducing the frequency of the corticosteroid drops to facilitate healing; suture repair (either at the slit lamp or in the operating room depending on the surgeon and patient's comfort level); and even conjunctival graft in extreme and rare circumstances. Compression sutures are sometimes successful in localizing a conjunctival defect and closing the aqueous leak, and can be a very helpful tool.[63]

A low IOP, with or without wound leak, is sometimes associated with a shallow or flat anterior chamber as well as choroidal effusions. Iridocorneal apposition can persist for some time without risk of corneal endothelial injury or permanent injury. However, IOL-corneal contact has a much greater risk of endothelial injury, and is an absolute indication for anterior chamber reformation with a viscoelastic agent.[64,75] This can be done in the office in most circumstances. A dilated fundus exam should be performed to document the presence and extent of choroidal effusions. Topical cycloplegic drops such as cyclopentolate, scopolamine, homatropine and atropine can also help to deepen the anterior chamber.

Overfiltration with leak: late (greater than 3 months postoperative)

Conservative attempts to close late bleb leaks may have limited success and depend on the degree of conjunctival ischemia in the leaking area. A large bandage contact lens may tamponade the leak and permit healing. Late leaks, which are usually associated with devitalized conjunctival tissue, most often require extensive bleb revision with creation of a new bleb surface. Late bleb leaks are also of great concern because of the increased risk of bleb failure, bleb infection and endophthalmitis. If there is no evidence of blepharitis or other factors that might predispose to endophthalmitis, there has been no previous occurrence of blebitis, and the IOP is normal (in the teens), the leak may be observed after educating the patient about signs and symptoms of infection and giving instructions to contact the doctor immediately if they occur. The patient may be given a prescription for a broad-spectrum antibiotic to use if signs and symptoms of infection arise until the doctor can be seen. Some surgeons have advised against the chronic prophylactic use of antibiotics in chronic bleb leaks because of the possibility of selecting for antibiotic resistant bacteria.

Overfiltration without leak: extensive bleb

Overfiltration may occur in the first few days following surgery as a result of inadequate scleral flap closure. (Most surgeons will ensure tight scleral flap closure, realizing that postoperative elevations of IOP can be treated with medications, paracentesis, or suture release rather than risk hypotony, which is more difficult to manage.) If overfiltration results in complications, such as choroidal detachment, shallow or flat anterior chamber, or hypotony maculopathy, management may include decreasing frequency of topical corticosteroids, deepening of the anterior chamber by

cycloplegics, pressure patch (with "torpedo" on the eyelid in the area of the filtering bleb) or injection of viscoelastic, resuturing of the scleral flap, and so on. The method and nature of management should be determined by the associated risks and the potential benefits of the treatment.

If hypotony is present beyond the normal period of resolution, and if reversible causes, such as choroidal detachment, and more permanent causes, such as cyclodialysis cleft, have been excluded, several management possibilities may be considered. Injection of autologous blood into the bleb, external local application of trichloroacetic acid, and treatment with cryotherapy have been effective in decreasing filtration.[65] Placement of a barrier suture across the filtering bleb can also limit the area of filtration and decrease bleb size.[63] Rarely, return to the operating room to place additional scleral flap sutures may be required.

In the absence of a bleb leak, hypotony may be observed without definitive treatment, as long as there are no complications. Many eyes will tolerate an IOP below 6 mm Hg indefinitely. Others may develop a choroidal detachment with an IOP as high as 10–12 mm Hg.

Overfiltration without leak: cyclodialysis cleft

Management of a cyclodialysis cleft may initially be attempted by use of topical cycloplegic eyedrops but may require laser treatment, cryotherapy, or transscleral suturing.[66,67]

Decreased ciliary body production of aqueous: cyclitis

This can be one of the most challenging problems associated with hypotony. Aggressive anti-inflammatory therapy may be helpful. This is a phenomenon that the authors have observed most commonly in patients of African ancestry. Hourly corticosteroid drops may need to be used for many weeks, sometimes also augmented with the use of oral prednisone. Reopening the conjunctival flap and resuturing the scleral flap to reduce or stop filtration may be necessary in rare circumstances.

Large uncomfortable bleb

Uncommonly, even though filtration provides excellent IOP control, the bleb size will cause discomfort or interfere with tear lubrication, and result in dellen formation or punctate corneal staining. This can be one of the most frustrating challenges for both the patient and the physician. Topical lubricants (drops during the day and ointment at bedtime) and topical nonsteroidal anti-inflammatory eyedrops may be helpful. Specialized techniques of laser treatment, use of trichloroacetic acid, and surface cryotherapy may improve comfort, though there is some risk of creating a bleb leak. Compression sutures have also been helpful. If all else has failed, bleb revision surgery can be considered with the risk that filtration will be compromised.[20,68–70]

Blebitis and endophthalmitis

Significant risk factors for blebitis and endophthalmitis include the presence of chronic blepharitis, poor hygiene, a thin-walled bleb, an avascular bleb, and a bleb leak. Patients should be alerted to the signs and symptoms of bleb infection, which are redness, discharge, pain, photophobia, and reduced vision, and they should be advised to contact their ophthalmologist immediately if they occur. If infection is limited to the bleb, a culture of the lids, conjunctiva, and bleb may be helpful in determining the etiologic agent. Intensive topical broad-spectrum antibiotic therapy may be curative. Evidence of more severe infection with hypopyon or vitreous involvement warrants more aggressive therapy that may include vitreous tap or vitrectomy and intraocular injection of antibiotics.[70]

■ CONCLUSION ■

Combined phacoemulsification and trabeculectomy is an excellent surgical technique for the management of coexisting glaucoma and cataract. The patient can benefit from decreased disability and morbidity by having one rather than two procedures performed. However, the surgeon must understand the appropriate indications and the special techniques required for intraoperative and postoperative care of these patients. This approach represents an exciting challenge for the surgeon with great potential for preserving visual function, increasing visual acuity, and improving quality of life.

References

[1] Spaeth GL, Sivalingam E. The partial-punch: a new combined cataract glaucoma operation. Ophthalmic Surg 1976;l7:53.

[2] Levene R. Triple procedure of extracapsular cataract surgery, posterior chamber lens implantation, and glaucoma filter. J Cataract Refract Surg 1986;12:385.

[3] Shields MB. Combined cataract extraction and guarded sclerectomy: reevaluation in the extracapsular era. Ophthalmology 1986;93:366.

[4] Shields M. Combined cataract extraction and glaucoma surgery. Ophthalmology 1982;89:231.

[5] Savage JA, Thomas JV, Belcher III CD, et al. Extracapsular cataract extraction and posterior chamber intraocular lens implantation in glaucomatous eyes. Ophthalmology 1985;92:1506.

[6] Vu MT, Shields MB. The early postoperative pressure course in glaucoma patients following cataract surgery. Ophthalmic Surg 1988;19:467.

[7] McCartney DL, Memmen JE, Stark WJ, et al. The efficacy and safety of combined trabeculectomy, cataract extraction, and intraocular lens implantation. Ophthalmology 1988;95:754.

[8] Krupin T, Feitl ME, Bishop KI. Postoperative intraocular pressure rise in open-angle glaucoma patients after cataract or combined cataract-filtration surgery. Ophthalmology 1989;96:579.

[9] Cohen JS, Greff LJ, Novack G et al. A placebo-controlled double-masked evaluation of mitomycin-C in combined glaucoma and cataract procedures. Ophthalmology 1996;103:1934.

[10] Carlson DW, Alward WLM, Barad JP, et al. A randomized study of mitomycin augmentation in combined phacoemulsification and trabeculectomy. Ophthalmology 1997;104:719.

[11] Budenz DL, Pyfer M, Singh K, et al. Comparison of phacotrabeculectomy with 5-fluorouracil, mitomycin-C, and without antifibrotic agents. Ophthalmic Surg Lasers 1999;30:367.

[12] Savage JA, Thomas JV, Belcher CD, et al. Extracapsular cataract extraction and posterior chamber intraocular lens implantation in glaucomatous eyes. Ophthalmology 1985;92:1506.

[13] McGuigan LJB, Gottsch J, Stark WJ, et al. Extracapsular cataract extraction and posterior chamber lens implantation in eyes with preexisting glaucoma. Arch Ophthalmol 1986;104:1301.

[14] Schwenn O, Burkhard Dick H, Krummenauer, et al. Intraocular pressure after small incision surgery: temporal sclerocorneal versus clear corneal incision. J Cataract Refract Surg 2001;27:421.

[15] Crichton ACS, Kirker AW. Intraocular pressure and medication control after clear corneal phacoemulsification and AcrySof posterior chamber intraocular lens implantation in patients with filtering blebs. J Glaucoma 2001;10:38.

[16] Seah SKL, Jap A, Prata Jr JA, et al. Cataract surgery after trabeculectomy. Ophthalmic Surg Lasers 1996;27:587.

[17] Murchison JF, Shields MB. An evaluation of three surgical approaches for coexisting cataract and glaucoma. Ophthalmic Surg 1989;20:383.

[18] Simmons ST, Litoff D, Nichols DA, et al. Extracapsular cataract extraction and posterior chamber intraocular lens implantation combined with trabeculectomy in patients with glaucoma. Am J Ophthalmol 1987;104:465.

[19] Hoskins Jr HD, Migliazzo C. Management of failing filtering blebs with the argon laser. Ophthalmic Surg 1984;15:731.

[20] Cohen JS, Shaffer RN, Hetherington Jr J, et al. Revision of filtration surgery. Arch Ophthalmol 1977;95:1612.

[21] Shin DH, Hughes BA, Song MS, et al. Primary glaucoma triple procedure with or without adjunctive mitomycin. Ophthalmology 1996;103:1925.

[22] Shingleton BJ, Wadhwani RA, O'Donoghue MW, et al. Evaluation of intraocular pressure in the immediate period after phacoemulsification. J Cataract Refract Surg 2001;27:524.

[23] Gressel MG, Parrish II RK, Folberg R. 5-Fluorouracil and glaucoma filtering surgery. I. An animal model. Ophthalmology 1984;91:378–383.

[24] Heuer DK, Parrish II RK, Gressel MG, et al. 5-Fluorouracil and glaucoma filtering surgery. II. A pilot study. Ophthalmology 1984;91:384–393.

[25] Heuer DK, Parrish II RK, Gressel MG, et al. 5-Fluorouracil and glaucoma filtering surgery. III. Intermediate follow-up of a pilot study. Ophthalmology 1986;93:1537–1546.

[26] Cohen JS. Combined cataract implant and filtering surgery with 5-fluorouracil. Ophthalmic Surg 1990;21:181–186.

[27] Budenz DL, Pyfer M, Singh K, et al. Comparison of phacotrabeculectomy with 5-fluorouracil, mitomycin-C, and without antifibrotic agents. Ophthalmic Surg Lasers 1999;30:367.

[28] Hennis HL, Stewart WC. The use of 5-fluorouracil in patients following combined trabeculectomy and cataract extraction. Ophthalmic Surg 1991;22:451.

[29] Wong PC, Ruderman JM, Krupin T. 5-Fluorouracil after primary combined filtration surgery. Am J Ophthalmol 1994;117:149.

[30] Chen C-W. Enhanced intraocular pressure controlling effectiveness of trabeculectomy by local application of mitomycin-C. Trans Asia-Pacific Acad Ophthalmol 1983;9:172.

[31] Palmer SS. Mitomycin as adjunct chemotherapy with trabeculectomy. Ophthalmology 1991;98:317.

[32] Carlson DW, Alward WLM, Barad JP, et al. A randomized study of mitomycin augmentation in combined phacoemulsification and trabeculectomy. Ophthalmology 1997;104:719.

[33] Cohen JS, Novack GD, Zhang LL. The role of mitomycin treatment duration and previous intraocular surgery on the success of trabeculectomy surgery. J Glaucoma 1997;6:3.

[34] Greenfield DS, Suner IJ, Miller MP, et al. Endophthalmitis after filtering surgery with mitomycin. Arch Ophthalmol 1996;114:943.

[35] Nuyts RM, Pels E, Greve EL. The effects of 5-fluorouracil and mitomycin C on the corneal endothelium. Curr Eye Res 1992;11:565.

[36] Sarraf D, Eezzuduemhoi RD, Cheng Q, et al. Aqueous and vitreous concentration of mitomycin C by topical administration after glaucoma filtration surgery in rabbits. Ophthalmology 1993;100:1574.

[37] Heaps RS, Nordlund JR, Gonzalez-Fernandez F, et al. Ultrastructural changes in rabbit ciliary body after extraocular mitomycin C. Invest Ophthalmol Vis Sci 1998;39:1971.

[38] Kee C, Pelzeki C, Kaufman PL. Mitomycin C suppresses aqueous humor flow in cynomolgus monkeys. Arch Ophthalmol 1995;113:239.

[39] Lederer Jr CM. Combined cataract extraction with intraocular lens implantation and mitomycin augmented trabeculectomy. Ophthalmology 1996;103:1025.

[40] Apt L, Isenberg SJ, Yoshimori R, et al. The effect of povidone-iodine solution applied at the conclusion of ophthalmic surgery. Am J Ophthalmol 1995;119:701.

[41] Broadway DC, Chang LP. Trabeculectomy, risk factors for failure and the preoperative state of the conjunctiva. J Glaucoma 2001;10:237.

[42] Tezel G, Kolker AE, Kass MA, et al. Comparative results of combined procedures for glaucoma and cataract. II. Limbus-based versus fornix-based conjunctival flaps. Ophthalmic Surg Lasers 1997;28:551.

[43] Frye LL. Pupil stretch maneuver, course #454 (Modern phacoemulsification/ ECCE implantation surgery: XII, Nov 11, 1992), Dallas, Tex: AAO.

[44] Miller KV, Keener Jr GT. Stretch pupilloplasty for small pupil phacoemulsification. Am J Ophthalmol 1994;117:107.

[45] Osher RH, editor. Video journal of cataract and refractive surgery, vol. 11(1). Cincinnati, Ohio: Cincinnati Eye Institute; 1995.

[46] Cohen JS, Osher RH. Releasable scleral flap sutures. In: Krupin T, Wax MB, editors. Ophthalmology Clinics of North America, new techniques in glaucoma surgery, vol. 1. Philadelphia: WB Saunders; 1988. p. 187.

[47] Kunesh MT, Cohen JS, Kunesh JC, et al. Releasable suture for trabeculectomy. Glaucoma 1993;15:185.

[48] Kolker AE, Kass MA, Rait JL. Trabeculectomy with releasable sutures. Arch Ophthalmol 1994;112:62.

[49] Hoskins HD, Migliazzo C. Management of failing filtering blebs with the argon laser. Ophthalmic Surg 1984;15:731.

[50] Savage JA, Condon GP, Lytle RA, et al. Laser suture lysis after trabeculectomy. Ophthalmology 1988;95:1631.

[51] McAllister JA, Wilson RP. Glaucoma. Boston: Butterworths; 1986. p. 243.

[52] Shin DH. Removable-suture closure of the lamellar scleral flap in trabeculectomy. Ann Ophthalmol 1987;19:51.

[53] Johnstone MS, Wellington DP, Ziel CJ. A releasable scleral flap suture for guarded filtration surgery. Arch Ophthalmol 1993;111:398.

[54] Wise JB. Mitomycin-compatible suture technique for fornix-based conjunctival flaps in glaucoma filtration surgery. Arch Ophthalmol 1993;111:992.

[55] Wyse T, Meyer M, Ruderman JM, et al. Combined trabeculectomy and phacoemulsification: a one-site vs a two-site approach. Am J Ophthalmol 1998;125:334.

[56] Sayyad FE, Helal M, El-Maghraby A, et al. One-site versus two-site phacotrabeculectomy: a randomized study. J Cataract Refract Surg 1999;25:77.

[57] Lundy DC, Sidoti P, Winarko T, et al. Intracameral tissue plasminogen activator after glaucoma surgery. Ophthalmology 1996;103:274.

[58] Traverso CE, Greenidge KC, Spaeth GL, et al. Focal pressure: a new method to encourage filtration after trabeculectomy. Ophthalmic Surg 1984;15:62.

[59] Mardelli PG, Lederer CM, Murray PL, et al. Slit-lamp needle revision of failed filtering blebs using mitomycin-C. Ophthalmology 1996;11:1946.

[60] Ewing RH, Stamper RL. Needle revision with and without 5-fluorouracil for the treatment of failed filtering blebs. Am J Ophthalmol 1990;110:254.

[61] Awan KJ, Spaeth PG. Use of Isobutyl-2-cyanoacrylate tissue adhesive in the repair of conjunctival fistula in filtering procedures for glaucoma. Ann Ophthalmol 1974;6:851.

[62] Weber PA, Baker ND. The use of cyanoacrylate adhesive with a collagen shield in leaking filtering blebs. Ophthalmic Surg 1989;20:284.

[63] Furgason TG, Perkins TW. A "clothesline" suture technique for the repair of a conjunctival tear during trabeculectomy. Ophthalmic Surg Lasers 1997;28:772–773.

[64] Osher RH, Cionni RJ, Cohen JS. Reforming the flat anterior chamber with Healon. J Cataract Refract Surg 1996;22:411.

[65] Wise J. Treatment of chronic postfiltration hypotony by intrableb injection of autologous blood. Arch Ophthalmol 1993;111:827.

[66] Stamper RL, Lieberman MF, Drake MV. Aqueous humor outflow. In: Becker-Shaffer's diagnosis and therapy of the glaucomas. 7th ed. St Louis: Mosby; 1999. p. 52.

[67] Stamper RL, Lieberman MF, Drake MV. Complications and failure of filtering surgery. In: Becker-Shaffer's diagnosis and therapy of the glaucomas. 7th ed. St Louis: Mosby; 1999. p. 632.

[68] Budenz DL, Chen PP, Yaffa KW. Conjunctival advancement for late-onset filtering bleb leaks. Arch Ophthalmol 1999;117:1014.

[69] Wadhwani RA, Bellows AR, Hutchinson BT. Surgical repair of leaking filtering blebs. Ophthalmology 2000;107:1681.

[70] Catoira Y, WuDunn D, Cantor LB. Revision of dysfunctional filtering blebs by conjunctival advancement with bleb preservation. Am J Ophthalmol 2000;130:574.

[71] Kahook MY, Schuman JS, Noecker RJ. Needle bleb revision of encapsulated filtering bleb with bevacizumab. Ophthalmic Surg Lasers Imaging 2006;37:148–150.

[72] Shingleton BJ, Campbell CA, O'Donoghue MW. Effect of pupil stretch technique during phacoemulsification on postoperative vision, intraocular pressure, and inflammation. J Cataract Refract Surg 2006;32:1142–1145.

[73] Osher RH. Pupil stretch technique. J Cataract Refract Surg 2007;33:362. [letter].

[74] Cohen JS, Osher RH, Weber F, Faulkner JD. Complications of extracapsular cataract surgery. The indications and risks of peripheral iridectomy. Ophthalmology 1984;91:826–830.

[75] Hoffman RS, Fine IH, Packer M. Stabilization of flat anterior chamber after trabeculectomy with Healon 5. J Cataract Refract Surg 2002;28:712–714.

Combined Cataract Extraction and Corneal Transplantation

Roger F. Steinert, MD

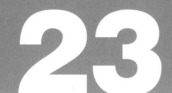

CONTENTS

CHAPTER HIGHLIGHTS

>> Evaluating the corneal endothelium preoperatively: combined procedure or not?

>> Combined phacoemulsification and endothelial transplantation

>> Special techniques for open-sky cataract extraction with penetrating keratoplasty

Successful combined cataract extraction and corneal transplantation requires appropriate preoperative assessment of suitable candidates[1-7] and attention to several specific surgical details of the combined procedure. This chapter reviews these particular issues. Mastery of corneal transplantation techniques, cataract surgery, and intraocular lens (IOL) implantation is assumed. This chapter emphasizes only those areas in which these techniques interact during the combined procedure.

◼ DECISION MAKING ◼

When a patient has a potentially optically significant corneal disorder simultaneous with a potentially optically significant cataract, the surgeon must assess the relative contribution of each.[8]

ASSESSMENT OF THE CATARACT

In the presence of an abnormal cornea, visualization of the cataract is impaired. Moderate corneal, epithelial, and stromal edema can be transiently cleared for diagnostic purposes with the application of several drops of 10% glycerin. This must be preceded with topical anesthetic drops to minimize patient discomfort. Some of the usual landmarks used to assess the optical significance of the cataract are reduced or eliminated. For example, the ability to see fundus details with a direct ophthalmoscope or the appearance of the media on red reflex does not distinguish between the contributions from the cornea and those from the lens. The status of the lens in the fellow eye is a useful clue if it can be visualized and if the patient has not had an ocular condition that might be expected to lead to unilateral cataract acceleration, such as inflammation or trauma. Pupillary dilation is mandatory to maximally visualize the lens. The surgeon must guard against extraction of a minimally brunescent but optically clear lens. The prognosis for rapid recovery of excellent vision is often best in a phakic eye. Moreover, cataract extraction performed after healing of the penetrating keratoplasty allows the surgeon the opportunity to adjust the refractive status with more accurate IOL power determination.[4,5] Conversely, a moderate cataract often will accelerate after uncomplicated penetrating keratoplasty.[9,10] Both the patient and the surgeon are frustrated when visual recovery after penetrating keratoplasty is progressively impaired by cataract progression just as the corneal optics improve. No study has been able to adequately resolve the relative stress to the corneal endothelium by cataract extraction following penetrating keratoplasty compared with a simultaneous combined procedure.

ASSESSMENT OF THE CORNEA

Corneal opacity itself can be assessed by the degree to which visualization of iris and crystalline lens detail is impaired. Surface irregularity is more deceptive. Slit-lamp biomicroscopy often will not disclose optically significant surface distortions. Corneal topography evaluation with a Placido disc, photokeratoscope, or computer-assisted topographic analysis will disclose the presence of irregularities but not their relative contribution to the visual impairment. A diagnostic hard contact lens refraction is invaluable in identifying and quantifying the extent of surface irregularity and its relationship to the total visual impairment. A frequent clinical dilemma is the decision about combining cataract extraction with corneal transplantation in a patient with dense corneal guttae in the absence of clinically evident microcystic epithelial edema or stromal edema. Many patients who exhibit severe central guttate changes in the central cornea can, nonetheless, undergo successful cataract extraction without subsequent corneal decompensation. Although dense guttae can sometimes cause a mild visual impairment, it is generally best to attempt cataract surgery alone in the absence of signs or symptoms of physiologic corneal endothelial corneal decompensation. Recovery from cataract extraction alone is much more rapid, and the patient is spared the lifelong problems associated with a corneal homograft. The patient and surgeon must have a frank discussion about the markedly increased chance of corneal decompensation postoperatively from the underlying corneal dystrophy to prevent later misunderstanding.

Conversely, if endothelial decompensation is inevitable after atraumatic cataract extraction, proceeding immediately to a combined procedure is warranted. Assessment of the endothelial reserve in a patient with significant guttate change is an inexact science at best. In taking the patient's history, the surgeon must be particularly alert to symptoms of early morning blur. Edema after lid closure throughout the night is often the first sign of frank decompensation. Slit-lamp biomicroscopic visualization of endothelial stria or microcystic edema is definitive evidence of early decompensation. Subtle microcystic edema can be particularly difficult to visualize in the presence of dense central guttae. Application of fluorescein will help demonstrate early microcystic epithelial changes.

Two special tests can be employed. Specular microscopy is often used in these circumstances, but it can be misleading. First, corneal endothelial decompensation occurs over a wide range of endothelial cell densities because endothelial pump function depends not only on the number of cells, but also on the number of pump sites per cell and the integrity of the cell membrane junctions, neither of which is assessed by specular microscopy. Second, in guttate dystrophy, interpretation of specular microscopy is impeded by masking of the endothelial cells that occurs because of the guttae. Corneal guttae appear dark on specular microscopy and prevent visualization of endothelium that may be covering the back of the excrescences of the Descemet's membrane. It has not been established whether endothelial cell density in the clearer corneal periphery can predict the status of the central endothelium.

The only readily available objective measure of physiologic endothelial pump function is pachymetry, either optical or ultrasonic. Normal corneas have a bell-shaped distribution of thickness and occasionally exceed 600 μm in thickness. As a general rule, pachymetry readings less than 600 μm indicate an adequately functioning endothelium for most patients, although a disparity between the same areas of the patient's two corneas exceeding 20 μm would raise suspicion of early edema in the thicker cornea. Pachymetry readings exceeding 650 μm strongly suggest the onset of physiologic endothelial decompensation, making combined penetrating keratoplasty and cataract extraction advisable even in the absence of frank corneal edema. Table 23-1 outlines the diagnostic steps in evaluating corneal endothelial function.

Table 23-1 Evaluation of corneal endothelial function

Morphologic evaluation
Specular microscopy
Confocal microscopy (research)

Physiologic function
Corneal thickness
    Ultrasonic pachymetry
    Light pachymetry
Evaluation of the diurnal curve (research) or recovery after patching (research)
Fluorophotometry

History
Morning blur
Glare complaints
Symptoms of variable contrast sensitivity impairment

■ COMBINED CATARACT REMOVAL AND LAMELLAR POSTERIOR ENDOTHELIAL TRANSPLANTATION (DSEK, DSAEK, DLEK, AND DMEK) ■

Lamellar transplantation of donor corneal endothelium is performed with several related techniques, most commonly descemet-stripping endothelial keratoplasty (DSEK) and descemet-stripping automated endothelial keratoplasty (DSAEK), but also including deep lamellar endothelial keratoplasty (DLEK) and descemet membrane endothelial keratoplasty (DMEK) techniques).

INDICATIONS

When the corneal endothelium is judged to have already failed, or to not be able to withstand even meticulous phacoemulsification cataract surgery, the surgeon has the option of combining cataract surgery with posterior endothelial transplantation under favorable circumstances. The key requirements are:

1. a clear cornea with good optical potential other than edema (e.g. no permanent scarring or irregularity)

2. a sufficiently low level of edema so that the surgeon can adequately visualize the lens to perform capsulorrhexis, nuclear phacoemulsification, cortical aspiration, and IOL placement into an intact capsular bag.

TECHNIQUE

Standard phacoemulsification cataract surgery is performed with the following special considerations:

1. The incision sizes and locations need to be compatible with both the surgeon's phacoemulsification technique and the lamellar endothelial transplant technique. For example, if the surgeon uses a 5 mm scleral incision for DSEK and typically locates that incision superiorly, but strongly prefers a temporal location for phacoemulsification, usually with a clear cornea

incision, then the best choice might be a temporal scleral tunnel for the combined surgery.

2. Use of a capsular dye such as trypan blue will facilitate visualization of the capsule through the hazy cornea. However, because the abnormal endothelium will uptake the dye as well, the surgeon should use a bolus of a highly cohesive ophthalmic viscosurgical device (OVD) (typically Healon 5 (AMO)) to fill the anterior chamber. The dye is then injected under the OVD and swept across the lens capsule, avoiding excess dye that would move anteriorly toward the backside of the cornea.

SPECIAL TECHNIQUES FOR COMBINED FULL-THICKNESS PENETRATING KERATOPLASTY AND CATARACT EXTRACTION

PREOPERATIVE PREPARATION

Obtaining a soft eye is critical to the success of an "open-sky" procedure. In addition to the administration of the usual dilating and antibiotic regimen employed for cataract surgery, softening of the globe and orbit begins with application of gentle pressure over the closed eyelids after administration of the peribulbar or retrobulbar block. An instrument such as the Honan balloon at 30 mm Hg should be applied for at least 20 min before beginning the procedure. Intravenous mannitol is administered over 1–2 min at the time of preparing and draping the patient. The dose should be adjusted according to the patient's body weight and medical status, taking particular care to avoid the patient with potential congestive heart failure. A typical dose for most adults is 50 mL of 25% mannitol. When administered at this time interval, the maximal hyperosmotic effect will occur at the time of opening the eye, in about 10–15 min. If the mannitol is administered earlier, the maximal pressure-lowering effect is sometimes lost.

TECHNIQUE FOR CATARACT REMOVAL

Some surgeons employ a phacoemulsification technique through a scleral tunnel limbal wound before the transplantation.[11] This has the advantage of the control inherent in a closed-chamber technique. It does require a separate wound and incurs the cost of the phacoemulsification tubing and tip. In many cases warranting a combined procedure, the corneal pathologic condition will impair the clear visualization necessary for phacoemulsification. In particular, visualization of the posterior capsule can be difficult.

Although open-sky extracapsular cataract extraction can be used routinely in conjunction with penetrating keratoplasty, the surgeon must be constantly aware of the risk of an open-sky procedure without protection against an expulsive suprachoroidal hemorrhage. Management of this potential complication is discussed later in the section on complications. An open-sky extracapsular extraction begins with the anterior capsulotomy. Manual retraction of the iris with an iris hook is often necessary because of an associated pathologic condition preventing wide dilation. A can-opener capsulotomy is usually satisfactory, as is a scissors capsulotomy. However, continuous curvilinear capsulorrhexis is ideal in terms of retaining a defined anterior capsular edge, facilitating cortical aspiration, and reliably implanting the IOL within the capsular bag. Obtaining an adequately sized anterior capsulotomy is critical to delivering the entire nucleus. In general, a diameter of 7 mm or larger is needed. Control of a capsulorrhexis tear at this diameter can be difficult. Because of the open-sky wound, some degree of positive pressure is inevitable. The posterior pressure on the nucleus tends to cause the capsulorrhexis to extend toward the equator. In addition to the critical decompression of the eye preoperatively (described earlier), positive pressure can be counteracted by using a spatula in the nondominant hand to apply posterior pressure on the center of the nucleus while the capsulorrhexis is being performed (Figure 23-1). If the tear begins to extend beyond 8 mm and cannot be recovered,

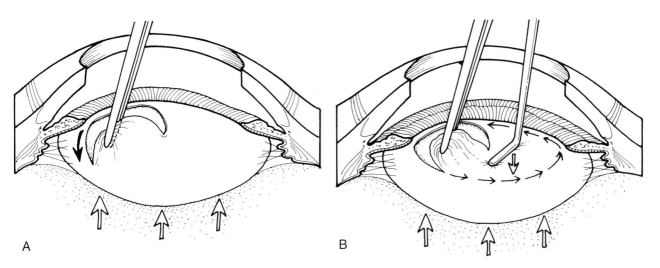

Figure 23-1 A, In the setting of penetrating keratoplasty, vitreous pressure is particularly likely to cause a circular tear capsulotomy to extend toward the equator and potentially around to the posterior capsule. B, In addition to preoperative maneuvers to soften the globe and to dehydrate the vitreous fluid, positive pressure intraoperatively can be counteracted by applying downward pressure on the nucleus itself while completing the circular tear anterior capsulotomy.

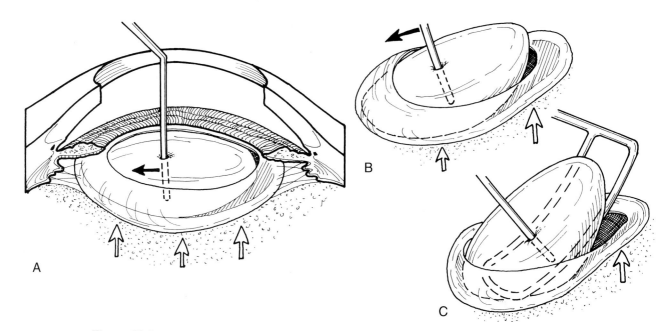

Figure 23-2 **A,** First step in delivering the nucleus is to rock the nucleus with an instrument such as a cyclodialysis spatula until one pole of the equator presents. Positive vitreous pressure usually facilitates this step; if the eye is particularly soft, gentle pressure on the sclera to create positive vitreous pressure can be helpful. **B,** Nucleus is tilted once the equatorial pole becomes exposed. **C,** A microsurgical lens loop can then be safely passed behind the nucleus and the nucleus delivered in its entirety.

it is best to discontinue the tearing maneuver and convert to a scissors capsulotomy to prevent further extension of the tear out to the equator and beyond.

The nucleus can be removed through several maneuvers. If the anterior capsular tear is continuous, hydrodissection can be safely employed. Hydrodissection is helpful in loosening the nucleus. If a fluid stream is directed under the anterior capsule, cortical cleaving hydrodissection may occur, greatly facilitating the later cortical cleanup (see Chapter 16). In the absence of hydrodissection, the nucleus can usually be loosened readily by rocking it with an impaled sharp instrument such as a 23-gauge hypodermic needle or the end of a fine dialysis spatula (Figure 23-2). When one edge of the nuclear equator can be visualized, a microsurgical loop is passed under the nucleus, and the nucleus is delivered though the center of the anterior capsulotomy. If the nucleus tends to fall back, very gentle placement of a small volume of viscoelastic agent behind the lens nucleus can lift it forward. Care must be taken not to create pressure posteriorly that would extend a capsular tear. Another alternative for delivering the lens nucleus is to place a cryoprobe on the central nucleus after removing as much loose anterior cortex as possible. If good adhesion is obtained, the nucleus is delivered in a "lollipop" maneuver.

Residual epinucleus and cortex are then aspirated. A conventional automated irrigation–aspiration unit can be used. In the open-sky situation, however, aspiration of air with resultant variation in pump function is inevitable. The large volumes of infusion fluid typical of automated units can be problematic in an open-sky setting. Furthermore, avoidance of aspiration of anterior capsular flaps and tearing of zonules can be difficult, particularly when there is any posterior pressure.

For these reasons, it is helpful to become comfortable with a manual irrigation–aspiration system such as the Simcoe or McIntyre systems. The so-called reverse Simcoe unit combines the advantages of each concept. An aspirating 3 mL syringe is attached to the unit directly. Because the irrigation–aspiration tip is flat and gently curved, it is particularly well suited to aspirating cortex in the presence of positive pressure with apposition of the anterior and posterior capsules (Figure 23-3).

Great care must be taken to avoid aspiration of the anterior capsule and tearing of zonules in the open-sky situation. All cortex must be cleaned to minimize postoperative inflammation that will be injurious to corneal transplantation.

After full removal of cortex, and polishing of the posterior capsule if needed, a posterior chamber IOL is placed. When placement within the capsular bag is ensured in an intact capsulorrhexis, my personal preference is a one-piece all-polymethylmethacrylate posterior chamber IOL with a haptic diameter of 12 mm. When sulcus fixation is possible or probable, a 13–14 mm haptic diameter is preferred to better ensure stability in the sulcus. A patient with a normal pupil can accept a 6 mm-diameter optic; if there is any pupillary abnormality, a 6.5 or 7 mm-diameter optic without any positioning holes is used.

The selection of an IOL power is problematic.[4,5,12,13] Axial length can be measured preoperatively, but penetrating keratoplasty will affect the keratometric contribution to the total optics. Some surgeons employ the patient's preoperative keratometry values to calculate IOL power. My personal preference is to use my "typical" value for corneal curvature after keratoplasty, which averages 45 diopters (D) for all patients. Each surgeon must determine his or her postoperative "personalized" keratometric value after corneal grafting. If a consistent surgical technique is employed, a keratoplasty surgeon will usually obtain repeatable results. Only occasionally will the postoperative power be sufficiently inaccurate that the anisometropia becomes symptomatic.

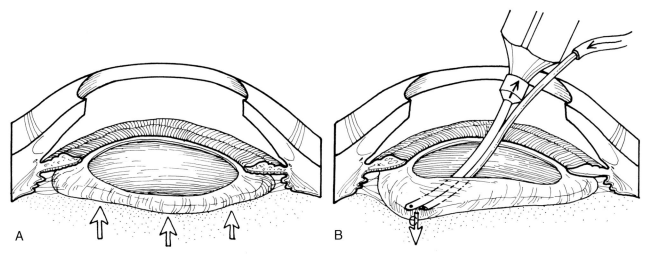

Figure 23-3 A, After nucleus delivery, the vitreous pressure flattens the capsular bag with apposition of the anterior and posterior capsules. B, Cortical clean-up can be performed with a variety of instruments. One device that is particularly well suited to the open-sky situation is the relatively flat and thin "reverse Simcoe" irrigation-aspiration needle. The tip can be gently slid between the anterior and posterior capsules, and then slight downward pressure separates the anterior and posterior capsules, allowing the equatorial cortex to be engaged and stripped safely.

■ COMPLICATIONS ■

POSITIVE PRESSURE AND VITREOUS LOSS

Positive pressure in the form of a bulging posterior capsule, but with maintenance of a normal red reflex, can be due to a variety of causes. The most common cause is transmitted lid and drape pressure through the lid speculum. To maximize the ability to resist such pressure on the open globe, a Schott or Smirmaul lid speculum provides excellent exposure while controlling pressure transmission to the eye. Wire lid specula are the most likely to transmit pressure to the globe. Whatever lid speculum is used in the presence of positive pressure, the surgeon must immediately check the lid speculum. Countersupport is provided if lifting or repositioning a lid speculum relieves the positive pressure.

If the positive pressure is extreme and threatens rupture of the posterior capsule or zonules, or both, the surgeon can attempt vitreous aspiration. With the open eye, however, a simple needle stab through the pars plana will generate even more positive pressure and ensure vitreous loss. Only an extremely delicate cutdown through the sclera with a sharp knife, such as a diamond knife, can minimize this risk. In many cases, the rapid progression of the positive pressure will not give the surgeon adequate time for this type of dissection.

The surgeon must always be alert for evidence of suprachoroidal hemorrhage or effusion. This much more threatening complication is discussed further on. Without signs of this additional complication, vitreous loss must be definitively addressed with vitrectomy. Automated mechanical vitrectomy with a guillotine-type cutter is preferred to minimize traction on the vitreous base. If a mechanical vitrectomy is not possible, an open-sky vitrectomy with cellulose sponge and scissors can be performed, taking care to minimize vitreous traction. At the completion of the vitrectomy, the anterior chamber must be carefully inspected, including wiping the pupillary aperture and iris face with a cellulose sponge to ensure removal of all vitreous. Residual vitreous in the anterior chamber will tend to become incarcerated in the keratoplasty wound, distorting the pupil, at a minimum, and often leading to further complications, such as cystoid macular edema.

SUPRACHOROIDAL HEMORRHAGE AND EFFUSION

With the corneal button removed, the eye is vulnerable to devastating suprachoroidal effusion and hemorrhage. The surgeon must always be alert to this possible complication and be prepared to deal with it immediately. Signs of suprachoroidal hemorrhage and effusion in an open-sky setting include positive pressure on an intact posterior capsule, rupture of the posterior capsule and zonules with vitreous loss, alteration in the red reflex, or a combination of these factors. If the patient is aphakic before the placement of the IOL, the retina may be directly visualized in detail through the operating microscope. An advancing smooth "roll" of elevated retina or normal color may represent effusion; if the advancing elevation is dark, suprachoroidal hemorrhage is likely. A slow hemorrhage is likely to lead to the expulsion of the intraocular contents if immediate action is not taken.

As soon as the suprachoroidal mass is recognized, the surgeon should immediately place a gloved index finger over the corneal opening. It is an excellent idea to have a clear lens available to maintain the globe when a suprachoroidal event is recognized. One such lens is the Cobo temporary keratoprosthesis, available from Ocular Instruments (Figure 23-4). This tapered lens can fit a wide range of trephine openings. This will stabilize the globe while the surgeon proceeds to a cutdown into the suprachoroidal space to remove the pressure.

One of the causes of suprachoroidal hemorrhage during penetrating keratoplasty is a lightly anesthetized patient under general anesthesia straining against the endotracheal tube. Because penetrating keratoplasty is relatively painless, little general anesthesia is needed, and many anesthesiologists progressively reduce the amount of general anesthetic during the

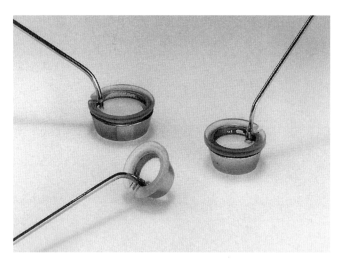

Figure 23-4 Cobo temporary keratoprosthesis (Ocular Instruments, Inc.) is highly valuable in controlling suprachoroidal effusion or hemorrhage in the vulnerable open-sky setting. (Courtesy Ocular Instruments, Inc., Bellevue, Wash.)

procedure to avoid hypotension. To avoid this complication, the anesthesiologist should be specifically instructed by the surgeon to use a paralytic agent.

INTRAOCULAR LENS IMPLANTATION AFTER VITREOUS LOSS

If vitreous loss has occurred, and the ability of the residual posterior capsule to support a posterior chamber IOL is in doubt, the surgeon faces three choices for IOL implantation: an anterior chamber IOL, an iris-sutured posterior chamber IOL, or a scleral suture-fixed posterior chamber IOL.

The literature does not show a clear-cut difference in outcomes among these three alternatives. If a posterior chamber IOL is desired, dissection of scleral flaps for scleral fixation is extremely difficult once the corneal button is absent. The surgeon can iris-fixate a posterior chamber IOL with midperipheral sutures (commonly referred to as "McCannel suture fixation") or, with a technique first described by Lane, use a scleral cutting technique that does not require dissecting scleral flaps. The latter can be performed using a posterior chamber IOL with a suturing hole in the haptic. A loop of permanent suture such as 10-0 or 9-0 polypropylene is passed through the positioning hole, and then each arm of the double-arm suture is passed through the sclera approximately 1 mm apart through the ciliary sulcus region. The suture is tied and cut. The knot is then rotated beneath the sclera. Conjunctiva is closed over the smooth loop of polypropylene. The smooth loop of external suture material will not erode through the conjunctiva. This technique is illustrated for a closed-chamber procedure in Figure 41-1.

References

[1] Lindstrom RL, Harris WS, Doughman DJ. Combined penetrating keratoplasty, extracapsular cataract extraction, and posterior chamber intraocular lens implantation. J Am Intraocul Implant Soc 1981;7:130–132.
[2] Hunkeler JD, Hyde LL. The triple procedure: combined penetrating keratoplasty, extracapsular cataract extraction, and posterior chamber intraocular lens implantation: an expanded experience. J Am Intraocul Implant Soc 1983;9:20–24.
[3] Kramer SG. Penetrating keratoplasty combined with extracapsular cataract extraction. Am J Ophthalmol 1985;100:129–133.
[4] Binder PS. The triple procedure: refractive results. 1985 Update. Ophthalmology 1986;93:1482–1488.
[5] Crawford GJ, Stulting RD, Waring GO et al. The triple procedure: analysis of outcome, refraction, and intraocular lens calculation. Ophthalmology 1986;93:817–824.
[6] Busin M, Arffa RC, McDonald MB et al. Combined penetrating keratoplasty, extracapsular cataract extraction, and posterior chamber intraocular lens implantation. Ophthalmic Surg 1987;18:272–275.
[7] Meyer RF, Musch DC. Assessment of success and complications of triple procedure surgery. Am J Ophthalmol 1987;104:233–240.
[8] Fine M. Therapeutic keratoplasty and Fuchs' dystrophy. Am J Ophthalmol 1964;57:371–378.
[9] Payant JA, Gordon LW, VanderZwaag R et al. Cataract formation following corneal transplantation in eyes with Fuchs' endothelial dystrophy. Cornea 1990;9:286–289.
[10] Martin TP, Reed JW, Legault C et al. Cataract formation and cataract extraction and penetrating keratoplasty. Ophthalmology 1984;101:113–119.
[11] Malbran ES, Malbran E, Buonsanti J et al. Closed-system phacoemulsification and posterior chamber implant combined with penetrating keratoplasty. Ophthalmic Surg 1993;24:403–406.
[12] Binder PS. Intraocular lens implantation after penetrating keratoplasty. Refractive Corneal Surg 1989;5:224–230.
[13] Flowers CW, McLeod SD, McDonnell PJ et al. Evaluation of intraocular lens power calculation formulas in the triple procedure. J Cataract Refract Surg 1996;22:116–122.

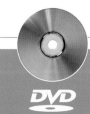

Control of Astigmatism in the Cataract Patient

Richard L. Lindstrom, MD, Douglas D. Koch, MD, Robert H. Osher, MD, Li Wang, MD, PhD and Mitchell P. Weikert, MD

24

CONTENTS

- Patient Selection and Evaluation
- The Cataract Incision
- Peripheral or Limbal Corneal Relaxing Incisions
- Conclusions

For over a century, it has been recognized that cataract incisions influence astigmatism.[1-3] Only in the past 15 years, however, have cataract surgeons mounted serious investigations aimed at measuring and minimizing astigmatism induced by cataract surgery. These efforts have paralleled but, until recently, have lagged behind the success of intraocular lenses (IOLs) in correcting the spherical refractive error precipitated by removal of the crystalline lens.

The term *refractive cataract surgery* has entered general ophthalmic usage. The term implies a coordinated and encompassing attention to both the spherical and astigmatic components of refraction. The current goal of refractive cataract surgery may or may not be to emmetropia; for some patients, the postsurgical target may be slight residual astigmatism, which contributes to depth of field. The critical difference between modern refractive cataract surgery and cataract surgery of a decade ago is the very existence of a target. Today's refractive cataract surgeon determines the starting point (the pre-existing astigmatic condition of the patient), knows the astigmatic effects of various approaches and selects a surgical plan that optimizes the refractive outcome for the individual patient. It is a degree of precision that was previously unattainable, requiring a depth of surgical planning that was previously unnecessary.

In addition to the cataract incision, whose size, location, and configuration help determine the astigmatic effects of surgery, the cataract surgeon now has two additional options in his armamentarium for correcting astigmatism: (1) corneal relaxing incisions (CRIs) and (2) toric IOLs. CRIs can be characterized as those made in the corneal mid-periphery, e.g. 6–8-mm zone, so-called "astigmatic keratotomy" (AK), and those made peripherally, so-called "peripheral or limbal corneal relaxing incisions" (PCRIs).

CRIs, particularly AK, were first studied purely for their corneal refractive effects.[2,4,5] In terms of both its nomenclature and the actual clinical practices that it incorporates, *refractive cataract surgery*, therefore, represents a true marriage of refractive and cataract surgical specialties.

This chapter describes the astigmatic effects of various cataract incisions, the techniques of PCRIs, two different approaches to AK, and toric IOLs. The reader will find no hard-and-fast rules herein. Depending on the cataract extraction technique employed, the degree and meridian of pre-existing astigmatism, and a host of other variables, the same patient might find effective treatment in a variety of ways. We hope to convey a sense of the general principles involved and to sketch out treatment approaches to the range of astigmatic errors that most cataract surgeons commonly encounter.

PATIENT SELECTION AND EVALUATION

People with over 0.5–0.75 diopters (D) of astigmatism usually require some kind of optical correction. Astigmatic errors of 1–2 D may reduce uncorrected visual acuity to the 20/30 or 20/50 level, whereas an astigmatic error of 2–3 D may correspond to visual acuity between 20/70 and 20/100.[6]

Up to 95% of eyes have some degree of naturally occurring astigmatic error. The incidence of clinically significant astigmatism reported in the literature varies between 7.5% and 75%.[6] From 3% to 15% of eyes may have astigmatic refractive errors greater than 2 D.[7] The incidence of postcataract surgery astigmatism greater than 2 D may be as high as 25% to 30%.[8,9]

Obviously, in a patient with little or no pre-existing astigmatism, cataract surgery should be designed to be as astigmatically neutral as possible. For patients with significant degrees of pre-existing astigmatism, two types of approaches can be employed as a function of the type of cataract incision. The surgeon can (1) operate on the steep corneal meridian and select the type of cataract incision that will produce the desired amount of against-the-wound flattening or (2) make a small incision at a favored location (e.g. clear corneal temporal incision), factor in the small amount of astigmatic change induced by this decision, and supplement it with either CRIs or implantation of a toric IOL. Obviously, CRIs can also be used postoperatively to further modify the result.

Careful patient selection is crucial in avoiding postoperative surprises and unhappy patients. As a rule of thumb, some form of astigmatic surgery should be considered in patients in whom a standard cataract operation will result in 1 D or more of postoperative astigmatism and whose fellow eye (1) has 1.5 D or less of astigmatism, (2) has astigmatism at a different meridian than that of the operative eye, or (3) has a similar amount and meridian of astigmatism and is itself an imminent surgical candidate.[10]

The rationale, surgical methods, and risks are discussed with the patient preoperatively. As noted previously, the target may be a slight undercorrection of the pre-existing astigmatism because some patients are bothered by the shift in astigmatic meridian brought about by an overcorrection, and a small amount of residual astigmatism can provide pseudophakic patients with reasonably good uncorrected near and distance vision.

The sections that follow address the cataract incision, CRIs (PCRIs and AK) and toric IOLs separately, and in greater detail. However, cataract incision manipulation and these other approaches are dual partners in the treatment of a wide range of astigmatism in people with varied personalities and lifestyle requirements.

ALIGNMENT

Accurate astigmatic surgery is highly sensitive to precise meridional alignment. Vector analysis demonstrates that a misalignment of only 15° results in a 50% reduction in the astigmatic correction. A 30° misalignment will maintain the preoperative astigmatism magnitude, but produce a large shift in the astigmatic axis. Misalignment errors in excess of 30° actually result in a net increase in the magnitude of the astigmatism.[11]

Various approaches can be taken to minimize alignment errors. Whenever possible we make small drawings of the patient's eyes when they are seen in the office preoperatively. The patient's head is carefully positioned to insure that it is vertically oriented in the slit lamp. We then look for prominent conjunctival, corneal, or iris features that are likely to be visible when the patient is dilated as seen in the operating room (Figure 24-1). It is particularly helpful to indicate landmarks that provide a clear indication of the 90° and 180° meridians, because these can be easily identified relative to the position of the vertical or horizontal slit-lamp beam.

An alternative approach is to mark the eye prior to entering the operating room. Topical anesthetic drops are administered, and the patient is asked to sit upright on the surgical stretcher. A marking pen is used to indicate either the 6:00 o'clock and 12:00 o'clock or 3:00 o'clock and 9:00 o'clock positions.

A third option is to mark the eyes as the patient is lying on the operating room table. For the majority of patients, this approach works extremely well. However, a small percentage of eyes rotate as the patient moves from an upright to a supine position. Swami et al.[12] demonstrated that 8% of eyes (20/240) had a deviation of greater than 10°.

A fourth option is to perform intraoperative keratoscopy to identify the major meridian and quantitate the amount, which should be consistent with the preoperative keratometry measurements and corneal topography. This can be achieved with

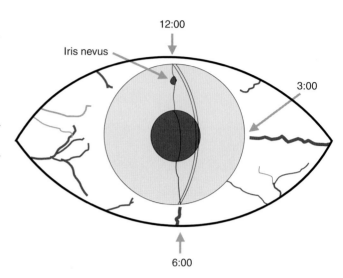

Figure 24-1 Identifying the steep meridian: find on the cornea, iris or conjunctiva one or more landmarks that are likely to be visible in surgery.

a device like the Hyde-Osher ruler manufactured by Ocular Instruments, which is accurate for identifying 1.5 D or more.

■ THE CATARACT INCISION ■

An incision of the cornea or sclera creates tissue gape. This gape causes corneal flattening along the meridian of the incision and steepening in the meridian 90° away (Figure 24-2), with

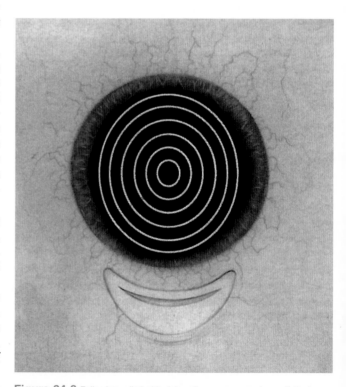

Figure 24-2 Following a limbal incision, tissue gape produces flattening along the meridian of the incision and steepening 90° away. (From Koch DD, Lindstrom RL. Controlling astigmatism in cataract surgery. Semin Ophthalmology 1992;7:224–233.)

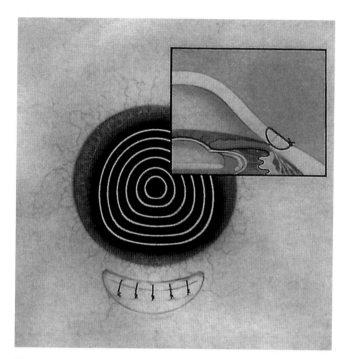

Figure 24-3 Sutures create peripheral flattening and central steepening along the meridian of the incision and steepening 90° away. (From Koch DD, Lindstrom RL. Controlling astigmatism in cataract surgery. Semin Ophthalmology 1992;7:224–233.)

Table 24-1 Induced corneal flattening along meridian of incision (scleral pocket incision) in eyebank eyes	
Incision length (mm)	**Mean flattening (standard deviation, D)**
2.0	0.07 (0.10)
2.5	0.10 (0.17)
3.0	0.24 (0.17)
3.5	0.47 (0.35)
4.0	0.74 (0.45)
4.5	1.00 (0.46)
5.0	1.07 (0.41)
5.5	1.40 (0.56)

From Samuelson SW, Koch DD, Kuglen CC. Determination of maximal incision length for true small-incision surgery. Ophthalmic Surg 1991;22:204–207.

the magnitude of this determined by several factors (see following two paragraphs). To compensate, wounds can be closed with sutures. Sutures produce local tissue compression, resulting in peripheral flattening and central steepening along the meridian of the incision and flattening 90° away (Figure 24-3).

The suture-induced net steepening persists for several months postoperatively. Over several years, however, progressive flattening occurs. The net result is an against-the-wound astigmatism.

Factors that affect the astigmatic change produced by a cataract incision include its length, meridional location, radial location (e.g. corneal, limbal or scleral), construction, and wound damage, such as thermal injury. With larger incisions, intrinsic patient factors can be important, as variations in wound healing can lead to markedly different astigmatic effects. Sutures have a temporary affect, but rarely produce changes that persist beyond 2 years, with the possible exception being those instances in which tissue is actually damaged or displaced by the sutures and heals in this new configuration.

Using scleral flap recessions of varying widths in eyebank eyes, Samuelson, Koch and Kuglen[13] have shown the direct relationship that exists between incision length and against-the-wound corneal flattening (Table 24-1). Notably, clinically significant flattening (0.5 D or more) occurred only in incisions longer than 3 mm.

SUTURE VERSUS SUTURELESS

Properly constructed scleral incisions up to 7 mm wide can be self-sealing in the absence of sutures. The key to watertightness is the anterior entry into the anterior chamber, which creates a valve effect as intraocular pressure compresses the mouth of the

incision closed. However, we suspect that sutured scleral incisions heal more rapidly and perhaps more completely than unsutured incisions. It is, therefore, possible that sutureless incisions are more prone to late wound sliding.

For corneal incisions, the vast majority can be left sutureless. However, unsutured clear corneal incisions may permit the ingress of surface fluid following minimal patient manipulation.[14,15] This may increase the risk of postoperative endophthalmitis, which has increased in frequency in the era of clear corneal cataract incisions.[16] We recommend suturing these incisions if they are greater than 4 mm in length or if the incision is not watertight at the conclusion of surgery.

INCISION LOCATION

As a general rule, for any given incision size and construction, the further the incision is from the center of the cornea, the less the surgically induced astigmatism. For small incisions, most surgeons have adopted the clear or near-clear corneal approach. Fortunately, these incisions are typically sufficiently small that they induce little astigmatism despite their anterior location. For incisions longer than 4°mm, the limbal and particularly scleral incisions offer greater astigmatic stability. Conversely, if against-the-wound drift is desired, these larger incisions can be placed more anteriorly in order to attempt to achieve the desired astigmatic change.

INCISION SIZE

Planned extracapsular Incisions

Curved scleral incisions concentric with the limbus and closed with interrupted 10-0 nylon or polyester sutures are recommended for planned extracapsular surgery.[10] Interrupted sutures are probably more prone to inducing excessive early steepness on the meridian of the incision, compared with continuous sutures. However, for these large incisions, interrupted sutures have two advantages: (1) they reduce the risk of excessive flattening along the meridian of the incision, and (2) they offer the opportunity to cut single sutures, which gives greater latitude in modifying astigmatism postoperatively. These incisions can typically drift 1–3 D in the first few years after surgery, and against-the-wound flattening of up to 5 D can, rarely, occur.

Enlarged phacoemulsification incisions

Incisions 6.5–7.5 mm wide are used for implantation of 6–7 mm polymethylmethacrylate (PMMA) optic lenses after phacoemulsification. The incisions may be curved, as with the extracapsular incision, or straight. An incision of this size can be expected to drift 1–2 D against the wound. If properly constructed, these incisions can be left unsutured, or they are closed with running shoelace suture, interrupted sutures, or a continuous horizontal suture. The advantage of a continuous horizontal suture is that it can be tightened sufficiently to provide watertight closure and perhaps to minimize late wound sliding without inducing excessive astigmatism. Long-term follow-up is needed to assess the stability of incisions closed in this manner. Additional techniques for suturing enlarged phacoemulsification incisions described by Masket and Shepherd (*Video Journal of Cataract and Refractive Surgery*, volume V, issue 3) are illustrated in Figures 24-4 and 24-5, respectively.

"Small-incision" cataract surgery

Incisions of 3 mm or less are used for insertion of foldable small-incision lenses after phacoemulsification. These incisions were originally made in the sclera or limbus, but clear or near-clear corneal incisions are now the most popular choice.

We have reviewed the ophthalmic literature regarding the astigmatic change induced by small scleral limbal and corneal

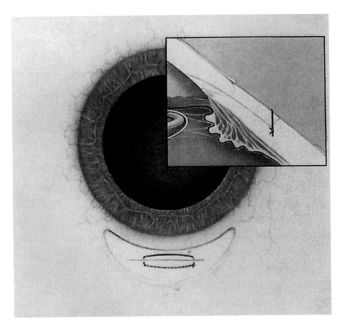

Figure 24-5 Technique for single vertical mattress suture. (From Koch DD, Lindstrom RL. Controlling astigmatism in cataract surgery. Semin Ophthalmology 1992;7:224–233.)

incisions, and the summary of these results are shown in Tables 24-2 and 24-3.[17–30] Interestingly, the results from these clinical studies mirror the results that were found in the cadaver eye study previously performed by Samuelson and Koch.

If we define true "small incision" surgery on an astigmatic basis such that less than 0.5 D is induced then this definition would pertain to scleral incisions measuring 4 mm and corneal incisions measuring 3.0–3.5 mm.

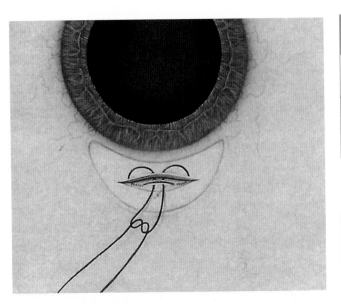

Figure 24-4 The Masket continuous horizontal suture closure consists of a posterior radial bite, two right-to-left bites concentric with the limbus, and an anterior-posterior radial bite. (From Koch DD, Lindstrom RL. Controlling astigmatism in cataract surgery. Semin Ophthalmology 1992;7:224–233.)

Table 24-2 Surgically induced astigmatism by scleral tunnel incisions

Incision length (mm)	Surgically induced astigmatism (D)
3.0–3.5	0.20–0.40
4.0	0.42–0.72
5.0–5.5	0.35–0.89

Table 24-3 Surgically induced astigmatism by clear corneal incisions

Incision length (mm)	Surgically induced astigmatism (D)
3.0–3.5	0.20–0.68
4.0	0.36–0.56
5.0–5.5	0.46–1.24

INCISION CONFIGURATION AND MANIPULATION

The configuration of the incision may also influence wound stability and eventual against-the-wound drift. A straight or frown-shaped incision appears to induce less against-the-wound astigmatic change than the traditional curved incision parallel to the limbus (Figure 24-6).

Pre-existing astigmatism can be reduced through the use of scleral flap recession on the steep corneal meridian. The approach has the advantages of (1) requiring only one incision (AK may be obviated), thereby minimizing wound-healing variables, and (2) avoiding the potential complications of corneal incisions, such as irregular astigmatism and glare.

To perform the technique, a trapezoidal scleral flap is made, centered meticulously on the steep meridian (Figure 24-7). The curvilinear base of the flap is located 2 mm behind the limbus, and the lateral walls of the flap are cut to within 0.5 mm of the cornea. The width of the flap at the limbus should slightly exceed the anticipated size of the incision into the anterior chamber (e.g. for a 6°mm incision, the flap measures 7°mm at the limbus and 8 mm posteriorly). The flap should be approximately two-thirds of the depth. As with standard incisions, the flap is dissected into clear cornea to enhance watertightness.

The flap is recessed and secured with a running 9-0 nylon suture anchored at each end and tied centrally. The suture pattern, shown in Figure 24-7, forms a barrier that prevents posterior migration of the flap and assures its stable fixation in the recessed position.[31]

With this technique up to 4–5 D of astigmatism can be corrected. Each 0.25 mm of recession produces about 1 D of astigmatic correction; the maximum recession is about 1 mm. The goal is to slightly overcorrect at surgery, as measured by qualitative or quantitative intraoperative keratometry. In the presence of significant undercorrection, the suture can be removed and the flap advanced an additional amount.

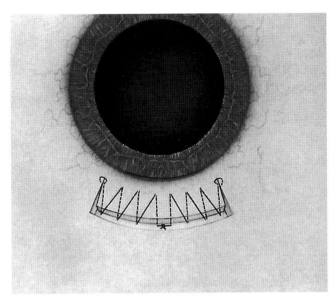

Figure 24-7 Configuration of the trapezoidal scleral flap and running suture closure for scleral flap recession. Note that the anterior edges of the flap are slightly lateral to the intended incision into the anterior chamber. Each suture bite exits in the bed of the flap to create a barrier that prevents posterior migration of the flap. (From Koch DD, Lindstrom RL. Controlling astigmatism in cataract surgery. Semin Ophthalmology 1992;7:224–233.)

Corneal relaxing incisions

The combination of CRI with cataract surgery (Figure 24-8) is fundamental to the current definition of *refractive cataract surgery*. A number of surgeons in the early 1980s, among them Fenzl, Lindstrom, Martin, Neumann, Nordan, Tate, Terry, and Thornton, began investigating surgical techniques to correct naturally occurring astigmatism. In 1983, Osher began a study that addressed the correction of pre-existing astigmatism by combining transverse relaxing incisions with cataract surgery. He presented preliminary results at general meetings from 1984 to 1990.[32]

Osher's original technique consisted of placing a single straight corneal relaxing incision in the periphery perpendicular to the steep meridian at the end of surgery and then adding a second parallel incision on a 7–10.5 mm-diameter optical zone. Maloney[33] described a more aggressive approach in which he placed two pairs of transverse incisions before phacoemulsification. Other surgeons attempted to quantify the effect of adding transverse corneal incisions to cataract surgery by varying incision length,[34] number of incisions,[35] optical zone size,[36] or incision depth.[37] Merlin[38] introduced arcuate incisions, and Thornton[39] and Lindstrom[40] became leading advocates while refining diamond blade technology.

Lindstrom[40] found that the *coupling ratio*, the amount of flattening in the incised meridian divided by the amount of steepening in the opposite meridian, was approximately 1:1 when a straight 3 mm keratotomy or a 45° to 90° arcuate keratotomy was used at 5–7 mm-diameter optical zones. The maximal effect of either straight or arcuate incisions occurred when incisions were placed around a 5–7 mm-diameter optical zone. Although most of the effect was achieved with the first pair of incisions, a 20% to 30% additional effect could be attained with a second pair of incisions. The effect could not be increased by placing more than four relaxing incisions in the cornea.

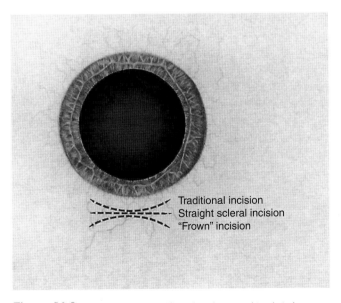

Figure 24-6 Induced astigmatic drift against the wound tends to be greatest with traditional curved incisions and least with frown-shaped incision configurations. (From Koch DD, Lindstrom RL. Controlling astigmatism in cataract surgery. Semin Ophthalmology 1992;7:224–233.)

Traditional incision
Straight scleral incision
"Frown" incision

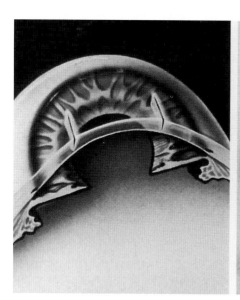
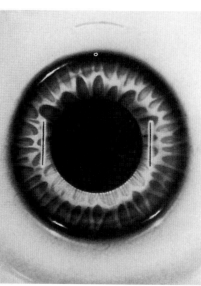

Figure 24-8 Transverse astigmatic keratotomy combined with cataract surgery. (From Osher RH. Transverse astigmatic keratotomy combined with cataract surgery. Ophthalmology Clin North Am 1992;5:717–725.)

Thornton[39] described what he believed was the geometric advantage of arcuate incisions, the use of which seems to be growing in popularity. He stated that true 1:1 coupling can occur only when the corneal circumference is unchanged, which is achieved only with short, concentric arcuate incisions. A straight transverse incision increases the overall corneal circumference, creating a flatter cornea and necessitating a compensatory addition of power to the IOL. Furthermore, a shorter arcuate incision achieves the same result as a longer straight incision.

■ PERIPHERAL OR LIMBAL CORNEAL RELAXING INCISIONS ■

Hollis and Gills first investigated the use of limbal relaxing incisions (LRIs) centered along the steep corneal meridian to correct pre-existing astigmatism during cataract surgery. As the single or paired relaxing incisions are placed just inside the limbal vessels, they are actually more appropriately called "peripheral corneal relaxing incisions" (PCRIs). Because they are placed at the peripheral cornea, a potential advantage of the incisions over AK is the minimal risk of inducing irregular astigmatism.

The criterion for PCRIs in conjunction with a temporal clear-corneal incision is pre-existing with-the-rule keratometric astigmatism of ≥0.75 D or pre-existing against-the-rule keratometric astigmatism of ≥1.25 D. This criterion was derived from a study of the astigmatic effect of a standard 3.2–3.5 mm temporal clear-corneal incision, which produces approximately 0.3 D of with-the-rule change. The length and number of PCRIs are determined according to a nomogram based on age and preoperative corneal astigmatism (Table 24-4). This nomogram is designed for use in combination with 3.2–3.5 mm temporal clear-corneal incision with PCRIs made near the end of the cataract surgery, and it is conservative in order to minimize the risk of overcorrections. PCRIs typically cause a mild hyperopic shift of approximately 0.2 D, and this should be taken into account when selecting IOL power.

Table 24-4 Nomogram for peripheral corneal relaxing incisions to correct keratometric astigmatism during cataract surgery (temporal 3.2 to 3.5 mm clear corneal incision)

Pre-operative astigmatism (D)	Age (year)	Number	Length
With-the-rule			
0.75–1.00	<65	2 (or 1 x 60°)	45°
	≥65	1	45°
1.01–1.50	<65	2	60°
	≥65	2 (or 1 x 60°)	50°
>1.50	<65	2	80°
	≥65	2	60°–70°
Against-the-rule			
1.00–1.25*	—	1 (or 2 x 30°)	35°–40°
1.26–2.00	—	1 (or 2 x 40°)	45°
≥2.00	—	2	45°

From Wang L, Misra M, and Koch DD. Peripheral corneal relaxing incisions combined with cataract surgery. J Cataract Refractive Surg 2003;29:712–722.

*Especially if cataract incision is not directly centered on steep meridian.

The location of the steep meridian is carefully determined as noted earlier in this chapter. Intraoperatively, the intended incision site is marked using one of many commercially available markers or even standard surgical calipers. The incision is made just inside the limbal vessels with a guarded diamond knife set at a depth of 600 μm (Figure 24-9). In eyes receiving paired incisions along the horizontal meridian (i.e. in eyes with pre-existing against-the-wound astigmatism), the groove of the temporal clear-corneal

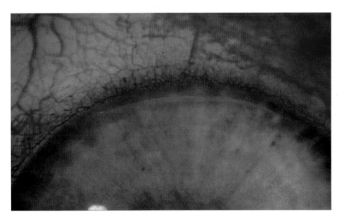

Figure 24-9 A view of a superior PCRI centered along 90° meridian on an eye 1 day after surgery.

incision is enlarged at the end of surgery to serve as the second peripheral relaxing incision, or the temporal peripheral relaxing incision can be made first by grooving at 600 μm depth to planned length and then entering the anterior chamber at the 50–75% depth of this incision. A PCRI at the cataract incision site can slightly destabilize the wound, so it is important to ensure that the incision is watertight at the conclusion of surgery.

Early studies with small number of cases showed that the PCRIs were an effective method of reducing pre-existing astigmatism during cataract surgery.[41,42] Recently, Wang, Misra, and Koch[43] reported the results in a large series of patients (93 eyes) who underwent combined clear corneal phacoemulsification and PCRIs. PCRIs significantly decreased pre-existing astigmatism, and the percentages of the eyes with keratometric astigmatism of ≤1 D increased from 6% preoperatively to 51% at 4 months postoperatively. Overcorrections of 1 D or more occurred in two eyes of two patients; both were over 80 years old. One of the two eyes had a corneal diameter of 10.5 mm, which might contribute to the overcorrection because of both the shorter distance between the PCRI and the center of the cornea and the longer arc length relative to the corneal circumference. For this reason, we recommend measuring PCRI length by degrees instead of millimeters. There were no ocular perforations in our series, suggesting a good safety profile for using a guarded diamond knife set at a depth of 600 μm when PCRIs are performed at the conclusion of cataract surgery.

We place PCRIs at the conclusion of the surgery because we had good success with this approach in our early cases and developed our first nomogram based on the results with these eyes. An advantage of performing the incisions at the conclusion of surgery is that these incisions can be omitted if there is some need to enlarge or change the site of the cataract incision. An obvious disadvantage is that there might be greater variability in corneal thickness and intraocular pressure at the conclusion of surgery, which could affect the depth of the incisions. We presume that incisions placed early in the surgery might have a greater effect and might also pose a greater risk of corneal perforation, particularly in older eyes with thinner corneas in the region of the limbus.

ASTIGMATIC KERATOTOMY

Lindstom and Koch's Technique

Manifest refraction, keratometry, and computerized videokeratography are performed preoperatively. For cataract patients, the surgical plan is formulated based on the intended incision and the pre-existing corneal astigmatism.

The standard nomograms shown in Tables 24-5 and 24-6 are used. The technique employs either a straight or arcuate keratotomy at the 6 mm and/or 7 mm zones. The nomogram, if adopted by others, needs to be adjusted to each surgeon's particular technique.

AK is performed at the end of the cataract procedure with the eye inflated. A smaller (5 mm or less) self-sealing incision is preferred when AK is combined with cataract surgery. When they are planning the AK, surgeons must factor in the expected against-the-would drift of the particular incision used.

Equipment includes an operating microscope, a Sinskey hook, 0.12 Colibri corneal fixation forceps, and various zone and incision markers. The Lindstrom arcuate marker (Katena Products, Denville, NJ) is preferred for arcuate incisions. Round 3 mm, 5 mm, and 7 mm radial keratotomy optical zone markers and 8-, 12-, and 16-cut radial keratotomy incision markers can be used to localize the incision location and length. A skin-marking pencil or stencil ink pad is used to clarify the marks. An ultrasonic pachymeter is used to measure corneal thickness intraoperatively. A surgical keratometer is useful but not essential for intraoperative monitoring.

A vertical-blade (push) diamond micrometer knife allows the surgeon good visibility while pushing through the length of the keratotomy. The knife is calibrated with the Mastel Retiscope (Mastel, Rapid City, SD) or a similar device. Extreme care should be taken in knife selection, calibration, and maintenance to assure reproducible cuts. Balanced salt solution and an irrigation cannula are used to keep the cornea moist and to irrigate incisions.

Topical anesthesia is particularly helpful in these patients, as it permits them to fixate the filament of the surgical microscope. This permits centration as demonstrated in Figure 24-10. For cataract patients who have been anesthetized with peribulbar or retrobulbar injection, the surgeon can accurately estimate the center of the pupil with the patient's eye adjusted to be perpendicular to the microscope. As with the method shown in Figure 24-10, the pupillary center is marked with a Sinskey hook or similar device.

The keratotomy optical zone is marked with a 7 mm marker (Figure 24-11). The steep meridian is marked with a skin-marking pen using intraoperative keratometry or preoperative landmarks and an axis marker (Figure 24-12). To mark the length of a 3 mm transverse keratotomy, a 3 mm circular zone marker is placed over the 7 mm zone mark (and also over the 5 mm zone mark if four cuts are planned) in the steep meridian (Figure 24-13). If arcuate keratotomy is preferred, the Lindstrom arcuate marker guides the performance of 45°, 60°, and 90° arcuate cuts (Figures 24-14 and 24-15). The use of a 16-ray, 12-ray, or 8-ray RK marker, respectively, can provide similar guidance (Figure 24-16). Arcuate incisions of more than 90° are not recommended.

Table 24-5 Arcuate keratotomy 6.0 mm optical zone nomogram*

			Surgical option			
Age (years)	1 x 30°	2 x 30° or 1 x 45°	1 x 60°	2 x 45° or 1 x 90°	2 x 60°	2 x 90°
20	0.60	1.20	1.80	2.40	3.60	4.80
21	0.62	1.23	1.85	2.46	3.69	4.92
22	0.63	1.26	1.89	2.52	3.78	5.04
23	0.65	1.29	1.94	2.58	3.87	5.16
24	0.66	1.32	1.98	2.64	3.96	5.28
25	0.68	1.35	2.03	2.70	4.05	5.40
26	0.69	1.38	2.07	2.76	4.14	5.52
27	0.71	1.41	2.12	2.82	4.23	5.64
28	0.72	1.44	2.16	2.88	4.32	5.76
29	0.74	1.47	2.21	2.94	4.41	5.88
30	0.75	1.50	2.25	3.00	4.50	6.00
31	0.77	1.53	2.30	3.06	4.59	6.12
32	0.78	1.56	2.34	3.12	4.68	6.24
33	0.80	1.59	2.39	3.18	4.77	6.36
34	0.81	1.62	2.43	3.24	4.86	6.48
35	0.83	1.65	2.48	3.30	4.95	6.60
36	0.84	1.68	2.52	3.36	5.04	6.72
37	0.86	1.71	2.57	3.42	5.13	6.84
38	0.87	1.74	2.61	3.48	5.22	6.96
39	0.89	1.77	2.66	3.54	5.31	7.08
40	0.90	1.80	2.70	3.60	5.40	7.20
41	0.92	1.83	2.75	3.66	5.49	7.32
42	0.93	1.86	2.79	3.72	5.58	7.44
43	0.95	1.89	2.84	3.78	5.67	7.56
44	0.96	1.92	2.88	3.84	5.76	7.68
45	0.98	1.95	2.93	3.90	5.85	7.80
46	0.99	1.98	2.97	3.96	5.94	7.92
47	1.01	2.01	3.02	4.02	6.03	8.04
48	1.02	2.04	3.06	4.08	6.12	8.16
49	1.04	2.07	3.11	4.14	6.21	8.28
50	1.05	2.10	3.15	4.20	6.30	8.40
51	1.07	2.13	3.20	4.26	6.39	8.52
52	1.08	2.16	3.24	4.32	6.48	8.64
53	1.10	2.19	3.29	4.38	6.57	8.76
54	1.11	2.22	3.33	4.44	6.66	8.88
55	1.13	2.25	3.38	4.50	6.75	9.00
56	1.14	2.28	3.42	4.56	6.84	9.12
57	1.16	2.31	3.47	4.62	6.93	9.24
58	1.17	2.34	3.51	4.68	7.02	9.36
59	1.19	2.37	3.56	4.74	7.11	9.48
60	1.20	2.40	3.60	4.80	7.20	9.60
61	1.22	2.43	3.65	4.86	7.29	9.72
62	1.23	2.46	3.69	4.92	7.38	9.84
63	1.25	2.49	3.74	4.98	7.47	9.96
64	1.26	2.52	3.78	5.04	7.56	10.08
65	1.28	2.55	3.83	5.10	7.65	10.20
66	1.29	2.58	3.87	5.16	7.74	10.32
67	1.31	2.61	3.92	5.22	7.83	10.44
68	1.32	2.64	3.96	5.28	7.92	10.56
69	1.34	2.67	4.01	5.34	8.01	10.68
70	1.35	2.70	4.05	5.40	8.10	10.80
71	1.37	2.73	4.10	5.46	8.19	10.92
72	1.38	2.76	4.14	5.52	8.28	11.04
73	1.40	2.79	4.19	5.58	8.37	11.16
74	1.41	2.82	4.23	5.64	8.46	11.28
75	1.43	2.85	4.28	5.70	8.55	11.40

From Richard L. Lindstrom, MD, Phillips Eye Institute, Minneapolis, Minnesota 55404, and Chiron IntraOptics, Irvine, CA.
*Find patient age, then move right to find result closest to refractive cylinder without going over.

Table 24-6 Arcuate keratotomy nomogram for males with 7.0 mm optical zone

	Surgical option						
Age (years)	1 x 45°	2 x 30°	1 x 60°	1 x 90°	2 x 45°	2 x 60°	2 x 90°
20	0.32	1.62	0.92	2.02	2.22	2.72	3.82
21	0.36	1.66	0.96	2.06	2.26	2.76	3.86
22	0.39	1.69	0.99	2.09	2.29	2.79	3.89
23	0.40	1.73	1.03	2.13	2.33	2.83	3.93
24	0.46	1.76	1.06	2.16	2.36	2.86	3.96
25	0.50	1.80	1.10	2.20	2.40	2.90	4.00
26	0.54	1.84	1.14	2.24	2.44	2.94	4.04
27	0.57	1.87	1.17	2.27	2.47	2.97	4.07
28	0.61	1.91	1.21	2.31	2.51	3.01	4.11
29	0.64	1.94	1.24	2.34	2.54	3.04	4.14
30	0.68	1.98	1.28	2.38	2.58	3.08	4.18
31	0.72	2.02	1.32	2.42	2.62	3.12	4.22
32	0.75	2.05	1.35	2.45	2.65	3.15	4.25
33	0.79	2.09	1.39	2.49	2.69	3.19	4.29
34	0.82	2.12	1.42	2.52	2.72	3.22	4.32
35	0.86	2.16	1.46	2.56	2.76	3.26	4.36
36	0.90	2.20	1.50	2.60	2.80	3.30	4.40
37	0.93	2.23	1.53	2.63	2.83	3.33	4.43
38	0.97	2.27	1.57	2.67	2.87	3.37	4.47
39	1.00	2.30	1.60	2.70	2.90	3.40	4.50
40	1.04	2.34	1.64	2.74	2.94	3.44	4.54
41	1.08	2.38	1.68	2.78	2.98	3.48	4.58
42	1.11	2.41	1.71	2.81	3.01	3.51	4.61
43	1.15	2.45	1.75	2.85	3.05	3.55	4.65
44	1.18	2.48	1.78	2.88	3.08	3.58	4.68
45	1.22	2.52	1.82	2.92	3.12	3.62	4.72
46	1.26	2.56	1.86	2.96	3.16	3.66	4.76
47	1.29	2.59	1.89	2.99	3.19	3.69	4.79
48	1.33	2.63	1.93	3.03	3.23	3.73	4.83
49	1.36	2.66	1.96	3.06	3.26	3.76	4.86
50	1.40	2.70	2.00	3.10	3.30	3.80	4.90
51	1.44	2.74	2.04	3.14	3.34	3.84	4.94
52	1.47	2.77	2.07	3.17	3.37	3.87	4.97
53	1.51	2.81	2.11	3.21	3.41	3.91	5.01
54	1.54	2.84	2.14	3.24	3.44	3.94	5.04
55	1.58	2.88	2.18	3.28	3.48	3.98	5.08
56	1.62	2.92	2.22	3.32	3.52	4.02	5.12
57	1.65	2.95	2.25	3.35	3.55	4.05	5.15
58	1.69	2.99	2.29	3.39	3.59	4.09	5.19
59	1.72	3.02	2.32	3.42	3.62	4.12	5.22
60	1.76	3.06	2.36	3.46	3.66	4.16	5.26
61	1.80	3.10	2.40	3.50	3.70	4.20	5.30
62	1.83	3.13	2.43	3.53	3.73	4.23	5.33
63	1.87	3.17	2.47	3.57	3.77	4.27	5.37
64	1.90	3.20	2.50	3.60	3.80	4.30	5.40
65	1.94	3.24	2.54	3.64	3.84	4.34	5.44
66	1.98	3.28	2.58	3.68	3.88	4.38	5.48
67	2.01	3.31	2.61	3.71	3.91	4.41	5.51
68	2.05	3.35	2.65	3.75	3.95	4.45	5.55
69	2.08	3.38	2.68	3.78	3.98	4.48	5.58
70	2.12	3.42	2.72	3.82	4.02	4.52	5.62
71	2.16	3.46	2.76	3.86	4.06	4.56	5.66
72	2.19	3.49	2.79	3.89	4.09	4.59	5.69
73	2.23	3.53	2.83	3.93	4.13	4.63	5.73
74	2.26	3.56	2.86	3.96	4.16	4.66	5.76
75	2.30	3.60	2.90	4.00	4.20	4.70	5.80

Subtract 0.37 from each predicted value for females.

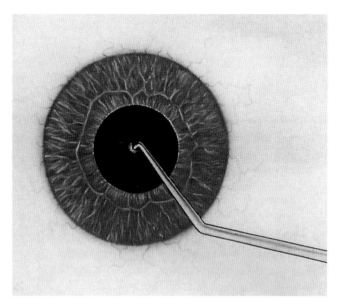

Figure 24-10 The center of the optical zone is determined by asking the patient to fixate on the microscope light, on a mark placed directly between the two oculars, or on the Mastel Aximeter (Mastel, Rapid City, SD). While the patient is properly fixating, the center of the entrance pupil is marked with a Sinskey hook. (From Koch DD, Lindstrom RL. Controlling astigmatism in cataract surgery. Semin Ophthalmology 1992;7:224–233.)

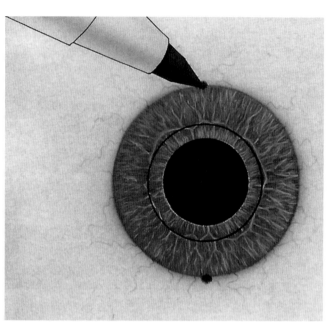

Figure 24-12 Marking the steep meridian. (From Koch DD, Lindstrom RL. Controlling astigmatism in cataract surgery. Semin Ophthalmology 1992;7: 224–233.)

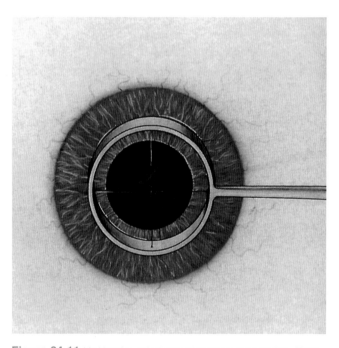

Figure 24-11 Marking the optical zone with a 7-mm zone marker. (From Koch DD, Lindstrom RL. Controlling astigmatism in cataract surgery. Semin Ophthalmology 1992;7:224–233.)

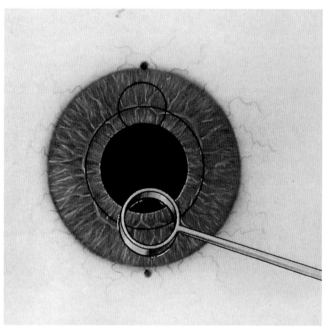

Figure 24-13 Use of a 3-mm zone marker to delineate the incision length. (From Koch DD, Lindstrom RL. Controlling astigmatism in cataract surgery. Semin Ophthalmology 1992;7:224–233.)

Intraoperative pachymetry is used at the appropriate optical zone in the steep meridian on one (for a single incision) or both sides of the cornea (Figure 24-17). The blade depth of the calibrated diamond knife is set at 100% of the thinnest paracentral pachymetry. If pachymetry is not available, setting the knife at 0.6 mm for a 7 mm optical zone incision appears to be safe and effective.

With the corneal fixation forceps held in the nondominant hand and used to grasp tissue at the limbus, the knife in the dominant hand is set into the cornea, pausing for 1 second. The knife is then guided slowly through the incision (Figure 24-18).

The completed incision is irrigated with balanced salt solution (Figure 24-19), and several drops of topical antibiotic are placed

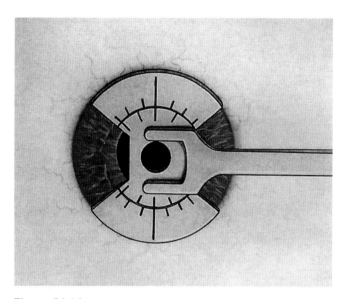

Figure 24-14 The Lindstrom arcuate marker (Katena Products) is placed on the cornea aligned with the steep meridian. (From Koch DD, Lindstrom RL. Controlling astigmatism in cataract surgery. Semin Ophthalmology 1992;7: 224–233.)

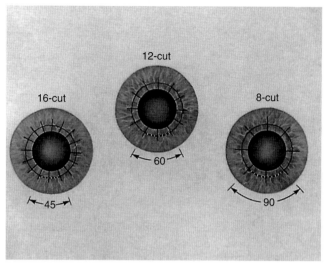

Figure 24-16 Left, Sixteen-ray RK marker is useful to delineate 45° arcuate keratotomy. Center, Twelve-ray RK marker is useful to delineate 60° arcuate keratotomy. Right, Eight-ray RK marker is useful to delineate 90° arcuate keratotomy. (From Koch DD, Lindstrom RL. Controlling astigmatism in cataract surgery. Semin Ophthalmology 1992;7:224–233.)

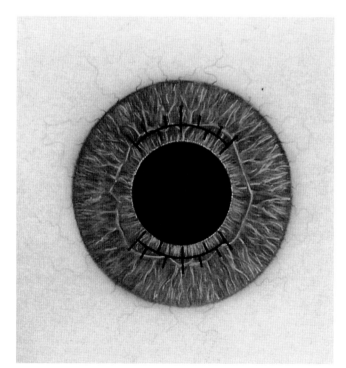

Figure 24-15 Cornea marked before astigmatic keratotomy. Perpendicular lines mark 45°, 60°, and 90° for arcuate cuts. (From Koch DD, Lindstrom RL. Controlling astigmatism in cataract surgery. Semin Ophthalmology 1992;7: 224–233.)

Osher's technique

Since beginning astigmatic keratometry combined with cataract surgery for the reduction of pre-existing astigmatism in 1983, Osher's technique has gone through several revisions. The initial examination had always included careful keratometry, and each new generation of corneal topography has been added. The amount of phakic or pseudophakic astigmatism in the fellow eye

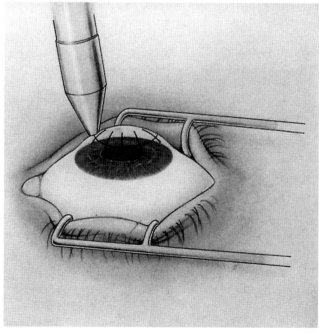

Figure 24-17 Corneal pachymetry is measured directly over the incision site; the blade is set at 90%–100% of the thinnest pachymetry reading. (From Koch DD, Lindstrom RL. Controlling astigmatism in cataract surgery. Semin Ophthalmology 1992;7:224–233.)

on the eye. Patching or cycloplegia is not routinely used. If a significant perforation occurs, subconjunctival antibiotic, topical cycloplegia, and a pressure patch are used; obviously, if chamber depth cannot be maintained, then the incision with the perforation is sutured. Perforations are extremely rare with the technique described.

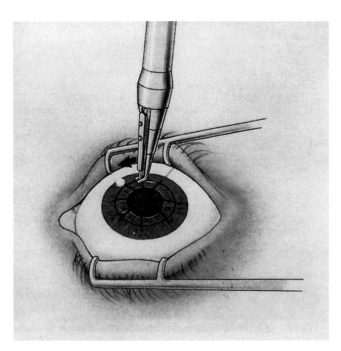

Figure 24-18 Marking the incision. (From Koch DD, Lindstrom RL. Controlling astigmatism in cataract surgery. Semin Ophthalmology 1992;7: 224–233.)

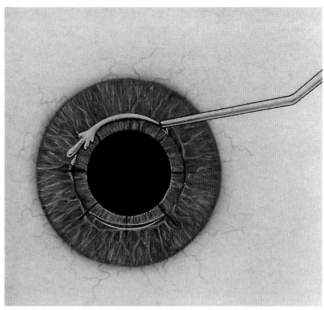

Figure 24-19 Irrigation with balanced salt solution. (From Koch DD, Lindstrom RL. Controlling astigmatism in cataract surgery. Semin Ophthalmology 1992;7:224–233.)

must be considered in determining candidacy. Patients with significant anterior membrane dystrophy or severe Fuch's endothelial dystrophy are excluded. An explanation of the surgical plan to reduce the astigmatism is given, and the patient is informed that this procedure is elective and inexact and may result in more ocular irritation than normal for several days following surgery (although this is usually not the case). Permission to perform the astigmatic keratometry is part of the routine informed consent form for cataract surgery.

Following the initial evaluation, an operative plan is formulated. The optical zone is selected, primarily based on the Osher nomogram (Table 24-7) while keeping the length, depth, and shape of the incisions constant.[44] Principles gained through experience, such as the greater response in eyes having against-the-rule cylinder, a large corneal diameter, increasing patient age, and the perceived effect of intraocular pressure are taken into consideration. The nomogram will need to be adjusted

according to each surgeon's particular technique. Since astigmatic keratotomy does not change *average* preoperative keratometric power, no change is needed in IOL power. After arriving at the optimal approach for the patient, a drawing is made on the chart, which is hung from the microscope next to the topography for easy reference. The drawing shows the size of the optical zone and the location of the incisions to assure proper orientation.

In the early years of performing this procedure, the major meridians of the eye were marked in the holding room prior to surgery with a drop of topical anesthetic and a cautery while the eye was in the primary position of gaze for distance fixation. This method has been replaced by quantitative intraoperative keratoscopy. A Hyde-Osher ruler made by Ocular Instruments has a series of spherical and astigmatic circles cut out of a metallic bar. This is held between the eye and the microscope and easily identifies the steep meridian of curvature, which is marked at the limbus with two spots 180° from each other using the coaptation cautery. With the eye coaxial with the microscope, the amount of cylinder is quantitated by neutralizing the progressive astigmatic openings in the bar until a circular reflex is observed. The measurements of the axis and amount of cylinder are usually consistent with the preoperative data. If the axis is off by several degrees, the intraoperative observations are favored. If a disparity greater than 10° or 15° exists, AK is not performed – a decision that is rarely necessary.

Although initially blade depth was determined by intraoperative pachymetry, for many years Osher has simply set the blade at 690 microns for an optical zone of 6mm or greater. Formerly, AK was performed at the conclusion of the procedure to maximize visualization during the cataract surgery, but currently the

Table 24-7 Osher nomogram for 3 mm T–cuts

Cylinder (D)	Optical zone (mm)
1.5	8.5
2.0	8.0
2.5	7.0–7.5
3.0	6.0–6.5
3.5	2 pair: 6 and 8.5

From Osher RH. Transverse astigmatic keratotomy combined with cataract surgery. Ophthalmology Clin North Am 1992;5:717–725.

incisions are made at the beginning of the procedure. The advantages include a firmer globe with a better epithelium, yielding more accurate intraoperative keratoscopy and incision depth. In addition, the healthier epithelium results in many fewer corneal abrasions, so the eye does not require patching.

The incision length is 3 mm. The globe is stabilized with a multiple dull-toothed forceps held in the fellow hand. Increasing experience has resulted in consistent incision depth between 80% and 95%, which is important in achieving effective results. A second pair of incisions is reserved for cylinder greater than 3.5 D. After the incisions are made, a 30 gauge cannula is used to confirm that the depth is adequate; it is then used to gently irrigate a stream of balanced salt solution into the incision to remove any trapped air bubbles or cellular debris. Complications include corneal abrasion in about 5% and microperforation in less than 1%. If a superficial abrasion occurs, a double pressure patch is applied at the conclusion of the procedure.

Astigmatic keratometry is performed in those 20% of patients, approximately, with pre-existing cylinder of $\geq$1.5 D. In a study of this conservative approach to AK using the same nomogram in which only the optical zone was varied, all eyes except one with amblyopia enjoyed a best-corrected visual acuity comparable to that of a controlled population not receiving AK.[32] However, the uncorrected vision was outstanding with acuity of 20/40 or better achieved in 76%. Certainly only a fraction of these patients would have achieved this visual result had their cylinder not been reduced by AK. Comparison of preoperative and postoperative keratometry measurement showed that the IOL selected would have been unchanged in 87% of eyes. Although 13% showed a power change of between 0.5 and 1 D, it was reassuring to find that the surgical change in the cornea influenced the IOL power less than 1 D in all cases.

Femtosecond laser-assisted arcuate keratotomy

With the advent of the femtosecond laser and its ability to produce both horizontal and vertical cleavage planes within the corneal stroma, several investigators have reported their use of the laser to create corneal incisions to reduce astigmatism. Harissi-Dagher and Azar[45] used a femtosecond laser to perform astigmatic keratotomy in two patients with high levels of corneal astigmatism following penetrating keratoplasty. The postoperative refractive cylinder measured 4.9 and 4.3 D, down from the preoperative levels of 8.5 and 7 D, respectively. The best-corrected visual acuities also improved from 20/100 and 20/200 before surgery to 20/30 and 20/60 after. No complications were seen in either case. Kymionis et al.[46] described their use of the femtosecond laser to correct irregular corneal astigmatism following penetrating keratoplasty. They used the keratoplasty software on the Intralase femtosecond laser (Abbot Medical Optics, Inc., location) to create a single arcuate side cut that was 6.5 mm in diameter. Six months following the procedure, the corneal astigmatism had decreased from 4 to 0.5 D and the best spectacle-corrected visual acuity had improved from 20/50 to 20/32.

Hoffart et al.[47] compared the effectiveness of a femtosecond laser to a mechanical method using the Hanna keratome (Moria, Inc., Anthony, France) in performing AK in 20 postkeratoplasty

eyes. The mean uncorrected and best-corrected acuities did not change significantly for either group. However, the mean refractive cylinder decreased from preoperative levels of 8.6 and 6.7 D to postoperative values of 3.9 and 4.7 D for the laser and mechanical methods, respectively. The Hanna group had a microperforation in one case and worse alignment, in general. Both treatments were found to be effective in reducing postkeratoplasty astigmatism, with the femtosecond laser showing some advantages over the mechanized method.

Although AK was performed in postkeratoplasty eyes in these cases, they do demonstrate the feasibility of using the laser to create corneal incisions that reduce astigmatism. The laser can be used in a similar fashion to create astigmatism-reducing corneal incisions following cataract surgery. Care must be taken to allow the corneal wounds to heal adequately before applying the suction ring required for use with the femtosecond laser. While the laser provides a very controlled and potentially repeatable method for performing AK, several disadvantages are associated with its use for AK: (1) there is an added expense for the disposable materials and treatment, (2) the treatment can not be performed at the time of cataract surgery, and (3) well-tested nomograms are needed.

TORIC INTRAOCULAR LENS

The toric IOL was devised by Shimizu, Misawa, and Suzuki[48] and has been used clinically since 1992. The first toric IOL introduced was a nonfoldable 3-piece posterior chamber lens; foldable toric single-piece IOLs are available currently. Advantages of astigmatism correction with toric IOLs over CRIs are reversibility and excellent optical quality with no induction of irregular astigmatism. The surgical technique of toric IOL implantation involves careful preoperative marking of the correct meridian for IOL alignment, as well as intraoperative rotation of the toric IOL to orient the its axis markings along the steep corneal meridian.

Staar toric IOL models (STAAR Surgical Company, Monrovia, CA) have a toric anterior surface, spherical posterior surface, two positioning marks along the long axis on the anterior surface, and two 1.15 mm fenestrations at the opposite ends (Figure 24-20). The lens is available in powers ranging from 9.5 to 28 D with cylindrical adds of 2 and 3.5 D, which theoretically correct 1.4

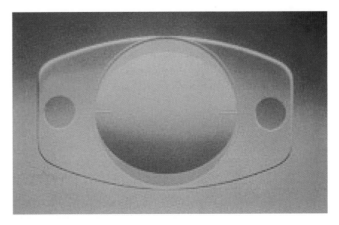

Figure 24-20 The Staar toric intraocular lens.

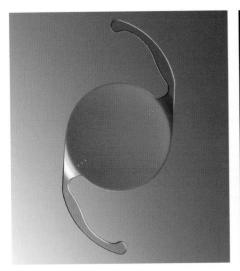
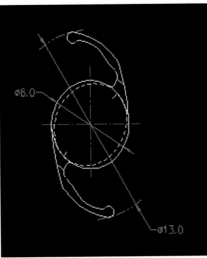

Figure 24-21 The Alcon Acrysof toric intraocular lens.

and 2.3 D of astigmatism at the corneal plane, respectively. Thus, patients with 1.5–3.5 D of regular pre-existing astigmatism are candidates for implantation of these lenses.

Postoperative rotation of this plate haptic toric IOL is a significant problem. Leyland et al.[49] reported that 18% (4 of 22) of IOLs rotated more than 30°. Sun et al.[50] reported that 18% rotated between 20° and 40°, and 7% rotated more than 40°. In the study by Till et al.[51] 6% of IOLs rotated more than 31°. This, presumably, results in a greater than 10% incidence of surgical reintervention to reposition the implants. Modifications in this plate haptic toric IOL design are needed to address this problem. An additional drawback in the use of this toric IOL is that the only cylindrical adds currently available are 2 and 3.5 D.

A one-piece acrylic toric IOL (Alcon Surgical, Inc.) was recently approved for use within the US. The lens design employs the widely used Acrysof single-piece platform with the toric correction on the posterior surface (Figure 24-21). The IOL is available in powers ranging from 5 to 30 D with three levels of cylindrical correction (1.5, 2.25, and 3 D), which correspond to 1.03, 1.55, and 2.06 D of astigmatism correction at the corneal plane, respectively. In the US FDA clinical trial, 494 eyes were randomized to implantation of the toric IOL or a standard spherical single-piece acrylic IOL. At 6 months following surgery, 420 eyes were available for analysis (211 with the toric IOL and 209 controls). Ninety-four percent of eyes receiving a toric IOL achieved monocular UCVA of 20/40 or better, compared to 79% of controls. Postoperative refractive cylinder was ≤0.50 D in 61% of toric patients and 19% of controls. The IOL showed excellent rotational stability with a mean postoperative rotation of 4°. Ninety-seven percent of the IOLs rotated less than 10°. In addition, 94% of patients receiving bilateral toric IOL implantation were spectacle-free for distance activities.

Several post-market studies have evaluated the performance of this toric IOL. Bauer et al.[52] looked at the outcomes of Acrysof toric IOL implantation in a prospective study of 53 eyes in 43 patients. Patients were somewhat evenly split between the T3 (16 eyes), T4 (14 eyes), and T5 (23 eyes). Thirteen eyes in the T5 group had the potential to be fully corrected, while 10 eyes had astigmatism levels that could only be partially corrected. Greater than 90% of eyes achieved uncorrected visual acuities of 20/40 or

better, while almost 80% had uncorrected visual acuities of 20/25 or better. Residual refractive astigmatism was less than 0.75 D in 74% of eyes and less than 1 D in 91%. The mean IOL misalignment was 3.5 ± 3°. Weinand et al.[53] found the rotational stability of the IOL to be excellent. They evaluated the IOL position using digital photographs taken immediately after implantation and 6 months later. By referencing features on the conjunctiva and IOL, they found a median postoperative IOL rotation of only 0.7° in a group of 17 eyes, with a maximum rotation of 1.8°. Chang[54] compared the rotational stability of the Acrysof toric IOL (100 eyes) to the Staar toric IOL (90 eyes). He found that 90%, 99%, and 100% of the Acrysof toric IOLs were aligned within 5, 10, and 15°, respectively. The Staar toric IOL had 70%, 90%, and 97% aligned within 5, 10, and 15°, respectively. The mean rotation of the Acrysof IOL was 3.35 ± 3.41°, while the mean rotation of the Staar toric IOL was 5.56 ± 8.49°. He concluded that both IOLs showed a small degree of postoperative rotation, with the Acrysof toric IOL demonstrating greater stability that was statistically significant.

Astigmatism correction with toric IOLs carries several advantages. Typically there is a need for only one surgical procedure. Also, the induction of irregular corneal astigmatism is avoided and the single-piece toric IOL demonstrates long-term stability. The most ideal way to manage residual astigmatism would be to modify the IOL after it has been implanted using a noninvasive approach. The Calhoun Vision silicone IOL, currently in development, may offer this possibility. The refractive power of this IOL can be modified with laser irradiation after implantation. Differential irradiation of the optic can alter its refractive power to correct astigmatism, as well as other higher-order aberrations. This IOL may have the potential to correct a wide variety of postoperative refractive errors.

CONCLUSIONS

Refractive cataract surgery requires meticulous planning and surgical technique in order to optimize the spherical and astigmatic refractive outcomes. Patient expectations are increasing; for many, excellent uncorrected visual acuity is a primary goal of surgery.[55] The development of multifocal and accommodating

IOLs heightens the clinical mandate for precision in reaching targeted refractive goals. The practitioner who has mastered the current tools and philosophies in dealing with astigmatism in cataract surgery may be in the best position to incorporate new technologies as they emerge.

Although no single best approach to astigmatism correction in cataract surgery has yet been established, it likely that evolving toric and adjustable IOL designs will ultimately provide the most consistent refractive results and superior optics. However, by incorporating the general principles outlined in this chapter, surgeons will be able to transition into the new subspecialty of refractive cataract surgery and greatly enhance their surgical outcomes using current technology. By paying meticulous attention to results, each surgeon will inevitably create his or her own nomograms, tailored not only to the technical aspects of a preferred surgical approach, but also to the visual demands of the individual patient.

References

[1] Schiotz HA. Ein fall von hochgradigem hornhautastigmatismus nach starrextraction. Besserung auf operativem wege. Arch Augenheilkunde 1885;15:178–181.

[2] Faber E. Operative behandelingf van astigmatisme. Ned Tijdschr Geneeskd 1895;2:495–496.

[3] Lans LJ. Experimentelle untersuchungen uber entstehung von astigmatismus durch nich–perforirende corneawunden. Albrect Con Graef's Arch Ophthalmol 1898;45:117–152.

[4] Bates WH. A suggestion of an operation to correct astigmatism. Arch Ophthalmol 1894;23:9–13.

[5] Frranks JB, Binder PS. Keratotomy procedures for the correction of astigmatism. J Refract Surg 1985;1:11–17.

[6] Duke-Elder SS, Abrams D. Ophthalmic optics and refraction. In: System of ophthalmology. Vol 5. St. Louis: CV Mosby; 1970. p. 274–295.

[7] Buzard K, Shearing S, Relyea R. Incidence of astigmatism in a cataract practice. J Refract Surg 1988;4:173.

[8] Axt JC. Longitudinal study of postoperative astigmatism. J Cataract Refract Surg 1987;13:381–388.

[9] Jampel HD, Thompson JR, Baker CC, et al. A computerized analysis of astigmatism after cataract surgery. Ophthalmic Surg 1986;17:786–790.

[10] Koch DD, Lindstrom RL. Controlling astigmatism in cataract surgery. Semin Ophthalmol 1992;7:224–233.

[11] Stevens JD. Astigmatic excimer laser treatment: theoretical effects of axis misalignment. Eur J Implant Ref Surg 1994;6:310–318.

[12] Swami AU, Steinert RF, Osborne WE, White AA. Rotational malposition during laser in situ keratomileusis. Am J Ophthalmol 2002;133:561–562.

[13] Samuelson SW, Koch DD, Kuglen CC. Determination of maximal incision length for true small-incision surgery. Ophthalmic Surg 1991;22:204–207.

[14] Herretes S, Stark WJ, Pirouzmanesh A, et al. Inflow of ocular surface fluid into the anterior chamber after phacoemulsification through sutureless corneal cataract wounds. Am J Ophthalmol 2005;140:737–740.

[15] Taban M, Sarayba MA, Ignacio TS, et al. Ingress of India ink into the anterior chamber through sutureless clear corneal cataract wounds. Arch Ophthalmol 2005;123(5):643–648.

[16] Taban M, Behrens A, Newcomb RL, et al. Acute endophthalmitis following cataract surgery: a systematic review of the literature. Arch Ophthalmol 2005;123(5):613–620.

[17] Pfleger T, Scholz U, Skorpik C. Postoperative astigmatism after no-stitch, small incision cataract surgery with 3.5 mm and 4.5 mm incisions. J Cataract Refract Surg 1994;20:400–505.

[18] Lyhne N, Corydon L. Two year follow-up of astigmatism after phacoemulsification with adjusted and unadjusted sutured versus sutureless 5.2 mm superior scleral incisions. J Cataract Refract Surg 1998;24:1647–1651.

[19] Huang FC, Tseng SH. Comparison of surgically induced astigmatism after sutureless temporal clear corneal and scleral frown incisions. J Cataract Refract Surg 1998;24:477–481.

[20] Dam-Johansen M, Olsen T. Induced astigmatism after 4 and 6 mm scleral tunnel incision. A randomized study. Acta Ophthalmol Scand 1997;75:669–674.

[21] Mendivil A. Frequency of induced astigmatism following phacoemulsification with suturing versus without suturing. Ophthalmic Surg Lasers 1997;28:377–381.

[22] Olsen T, Dam-Johansen M, Bek T, Hjortdal JO. Corneal versus scleral tunnel incision in cataract surgery: a randomized study. J Cataract Refract Surg 1997;23:337–341.

[23] Haubrich T, Knorz MC, Seiberth V, Liesenhoff H. Vector analysis of surgically-induced astigmatism in cataract operation with 4 tunnel incision techniques. Ophthalmologe 1996;93:12–16.

[24] Gross RH, Miller KM. Corneal astigmatism after phacoemulsification and lens implantation through unsutured scleral and corneal tunnel incisions. Am J Ophthalmol 1996;121:57–64.

[25] Beltrame G, Salvetat ML, Chizzolini M, Driussi G. Corneal topographic changes induced by different oblique cataract incisions. J Cataract Refract Surg 2001;27:720–727.

[26] Lyhne N, Krogsager J, Corydon L, Kjeldgaard M. One year follow-up of astigmatism after 4.0 mm temporal clear corneal and superior scleral incisions. J Cataract Refract Surg 2000;26:83–87.

[27] Pfleger T, Skorpik C, Menapace R, Scholz U, Weghaupt H, Zehetmayer M. Long-term course of induced astigmatism after clear corneal incision cataract surgery. J Cataract Refract Surg 1996;22:72–77.

[28] Kohnen T, Dick B, Jacobi KW. Comparison of the induced astigmatism after temporal clear corneal tunnel incisions of different sizes. J Cataract Refract Surg 1995;21:417–424.

[29] Nielsen PJ. Prospective evaluation of surgically induced astigmatism and astigmatic keratotomy effects of various self-sealing small incisions. J Cataract Refract Surg 1995;21:43–48.

[30] Vass C, Menapace R, Rainer G, Findl O, Steineck I. Comparative study of corneal topographic changes after 3.0 mm beveled and hinged clear corneal incisions. J Cataract Refract Surg 1998;24:1498–1504.

[31] Koch DD, Del Pero RA, Wong TC, et al. Scleral flap surgery for modification of corneal astigmatism. Am J Ophthalmol 1987;104:259–264.

[32] Osher RH. Paired transverse relaxing keratotomy: A combined technique for reducing astigmatism. J Cataract Refract Surg 1989;15:32–37.

[33] Maloney WF. Refractive cataract replacement: a comprehensive approach to maximize refractive benefits of cataract extraction. Annual Meeting of the American Society of Cataract and Refractive Surgery, Los Angeles, 1986.

[34] Shepherd JR. Induced astigmatism in small incision surgery. J Cataract Refract Surg 1989;15:85–88.

[35] Davison JA. Transverse astigmatic keratotomy combined with phacoemulsification and intraocular lens implantation. J Cataract Refract Surg 1989;15:38–44.

[36] Hall GW, Campion M, Sorenson CM, et al. Reduction of corneal astigmatism at cataract surgery. J Cataract Refract Surg 1991;17:407–414.

[37] Gills JP. Relaxing incisions reduce postop astigmatism. Ophthalmology Times November 1991;15:11.

[38] Merlin U. Corneal keratotomy procedure for congenital astigmatism. J Refract Surg 1987;3:92–97.

[39] Thornton SP. Theory behind corneal relaxing incision/Thornton nomogram. In: Gills JP, Martin RG, Sanders DR, editors. Sutureless cataract surgery. Thorofare, NJ: Slack Inc; 1992. p. 123–144.

[40] Lindstrom RL. The surgical correction of astigmatism: A clinician's perspective. J Cataract Corneal Surg 1990;6:441–454.

[41] Budak K, Friedman NJ, Koch DD. Limbal relaxing incisions with cataract surgery. J Cataract Refractive Surg 1998;24:503–508.

[42] Müller-Jensen K, Fischer P, Siepe U. Limbal relaxing incisions to correct astigmatism in clear corneal cataract surgery. J Refract Surg 1999;15:586–589.

[43] Wang L, Misra M, Koch DD. Peripheral corneal relaxing incisions combined with cataract surgery. J Cataract Refractive Surg 2003;29:712–722.

[44] Osher RH. Transverse astigmatic keratotomy combined with cataract surgery. In: Robert Stamper M, editor. Ophthalmology clinics of North America: contemporary refractive surgery. Philadelphia, PA: W.B. Saunders Co; 1992. p. 717–725.

[45] Harissi-Dagher M, Azar DT. Femtosecond laser astigmatic keratotomy for postkeratoplasty astigmatism. Can J Ophthalmol 2008;43:367–369.

[46] Kymionis GD, Yoo SH, Ide T, Culbertson WW. Femtosecond-assisted astigmatic keratotomy for post-keratoplasty irregular astigmatism. J Cataract Refract Surg 2009;35:11–13.

[47] Hoffart L, Proust H, Matonti F, Conrath J, Ridings B. Correction of postkeratoplasty astigmatism by femtosecond laser compared with mechanized astigmatic keratotomy. Am J Ophthalmol 147:779–787 [Published online 20 Feb 2009].

[48] Shimizu K, Misawa A, Suzuki Y. Toric intraocular lenses: correcting astigmatism while controlling axis shift. J Cataract Refractive Surg 1994;20:523–526.

[49] Bauer NJC, de Vries NE, Webers CA, et al. Astigmatism management in cataract surgery with the Acrysof toric intraocular lens. J Cataract Refract Surg 2008;34(9):1483–1488.

[50] Weinand F, Jung A, Stein A, et al. Rotational stability of a single-piece hydrophobic acrylic intraocular lens: New method for high-precision rotation control. J Cataract Refract Surg 2007;33(5):800–803.

[51] Chang DF. Comparative rotational stability of single-piece open-loop acrylic and plate-haptic silicone toric intraocular lenses. J Cataract Refract Surg 2008;34(11):1842–1847.

[52] Leyland M, Zinicola E, Bloom P, Lee N. Prospective evaluation of a plate haptic toric intraocular lens. Eye 2001;15:202–205.

[53] Sun XY, Vicary D, Montgomery P, Griffiths M. Toric intraocular lenses for correcting astigmatism in 130 eyes. Ophthalmology 2000;107:1776–1781.

[54] Till JS, Yoder PR Jr, Wilcox TK, Spielman JL. Toric intraocular lens implantation: 100 consecutive cases. J Cataract Refract Surg 2002;28:295–301.

[55] Osher RH. Evolution of refractive cataract surgery. In: Bruce Wallace R, editor. Refractive cataract surgery and multifocal IOLs. Thorofare, NJ: Slack Inc; 2001.

Cataract Surgery in Uveitis Patients

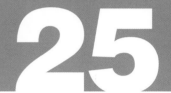

Michael B. Raizman, MD

CONTENTS

CHAPTER HIGHLIGHTS

>> Pre- and postoperative drug regimens

>> Operative techniques in uveitis

>> When an intraocular lens is contraindicated

Most of the medical literature on cataract extraction in patients with uveitis dates from the 1960s, 1970s, and 1980s.[1] Predictably, the tone of these articles is pessimistic and cautionary. Since the late 1980s, there has been a shift in belief and a new consensus has arisen, one that recognizes the utility and safety of cataract extraction and intraocular lens (IOL) implantation in the majority of patients with uveitis.[1–8] This change is largely a result of improvements in surgical techniques and, to some extent, a greater recognition of the need to aggressively control inflammation in the eyes of these patients before and after surgery.

Only a small portion of the cataract extractions performed in an average practice will be on eyes with uveitis. However, nearly every ophthalmologist faces such cases periodically. Cataracts may be induced by the inflammation or the corticosteroid therapy prescribed to control the inflammation. Of course, patients with uveitis may also experience age-related (not uveitis-related) cataracts that require removal. In certain conditions – especially intermediate uveitis (pars planitis), Fuchs' heterochromic iridocyclitis, and juvenile rheumatoid arthritis with uveitis – the majority of eyes will develop cataract.[9–11] Cataract extraction in such situations can be challenging. The strategies outlined in this chapter will allow consistently successful management of cataracts in uveitis patients.

PATIENT SELECTION

Given the greater inherent risks of operating on an eye with uveitis, cataract surgery is generally deferred longer in these cases than in a case of uncomplicated cataract. In many cases, the posterior pole cannot be seen to assist in determining visual potential. Current techniques for assessing visual potential, such as a potential acuity meter, laser interferometry, or entoptic phenomena, can be helpful, but are limited.[12] Fluorescein angiography and ultrasonography can occasionally provide useful information. Before surgery, patients must realize that visual potential may be restricted by the pre-existing complications of uveitis, such as cystoid macular edema (CME), epiretinal membranes, or glaucomatous optic neuropathy. For less opaque cataracts, preoperative optical coherence tomography (OCT) may be helpful.

The cause of the inflammation should be ascertained whenever possible. This can help in determining a prognosis and whether to implant an IOL. In some conditions, clinical findings will permit a diagnosis (e.g., heterochromia in Fuchs' iridocyclitis or pars planitis "snowbanks" in intermediate uveitis). Other cases will require laboratory evaluations. Depending on the clinical setting, useful laboratory studies may include a complete blood count, a fluorescent treponemal antibody absorption test (FTA-Abs), a chest X-ray, screening for angiotensin-converting enzyme and HLA-B27, and urinalysis.

Cataract surgery may be performed successfully regardless of the cause of the uveitis. However, some conditions pose a relative contraindication to lens implantation.[1–4] In general, patients with juvenile rheumatoid arthritis, Vogt-Koyanagi-Harada or Harada syndrome, sympathetic ophthalmia, or recurrent granulomatous uveitis of any cause with extensive synechia formation are poorer candidates for lens implantation (Figure 25-1).[13–16] Some controversy exists regarding the placement of an IOL in patients with juvenile rheumatoid arthritis. The preponderance of the literature suggests that IOLs should be avoided in most of these eyes, but aggressive management of inflammation before and after surgery may allow better tolerance of the IOL.[17–21] IOL implantation may also present a problem in patients with any form of uveitis that is difficult to control (Figure 25-2). Certain uveitis patients do especially well after cataract extraction with

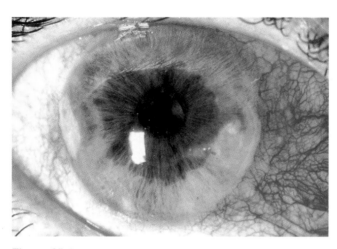

Figure 25-1 This cataract, in a patient with chronic iritis associated with juvenile rheumatoid arthritis, is probably best removed in combination with a vitrectomy. Eyes such as these usually do poorly with an intraocular lens. Note the band keratopathy and posterior synechiae, characteristic ocular features of juvenile rheumatoid arthritis with uveitis.

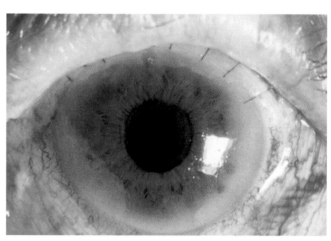

Figure 25-2 Excessive postoperative inflammation with fibrinous membranes across the intraocular lens is apt to occur when surgery is performed in an eye with chronic, uncontrolled inflammation, as in this case.

lens implantation. In particular, patients with Fuchs' heterochromic iridocyclitis almost always have a good outcome,[10,25] as do patients whose uveitis has been quiet for more than 1 year without the use of medication. In one study, after posterior chamber IOL implantation in eyes with uveitis, uveitis recurred in 41%, CME in 33%, and posterior synechiae in 8%.[26] In every case, good clinical judgment is needed to determine whether lens implantation is appropriate.

Some patients with uveitis and glaucoma may do well with combined cataract extraction, lens implantation, and filtering surgery. Glaucoma should be controlled as well as possible before surgery. The use of antimetabolites is common in eyes with uveitis and may reduce the chance of filter failure.[27] Some surgeons prefer to place a seton in eyes with uveitis and glaucoma.

PREOPERATIVE MANAGEMENT

One of the most important determinants of successful cataract extraction in a patient with uveitis, is the ability to control the inflammation before surgery. Elimination of intraocular inflammation for at least 3 months (and preferably longer) before surgery is desirable. Elimination of flare may be impossible in patients with long-standing inflammation, so the emphasis should be on the absence of cells in the anterior chamber and the absence of "active," mobile cells in the vitreous. The mainstay of preoperative anti-inflammatory therapy is topical corticosteroids. Potent topical corticosteroids, such as prednisolone acetate or prednisolone sodium 1% or dexamethasone 0.1%, should be used as often as needed for the months before surgery to reduce all inflammation. A typical patient might require one drop two to four times a day. For patients with severe uveitis that requires more intensive therapy, cataract surgery should be postponed.

In unusual situations, cataract surgery may be required despite active uveitis. Such cases arise, for example, when surgical intervention for vitreoretinal diseases cannot be accomplished without cataract removal. In these circumstances, intraorbital injections of corticosteroids or oral prednisone may be used. Rarely, other

immunosuppressive agents such as cyclosporine, methotrexate, azathioprine, cyclophosphamide, or TNF-α blockers are required to control inflammation. This therapy should be coordinated with a rheumatologist, hematologist, or other practitioner experienced in the use of these drugs.

It is helpful to treat all uveitis patients with oral prednisone for 3 to 7 days before surgery. A daily dose of 60 mg is reasonable for most individuals. The risks of this therapy must be discussed with the patient, although short-term use of prednisone is relatively safe. The use of oral nonsteroidal agents has been advocated in the preoperative period, but their efficacy has not been clearly demonstrated.

CATARACT EXTRACTION

SURGICAL APPROACH

Phacoemulsification is the preferred approach for the removal of most cataracts in eyes with uveitis. The small incision, reduction of iris trauma from prolapse into the wound, reduction of iris stretch with nucleus expression, and capsulorrhexis all favor phacoemulsification. Studies confirm the reduction in inflammation with a smaller incision,[28,29] but the issue has not been well studied specifically in eyes with uveitis. Nevertheless, excellent results can be obtained with nucleus expression, and surgeons may use either approach.

There are advocates for the removal of the cataract through a limbal approach and advocates of a pars plana approach. Pars plana vitrectomy and lensectomy are preferable when posterior segment disease must be addressed surgically, and complete removal of the cataract and capsule is desired.[30–34] In such cases, lens implantation is not performed. The most common setting for this surgery is in a patient with juvenile rheumatoid arthritis.[35–37] These eyes often do poorly with IOLs. In addition, leaving the posterior capsule in place may provide a scaffold for cyclitic membrane formation. For these individuals, pars plana vitrectomy and lensectomy are preferred.

When vitreous debris is present, limiting vision along with the cataract, a reasonable approach is to perform cataract extraction via the limbus and vitrectomy through the pars plana, allowing the placement of an IOL in the capsular bag.[38] Vitrectomy may be performed at the same sitting or as a second surgical procedure. It is possible that removal of the vitreous may reduce subsequent inflammation in the posterior segment.[39] This is hard to confirm, and vitrectomy probably should not be performed unless the vitreous opacity limits vision.

In the special circumstance of lens-induced uveitis following trauma or resulting from a hypermature lens, extracapsular surgery by phacoemulsification or expression is safe and effective. IOLs are well tolerated in most of these eyes. Intracapsular extraction is not longer the treatment of choice.

Clear corneal incisions may produce less inflammation than scleral tunnel incisions,[40,41] but this advantage has not been well documented in eyes with uveitis.

MANAGEMENT OF THE PUPIL

Poor dilation can be a problem in eyes with uveitis. The pupil may be held in place by synechiae to the lens at the pupil or anywhere on the posterior surface of the iris (Figures 25-3 and 25-4). In addition, fibrous bands on the pupil and around the sphincter may prevent dilation. On occasion, fibrous bands at the pupil can be stripped off with a forceps or gently excised with scissors, allowing dilation. Any of the techniques mentioned in Chapter 21 can be used in these individuals. Whatever technique is used to enlarge the pupil, it is important to minimize trauma to the iris and to avoid cutting iris vessels if possible. Synechiae should be gently lysed with a spatula placed under the iris through the pupil. A collar button or similar hook can be used to push and pull the pupil to free synechiae. Stretching the pupil with two instruments placed 180° apart at the pupil margin can help break circumferential fibrous bands. Injection of balanced salt solution containing epinephrine can help, as can placement of viscoelastic material in the anterior chamber and under the iris. At this point the pupil may be large enough to permit the capsule to be opened.

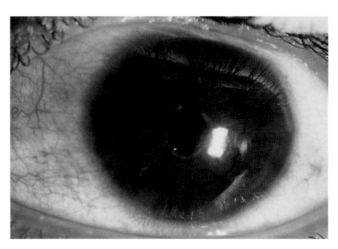

Figure 25-4 With some cases of chronic inflammation, as in this example of uveitis with Vogt-Koyanagi-Harada disease, a fibrous band forms at the pupil. This must be excised or transected to allow dilation of the pupil. Stretching maneuvers or the use of iris hooks do not succeed until the integrity of the fibrous ring is disrupted.

If the pupil is still too small, iris hooks may be inserted. They provide good visualization and are less likely to transect iris vessels than are multiple sphincterotomies or a radial iridotomy. Excessive stretch from the iris hooks can lead to postoperative inflammation and permanent distortion of the pupil. Just enough dilation for adequate exposure should be achieved.

Peripheral iridectomies are not needed in most patients with uveitis, although controversy about this exists. Creating a peripheral iridectomy increases inflammation but reduces the risk of postoperative iris bombé and angle-closure glaucoma. Most cases of iris bombé can be managed with yttrium-aluminum-garnet (YAG) laser iridectomy. Given the low rate of iris bombé after cataract surgery, even in patients with uveitis, routine iridectomies are probably not needed. Certainly, in cases of severe inflammation or narrow angles, performing an iridectomy is prudent.

CAPSULORRHEXIS AND CATARACT EXTRACTION

A round capsulorrhexis is preferred in patients with uveitis. Synechiae are less likely to form with a smooth capsulorrhexis edge than with a ragged, torn capsular edge. In addition, a rhexis smaller than the optic diameter prevents adhesions from the iris to the posterior capsule, a problem with capsule tears that extend beyond the optic. With a rhexis of 4–5 mm, the pupil may be kept dilated after surgery, significantly reducing the formation of posterior synechiae. Another alternative is to create a 7 mm rhexis and avoid dilation after surgery. Pigment on the anterior lens capsule can impede or divert the capsulorrhexis. This pigment can usually be removed with forceps or a spatula before creating the capsulorrhexis.

Removal of the nucleus and cortex is the same as in an eye without uveitis. However, it is optimal to remove all cortical material to prevent postoperative phacogenic inflammation. The bag should be carefully inspected, with retraction of the iris to ensure complete cortical removal.

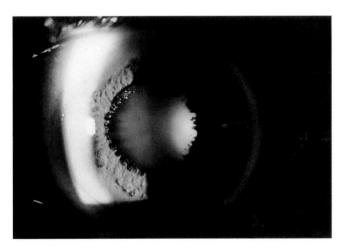

Figure 25-3 Posterior synechiae can usually be easily lysed with a spatula or hook, providing adequate visualization for capsulotomy and phacoemulsification.

After placement of the posterior chamber IOL in the capsular bag, the pupil may be pharmacologically constricted or dilated, depending on size of the capsulorrhexis and the degree of anticipated inflammation. Topical and subconjunctival corticosteroids administered at the conclusion of the case are helpful. Intravitreal corticosteroids may be of value, especially in patients who cannot tolerate systemic corticosteroids.[42]

INTRAOCULAR LENS IMPLANTATION

There may be, theoretically, an advantage to lenses made wholly of polymethylmethacrylate (PMMA) over those with Prolene haptics. Prolene may induce complement activation and has been associated with a slightly higher rate of endophthalmitis, including anaerobic infections.[43–45] Prolene haptics are no longer present on most IOLs. Silicone lenses with silicone or PMMA haptics have been used in patients with uveitis. Acrylic lenses appear to be well tolerated, as well.[46–48] Several controlled studies support the effectiveness of surface-modified IOLs, though the clinical significance remains unclear.[49–53]

Every effort should be made to place the lens in the capsular bag. This eliminates contact of the lens with other ocular structures, especially the iris and ciliary body. Contact of the lens with these structures in an eye with pre-existing uveitis can lead to uncontrollable inflammation, deposition of inflammatory debris on the implant, and, rarely, hyphema and glaucoma, even with posterior chamber placement.[54,55] Many patients do well despite placement of the lens in the ciliary sulcus.[56] Problems with anterior chamber lenses in eyes with uveitis occur frequently enough to contraindicate their use in such cases. If complications arise during surgery and it is not possible to place the implant in the capsular bag, it is probably best to leave the eye aphakic. In some cases of mild uveitis, including eyes that have been quiet without medication for more than 1 year, sulcus placement or suturing the lens to the sclera may be acceptable. This should be performed with caution, bearing in mind that it is possible to return at a later date for secondary lens placement in the same site if the patient does not tolerate aphakic spectacles or a contact lens.

■ POSTOPERATIVE MANAGEMENT AND COMPLICATIONS ■

Topical corticosteroids should be used as often as every hour, if necessary, to control inflammation after surgery. Prednisone should be tapered over 7–10 days after surgery. If hourly corticosteroid drops are inadequate to control inflammation, prednisone should be continued. Alternatively, intraorbital injections of 1 mL triamcinolone (Kenalog) 40 mg/mL may be performed weekly or as needed. Systemic immunosuppression besides prednisone is rarely necessary, but occasionally a patient who is intolerant of prednisone or who has uncontrollable pressure elevation from corticosteroids will benefit from alternative systemic immunosuppressive agents, as mentioned above.

Cycloplegia need not be routine but can be useful in eyes with fibrin in the anterior chamber and in any eye with even a hint of synechia formation.

Patients with uveitis are more likely to experience inflammatory glaucoma and iris bombé. It is best to avoid pilocarpine therapy in

these eyes. YAG laser iridectomy is usually effective in eyes with iris bombé. Treatment first with argon laser to close vessels, followed by a large YAG laser iridectomy, is most likely to ensure patency. In some eyes, repeat closure of laser iridectomies will be best managed by surgical iridectomy.

Prophylactic therapy of CME is controversial. Many of these eyes have pre-existing macular edema from long-standing uveitis. It is reasonable to use topical nonsteroidal agents following cataract extraction in all patients with uveitis. When CME develops, standard therapy, as outlined in Chapter 54, applies, but it is also essential to eliminate all intraocular inflammation.

Hypotony and cyclitic membrane formation after cataract extraction are quite unusual and usually require pars plana vitrectomy and membranectomy. Macular pucker and membranes can be treated surgically in selected cases. Pupillary membranes or membranes around the IOL that do not respond to corticosteroids and recur following YAG laser therapy necessitate removal of the IOL.

Iris capture of an IOL with excessive lens deposits and inflammation can be managed, in some cases, by repositioning the lens and eliminating iris contact. However, some cases require lens removal.[57] Other postoperative problems are discussed in Chapters 43 through 57 (in particular, see Chapter 57, Prolonged Intraocular Inflammation).

References

[1] Hooper PL, Rao NA, Smith RE. Cataract extraction in uveitis patients. Surv Ophthalmol 1990;35:120–144.
[2] Foster CS, Fong LP, Singh G. Cataract surgery and intraocular lens implantation in patients with uveitis. Ophthalmology 1989;96:281–288.
[3] Foster RE, Lowder CY, Meisler DM, et al. Extracapsular cataract extraction and posterior chamber intraocular lens implantation in uveitis patients. Ophthalmology 1992;99:1234–1241.
[4] Chung YM, Yeh TS. Intraocular lens implantation following extracapsular cataract extraction in uveitis. Ophthalmic Surg 1990;21:272–276.
[5] Anderson W. IOLs in uveitis patients. Ophthalmology 1994;101:625–626.
[6] Alio JL, Chipont E. Surgery of cataract in patients with uveitis. Dev Ophthalmol 1999;31:166–174.
[7] Rahman I, Jones NP. Long-term results of cataract extraction with intraocular lens implantation in patients with uveitis. Eye 2005;19:191–197.
[8] Elgohary MA, McCluskey PJ, Towler HM, et al. Outcome of phacoemulsification in patients with uveitis. Br J Ophthalmol 2007;91:916–921.
[9] Michelson JB, Friedlander MH, Nozik RA. Lens implant surgery in pars planitis. Ophthalmology 1990;97:1023–1026.
[10] Rutzen AR, Raizman MB. Fuchs' heterochromic iridocyclitis. In: Albert DM, Jakobiec FA, editors. Principles and practice of ophthalmology. Philadelphia: WB Saunders; 1994. p. 503–516.
[11] Wolf MD, Lichter PR, Ragsdale CG. Prognostic factors in the uveitis of juvenile rheumatoid arthritis. Ophthalmology 1987;94:1242–1248.
[12] Palestine AG, Alter GJ, Chan CC, et al. Laser interferometry and visual prognosis in uveitis. Ophthalmology 1985;92:1567–1569.
[13] Akova YA, Foster CS. Cataract surgery in patients with sarcoidosis-associated uveitis. Ophthalmology 1994;101:473–479.
[14] Moorthy RS, Rajeev B, Smith RE, et al. Incidence and management of cataracts in Vogt-Koyanagi-Harada syndrome. Am J Ophthalmol 1994;118:197–204.
[15] Ganesh SK, Sundaram PM, Biswas J, et al. Cataract surgery in sympathetic ophthalmia. J Cataract Refract Surg 2004;30:2371–2376.
[16] Ganesh SK, Padmaja BK, et al. Cataract surgery in patients with Vogt-Koyanagi-Harada syndrome. J Cataract Refract Surg 2004;30:95–100.
[17] Harris Jr DJ. Causes of reduced visual acuity on long-term follow-up after cataract extraction in patients with uveitis and juvenile rheumatoid arthritis. Am J Ophthalmol 1993;115:682–684.
[18] Probst LE, Holland EJ. Intraocular lens implantation in patients with juvenile rheumatoid arthritis. Am J Ophthalmol 1996;122:161–170.
[19] Holland GN. Intraocular lens implantation in patients with juvenile rheumatoid arthritis-associated uveitis: an unresolved management issue. Am J Ophthalmol 1996;122:255–257.
[20] BenEzra D, Cohen E. Cataract surgery in children with chronic uveitis. Ophthalmology 2000;107:1255–1260.
[21] Lundvall A, Zetterstrom C. Cataract extraction and intraocular lens implantation in children with uveitis. Br J Ophthalmol 2000;84:791–793.
[22] Lam LA, Lowder CY, Baerveldt G, et al. Surgical management of cataracts in children with juvenile rheumatoid arthritis-associated uveitis. Am J Ophthalmol 2003;135:772–778.
[23] Kotaniemi K, Penttila H. Intraocular lens implantation in patients with juvenile idiopathic arthritis-associated uveitis. Ophthalmic Res 2006;38:316–317.
[24] Nemet AY, Raz J, Sachs D, et al. Primary intraocular lens implantation in pediatric uveitis: a comparison of 2 populations. Arch Ophthalmol 2007;125:354–360.
[25] Avramides S, Sakkias G, Traianidis P. Cataract surgery in Fuchs' heterochromic iridocyclitis. Eur J Ophthalmol 1997;7:149–151.
[26] Estafanous MF, Lowder CY, Meisler DM, et al. Phacoemulsification cataract extraction and posterior chamber lens implantation in patients with uveitis. Am J Ophthalmol 2001;131:620–625.
[27] Patitsas CJ, Rockwood EJ, Meisler DM, et al. Glaucoma filtering surgery with postoperative 5-fluorouracil in patients with intraocular inflammatory disease. Ophthalmology 1992;99:594–599.

[28] Chee S-P, Ti S-E, Sivakuma M, et al. Postoperative inflammation: extracapsular cataract extraction versus phacoemulsification. J Cataract Refract Surg 1999;25:1280–1285.

[29] Dowler JG, Hykin PG, Hamilton AM. Phacoemulsification versus extracapsular cataract extraction in patients with diabetes. Ophthalmology 2000;107:457–462.

[30] Diamond JG, Kaplan HJ. Lensectomy and vitrectomy for complicated cataract due to uveitis. Arch Ophthalmol 1978;96:1798–1804.

[31] Dangel ME, Stark WJ, Michels RG. Surgical management of cataract associated with uveitis. Ophthalmic Surg 1983;14:145–149.

[32] Nobe JR, Kokoris N, Diddle KR, et al. Lensectomy-vitrectomy in chronic uveitis. Retina 1983;3:71–76.

[33] Petrilli AM, Belfort Jr R, Abre MT, et al. Ultrasonic fragmentation in of cataract in uveitis. Retina 1986;6:61–65.

[34] Girard LJ, Rodriguez J, Mailman ML, et al. Cataract and uveitis management by pars plana lensectomy and vitrectomy by ultrasonic fragmentation. Retina 1985;5:107–114.

[35] Flynn Jr HW, Davis JL, Culbertson WW. Pars plana lensectomy and vitrectomy for complicated cataracts in juvenile rheumatoid arthritis. Ophthalmology 1988;95:1114–1119.

[36] Fox GM, Flynn Jr HW, Davis JL, et al. Causes of reduced visual acuity on long-term follow-up after cataract extraction in patients with uveitis. Am J Ophthalmol 1992;114:708–714.

[37] Androudi S, Ahmed M, Fiore T, et al. Combined pars plana vitrectomy and phacoemulsification to restore visual acuity in patients with chronic uveitis. J Cataract Refract Surg 2005;31:472–478.

[38] Foster RE, Lowder CY, Meisler DM, et al. Combined extracapsular cataract extraction, posterior chamber intraocular lens implantation, and pars plana vitrectomy. Ophthalmic Surg 1993;24: 446–452.

[39] Diamond JG, Kaplan HJ. Uveitis: Effect of vitrectomy combined with lensectomy. Ophthalmology 1979;86:1320–1327.

[40] Dick HB, Schwenn O, Krummenauer F, et al. Inflammation after sclerocorneal versus clear corneal tunnel phacoemulsification. Ophthalmology 2000;107:241–247.

[41] Rauz S, Stavrou P, Murray PI. Evaluation of foldable intraocular lenses in patients with uveitis. Ophthalmology 2000;107:909–919.

[42] Okhravi N, Morris A, Dowler GF, et al. Intraoperative use of intravitreal triamcinolone in uveitic eyes having cataract surgery: Pilot study. J Cataract Refract Surg 2007;33:1278–1283.

[43] Tuberville AW, Galin MA, Perez HD, et al. Complement activation by nylon- and polypropylene-looped prosthetic intraocular lenses. Invest Ophthalmol Vis Sci 1982;22:727–733.

[44] Mondino BJ, Nagata S, Glovsky MM. Activation of the alternative complement pathway by intraocular lenses. Invest Ophthalmol Vis Sci 1985;26:905–908.

[45] Menikoff JA, Speaker MG, Marmor M, et al. A case-control study of risk factors for postoperative endophthalmitis. Ophthalmology 1991;98:1761–1768.

[46] Alio JL, Chipont E, BenEzra D, et al. Comparative performance of intraocular lenses in eyes with cataract and uveitis. J Cataract Refract Surg 2002;28:2096–2108.

[47] Abela-Formanek C, Amon M, Schauersberger J, et al. Results of hydrophilic acrylic, hydrophobic acrylic, and silicone intraocular lenses in uveitic eyes with cataract: comparison to a control group. J Cataract Refract Surg 2002;28:1141–1152.

[48] Abela-Formanek C, Amon M, Schild G, et al. Inflammation after implantation of hydrophilic acrylic, hydrophobic acrylic, or silicone intraocular lenses in eyes with cataract and uveitis: comparison to a control group. J Cataract Refract Surg 2002;28:1153–1159.

[49] Rose GE. Fibrinous uveitis and intraocular lens implantation: surface modification of polymethylmethacrylate during extracapsular cataract surgery. Ophthalmology 1992;99:1242–1247.

[50] Lin CL, Wang AG, Chou JC, et al. Heparin-surface-modified intraocular lens implantation in patients with glaucoma, diabetes, or uveitis. J Cataract Refract Surg 1994;20:550–553.

[51] Lardenoye CW, van der LA, Berendschot TT, et al. A retrospective analysis of heparin-surface-modified intraocular lenses versus regular polymethylmethacrylate intraocular lenses in patients with uveitis. Doc Ophthalmol 1996;92:41–50.

[52] Trocme SD, Li H. Effect of heparin-surface-modified intraocular lenses on postoperative inflammation after phacoemulsification: a randomized trial in a United States patient population: heparin-Surface-Modified Lens Study Group. Ophthalmology 2000;107:1031–1037.

[53] Ravalico G, Baccara F, Lovisato A, et al. Postoperative cellular reaction on various intraocular lens materials. Ophthalmology 1997;104:1084–1091.

[54] Van Liefferinge T, Van Oye R, Kestelyn P. Uveitis-glaucoma-hyphema syndrome: a late complication of posterior chamber lenses. Bull Soc Belge Ophthalmol 1994;252:61–66.

[55] Aonuma H, Matsushita H, Nakajima K, et al. Uveitis-glaucoma-hyphema syndrome after posterior chamber intraocular lens implantation. Jpn J Ophthalmol 1997;41:98–100.

[56] Holland GN, Van Horn SD, Margolis TP. Cataract surgery with ciliary sulcus fixation of intraocular lenses in patients with uveitis. Am J Ophthalmol 1999;128:21–30.

[57] Foster RE, Stavrou P, Zafirakis P, et al. Intraocular lens removal from patients with uveitis. Am J Ophthalmol 1999;128:31–37.

POSTOPERATIVE MANAGEMENT AND COMPLICATIONS

Surgical Management of Pediatric Cataracts and Aphakia

Howard V. Gimbel, MD, MPH, Brian M. DeBroff, MD, Jennifer A. Dunbar, MD and Bharti R. Nihalani, MD

26

CONTENTS

CHAPTER HIGHLIGHTS

>> Capsule and zonule differences from adult lens require different techniques

>> Management of inflammation and reactive membranes

>> Intraocular lens (IOL) power calculation and strategies in growing eyes

>> Secondary IOL implantation in children

Pediatric cataract is one of the leading causes of treatable childhood blindness, accounting for 7–20% of blindness in children worldwide.[1,2] A prospective collaborative project conducted by 12 US universities reported the prevalence of infantile cataract as 13.6/10,000 infants.[3] In 2003, Holmes et al. reported, in a retrospective population-based medical record retrieval in the US population, that the birth prevalence of visually significant cataracts was 3.0 to 4.5 /10,000.[4]

Because of the high incidence and treatable nature of the condition, an improved approach to the management of childhood cataracts would have a large impact on childhood blindness as a whole.

Cataract extraction with lens implantation in children has undergone dramatic changes during the past 40 years, largely as a result of advances in technology and microsurgical techniques.[5–11] Managing cataracts in children remains a challenge; treatment is often difficult and tedious and requires a dedicated team effort. The timing of surgery, the surgical technique, the choice of the intraocular lens (IOL), and the management of amblyopia are of the utmost importance for achieving good visual results in children.[7,12–15] Other challenges in the management of cataracts in infants and children include the difficulties in examining this particular group, the risks of general anesthesia, poor preoperative pupillary dilation, and the management of postoperative inflammation and fibrin formation. Children are at higher risk for postoperative pupillary capture, posterior synechiae, IOL precipitates, fibrinous uveitis, corectopia, pupillary block glaucoma, and peripheral iris erosion.[16] Many ophthalmologists lack surgical experience of this particular group of patients. The development of continuous curvilinear capsulorrhexis (CCC)[17] and viscoelastic agents, advances in posterior chamber IOL designs, and the use of the neodymium:yttrium-aluminum-garnet (Nd:YAG) laser have brought the pediatric cataract surgical technique closer to the adult procedure. With advancements in surgical techniques, improved intraocular lenses and better understanding of the growth of the pediatric eyes, primary implantation of intraocular lenses is becoming popular even in the youngest of patients.

There are many nuances of pediatric surgery – including preoperative evaluation, timing of surgery, operative technique, and postoperative management – which this chapter will attempt to elucidate. The evolution of techniques in pediatric cataract surgery will be emphasized, including the trend toward anterior and posterior CCC, anterior vitrectomy, placement of posterior chamber lenses in the capsular bag, and methods to reduce the formation of secondary cataracts.

ETIOLOGY OF CONGENITAL CATARACT

The most common cause of bilateral congenital cataract is idiopathic. About one-third of cases are hereditary, without a systemic disease. Other causes include metabolic disorders, intrauterine infections, systemic abnormalities and a few ocular conditions. In contrast, unilateral cataract in most cases is idiopathic.[18]

■ PREOPERATIVE EVALUATION ■

A preoperative assessment is essential to adequately evaluate the size, density, location, and visual impact of the cataract; to evaluate for other ocular abnormalities; and to properly plan the surgical procedure. A history from the parents is often helpful in clarifying whether the cataract is congenital, developmental, or traumatic, and to ascertain if there was any maternal drug use, infections, or exposure to ionizing radiation during pregnancy. Infants with bilateral congenital cataracts demonstrate decreased visual interest and may have delayed developmental milestones.[19] Past or present illness and a history of medication use may give a clue as to the cause of the cataract. Past ocular history and a family history of ocular diseases may reveal other possible causes.

The value of counseling the parents cannot be overstressed. Parents should understand that treatment of the child continues well after surgery. They need to come for regular follow-up visits and help ensure that the child wears glasses or contact lenses despite IOL implantation; the child may also need occlusion therapy following surgery. In addition, further interventions such as a secondary procedure to clear the visual axis or strabismus surgery may be required.

Complete examination of infants and young children with fully dilated pupils, done, if necessary, under sedation or even general anesthesia, is mandatory in both the eyes. Although there may be variations in the baseline ophthalmic assessment because of the age and compliance of the pediatric cataract surgery patient, a full anterior and posterior segment examination is essential in all patients preoperatively. An assessment of the best corrected visual function is performed by testing the patient's ability to fix and follow (in infants), progressing to picture cards, illiterate Es, and Snellen letter charts in older children. Cycloplegic refraction by retinoscopy, autorefractor, or even trial lenses is important to determine the best correction. Binocularity, fusion, and stereopsis testing preoperatively give the ophthalmologist an idea of how well the eyes function together. Strabismus evaluation should involve cover–uncover and alternative cover testing for both distance and close up. Any restrictions of extraocular movements should be noted. The presence of nystagmus is an ominous sign, indicating poor vision resulting from sensory deprivation.[20] Pupils should be evaluated for the presence of an afferent pupillary defect.

An anterior segment examination, preferably by slit-lamp microscopy, may reveal potential challenges to surgery, including iris deformities, synechia, zonulolysis, posterior lentiglobus, intumescent cataract, pre-existing posterior capsule defect, anterior or posterior capsule plaques, or evidence of past trauma. The extent and location of the cataract must be evaluated. Small anterior polar cataracts often do not require lens extraction, whereas nuclear and, especially, posterior opacities tend to be more visually significant.

When the clarity of the media permits, indirect ophthalmoscopy will reveal any posterior segment abnormalities or pathologic condition that may have an impact on postoperative vision. Axial length and corneal curvature are essential measurement for IOL power determination. To measure the axial length of an eye in a child as young as 2 years old, a hand-held A-scan and keratometry can be performed without sedation so that the child can fixate on a target object. However, both A-scan and keratometry may be performed in the operating room under general anesthesia prior to cataract extraction or during an examination under anesthesia. In the event of a traumatic cataract in which the A-scan is unattainable, the patient's other eye may be used for proxy measurements on which to base IOL power calculations. Corneal diameter measurement helps rule out microcornea. Measurement of intraocular pressure can be accomplished by Tonopen, Shiotz tonometry, or pneumotonometry under anesthesia in infants or by applanation tonometry in older children. If the cataract is very dense with no view of the fundus, a B-scan will help evaluate any posterior segment abnormalities. Also, electrophysiological testing, including electroretinography and visual-evoked potential, may be performed to assess the neurological function of the retina and to detect stimulus deprivation and amblyopia.[21]

Consultation with a pediatrician is essential for infants with congenital cataracts. Some laboratory tests that may be considered include urine evaluation for reducing substances; toxoplasmosis, rubella, cytomegalovirus, and herpes simplex titer; serum screen for galactosemia; and a serum calcium screen to evaluate for hypoparathyroidism.[22] Also, it is important to observe for any systemic processes that may be coexistent, especially in children with bilateral cataracts. Genetic testing should be considered for infants with congenital cataracts.[23]

■ TIMING OF SURGERY ■

The timing for surgical intervention in pediatric cataracts was profoundly influenced by the work of Hubel and Weisel and later by von Noorden who established that sensory deprivation in the first few months of life is the critical period for visual development and that sensory deprivation during this period results in both irreversible anatomical changes in the lateral geniculate bodies and decreased activity in the occipital cortex upon visual stimulation.[13,23,24] Congenital monocular complete cataracts should be removed within the first few months of life and, preferably, in the first few days or weeks of life.[25–27] If surgery is performed within the first 4 months of life, deprivation amblyopia can still be reversed.[14,22,28] Bilateral complete congenital cataracts should be removed within the first few months of life, first in the eye with the more opaque lens opacity and approximately 1 week later in the other eye. In children who are at an age at which they are at risk for the development of amblyopia, a monocular cataract should be operated on when the best corrected visual acuity is 20/70 or worse.[29] Recommendation for surgery in children with bilateral cataracts is often made when the vision in the worse eye is 20/70 or poorer. In children older than 8 years, who are no longer at much risk for amblyopia, cataract surgery is recommended when the child has difficulty functioning in school or in sports, or has problems with normal daily activities. Indications for cataract surgery include visually significant central cataracts larger than 3 mm in diameter, dense nuclear cataracts, cataracts obstructing the examiner's view of the fundus and cataracts associated with strabismus. Certain cataracts like anterior polar, sutural, lamellar or blue dot cataracts may be compatible with good vision and may be followed up to watch for any progress. Although surgical removal is the definitive therapy for the vast majority of congenital cataracts when visual function is jeopardized, visual acuity in many children with small cataracts may be improved by first maintaining dilation of the pupil. When cycloplegia is used, however, photophobia is often aggravated and reading glasses are often necessary.[20,30]

■ ARE PEDIATRIC EYES DIFFERENT? ■

In comparison with adult eyes, pediatric eyes have greater elasticity of the capsule, lower scleral rigidity and more mitotically active lens epithelial cells, leading to higher incidence of posterior capsule opacification necessitating primary management of the posterior capsule. They also have a thick vitreous gel which may give more protection against cystoid macular edema.

■ REVIEW OF PEDIATRIC SURGICAL TECHNIQUES ■

THE EARLY YEARS

Several different surgical techniques for the management of cataracts in pediatric patients have been advocated in the past, including discission or needling, linear extraction, or a combination of discission and displacement of lens fragments into the anterior chamber by irrigation without IOL implantation.[31–34] In the early 1960s the aspiration procedure, as popularized by Scheie and associates,[35] with the widespread use of the operating microscope became the accepted technique for extracting cataracts in infants and children.[35,36] With the aspiration technique, the lens material was suctioned by a push–pull technique using a needle with a syringe attached. Using this method, surgical complications associated with earlier techniques were dramatically reduced. Significant intraoperative risks, however, such as anterior chamber collapse and vitreous loss remained prevalent.[35,36] The Scheie technique, which leaves the posterior capsule intact, led to an extremely high incidence of secondary membranes and the development of synechiae between the iris and the remaining capsular bag. A sector iridectomy was necessary to prevent iris bombé and secondary glaucoma.[31,35,37–40] Often, additional operations using general anesthesia were required. The delay in amblyopia therapy became significant and was undoubtedly part of the poor visual results seen in patients with unilateral and bilateral congenital cataracts.

In the mid-1960s, the next development that changed pediatric cataract surgery was the introduction of a double-barreled cannula, one for aspiration and one for irrigation.[41] The irrigation–aspiration technique enabled the ophthalmologist to maintain anterior chamber depth during cataract aspiration while keeping the posterior capsule intact. Unfortunately, in many pediatric cases, residual lens epithelial cells would still relentlessly grow in from the periphery and cover the posterior capsule surface, resulting in an opaque membrane.[37] The incidence of postoperative secondary membrane formation with aspiration techniques remained high,[37,42] necessitating a secondary surgical procedure weeks or months later to open the posterior lens capsule.[43]

The 1970s witnessed the introduction of phacoemulsification in pediatric cataract surgery.[44,45] Although many pediatric cataracts can be removed using the irrigation–aspiration handpiece alone or by using the phacoemulsification handpiece with no ultrasound power, in some cases short bursts of phacoemulsification may be required. Pediatric cataracts vary dramatically in type, ranging from the very soft to the very hard and calcified. Nuclei that are too hard to be simply aspirated can be fragmented using phacoemulsification. Thus, phacoemulsification in pediatric surgery allows a wider application of the basic aspiration technique.[46,47] In addition, the closed phacoemulsification system incorporates the principles of controlled infusion to maintain intraocular pressure and variable and controlled suction or aspiration. Even with phacoemulsification and meticulous polishing of the anterior and posterior capsule, however, the incidence of posterior capsule opacification remained significantly high.[48–50]

PEDIATRIC INTRAOCULAR LENS IMPLANTATION

The options for optical correction following congenital cataract surgery are primary intraocular lens implantation, aphakic glasses, contact lenses and secondary intraocular lens implantation.

Aphakic spectacles are severely debilitating visually, cosmetically, and psychologically. Contact lenses have proved to be a good option. Contact lenses also provide an answer to the problem of the changing refraction that often accompanies IOL implantation in children. However, contact lenses are successful in a relatively small number of pediatric cases over a long period, are emotionally stressful both for the child and the family, and are economically beyond the reach of many patients, particularly those in developing countries.[51,52] Epikeratophakia is no longer practiced in pediatric eyes. It requires intensive postoperative management and may be associated with decreased corneal lenticular clarity, irregular astigmatism, spherical error, and a prolonged period until visual rehabilitation is achieved.[53–55] Such difficulties with aphakic spectacles, contact lenses and epikeratophakia, combined with more experience with IOLs, viscoelastics, improved IOL design, and improved surgical techniques, have increased the popularity and diminished the controversy over IOL implantation. Pseudophakia offers the method of optical correction that requires the least compliance and induces minimal aniseikonia and astigmatism.[56]

Intraocular lens implants were first advocated by anterior segment surgeons as early as 1955.[5,57–60] Early IOL implantation in children involved anterior chamber and iris-supported IOLs.[59] The first published implantation of an IOL in a child was by Choyce in 1955, using an anterior chamber lens.[61] Anterior chamber lenses may stimulate an inflammatory response as a result of their contact with vascular tissues and are associated with long-term complications in adults.[6,62] Endothelial cell loss over many years is a concern, especially with children who tend to rub their eyes frequently. Trauma to an eye with an anterior chamber lens may lead to iris or ciliary body rupture. Binkhorst and Gobin implanted an iridocapsular fixated IOL in 1959 (Figure 26-1).[63] When fixed and stable in the capsule, the iridocapsular IOLs were very successful. Some, however, were associated with complications, including iris sphincter erosion, hyphema, anterior synechiae, iris bombé, iritis, and pupillary fibrotic membranes. Also, lens dislocation, pseudophakodonesis, and corneal endothelial trauma were possible when capsule fixation was not achieved.

These complications, which were secondary to inferior lens design and primitive microsurgical techniques, had at one point made IOL implantation in children a very controversial subject.

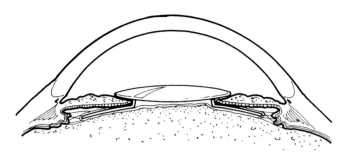

Figure 26-1 Capsule-fixated Binkhorst two-loop iridocapsular lens.

Additional negative opinion toward implantation of IOLs in children resulted from the concern of the possible long-term risk of the eye reacting to polymethylmethacrylate. The observation times in most pediatric IOL series are short in relation to a child's life expectancy.[5,9,52,64–68] Also, many ophthalmologists were concerned that an intense inflammatory reaction might be incited by placement of implants in infants. Histopathological studies, however, have subsequently revealed that the eyes of children could tolerate IOLs in a manner similar to that of adult eyes.[69] Work by Hiles in the 1970s and 1980s helped demonstrate the safety and effectiveness of aphakic rehabilitation of children with IOLs, especially in cases of traumatic or unilateral infantile cataracts.[6,70]

Intraocular lens implantation is now becoming the preferred method of pediatric aphakic rehabilitation, especially for children over 1 year of age.[6,26,49,52,56,58,71–77] With IOL implantation, there is almost immediate postoperative visual rehabilitation, which maximizes the treatment of amblyopia. In addition, the technique of CCC developed in the 1980s providing assurance of in-the-bag placement of the IOL, and the development of improved lens designs, have helped avoid many complications associated with early lens implantation in children. Relative contraindications do exist for IOL implantation. They include glaucoma, persistent or recurrent uveitis, aniridia, severe microphthalmia, persistent hyperplastic primary vitreous, other ophthalmic defects that preclude useful vision, and cases of inadequate capsular support.[6] Recent studies have shown that good results can be achieved in microphthalmic eyes, and this problem is now becoming less of a concern.[78,79] Capsular tension rings with artificial irides may provide improved quality of vision in patients with aniridia.

Some ophthalmologists consider patient age of less than 1 year to be a relative contraindication for IOL implantation. The youngest age at which implants can be safely and effectively used has not yet been clearly established. Many ophthalmologists prefer aphakia for bilateral congenital cataracts with the plan of secondary implants within a couple of years. In children older than 2 years of age, lens implantation into the capsular bag may be routinely achieved in monocular or bilateral congenital, developmental, or traumatic cases using current surgical techniques, including continuous curvilinear capsulorrhexis, and viscoelastic materials. Experts in the field of infantile cataract extraction have recently been implanting posterior chamber IOLs in infants as early as 2 months old.[80,81] Proponents of IOL implantation for treatment of unilateral infantile aphakia claim that this is the best available method to reduce the incidence of irreversible amblyopia.[80–82] Recent studies have shown the effectiveness of bilateral implants in children over the age of 2,[83] and other studies have

demonstrated excellent results in children between the ages of 4–6 months of age.[84] More recently, O'Keefe et al found bilateral IOL implantation safe and produced good visual results in children of all ages including infants.[85] Peterseim and Wilson have also published encouraging results.[86] Because the infant eye has a rapidly changing refraction during the first year of life, controversy surrounds the correct choice of lens power for implants in infants.[81]

The development of the eye necessitates initial under-correction to avoid permanent over-correction. The growth of the anterior segment of the eye is generally completed at the end of the second year of life.[87] Therefore, little adaptation of the size and power of the IOL is needed in the eyes of children older than 2 years. Under power of the IOL targeting hyperopia is often desired in younger children, although anisometropia should be minimized to promote binocular function. The final hyperopia desired should be correlated to the child's age. Because the greatest change in axial length and keratometry readings occurs in the first 2 years of life, it is wiser to choose an IOL that will initially correct only 80% of the aphakia in infants. In order to minimize the need to exchange IOLs, it is preferable to under-correct young children by 10 to 20%. In infants, greater degrees of initial hypermetropia are required because the greatest degree of eye growth occurs before 2 years of age. Over 6 diopters (D) of average myopic shift has been documented in pseudophakic infants over a minimum 2-year follow-up.[88] Aiming for emmetropia in infants would create a large myopic shift that can be amblyogenic itself and may require an IOL exchange, or piggyback IOL such as an implantable corrective lens (ICL) or corneal refractive surgery, when age permits.[89,90] An infant should receive 80% of the IOL power needed for emmetropia.[88] The initial hypermetropia can be corrected with spectacles or contact lenses and adjusted as the eye grows, to prevent amblyopia. Dr. M. Edward Wilson has developed a technique of piggyback IOL for infants with a planned removal of an IOL later in life after eye growth.[91] The permanent IOL is placed within the capsular bag and the temporary IOL is placed within the ciliary sulcus. On average a 26.5 D IOL is placed in the bag and an 11 D lens in the sulcus. In the future ICL lenses may be considered for this technique. This approach may be most appropriate for families less likely to comply with scheduled follow-up visits or wearing glasses full time. In children aged 2–5 years, a postoperative hyperopic spherical equivalent of 2.5 D is desired. Preschoolers are usually able to tolerate small amounts of residual hyperopia and astigmatism quite well without the need for spectacle correction. Higher residual refractive errors can be corrected with glasses, which are adjusted as necessary during childhood. Using this method, the patients are initially hyperopic. As the eye grows, emmetropia is approached, and by adolescence moderate myopia is common. Eye growth with progressively decreasing hyperopia appears to run its normal course in the eye with an IOL provided that the eye attains sufficient visual acuity.[87,92] In children who have already started school, the desired postoperative refraction should approach emmetropia. Bifocal lenses are often required for near vision.

Compared to the other currently available methods, postoperative amblyopic therapy is best maximized by the immediate visual rehabilitation afforded by IOL implantation.[49,50,93] Better visual outcomes in children with IOLs are probably related to the uninterrupted and permanent optical correction provided by the lens implant. Strict compliance with amblyopic treatment, however, is still necessary.[94] It is undeniable that in young children in need of amblyopic treatment, implantation of IOLs has far-reaching advantages, including immediate correction of the major portion of the refractive error. IOL implantation with patching of the nonoperated eye is most readily accepted by children and parents, and it maximizes postoperative visual acuity.[51]

Primary implantation of an IOL after cataract removal is gaining popularity, even in infants and young children.[95] A large randomized clinical trial, the Infant Aphakia Treatment Study (IATS), is currently underway to compare primary IOL implantation with contact-lens correction in children undergoing unilateral cataract surgery in the first year of life. A current trend among high-volume cataract surgeons dealing with pediatric cataracts and many pediatric ophthalmologists is to consider IOL implantation as a viable option on a selective basis in children who are under 2 years.

■ CURRENT SURGICAL TECHNIQUES ■

In cataract surgery on a child's eye the surgeon should strictly adhere to the principles of the closed-chamber technique, such as valvular incision, injection of viscoelastic before removing any coaxial instrument from the eye, bimanual irrigation–aspiration, and two port anterior vitrectomy.

PARS PLANA VS. LIMBAL APPROACH

In addition to successfully managing secondary membranes and vitreous loss, vitrectomy instruments have allowed surgeons to perform cataract procedures via a pars plana approach.[96–98] Both the limbal and pars plana approaches have their advocates and opponents.[51,94,99,100] The main advantages of the pars plana approach are the reduced incidence of vitreous prolapse into the wound and retinal traction when performing an anterior vitrectomy,[101] the facilitation of reaching lenticular material in the periphery, and less damage to corneal endothelium and iris tissue.[99,102] The principal disadvantage of the pars plana approach is the loss of integrity of the capsular bag. Removal of the entire cataract by a pars plana approach takes away the majority of capsular bag support for IOL placement and virtually eliminates the possibility of in-the-bag IOL placement.[99,53] Implantation of a posterior chamber lens in the sulcus, although possible after pars plana lensectomy, is less certain and advantageous.[103] An IOL placed in the sulcus has the disadvantage of contact with vascular tissue and the possibility of inducing a chronic inflammatory response. Thus, the pars plana approach limits the safety of IOL placement and decreases the options for optical rehabilitation if contact lenses cannot be worn or if epikeratophakia fails. The pars plana approach also increases the risk for iatrogenic retinal dialysis or ciliary body detachment.[96] Perhaps the only true indication of pars plana lensectomy is a small eye with microcornea, microphthalmos, or small pupil.

The risk of retinal detachment, however, has persuaded many ophthalmologists to use the limbal approach.[104] Keech et al. report one case of retinal detachment 6 years after translimbal lensectomy and anterior vitrectomy.[104] Studies, however, have shown no statistically significant differences between the limbal

and pars plana approach.[105] Increasing preference for the limbal surgical approach for pediatric cataract extraction also occurred with the introduction of higher viscosity viscoelastic agents including Healon GV and Healon 5. These agents have facilitated the maintenance of the anterior chamber, the performance of anterior and posterior capsulotomies, the manipulation of instruments within the anterior chamber, and the placement of IOLs into the capsular bag, while protecting the corneal endothelium.[18] The limbal approach allows CCC, complete removal of the cataract, PCCC, optic capture and or anterior vitrectomy and implantation of an IOL in the capsular bag. As pediatric surgical techniques and intraocular implants have continued to be refined, more interest has shifted to posterior chamber IOLs placed through a limbal incision into the capsular bag as a means of aphakic correction in children of younger ages and even infants.

Some surgeons prefer a combined approach using a limbal approach for performing an anterior CCC and implantation of IOL in the bag and subsequently perform posterior capsulotomy and anterior vitrectomy using parsplana incision.

Paracentesis Incision

A paracentesis incision should be created in the clear cornea 30° on either side of the main incision. Some surgeons prefer two paracentesis incisions, for instance at 12 and 6 o' clock if the main incision is made temporally. The anterior chamber should be inflated with a high-viscosity viscoelastic agent before creating the main entry. The small tunnel paracentesis incisions of 0.9–1.2 mm width are adequate to allow insertion of irrigation–aspiration cannulas and vitrectomy probe. Bimanual irrigation–aspiration is preferred in pediatric cataract surgery because it maintains a stable anterior chamber and allows thorough removal of cortical material, which helps to reduce the incidence of postoperative inflammation and secondary cataract formation. Since there is a tendency in the pediatric population for the paracentesis to leak, some surgeons attempt to eliminate their use, or make them with a longer tunnel length to prevent leakage. The paracentesis incisions may be helpful in breaking the anterior synechiae and for assisting in the placement of an IOL. A paracentesis is also helpful to re-form the anterior chamber and obtain and test the seal of the main incision.

Limbal Incision

A 2.6–3 mm wide limbal valvular incision with 1–1.5 mm internal entry is preferred. Some surgeons prefer to place the incision in the steep meridian obtained by keratometry. The sclera in a young child is elastic, encouraging the use of the smallest possible incision, which also helps to prevent iris prolapse. For a scleral tunnel incision, a small scleral scratch incision is made approximately 2 mm from the limbus and is dissected as a 3 mm or 5.5–6.5 mm wide scleral tunnel depending on the IOL selected using a crescent blade (Figure 26-2).

Capsulorrhexis

Achieving an intact and identifiable continuous capsular rim with the CCC technique is an important step in pediatric implantation procedures because it facilitates lens extraction and assures in-the-bag placement of the IOL. A high-viscosity viscoelastic,

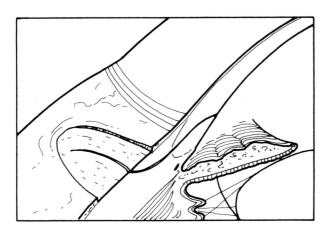

Figure 26-2 Scleral tunnel incision (cross-sectional view).

preferably Healon GV or Healon 5 is used to counteract the intralenticular forces that cause the CCC's tendency to turn toward the equator. Manual CCC may be achieved using a bent needle, cystotome, forceps, or a combination of these. A forceps is often necessary for control of the elastic capsule encountered in children. Because of the increased elasticity of the pediatric capsule,[106] any discontinuity that occurs in the rim during a capsulotomy can easily extend as a tear out to the equator. When this happens, the edges of the capsule may retract, making it extremely difficult to ascertain, with confidence, that the lens loops are positioned in the capsular bag. Also, anterior capsule tears that extend into the posterior capsule present the greatest intraoperative challenge for nucleus removal, and they compromise in-the-bag or even sulcus IOL placement.

When attempting CCC in a pediatric patient, the tip of an irrigating cystotome, bent needle, or capsulorrhexis forceps is used to make a small central puncture (Figure 26-3). The elastic pediatric

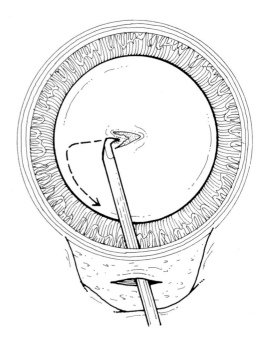

Figure 26-4 Cystotome guiding tear radially to start continuous curvilinear capsulorrhexis.

lens capsule requires a distinct pressure point to achieve a central puncture. Once the central puncture is made, the cystotome or forceps guides the tear radially out to the desired circumference at the 3 o'clock position (Figure 26-4). If the tear is not easily guided because of the elasticity of the capsule, forceps are more effectively used to grasp at the leading edge of the tear (Figure 26-5). To overcome the stretchability of the capsule,

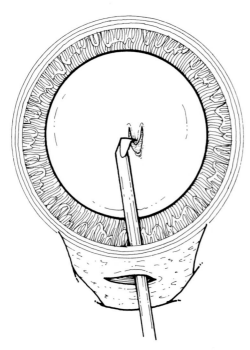

Figure 26-3 Cystotome makes a central puncture in anterior capsule.

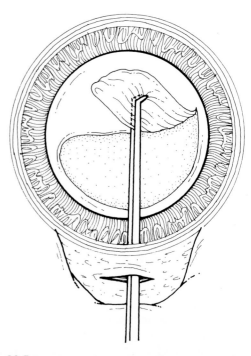

Figure 26-5 Capsulorrhexis forceps is used for better control of progressing curvilinear tear.

several repeated grasps at the leading edge of the tear are recommended for maximal control of the tear. With these small regrasping maneuvers at the leading edge of the tear, capsulorrhexis is directed to achieve the desired diameter. Viscoelastic material is added as required. The capsulorrhexis should be kept relatively small because the elasticity of the child's lens capsule can create a capsular opening that is larger than expected or desired. The pediatric capsule acts like a thin rubber sheet that retracts toward the periphery after anterior capsulotomy. This elasticity necessitates frequent relaxing and regrasping of the leading edge of the capsular tear with careful observation and direction of vector forces to ensure that radial extensions are prevented. During capsulorrhexis, the internal pressure or anterior chamber depth needs to be well maintained by injecting a viscous viscoelastic agent such as Healon GV or Healon 5. A central capsulorrhexis of about 4.5–5 mm is usually adequate so that it covers the IOL optic in all directions.

Alternative techniques currently available include vitrectorrhexis, radio-frequency diathermy and Fugo plasma blade. Vitrectorrhexis has proved to be a good alternative to manual CCC for young children, especially in the first 2 years of life when the capsule is very elastic and difficult to control. Vitrectorrhexis is easier to perform and is a good option for children when anterior vitrectomy is performed as part of primary management. In contrast, a diathermy-cut capsulotomy, even when performed perfectly, can be seen to have coagulated capsular debris along the edge.[107] In addition, this edge has been shown experimentally to be less elastic than a manual CCC. The Fugo blade is a unique cutting instrument that uses plasma for ablating tissue.[108,109] The Fugo blade helps to create a perfectly controlled anterior capsulotomy of any size, without the risk of a radial tear. The peculiar structure of the cut edge ensures that even if a deliberate radial cut is made in the capsulotomy, it will not spontaneously extend towards the equator. Radio-frequency diathermy and the Fugo blade are recommended when fibrotic capsules are encountered or in white mature cataracts with the absence of the red reflex, if trypan blue is not available. All these alternative methods may not leave as much of a tear-resistant capsular edge as manual CCC, which is especially important for performing optic capture. Wilson has compared five different anterior capsulotomy techniques using a porcine model.[110] Extensibility and edge characteristics were reviewed with each technique. Manual CCC was found to produce the most extensible capsulotomy with most regular edge.

If the cataract is intumescent, trypan blue is used to stain the capsule, then a sharp needle is used to make the central puncture in the capsule (Figure 26-6), and any liquid cortex is aspirated prior to capsulorrhexis (Figure 26-7). Intumescent cataracts have high intralenticular pressure; hence, the surgeon should always aim for a small capsulorrhexis. The capsulorrhexis can be enlarged using the two-stage CCC technique (initial small and definitive large rhexis just before IOL implantation).[111] If poor visualization prevents a CCC from being performed, a can-opener capsulotomy is best achieved using several small bites with a needle or a cystotome (Figure 26-8). Liquid lens material may then be aspirated using a 25-guage cannula through a paracentesis and a chamber maintainer through another and, if necessary, the remaining nucleus is removed with an irrigation–aspiration or ultrasound hand piece. The can-opener capsulotomy is converted

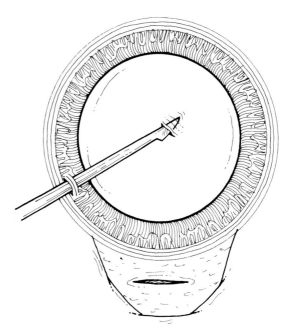

Figure 26-6 Sharp needle is used to make central puncture in anterior capsule of intumescent lens.

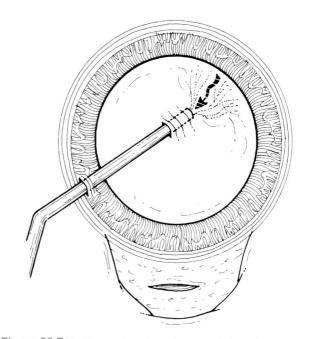

Figure 26-7 Liquid cortex is aspirated from capsular bag of intumescent lens.

to a CCC using the two-stage CCC technique prior to IOL implantation (Figures 26-9–26-12).[112]

Irrigation–Aspiration and Ultrasound

Separate irrigation–aspiration minimizes the anterior chamber fluctuations and aids in thorough removal of cortex, which is especially crucial in these small eyes. Most nuclei are too soft to be fractured and

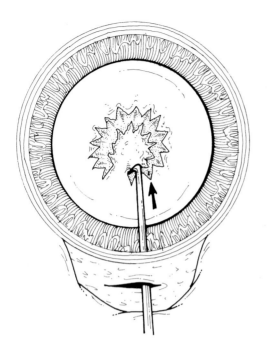

Figure 26-8 Can-opener capsulotomy necessitated by poor visualization in intumescent lens.

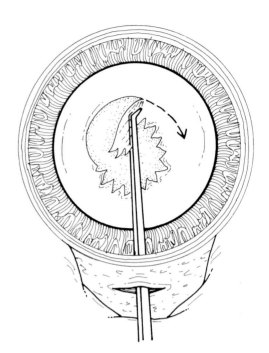

Figure 26-10 Forceps continues the conversion.

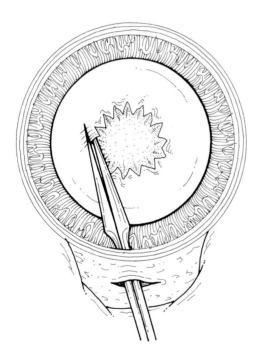

Figure 26-9 A scissor cut begins the two-stage continuous curvilinear capsulorrhexis technique to convert can-opener capsulotomy to continuous curvilinear capsulorrhexis.

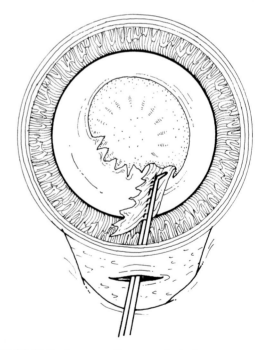

Figure 26-11 Continuous curvilinear capsulorrhexis progresses.

the lens removal can be accomplished using bimanual irrigation–aspiration. In rare cases, the harder nuclei may require short bursts of ultrasound energy using the phacoemulsification handpiece.

Posterior Continuous Curvilinear Capsulorrhexis

A planned primary posterior capsule opening, created either in an attempt to prevent inevitable secondary cataract formation or to remove a posterior plaque, should be achieved using the PCCC technique. PCCC can also be used as a method of preventing the extension of a tear when a small linear or triangular posterior capsular rupture inadvertently occurs. Posterior capsulorrhexis requires the use of viscoelastic agents and may be performed before or after posterior chamber IOL in-the-bag implantation.[113] Primary posterior capsulotomy is the preferred choice in children up to 6–8 years of age. Primary capsulotomy is combined

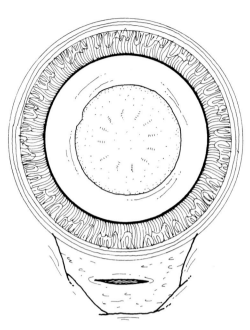

Figure 26-12 Two-stage continuous curvilinear capsulorrhexis conversion is completed.

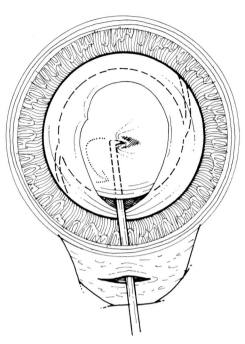

Figure 26-14 Posterior continuous curvilinear capsulorrhexis (CCC) is extended toward 3 o'clock; this technique is similar to that used with CCC.

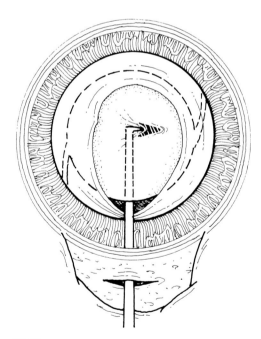

Figure 26-13 Posterior continuous curvilinear capsulorrhexis is started using a cystotome to create a central puncture of the posterior capsule posterior to the posterior chamber intraocular lens.

towards the surgeon and at the same time initiates the puncture. Pushing the margin of the puncture inferiorly creates a small flap. The flap is then held with capsulorrhexis forceps and a PCCC is accomplished aiming at a size of 3.5–4 mm by using the ACCC principles and strategies. Additional viscoelastic material can be placed through the central puncture of the posterior capsule to push the vitreous face away (Figure 26-14). Care should be taken that the viscoelastic agent does not push the flap posteriorly, thus making it difficult to grasp the posterior capsule tag. Also, if too much viscoelastic material is pushed through the opening, it may extend the tear in an unpredictable fashion. The end result should be a well-centered PCCC concentric to and smaller than the ACCC. PCCC resists the peripheral extension of the tear and holds the vitreous in place. The IOL can be supported over the capsule. PCCC can also be performed after the placement of an IOL. This ensures IOL fixation in the desired plane. However, performing PCCC and anterior vitrectomy becomes more difficult with this method and may require a pars plana approach. Moreover, manual capsulorrhexis is believed to yield a stronger margin than the vitrector-assisted capsulotomy.

Anterior Vitrectomy

The anterior vitreous is more reactive in infants and young children. Inflammatory response in small children is severe and fibrous membranes may form on an intact vitreous face. This acts as a scaffold for lens epithelial cell (LEC) migration and proliferation. Hence anterior vitrectomy along with posterior capsulotomy is advocated in infants and young children up to 2 years of age.

The aim of vitrectomy is to remove the central anterior vitreous without complete peripheral vitrectomy. For this limited purpose, most surgeons prefer the anterior approach through two limbal

with vitrectomy depending on the IOL material and design and the age of the child at surgery.

After aspiration of the lens matter, the capsule bag and the anterior chamber are filled with high-viscosity viscoelastic agent sodium hyaluronate. A 26-gauge cystotome or bent tip of a disposable needle makes the initial puncture (Figure 26-13). For this, the cystotome or needle engages the central capsule, lifts it (corneal) ports. Removal of subincisional vitreous is accomplished thoroughly by exchanging the ports. The main valvular incision seals itself and maintains the stability of anterior chamber, reducing the fluctuations of iris-lens diaphragm and uveal trauma. The vitrectomy probe is kept steady with the port directed posteriorly within the area of PCCC. A central anterior vitrectomy up to the depth of 2 mm is adequate. The recommended parameters are 30 cc flow rate, 300–400 cc vacuum and 400–800 cut rate.

Intraocular Lens Implantation

IOL fixation, material and size are important determinants of immediate and long-term outcome. In-the-bag fixation is the most preferred site of IOL implantation. Regarding IOL material, polymethyl methacrylate (PMMA) is the material that has undergone the most historical testing and of which surgeons have the most experience. An exaggerated capsular and inflammatory response, however, has remained a problem with PMMA material. Despite meticulous surgical technique, problems like visual axis opacification, inflammatory cell deposits, synechiae and pupil capture are often encountered in the early postoperative period. Moreover, PMMA is a rigid material, which requires an incision as large as the IOL optic diameter for implantation. Kugelberg and co-authors in their animal studies have showed that implantation of a regular-sized PMMA IOL retards eye growth in newborn rabbit eyes. Modification of PMMA surface was advocated to render IOL more biocompatible. Heparin surface modification was found to lower the incidence of inflammatory cell deposit formation. However, it did not alter the capsular behavior. PMMA IOLs are, therefore, gradually losing their popularity.

AcrySof is representative of the group of foldable IOLs made from flexible hydrophobic acrylic material (Alcon Laboratories, Fort Worth, TX). Acrysof is available as either a three-piece or a single-piece lens. The current opinion favors the use of AcrySof IOLs.[95] With AcrySof, the type of PCO is predominantly proliferative. PCO sets in at a later stage, typically at 14–16 months. Visual axis obscuration produced with AcrySof is less severe than PMMA and is, therefore, less amblyogenic. The preliminary results of single-piece AcrySof have been encouraging. Trivedi and Wilson believe that single-piece AcrySof SA series would be ideal for children. Kugelberg and colleagues also found that SA30AL maintained good centration, produced minimal inflammation and was well tolerated in pediatric eyes. Nihalani BR and Vasavada AR conducted a prospective observational study of 134 eyes of children aged 2–15 years with congenital and developmental cataracts, and found that SA30AL produced satisfactory visual axis clarity, acceptable inflammatory response and maintained good centration. Single piece AcrySof has extremely flexible haptics, combined with excellent memory, which makes the lens easy to implant and not prone to deformation. As the haptics unfold slowly, it is easier to manipulate IOLs in the bag even in the presence of PCCC. One-piece construction is believed to be robust in resisting capsule contracting forces. Also, single-piece AcrySof adapts to the smallest capsular bag without becoming decentered. These unique characteristics have led some surgeons to prefer single-piece over three-piece AcrySof for pediatric cataract surgery. However, long-term clinical experience is necessary to derive firm conclusions regarding the biocompatibility of single-piece AcrySof in pediatric eyes.

Single-piece Acrylic IOLs may not be as effective in preventing epithelial pearls from escaping onto the vitreous face and obscuring the visual axis as are the three-piece Acrylic IOLs because of the wide haptic-optic junctions.

Recently, multifocal IOLs have been suggested for pediatric implants with potential benefits of compensation for presbyopia, functional vision over a broader range of distances, and greater spectacle independence.[114] Some concerns with the placement of multifocal IOLs in children include centration problems, IOL power calculations, the use of silicone IOLs, the amblyogenic effect of multiple overlapping images and decreased contrast, and the tolerability of glare.[115] Caution should be used when considering the insertion of multifocal IOLs in children outside of research protocols at the present time.

Posterior Capsule Capture

Posterior capture of the IOL optic may be carried out after suturing of the incision but before the viscoelastic material is removed. Under and through the viscoelastic, one side and then the other of the IOL optic, 90° form the haptic optic junctions are slipped through the PCCC by means of a spatula or cannula. The haptics remain in the bag (Figure 26-15). Viscoelastic material behind the IOL is left in place, whereas that remaining in the anterior chamber is slowly and carefully removed. Simultaneous irrigation of balanced salt solution (BSS) (preferably with a chamber maintainer) is performed while aspirating the viscoelastic material to maintain a deep chamber and prevent vitreous and the IOL from moving forward. If the PCCC is not 1.5 mm smaller than the optic the capture may be lost by the forward movement of the lens as the viscoelastic is removed and before the chamber pressure is restored with BSS. An anterior vitrectomy may be necessary if vitreous herniates at the time of PCCC.

Posterior capsulorrhexis with posterior capsular optic capture is a technically challenging procedure. The posterior capsule is thinner than the anterior capsule, adding to the difficulty of achieving a circular opening that is small and concentric to the

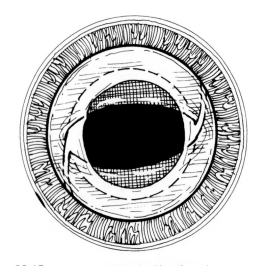

Figure 26-15 Posterior capsulorrhexis with optic capture.

pupil. In order to have a well-positioned posterior capsulorrhexis captured optic, the PCCC must be reasonably well centered. The lens loops, being in the bag, will exert a strong centering force. The vaulting of the intraocular optic through the PCCC requires cautious manipulation as the posterior capsule is thin. The PCCC seems to have the same stretching capacity as the anterior CCC.[96,116,117] The disadvantage of this technique is that it requires skill to avoid peripheral tears in the posterior capsule, which could destroy the integrity of the capsular bag. If the bag integrity is lost before the IOL is placed in the bag a lens may be fixed to the capsule using Rhexis Fixation which is CCC optic capture of a sulcus placed IOL. If, after the IOL is in the bag, the integrity of the posterior is lost for PCCC optic capture and bag fixation is unstable the loops may be left behind the CCC and the optic pulled out through the CCC to capture it and achieve stable capsule fixation. So the PCCC may be done either before the IOL is placed or after the lens is in the bag.

Closure

Most surgeons prefer to suture all the incisions in view of the low scleral rigidity and a child's tendency to rub the eyes (Figure 26-16). Small incisions for foldable IOLs may still require a suture in very young eyes to obtain a watertight closure or to ensure that the wound does not reopen with blinking or eye rubbing. Currently, the most popular suture material for closing corneoscleral incisions in children is 10-0 nylon, 9-0 Vicryl, or 10-0 Vicryl suture.[118] One or more interrupted 10-0 nylon sutures may be required to close the paracentesis site. Peripheral iridectomy is not routinely performed. The chamber is re-deepened after wound closure, and the wound is checked for water tightness. The internal portion of the wound is also checked for gaping or fish mouthing with a sterile Posner gonioscopy mirror (Figure 26-17). Full-thickness corneal sutures of 10-0 nylon are placed as necessary to close the internal wound.

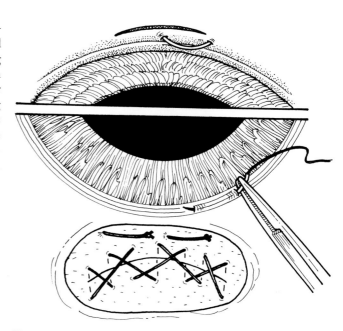

Figure 26-17 Suture technique for repair of fish-mouthing of internal wound.

■ POSTOPERATIVE TREATMENT ■

Postoperatively, a child's eye will tend to react with more inflammation than will that of an adult.[6,51,119,120] The inflammatory response can usually be managed well with intensive topical steroid therapy including atropinization.

After cataract surgery in infants, administration of topical steroids and antibiotic drops should be administered using the same routine as in adults. Cycloplegia is gradually tapered off over the ensuing weeks. By 4–6 weeks postoperatively, the child is no longer receiving any eye medication. Suture removal is performed within 2–3 months postoperatively, using general anesthesia if the child is too young to cooperate at the slit lamp, unless absorbable suture has been used. The refractive status can be evaluated at the same time. Amblyopia treatment starts within 1 week postoperatively when the media is clear. Close follow-up by a pediatric ophthalmologist is mandatory until the patient is 10–12 years of age.

Postoperative treatment in children older than 2 years of age should begin immediately at the end of surgery with the instillation of a combination ointment of antibiotic and corticosteroids. Atropine (1%) or homatropine (5%) is also instilled, and the eye is patched until the child fully recovers from the anesthesia. Cycloplegia is continued for up to 1 month after surgery to minimize fibrin deposition.[30] Also, corticosteroid drops are used postoperatively on a tapering schedule for up to 3 months.

In both infants and children, the peak inflammatory reaction does not appear until a day or two after surgery. The surgeon should not be deceived by a very quiet eye the first day after surgery but should remain vigilant in the management of postoperative inflammation in pediatric patients. Because the inflammatory response may be subtle, with few symptoms and only mild ciliary congestion, frequent postoperative visits are recommended.[62] Postoperative synechiae formation is also possible, even though

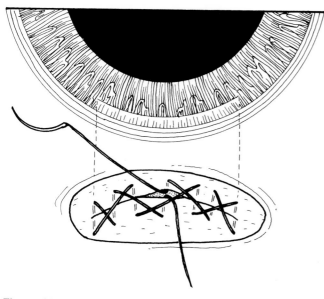

Figure 26-16 Shoelace suturing techniques.

the eye may appear to be quiet. The Nd:YAG laser may be used to break up fibrin strands and to disperse anterior and posterior keratic precipitates on the IOL.

Despite recent advances in pediatric surgical techniques, inadequate preoperative evaluation and postoperative treatment of amblyopia may limit the ultimate visual success in pediatric cases, especially those involving monocular cataract.[120–123] Vigorous occlusion therapy is instituted as early as possible in all cases of unilateral cataract extraction in infancy. Alternate patching may be recommended in patients with bilateral correction.

■ COMPLICATIONS OF PEDIATRIC SURGERY ■

POSTERIOR CAPSULE OPACIFICATION

Posterior capsule opacification is one of the most serious complications because it can lead to irreversible deprivation amblyopia, caused by the insidious formation of retro-pseudophakic membranes. The management and prevention of secondary cataracts, including the proposal of a new technique, are discussed in the section Review of Pediatric Surgical Techniques.

Pharmacological Method to Reduce the Incidence of Secondary Cataract Formation

Tissue plasminogen activator can be used to decrease fibrin following cataract surgery.[124,125] Experimentally, hirudin has been evaluated for preventing postoperative fibrin formation.[126] Heparin-surface-modified IOLs and even heparin infusion at a concentration of 5 IU/mL of infusion of fluid may help prevent secondary membrane.[127,128] Other experimental methods to reduce secondary membrane formation include antimetabolites, including mitomycin and caffeine acid, phenyl ester, immunotoxins including one in a phase III clinical trial, anti-growth factor agents, agents which inhibit binding of lens epithelial cells to the capsule, and even a gene therapy involving a replication–defective recombinant adenovirus. If toxicity issues can be overcome and these agents can be shown to affect lens epithelial cells (proliferation, migration, adhesion to the capsular bag, and fibrous metaplasia) without collateral damage to ocular tissues, this may represent the future in prevention of secondary membranes. Such agents may in the future be given by single injections, combined with viscoelastic, sustained relapse, or via coating the IOL. The most promising are either gene therapy or specific monoclonal antibodies which selectively target lens epithelial cells.

Sealed-capsule irrigation device has a potential clinical usefulness in reducing visual axis opacification in pediatric eyes. It isolates the interior of the capsular bag from the anterior segment, permitting isolated targeting of lens epithelial cells in vivo using pharmacologic agents while minimizing the risk of damage to other intraocular structures. Early results using demineralized water and Triton X 100 in a histological study in rabbit eyes and some human eyes have been encouraging.[129,130]

New Techniques to Reduce the Incidence of Secondary Cataract Formation

One of the major concerns in pediatric IOL implantation surgery has been the high incidence of postoperative opacification of the posterior capsule and retro-pseudophakic membrane formation.[37,63,131] Residual lens capsule epithelial cells transform to fibroblasts and Elschnig pearls, which proliferate using the posterior capsule, anterior vitreous face, and anterior and posterior surfaces of the IOL as a scaffold.[132,133] Secondary membranes form, re-occlude the visual axis, and can lead to irreversible deprivation amblyopia. In general, with decreasing age there is an increasing aggressiveness of secondary cataract formation.[134] Different techniques to avoid or reduce postoperative fibrosis or Elschnig pearl formation have been proposed, including primary posterior capsulotomy and anterior vitrectomy, pars plana posterior capsulotomy, and PCCC with posterior optic capture.[32–34,41,135–138]

With the development of automated vitrectomy instruments in the 1970s, cutting and aspirating capabilities added a new dimension to the treatment of pediatric cataracts.[60] By performing a posterior capsulotomy and anterior vitrectomy at the time of cataract extraction, a clear optical axis resulted, whereas the need for secondary surgical procedures was minimized. Controversy exists regarding the advisability of performing a primary posterior capsulotomy and anterior vitrectomy versus a posterior capsulotomy at a later date.[43,117]

The eye in children older than 5 years of age responds to surgery with less inflammation and posterior capsule opacification than does the infant's eye.[49] Also with the development of modern microsurgical techniques and the availability of the Nd:YAG laser, routine primary posterior capsulotomy openings are unnecessary in this population. Leaving the posterior capsule intact for posterior chamber in-the-bag IOL implantation, with the option of Nd:YAG posterior capsulotomy at a later date, may be the best approach in older children and provides the best visual results with the least risk.[62] Secondary Nd:YAG capsulotomy has been demonstrated to be successful in children older than 6 years of age with posterior capsular opacity.[93,139]

For children younger than 5 or 6 years of age, less cooperative children, and infants, an Nd:YAG laser vertically mounted in the operating room can be used to perform posterior capsulotomies in infants and children either at the time of surgery or weeks to months after the cataract procedure. Laser capsulotomy in the pediatric population, however, requires high energy, and some membranes are too dense to allow penetration of the membrane or a large enough opening. General anesthesia is required, and the recurrence of the membrane is possible because the anterior vitreous face remains as a scaffold for secondary membrane formation.

Studies have demonstrated an inevitable development of secondary cataracts in younger children unless the posterior capsule is opened generously and an anterior vitrectomy is performed at the time of cataract extraction and IOL implantation.[140–142] Many pediatric ophthalmologists currently perform a posterior capsulotomy and a shallow anterior vitrectomy routinely at the time of cataract extraction, prior to insertion of the IOL.[51,80] Special instruments have been developed to perform a PCCC underneath a posterior chamber IOL.[143] Higher viscous viscoelastics including Healon 5 make this a safer and technically less difficult procedure. One modification involved removing the cataract through a scleral tunnel incision with implantation of a posterior chamber IOL and then, during the same procedure, performing a pars plana posterior capsulotomy and pars plana anterior vitrectomy.[63,134] It was believed to ensure proper positioning of the IOL prior to performing the capsulotomy, and it was possible to achieve large capsular openings. One disadvantage of primary capsulotomy and anterior vitrectomy is dislocation of the IOLs, which has been demonstrated in 3–20% of cases.[134,144–146] In addition, there have been reports of cystoid macular edema following pediatric cataract extraction with anterior vitrectomy.[147] Subsequent studies, however, have found the risk of this complication to be quite minimal.[16,49,50,141,142,148–151] Anterior vitrectomy may also be associated with vitreous incarceration in the wound and vitreous adhesions that increase the risk of retinal detachment.[56] Finally, even after primary posterior capsulectomy with vitrectomy, many children's visual axes still become re-occluded by secondary membranes,[134,139,152] necessitating repeated capsulotomies and sometimes pars plana membranectomy.[49,71]

Other techniques have been proposed to prevent posterior capsular and vitreous face membrane formation while reducing the risk of dislocation of the IOL. One such technique involves placing the IOL anterior to the entire capsular bag. This creates a tight adhesion between the anterior and posterior capsule and helps prevent lens epithelial cells from migrating, proliferating, and forming Elschnig pearls.[46–49] Another new technique called "bag-in-the-lens" technique described by Marie-José Tassignon and performed in a limited number of cases with excellent results involves a newly designed IOL that fits within an anterior and posterior CCC and sandwiches the capsule leaflets in a peripheral circumferential concavity of the IOL. Successful implantation was achieved in 95% of the cases. At a mean follow-up of 22.7 months, lens epithelial cell proliferation was mild, confined to peripheral capsular bag and bag-in-the-lens optic remained clear.[153]

Posterior Capsulorrhexis with Optic Capture

To further reduce or eliminate opacification of the posterior capsule in pediatric cases while reducing the need for anterior vitrectomy, a technique of posterior capsulorrhexis with optic capture has been shown to be beneficial.[135–138] This technique involves primary posterior continuous curvilinear capsulorrhexis and placement of the optic of the IOL through the posterior capsulorrhexis opening with resultant optic capture while the haptics remain in the bag.[45,47] This is a technique that has been used in pediatric cases since April 1993 with promising results. The technique for performing posterior capsulorrhexis with optic capture is described later in *Current Surgical Techniques*.

Primary PCCC with posterior capsule optic capture helps to maintain a clear visual axis, reducing the need for subsequent intervention because of the apposition of anterior and posterior capsule leaflets anterior to the IOL. These capsule leaflets are apposed and anterior to the IOL for 360°, except at the haptic-optic junctions. This causes release of Elschnig pearls to occur anterior to the IOL, where they will be removed by the aqueous (Figure 26-18). Any possible adhesion of protein on the anterior surface of the IOL may be cleared away with the Nd:YAG laser. The benefit of this technique is that it provides excellent IOL fixation and ensures centration of the IOL. The tight barrier which is created prevents vitreous from moving forward. The disadvantages are that the

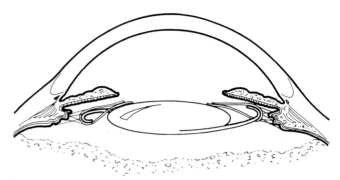

Figure 26-18 Posterior capsulorrhexis with optic capture.

procedure is technically challenging, requires precise and controlled capsulotomies, and makes IOL exchange difficult.[154,155] Piggyback IOL placement is possible, however. Koch has described that performing this technique in conjunction with anterior vitrectomy is beneficial in preventing posterior capsule opacifications.[154] Primary PCCC with posterior capsule optic capture represents a technique that serves to keep the optical axis clear while maintaining excellent support and centration of the implant.

Double Optic Capture with Capsular Fusion

Dr. DeBroff has developed a new technique for infantile cataracts when the surgeon is planning on placing an IOL at the time of surgery. IOL implantation is becoming more accepted for not only unilateral cataracts in infants, but also some cases of bilateral infantile cataracts. This new technique is becoming more frequent with parents who, for financial reasons or because of a lack of dexterity, are unable to maintain contact-lens correction. The high rate of visual axis opacification has been the reason why many surgeons are reluctant to place IOLs in infants. Posterior capsulorrhexis with optic capture has been shown to be an effective technique in children over 2 years of age that effectively creates an apposition of the anterior and posterior capsule leaflets anterior to the IOL, enabling effective sealing of the capsular bag. This technique is very challenging in infants because of the very small size of the eye, the extreme elasticity of the anterior and posterior capsules, and the overall size of the capsular bag.

The technique of double optic capture with capsular fusion involves capturing the optic and, thus, sequestering lens epithelial cells, fixating the IOL optic, preventing IOL movement and decreasing uveal rub. The technique involves performing an anterior CCC, removing the cataract, and performing a primary posterior capsulotomy and anterior vitrectomy using an anterior vitrectomy handpiece. The posterior capsulotomy is enlarged with the vitrectomy handpiece to closely match the size of the anterior capsulorrhexis opening. The ideal size of the capsulotomies would be 1–2 mm smaller than the diameter of the IOL optic that is to be implanted. The IOL is placed in the sulcus and the optic is captured through both the anterior capsulorrhexis opening and the posterior capsulotomy opening. In such a manner, double optic capture occurs with the IOL optic posterior to both capsulotomy openings, allowing the capsule leaflets to fuse 360° anterior to the IOL optic. This technique has been utilized for 18 months with no evidence of secondary membranes in 10 eyes and no evidence of increased inflammation, IOL dislocation, or elevated IOP. In addition, the technique of performing the posterior capsulotomy with the vitrector handpiece is technically less difficult than performing a PCCC, but still offers a tear resistant edge in infantile eyes that is amenable to optic capture. Further studies and longer-term follow-up with this technique are planned.

■ GLAUCOMA ■

Glaucoma is a recognized complication after pediatric cataract surgery. Despite improved surgical techniques, the incidence of glaucoma following successful cataract removal remains high. A significant number of surgeons regard aphakia as a cause of glaucoma. This glaucoma is, however, described as 'glaucoma in aphakia and pseudophakia'. The most common type of glaucoma to develop following congenital cataract surgery is open-angle glaucoma. The risk factors include age at surgery; pre-existing ocular abnormalities; type of cataract; and the effect of lens particles, lens proteins, inflammatory cells and retained lens material. In addition, microcornea, secondary surgery, chronic postoperative inflammation, the type of lensectomy procedure or instrumentation, pupillary block and the duration of postoperative observation have been found to influence the likelihood of glaucoma after pediatric cataract surgery. Certain eye diseases are associated with both cataracts and glaucoma (e.g., Lowe syndrome and congenital rubella). Undergoing lensectomy at a very young age, especially in the first year of life, may be a risk factor for development of glaucoma. It has been suggested that the immaturity of the developing infant's angle leads to increased susceptibility to secondary surgical trauma. Hence some surgeons believe it to be prudent to consider delaying surgery until the infant is 4 weeks old in bilateral cases. Glaucoma can occur at any time after congenital cataract surgery. Therefore, pediatric aphakic and pseudophakic patients should be routinely monitored for glaucoma throughout their lives. The incidence of pediatric pseudophakic glaucoma seems to be less than the incidence in pediatric aphakic glaucoma if the IOL is in the bag or separating the anterior and posterior compartments.

UVEAL INFLAMMATION

Intense uveal inflammation or severe fibrinoid reaction is a concern, particularly in infants and younger children. The addition of heparin to the irrigating solution has been suggested to reduce postoperative inflammatory reaction and related complications such as synechiae, pupil irregularity and IOL decentration. Atraumatic surgical techniques and in-the-bag fixation are most important contributors which may help to reduce the inflammatory response. Atropine, rather than shorter acting cycloplegics, helps to prevent this fibrinoid reaction that may not be present on the first day or two after surgery, but more typically on the third or fourth day if atropine is not used.

ENDOPHTHALMITIS

Endophthalmitis is the most serious eye complication after surgery. The incidence has been reported to be 0.07%, which is similar to that reported in the adult population.[156] This complication

is the strongest argument against synchronous bilateral surgery in children with bilateral cataracts.[157] Absolute sterility must be maintained and excellent wound closure achieved. Upper-respiratory-tract infection and nasolacrimal duct obstruction should be treated prior to cataract surgery.[157] Careful follow-up of the patient is necessary to observe for any signs of infection, especially in cases of cataracts induced by trauma. Because children and infants are often unable to appreciate or recognize the importance of sudden decreased vision, careful follow-up is essential.

WOUND LEAK

Children often rub their eyes and are often involved in activities of physical contact that can lead to eye trauma. It is important to tightly suture the wound and have the child wear an eye shield until the wound is well healed.

STRABISMUS

Strabismus is the most common complication following pediatric cataract extraction.[22] The interruption of fusion caused by the lens opacification and possible anisometropia and aniseikonia that follows aphakic correction leads to a 66–86% incidence of strabismus in children who are treated for cataracts.[158,159] Approximately one-quarter of pediatric patients undergoing cataract surgery may require strabismus surgery.[22]

AMBLYOPIA

Amblyopia is more often associated with monocular than bilateral cataracts. Occlusion therapy, carried out during the postoperative period, is essential.

NYSTAGMUS

The presence of nystagmus indicates poor vision resulting from sensory deprivation[17] and usually will be present if a congenital cataract is not removed by the fourth month of life. If nystagmus is present, the best visual acuity after cataract surgery will usually be less than 20/50.

RETINAL DETACHMENT

The incidence of retinal detachment after pediatric cataract surgery has been found to be between 1% and 1.5%.[104,160] With older techniques, such as lens needling, the incidence was as high as 10%.[161] Although the pathogenesis of retinal detachment in pseudophakic patients is not fully understood, secondary changes of the vitreoretinal interface may be important factors.[162,163] Retinal detachment may occur many years after surgery. The mean age in one series was 31.9 years.[164]

The incidence of retinal detachment after pediatric cataract surgery using PCCC and optic capture, bag-in-lens or Stegmann's optic entrapment (all of these techniques without vitrectomy), has not been studied in large enough series to compare the incidence in cases where primary vitrectomy or later Nd: YAG capsulotomy is used.

■ CHALLENGES ■

SMALL PUPIL

Even with mydriatics, the pupils of children especially infants may remain small. This is especially true with cataracts caused by rubella.[101] In addition, use of phenylephrine drops is often contraindicated in infants. Difficulties in performing CCC may be encountered with small pupils. Healon 5 helps to expand a pupil that is not fibrotic. A smooth-edged capsular border can be made larger than the diameter of the small pupil by guiding the tear under the iris while observing the folded edge of the capsular flap. To improve visualization during this procedure, the surgeon may stretch the iris in the quadrant of the advancing tear, using the shaft of the cystotome or a bent needle, or by using a second instrument such as a Y hook or cyclodialysis spatula (Figure 26-19).[165] If emulsification of the cataract is necessary, it should be performed in the central part of the small pupil where visualization is adequate and where the risk of touching the iris or capsule with the tip of the instrument is minimized. Iris trauma should be minimal as the pediatric eyes react in the form of severe postoperative inflammatory response. Iris hooks may be necessary in very small pupil cases.

MAINTAINING THE INTRAOCULAR LENS CENTRATION

A precise CCC that preserves the architecture of the capsular bag is proving to be one of the most important advances in pediatric cataract surgery. The CCC technique increases the probability of safe and secure in-the-bag IOL placement because it maintains the relative integrity of the capsular bag. The visible, flexible rim of a CCC always makes it possible to verify the placement of IOL haptics within the bag and, therefore, guarantees centration (Figure 26-20). Performing CCC in the pediatric population

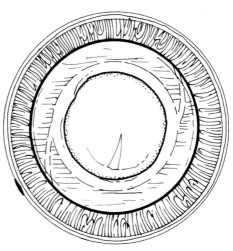

Figure 26-20 Continuous curvilinear capsulorrhexis ensures centration and verification of the intraocular lens haptics in the bag.

is more challenging than in adults because of the elastic nature of the child's capsule and zonules. Because of the zonular elasticity, centration and size of the CCC may be deceiving. It may be necessary to release the forceps from the anterior capsule as the tear is progressing to allow the lens to assume its natural position. Reinspection is important to ascertain if the tear is progressing in a manner that will create an appropriately sized central capsulorrhexis opening.

Late decentration of in-the-bag posterior chamber IOL implants is a potential problem with pediatric lens implants. Some contraction of the bag always occurs postoperatively, primarily along the torn edge of the anterior capsule because of fibrous metaplasia of lens epithelial cells and the subsequent contracture of the fibrous membrane attached to the capsule. Anterior capsulectomy techniques, such as the can-opener capsulotomy, the Christmas tree technique, the scissors technique, or any opening that has edge discontinuity, increases the chances of an asymmetrical contracture of the rim. This results in uneven tension on the capsular bag and zonules. Significant decentration is likely to occur if one loop is in the bag and the other is in the sulcus. With CCC, the contracture is symmetrical if the capsular opening is circular, central, and smaller than the optic of the IOL. If the CCC is outside the edge of the optic on one side of the optic the adhesion of the CCC edge there to the posterior capsule may progressively nudge the IOL to the other side and result in eccentricity of the IOL, even though it was once centered and it is still in the bag.

If a short anterior capsule tear occurs in the pediatric anterior capsule CCC border without extension to the equator, it can be blunted or turned back toward the CCC by using forceps (Figure 26-21). The opening will be eccentric, but the smooth continuous rim prevents radial extensions of tears in elastic pediatric capsules. If a longer anterior capsule tear occurs, care must be taken during cataract removal to prevent excessive pressure that could extend the tear past the equator and into the posterior capsule (Figure 26-22). In such cases, the irrigation–aspiration or ultrasound should be carried out with the handpiece kept centrally over the capsulotomy, avoiding stress to the anterior capsule rim. The irrigation–aspiration should be slow with fewer movements for vacuuming of cortical material.

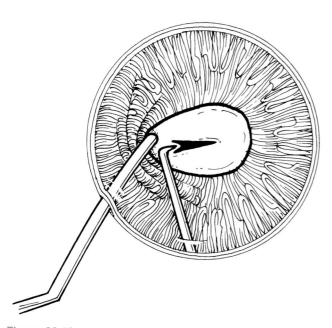

Figure 26-19 Improving visualization for continuous curvilinear capsulorrhexis in a small pupil case by stretching the iris with a second instrument.

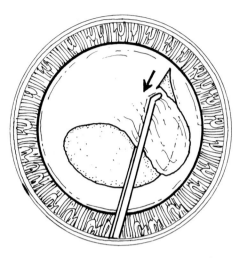

Figure 26-21 Turning back a radial extension of the continuous curvilinear capsulorrhexis tear.

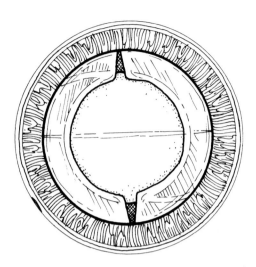

Figure 26-23 Anterior capsular tear matched with second anterior capsular tear 180° away to ensure symmetric tension on the anterior capsular rim.

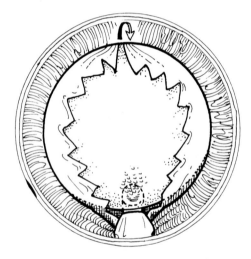

Figure 26-22 Pressure during phacoemulsification in the presence of an anterior capsular radial tear causing extension of the tear.

weakened zonules or after trauma in any age group, significant contraction of the capsule may occur along the edge of the tear a few months postoperatively. Unlike the situation after irregularly torn capsulotomies, this contracture rarely leads to any significant degree of IOL decentration, as there is usually a symmetrical contracture of the CCC. Anterior capsule ring contracture can be released using the Nd:YAG laser. Radial peripheral placement of Nd:YAG pulses in the contracted anterior capsule releases the contracture of the capsule and prevents early or late decentration of the IOL. The Nd:YAG successfully releases this anterior capsule purse-string effect.[49]

POSTERIOR CAPSULAR TEARS

PCCC may be employed in the making of a primary posterior capsulectomy, as previously described. It may also be used when a small linear or triangular tear inadvertently occurs in the posterior capsule; even though the posterior capsule is resistant to radial tears and, thus, maintains capsular bag integrity (Figure 26-24).[166] Tears of the posterior capsule that have not extended as

When an anterior capsule tear occurs, cohesive viscoelastic agents may be useful to help avoid an extension around to the posterior capsule during IOL insertion. However, the viscoelastic agent should be injected carefully, adding a little above and then below the torn edge to sandwich it within the viscoelastic material. If the capsular bag is filled without significant viscoelastic material above the capsule, the pressure within the bag can extend the tear. The IOL haptics should be oriented perpendicular to the tear. In addition, the anterior capsule tear can be matched by creating a second anterior capsule tear 180° away from the first. This precaution ensures symmetrical tension on the anterior capsule rim as the capsule contracts postoperatively (Figure 26-23). Consistent in-the-bag IOL centration can be achieved by analyzing the configuration and locating the anterior capsule defects.

ANTERIOR CAPSULE RING CONTRACTURE

Although there are multiple advantages of CCC, there is one potential complication peculiar to the technique. In adults with

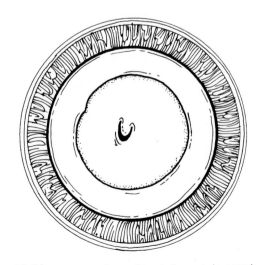

Figure 26-24 Appearance of a small tear in the posterior capsule.

far as the capsular equator are candidates for PCCC. The rounding off of a posterior capsule tear or completing it full circle usually prevents extension of the tear, which can frequently occur during anterior vitrectomy or lens placement. Thus, PCCC should be performed prior to anterior vitrectomy or lens insertion when a small posterior capsule tear has occurred. Also, if a stalk of a persistent hyaloid membrane is present, Vannas scissors can be used to sever it after completing PCCC.

The goal is to direct the advancing tear into a circle that encompasses the entire extent of the tear. Alternatively, one or both ends of a linear tear may be rounded and blunted by means of PCCC techniques. For maximal control when redirecting a tear of the posterior capsule, capsulorrhexis forceps are used to grasp the capsule flap near one point of the tear and to turn the tear in the desired direction (Figures 26-25, 26-26). The PCCC is kept as small as possible to preserve maximal integrity of the posterior capsule.

PRE-EXISTING POSTERIOR CAPSULE DEFECTS AND POSTERIOR LENTIGLOBUS

Posterior lentiglobus tends to distort the preoperative retinoscopy reflex – a condition that makes optical correction of refractive errors difficult.[10,167–169] Early detection of this condition and other conditions that produce higher-order optical aberrations will be facilitated by the more general availability of wavefront sensing instruments. Cataract extraction should be performed as soon as any decrease in visual acuity occurs that is unamenable to optical correction and amblyopia therapy.[150] Because the posterior capsule in these patients is thinned and weakened centrally, hydrodissection should never be performed, as this can create a posterior capsule rupture. "Hydro-free" fluidless dissection can be used to aid in dissection of the cortex from the anterior capsule prior to aspiration or phacoemulsification of the lens (Figures 26-27, 26-28).[170,171]

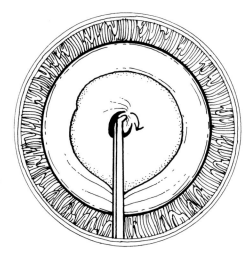

Figure 26-25 Posterior continuous curvilinear capsulorrhexis (CCC) technique for blunting small tears in the posterior capsule is identical to anterior CCC.

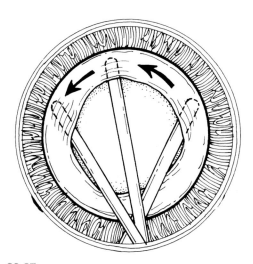

Figure 26-27 Hydro-free dissection: achieving dissection of the cortex from the capsule without injecting fluid inferiorly.

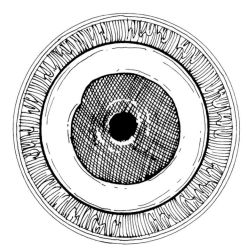

Figure 26-26 Posterior tear cannot enlarge after completion of posterior continuous curvilinear capsulorrhexis.

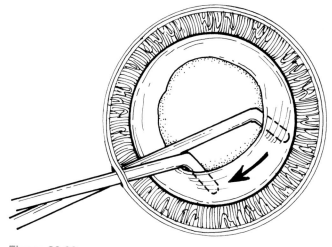

Figure 26-28 Hydro-free dissection superiorly through the paracentesis wound.

Pre-existent defects or splits in the posterior capsule (as in posterior lentiglobus or perforating trauma) may also be managed by PCCC. Complete PCCC may not be possible, depending on the configuration and extent of the split of the lentiglobus. However, the technique may still possibly be used to round off the points of the leading tears. Pre-existing defects may be associated with degenerated vitreous which needs to be removed with vitrectomy. The capsule is weak in most of these cases, in which case the IOL should be placed in the sulcus. Sometimes an IOL may be placed in the bag with its loops perpendicular to the tear. If the IOL is not stable and secure in the capsular bag with this method, the optic should be pulled out through the CCC for optic capture (reverse rhexis fixation) or it should be removed from the bag and placed in the sulcus. To assure centration following this maneuver and to avoid late complications such as transillumination defects, glaucoma and hyphema, especially when Soemmering's rings develop, the optic should then be pushed through the anterior CCC into the bag.[172]

POSTERIOR CAPSULE PLAQUES

PCCC can also be employed for the removal of thickened fibrotic posterior capsule plaques. In these cases, the PCCC is made as a controlled circle that encompasses the central opacity and results in a posterior capsule opening that resists extension to the equator. This capsular opening can be made before or after the IOL is implanted in the capsular bag. By nudging the IOL eccentrically and slipping a barbed needle on a syringe of viscoelastic material under the lens, PCCC is achieved. This technique was successfully used in 1987 for the removal of dense plaque from the posterior capsule of a 7-year-old boy who had acquired a cataract secondary to irradiation for rhabdomyosarcoma.[112] If the posterior capsule plaque is too large involving the entire posterior capsule, a central nick should be placed in the central posterior capsule with a slit knife and the plaque can be cut with scissors and/or a vitrectome with the port facing superiorly. The Fugo blade is another option.

EYE GROWTH AND CHANGING REFRACTION

Predicting axial growth, and the refractive changes that accompany it, are major challenges for the long-term care following pediatric cataract surgery. This is especially true with the widespread acceptance of fixed-power IOL implantation. Unless the growth of the eye can be accurately predicted, selection of IOL power is a difficult task.

Axial growth after cataract surgery can be attributed to normal eye growth and other factors, including age at surgery, visual input, the presence or absence of IOL, laterality and genetic factors. The interocular axial length difference was found to be another important variable influencing axial growth. Understanding pediatric eye growth will help in IOL power calculation and the prediction of refractive changes after IOL implantation.

SECONDARY INTRAOCULAR LENSES IN CHILDREN

The need for secondary IOLs in children occurs frequently because many infants are left aphakic following cataract surgery due to their small size and young age, and because of the

Table 26-1 Secondary intraocular lenses in children

I. Indications
  a. Failure of contact lens
  b. Nystagmus

II. Preoperative considerations
  a. IOL calculation and measurements
    i. Patient cooperation
    ii. A scan
    iii. Keratometry
    iv. Cycloplegic refraction
    v. Refraction goal
  b. Capsular support

III. Technique
  a. In the bag
    i. Technique – Wilson et al
  b. Sulcus fixated lens
    i. Simple
    ii. Optic capture
    iii. Capsular membrane sutured lens
  c. Iris fixated lens
  d. Scleral sutured lens

IV. Complications
  a. Vision decrease (5.8%)
  b. IOL decentration (Crnic 5%) (Trivedi & Wilson 5%)
  c. Wound leak (5%)
  d. Secondary membrane (Crnic 9%) visual axis opacification (5.2% Wilson)
  e. Pupillary block glaucoma (2%)
  f. Ptosis (2%)
  g. Glaucoma
  h. Dislocation of IOL (2.6% Wilson)
  i. Pupillary capture (1.3% Wilson)
  j. Decentration with simple sulcus-fixated foldable IOL – inferior in males? not seen in PMMA, worse if axial length >23 mm (28.6% Wilson)

difficulty of using aphakic contact lenses in children (Table 26-1). In addition, secondary IOLs may be needed in children left aphakic after traumatic cataracts. Some pediatric IOLs may require removal and replacement with a secondary IOL because of Nd:YAG pitting or subluxation. Older children and young adults may find the optical aberrations of aphakic spectacles disabling. Children with nystagmus may not tolerate aphakic spectacles or contact lenses. The effective use of secondary IOLs in children has been described.[173–179]

Careful preoperative planning optimizes results. Preoperative considerations include the ability of the child to cooperate with sitting for axial length and keratometry measurements. If a child cannot cooperate in the clinic setting, then these must be planned under a separate sedation or under general anesthesia at the time of the procedure. Cycloplegic refraction and the goal refraction for the operated eye are considered. Refraction in the sound eye should also be performed to help avoid anisometropia, which may be amblyogenic. The surgeon should also evaluate the patient for the presence of adequate capsular support and the presence of synechiae, which may make positioning of a lens difficult.

Finally, the type of procedure and the lens appropriate for the procedure are chosen. Patients with adequate capsular support may be well-served by a variety of procedures. In-the-bag placement, membrane optic capture, or IOL membrane suture fixation is always desirable for improved centration, sequestration of the lens from uveal elements, and the long-term stability needed for the decades to come in these young children. When possible, the authors employ a technique independently described by Wilson et al. for in-the-bag secondary IOL placement for patients with a Soemmering's ring. The anterior capsule near the apposed edge of the capsular leaflets is opened, followed by aspiration of the epithelial elements between the leaflets. The IOL is then placed in the bag, between the opened leaflets of the Soemmering's ring.[176]

Optic capture is another method affording excellent centration and long-term stability for secondary IOL placement.

In patients with membrane support, but not an appropriate opening for membrane optic capture the authors consider suturing the IOL to the capsular membrane for stable fixation and to avoid iris contact.

In patients without adequate capsular support, a scleral or iris-sutured secondary IOL may be considered. Iris-fixated lenses are demonstrating their effectiveness and a reduction in the risk of endophthalmitis that may occur with scleral-sutured posterior chamber IOL.

Because support for the IOL is more difficult to achieve, one of the most significant complications of secondary simple sulcus IOL placement is IOL decentration, which occurs in about 5% of cases.[178,179] In none of these reported cases was optic capture, membrane suturing, or Soemmering's ring bag placement used. In a series by Trivedi and Wilson, all decentrations occurred in sulcus-fixated foldable IOLs and none occurred in sulcus-fixated PMMA lenses. Males with axial length of >23 mm were especially susceptible in this series.

Other reported complications include vision decrease (5.8%), wound leak (5%), secondary membrane (9%: Crnic), visual axis opacification (5.2%: Wilson), pupillary block glaucoma (2%), ptosis (2%), dislocation of IOL (2.6%: Wilson), and pupillary capture (1.3%: Wilson).

FUNCTIONAL OUTCOME

Congenital cataracts cause visual deprivation that results in severe amblyopia. Changing refraction with amblyopia poses a grave challenge to visual rehabilitation. Strabismus is another factor influencing visual rehabilitation following pediatric cataract surgery. Despite a satisfactory technical outcome, functional outcome remains unpredictable.

■ CONCLUSIONS ■

Given the characteristics of children's eyes, pediatric cataract surgery is technically challenging. Tissue elasticity, a propensity for postoperative inflammation, and a high rate of secondary cataract formation are matters of concern. The surgical techniques are more demanding and there is less room for error. Also, diligent

preoperative and postoperative management is essential for satisfactory visual results. The timing of surgery is often crucial to prevent deprivational amblyopia and to attempt the preservation or restoration of binocular vision. The surgeon must be cognizant of the many complications that may occur in pediatric cataract surgery and must be prepared to manage any that do arise.

Longer-term follow-up of larger IOL series should continue to support the safety and efficacy of posterior chamber IOL implantation after cataract extraction in infants and children. With continued improvements in surgical and laser techniques, IOL designs, anti-inflammatory agents, and amblyopia therapy, the refractive and visual outcomes in pediatric cataract surgery should continue to improve, whereas the need for secondary procedures should diminish.

References

[1] Gilbert C, Foster A, Negrel AD, et al. Childhood blindness: a new form for recording causes of visual loss in children. Bull WHO 1993;71:485–489.

[2] Foster A, Gilbert C, Rahi J. Epidemiology of cataract in childhood: a global perspective. J Cataract Refract Surg 1997;23:601–604.

[3] San Giovanni JP, Chew EY, Reed GF, et al. Infantile cataract in the colloborative perinatal project: prevalence and risk factors. Arch Ophthalmol 2002;120:1559–1565.

[4] Holmes JM, Leske DA, Burke JP, et al. Birth prevalence of visually significant infantile cataract in a defined U.S population. Ophthal Epidemiol 2003;10:67–74.

[5] Maida JW, Sheets JIII. Pseudophakia in children: a review of results of eighteen implant surgeons. Ophthalmic Surg 1997;10:61–66.

[6] Hiles DA. Intraocular lens implantation in children with monocular cataracts 1974–1983. Ophthalmology 1984;91:1231–1237.

[7] Juler F. Visual acuity after traumatic cataract in children. Trans Ophthalmol Soc UK 1921;41:129.

[8] McKinna AJ. Results of treatment of traumatic cataract in children. Am J Ophthalmol 1961;52:43.

[9] Menezo JL, Taboada JF, Ferrer E. Complications of intraocular lenses in children. Trans Ophthalmol Soc UK 1985;104:546–552.

[10] Crouch ER, Parks MM. Management of posterior lenticonus complicated by unilateral cataract. Am J Ophthalmol 1978;85:503–508.

[11] Nelson LB. Diagnosis and management of cataracts in infancy and childhood. Ophthalmic Surg 1984;15:688–697.

[12] Wiesel TVN, Hubel DH. Effects of visual deprivation on morphology and physiology of cells in the cat's lateral geniculate body. J Neurophysiol 1963;26:978–993.

[13] von Noorden GK. Experimental amblyopia in monkeys: Further behavioral observations and clinical correlations. Invest Ophthalmol Vis Sci 1973;12:721–726.

[14] Vaegan Taylor D. Critical period for deprivation amblyopia in children. Trans Ophthalmol Soc UK 1979;99:432–439.

[15] Robb RM, Mayer DI, Moore BD. Results of early treatment of unilateral congenital cataracts. J Pediatr Ophthalmol Strabismus 1987;24:178–181.

[16] Sharma N, Pushker N, Dada T, et al. Complications of pediatric cataract surgery and intraocular lens implantation. J Cataract Refract Surg 1999;12:1585–1588.

[17] Gimbel HV, Neuhann T. Development, advantages, and methods of the continuous circular capsulorhexis technique. J Cataract Refract Surg 1990;16:31–37.

[18] Zetterstrom C, Lundvall A, Kugelberg M. Cataracts in children. J Cataract Refract Surg 2005;31:824–840.

[19] Parks MM. Visual results in aphakic children. Am J Ophthalmol 1982;94:441–449.

[20] Crawford JS, Morin JD. The lens. In: Crawford JS, Morin JD, editors. The eye in childhood. New York: Grune & Stratton; 1982. p. 259–287.

[21] Ohzeki T. The value of electro-physiological testing in assessment of visual function in children. Eur J Implant Refract Surg 1990;2:249–252.

[22] Del Monte MA. Diagnosis and management of congenital and developmental cataracts. Ophthalmol Clin North Am 1990;3:205–219.

[23] Awaya S. Stimulus vision deprivation amblyopia in humans. In: Reinecke RD, editor. Strabismus. Proceedings of the Third Meeting of the International Strabismological Association. May 10–12,1978, Kyoto. Japan. New York: Grune & Stratton; 1978. p. 31–44.

[24] Beller R, Hoyt CS, Marg E, Odom JV. Good visual function after neonatal surgery for congenital monocular cataracts. Am J Ophthalmol 1981;91:599–565.

[25] Hoyt CS. Treatment of congenital cataracts. In: Davidson SI, editor. Recent advances in ophthalmology. New York: Churchill Livingstone; 1987.

[26] Gelbert SS, Hoyt CS, Jastrebski G, Marg E. Long-term visual results in bilateral congenital cataracts. Am J Ophthalmol 1982;93:615–621.

[27] Stark WJ, Taylor HR, Michels RG, et al. Management of congenital cataracts. Ophthalmology 1979;86:1571–1578.

[28] Taylor D. Choice of surgical technique in the management of congenital cataract. Trans Ophthalmol Soc UK 1981;101:114–117.

[29] Nelson LB, Ullman S. Congenital and developmental cataracts. In: Tasman W, Jaeger EA, editors. Duane's clinical ophthalmology, vol. 1. Philadelphia: JB Lippincot; 1992. p. 1–10.

[30] Palmer EA. How safe are ocular drugs in pediatrics? Ophthalmology 1986;93:1038–1040.

[31] Moncrieff WF. Contributions to the surgery of congenital cataract. I. Modification of discission in the preschool age group. Am J Ophthalmol 1946;29:1513–1522.

[32] Chandler PA. Surgery of congenital cataracts. Am J Ophthalmol 1968;65:663–674.

[33] Jones IS. The treatment of congenital cataracts by needling. Am J Ophthalmol 1961;52:347–355.

[34] Dordes FH. A linear extraction of congenital cataract surgery. Am J Ophthalmol 1961;52:355–360.

[35] Scheie HG, Rubenstein RA, Kent RB. Aspiration of congenital or soft cataracts: Further experience. Am J Ophthalmol 1967;63:3–8.

[36] Scheie HG. Aspiration of congenital or soft cataracts: a new technique. Am J Ophthalmol 1960;50:1048–1056.

[37] Parks MM, Hiles DA. Management of infantile cataracts. Am J Ophthalmol 1967;63:10–19.
[38] Francois J. Late results of congenital cataract surgery. Trans Am Acad Ophthalmol Otolaryngol 1979;86:1586–1598.
[39] Francois J. Glaucoma and uveitis after congenital cataract surgery. Ann Ophthalmol 1971;3:131–135.
[40] Phelps CD, Arafat NJ. Open angle glaucoma following surgery for congenital cataracts. Arch Ophthalmol 1977;95:1985–1987.
[41] Ferguson AC. A modified instrument for aspiration and irrigation of congenital and soft cataract. Am J Ophthalmol 1964;57:596–600.
[42] Sheppard RW, Crawford JS. The treatment of congenital cataracts. Surv Ophthalmol 1973;17:340–347.
[43] Parks MM. Posterior lens capsulectomy during primary cataract surgery in children. Ophthalmology 1983;90:344–345.
[44] Hiles DA, Hurite FG. Results of the first year's experience with phaco-emulsification. Am J Ophthalmol 1973;75:473.
[45] Hiles DA, Wallan PH. Phacoemulsification versus aspiration in infantile cataract surgery. Ophthalmic Surg 1974;5:13–26.
[46] Hiles DA, Carter DT, Chotnier D. Phacoemulsification of infantile cataracts. Trans Pa Acad Ophthalmol Otolaryngol 1978;31:30–37.
[47] Callahan MA. Technique of congenital cataract surgery with the Kelman cavitron phaco emulsifier. Ophthalmology 1979;86:1994–1998.
[48] Hiles DA. Phacoemulsification of infantile cataracts. Int Ophthalmol Clin 1977;17:83–102.
[49] Gimbel HV. Implantation in children. J Pediatr Ophthalmol Strabismus 1993;30:69–79.
[50] Sinskey RM, Stoppel JO, Amin P. Long-term results of intraocular lens implantation in pediatric patients. J Cataract Refract Surg 1993;19:405–408.
[51] Hemo Y, BenEzra D. Traumatic cataracts in young children. Correction of aphakia by intraocular lens implantation. Ophthalmic Paediatr Genet 1987;8:2032–2207.
[52] Hiles DA. Indications, techniques and complications associated with IOL implantation in children. In: Hiles DA, editor. Intraocular lens implants in children. New York: Grune & Stratton; 1980. p. 189.
[53] Morgan KS, McDonald MB, Hiles DA, et al. The nationwide study of epikeratophakia for aphakia in children. Am J Ophthalmol 1987;103:366–374.
[54] Steinert RF, Grene RB. Postoperative management of epikeratoplasty. J Cataract Refract Surg 1988;14:255–264.
[55] Kelley CG, Keates RH, Lembach RG. Epikeratophakia for pediatric aphakia. Arch Ophthalmol 1986;104:680–682.
[56] Koenig SB, Ruttum MS, Lewandowsit MF, Schultz RD. Pseudophakia for traumatic cataracts in children. Ophthalmology 1993;100:1218–1224.
[57] Binkhorst CD, Gobin MH. Treatment of congenital and juvenile cataract with intraocular lens implants (pseudophakos). Br J Ophthalmol 1970;54:759–765.
[58] Binkhorst CD, Gobin MH. Congenital cataract and lens implantation. Ophthalmologica 1972;164:392–397.
[59] Hiles DA. The need for intraocular lens implantation in children. Ophthalmic Surg 1977;8:162–169.
[60] Binkhorst CD. The irido-capsular (two-loop) lens and the iris-clip (four-loop) lens in pseudophakia. Trans Am Acad Ophthalmol Otolaryngol 1973;77:589–617.
[61] Choyce DP. Correction of uni-ocular aphakia by means of anterior chamber acrylic implants. Trans Ophthalmol Soc UK 1958;78:459–470.
[62] Sinskey RM, Karel F, Dal Ri E. Management of cataracts in children. J Cataract Refract Surg 1989;15:196–200.
[63] Binkhorst CD, Gobin MH. Injuries to the eye with lens opacity in young children. Ophthalmologica 1964;148:169–183.
[64] Hiles DA. Intraocular lens implantations in children. Ann Ophthalmol 1977;9:789–797.
[65] Binkhorst CD, Greaves B, Kats A, Birmingham AK. Lens injury in children with iridocapsular supported intraocular lenses. J Am Intraocular Implant Soc 1978;4:34.
[66] Choyce DP. Anterior chamber lens implantation in children under eighteen years. In: Hiles DA, editor. Intraocular lens implants in children. New York: Grune & Stratton; 1980. p. 179.
[67] Fyodorov SN. The results of intraocular lens correction of aphakia in children. In: Hiles DA, editor. Intraocular lens implants in children. New York: Grune & Stratton; 1980. p. 41.
[68] Helveston EM, Saunders RA, Ellis FD. Unilateral cataracts in children. Ophthalmic Surg 1980;11:102–108.
[69] Reynolds JD, Hiles DA, Johnson BL, Biglan AW. A histopathological study of bilateral aphakia with a unilateral intraocular lens in a child. Am J Ophthalmol 1982;93:289–293.
[70] Hiles DA. Visual acuities of monocular IOL and non-IOL aphakic children. Ophthalmology 1980;87:1296–1300.
[71] Gimbel HV, Ferensowicz M, Ranaan M, Deluca M. Implantation in children. J Pediatr Ophthalmol Strabismus 1993;19:405–408.
[72] van Balen ATM. Binkhorst's method of implantation of pseudophakoi in unilateral traumatic cataract. Ophthalmologica 1972;165:490–494.
[73] Sinskey RM, Patel J. Posterior chamber intraocular lens implants in children: report of a series. J Am Intraocular Implant Soc 1983;9:157–160.
[74] Fyodorov SN, Egorova EV, Zubareva LN. 1004 cases of traumatic cataract surgery with implantation of an intraocular lens. J Am Intraocular Implant Soc 1981;7:147–153.
[75] Sheets JH. Indications for Intraocular Lens Implantations in Children. New York: Grune & Stratton; 1980.
[76] Aron JJ, Aron-Rosa D. Intraocular lens implantation in unilateral congenital cataract. A preliminary report. J Am Intraocular Implant Soc 1983;9:306–308.
[77] Gupta AK, Grover AK, Gurha N. Traumatic cataract surgery with intraocular lens implantation in children. J Pediatr Ophthalmol Strabismus 1992;29:73–78.
[78] Dahan E. Lens implantation in microphthalmic eyes of infants. Eur J Implant Refract Surg 1989;1:9–11.
[79] Sinskey RM, Stoppel J. Intraocular lens implantation in microphthalmic patients. J Cataract Refract Surg 1992;18:480–484.
[80] Dahan E, Salmenson BD. Pseudophakia in children: precautions, technique and feasibility. J Cataract Refract Surg 1990;16:75–82.
[81] Dahan E, Welsh NH, Salmenson BD. Posterior chamber implants in unilateral congenital and developmental cataracts. Eur J Implant Refract Surg 1990;2:295–302.
[82] Lambert SR, Lynn M, Drews-Botsch C, et al. A comparison of grading visual acuity, strabismus, and reoperation outcomes among children with aphakia and pseudophakia after unilateral cataract surgery using the first six months of life. J Pediatr Ophthalmol Strabismus 2001;5:70–75.
[83] Gimbel HV, Basti S, Ferensowicz M, DeBroff BM. Results of bilateral cataract extraction with posterior chamber intraocular lens implantation in children. Ophthalmology 1997;104:1737–1743.
[84] Metge P, Cohen H, Chemila JF. Intercapsular implantation in children. Eur J Implant Refract Surg 1990;2:319–328.
[85] O'Keefe M, Mulvihill A, Yeoh PL. Visual outcome and complication of bilateral intraocular lens implantation in children. J Cataract Refract Surg 2000;26:1758–1764.
[86] Peterseim MW, Wilson ME. Bilateral intraocular lens implantation in the pediatric population. Ophthalmology 2000;107:1261–1266.
[87] van Balen AT, Koole FD. Lens implantation in children. Ophthalmic Pediatr Genet 1988;9:121–125.
[88] Dahan E, Drusedau MUH. Choice of lens and dioptric power in pediatric pseudophakia. J Cataract Refract Surg 1997;23(Suppl.):S618–S623.
[89] Koro Y, Shimisu K, Inatomi M, et al. Eye growth after cataract extraction and intraocular lens implantation in children. Ophthalmic Surg 1993;24:467–475.
[90] Huber C. Increasing myopia in children with intraocular lenses (IOL): an experiment in form deprivation myopia? Eur J Implant Refract Surg 1993;5:154–158.
[91] Wilson ME, Peterseim MW, Englert JA, et al. Pseudophakia and polypseudophakia in the first year of life. J AAPOS 2001;5:238–245.
[92] Rabin J, Van Sluyters RC, Malach R. Emmetropization: a vision dependent phenomenon. Invest Ophthalmol Vis Sci 1981;20:561–564.
[93] Kora Y, Inatomi M, Yoshinao F, et al. Long-term study of children with implanted intraocular lenses. J Cataract Refract Surg 1992;18:485–488.
[94] BenEzra D, Paez JH. Congenital cataract and intraocular lenses. Am J Ophthalmol 1983;96:311–314.
[95] Vasavada AR, Nihalani BR. Pediatric cataract surgery. Curr Opin Ophthalmol 2006;17:54–61.
[96] Calhoun JH, Harley RD. The roto-extractor in pediatric ophthalmology. Trans Am Ophthalmol Soc 1975;73:292–305.
[97] Peyman GA, Raichand M, Goldberg MF. Surgery of congenital and juvenile cataracts: A pars plicata approach with the vitrophage. Br J Ophthalmol 1978;62:780–783.
[98] Calhoun JH. Cataracts. In: Harley RD, editor. Pediatric ophthalmology. 2nd ed. Philadelphia: WB Saunders Co; 1983. p. 558.
[99] BenEzra D. The surgical approaches to paediatric cataract. Eur J Implant Refract Surg 1990;2:241–244.
[100] BenEzra D, Rose L. Intraocular versus contact lenses for the correction of aphakia in unilateral congenital and developmental cataract. Eur J Implant Refract Surg 1990;2:303–307.
[101] Cheah WM. A review of the management of congenital cataract. Asia-Pacific J Ophthalmol 1989;1:22–26.
[102] Green BF, Morin JD, Grant HP. Pars plicata lensectomy/vitrectomy for developmental cataract extraction: surgical results. J Pediatr Ophthalmol Strabismus 1990;27:229–232.
[103] Tablante RT, Cruz EDG, Lapus JV, Santos AM. A new technique of congenital cataract surgery with primary posterior chamber intraocular lens implantation. J Cataract Refract Surg 1988;14:139–157.
[104] Keech RV, Tongue AC, Scott WE. Complications after surgery for congenital and infantile cataracts. Am J Ophthalmol 1989;108:136–141.
[105] Ahmadieh H, Javadi MA, Ahmady M, et al. Primary capsulectomy, anterior vitrectomy, lensectomy, and posterior chamber lens implantation in children: limbal versus pars plana. J Cataract Refract Surg 1999;25:768–775.
[106] Andreo LK, Wilson E, Apple DJ. Elastic properties and scanning electron microscopic appearance at manual continuous curvilinear capsulorhexis and vitrectorhexis in an animal model of pediatric cataract. J Cataract Refract Surg 1999;25:534–539.
[107] Morgan JE, Ellingham RB, Young RD, et al. Mechanical properties of a human lens capsule following capsulorhexis or radiofrequency diathermy capsulotomy. Arch Ophthalmol 1996;114:1110–1115.
[108] Fugo RJ, DelCampo DM. The Fugo blade: the next step after capsulorhexis. Ann Ophthalmol 2001;33:12–20.
[109] Singh D. Use of Fugo blade in complicated cases. J Cataract Refract Surg 2002;28:573–574.
[110] Wilson Jr ME. Anterior lens capsule management in pediatric cataract surgery. Trans Am Ophthalmol Soc 2004;102:391–422.
[111] Vasavada AR, Shastri L. Initial and definitive capsulorhexis:an extended application. J Cataract Refract Surg 2000;26:634.
[112] Gimbel HV. Two-stage capsulorhexis for endocapsular phacoemulsification. J Cataract Refract Surg 1990;16:246–249.
[113] Gimbel HV. Posterior capsule tears using phacoemulsification. Causes, prevention and management. Eur J Implant Refract Surg 1990;2:63–69.
[114] Jacobi PC, Dietlein TS, Konen W. Multifocal intraocular lens implantation in pediatric cataract surgery. Ophthalmology 2001;108:1375–1380.
[115] Hunter DG. Multifocal intraocular lenses in children (guest editorial). Ophthalmology 2001;108:1373–1374.
[116] Machamer R, Parel J, Buettner H. A new concept for vitreous surgery. Instrumentation. Am J Ophthalmol 1972;73:1–7.
[117] France TD. Management of the posterior capsule in congenital cataracts. J Pediatr Ophthalmol Strabismus 1984;21:116–117.
[118] Lavrich JB, Goldberg DS, Nelson LB. Suture use in pediatric cataract surgery. A survey. Ophthalmic Surg 1993;24:554–555.
[119] Blumenthal M, Yalon M, Treister G. Intraocular lens implantation in traumatic cataract in children. J Am Intraocular Implant Soc 1983;9:40–41.
[120] Maltzman BA, Wagner RS, Caputo AR. Neudymium:YAG laser surgery: The treatment of pediatric cataract disease. Ann Ophthalmol 1986;18:245–246.
[121] Catalano RA, Simon JW, Jenkins PL, Kandel GL. Preferential looking as a guide for amblyopia therapy in monocular infantile cataracts. J Pediatr Ophthalmol Strabismus 1987;24:56–63.
[122] Cheng KP, Hiles DA, Biglan AW, et al. Visual results after early surgical treatment of unilateral cataracts. Ophthalmology 1991;98:903–910.
[123] Pratt-Johnson JA, Tillson G. Unilateral congenital cataracts: Binocular status after treatment. J Pediatr Ophthalmol Strabismus 1989;26:72–75.
[124] Lesser GR, Osher RH, Whipple D, et al. Treatment of anterior chamber from fibrin following cataract surgery with tissue plasminogen activator. J Cataract Refract Surg 1993;19:301–305.
[125] Klais CM, Hattenbach L, Steinkamp GWK, et al. Intraocular recombinant tissue-plasminogen activator fibrinolysis of fibrin formation after cataract surgery in children. J Cataract Refract Surg 1999;25:357–362.
[126] Mittra RA, Dev S, Nasir MA, Toth CA. Recombinent hirudin prevents postoperative fibrin formation after experimental cataract surgery. Ophthalmology 1997;104:558–561.
[127] Johnson RN, Blankenship GA. A prospective, randomized clinical trial of heparin therapy for postoperative intraocular fibrin. Ophthalmology 1988;95:312–317.
[128] Basti S, Aasuri M, Reddy MK, et al. Heparin-surface-modified intraocular lenses in pediatric cataract surgery: propspective randomized study. J Cataract Refract Surg 1999;25:782–787.
[129] Maloof AJ, Pandey SK, Neilson G, et al. Selective death of lens epithelial cells using demineralized water and Triton X 100 with PerfectCapsule sealed capsule irrigation – a histological study in rabbit eyes. Arch Ophthalmol 2005;123:1378–1384.
[130] Crowston JG, Healey PR, Hopley C, et al. Water mediated lysis of lens epithelial cells attached to lens capsule. J Cataract Refract Surg 2004;30:1102–1106.

[131] Binkhorst CD. Iris-clip and irido-capsular lens implants (pseudophakoi); personal techniques of pseudophakia, Br J Ophthalmol 51:767–771.

[132] Cobo LM, Ohsawa E, Chandler D, et al. Pathogeneses of capsular opacification after extracapsular cataract extraction. An animal model. Ophthalmology 1984;91:857.

[133] Nishi O. Fibrinous membrane formation on the posterior chamber lens during the early postoperative period. J Cataract Refract Surg 1988;14:73–77.

[134] Buckley E, Kombers L, Seaber J, et al. Management of posterior capsule during pediatric intraocular lens implantation. Am J Ophthalmol 1993;115:722–728.

[135] Gimbel HV, DeBroff BM. Posterior capsulorhexis with optic capture: maintaining a clear visual axis after pediatric cataract surgery. J Cataract Refract Surg 1994;20:658–664.

[136] Gimbel HV. Posterior capsulorhexis with optic capture in pediatric cataract and intraocular lens surgery. Ophthalmology 1996;103:1871–1875.

[137] Gimbel HV. Posterior continuous curvilinear capsulorhexis and optic capture of the intraocular lens to prevent secondary opacification in pediatric cataract surgery. J Cataract Refract Surg 1997;23:652–656.

[138] Gimbel HV, DeBroff BM. Management of lens implant and posterior capsular with respect to prevention of secondary cataract. Op Tech Cataract Refract Surg 1998;1:185–190.

[139] Hiles DA, Hered RW. Modern intraocular lens implants in children with new age limitations. J Cataract Refract Surg 1987;13:493–497.

[140] McDonnell PJ, Zarbin MA, Green WR. Posterior capsule opacification in pseudophakic eyes. Ophthalmology 1983;90:1548–1553.

[141] Hiles DA, Johnson DL. The role of the crystalline lens epithelium in postpseudophakos membrane formation. J Am Intraocular Implant Soc 1980;34:365.

[142] Morgan KS, Karcioglu ZA. Secondary cataracts in infants after lensectomies. J Pediatr Ophthalmol Strabismus 1987;24:45–48.

[143] Lischetti P. New technique for posterior capsulotomy. Eur J Implant Refract Surg 1990;2:77–79.

[144] Hiles DA, Watson BA. Complications of implant surgery in children. J Am Intraocular Implant Soc 1979;5:24–32.

[145] Burke JP, Willshaw HE, Young JDH. Intraocular lens implants for uniocular cataracts in childhood. Br J Ophthalmol 1989;73:860–864.

[146] Dutton JJ, Baker JD, Hiles DA, Morgan KS. Visual rehabilitation of aphakic children. Surv Ophthalmol 1990;34:365.

[147] Hoyt CS, Nickel B. Aphakic cystoid macular edema: Occurrence in infants and children after transpupillary lensectomy and anterior vitrectomy. Arch Ophthalmol 1982;100:746–749.

[148] Morgan KS, Franklin RM. Oral fluorescein angioscopy in aphakic children. J Pediatr Ophthalmol Strabismus 1984;21:33–36.

[149] Poer DV, Helveston EM, Ellis FD. Aphakic cystoid macular edema in children. Arch Ophthalmol 1981;99:249–252.

[150] Cheng KP, Hiles DA, Biglan AW, Pettapiece MC. Management of posterior lenticonus. J Pediatr Ophthalmol Strabismus 1991;28:143–149.

[151] Rao SK, Ravishankar K, Sitalakshmi G, et al. Cystoid macular edema after pediatric intraocular lens implantation: fluorescein angioscopy results and literature review. J Cataract Refract Surg 2001;27:432–436.

[152] Wright KW, Christensen LE, Noguchi BA. Results of late surgery for presumed congenital cataracts. Am J Ophthalmol 1992;114:409–415.

[153] DeGroot V, Leysen I, Neuhann T, Gobin L, Tassignon MJ. One year followup of bag-in-the-lens intraocular lens implantation in 60 eyes. J Cataract Refract Surg 2006;32:1632–1637.

[154] Koch DD, Kohnen T. Retrospective comparison of techniques to prevent secondary cataract formation after posterior chamber intraocular lens implantation in infants and children. J Cataract Refract Surg 1997;23:657–663.

[155] DeVaro JM, Buckley EG, Awner S, Seaber J. Secondary posterior chamber intraocular lens implantation in pediatric patients. Am J Ophthalmol 1997;123:24–30.

[156] Wheeler DT, Stager DR, Weakley DR. Endophthalmitis following pediatric intraocular surgery for congenital cataracts and congenital glaucoma. J Pediatr Ophthalmol Strabismus 1992;29:139–141.

[157] Lloyd IC, Goss-Sampson M, Jeffrey BG, et al. Neonatal cataract: Aetiology, pathogenesis, and management. Eye 1992;6(Pt 2):184–196.

[158] France TD, Frank JW. The association of strabismus and aphakia in children. J Pediatr Ophthalmol Strabismus 1984;21:223–226.

[159] Lambert SR, Amaya L, Taylor D. Detection and treatment of infantile cataracts. Int Ophthalmol Clin 1989;29:51–56.

[160] Chrousos GA, Parks MM, O'Neill JF. Incidence of chronic glaucoma, retinal detachment and secondary membrane surgery in pediatric aphakic patients. Ophthalmology 1984;91:1238–1241.

[161] Shephard CD. Retinal detachment in aphakia. Trans Ophthalmol Soc UK 1934;54:176.

[162] Jagger JD, Cooling RJ, Fison LG, et al. Management of retinal detachment following congenital cataract surgery. Trans Ophthalmol Soc UK 1983;103:103–107.

[163] DeJuan Jr E. The treatment of pediatric retinal detachments. Arch Ophthalmol 1993;111:599.

[164] Toyofuku H, Hirose T, Schepens CL. Retinal detachment following congenital cataract surgery. I. Preoperative findings in 114 eyes. Arch Ophthalmol 1980;98:669–675.

[165] Gimbel HV. Nucleofractis phacoemulsification through a small pupil. Can J Ophthalmol 1992;27:115–119.

[166] Castaneda VE, Ulrich FC, Legler MD, et al. Posterior continuous curvilinear capsulorhexis. Ophthalmology 1992;99:45–50.

[167] Butler TH. Lenticonus posterior. Arch Ophthalmol 1930;3:425–436.

[168] Franceschetti A, Rickli H. Posterior (eccentric) lenticonus. Arch Ophthalmol 1954;51:499–508.

[169] March EJ. Slit-lamp study of posterior lenticonus. Arch Ophthalmol 1927;56:128–136.

[170] Gimbel HV. Hydro-free dissection. Video presentation at the 1992 ASCRS film festival in San Diego.

[171] Gimbel HV. Evolving techniques of cataract surgery; continuous curvilinear capsulorhexis, down-slope sculpting and nucleofractis. Semin Ophthalmol 1992;7:193–207.

[172] Neuhann TH. The rhexis-fixation lens [Film]. Boston: American Society of Cataract Refractive Surgery; 1991.

[173] Biglan AW, Cheng KP, Davis JS, Gerontis CC. Results following intraocular lens implantation in children. Trans Am Ophthalmol Soc 1996;94:353–373.

[174] Sharma A, Basti S, Gupta S. Secondary capsule-supported intraocular lens implantation in children. J Cataract Refract Surg 1997;23(Suppl. 1):675–680.

[175] DeVaro JM, Buckley EG, Awner S, Seaber J. Secondary posterior chamber intraocular lens implantation in pediatric patients. Am J Ophthalmol 1997;123:24–30.

[176] Wilson ME, Englert JA, Greenwald MJ. In-the-bag secondary intraocular lens implantation in children. J AAPOS 1999;3:350–355.

[177] Jacobi PC, Dietlin TS, Jacobi FK. Scleral fixation of secondary foldable multifocal intraocular lens implants in children and young adults. Ophthalmology 2002;109:1215–1224.

[178] Crnic T, Weakley Jr dR, Stager Jr D, Felius J. Use of AcrySof acrylic foldable intraocular lens for secondary implantation in children. J AAPOS 2004;8:151–155.

[179] Trivedi RH, Wilson Jr ME, Facciani J. Secondary intraocular lens implantation for pediatric aphakia. J AAPOS 2005;9:346–352.

Further Reading

Asrani S, Friedman S, Hasselblad V, et al. Does primary intraocular lens implantation prevent "aphakic" glaucoma in children? J Pediatr Ophthalmol Strabismus 2000;4:33–39.

Mackool R, Chhatiawala H. Pediatric cataract surgery and intraocular lens implantation: a new technique for preventing or excising postoperative secondary membranes. J Cataract Refract Surg 1991;17:62–66.

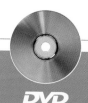

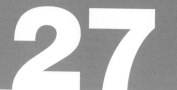

The Intumescent Cataract

Roger F. Steinert, MD

27

CHAPTER HIGHLIGHTS

>> Hydration changes in the lens capsule

>> Techniques for capsular dye staining

>> Issues with zonules and the nucleus

Surgical removal of an intumescent lens presents several special challenges to the surgeon. An intumescent lens is a lens that has begun to lose structural integrity; the protein is denatured to the point that the lens is becoming hydrating. The capsule is thinner and more fragile, the red reflex is absent, zonules may be weakened or absent, and the nucleus is often large and hard if the intumescence occurs in an age-related cataract.

CLINICAL PRESENTATION

A crystalline lens in which the cortex has become extensively hydrated, with white opacification, is historically known as a mature cataract. A mature lens that is swollen to the point of obstructing aqueous flow through the pupil and/or physically crowding the anterior chamber and angle is causing phacomorphic glaucoma. If the nucleus has sunk off-center in the lens as a result of liquefaction of the cortex, it is known as morgagnian. If the process is so advanced that some hydrated and denatured protein has begun to slowly leave the capsular bag, resulting in wrinkles in the no longer distended bag, the cataract is called hypermature. If the capsule loses integrity so that macrophages

are attracted to scavenge the lens protein that has been released out of the capsular bag, phacolytic glaucoma may result from obstruction of the trabecular outflow. Severe inflammation caused by the released lens protein is called phacoanaphylaxis.

Some cases of intumescent cataract are due to physical damage to the capsule. A frank traumatic break in the capsule will result in rapid hydration and opacification of the cortex. A small break, particularly a puncture, will occasionally seal itself and result in only a local opacity. Physical damage to the capsule usually occurs in the setting of a perforating or severe blunt trauma or from intraocular surgery, particularly pars plana vitrectomy. Zonules are often damaged in this same process.

In mature and hypermature cataracts, the anterior capsule may undergo degeneration, with deposition of calcium or development of focal dense plaques. Dense postinflammatory plaques are particularly common after blunt trauma that triggers an intumescent cataract (Figure 27-1). If present, these areas will interfere with a normal capsulorrhexis tear. The surgeon will need to direct the tear around these abnormalities, if possible, or use another technique, such as a Gills-Vannas scissors, to cut across these densities.

As part of the preoperative evaluation of a patient with an intumescent cataract, the surgeon should ask about past ocular history that might alter the surgical approach, obtain past medical records if possible, perform further nonroutine preoperative testing, and discuss with the patient that the potential for surgical complications is increased and the prognosis for full recovery of vision is uncertain. In particular, the surgeon must try to answer the questions: "Why did the patient wait so long before presenting?" Is the eye densely amblyopic, or was useful vision lost years earlier to a process such as a retinal vascular occlusion or retinal detachment? Did the patient suffer traumatic maculopathy or optic neuropathy? In most cases of an intumescent lens, where the fundus cannot be seen, a B-scan ultrasound is indicated. Other helpful evaluations include testing for entoptic imagery, perception of colored lights, gross visual field examination with a point light source, and bright flash visual-evoked response. Usually these tests do not provide a highly accurate prognosis of visual potential, but they may help determine the potential value of surgery in patients with questionable past histories.

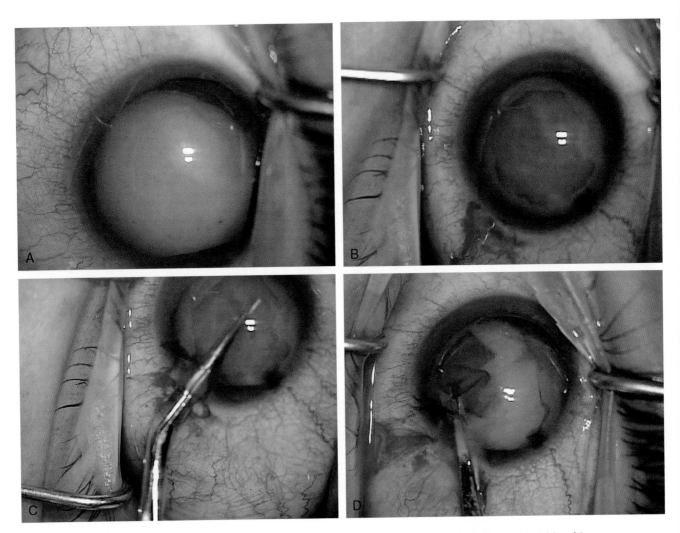

Figure 27-1 **A,** Intumescent traumatic cataract. Note the loss of zonules in the upper right. **B,** Trypan blue staining of the anterior capsule reveals a dense, darker staining plaque on the anterior capsule that will not tear with a conventional capsulorhexis technique. **C** and **D,** Gills-Vannas scissors must be used to cut through the anterior capsular plaque.

■ ABSENCE OF THE RED REFLEX ■

The largest challenge in removal of the intumescent cataract is the absence of a red fundus reflex when the cataract is viewed through the operating microscope.[1] If the surgeon intends to perform phacoemulsification with placement of an intraocular lens (IOL) in the capsular bag, an intact capsulorrhexis is critical in maintaining structural integrity.[2] If the surgeon's intention is to perform an extracapsular cataract extraction and express the nucleus, then a can-opener style of anterior capsulotomy may be acceptable. Even then, however, it is nearly impossible to avoid large capsule flaps and the potential for equatorial and posterior tears unless the anterior capsule can be visualized.

Surgeons have used several approaches to improve visualization of the anterior capsule in the absence of the red reflex, most notably employing oblique illumination from another instrument such as a fiberoptic light pipe.[3] In addition, when the anterior capsule is opened and white cortex clouds the surgeon's view, the surgeon should pause the capsulotomy and improve the view, either by adding more viscoelastic or using the irrigation–aspiration device to remove the obscuring cortex while taking care not to engage the capsule.

The most important advance in managing the anterior capsule in the absence of a red reflex is the use of an anterior capsule stain. Surgeons have attempted to stain the anterior capsule with a variety of substances. Fluorescein sodium 2% weakly stains the anterior capsule on the exterior surface and has slightly stronger uptake on the inner (epithelial) surface if it is injected after an initial opening into the capsular bag.[4] Cobalt blue illumination, not generally available on most operating microscopes, may be necessary to visualize the stain.[5] Some other commonly available stains, such as methylene blue and gentian violet, are toxic to the endothelium, at least in many common formulations.[6] The patient's own blood has been applied to the capsule as a method of staining as well.[7]

Two dyes are available that have been proven safe and effective for staining the anterior capsule. Horiguchi et al.[8] elegantly demonstrated both the endothelial safety and also the effective technique for safely dissolving, diluting, and applying indocyanine green to the anterior capsule. Melles et al.[9] have developed a commercial preparation of trypan blue (VisionBlue, DORC, Zuidland, Holland) that is also safe and effective. In the original version of these techniques, the dye is applied under an air bubble that fills the anterior chamber, in order not to dilute the dye. The dye is applied as one or two microdrops wiped across the anterior capsule under the air bubble from a 27- or 30-gauge cannula. The air bubble itself, although preventing dye dilution by aqueous humor in the anterior chamber, prevents the dye from contacting the anterior capsule; therefore, the cannula is used to wipe the dye under the air bubble and across the anterior capsule. The air bubble is then replaced with viscoelastic, and the capsulotomy is performed in the usual manner (Figure 27-2).

An alternative to the air bubble technique is the use of a high concentration cohesive ophthalmic viscoelastic device, most commonly Healon 5 (Advanced Medical Optics). The surgeon must avoid injection of more than the minimum amount of dye necessary to stain the capsule. Otherwise, free dye in the anterior chamber surrounding the bolus of Healon 5 may obscure visualization of the anterior capsule and require washout of the anterior chamber and reinstillation of viscoelastic to perform the capsulorrhexis. However, in the author's experience, Healon 5 allows better contact of the dye with the anterior capsule compared with an air bubble (Figure 27-3). More intense anterior capsule staining results. In addition, there is no need to perform the steps of injecting air and later exchanging the air bubble for the viscoelastic agent to perform the anterior capsulotomy.

Some surgeons simply inject enough trypan blue into the anterior chamber to overcome initial dilution and thereby directly stain the capsule. The surgeon must be aware that if the corneal endothelium is diseased, however, especially in Fuch's dystrophy, the posterior cornea will take up the dye and impair the surgeon's view of the cataract.

With either the air bubble or Healon 5 technique, the dye should be left in contact with the anterior capsule for at least 1 min before performing the anterior capsulotomy to obtain adequately intense staining of the anterior capsule.

In addition to facilitating the capsulotomy, the dye-enhanced visualization of the capsule often proves helpful in avoiding operative trauma to the capsulorrhexis edge by the phacoemulsification instruments (see Figure 27-2E and F).

THINNING AND WEAKENING OF THE POSTERIOR CAPSULE

Many clinicians have the clinical impression that the posterior capsule presents increased challenges in the surgery of an intumescent lens. More prolonged phacoemulsification time and manipulation of a large and hard nucleus explain only part of the reason for increased frequency of posterior capsule complications.

The posterior capsule is often thinned and stretched by the expanded intumescent lens. As a result, the surgeon is faced with a posterior capsule that is not only weak but also flaccid, with wrinkles and a laxity that makes it prone to come up to the phaco tip and be ruptured. This problem is worsened by the absence of

any epinucleus that protects the posterior capsule. A useful step is to inject a dispersive, noncohesive viscoelastic behind the nucleus one or more times during the phacoemulsification. This will provide an artificial epinucleus to keep the posterior capsule back from the operative plane and also stabilize the nucleus against tumbling.

WEAK OR ABSENT ZONULES

Zonular weakness or frank absence of zonules sometimes presents a challenge during surgery on an intumescent cataract. Usually this occurs either because the patient is elderly, when zonules typically weaken as part of the aging process, or because the cataract has been induced by trauma.

As soon as clinically significant zonular weakness is suspected, placement of a Witschell capsular tension ring (Morcher GmbH) is advised. If the loss of zonules is severe, with major instability of the capsular bag, then the Cionni modification of the capsule tension ring allows the surgeon to directly add stabilization with an ab interno polypropylene transscleral suture (see Chapter 29).

If the capsular bag and/or sulcus are/is compromised to the point where the ability to support an IOL long term is uncertain, then a transscleral sutured posterior chamber IOL or an anterior chamber IOL should be implanted (see Chapter 41).

THE NUCLEUS

In a relatively young patient with an intumescent lens, the hydration that opacifies the cortex will also lead to softening of the immature nucleus. The nucleus will then aspirate or require minimal ultrasound for removal. In elderly patients, however, the nucleus is often quite sclerotic and large. Because the cortex is already hydrated, hydrodissection and hydrodelineation are unnecessary. The removal of a large, hard nucleus is covered in Chapter 28 and is not discussed here. Caution must be taken in view of the weak posterior capsule and zonules.

In some advanced cases of intumescence, the nucleus itself will begin to hydrate slightly. These mildly hydrated nuclei typically have a characteristic golden haze rather than the dark brown, molasses color of a dense and aged nucleus. Although the nucleus will not soften to the point of being removable with aspiration alone, it will split more readily with chopping or cracking techniques and not be encumbered by a leathery posterior epinucleus, unlike a dark brown nucleus.

CONCLUSION

The intumescent cataract presents some special surgical challenges, most notably in visualizing the anterior capsule and protecting potentially weakened zonules and posterior capsule.

With the advent of staining of the anterior capsule to ensure visibility during surgery and with increasingly atraumatic phacoemulsification techniques, supplemented by use of viscoelastics, capsule tension rings, and transscleral sutures, the removal of an intumescent cataract is a surgical challenge that frequently has a successful outcome.

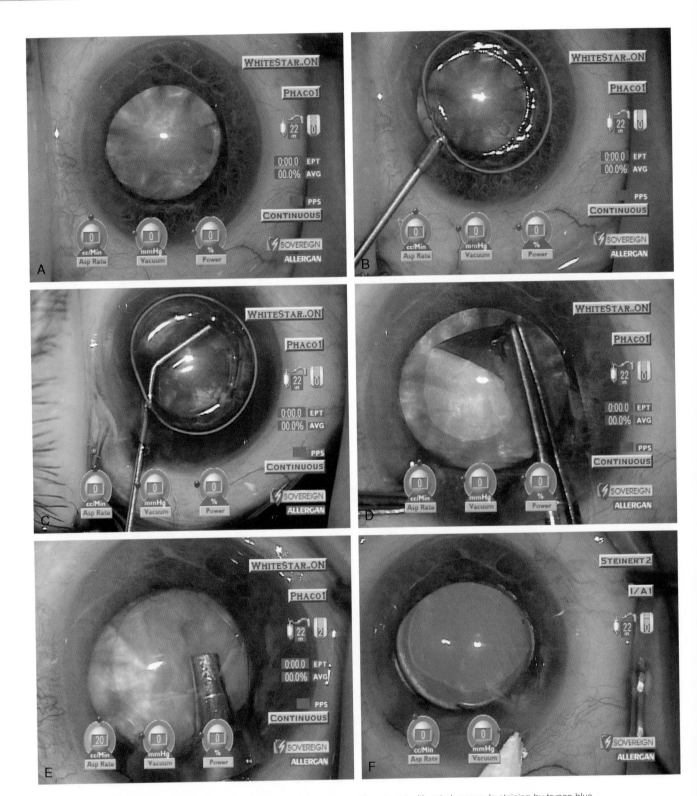

Figure 27-2 **A**, Intraoperative photographs of a mature white cataract with anterior capsule staining by trypan blue. **B**, Injection of air bubble through paracentesis. **C**, Trypan blue dye is applied under an air bubble filling the anterior chamber, using a blunt-tip cannula to inject and wipe the stain across the anterior capsule. **D**, Capsulorrhexis proceeds normally, with clear visualization as a result of the staining. **E**, During phacoemulsification, the surgeon can visualize the stained anterior capsule edge, reducing the potential for inadvertent damage by the phaco tip. **F**, After intraocular lens (IOL) implantation, the stained anterior capsule can be seen overlying the IOL optic.

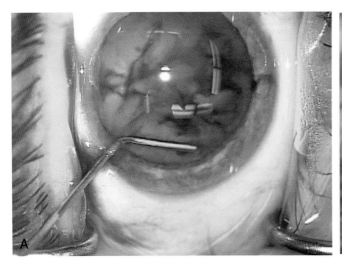
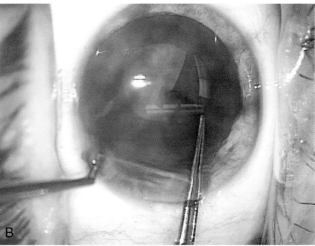

Figure 27-3 Application of trypan blue stain under a dome of Healon 5. **A,** Cannula is wiped across the anterior capsule while the stain is injected into the space created between the capsule and the Healon 5. **B,** If the dye does not mix with the solid mass of Healon 5 and the surgeon avoids injecting excess dye, visualization is adequate to proceed with the capsulorrhexis without washing out the Healon 5 and replacing it.

References

[1] Gimbel HV, Willerscheidt AB. What to do with a limited view: the intumescent cataract. J Cataract Refract Surg 1993;19:657–661.
[2] Gimbel HV, Neuhann T. Development, advantages, and methods of the continuous circular capsulorrhexis technique. J Cataract Refract Surg 1990;16:31–37.
[3] Mansour AM. Anterior capsulorrhexis in hypermature cataracts. J Cataract Refract Surg 1993;19:116–117. [letter].
[4] Hoffer KJ, McFarland JE. Intracameral subcapsular fluorescein staining for improved visualization during capsulorrhexis in mature cataracts. J Cataract Refract Surg 1993;19:566. [letter].
[5] Fritz WL. Fluorescein blue light-assisted capsulorrhexis for mature or hypermature cataract. J Cataract Refract Surg 1998;24:19–20.
[6] Perez AR, Vainer AI. Capsular dyes. Video presentation at the Symposium on Cataract, IOL, and Refractive Surgery, San Diego, Calif. April 1998.
[7] Cimetta DJ, Gatti M, Lobianco G. Haemocoloration of the anterior capsule in white cataract CCC. Eur J Implant Refract Surg 1995;7:184–185.
[8] Horiguchi M, Miyake K, Ohta I et al. Staining of the lens capsule for circular continuous capsulorrhexis in eyes with white cataract. Arch Ophthalmol 1998;116:535–537.
[9] Melles GRJ, de Waard PWT, Pameyer JH et al: Trypan blue capsule staining to visualize the capsulorrhexis in cataract surgery. J Cataract Refract Surg 1999;25:7–9.

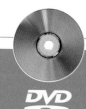

Dense Brunescent Cataract

Roger F. Steinert, MD

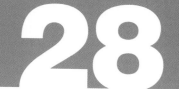

	CHAPTER HIGHLIGHTS

>> Selecting the best ophthalmological viscosurgical device to protect the cornea

>> The "Visco Vault" to protect the posterior capsule

>> Surgical maneuvers for the leathery posterior nucleus

A darkly brunescent nucleus, with the color of molasses or a cola soft drink, presents special surgical challenges. First the surgeon must select the basic surgical strategy. Depending on a surgeon's experience, the details of the patient's pathologic condition, and the treatment goals, the patient may be best served by phacoemulsification, by extracapsular cataract extraction, or by referral to a surgeon with experience and good results in phacoemulsification of dense nuclei.

Paradoxically, patients with particularly strong indications for small-incision phacoemulsification are often the patients who present with these advanced, technically challenging cataracts. A common clinical scenario is a patient with one functional eye who was told by an eye doctor decades earlier, "Don't let anyone touch your good eye." Today, such a patient is often better served by small-incision phacoemulsification surgery under topical anesthesia, retaining the use of the good eye. Other patients with a particular indication for small-incision cataract surgery include high myopes, at risk for scleral collapse or with liquefied vitreous inhibiting nuclear expression in extracapsular extraction, and high hyperopes who may have microphthalmos or nanophthalmos, with increased risk for positive pressure vitreous loss and/or choroidal effusion (see Chapter 33).

If phacoemulsification is thought to be the best alternative for the lens extraction, several special aspects of cataract surgery in this setting are important to maximize the probability of a successful outcome in the presence of a densely brunescent cataract.

ANTERIOR CAPSULAR STAINING

Staining the anterior capsule is a critical step in performing successful phacoemulsification cataract surgery in situations in which the red reflex is insufficient to allow adequate visualization of the anterior capsule edge. In addition, a stained peripheral anterior capsule facilitates later phacoemulsification. The surgeon who can see the anterior capsule edge is less likely to nick it with the ultrasound tip or misplace a phaco chopping instrument on top of the anterior capsule.

The technique for anterior capsule staining is illustrated in detail in the chapter on the intumescent cataract (see Chapter 27).

PROTECTING THE ENDOTHELIUM AND THE POSTERIOR CAPSULE (THE "VISCO VAULT")

The protection of the corneal endothelium is especially important in phacoemulsification of dense nuclei, for which the surgery is prolonged, more manipulation is required, and more ultrasound power is employed. The corneal endothelium in such cases is often clinically "stressed" on the first postoperative day, with striae of Descemet's membrane and stromal edema.

In addition to meticulous surgical technique, protection of the endothelium is best achieved by a dispersive, retentive ophthalmic viscosurgical device (OVD) (see Chapter 6).

Cohesive viscoadaptive devices, typically high-molecular-weight hyaluronic acid, often are flushed out of the anterior chamber within several seconds of initiating phacoemulsification. The dispersive agents (most commonly Viscoat [Alcon] and Healon D [AMO]) are more likely to be retained as a protective layer against the endothelium.

Dispersive, retentive viscoadaptive agents can also be used to create an artificial epinucleus to protect the posterior capsule. A dense brunescent cataract usually has little to no epinucleus;

the epinucleus has stiffened and become part of the nucleus. The posterior capsule, therefore, has no protective layer to guard against laceration from the sharp and bulky nuclear fragments. In addition, the posterior capsule is usually thinner and more vulnerable because the advanced cataract has stretched the capsule as the cataract expanded.

A helpful maneuver is to pause the phacoemulsification once enough of the nucleus has been removed to expose a small portion of the posterior capsule, heralded by the appearance of a "window" of bright red reflex. The viscoadaptive agent is injected between the posterior capsule and remaining nucleus. This creates an artificial epinucleus, physically separating the posterior capsule from the nucleus undergoing phacoemulsification. I call this maneuver the "visco vault" because the OVD acts like a protective wall, or "vault," to protect the posterior capsule.

In addition, the viscoadaptive agent stabilizes the remaining nucleus, reducing tumbling of the nuclear fragments (Figure 28-1). The OVD also will elevate the remaining nuclear fragments toward the phaco tip, facilitating access of the phaco tip to a favorable edge of nucleus that can then be engaged and removed.

THE "LEATHERY" POSTERIOR NUCLEUS ■

A frequent surgical observation during phacoemulsification of a dense brunescent nucleus, whether by quadrant cracking or phaco chop technique, is that split fragments will, nevertheless, resist being drawn into the mid-anterior chamber for complete destruction and aspiration by the ultrasound needle. The reason for this problem is that tough elastic strands, with a "leathery" quality and appearance, span across and connect the split nuclear fragments on their posterior surface.

These leathery strands emanate from the epinuclear layer, which, in advanced brunescence, is stiffened and becomes more tightly adhered to the nucleus.

These strands on the posterior surface will challenge the surgeon attempting to mobilize nuclear pieces in a controlled manner. The best technique to address these strands is to transect them with an instrument. The nuclear fragment is engaged and stabilized by the vacuum of the phaco tip. While the nuclear fragment is partially drawn anteriorly, but not to the point of breaking the vacuum hold, the second instrument is used to transect the strands. The author prefers the phaco chopper as the second instrument. The handle is rotated so that the chopper is parallel to the posterior capsule, and the chopper is drawn across the strands. As long as the chopper is parallel to the posterior capsule, and the surgeon maintains an infusion of balanced salt solution (phaco foot position 1 or higher), the posterior capsule will not be endangered (Figure 28-2).

The surgeon must be patient in dealing with these many strands, but, ultimately, the nucleus can be successfully divided and emulsified.

When the remaining nucleus is small enough, sometimes the surgeon can safely "flip" the nucleus within the capsular bag. If this can be accomplished, the remaining leathery strands will be anterior, where the surgeon can visualize them and directly emulsify them. The author does not recommend, however, that the surgeon use a "phaco flip" technique where the large nucleus is delivered above the capsule. The large amount of ultrasound power that would need to be employed, combined with the proximity to the endothelium, increases the risk of corneal edema.

SPECIAL INSTRUMENTS ■

When confronted with a particularly challenging case, the surgeon generally should not attempt a new, unfamiliar technique. However, for surgeons who routinely employ phaco chop (see Chapter 17), a small adjustment can be helpful. Most phaco chopping instruments have a distal tip length of 1.25–1.5 mm. This is sufficient to reach the middle of an average nucleus. Having the tip of the chopper reach the middle of the nucleus is important in achieving a reliable chop.

Some choppers have a longer tip for use with dense nuclei. Elongating the tip to only 1.75 mm is sufficient to dramatically

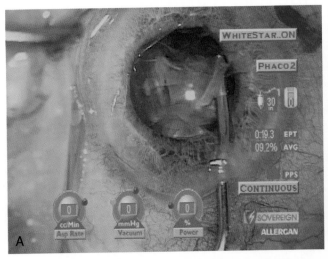
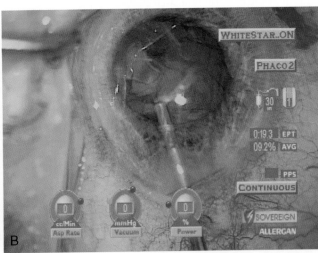

Figure 28-1 **A,** When the red reflex becomes visible, injection of a retentive viscoadaptive device behind the remaining nucleus will create an artificial epinucleus, protecting the posterior capsule and stabilizing the remaining nucleus. **B,** Later in the procedure, injection of further retentive viscoadaptive agent behind the nucleus helps preserve the protection of the posterior capsule.

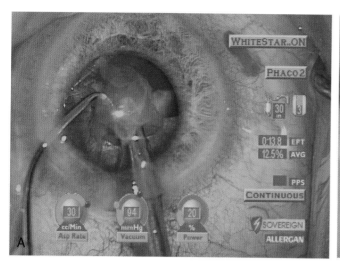

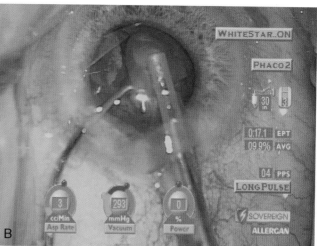

Figure 28-2 A, Chopping instrument can be oriented horizontally and used to cut across posterior leathery nuclear strands. **B,** Posterior strand cutting must continue across the apex of the nuclear wedge centrally.

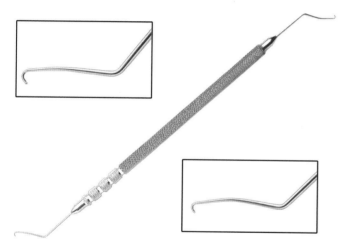

Figure 28-3 Chopping a dense, 4-plus nucleus is facilitated by a longer chopping tip, such as 1.75 mm (top left), compared with the more common 1.5 mm length chopping tip used for average-sized nuclei (bottom right). (Photo courtesy Rhein Medical, Tampa, Fla.)

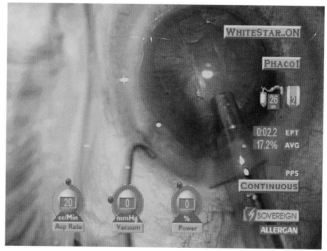

Figure 28-4 Creation of a groove in a dense nucleus facilitates chopping by thinning the nucleus and creating a weak zone, similar to the grooves that facilitate cracking a chocolate candy bar.

improve the reliability of successfully transecting a thicker, dense nucleus. Although such an instrument will look large inside the eye, the nuclear thickness that often approaches 4 mm or more means that the posterior capsule is not endangered (Figure 28-3). Alternatively, creation of a preparatory groove will reduce the nuclear thickness and create a weak zone more likely to crack (Figure 28-4).

Manufacturers are devoting increased attention to modulation of the delivery of ultrasound energy and control of fluidics (see Chapter 7).

These advances enhance the surgeon's ability to deal with challenging dense nuclei, as well as more routine cataracts.

Further Reading

Mehta KR. Simplified and safe phacoemulsification of supra hard cataracts. In: Agarwal A, Agarwal S, Sachdev MS, et al., editors. Phacoemulsification, laser cataract surgery, and foldable IOLs. New Delhi: Jaypee; 1998. p. 210–211.

Vanathi M, Vajpayee RB, Tandon R et al. Crater-and-chop technique for phacoemulsification of hard cataracts. J Cataract Refract Surg 2001;27:659–661.

Vasavada A, Singh R. Surgical techniques for difficult cataracts. Curr Opin Ophthalmol 1999; 10:46–52.

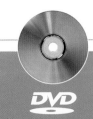
Capsule Tension Rings and Segments

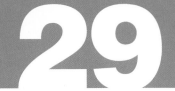

Robert J. Cionni, MD

CONTENTS

- Capsular Tension Rings
- Preoperative Evaluation
- Surgical Technique
- Conclusion

CHAPTER HIGHLIGHTS

>> Indications for capsule tension rings and segments

>> Styles of capsule stabilizing devices

>> Surgical technique

The management of weak or missing zonules can be quite challenging. Such zonular compromise can result from trauma, itatrogenic or otherwise, progressive diseases, such as pseudo-exfoliation syndrome, or congenital disorders such as in Marfan syndrome, homocystinuria, Weill–Marchesani syndrome, hyperlysinemia, or sulfite oxidase deficiency (Figure 29-1). Even without the development of cataract, subluxation of the crystalline lens can induce significant symptoms such as large refractive errors, anisometropia and marked visual disturbances. Such disturbances in a child undergoing visual development will often result in amblyopia. Therefore, intervening quickly in young children with significant lenticular subluxation is important so that amblyopia can be prevented or amblyopia therapy can be started.

Historically, surgical removal of the congenitally subluxated lens has been undertaken with great caution because of numerous reports of complications and poor visual outcomes.[1–3] Until recently, the surgical management was limited to iridectomy, laser iridotomy, discission, or intracapsular extraction.[4] After intracapsular surgery, the patients were usually left aphakic, requiring aphakic spectacles or aphakic contact lenses. Alternatively, these eyes received epikeratophakia or, in older patients, an anterior chamber intraocular lens (AC IOL). These patients often ended up with graft rejection, retinal detachments, glaucoma, vitreous loss, and poor visual outcomes after surgery. Similarly, trauma or disease-induced cases

of compromised zonules were fraught with higher risks of complications and resultant poor outcomes.

Many advances have been made in the ability to surgically treat patients with weak or missing zonules. With the introduction of small-incision cataract surgery and vitreous cutting devices, the success rate has dramatically increased. Pars plana vitrectomy and lensectomy, combined with aphakic contact lens wear or in the older patient an AC IOL, is a viable surgical option. The ability to suture a posterior chamber intraocular lens (PC IOL) into the ciliary sulcus or to the posterior aspect of the iris[5] provides yet more options. Some surgeons are favoring sutured PC IOLs even in children.[6] Even more recently, capsular tension rings (CTRs), modified capsular tension rings (MCTRs) and capsular tension segments (CTSs) have provided the opportunity to perform small-incision phacoemulsification and in-the-bag implantation of a PC IOL.[7–10]

CAPSULAR TENSION RINGS

In 1993, Legler and Witschel[11] showed us that the CTR could provide both intraoperative and postoperative stabilization of the capsular bag and IOL in patients with zonular dialysis. Since its introduction, many surgeons have come to depend on the CTR for their patients with zonular compromise. These polymethylmethacrylate (PMMA) rings can be inserted into the capsular bag at any point after the capsulorrhexis has been completed. The effect is a dramatic expansion and stabilization of the capsular bag.

Although the CTR has helped surgeons manage patients with a moderate loss of zonular support, eyes with profound zonular compromise or lens subluxation may still not obtain adequate stabilization or centration despite CTR placement. Additionally, patients with progressive zonular disease such as pseudoexfoliation syndrome may develop late dislocation of the capsular bag/IOL/ CTR complex.[12] Several surgeons have devised techniques for suturing the CTR to the scleral wall for better support and centration. Osher[13] demonstrated the technique of suturing the CTR to the scleral wall by straddling the CTR with 10-0 Prolene suture, double-armed with CIF-4 needles. This technique may work well yet involves passing needles through the peripheral capsular bag, risking rupture of the bag because it is under stretch from the presence of the CTR. Pfeifer[14] preferred to fashion a small peripheral

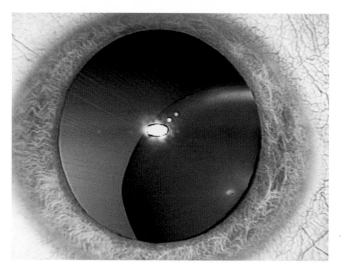

Figure 29-1 Subluxated lens in a young boy with Marfan syndrome.

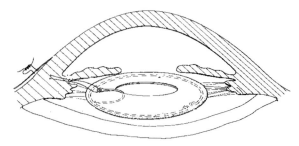

Figure 29-3 Diagram showing how the modified capsular tension ring can be sutured through the ciliary sulcus and to the scleral wall to induce bag centration and stabilization.

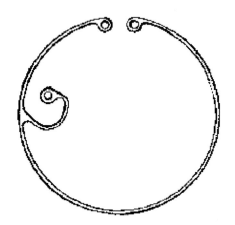

Figure 29-4 Modified capsular tension ring (Model 2-C) can be used with the Geuder shooter.

capsulorrhexis through which a similar passage of suture could be made. Both techniques provide a solution to the bag that remains displaced after insertion of the CTR. However, both involve violating the integrity of the peripheral capsular bag and may risk rupture of the bag after placement of the CTR.

The MCTR, designed by Dr. Robert Cionni, incorporates a unique fixation hook to provide scleral fixation without violating the integrity of the capsular bag[15] (Figure 29-2). The MCTR is manufactured by Morcher GmbH (Stuttgart, Germany). Like the original CTR, it consists of an open, flexible PMMA filament. However, the MCTR has a fixation hook that courses anteriorly and centrally in a second plane. The hook wraps around the capsulorrhexis edge and rests on the residual anterior capsular rim. At the free end of the hook is an eyelet through which a suture can be passed to allow scleral fixation (Figure 29-3). Currently, there are three MCTR models. Model 1-L has a single fixation hook distant from the insertion end of the ring. Model 2-C has a single fixation hook near the insertion end of the ring, allowing it to be implanted with the Geuder shooter (Figure 29-4). Model 2-L has two fixation hooks (Figure 29-5). This model is useful in patients with very

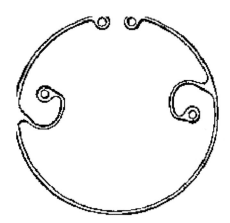

Figure 29-5 Modified capsular tension ring (Model 2-L) has two fixation hooks for maximal stabilization of the most significantly loose lenses.

significant generalized zonular weakness. The CTS is a shortened version of the MCTR, designed by Dr. Ike Ahmed. The CTS can be used to stabilize a quadrant of zonular compromise without expanding the capsular bag circumferentially.

■ PREOPERATIVE EVALUATION ■

Before surgery, the surgeon should characterize the areas of zonular weakness in terms of degrees of loss, location of the defect, presence or absence of vitreous prolapse, and the presence or absence of phacodonesis. Phacodonesis is more noticeable and dramatic

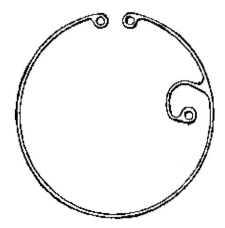

Figure 29-2 Diagram of the Cionni modified capsular tension ring (MCTR) (Model 1-L).

before dilation because dilation often stabilizes the ciliary body and iris, dampening any iris or lens movement. The surgeon should be wary of the inferiorly subluxated lens, especially if congenital. Inferior subluxation of a congenitally subluxed lens may indicate 360° of very significant zonular weakness combined with the effect of gravity. Such significant generalized zonular weakness makes it unlikely that the surgeon will be able to remove the lens while maintaining the capsular bag for PC IOL support. Pars plana lensectomy should be considered in these eyes. On the other hand, if the etiology of the inferior subluxation is trauma, there will often be strong inferior zonules remaining making the chance for successful implantation of an in-the-bag PCIOL more likely.

The presence or absence of additional ocular pathologic conditions that might affect the visual outcome must be considered and the patient counseled accordingly. Many patients with Marfan syndrome have significant systemic problems, which increase the risk of death or morbidity. These patients need to be evaluated by their primary medical doctor or cardiologist before surgery. Patients taking anticoagulant medicine for heart, vessel, and/or valvular abnormalities need to be counseled in detail concerning the implications of discontinuing anticoagulants versus undergoing surgery while anticoagulated.

■ SURGICAL TECHNIQUE ■

The surgeon should attempt to make the incision away from the area of zonular weakness. This will help reduce the stress placed on the existing zonules during phacoemulsification. Unfortunately, some patients may have generalized zonular weakness. The surgeon should then try to place the incision over the quadrant of subluxation because the zonules in the opposite quadrant have proven to be the weakest. However, the surgeon should not compromise his or her surgical abilities by operating at a meridian that is uncomfortable. The surgeon should always work through the smallest incision possible without compromising his or her ability to perform the necessary maneuvers. Doing so will minimize fluid egress through the incision and, therefore, will help to limit anterior chamber collapses. The initial anterior chamber entry should be made just large enough to insert the viscoelastic cannula and place a generous amount of a dispersive viscoelastic over the area of zonular dialysis to tamponade vitreous. Next, a cohesive viscoelastic is injected to maintain a deep anterior chamber.

The surgeon should start the capsulorrhexis in an area remote from the dialysis and use the countertraction provided by the remaining healthy zonules (Figure 29-6). A second blunt instrument, such as the Osher Nucleus Manipulator (Duckworth and Kent, St. Louis, Mo.), may be used for countertraction or to push the lens into view if it is significantly decentered under the iris. With extensive zonular loss or weakness, it may be necessary to begin the tear by cutting the anterior capsule with a sharp-tipped 15° blade or a diamond blade. A 5.5–6 mm capsulorrhexis should allow the surgeon to more easily manipulate the nucleus. The capsulorrhexis can be made "off-center" as bag recentration with a CTR or MCTR will change what appears to be the center of the anterior capsule. If a complete and intact capsulorrhexis is not obtained, CTR or MCTR placement should not be attempted as the expansile force of these rings will likely induce complete bag rupture. The same holds true for a posterior capsule tear that

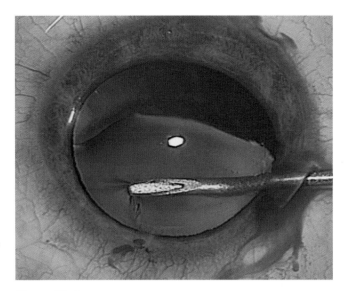

Figure 29-6 Remaining "strong zonules" provide the necessary countertraction to begin capsulorrhexis with a 22-gauge bent needle.

cannot be converted into a posterior capsulorrhexis. However, it may be possible to place a CTS in these cases as the CTS does not induce an expansile force. Although a CTR or MCTR could be placed into the capsular bag immediately following capsulorrhexis, the bulk of the nucleus can make placement of these devices difficult.[16] In addition, visualization during insertion is better if the nucleus is removed first. Instead, the author prefers to stabilize the capsular bag by grasping the capsulorrhexis edge with one to three disposable nylon iris retractors placed through limbal stab incisions[17] (Figure 29-7). Alternatively a CTS can be used at this point to stabilize the capsular bag. Hydrodissection is performed carefully, yet thoroughly, to maximally free the nucleus and thereby decrease zonular stress during manipulation of the nucleus. If the

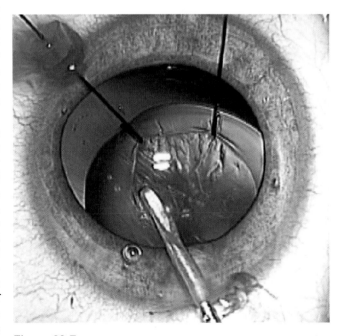

Figure 29-7 Two iris hooks are used to grasp the capsulorrhexis edge for stabilization.

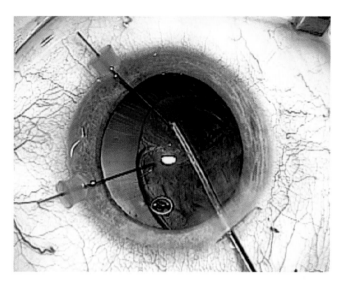

Figure 29-8 Viscodissection of anterior and peripheral cortex before placing modified capsular tension ring.

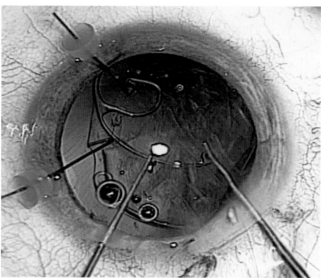

Figure 29-9 Modified capsular tension ring (Model 1-L) is dialed into the capsular bag with an Osher Y-hook and an Osher nucleus manipulator.

epinucleus is soft, hydrodissection completely into the anterior chamber is preferred. Doing so will greatly simplify its removal via automated aspiration or phacoemulsification and will virtually eliminate zonular stress during phacoemulsification.[18]

Phacoemulsification should be performed using low vacuum and aspiration settings to keep the bottle height at a minimum.[19] High bottles cause high inflow rates, which can force fluid through the areas of zonular weakness and thereby induce positive pressure, anterior chamber shallowing, and vitreous prolapse. However, it is important to not lower the bottle so much as to allow outflow to outpace inflow as this situation can also lead to vitreous prolapse due to anterior chamber shallowing.

For the denser nucleus, divide or chop techniques are preferred. These techniques will minimize zonular stress during phacoemulsification if the surgeon is careful to apply equal forces in opposing directions to avoid displacing the nucleus. It is very helpful to "viscodissect" the nuclear halves or quadrants free from the cortex in areas of zonular weakness.[20] Viscoelastic injected between the nuclear quadrants and peripheral capsular bag will lift the nuclear fragments while expanding and stabilizing the bag.

Before inserting a CTR or MCTR, the surgeon should place viscoelastic just under the surface of the residual anterior capsular rim to create a space for the ring and to dissect residual cortex away from the peripheral capsule, making cortical entrapment by the ring less likely (Figure 29-8). The CTR can be inserted manually or with a CTR injector. When using a MCTR, one should preplace a double-armed suture through the eyelet of the fixation hook before inserting the ring into the capsular bag. Alternatively, the suture can be single-armed and the free end of the suture tied to the fixation hook eyelet. Cases of late suture breakage when using 10.0 Prolene suture for this purpose has led to the current recommendation of 9.0 Prolene or 8.0 Gortex suture for MCTR fixation. The MCTR is inserted with smooth forceps through the main incision and dialed into the capsular bag with a Y-hook (Figure 29-9). The fixation hook will often "capture" anterior to the capsulorrhexis edge. If it does not do so, the hook is easily manipulated anteriorly with a Y-hook (Osher Y-Hook,

Duckworth and Kent, St. Louis, Mo.) and a second dull instrument to retract the capsulorrhexis edge. The Y-hook is used to "dial" the MCTR until the eyelet is centered at the site of zonular dehiscence or zonular weakness. The same hook can then be used to push the fixation hook to the scleral wall to be certain that the chosen location will result in bag centration (Figure 29-10). A scleral flap is fashioned at this site so that, once the suture is tied, the knot can be covered. Viscoelastic is then used to create space between the undersurface of the iris and the anterior capsule in preparation for needle passage. The needles are placed through the incision, into the pupil, and behind the iris. The needle and suture should remain anterior to the anterior capsule at all times (Figure 29-11). This needle pass is then continued out through

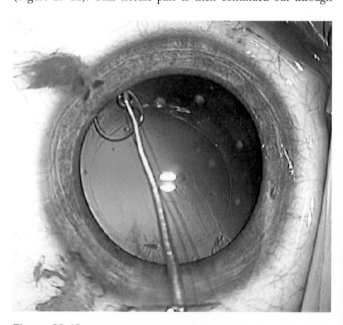

Figure 29-10 Osher Y-hook pushes the fixation hook to the scleral wall to determine the correct meridian of hook fixation to achieve bag centration before needle passage.

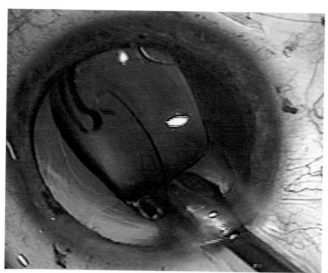

Figure 29-13 AcrySof SN 60WF is injected into the capsular bag through a 2.2 mm incision.

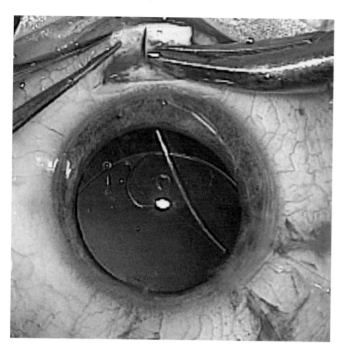

Figure 29-11 Needle is placed through the incision, between the anterior capsule and the undersurface of the iris and out through the ciliary sulcus and scleral wall.

the scleral wall at the site of the fixation hook. The needles should exit the scleral wall approximately 1.5 mm posterior to the corneal–scleral junction. This will position the fixation hook posterior enough to prevent postoperative iris chaffing. Prior to removing the needle from the scleral wall, the author will often enlarge the needle tract with a 15° blade to lessen the effort required to rotate and bury the knot. An ab externo approach to passing the suture, as described by Drs. Alan Crandal and Ike Ahmed, will eliminate a "blind-pass" of the needle as it disappears into the iris.[21] The sutures are cinched-up until centration is obtained and a knot tied (Figure 29-12). The knot can be rotated beneath the sclera or the knot tails cut long and left buried beneath the scleral flap. If a single-armed suture is used, the needle is passed partial thickness through scleral bed beneath the scleral flap, and the suture is then

tied to itself. After CTR placement or suture fixation of the MCTR, any remaining cortex can be aspirated. The capsular bag is then reinflated with viscoelastic before PC IOL insertion. The author has found it easiest to insert a foldable-style single-piece acrylic PC IOL into the capsular bag in these cases (Figure 29-13).

If the two-hook MCTR (2-L) is used, the fixation site for each hook must be ascertained by displacing each hook to the scleral wall before suturing. Depending on the size of the capsular bag, the best centration may be obtained with the hooks less than 180° apart (Figure 29-14). Viscoelastic is removed manually

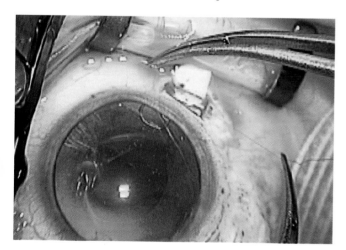

Figure 29-12 The 9-0 Prolene suture is tightened, and a temporary knot is tied to recenter and stabilize the capsular bag.

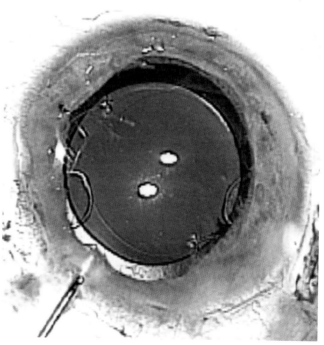

Figure 29-14 Modified capsular tension ring (Model 2-L) with a nicely centered AcrySof MA60 in a young boy with Marfan syndrome.

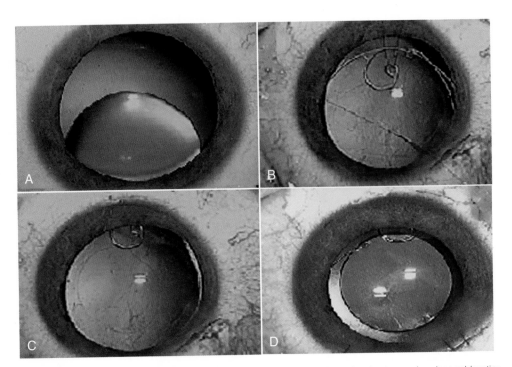

Figure 29-15 An 11-year-old boy with Marfan syndrome. **A,** Preoperative photo showing tremendous lens subluxation. **B,** After placement of the modified capsular tension ring (MCTR) (Model 2-C) and before tightening the Prolene sutures, the bag is expanded yet remains decentered. **C,** Tightening the MCTR's Prolene sutures centers the expanded capsular bag. **D,** With the MCTR secured in place, the capsular bag and PC IOL are well centered and stable at the end of the case. The patient's vision after 24 hours measured 20/25 without glasses.

through the side-port incision or with an automated irrigation–aspiration handpiece. Acetylcholine (Miochol) is instilled to ensure that the pupil rounds and that the anterior chamber is free of vitreous. Conjunctiva is reapproximated over the scleral flap and the near-clear corneal incision is hydrated and checked to be certain that it is watertight.

If vitreous presents at any time during the procedure, it should be carefully and completely removed from the anterior chamber. Small amounts of vitreous can be removed by using a "dry" vitrectomy technique with an automated vitrector and an anterior chamber filled with viscoelastic.[22] For significant vitreous prolapse, a bimanual vitrectomy should be performed. This is best accomplished by using a side-port incision for irrigation with a 25- or 27-gauge cannula. The vitrectomy handpiece can be inserted through the initial incision or through a pars plana sclerotomy.[23]

■ CONCLUSION ■

The management of the significant zonular weakness remains challenging. However, newer surgical techniques now afford us the possibility of saving the capsular bag, recentering the capsular bag, and even placing a PC IOL within the capsular bag (Figure 29-15). This allows the surgery to be performed through

a 2.2 mm incision, giving the patient a rapid visual recovery. This is most important in young children because prolonged visual deprivation could result in dense amblyopia.

References

[1] Jensen A, Cross H. Surgical treatment of dislocated lenses in Marfan's syndrome and homocystinuria. Trans Am Acad Ophthalmol Otolaryngol 1972;76:1491–1499.
[2] Varga B. The results of my operations improving visual acuity of ectopia lentis. Ophthalmologica 1971;162:98–110.
[3] Maumenee IH. The eye in Marfan's syndrome. Trans Am Acad Ophthalmol Soc 1981;79: 684–733.
[4] Straatsma B, Allen R, Pettit T, et al. Subluxation of the lens with iris photocoagulation. Am J Ophthalmol 1966;61:1312–1324.
[5] Gimbel H, Condon G, Kohnen T, Olson R, Halkiadakis I. Late in-the-bag intraocular lens dislocation: incidence, prevention, and management. J Cataract Refract Surg 2005;11:2193–2204.
[6] Zetterstrom C, Lundvall A, Weeber Jr H, et al. Sulcus fixation without capsular support in children. J Cataract Refract Surg 1999;25:776–781.
[7] Cionni R, Osher R. Endocapsular ring approach to the subluxated cataractous lens. J Cataract Refract Surg 1995;21:245–249.
[8] Cionni R, Osher R. Management of profound zonular dialysis or weakness with a new endocapsular ring designed for scleral fixation. J Cataract Refract Surg 1998;10:1299–1306.
[9] Cionni R, Osher R, Marques D, Marques F, Snyder M, Shapiro S. Modified capsular tension ring for patients with congenital loss of zonular support. J Cataract Refract Surg 2003;9:1668–1673.
[10] Hasanee K, Butler M, Ahmed I. Capsular tension rings and related devices: current concepts. Curr Opin Ophthalmol 2006;17:31–41.
[11] Legler U, Witschel B, et al. The capsular tension ring, a new device for complicated cataract surgery. Presented at the American Society of Cataract and Refractive Surgery, Seattle, Wash, May 1993.
[12] Ahmed I, Chen S, Kranemann C, Wong T. Surgical repositioning of dislocated capsular tension rings. Ophthalmology 2005;112:1725–1733.
[13] Osher R. Synthetic zonules. J Cataract Refract Surg 1997;8. [video].
[14] Pfeifer V. Video presentation at the American Society of Cataract and Refractive Surgery, San Diego, Calif, April 1998.
[15] Cionni R, Osher R. Management of profound zonular dialysis or weakness with a new endocapsular ring designed for scleral fixation. J Cataract Refract Surg 1998;24:1299–1306.

[16] Ahmed I, Cionni R, Kranemann C, Crandall A. Optimal timing of capsular tension ring implantation: Miyake-Apple video analysis. J Cataract Refract Surg 2005;9:1809.

[17] Merriam J, Zheng L. Iris hooks for phacoemulsification of the subluxated lens. J Cataract Refract Surg 1997;23:1295.

[18] Maloney W. Supracapsular phaco: achieving greater efficiency with phaco outside of the capsular bag – a 3-year experience. Presented at the American Society of Cataract and Refractive Surgery, Seattle, Wash, April, 1999.

[19] Osher R. Slow motion phacoemulsification approach. J Cataract Refract Surg 1993;19:667. [letter].

[20] Cionni R, Osher R. Complications of phacoemulsification. In: Weinstock FJ, editor. Management and care of the cataract patient. Cambridge, Mass: Blackwell Scientific; 1992. p. 209–210.

[21] Ahmed I, Crandall A. Ab externo scleral fixation of the Cionni modified capsular tension ring. J Cataract Refract Surg 2001;7:977.

[22] Osher R. Dry vitrectomy. J Cataract Refract Surg 1992;8. [video].

[23] Snyder ME, Cionni RJ, Osher RH. Management of intraoperative complications. In: Gills JP, editor. Cataract surgery: the state of the art. Thorofare, NJ: Slack; 1998. p. 149–152.

CONCLUSION

Techniques and Principles of Surgical Management for the Traumatic Cataract

Michael E. Snyder, MD and Robert H. Osher, MD

30

CONTENTS

CHAPTER HIGHLIGHTS

>> Preoperative assessment and surgical planning

>> Modifications in surgical technique

>> Use of hooks, rings, and segments

>> Case studies

■ INTRODUCTION ■

Management of the patient with a traumatized anterior segment often poses challenges both at initial evaluation and in the operating room. Traumatic cataract commonly occurs with severe penetrating ocular trauma, but may also result from blunt injury by, for example, snowballs, waterballoons,[1] and airbags.[2] Athletic events and other seemingly harmless everyday activities may also give rise to traumatic cataracts. In a particularly peculiar case, a golfer sustained a large corneal laceration teeing off when a bird flew into his eye! Traumatic injuries are thus, by their very nature, highly variable and the extent of damage can be difficult to determine at the initial presentation. The anterior segment injury may appear either much less or much greater than it actually is. Furthermore, concurrent posterior segment damage may require vitreo-retinal intervention which may precede, follow or be concurrent with the cataract operation, necessitating communication

and coordination with the vitreoretinal surgeon. Traumatic cataracts are among the most technically demanding cases that the anterior segment surgeon may face. As with all surgeries, preparation and planning for any anticipated or unanticipated intraoperative events will serve to maximize both the patient's outcome and the surgeon's comfort with the operative procedure.

In acute, severe injuries, preparation may include delving a bit into the psyche of the injured patient, allowing the surgeon to provide appropriate counseling, emphasizing the unpredictable nature of these cases and the reasonable short-term and long-term expectations. The patient began with "normal vision" and may anticipate returning to pre-injury status; however, this may or may not be possible in any given case. While it is important to offer reasonable hope, the authors would advocate the "underpromise and overdeliver" philosophy.

The goal of this chapter is to outline a careful, systematic approach to surgery for traumatic cataract and to describe several surgical techniques which may be helpful in these challenging settings.

■ CLINICAL EVALUATION ■

Careful preoperative evaluation of the patient with a traumatic cataract is essential in gaining a complete understanding of the disrupted ocular anatomy and for anticipating events which may occur in the operating room. The goal of the preoperative evaluation is to assess the degree of ocular damage, formulate an operative plan, and determine all potentially needed instruments, equipment, sutures, and implants in advance. Careful preoperative planning should reduce the number and degree of intraoperative surprises, thereby enhancing the surgeon's comfort with the operation and maximizing patient's visual outcome.

■ HISTORY OF THE INJURY ■

In the acute setting, the preoperative evaluation should include a careful history of how the injury occurred. The force and mechanism of the injury may give clues as to whether an occult perforation or intraocular foreign body may exist or whether coexisting posterior segment damage should be anticipated. Metal-on-metal injuries should raise suspicions of an iron-containing intraocular foreign body. In cases of an open globe, inquiry about the environment where the injury occurred may provide clues as to the presence of potentially infectious or inflammatory material. Keep in mind that the history of events surrounding the injury may be unreliable when provided by children. In our experience, children and adolescents may not be entirely forthright initially and often the real story is not disclosed for weeks or months. The implication for the clinician is the need to maintain a high degree of vigilance and refrain from eliminating any possibilities based on the history provided by a child.

Some cases of traumatic cataract will present months, years, or even decades after the injury; the patient may have long forgotten the details or even the occurrence of the injury and may remember details only after the surgeon has posed several probing questions.

■ EXAMINATION ■

This section will review those components of the ophthalmic examination that are particularly relevant to cases of traumatic cataract.

ASSESSING VISUAL FUNCTION

The examination should, of course, always begin with an assessment of visual acuity. Ideally, this will be a best-corrected Snellen visual acuity tested in the controlled setting of the office environment. Of course in acute trauma this ideal situation may not present itself. When testing reveals hand motions or light perception vision, the ability to identify colored light gives some prognostic information about macular function. Confrontational visual fields give very helpful information, but are not possible in eyes with mature cataracts. The patient's response to the Purkinje phenomenon may provide indirect evidence about whether the retina is attached or detached or if glaucomatous or visual field loss may be present. The authors once examined a patient with a mature cataract who noted the Purkinje phenomenon only in the nasal visual field. An MRI disclosed an otherwise asymtomatic pituitary tumor! Simlarly, Carp et. al. reported a patient who presented 3 months after an ocular injury with a monocular nasal hemianopia confirmed by Humphrey 24-2 testing. The hemianopia resolved completely following extraction of a posterior subcapsular cataract.[3] Purkinje testing is contraindicated in the presence of an open penetrating wound.

For evaluations performed in the emergency room formal Snellen assessments may not be possible. It is possible, however, to document light perception, hand motions, count fingers . . . all the way up to "recognizes faces" or even "reads 14 point print on hospital consent form." Though visual acuity measurements can underestimate visual potential in the setting of acute penetrating trauma, proper documentation and patient/family counseling may protect the surgeon from inaccuracies in a patient's or family's subsequent recollections of the severity of the initial injury.

As the only objective measure of visual function, assessment for an afferent pupillary defect should always be ascertained. While assessment of the pupillary response can be extremely helpful in predicting prognosis, it is not always easily performed in the acute setting on an anxious patient with an open globe. Since traumatic mydriasis, miosis, and frank iris tears or incarceration may limit the function of the involved pupil, the ophthalmologist should always

remember that visualization of only one pupil is required to determine the presence or absence of an afferent pupillary defect. Significant efforts to simultaneously open both lids should be avoided if it is likely to result in the patient squeezing them closed.

BIOMICROSCOPY

Slit-lamp biomicroscopy provides extremely helpful information for the operative intervention. First, the anterior chamber may be studied for possible vitreous prolapse or retained intraocular foreign body. The presence and degree of iris damage or loss can be assessed and, of course, the crystalline lens can be scrutinized. In fact, the traumatic origin of cataract is sometimes revealed by noting the subtle findings of a gap between the iris margin and lens surface or decentration of the Y-sutures relative to the pupil center. Phacodonesis, frank decentration, and zonular loss should be carefully documented in both location and degree. When the lens capsule is visibly damaged, the extent of a tear should be carefully delineated and recorded. A corrugated appearance to the lens capsule may indicate compromised capsular or zonular integrity. The anterior lens capsule can be ruptured even in cases of blunt (non-penetrating) trauma.[4] The surgeon should already be thinking about how a capsulorrhexis might be able to incorporate the defect. An anterior capsule tear will typically enlarge as the lens material swells. Therefore, if a defect is near the margin to which it could be incorporated into a capsulorrhexis, intervention might be expedited. Posterior capsular breaks can, similarly, occur with either penetrating or blunt trauma;[5] though this may not be apparent on clinical exam, since cataract formation may limit the examiner's view.

Some biomicroscopic findings may be fairly obvious in some cases. Netland and colleagues describe a case of dislocation of the crystalline lens into the anterior chamber following blunt injury.[6]

In the setting of an open corneoscleral laceration, careful preoperative evaluation at the slit lamp may be either impractical or impossible, making surgical planning much more challenging.

OPHTHALMOSCOPY

Funduscopic evaluation (when view permits) should include an evaluation for retinal holes, tears, or commotio. Subretinal or suprachoroidal hemorrhage may portend a more guarded prognosis. When any suprachoroidal hemorrhage is present, the surgeon should expect positive posterior pressure in surgery.

SPECIAL TESTING

When a "mature," opaque cataract is present, B-scan ultrasonography is instrumental in the surgical planning. First, the B-scan can provide crucial information about the status of the posterior lens capsule. In one case of mature cataract following penetrating injury, B-scan ultrasonography confirmed a displaced rupture of the posterior lens capsule (Figure 30-1). In addition to confirming the posterior segment status, B-scan information may alter the surgeon's approach to removing the cataract. When a suprachoroidal hemorrhage is detected, for example, the anterior segment surgeon should exercise caution in considering a pars plana approach for anterior vitrectomy. If possible, intervention should be delayed until the hemorrhage has resolved. If a large

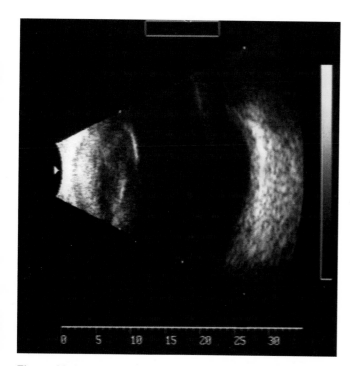

Figure 30-1 This B-scan ultrasound demonstrates a full thickness laceration of the lens with discontinuity of the two hemispheres. This case is described in detail in Demonstrative case number one at the end of the chapter.

suprachoroidal hemorrhage is present, vitreoretinal consultation is recommended, since drainage may be required. Though the drainage procedure is not particularly difficult, subsequent retinal detachment may occur as the choroidal mounds flatten. Ultrasound testing can also demonstrate vital features in the anterior segment. Sathish and colleagues reported a patient who sustained an anterior scleral rupture with ultrasound-documented dislocation of the crystalline lens into the subconjunctival space.[7]

If the surgeon suspects an intraocular or intraorbital foreign body, CT scan imaging of the orbits with thin slices is indicated. CT scanning may have some role in diagnosing traumatic cataract in the setting of acute trauma. One study reports that a low attenuation of the lens is diagnositic of current or near-term development of visually significant cataract.[8] In that study, no patients with normal attenuation developed cataract within 1 year. The ophthalmologist should be aware of another study which demonstrated that an intumescent cataract may appear invisible on CT scan, giving a false impression of traumatic aphakia.[9] MRI scanning is not particularly helpful in the management of the traumatic cataract patient and could cause serious damage if a ferromagnetic foreign body is present in the eye or orbit.

◼ CATARACT SURGERY IN THE ACUTELY TRAUMATIZED GLOBE ◼

While some articles advocate primary cataract extraction at the time of an open globe repair,[10] there are advantages to a staged approach. First, there are many instances where corneal clarity, anterior chamber hyphema, clot or disorganization of the anatomy may obscure the view of anterior segment structures and may lead to unanticipated complications. Further examination and testing after repair

of the primary laceration can lead to more accurate surgical planning. Second, at the time of an open globe injury, keratometry and biometry of the affected eye are virtually impossible, and usually the patient is unable to cooperate maximally for accurate A-scan and keratometry measurements of the contralateral eye. This may lead to a greater likelihood of significant ammetropia or anisometropia in what might be an otherwise optimal visual result.

Occasionally, the degree of injury to the lens may appear greater at the initial presentation, but, in fact, it may not require cataract extraction. One patient presented emergently to the authors with a full-thickness central corneal laceration that penetrated the anterior capsule of the lens. The cornea was closed primarily and cataract extraction was not performed. The lens capsule sealed over and developed only a small, focal cataract. The patient retained 20/20 vision and was asymptomatic. Pieramici and colleagues reported five cases in which peripheral lens perforation occurred and lens clarity was maintained using a lens-sparing approach for intraocular foreign body removal.[11] They noted that some inert (glass) foreign bodies were well tolerated without removal. Conversely, any potentially iron-containing foreign body should be removed since an iron-containing intralenticular foreign body may result in ocular siderosis with potentially devastating visual consequences.[12]

◼ CATARACT SURGERY AND THE ACUTE OPERATIVE INTERVENTION ◼

There are, of course, certain occasions where cataract surgery at the time of primary open-globe repair is absolutely indicated. First, when traumatic cataract obscures the view for removal of a known intraocular foreign body, cataract extraction should be immediate, particularly when the foreign body may carry vegetable or other contaminated material. Delayed treatment of an intraocular foreign body significantly reduces the chances of a favorable outcome.[13] If the foreign body is in the posterior segment, the anterior segment surgeon should work in combination with a vitreoretinal surgeon. Preferably, the traumatic cataract should be removed using an anterior approach. Pars plana lensectomy leads to more capsular damage and may commit the patient to aphakia unnecessarily or result in the need for a sutured posterior chamber intraocular lens (PC IOL). If the posterior segment surgeon feels strongly that a pars plana approach lensectomy is required for vitreoretinal reasons, efforts should be made to retain as much capsular support as possible.

Also, some patients may have medical conditions which may significantly increase their anesthetic risks, making a single general anesthetic episode more desirable. In these instances an expeditious primary extraction is appropriate, though the surgeon should remember that the alternative of a secondary procedure may often be performed under regional anesthesia with a lesser anesthetic risk.

Preoperative patient counselling should be directed at setting realistic expectations based on the available prognostic information.

◼ SURGICAL PLANNING AND TECHNIQUE ◼

Ideally, the surgeon should be able to plan the case well in advance so that the operative procedure is one that has been mentally rehearsed. This means anticipating each surgical step to the best degree possible preoperatively. The first decision in any operative plan is the selection of the anesthetic approach. In traumatic cataract cases, the surgeon will usually be choosing between general and local anesthesia. For open-globe situations, general anesthesia usually provides greater safety. In the setting of a secure globe, the decision about regional or general anesthesia may be based on factors relating to the patient's ability to cooperate and the anticipated length of the procedure. Topical anesthesia should be reserved for only the most straightforward traumatic cataract cases. If significant posterior pressure is anticipated, intravenous mannitol administered in the holding room may be helpful. Though some informal, anecdotal teachings suggested a link between intravenous mannitol and suprachoroidal hemorrhage, formal studies have not identified mannitol as an independant risk factor. Traumatic eye injury, though, is a well-documented risk for suprachoroidal hemorrhage.[14,15]

SELECTION OF WOUND LOCATION

Once anesthetic concerns have been addressed, the surgeon needs to select the planned location of the scleral or corneal wound. The wound should preferably be positioned in the area of the most normal anterior segment anatomy. A cataract incision placed over a zonular dialysis will make scleral suturing of a modified, Cionni capsular tension ring or sutured posterior chamber implant unnecessarily more difficult. Furthermore, the surgeon will be working directly over an exposed hyaloid face, increasing the chances of disturbing the vitreous. Sometimes a steep orbital rim will mandate a temporal approach, though if the traumatic wound crosses the temporal limbus, this area should be strictly avoided for the cataract incision. In such a case, an inferior incision may be considered. If the factors described above do not limit the surgeon's choices of wound location, then astigmatic considerations may be taken into account. The planned wound location will usually dictate the most appropriate orientation of the surgeon's operating position.

MANAGING THE CONJUNCTIVA

Often in traumatic cases, the additional strength of a scleral tunnel wound is preferable, since a larger incision may be required if the surgeon has selected a polymethylmethacrylate (PMMA) implant. While the conjunctival incision is not the most glamorous part of the procedure, careful consideration should be given to the location and extent of the peritomy. The conjunctival openings should allow ample access to the planned scleral tunnel wound sites and, additionally, should include access for a pars plana sclerotomy or a site for scleral suturing of a PC IOL or modified, Cionni capsular tension ring. While adequate access is of vital importance, uninvolved conjunctiva should be respected, since several traumatic cataract cases may find themselves seeing a glaucoma specialist at some point in the future.

VISCOELASTIC OPTIONS

Selection of the viscoelastic agent for a traumatic cataract case depends on several factors. In some cases more than one agent may be appropriate. When the intact hyaloid face is partly exposed, a dispersive viscoelastic agent such as Viscoat (Alcon, Fort Worth, Texas) or Healon D (AMO, California) may tamponade the vitreous and keep it back[16] (Figure 30-2). The highly

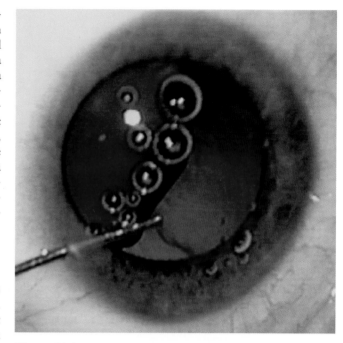

Figure 30-2 A dispersive viscoelastic can create a "plug" to protect an exposed hyaloid face.

retentive agents are also excellent endothelial protectants. This may be particularly relevant to cases in which the endothelial cell density has been reduced by the trauma.[17] The space-retaining qualities and ease of removal typical of highly cohesive viscoelastic agents, such as Healon GV and Healon 5 (AMO, California), make these agents more facile for the lens implantation stage of a procedure. In some cases one may choose the "soft shell" technique,[18] which combines the added endothelial protection of a highly dispersive agent with the space-maintaining abilities, ease of removal, and clarity of the cohesive agents. The "soft shell" is created by loosely filling the corneal dome with a dispersive viscoelastic, then instilling a cohesive viscoelastic just in front of the crystalline lens. This presses the dispersive agent against the corneal endothelium, creating a thin protective layer. The soft shell approach should be used cautiously when vitreous tamponade is desired since the cohesive agent may thin or displace the protective "plug" in front of the vitreous.

Some surgeons prefer a "pseudoplastic" agent such as Healon 5 with outstanding space-maintaining properties. At higher aspiration flow rates, the cohesive agent sheers, providing properties similar to the dispersive materials. Healon 5 holds promise for use in traumatic cataracts; however, the authors' experience in this setting is still in the early stages and any surgeon should be alerted to the possibility of greater intraocular pressure elevation if any agent remains in the globe at the completion of the procedure.

DisCoVisc ® (Alocn, Fort Worth, Texas) has recently been added to the authors' ophthalmic viscosurgical device (OVD) armamentarium. This agent contains a mixture of hyaluronic acid and chondroitin sulfate and, accordingly, maintains significant dispersive and cohesive properties of each.

When "dry" lens material aspiration under viscoelastic is anticipated,[19] highly dispersive viscoelastics tend to clog the cannula for manual aspiration techniques while Healon GV and Healon

5 tend to follow into the tip of the cannula preferentially to the lens material and, in fact, can inhibit aspiration of cortex. In this setting, Healon, Provisc, and Discovisc may be more suitable.

THE CAPSULOTOMY

The anterior capsulotomy often determines the ease or difficulty of the cataract removal. Sometimes, the traumatic injury may have caused either an anterior capsular defect either from a blunt rupture or a sharp laceration. The opening may provide direct access to the lens material, yet every effort should be made to convert the capsular tear into an intact capsulorrhexis. A complete capsulorrhexis has far superior mechanical integrity to either a can-opener capsulotomy or a partial capsulorrhexis[20] and will improve the safety of each subsequent step of the operative procedure.

Microinstrumentation 23- and 25-gauge forceps are available in both reusable and disposable formats, and can be very helpful in completing a capsulorrhexis through a paracentesis, perhaps placed in an area of particularly tough or thickened capsule.

Occasionally, a vitrector may be useful in creating an anterior capsular opening. This type of capsulotomy has a greater structural integrity than a can-opener, but is not as desirable as a complete capsulorrhexis.[21] The vitrectorrhexis technique can be less facile in practice than in theory since the lens capsule is not always easily aspirated to the cutting port. Moreover, when the capsule is engaged in the port, marginal zonules may be compromised.

Visualization for the capsulorrhexis may be much more difficult in cases of traumatic cataract, particularly when the capsule is torn or the cortex is opaque. Several dyes have been recommended to aid in visualization of the anterior capsule, including fluorescein,[22] methylene blue, gentian violet,[23] crystal violet, trypan blue,[24] and indocyanine green (ICG).[25] Clinically, ICG (IC Green, Akorn, NJ) and trypan blue (Vision Blue, Dutch Ophthalmic Research Corporation, Netherlands) are extremely helpful and have acceptable safety profiles[26] (Figure 30-3). The initial descriptions of ICG recommended instillation under air. However, the authors have found that when the capsule is intact, gently painting a drop of ICG or trypan blue across the anterior capsule under viscoelastic is equally effective. The "three step" technique stains the capsule by creating a fluid layer of BSS over the capsule and under the OVD-filled anterior chamber.[27] The stain may even delineate the edges of a torn capsule. Trypan blue has an impressive safety profile and may be directly irrigated into the anterior chamber, then diluted with balanced salt solution (BSS). In the presence of a zonular dialysis, however, trypan blue entrance into the vitreous cavity can reduce or eliminate the red reflex. Focal placement of DisCoVisc over the dialysis can create a "plug" and prevent inadvertent migration of the dye into the posterior segment. Fluorescein has a high index of safety, but stains the capsule only weakly and tends to cause a diffuse yellow appearance of the operative field which may limit visualization of subsequent steps. Methylene blue and gentian violet have a known cytotoxicity.[28]

Tangential illumination of the anterior capsule using a sterile endoilluminator probe may also facilitate visualization for capsulotomy with a white lens. Metz[29] and, subsequently, Gimbel and Willerscheidt[30] reported aspirating liquified, white cortical material through a tiny, central capsular opening to decompress the capsular bag in cases of intumescent white cataract. This may decrease the tendancy for peripheral extension by lowering the endocapsular pressure.

The surgeon should exercise meticulous technique in creating a capsular tear in traumatized lenses. Zonular countertraction may not be uniform so the physics of creating the tear are slightly different to the usual case. The surgeon should make special efforts to have the leading edge of the capsular flap *folded over* in order to control the path of the tear more predictably (Figure 30-4).

If significant zonular instability is present, the surgeon may use a side port instrument to stabilize the lens nucleus during

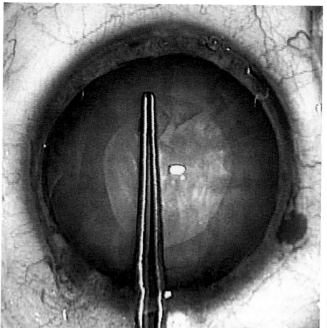
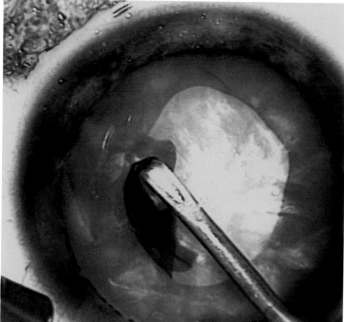

Figure 30-3 Indocyanin green (ICG) (left) or trypan blue (right) can be used to stain the anterior capsule for greater visibility in the white cataract.

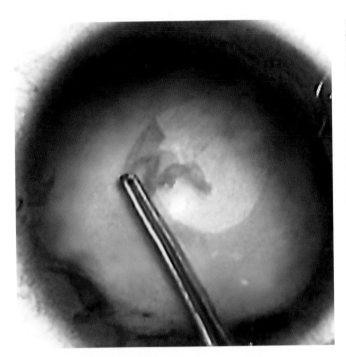

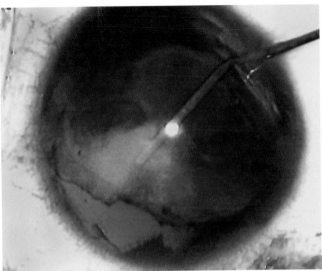

Figure 30-5 The remaining white cortical material within the capsular bag is aspirated manually with a 27-gauge cannula in a "dry" fashion. Viscoelastic material protects the exposed hyaloid face in an area of pre-existing posterior capsular tear seen just up and to the left of the cannula tip.

Figure 30-4 If the anterior capsular flap is folded over, the surgeon will have greater control over the direction of the capsular tear. Indocyanin green (ICG) was used in this case to better demonstrate the capsular flap. In this case, the ICG was administered under viscoelastic and some residual dye is visible within the viscoelastic material.

capsulorrhexis. A "pincushion" appearance of the anterior capsule noted before the cystotome penetrates through the capsule is an indicator of diffuse zonular laxity. The anterior capsulorrhexis in children with traumatic cataract may be even more challenging than their adult counterparts since the pediatric lens capsule has a stronger and more elastic consistency. For these patients it may be easier to plan to make the capsulorrhexis smaller initially and enlarge it later if needed, since these capsules have a greater tendency toward peripheral extension of the circular tear.

NUCLEUS REMOVAL

Removal of the lens nucleus can be addressed by a number of different techniques, each of which has potential advantages and disadvantages, depending on the setting. In a young patient the nucleus is usually very soft and is amenable to many different options. For a patient with an intact capsulorrhexis, phaco-aspiration of the nucleus is typically safe and expeditious. If an anterior or posterior capsular tear is present, then manual aspiration with a Simcoe-style cannula affords greater control (Figure 30-5). "Dry" aspiration of the soft nucleus under viscoelastic material offers exquisite control, especially in the most complicated cases.[15]

Since the nucleus is denser in older patients, its removal will require a more challenging disassembly. The superior control of a small incision, closed-system approach to nucleus removal shines particularly brightly in cases with distorted anatomy and potentially weakened zonules. Since traumatized eyes are at greater risk for suprachoroidal hemorrhage, maintaining a closed system reduces the chances of the catastrophic expulsive consequences. Furthermore, a closed system allows compartmentalization within the anterior segment. If the posterior capsule is broken or if a zonular

dehiscence is present, viscoelastic tamponade of the vitreous can be best maintained in the setting of a closed system. Manual extracapsular cataract extraction and manual phacosection techniques require an open wound and thereby compromise an important degree of control over the intraocular environment.

The technique of phacoemulsification may vary somewhat depending on the surgeon's usual approach, though some important principles should be incorporated into these special traumatic cases. A cautious respect for the zonular support in the traumatic cataract should guide the surgeon away from choosing a "phaco-flip," "chip-and-flip" or other technique which may exert trampoline-like pressure to the zonular apparatus, even when no frank zonulodialysis is detected preoperatively. Many variations of gentle divide and conquer techniques or phaco-chop techniques can be modified to incorporate the principles of "slow motion phaco."[31]

PHACOEMULSIFICATION IN THE PRESENCE OF ZONULAR COMPROMISE

In some patients with very weak zonules, grooving for a divide and conquer, and other endocapsular manipulations, may stress the already compromised capsular support. A relatively large capsulorrhexis will facilitate viscoexpression of the nucleus into the anterior chamber. Alternatively, a very gentle chopping procedure is protective to the remaining intact zonules since all applied forces are borne by the chopper instrument, the nucleus, and the countertraction of the phacoemulsification handpiece.

When severe zonular damage is present, the surgeon can use a capsular tension ring to help stabilize the lens nucleus before phacoemulsification begins. In order to facilitate endocapsular ring placement, cortical cleaving viscodissection will create the potential space for the ring to pass into the capsular bag. When more than 4 clock hours of zonular damage is present, the modified Cionni capsular tension ring (Morcher, Germany) adds suture fixation to the area of greatest zonular weakness[32] (Figure 30-6). The authors

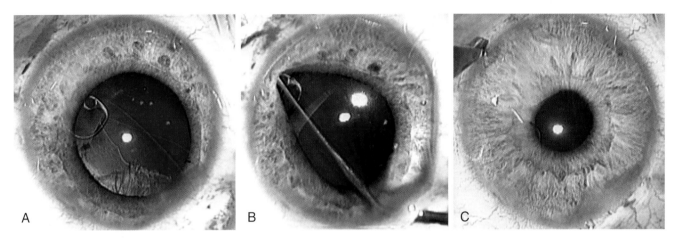

Figure 30-6 A, A modified (Cionni) capsular tension ring in situ within the capsular bag. The fixation eyelet courses in front of the capsulorrhexis margin. The sutures have not yet been passed through the sclera. **B,** The position of the fixation element is seen after the fixation sutures have been tightened. The second light reflex is the second Purkinje-Sanson image from the front surface of the well centered intraocular lens. **C,** The appearance of the eye at the end of the procedure.

have found that it is easiest to load the suture through the fixation eyelet prior to ring implantation, then to pass the transcleral sutures in an ab-interno fashion once the fixation element has been guided into the proper meridion. Suture fixation improves the lens stability for the remainder of the case. If the lens nucleus is particularly large and dense, it may be difficult or impossible to place the endocapsular ring prior to phacoemulsification. In such cases the surgeon can temporarily augment the native zonular support with flexible nylon "iris" retractors placed through a limbal incision to engage the capsulorrhexis margin (Figure 30-7). The retractor can be placed through a paracentesis tract, though a pathway may be created with a curved S-14 spatula needle placed

perpendicular at the conjunctival insertion, entering the anterior chamber just above the iris insertion. This method of placement creates less anterior movement of the lens–capsular complex, thereby providing a deeper anterior chamber to work in. The tract of an S-14 needle is self-sealing. Once the nucleus is emulsified, the endocapsular ring may be placed with greater ease.

Though not yet available in the United States, the Ahmed segment (Morcher GmbH, Germany) is an excellent approach to stabilize the loose lens either prior to or after the phacoemulsification of the nucleus.[33,34] The Ahmed segment has the same fixation element as the Cionni CTRs, but is only a 120° arc instead of a complete ring. Its smaller size makes it more facile to insert into the capsular bag, particularly when the bag still contains nuclear material.

Theoretically, the capsular tension ring could be inserted after a posterior capsular break if both an intact anterior and posterior capsulorrhexis were present. Capsular tension ring placement should *not* be considered with any other setting of anterior or posterior capsular break. If a capsular tear or break were to occur with the endocapsular ring in situ, the device should be promptly retrieved from the anterior segment since its stability is no longer guaranteed.

CORTICAL REMOVAL

Once the lens nucleus has been successfully removed, the capsular bag should be inspected carefully for integrity. Isolated posterior capsule rupture has been reported as a result of blunt injury.[35–38] When the capsular bag and zonular apparatus are intact, cortical removal can be routine, but when zonular damage is present, the cortex is best removed by a very gentle, controlled technique. Some of the principles discussed above for soft nuclei apply particularly well to cortical removal and will be reviewed in more detail here. If cortical cleaving hydrodissection was performed at the beginning of the case, this step may be much easier. If hydrodissection was incomplete or not performed, viscodissection can gently separate cortical material from the capsular bag[39] (Figure 30-8). When an automated irrigation–aspiration method is used, teasing the cortical strands parallel to the zonular dialysis will be less likely to cause the intact zonules to unzip. The same

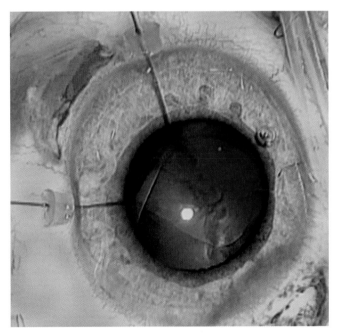

Figure 30-7 Flexible "iris" retractors can be placed to stabilize the capsular bag for phacoemulsification when zonular support is compromised. After the phacemulsification, the capsular tension ring can be more easily inserted.

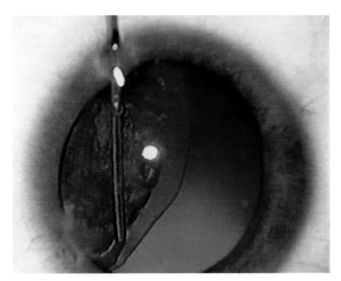

Figure 30-8 Cortical cleaving "viscodissection" can separate the lens material from the capsular bag, making the cortex easier to remove.

principle applies to manual aspiration with a Simcoe-type cannula, which offers a greater degree of control within a stable chamber. If a posterior capsular break is present, a viscoelastic tamponade of the intact hyaloid face, combined with a manual "dry" aspiration with a 25- or 27-gauge cannula on a 3 cc syringe in a chamber filled with viscoelastic material, can facilitate complete cortical removal without vitreous loss. The exquisite control of the dry aspiration technique offsets the more tedious and time-consuming nature of this approach.[23]

REMOVAL OF LENS MATERIAL WITH VITREOUS PROLAPSE

Vitreous in the anterior segment alone or admixed within the lens material increases the risk of posterior segment complications. It is not uncommon for penetrating injuries to go through the lens and into the vitreous. If the penetrating object is withdrawn, vitreous may be pulled into or through the lacerated crystalline lens. The surgeon should always try to avoid aspirating any vitreous material. Any traction on the firm attachments of the anterior vitreous to the vitreous base can create a retinal break and subsequent retinal detachment. If there is extensive loss of zonular support and the capsular remnants are severely lacerated, a pars plana lensectomy with vitrectomy may be the most appropriate course.

When vitreous is identified within the lens material but the lens support and peripheral lens anatomy are relatively intact, some special anterior segment approaches are indicated. First, any vitreous which has prolapsed through the laceration or surgical wound should be removed with an automated vitreous cutter. A dry vitrectomy can be performed at the wound site by placing the cutting port against the scleral or corneal opening. This will effectively remove any external vitreous without creating traction. The machine settings should have relatively low flow and low vacuum.

Next, the vitreous cutter can be placed into the anterior chamber and a gentle anterior vitrectomy can be performed to remove the vitreous material from the anterior segment and sever any incarcerations or attachments to the anterior segment wounds. Coaxial irrigation on the vitrector handpiece can blow the vitreous away from the cutting port and thus cause unneccessary flow through the anterior chamber. Bimanual or split infusion via a separate paracentesis site is preferable using a 21-guage butterfly or blunt cannula to allow control of the direction of the irrigation stream.

When the anterior chamber is clear of vitreous, attention is turned to the removal of the lens material. When the lens material is soft, it may be aspirated via the vitrector handpiece on "I/A cutter" settings so that the instrument behaves as an I/A device until foot position three, in which cutting action is engaged. Use of the vitrector handpiece adds additional safety when vitreous may be admixed with lens material since, if an errant strand of vitreous finds its way to the aspiration port, cutting may be immediately initiated, thereby releasing vitreous traction.

DRY CORTICAL ASPIRATION

If zonular damage is present and exquisite control is required, a "dry "aspiration technique under a chamber filled with viscoelastic can be carefully performed. A moderately cohesive viscoelastic agent can be injected to deepen the chamber. Special caution should be used to place the viscoelastic agent at the wound first and not to overfill the chamber. If too much viscoelastic material is injected, the increase in the intraocular pressure may cause vitreous to prolapse through the wound during instillation. The aspiration is most effective introducing a 25- or 27-gauge cannula *into* the soft lens material with the cannula tip placed as far from the capsular break as possible. The lens material can be carefully stripped and aspirated, working from the area most distal to the capsular break. If vitreous is engaged at any point it must be immediately released and additional vitrectomy is performed.

DENSE CAPSULAR PLAQUES

Not infrequently, capsular plaques may line either the posterior capsule or, occasionally, the entire internal circumference of the capsular bag. Once an edge of the plaque is elevated, viscodissection, blunt dissection, and peeling of the plaque may result in a clear posterior capsule and clean capsular bag (Figure 30-9). Other times, a posterior capsulorrhexis may be created or, alternatively, YAG laser capsulotomy may be performed after surgery.

DENSE NUCLEUS AND AN OPEN POSTERIOR CAPSULE

In the presence of dense cataractous lens material, phacoemulsification may be required. If the anterior segment has been entirely cleared of vitreous, an anterior chamber phaco over a bed of dispersive viscoelastic or a Sheets glide may be cautiously considered. In this setting, a side-port instrument should be used to support the lens material. Sheets glide placement technique should be meticulous, since inaccurate insertion can engage or tear remaining capsular support. The surgeon should consider that a Sheets glide can be very difficult to place from a clear corneal wound.

Preferentially, if a complete anterior capsulorrhexis can be achieved, slightly smaller than the IOL optic, then the nuclear

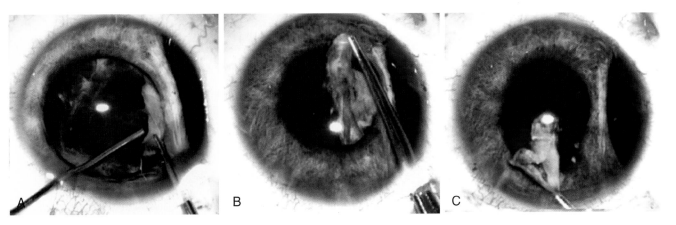

Figure 30-9 **A,** A dense capsular plaque is viscodissected from the capsular bag. The plaque encompasses the entire internal lining of the intact bag. **B,** Once the tightest adhesins have been lysed, the plaque can be peeled away from the capsule. **C,** The plaque is removed *en bloc,* leaving an intact and clear capsular bag.

fragments can be placed on the iris leaflet anteriorly, the cortex can be manually aspirated in a "dry" fashion, and the IOL can be placed in the ciliary sulcus. With posterior capture of the implant optic through the capsulorrhexis, the barrier between the anterior and posterior segments has been reestablished and anterior chamber phaco can be performed without concern for posterior dislocation of lens fragments (Figure 30-10).

Kelman has proposed a technique which he calls "posterior assisted levitation" in which nuclear material is supported from behind via a second instrument placed through the pars plana.[40] With this technique the surgeon should be vigilant in watching for vitreous at the port of the phacoemulsification handpiece. The surgeon should always avoid manual manipulation of the vitreous gel, since traction on the anterior vitreous base may lead to serious retinal sequellae.

ANTERIOR SEGMENT CLEAN-UP

Once the lens material is removed, careful re-evaluation of the anterior segment for any anteriorly displaced vitreous should be carried out. If vitreous is identified, further vitrectomy should be performed. Once the anterior segment media permits a view through the pupillary space, vitrectomy through a pars plana incision, again with a split, anterior infusion can be utilized. The vitrector handpiece is placed through a sclerotomy created 3 mm posterior to the limbus by a 20-gauge V-lance blade (Figure 30-11). Some 25-gauge vitreous cutters utilize a trocar system with equal effectiveness. The pars plana approach has several advantages over limbal vitrectomy. First, the vitreous material is aspirated posteriorly away from the anterior segment wounds. With anterior–irrigation and posteriorly placed vitrector aspiration, a localized pressure gradient occurs creating a flow from anterior to posterior, as desired. Pulling the vitreous back into the vitreous cavity creates less traction on the vitreous base and allows better access to subincisional vitreous, which may be coursing around the iris margin.[41] Furthermore, when the vitrector handpiece is placed through the cataract incision, the corneal dome is more likely to be distorted, leading to suboptimal visualization. With the pars plana approach, the view through the

cornea is excellent. Once an adequate vitrectomy has been completed, the 20-gauge sclerotomy should be cleaned externally (as described above) and then closed with a suture, for example, a figure of eight, 7-0 vicryl suture. Although the 25-gauge trocar opening can be left unsutured, but may result in transient undesired hypotony in a globe with at least one risk factor (trauma) for suprachoroidal hemorrhage.

MANAGING THE COMPROMISED CAPSULE

When all lens material and any offending vitreous have been safely removed, the surgeon can breathe only a brief sigh of relief; they must then move on to assessing the degree of zonular and capsular support that remains. After filling the anterior segment with viscoelastic, the surgeon may gently retract the iris in order to directly visualize the underlying anatomy. When the anterior capsulorrhexis is intact, but a posterior capsular break is present, a few different options exist. Ideally, if the posterior capsular tear is small, some viscoelastic can be placed through the opening to retroplace the vitreous and the posterior tear may be converted into a posterior capsulorrhexis. This can preserve the capsular strength for endocapsular placement of a posterior chamber implant (Figure 30-12).

The experienced surgeon may be able to implant the IOL into the torn capsular bag even when the posterior tear cannot be safely converted to a capsulorrhexis, yet it may be safer to place the haptics of a three-piece posterior chamber implant into the ciliary sulcus. If the anterior capsulorrhexis is intact and measures 5 mm or less, the lens optic can be prolapsed into the capsular bag, providing addition support and centration. In this setting, the implant power would be chosen as usually calculated. If both the optic and the haptics are in the plane of the ciliary sulcus, 0.5 diopter should be subtracted from the calculated implant power. (Unpublished data presented at American Society of Cataract and Refractive Surgeons Annual Meeting, 1984.)

If significant capsular damage exists, a determination should be made as to whether there is enough support for the placement of a posterior chamber implant in the ciliary sulcus. The torn posterior capsular bag will often provide long-term fixation of an IOL,

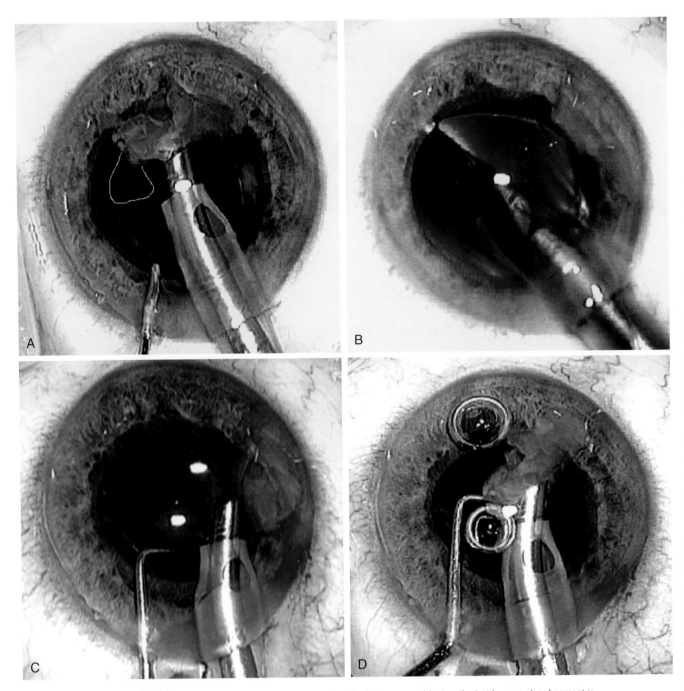

Figure 30-10 A, A posterior capsular break (outlined in yellow) becomes evident as the last large nuclear fragment is held at the phacoemusification tip. The anterior chamber and bag were filled with viscoelastic material, tamponading the hyaloid face. The fragment was placed on the iris leaflet. B, The posterior chamber intraocular lens (PC IOL) was inserted into the ciliary sulcus. C, The optic was captured into the capsulorhexis reestablishing a barrier between the anterior segment and the vitreous. D, The nuclear fragment is safely emulsified without risk of posterior dislocation.

yet the surgeon must be capable of modifying the implantation technique in order to safely insert the lens without further damaging the capsular remnants. Special attention should be given to the inferior support since gravity may gradually rotate a horizontally oriented implant. When the lens is placed and found to be centered, the "Osher bounce test" can confirm stability.

The optic is gently decentered toward each haptic, then released; the implant should spontaneously recenter. If capsular support is absent or deemed to be inadequate, the surgeon should consider scleral or iris suture fixation of one or both haptics of the posterior chamber implant. The techniques for this are covered in detail in Chapter 16.

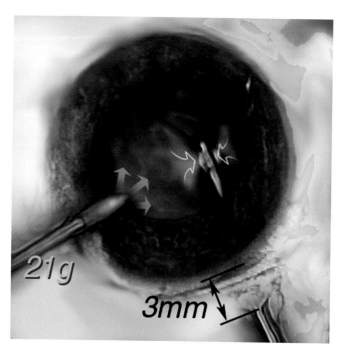

Figure 30-11 Anterior vitrectomy is achieved via a pars plana approach. The automated vitrector is placed through a 20-gauge opening 3 mm posterior to the limbus. Irrigation fluid is infused (blue arrows) through a 21-gauge butterfly needle placed through a corneal paracentesis tract. The prolapsed vitreous material is pulled back into the vitreous cavity and removed with the automated cutting device (open white arrows).

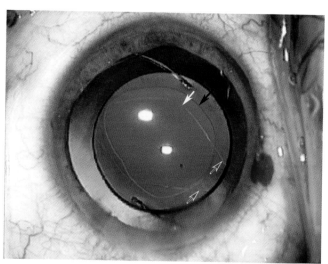

Figure 30-12 A three-piece acrylic posterior chamber intraocular lens (PC IOL) is placed wihin the capsular bag following posterior capsulorrhexis (PCCC). The anterior capsulorrhexis (black arrow) maintains its usual round appearance, while the PCCC (white arrow) becomes ovoid from the tension of the haptic on the fornices of the bag, inducing some striae (open white arrows) in the posterior capsule.

INTRAOCULAR LENS OPTIONS

Once the cataract has been safely removed from the eye, the surgeon should consider the guidelines in the selection of an appropriate implant lens design and material. First, silicone-based lenses may increase the difficulty of future vitrectomy surgeries; therefore, they are a suboptimal choice if the injury has included the posterior segment.[42,43] Both PMMA and acrylic lenses are well tolerated by the eye and are preferred by the vitreoretinal surgeons.

Since traumatic cataracts are not uncommonly associated with some degree of traumatic mydriasis, a 6 mm or larger diameter IOL optic seems prudent. Large optic diameters are also more forgiving in implant decentrations, which may be more likely in traumatic cataract cases.

When a sutured implant is required, a rigid, one-piece PMMA implant may provide additional stability and can be attached to the sclera with two- or four-point fixation, the latter decreasing the likelihood of tilt. A rigid implant, however, requires a larger incision. An implant with a fixation element on the apex of each haptic is preferable. Foldable acrylic lenses can be sutured to the ciliary sulcus as well, though with currently available implants only one suture can be affixed to each haptic, achieving just two points of fixation. An implant haptic and suture guard (patented by Michael E. Snyder, MD, Cincinnati, Ohio) will facilitate easier four-point fixation of a foldable PC IOL. This design has not yet been incorporated into a commercially available IOL.

One-piece acrylic lenses are suitable only for in-the-bag fixation. The surgeon should always consider the overall length of the IOL, since sulcus support cannot be predictably achieved using IOLs designed for endocapsular fixation, which have shorter overall lengths.

In cases where glaucoma is present and preservation of conjunctiva for an existing or future filtering bleb is paramount, the surgeon may consider an acrylic lens with a clear corneal incision.

Some experts discourage the use of anterior chamber implants, especially in the setting of a traumatized eye, since "modern" angle-fixated implants, even when perfectly positioned, will have some contact with the delicate uveal tissue of the ciliary body band and may induce a low-grade chronic cyclitis and, perhaps, cystoid macular edema. Moreover, the relationship to the trabecular meshwork is of concern when traumatic glaucoma is present. A recent study reported *delayed-onset* pupil deformity in 58% of patients with a Kelman-style anterior chamber implant.[44] This may represent a chronic inflammatory or ischemic response. Furthermore, the anterior chamber implant lens optics may be smaller than the preferred 6 mm or larger diameter. These angle-fixated lenses vault anteriorly in front of the iris plane, making the effective coverage of the entrance pupil even smaller yet, thereby accentuating the possibility of unwanted visual phenomena (such as halos, arcs, and edge glare). In some countries outside of the United States anterior chamber iris fixated "claw" lenses are popular (Artisan, Ophtec, Groningan, Netherlands).

The patient with a traumatic cataract who also has a reasonably good visual prognosis should not be dismissed from consideration for acrylic-based presbyopia-correcting IOLs.

Plate haptic silicone implants should be avoided in traumatic cataract patients. They are unforgiving in cases of capsular and zonular asymmetry, which may not be apparent at the time of surgery and, should YAG capsulotomy be required, the small size of the posterior capsule opening desired to prevent posterior dislocation[45] may afford an inadequate view of the retinal periphery.

INTRAOCULAR LENS PLACEMENT

If the capsular bag retains its integrity, intracapsular placement of the implant is desirable. Even in the face of zonular damage, a few options exist for capsular fixation of the implant lens. As described previously, the capsular tension rings can be inserted at any stage of the procedure, providing that there is an intact anterior capsulorrhexis and the capsular bag is intact. If the ring is placed before complete cortical removal, special effort should be taken to avoid trapping cortical fibers in the fornix of the bag since they can be extremely difficult to remove. This is less problematic when the Ahmed segment is utilized, as the cortex can usually be stripped around either side of the 120° arc. If an endocapsular ring or segment is not available and only a small area of zonular dehiscence is present, one can orient the haptics of the implant along the axis of the weakness, unless it is obvious that the best centration is achieved in a different axis. Slowly unfolding the implant or gently placing a rigid lens will minimize the stress on the intact zonules.

Ciliary sulcus placement of a posterior chamber implant is still possible in the setting of a posterior capsular tear or zonular dialysis. If the anterior capsulorrhexis is intact, yet a severe posterior capsule break exists, the haptics should be placed in the sulcus and it may be possible to capture the lens optic posteriorly into the capsulorrhexis. This will provide adequate support and will prevent the lens from subsequently dislocating. If the capsulorrhexis is incompetent or larger than the implant optic then simple sulcus fixation with a large diameter implant can be utilized. If an inferior zonulolysis is present and capture within the rhexis is not possible, then suture fixation can add additional safety, since gravity may induce inferior lens migration over time (Figure 30-13).

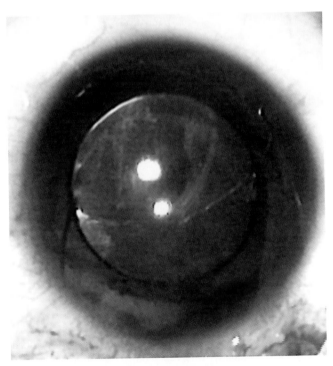

Figure 30-13 The posterior chamber intraocular lens (PC IOL) optic is captured within the capsulorrhexis. The capsule was stained with indocyanin green (ICG). The lower haptic is fixated to the sclera by a suture. With this double fixation method the implant was well entered and secure.

INTRAOCULAR LENSES AND CHILDREN

While many surgeons now commonly place intraocular lenses in children, the correction of aphakia in children remains somewhat controversial. Traumatic injuries typically affect only one eye and in uniocular aphakia, contact lens compliance may be even more poorly tolerated than in bilateral aphakes. Intraocular lenses can be safely tolerated in most children, even following trauma.[46] Intraocular lens implantation may be significantly easier at the time of cataract extraction than at a later date, since iridocapsular adhesions and fusion of the anterior and posterior capsular flaps make a subsequent secondary implant procedure more challenging. In cases where the posterior capsule remains intact, the presence of an implant may reduce the risk of posterior capsular opacity[47] and, should YAG laser capsulotomy be required, the implant will also prevent vitreous prolapse into the anterior segment. Furthermore, if we can extrapolate from the literature addressing implants in uveitic patients, an intraocular lens may decrease the chances of significant posterior synechiae.[48] Scleral sutured posterior chamber implant lenses have been used successfully in children, although the long-term integrity of prolene sutures is still unknown.[49] While the authors favor the use of implants in children, each surgeon must evaluate the merits of each implant option for each case. The informed consent discussion with the parent or guardian should include the fact that most intraocular lenses are still not approved by the FDA for use in children.

Some investigators in China have advocated the use of epikeratophakia for correction of pediatric aphakia following surgery for traumatic cataract. While they have had some promising successes, worldwide exprience with this approach is still limited. Epikeratophakia lenticules are currently not available in the United States.[50] The authors feel that, currently, intraocular lenses remain the best option for the pediatric aphakia.

IRIS REPAIR AND REPLACEMENT

Unless the iris damage is extensive, preventing access to the lens or interfering with the operative procedure, the repair of iris defects can follow cataract extraction and lens implantation steps. The pseudophakos is significantly thinner than the intumescent cataract and, therefore, the anterior chamber is deeper allowing for more working space. Also, the long needles used for iris repair may inadvertently engage lens capsule, cortex, or vitreous if the passes are placed early in the operative procedure. Gentle lysis of iridocapsular adhesions can be performed early; however, when the zonules are damaged, the iridocapsular adhesions may provide extra support during the capsulorrhexis and phacoemulsification.

Five types of iris injury can be present with trauma: holes, sphincter tears, iridodialyses, traumatic mydriasis, and partial or total loss of iris tissue. Repair of iris defects can be accomplished with transcameral 10-0 prolene sutures. A paracentesis location and orientation are selected so that passage of a long, curved needle can be easily directed toward the iris defect. The needle is gently wiggled into the paracentesis, taking care not to catch any stromal fibers. The tip of the needle engages one edge of the iris at the proximal margin of the tear. The tip then engages the distal iris leaflet (from the underside) and the needle is passed through the peripheral cornea. For iris sphincter tears, it is best to

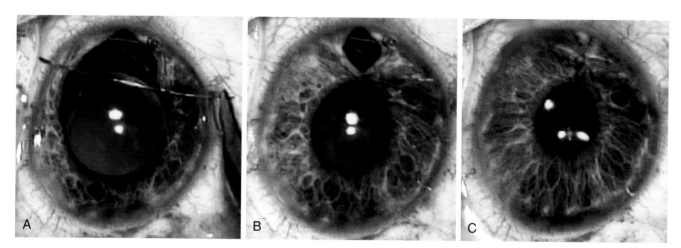

Figure 30-14 The cut margin of the iris sphincter is identified. **A,** A 10-0 prolene suture on a long, curved needle is passed through the iris margin of each iris leaflet and then passed out the distal limbus. **B,** As the suture knot is secured, the pupil begins to return to a more normal shape.

identify the cut margin at each side and to take a healthy bite of iris tissue (Figure 30-14). The suture can be tied within the anterior chamber with the sliding knot technique, as described by Steven Siepser, MD.[51] Orientation of the suture ends is particularly important so that the suture will create a knot and not just a twist as the two ends are drawn together (Figure 30-15). We typically will use a double throw followed by a single throw. A locking knot can be achieved by alternate suture throw orientation.[52] It is also possible to close an iris defect via a limbal incision using the basic technique described by McCannel.[53]

Iridodialysis can be repaired by passing each needle of a double armed 10-0 prolene suture through the disinserted peripheral iris, then out the scleral wall at the iris root.[54,55] The knot can be tied externally and rotated internally (Figure 30-16).

Traumatic mydriasis may result in postoperative glare from edge-related symptoms. A cerclage-type procedure can be performed to reduce the pupillary aperture.[56,57] While different techniques may be used to pass the suture through the iris tissue, each approach attempts to create either a segmental or circumferential purse-string of the iris margin.

When significant iris tissue has been lost, implantation of a diaphragm intraocular lens (Morcher and Ophtec), intracapsular iris rings (Morcher), occluding ring segments (Morcher), or the multipiece iris prosthetic system of Hermeking (Ophtec) should be considered. Details of iris supplements are beyond the scope of this chapter.

MEMBRANOUS CATARACT AND LONGSTANDING CHANGES

Occasionally, a patient may present for evaluation of a white or brunescent cataract many years after a penetrating injury has occurred. In some of these cases, a significant portion of the lens material may have been resorbed; thus, leaving little separation between the anterior and posterior capsules. Special caution will prevent inadvertent entry into the vitreous cavity. The surgeon may occasionally encounter a fibrotic or calcified capsule or lens

remnant requiring sharp incision and scissors dissection, and removal of the tough capsular material with the vitrector handpiece. Of benefit to the surgeon is the knowledge that longstanding traumatic capsular tears do not readily extend, as acute capsular tears tend to do.

■ DEMONSTRATIVE CASES ■

CASE ONE

A 14-year-old boy accidentally struck his right eye while cutting a piece of rubber with a carpet knife. He had a corneoscleral laceration extending from the superior limbus through cornea, iris, and lens. The laceration deviated paracentrally 1.5 mm around the corneal apex, severed the inferior limbus and ciliary body, and extended to just before the inferior rectus insertion. Vitreous was present at the limbus. The laceration was repaired primarily with automated vitrectomy performed at the scleral opening. Primary cataract extraction was not performed.

His clinical evaluation the next day revealed light perception vision with brisk identification of colored lights. The Purkinje phenomenon was present and no afferent defect was noted. The corneal wound was secure and the superior and inferior iris leaflets were bisected. A small amount of vitreous prolapse was noted at the inferior iris break. The anterior lens capsule was torn from the superior to inferior equatorial regions. B-scan ultrasonography showed a displaced rupture of the posterior crystalline lens (see Figure 30-1).

Problem list:

- Intumescent traumatic cataract
- Ruptured anterior capsule
- Ruptured posterior capsule
- Vitreous prolapse
- Lacerated iris
- Corneoscleral and ciliary body laceration (repaired).

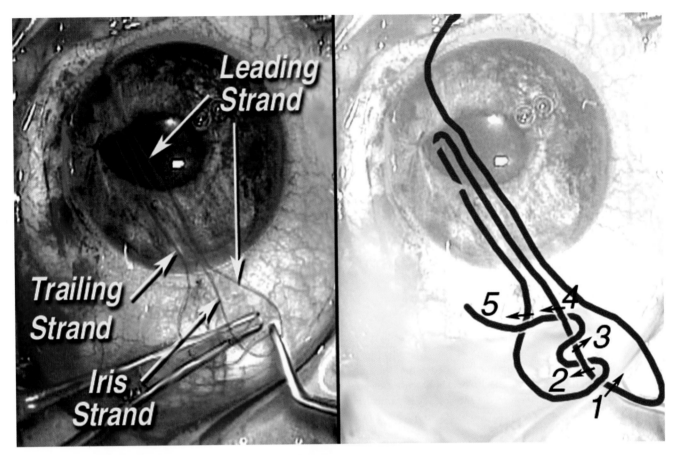

Figure 30-15 Tying the sliding suture knot requires meticulous attention to suture orientation. First, the suture loops should be laid out on the globe as shown with the strand coming from the iris margin (iris strand) adjacent to the free (trailing strand) end. The free end of the trailing strand is passed *down through* the retrieved loop (1), *under* the iris strand (2), *down through* the loop again (3), *under* the strand again (4), then *over* the trailing strand (5). The distal and proximal ends are pulled and the knot slides into the anterior chamber without causing any tension on the iris tissue. The knot is secured by a second retrieval and single or double throw.

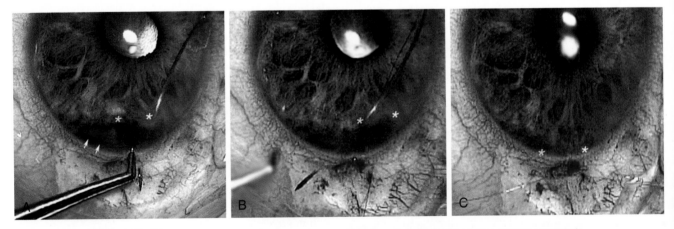

Figure 30-16 A, A double-armed 10-0 prolene suture on a long, curved needle is passed via a corneal paracentesis through the disinserted peripheral iris at the junction between the middle and outer thirds, then out at the level of the iris insertion at the scleral wall. The white asterisk identified the site of the first suture pass; the yellow asterisk identifies the intended site of the second pass. Note that the peripheral iris anatomy is distorted by the needle during the suture pass. B, The second arm of the suture is similarly passed, a few milimeters from the first. C, As the suture ends are pulled, the suture loop is pulled into and across the anterior chamber. D, The suture is tied, achieving closure of the iridodialysis.

The patient was brought back to the operating room 5 days later. A temporal wound site was chosen (the area of most normal anatomy). The corneal dome was filled with Viscoat Alcon, Fort Worth, Texas) and the anterior chamber was gently deepened with Healon (Pharmacia, Monrovia, California) in the "soft shell" technique. A 19-gauge cannula was placed via the superotemporal paracentesis site and the tip was placed into the peripheral lens material nasally where the lens anatomy was not damaged. Manual aspiration of lens material was undertaken in a "dry" fashion. Additional Healon was added serially to maintain the anterior chamber. The peripheral lens material was similarly removed from the temporal area via a nasal paracentesis. Viscoat was used to tamponade the anterior hyaloid centrally, allowing aspiration of the remaining central lens material. In this young boy, the soft lens nucleus was easily aspirated with a cannula alone. The area inferiorly around the prolapsed vitreous was carefully avoided. An inferotemporal pars plana sclerotomy was created and an automated vitrectomy was performed locally using irrigation via the superior paracentesis site. The small knuckle of vitreous was pulled back posteriorly and removed with the cutter device. The small bit of lens material in this region was removed with the vitrector handpiece. An acrylic foldable lens (MA60BM Acrysof, Alcon, Fort Worth, Texas) was placed into the ciliary sulcus, oriented horizontally, with excellent support. The iris was then repaired in a "closed chamber" sliding-knot technique. The viscoelastic was removed with the vitrector handpiece. Postoperative uncorrected visual acuity improved to 20/40.

CASE TWO

A 25-year-old man presented with light perception vision in his left eye after hammering a nail that hit his left eye. Examination showed vague light perception vision and a questionable afferent pupillary defect. Testing was limited by poor cooperation. Brief glimpses at the slit lamp showed a central corneal full-thickness laceration. The anterior chamber was deep with an admixture of fibrin, heme, and, possibly, vitreous. The pupillary outline was irregular, but central. The status of the lens could not be ascertained.

Problem list:

* Central corneal laceration
* Vitreous prolapse?
* Lens status?
* Status of anterior choroid/pars plana?

The patient was brought to the operating room and the corneal wound was closed under general anesthesia. Vitreous was present outside the corneal wound and was carefully removed at the level of the laceration with the automated cutter. The lens was not removed.

The following day, vision was counting fingers and the corneal wound was secure. Vitreous streamed through the inferior portion of the lens to the back of the cornea. Condensing fibrin filled the anterior chamber. The crystalline lens was obviously lacerated and was starting to turn white. B-scan showed a clear vitreous, an attached retina, and no suprachoroidal hemorrhage. Steroids, cycloplegics, and antibiotics were administered. A-scan

ultrasonography was performed on each eye and keratometry readings were obtained.

Problem list:

* Repaired central corneal laceration
* Vitreous through lens to posterior cornea
* Traumatic, lacerated cataract.

On post-injury day 4 the patient was brought to the operating room for cataract extraction, PC IOL implantation, and vitrectomy. A supero-temporal wound site was selected. The anterior segment anatomy was most normal superiorly and, additionally, a superotemporal incision would best offset the probability of future induced astigmatism from the corneal wound. (Typically, the steep axis will be perpendicular to the sutured laceration.) Two paracenteses were created, one superonasally and the other temporally. A bimanual (split irrigation) anterior vitrectomy was performed via these two sites to sever the bands of vitreous going to the corneal wound and to clear the vitreous from the anterior chamber. Healon GV was used to maintain the anterior chamber and for endothelial protection. The cataract material in the area of the lens laceration was removed with the vitrector handpiece on irrigation–aspiration cutter mode. This successfully cleared a view through the pupillary space. A pars plana sclerotomy was then created 3 mm posterior to the limbus and the remaining vitreous material was cleared from the pupillary and retropupillary space. The remaining lens material was removed with the vitrector on irrigation–aspiration cutter mode. Examination of the capsular remains showed no support inferiorly and inferonasally. It was elected to suture a 6 mm optic, single piece, PMMA posterior chamber implant to the ciliary sulcus. Miochol was instilled. The vitrector was used to remove the viscoelastic material from the anterior chamber.

The postoperative course was unremarkable and the patient achieved a suture-out 20/25 result with a $-3.25+3.25 \times 090$ correction, despite the central, apical corneal laceration. Topographic astigmatism was regular. Neither corneal transplant nor contact lens was required.

CASE THREE

A 66-year-old man sustained a blunt injury when a softball struck his right eye 2 years prior to evaluation. At his initial presentation, his right eye vision was counting fingers at 6 feet and his intraocular pressure was elevated to 36 mm Hg. An afferent pupillary defect was present. The slit-lamp finding showed a subluxated dense nuclear, cortical, and PSC cataract with obvious phacodonesis. Zonules were absent from 10 o'clock to 4 o'clock positions. Vitreous was prolapsed anteriorly around the lens equator and into the anterior chamber. A fundus exam showed a pale optic nerve head with no posterior segment details. Gonioscopy revealed 7 clock-hours of angle recession.

Problem list:

* Subluxated, dense traumatic cataract
* Vitreous prolapse
* Angle recession glaucoma.

The patient chose to undergo cataract extraction with endocapsular ring placement, IOL implantation, pars plana approach

CONCLUSION

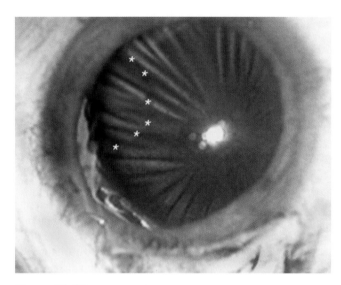

Figure 30-17 In this case of traumatic cataract, vitreous is prolapsed around the lens equator and into the anterior chamber. Asterisks outline pigment clumps along the edge of the prolapsed knuckle of vitreous *anterior* to the crystalline lens. The vitrector is placed behind the lens and the vitreous is pulled posteriorly out of the anterior chamber and removed with the cutter device. Folds in the lens capsule are not uncommon in cases of traumatic cataract.

anterior vitrectomy, and trabeculectomy. First, the trabeculectomy site was prepared with a fornix-based flap. A superonasal paracentesis was created for anterior–irrigation. A pars plana sclerotomy was performed 3 mm posterior to the 10:30 limbus. The prolapsed vitreous material was removed with the automated vitrector, pulling the vitreous back into the vitreous cavity (Figure 30-17). Viscoat (Alcon, Fort Worth, Texas) was placed to tamponade the remaining vitreous posterior to the lens. A capsulorrhexis was then performed and the lens nucleus was meticulously emulsified with a phaco-chop technique. The cortical material was aspirated with a Simcoe cannula and dry cortical stripping was performed. An endocapsular ring was placed. This resulted in nice recentration of the capsular bag. An acrylic implant (Acrysof MA60BM, Alcon, Fort Worth, Texas) was placed intracapsularly. The scleral tunnel was then pedunculated to create a scleral flap and several punches were taken from the posterior scleral rim. The flap was secured with releasable sutures and conjuctiva was closed. The final postoperative vision was 20/20 and intraocular pressure was 16 mm Hg. The patient retained this result at 2 year follow-up.

■ CONCLUSION ■

Traumatic cataracts vary widely in nature, presentation, and degree of ocular comorbidity. With careful clinical evaluation and meticulous attention to surgical technique, these cases can often yield excellent visual, functional and cosmetic results. In fact, rehabilitation of these challenging cases can often be among the most gratifying services provided to patients.

References

[1] Bulluck JD, Ballal DR, Johnson DA, et al. Ocular and orbital trauma from water balloon slingshots. A clinical, epidemiological, and experimental study. Ophthalmology 1997;104:878–887.
[2] McDermott ML, Shin DH, Hughes BH, et al. Anterior segment trauma and air bags. Arch Ophthalmol 1995;113:1567–1568.
[3] Karp CL, Fazio JR. Traumatic cataract presenting with unilateral nasal hemianopsia. J Cataract Refract Surg 1999;25:1302–1303.
[4] Zabriskie NA, Hwang IP, Ramsey JF, et al. Anterior lens capsule rupture caused by air bag trauma. Am J Ophthalmol 1997;123:832–833.
[5] Angra SK, Vajpayee RB, Titiyal JS, et al. Types of posterior capsular breaks and their implications. Opthalmic Surg 1991;22:388–391.
[6] Netland KE, Martinez J, LaCour 3rd OJ, Netland PA. Traumatic anterior lens dislocation: a case report. J Emerg Med 2000;19:73–74.
[7] Sathish S, Chakrabarti A, Prajna V. Traumatic subconjunctival dislocation of the crystalline lens and its surgical management. Ophthalmic Surg Lasers 1999;30:684–686.
[8] Boorstein JM, Titelbaum DS, Patel Y, et al. CT diagnosis of unsuspected traumatic cataract in patients with complicated eye injuries: significance of attenuation value of the lens. Am J Roentgenol 1995;164:181–184.
[9] Almog Y, Reider-Grosswasser I, Goldstein M, et al. "The disappearing lens": failure of CT to image the lens in traumatic intumescent cataract. J Comput Assist Tomogr 1999;23:354–356.
[10] Rubsanen PE, Irvine WD, McCuen BW, et al. Primary intraocular lens implantation in the setting of penetrating ocular trauma. Ophthalmology 1995;102:101–107.
[11] Pieramici DJ, Capone A, Rabsame PE, et al. Lens preservation after intraocular foreign body injuries. Ophthalmology 1996;103:1563–1567.
[12] O'Duffy D, Salmon JF. Siderosis bulbi resulting from an intralenticular foreign body. Am J Ophthalmol 1999;2:218–219.
[13] Jonas JB, Budde WM. Early versus late removal of retained intraocular foreign bodies. Retina 1999;19:193–197.
[14] Speaker MG, Guerriero PN, Met JA, et al. A case controlled study of risk factors for intraoperative suprachoroidal expulsive hemorrhage. Ophthalmology 1991;98:202–209.
[15] Arnold PN. Study of acute intraoperative suprachoroidal hemorrhage. J Cataract Refract Surg 1992;18:489–494.
[16] Osher RH. Complications – the torn posterior capsule: management principles. Video J Cataract Refract Surg 1991;8.
[17] Fukagawa K, Tsubota K, Kimura C, et al. Corneal endothelial cell loss induced by air bags. Ophthalmology 1993;100:1819–1823.
[18] Arshinoff SA. Dispersive-cohesive viscoelastic soft shell technique. J Cataract Refract Surg 1999;25:167–173.
[19] Osher RH, Cionni RJ. The torn posterior capsule: its intraoperative behavior, surgical management, and long-term consequences. J Cataract Refract Surg 1990;16:490–494.
[20] Krag S, Thim K, Corydon L, et al. Biomechanical aspects of the anterior capsulotomy. J Cataract Refract Surg 1994;20:410–416.
[21] Andreo LK, Wilson ME, Apple DJ. Elastic properties and scanning electron microscopic appearance of manual continuous curvilinear capsulorrhexis and vitrectorrhexis in an animal model of pediatric cataract. J Cataract Refract Surg 1999;25:534–539.
[22] Fenzl R. Avoiding the complication cascade. In: Gills JP, editor. Cataract surgery: the state of the art. Thorofare, NJ: Slack, Inc.: 1998. p. 130–131.
[23] Prieto I, Cabral I, Rogue J. Capsular staining–Gentian violet. Vid J Catarct Refract Surg 1999;XV(2).
[24] Melles GR, deWaard PW, Pameyer JH, et al. Trypan blue capsule staining to visualize capsulorrhexis in cataract surgery. J Cataract Refract Surg 1999;25:7–9.
[25] Horiguchi M, Miyake K, Ohta Y, et al. Staining of the lens capsule for continuous circular capsulorrhexis in eyes with white cataract. Arch Ophthalmol 1998;116:535–537.
[26] Newsom TH, Oetting TA. Indocyanine green staining in traumatic cataract. J Cataract Refract Surg 2000;26:1691–1693.
[27] Marques DM, Marques FF, Osher RH. Three-step technique for staining the anterior lens capsule with indocyanine green or trypan blue. J Cataract Refract Surg 2004;30:13–16.
[28] Wainwright M, Phoenix DA, Rice L, et al. Increased cytotoxicity and phototoxicity in the methylene blue series via chromophore methylation. J Photochem Photobiol B 1997;40:233–239.
[29] Metz G. Lens induced glaucoma. J Catarct Refract Surg 1986;2. [audiovisual].
[30] Gimbel HV, Willerscheidt AB. What to do with limited view: the intumescent cataract. J Cataract Refract Surg 1993;19:657–661.
[31] Osher RH. Slow motion phacoemulsification approach [letter; comment]. J Cataract Refract Surg 1993;19:667.
[32] Cionni RJ, Osher RH, Solomon K. The Cionni ring. Vid J Catarct Refract Surg 1998;14.
[33] Hasanee K, Butler M, Ahmed II. Capsular tension rings and related devices: current concepts. Curr Opin Ophthalmol 2006;17:31–41. [review].
[34] Ahmed II, Chen SH, Kranemann C, Wong DT. Surgical repositioning of dislocated capsular tension rings. Ophthalmology 2005;112:1725–1733.
[35] Camponella PC, Aminlari A, DeMaio R. Traumatic Cataract and Weigert's ligament. Ophthalmic Surgery and Lasers 1997;28:422–423.
[36] Yasukawa T, Kita M, Honda Y. Traumatic cataract with a ruptured posterior capsule from a non-penetrating ocular injury. J Cataract Refract Surg 1998;24:868–869.
[37] Thomas R. Posterior capsular rupture after blunt trauma. J Cataract Refract Surg 1998;24:283–284.
[38] Rao SK, Parikh S, Padhmanabhan P. Isolated posterior capsule rupture in blunt trauma: pathogenesis and management. Ophthalmimc Surgery and Lasers 1998;29:338–342.
[39] Osher RH. Surgery of the loose cataract. Vid J Catarct Refract Surg 1989;5.
[40] Kelman C. Posterior capsular rupture: PAL Technique. Vid J Catarct Refract Surg 1996;12.
[41] Eller AW, Barad RF. Miyake analysis of anterior vitrectomy techniques. J Cataract Refract Surg 1996;22:213–217.
[42] Khawly JA, Lambert RJ, Jaffe GJ. Intraocular lens changes after short- and long-term exposure to intraocular silicone oil. An in vivo study. Ophthalmology 1998;105:1227–1233.
[43] Bartz-Schmidt KU, Kirchhof B, Heimann K. Condensation on IOL's during fluid–air exchange. Ophthalmology 1996;103:199. [letter].
[44] Sawada T, Kimura W, Kimura T, et al. Long-term follow-up of primary anterior chamber intraocular lens implantation. J Cataract Refract Surg 1998;24:1515–1520.
[45] Dick B, Schwenn O, Stoffelns B, et al. Late dislocation of a plate haptic silicone lens into the vitreous body after Nd:YAG capsulotomy. A case report. Ophthalmologe 1998;95:181–185.
[46] Churchill AJ, Noble BA, Etchells DE, George NJ. Factors affecting visual outcome following uniocular traumatic cataract. Eye 1995;9:285–291.
[47] Ram J, Apple DJ, Peng Q, et al. Update on fixation of rigid and foldable posterior chamber intraocular lenses. Part II: choosing the correct haptic fixation and intraocular lens design to help eradicate posterior capsule opacification. Ophthalmology 1999;106:891–900.
[48] Holland GN, Van Horn SD, Margolis TP. Cataract surgery with ciliary sulcus fixation of intraocular lenses in patients with uveitis. Am J Ophthalmol 1999;128:21–30.

[49] Lam SC, Joan SK, Fan DS, et al. Short-term results of scleral sutured intraocular lens fixation in children. J Cataract Refract Surg 1998;24:1474–1479.

[50] Feng C, Chen J, Liu H, Chen L, Chen H. The preliminary report of epikeratophakia in the treatment of pediatric aphakia after traumatic cataract extraction. Yan Ke Xue Bao 1997;13:38–40.

[51] Seipser SP. The closed chamber slipping suture technique for iris repair. Ann Ophthalmology 1994;26:71–72.

[52] Osher RH, Snyder ME, Cionni RJ. Modification of the Siepser slip-knot technique. J Cataract Refract Surg 2005;31:1098–1100.

[53] McCannel M. A retrievable suture idea for anterior uveal problems. Ophthalmic Surg 1976;7:98–103.

[54] Wachler BB, Krueger RR. Double-armed McCannel suture for repair of traumatic iridodialysis. Am J Ophthalmol 1996;122:109–110.

[55] Kaufman SC, Insler MS. Surgical repair of traumatic iridodialysis. Ophthalmic Surg and Lasers 1996;27:963–966.

[56] Osher RH. Consultation section. J Cataract Refract Surg 1994;20:665–669.

[57] Ogawa GS. The iris cerclage suture for permanent mydriasis: a running suture technique. Ophthalmic Surg Lasers 1998;29:1001–1009.

CONCLUSION

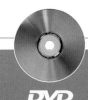

Iris Repair

Michael E. Snyder, MD, Roger F. Steinert, MD, Christopher Khng, MD and Scott E. Burk, MD, PhD

31

IRIS RECONSTRUCTION

CONTENTS

CHAPTER HIGHLIGHTS

Iris abnormalities that present in conjunction with cataract or intraocular lens (IOL) surgery are usually the result of accidental or surgical trauma. Less commonly, the iris abnormalities may be congenital, such as an iris coloboma or corectopia, or the abnormality may be the result of a later-onset degenerative process.

Penetrating injuries of the cornea or anterior sclera may result in iris injury from direct laceration or as a consequence of iris prolapse through the wound. Blunt, nonpenetrating trauma to the anterior segment may also injure the iris.[1-3] The most common patterns of iris injury after severe blunt trauma are localized sphincter tears, generalized sphincter paralysis, and dialysis of the iris root.[4]

Preservation of iris tissue and restoration of normal iris architecture are important for two principal reasons. Most importantly, the optical performance of the eye is highly dependent on the pupillary aperture. Higher order optical aberrations and lens edge effects, in particular, are more prominent at larger pupil apertures.

A large and nonreactive pupil results in photophobia and glare. In addition, aberrations from the peripheral cornea, as well as the peripheral IOL and/or exposed capsule, can be highly disturbing to the functional vision of a patient. Pupillary distortions are better tolerated by a patient with a clear crystalline lens than a pseudophakic patient because the IOL has a substantially smaller optical diameter than the crystalline lens.

The first step in the management of traumatic iris abnormalities is, therefore, to minimize further damage to the iris and to preserve as much iris tissue as possible. Prolapsed iris tissue does not necessarily need to be excised; the surgeon performing the primary repair must judge the likelihood of microbial contamination of the iris before sacrificing a prolapsed iris.

■ IRIS RECONSTRUCTION ■

SURGICAL PRINCIPLES OF IRIS SUTURING

Although iris deformities have an infinite number of possible configurations, the basic principles of surgical repair can be summarized in a few basic techniques.

Principle 1: Mobilization

The first principle is to free up and mobilize as much iris tissue as possible. Synechia to the cataract or capsule should be bluntly dissected. Most iridocapsular adhesions are strongly attached only at the sphincter edge. Often there is some proliferation of iris pigment epithelium from the posterior iris surface to the capsule involving the more peripheral iris, but these adhesions are weak and can be easily separated with an instrument such as a cyclodialysis spatula or a cannula with viscoelastic agent. If iridocapsular adhesions cannot be bluntly dissected, then careful excision with a scissors or blade should be performed, preserving as much iris tissue as possible by taking care not to excise any iris tissue that is salvageable.

After freeing up all iridocapsular adhesions, the surgeon should then release any peripheral adhesions. Peripheral anterior synechia usually can be released with traction using forceps or a pointed hook such as a Sinskey hook or Osher Y hook or by sweeping maneuvers with a spatula. In addition, inflammation sometimes causes the iris stroma to form adhesions internally, causing contraction of the iris in a manner similar to accordion pleats. Again, gentle traction can release many of these adhesions and produce a surprising amount of iris tissue necessary for the subsequent repair. Mobilization of iris tissue from peripheral synechiae is illustrated later in Case Studies 1, 2, and 5.

Principle 2: Intraocular Suturing and Knot Tying

The second fundamental principle is the method for suturing iris and tying knots within the eye. Often the knot is central, and traction to bring the iris with the knot to a limbal wound will damage the iris repair. Figure 31-1 illustrates the basic technique for passing the suture into the anterior chamber via a paracentesis, through a radially oriented iris defect, and then out through the peripheral cornea on the opposite side of the paracentesis. In all cases, a non-biodegradable suture material should be used. The most common suture employed is 10-0 polypropylene (Prolene). A long, gently curved needle is typically used. The Ethicon CIF-4 needle is strong and relatively easy to control. Although it has a noncutting needle tip, the bulk of the needle has the disadvantage of leaving a small

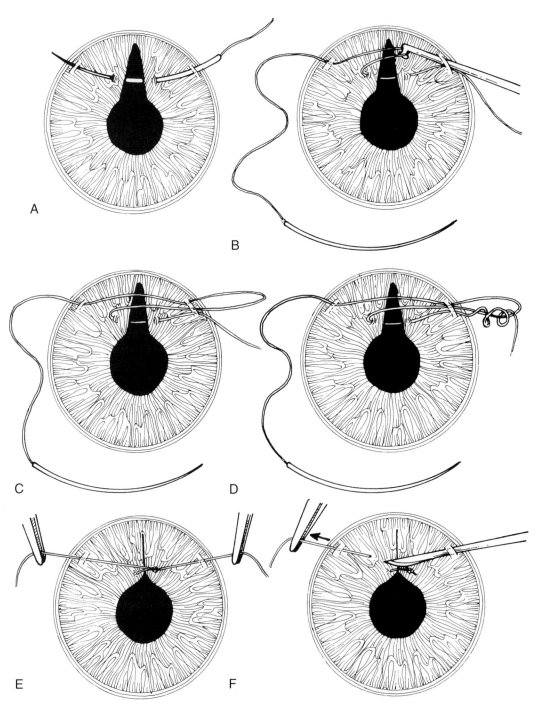

Figure 31-1 A, Long needle enters through a paracentesis, across the iris defect, and exits by puncturing through the peripheral cornea. **B,** Hook such as a Kuglen hook retrieves a loop of the distal arm of the suture, making sure that the needle end of the suture remains external to the eye. **C,** Loop is now external through the paracentesis. **D,** Proximal end of the suture is wrapped around the suture loop twice, creating one throw of what will become the knot. **E,** Tension on each end of the suture draws the knot into the eye and tightens it. **F,** After four throws, the suture ends are cut with a thin sharp knife such as a Wheeler blade. (Technique credited to Steven Siepser, MD.)

new iris puncture defect in its path. Finer needles that create less of an iris defect but are correspondingly more difficult to handle are the Ethicon CTC-6 (curved) and STC-6 (straight).

A flaccid iris and a knot close to a wound may allow the surgeon to tie the knot at the limbus without undue iris damage. Successful completion of many cases of iris reconstruction requires that no additional traction be placed on the iris, however. The knot must be advanced into the eye and tied internally. One method to accomplish a knot deep inside the anterior chamber is to form the knot loop externally and then use a hook such as a Kuglen hook to advance the loop into the eye and make it snug. The procedure is repeated three or four times, achieving a secure knot at completion. The disadvantage of this technique is that it requires a skilled assistant, as it is necessary to maintain gentle traction on each of the suture ends while simultaneously advancing the knot with the hook. Three skilled hands are, therefore, needed.

Figure 31-1 illustrates an alternative two-handed technique popularized by Stephen Siepser, MD. In this variation, the knot is tied by passing loops externally, but the two ends of the suture can then be tightened, which draw the knot internally into the eye. This technique is elegant and does not require the third hand of a skilled assistant. A second throw is typically placed. In the original description by Seipser, the second throw creates a "granny" knot. Osher teaches a true locking knot in which the second throw is passed either in mirror image of suture orientation or in the opposite direction around the suture loop to create a more "square" locking knot.[5] Once the knot is tied, the suture may be cut using micro scissors through an unenlarged paracentesis, or with Vannas' scissors through a slightly enlarged limbal incision.

Principle 3: Reattachment of Iris to Sclera

The third principle is the technique for repair of a peripheral iris defect with the use of horizontal mattress sutures. A double-armed suture is employed. The mattress suture brings the iris back to its origin, if possible (Figure 31-2), or closes a peripheral defect using available adjacent iris tissue (Figures 31-3A and B). The knot is tied externally but then rotated below the surface so

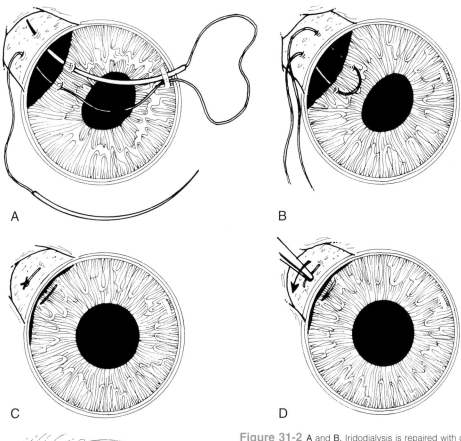

A

B

C

D

E

Figure 31-2 A and B, Iridodialysis is repaired with one or more mattress sutures of double-armed 10-0 polypropylene sutures tied externally under a conjunctival flap. Both arms of the polypropylene suture are introduced through a paracentesis opening on the opposite side of the anterior chamber. The dialyzed edge of iris is engaged by each needle in turn, and the needle is passed through the sclera. C, Mattress suture is tied. D, Knot is rotated below the surface of the sclera, preventing later suture erosion through the conjunctiva. E, Conjunctival flap is then closed over the polypropylene mattress suture with corner sutures of 8-0 Vicryl or other absorbable suture material.

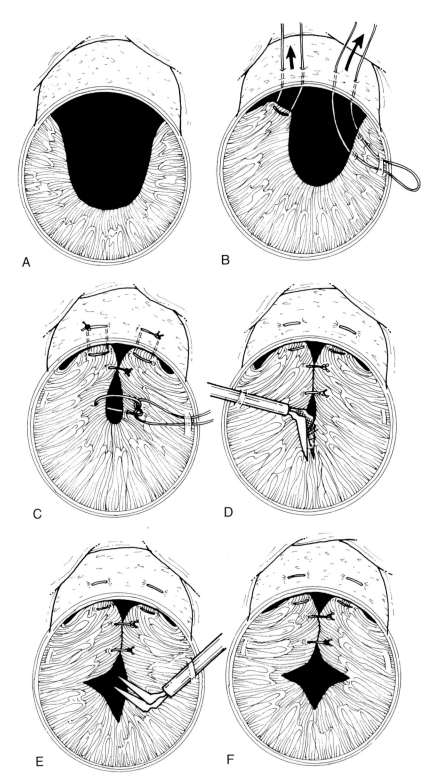

Figure 31-3 A, Conjunctival flap is recessed in the area of a sector iris defect. **B,** Horizontal mattress sutures bring midperipheral iris tissue into the basal area without iris. **C,** Interrupted sutures close the midperipheral space. **D–F,** "Sphincterotomies" in the central zone create a new pupillary aperture.

that only a smooth loop of external suture remains. By using this technique of suture rotation and burying the knot, identical to the concept used in transscleral suturing of secondary posterior chamber (PC) IOLs (see Chapter 41, Figure 41-2), only a smooth loop of suture material remains. A scleral flap does not need to be dissected, and conjunctiva alone provides adequate coverage of the suture material. Alternatively, if it is desired that both suture material and knot lie below the scleral surface, then creating a scleral groove with a beaver blade before placement of the sutures can be helpful. This allows the suture material to lie in a trench beneath the scleral surface when the knot is tied. The knot can similarly be rotated into the sclera. A large iridodialysis will require several adjacent horizontal mattress sutures. The size of each suture "bite" of iris should be about 1½ clock hours.

A large defect may require a combination of these techniques (see Figure 31-3). Typically the repair begins by using horizontal mattress sutures to create as much coverage of the peripheral and midperipheral cornea as possible (see Figures 31-3A and B). Often, this results in a distortion of the pupil itself (see Figure 31-3C). A new pupil is constructed by judicious incisions in the iris and placement of additional sutures (see Figures 31-3C–F). Case Studies 3 and 4 particularly illustrate these techniques. The iris is highly visible in some individuals and often important to the patient cosmetically.

In general, the surgeon should err on the side of leaving a pupil too small rather than too big. Postoperatively, a surgeon can use the neodymium:yttrium-aluminum-garnet (Nd:YAG) laser to expand the pupil by performing sphincterotomies with Nd:YAG laser pulses. The technique is similar to peripheral iridectomies with the Nd:YAG laser. A focusing contact lens is helpful. The laser setting is typically 6 mJ.

Principle 4: Pupil Repair

Blunt trauma often causes injury to the iris sphincter. An isolated rupture of the sphincter muscle is repaired with single interrupted sutures, similar to the technique illustrated in Figures 31-1 and 31-2. Case Study 1 illustrates the repair of local sphincter damage with interrupted sutures. When there is more generalized damage to the iris sphincter, caused by either multiple ruptures or ischemia, a different technique is needed. The surgeon can generally determine by careful preoperative inspection whether generalized iris sphincter injury has occurred. At the slit lamp examination, while varying the illumination through the pupil, the surgeon can inspect whether there is reactivity of the iris sphincter. In addition, the iris sphincter architecture is carefully inspected. When the iris sphincter architecture is not preserved and there is little to no reactivity, then a larger-scale repair of the pupil is needed.

The surgeon has two choices. The simpler choice is to place multiple interrupted sutures. This will typically result in a square or diamond-shaped pupil (Figure 31-4). Although cosmetically suboptimal, the optical benefit to the patient is substantial.

Alternatively, the surgeon can perform a 360° purse-string suture. This procedure was originally demonstrated by Dr. Pius Bucher of Austria and is illustrated in Case Study 6. The placement of the suture occurs after the completion of any cataract removal and IOL placement, of course. In the iris cerclage purse-string suture technique, a 10-0 Prolene suture on a CTC-6 needle (Ethicon) is recommended. In addition to the larger principal incision used for the cataract and IOL surgery, the surgeon should place two or three paracentesis openings at approximately equally spaced intervals. The needle is introduced through the principal incision and is passed in and out of the midperipheral iris stroma, typically for three or four passes. The needle is then passed out of the paracentesis by "docking" the needle tip into the end of a blunt 27-gauge irrigating cannula that has been passed through the paracentesis into the anterior chamber. In this manner, the pointed needle can be externalized without engaging the corneal tissue around the paracentesis. The needle is then regrasped with the needle holder and reintroduced into the eye, repeating the process for another quadrant or third of the iris. In reintroducing the needle through the paracentesis, great care must be taken not to inadvertently engage the lip of Descemet's membrane or any of the stroma. It is of great help during needle reintroduction to wiggle and side-sweep the needle tip while advancing the needle within the paracentesis to ensure that no corneal stromal fibers are engaged. If the

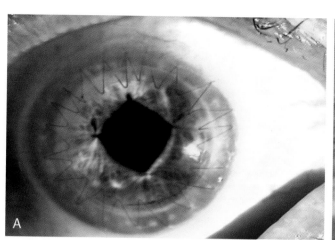
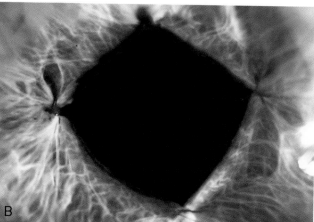

Figure 31-4 A, Diamond-shaped appearance of the pupil after four interrupted sutures reduced a large atonic pupil at the time of penetrating keratoplasty. **B,** High magnification shows the four polypropylene suture knots.

surgeon encounters difficulty passing the tip of the needle through the paracentesis cleanly, placement of some viscoelastic in the paracentesis can be a great aid in opening the passageway.

In one approach the bites of the cerclage suture are placed in the midperipheral iris, not close to the pupillary margin. The reason is that, once the suture is tightened, the suture between each of the bites will tighten and constrict. If the suture bites are near the pupillary edge, the suture material will be pulled into the pupillary opening, resulting in scalloping and a petalloid appearance to the pupil border. In contrast, if the suture material is kept in the midperiphery, the suture material itself will not be able to cross over the pupillary zone itself. In an alternate approach, the sutures bite are passed near the sphincter margin in a "spiral or baseball" stitch fashion in which the majority of the bites are placed through the iris tissue from the underside, then the needle tip is wrapped around the pupil margin and the next bite is taken. Both approaches result in an excellent cosmetic and functional result. If there is any difficulty controlling the passage of the needle through the iris tissue, micro forceps, such as those used for bi-axial microincision surgery, introduced through a paracentesis may be helpful by grabbing iris tissue during the needle pass.

After completing the 360° passage of the suture, the knot is carefully tied through the principal limbal incision. Alternatively, the needle can be passed out through a paracentesis, and the suture tied through the main incision using the Siepser sliding knot technique. The pupil is drawn down to a size of 3–4 mm, which is a good compromise between cosmetic and functional result, and fundus visualization. During knot tying, pulling on the suture ends often results in a smaller than desired pupil size, and it is often helpful to deliberately start with a pupil size that is larger than required, and then draw it down to size, The postoperative appearance of the pupil is usually circular or only slightly irregular.

If a major retinal problem occurs subsequently, such as retinal detachment, the iris cerclage suture can be released with either laser spots or intraoperatively by cutting the suture.

Adjunctive pupil repair techniques are useful in situations where the pupil is distorted or eccentric. Pupil distortion and ovalization may occur resulting from trauma itself, or sometimes after repair of an iris dialysis. This may be remedied by the strategic placement of an interrupted suture to the pupil margin, with or without pupil sculpting techniques to round it off. Pupil reshaping may be achieved with a vitrector on the lowest available cut rate and moderate vacuum, or by using intraocular scissors. If the pupil is markedly eccentric, the pupil may be translocated by opening up a new pupil in the center with a vitrector, and closing the peripheral one with one or more interrupted sutures.

■ CASE STUDIES IN IRIS RECONSTRUCTION ■

CASE 1: TRAUMATIC MYDRIASIS CAUSED BY LOCALIZED SPHINCTER RUPTURE

This patient had blunt trauma from a paintball gun injury, resulting in cataract and traumatic mydriasis (Figure C1-1). Preoperative slit-lamp examination showed that the sphincter muscle had ruptured temporally with atrophy of the sphincter in that region and that the remainder of the sphincter muscle reacted normally to light. After cataract surgery and IOL implantation, a Y-hook was used to bring the iris tissue out of the angle (Figure C1-2). Repair of the temporal iris consisted of placing two interrupted 10-0 polypropylene sutures (Figures C1-3–C1-6, surgeon's view temporally). One day after surgery, a reasonably well-centered pupil was present, centered over the IOL (Figure C1-7, slit-lamp view).

CASE 2: AIRBAG INJURY

A severely eccentric pupil and cataract resulted from an airbag injury in a motor-vehicle accident. The iris appeared absent inferotemporally (Figure C2-1). Preoperative gonioscopy showed that the iris appeared bunched up into the angle of the area corresponding to the pupil abnormality (Figure C2-2). The surgical photos are from the surgeon's perspective, sitting superiorly. At surgery, the severely subluxated lens had been removed by pars plana lensectomy and vitrectomy (Figure C2-3). A posterior chamber IOL with a 7 mm optic was secured through transscleral

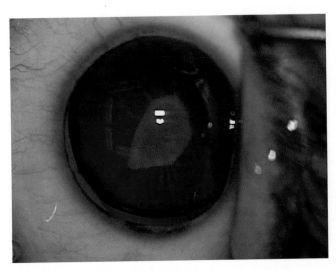

Figure C1-1

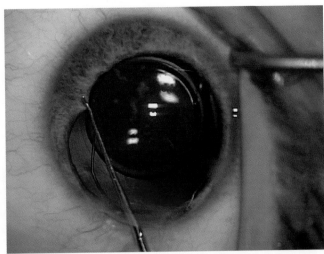

Figure C1-2

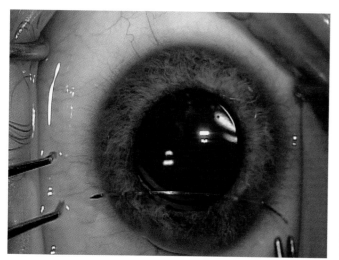

Figure C1-3

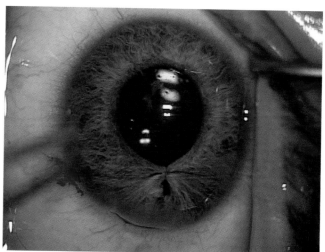

Figure C1-4

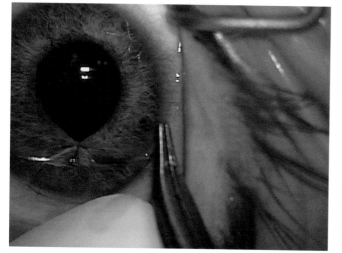

Figure C1-5

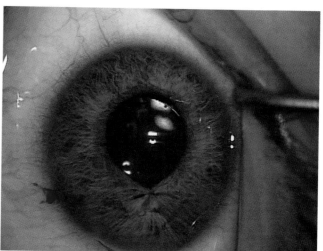

Figure C1-6

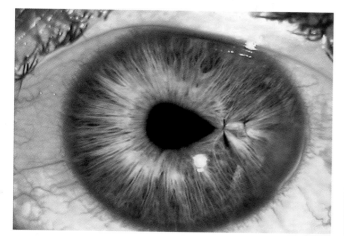

Figure C1-7

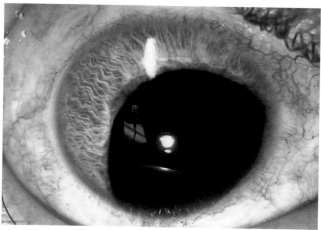

Figure C2-1

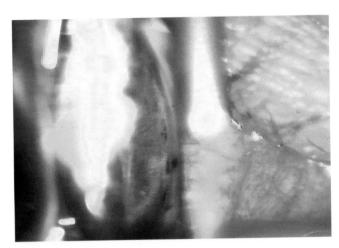

Figure C2-2

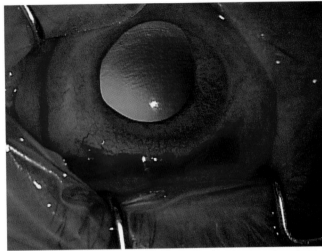

Figure C2-3

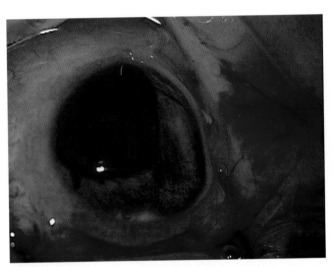

Figure C2-4

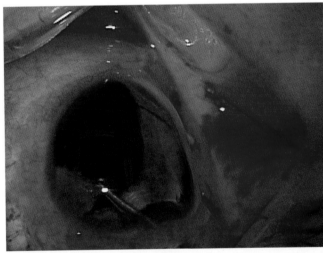

Figure C2-5

sutures, deliberately decentered in the direction of the pupil deformity in case the pupil cannot be fully shifted centrally (Figure C2-4). Repair of the iris began with traction on the peripheral iris to release adhesions, taking care to avoid dialysis of the iris root (Figures C2-5–C2-7), markedly improving the amount of peripheral iris tissue, but leaving a nonreactive pupil that was still large enough to cause glare (Figure C2-8). A single interrupted suture across the inferotemporal pupil (Figure C2-9) reduced the pupil to an acceptable size and shape (Figure C2-10).

CASE 3: SECTOR IRIS DEFECT AFTER MELANOMA EXCISION

A slowly expanding iris melanoma, observed and documented for over a decade, threatened to invade the angle in a patient with developing cataract (Figures C3-1 and C3-2). The surgeon sat superiorly (Figure C3-3) to have a better angle of access for

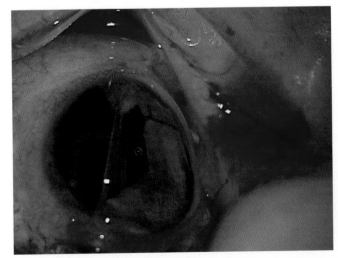

Figure C2-6

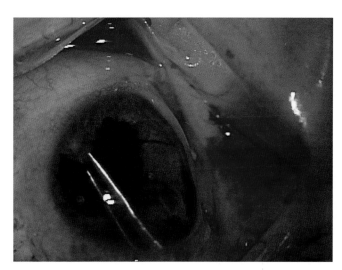

Figure C2-7

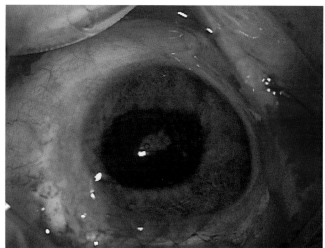

Figure C2-8

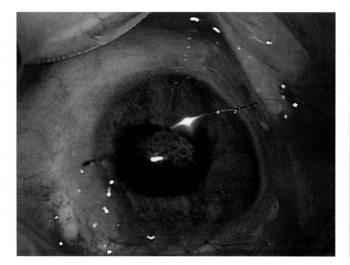

Figure C2-9

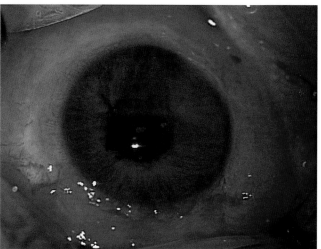

Figure C2-10

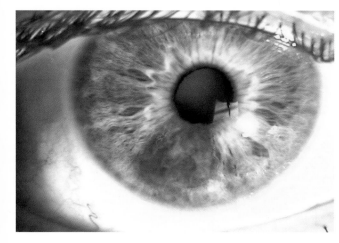

Figure C3-1

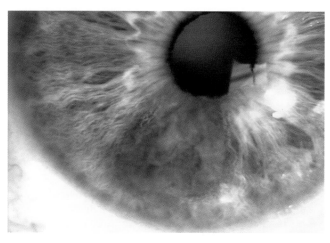

Figure C3-2

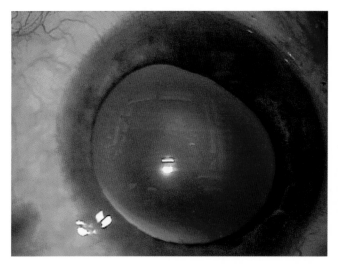

Figure C3-3

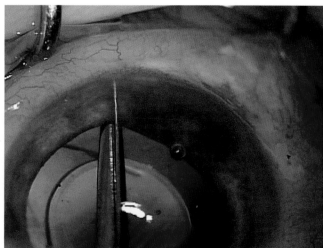

Figure C3-4

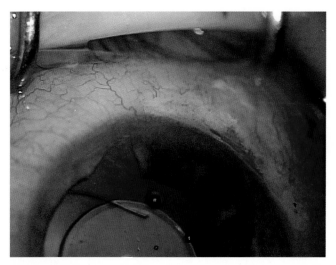

Figure C3-5

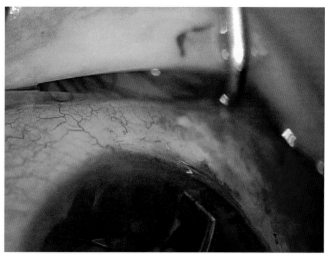

Figure C3-6

excising the tumor after phacoemulsification cataract extraction and capsular bag placement of a PC IOL in this right eye.

The melanoma was isolated first with radial incisions by a Gills-Vannas scissors, with a small margin of normal iris (Figures C3-4 and C3-5). The basal iris was excised as close as possible to the angle using horizontal vitreous scissors (Figures C3-6 and C3-7) and the tumor placed on a sterile tongue blade (Figure C3-8) to maintain a flat orientation for pathologic examination.

The reconstruction began with a 10-0 polypropylene suture reapproximating the sphincter edges (Figures C3-9 and C3-10). Note how much larger the defect became because of relaxations of the iris, compared with the original area of excision (Figure C3-4). A second suture added reinforcement (Figures C3-11 and C3-12), but it became apparent that a large basal defect would persist that, given the exposed inferior location, would be a source of glare.

To close the basal defect, a double-armed 10-0 polypropylene suture was passed in a horizontal mattress orientation (Figures C3-13 and C3-14) through the iris and the limbus, which closed

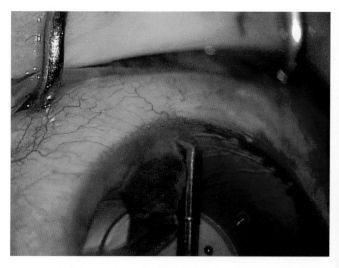

Figure C3-7

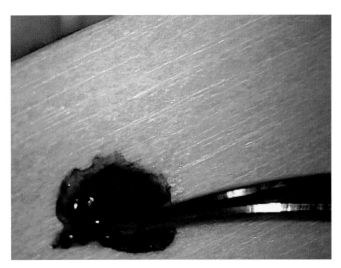

Figure C3-8

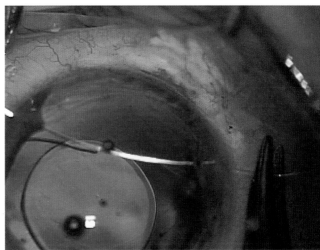

Figure C3-9

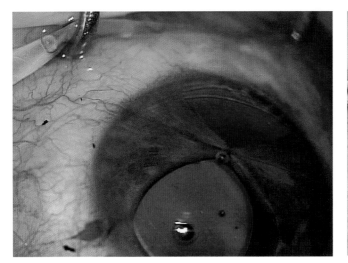

Figure C3-10

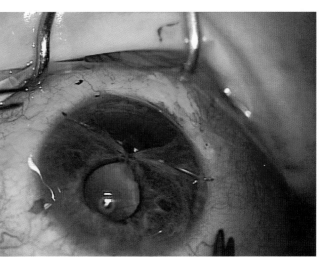

Figure C3-11

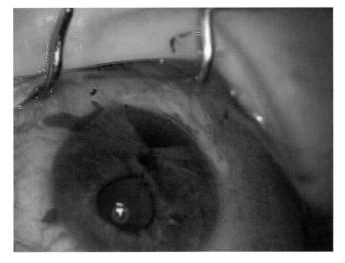

Figure C3-12

the basal defect when tied (Figure C3-15). The knot was rotated beneath the scleral surface to prevent later erosion through the conjunctiva (Figure C3-16).

As a consequence, the pupil was shifted eccentrically. Two additional sutures closed the eccentric opening (Figures C3-17 and C3-18), restoring a nearly round and well-centered pupil (Figure C3-19). The appearance on the first postoperative day showed a somewhat small pupil (Figure C3-20), but the patient had no complaints of dark vision. It is better to err on the side of leaving the pupil too small at the time of the surgical repair, as later expansion of the pupil can be achieved easily with laser sphincterotomies (see Chapter 52) and/or lysis of a suture.

CASE 4: IRIS LOSS AT CATARACT SURGERY

This patient experienced iris prolapse and subsequent bleeding from the iris root during an attempted implantation of a phakic

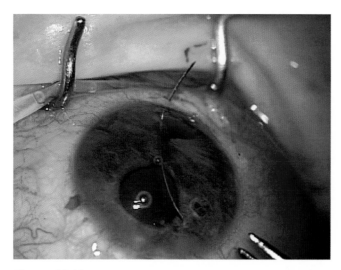

Figure C3-13

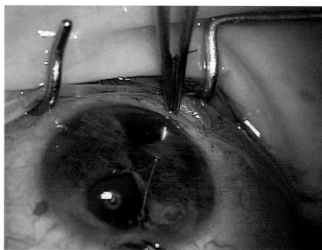

Figure C3-14

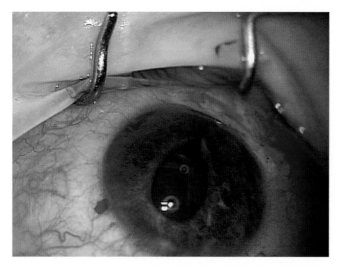

Figure C3-15

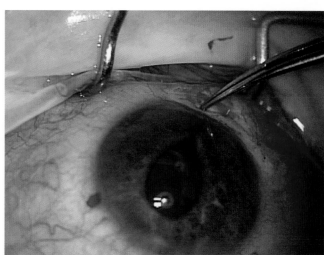

Figure C3-16

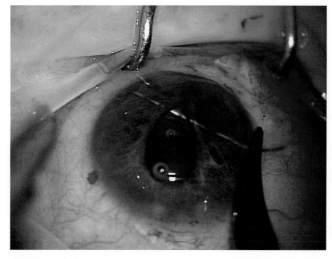

Figure C3-17

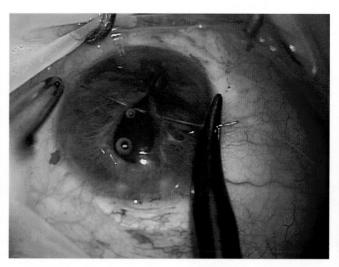

Figure C3-18

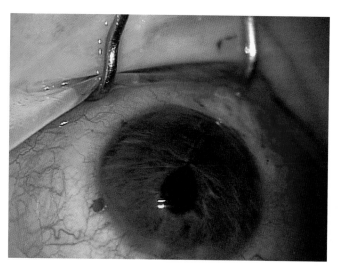

Figure C3-19

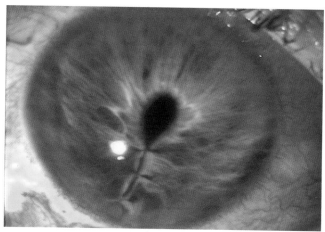

Figure C3-20

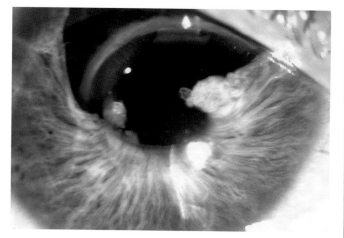

Figure C4-1

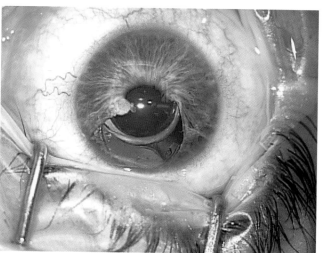

Figure C4-2

IOL for the correction of high hyperopia. A secondary cataract developed, and uncomplicated cataract surgery with PC IOL implantation was performed. The patient complained about severe glare postoperatively resulting from exposure of the IOL edge (Figure C4-1). An artificial prosthetic iris was recommended, but the patient was unhappy with the prospect of implantation of an investigational device and sought other surgical remedies.

From the surgeon's perspective seated superiorly (Figure C4-2), the first area to be addressed was the loose stub of iris tissue. A double-armed 10-0 polypropylene suture was passed as a horizontal mattress closure (Figures C4-3 and C4-4) that provided partial coverage when the suture was tightened (Figure C4-5).

The inferior pupil appeared to be too superior after the horizontal mattress suture, and an inferior sphincterotomy was performed with Gills–Vannas scissors (Figure C4-6). The superior gape was closed with two interrupted sutures (Figures C4-7–C4-9). The pupil appeared too small, with a vertical slit configuration. Small

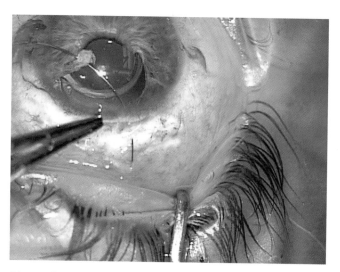

Figure C4-3

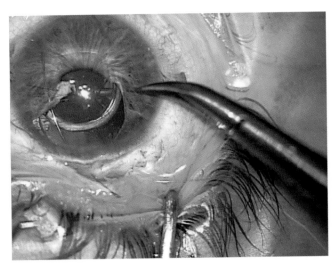

Figure C4-4

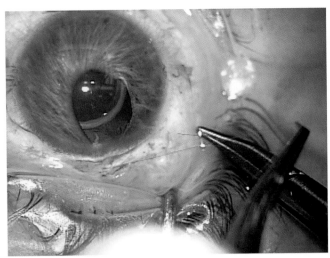

Figure C4-5

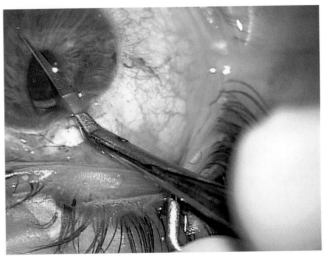

Figure C4-6

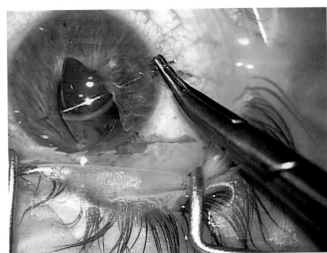

Figure C4-7

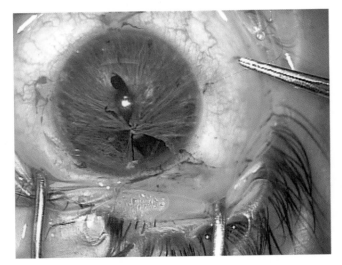

Figure C4-8

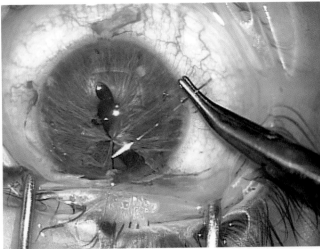

Figure C4-9

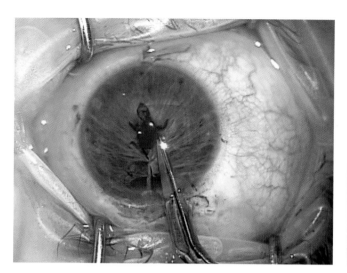

Figure C4-10

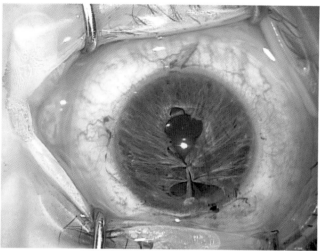

Figure C4-11

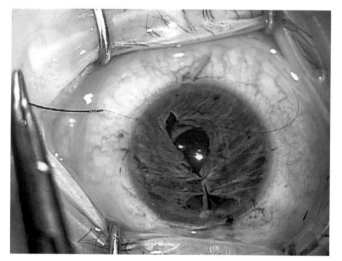

Figure C4-12

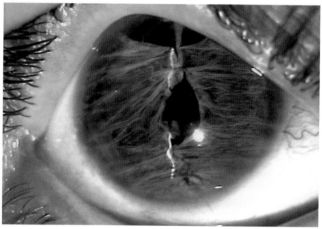

Figure C4-13

sphincterotomies were then placed horizontally to the left and to the right (Figure C4-10).

At this point, the original inferior sphincterotomy shown in Figure C4-6 appeared excessive, with exposure of the inferior edge of the capsulorrhexis margin (Figure C4-11). The exposure was remedied with an interrupted suture (Figure C4-12). Postoperatively, the patient reported elimination of the glare and was pleased by the improvement in the appearance of her highly visible iris (Figure C4-13). The upper lid in its natural position covered the remaining superior peripheral iris defect.

CASE 5: ANTERIOR CHAMBER INTRAOCULAR-LENS-INDUCED PUPILLARY DISTORTION

The patient was experiencing both severe glare and loss of vision caused by cystoid macular edema associated with iris tuck 6 months after secondary implantation of flexible open-loop

anterior chamber IOL. The view of the surgeon sitting superiorly is shown in Figure C5-1. Simple removal of the misplaced haptics that caused the iris tuck did not relieve the pupillary distortion (Figure C5-2).

After thorough vitrectomy and placement of a transscleral suture-fixated PC IOL, traction on the peripheral iris released some peripheral synechiae (Figure C5-3). Next, the large iridectomy was closed with a single interrupted suture (Figure C5-4).

The pupillary aperture was then reduced with interrupted sutures nasally and temporally (Figures C5-5 and C5-6). To create a rounder pupil, small sphincterotomies were added inferiorly (Figure C5-7) and superiorly (Figure C5-8). On the first postoperative day, the view was mildly hazy because of the inflammatory reaction, but the slit-lamp appearance showed a reasonably sized central pupil (Figure C5-9). Over 3 months the cystoid macular edema resolved with improvement of best-corrected visual acuity and full relief from glare.

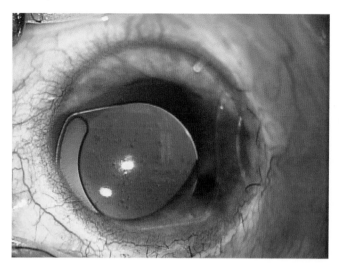

Figure C5-1

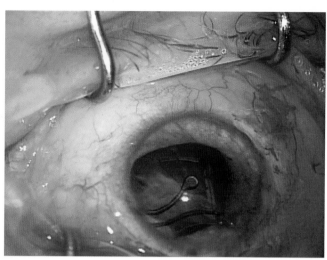

Figure C5-2

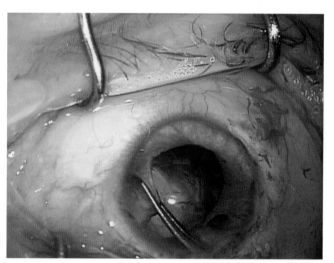

Figure C5-3

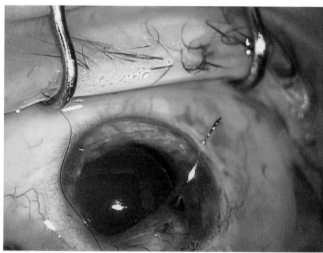

Figure C5-4

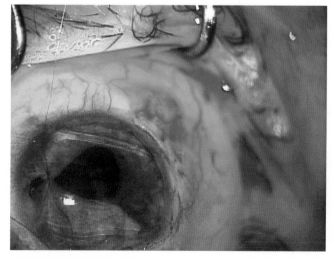

Figure C5-5

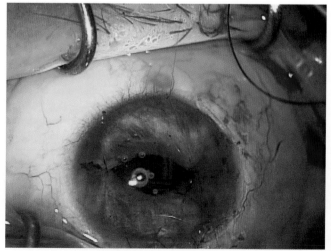

Figure C5-6

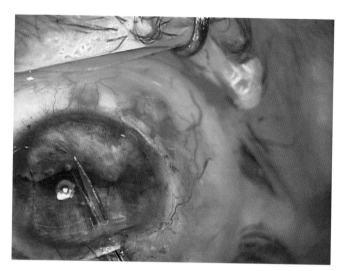

Figure C5-7

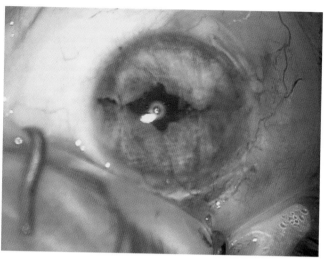

Figure C5-8

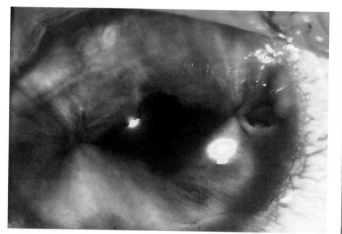

Figure C5-9

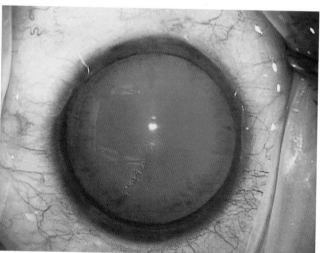

Figure C6-1

CASE 6: ATONIC PUPIL CORRECTED WITH IRIS CIRCLAGE PURSE-STRING SUTURE

This patient requiring cataract surgery had a lifelong history of isolated bilateral atonic pupils that measured 8 mm without dilation and nonreactive to light. His clinical presentation is more commonly seen after blunt trauma leading to generalized atrophy of the sphincter muscle. Glare symptoms will be worsened after cataract surgery because the IOL optic edge will not be covered by iris.

The appearance of the pupil at the start of surgery is shown in Figure C6-1. The appearance after completion of phacoemulsification and PC IOL implantation through a temporal clear corneal incision is shown in Figure C6-2. Two additional paracentesis openings were made at 4 o'clock and 8 o'clock positions relative to the principal incision (120° spacing).

A 10-0 polypropylene suture on a CTC-6 (Ethicon) needle initially made three full-thickness bites in the midperipheral iris

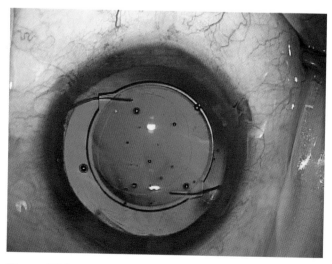

Figure C6-2

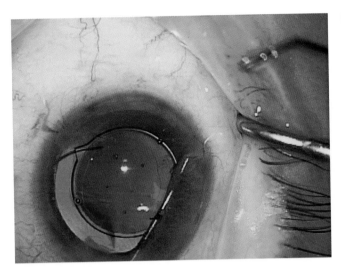

Figure C6-3

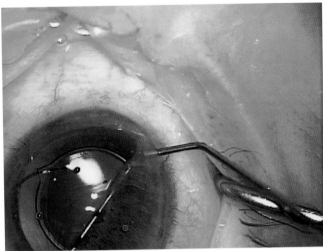

Figure C6-4

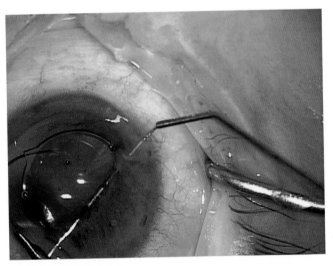

Figure C6-5

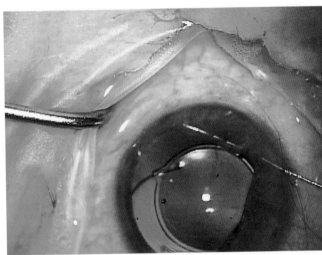

Figure C6-6

(Figure C6-3), moving from the principal incision toward the first paracentesis. For the needle tip to exit the paracentesis without engaging any corneal tissue, a blunt-tip 27-gauge cannula was inserted into the anterior chamber, and the needle tip "docked" inside the cannula (Figure C6-4). The needle and cannula were then externalized as a unit (Figure C6-5). The needle was reinserted through the paracentesis, taking care to make sure that no corneal tissue was engaged, and the purse-string iris suture technique was repeated in each remaining sector, ending at the original incision (Figures C6-6 and C6-7).

The suture ends were then tied externally, and the knot was advanced into the eye with a Kuglen hook while the surgeon and assistant maintained gentle tension on each suture end (Figure C6-8). After four throws, the suture ends were cut with a Gills–Vannas scissors, leaving a central, normal-sized pupil (Figure C6-9).

Postoperatively, the appearance of the pupil was grossly normal, for the first time in the patient's life (Figure C6-10).

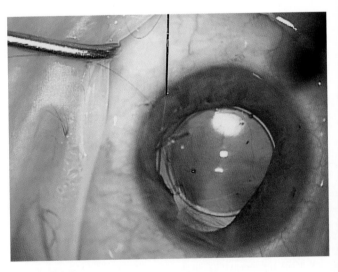

Figure C6-7

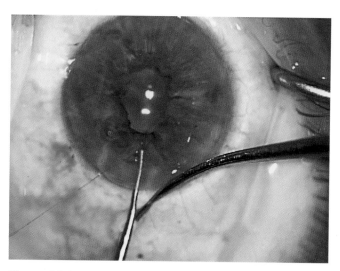

Figure C6-8

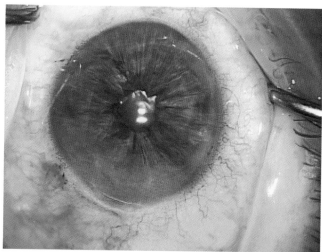

Figure C6-9

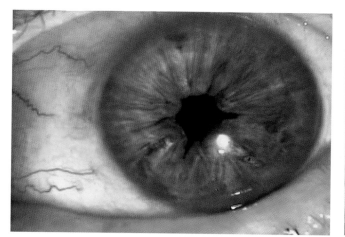

Figure C6-10

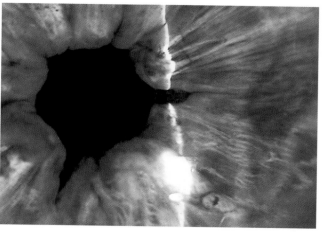

Figure C6-11

High-magnification inspection revealed two barely visible strands of the polypropylene suture across small gaps in the gathered-up iris (Figure C6-11). Although this is of no optical consequence, it illustrates the importance of placing the suture bites in the mid-peripheral iris rather than near the sphincter edge. Suture bites near the sphincter margin will result in more gaps with exposed suture and a more irregularly bordered pupil.

CASE 7: PRESERVATION OF IRIS

This complex multistep case is presented in summary form to illustrate the critical importance of never sacrificing iris tissue that may be salvaged for reconstruction. This 37-year-old man suffered massive accidental blunt trauma that ruptured the superior limbus and dialyzed all iris attachments except 2–3 clock hours inferiorly. Emergency repair closed the superior wound with iris prolapse covered by conjunctiva and no visible pupil (Figure C7-1). The patient was referred for repair.

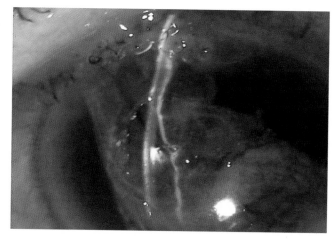

Figure C7-1

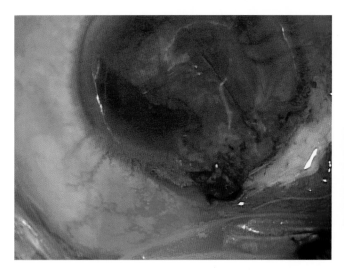

Figure C7-2

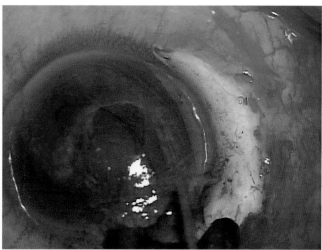

Figure C7-3

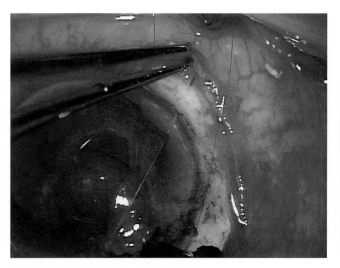

Figure C7-4

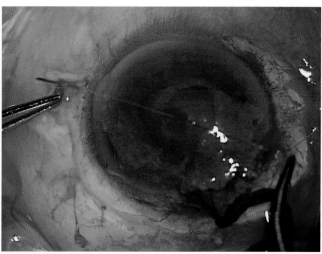

Figure C7-5

At surgery, a conjunctival flap was dissected back, exposing a large amount of prolapsed iris tissue (Figure C7-2). Viscoelastic agent infusion separated the iris pillars, revealing the original pupillary space (Figure C7-3). The iris pillars were reattached to the sclera with multiple, horizontal, mattress, double-armed sutures (Figures C7-4 and C7-5).

The result was a marked improvement, particularly in the critical areas inferiorly, nasally, and temporally, where most glare originates (Figure C7-6). If glare proves to be a problem, despite any maximal reconstruction of available iris, then subsequent implantation of a prosthetic iris device can be considered.

■ IRIS PROSTHESES ■

Every effort should be made to reconstruct the natural iris. However, some patients do not have adequate residual iris tissue to prevent glare and other optical aberrations. In general, iris

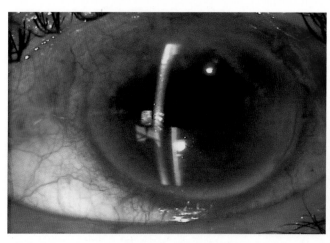

Figure C7-6

prosthesis is required when more than a quadrant of iris tissue is missing. Iris defects spanning less than 3 clock hours can usually be repaired with imbrication suture techniques, such as those described earlier in this chapter. In some patients, although iris tissue is not actually missing, the quality of the iris stroma present may be too poor to function properly and to repair. Examples include the iris in uveitic patients or iridocorneal endothelial (ICE) syndrome. Similarly, in patients with ocular albinism, the pigment layer can be either transparent or highly dysfunctional, depending on whether the patient is tyrosinase positive or negative. Under these circumstances, the surgeon has two principal options. The first is to attempt to fit the patient with a "narcissus" contact lens with an "artificial iris" peripheral pigmentation painted on it. Some patients have been greatly helped by these devices, but these lenses are expensive and need periodic replacement. In the absence of the contact lens, the patient has a return of the visual impairment.

Alternatively, IOL and polymer technology have permitted the development of pigmented materials that can be permanently implanted as iris prostheses within the eye.

The artificial iris implant was first introduced and published in Europe by Sundmacher, Reihnhard, and Althaus[6–8] in 1994. They reported using a single-piece black diaphragm IOL in cases of traumatic or congenital aniridia. The first use of small-incision artificial iris ring implants was reported at the Welch (Man named Welch) Cataract Congress by Kenneth Rosenthal in 1996. Subsequently, two independent series of cases have been reported, demonstrating the safety and efficacy of both the single-piece black diaphragm IOL and the endocapsular prosthetic iris rings.[9,10]

When contemplating use of a prosthetic iris device, the surgeon must first define the clinical situation and choose the appropriate device based on the relevant anatomy. Currently there are two main categories of prosthetic iris implant available, each with specific indications.

The single-piece black diaphragm IOL (Figure 31-5) available from Morcher GmbH provides a full iris diaphragm and IOL

that can be placed in the ciliary sulcus on capsular support or transsclerally sutured. However, a significant drawback of the single-piece diaphragm IOL is that it requires a relatively large incision size, which is associated with delayed visual rehabilitation, increased astigmatism, and increased risk of intraoperative suprachoroidal hemorrhage. When implanting the Morcher single-piece iris diaphragm IOL, care must be taken while manipulating the haptics, because they are brittle and easily broken. Other manufacturers, such as Ophtec BV, also produce single-piece diaphragm IOLs, and these are available in a variety of colors in an attempt to more closely match that of the native iris. The colors available are light blue, light green, mid brown and black. The Ophtec model 311 requires a slightly smaller 9 mm incision than the 10 mm for the Morcher implant, and also has haptics that are less susceptible to fracturing. The black IOL is made of a polycarbonate material, while the other colored IOLs are made of polymethyl methacylate (PMMA). The Morcher device has a 5 mm aperture, while the Ophtec device has a 4 mm "pupillary" opening. They also differ in edge configuration of the optic. The Morcher 67-series devices have a squared-edged optic fused to the black carrier material, while the Ophtec 311 device's optic has a round edge which is inset into a rounded notch in the carrier device.

Morcher GMBH has recently introduced a 30-B series that consists of a clear PMMA diaphragm backbone with an opaque, colored film applied to the anterior surface (see Figure 31-6). The colors are merged from pixilated multicolored dots within the film (see Figure 31-7). This far, one case in the US has been presented by Sam Masket, MD at ASCRS, San Francisco 2009.

Another category of iris prosthetic devices is designed specifically for endocapsular fixation. One type currently available is the Morcher 50-series endocapsular rings with iris diaphragm designed around a standard capsular tension ring, developed by Volker Rasch of Potsdam, Germany. The other endocapsular device is the Iris Prosthetic System (IPS) from Ophtec BV. Neither of these endocapsular aniridia devices have an optical portion and, therefore, can be inserted through a small incision. Slight

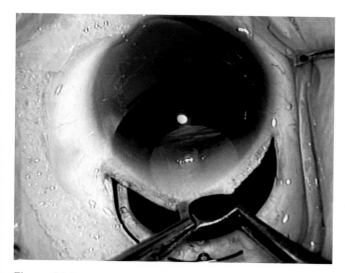

Figure 31-5 Intraocular lens (IOL) with a peripheral pigment skirt for cases of aniridia or other generalized absence of iris tissue. Implantation of this large IOL requires an incision of at least 10 mm.

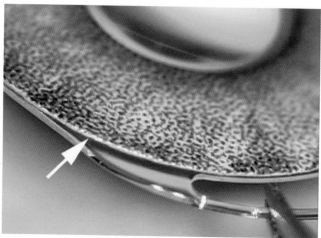

Figure 31-6 The Morcher 30-B device has an opaque, colored film (seen on edge here) applied to the PMMA backbone.

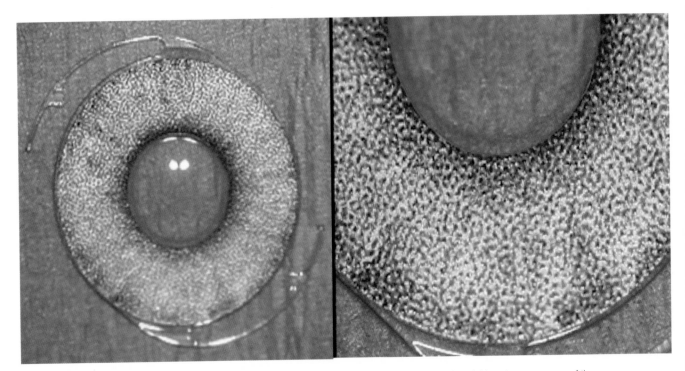

Figure 31-7 The Morcher 30-B device is seen here at low mag (left) and high mag (right). Note the appearance of the colored flecks under low mag which blend to create the desired effect when viewed with the naked eye.

enlargement of the incision may be necessary, depending on the specific implant chosen. The Morcher 50-C can be placed through a 3 mm incision, while the 50D, E, or F may require a slightly larger incision depending on the desired pupil size. The Ophtec "IPS" multipiece device requires an approximately 5 mm incision.

There are two styles of Morcher iris endocapsular ring devices. One style consists of a ring with a single fin (Type 96F) and is used for sectoral iris atrophy or loss, and each fin will cover up to 3 clock hours of loss (Figure 31-8). Two or more rings may be used to cover

larger defects. The other style consists of two rings, each with multiple fins that interdigitate (Morcher Types 50C, D, E, and F), and are used to create a full iris diaphragm (Figure 31-9). The Type 50C rings produce an iris diaphragm with a pupil size of approximately 6 mm, which reduces the stray light entering the eye by 75% yet provides an aperture compatible with excellent fundus viewing postoperatively. If a smaller pupil size is desired, newer models 50D, E, and F are available with pupil sizes of 4, 3.5, and 4 mm respectively. The 50F device has less space between the interdigitating fins, making alignment of the two pieces more facile.

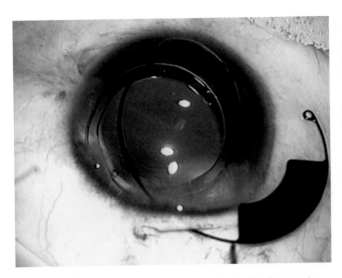

Figure 31-8 Segment of single-fin opaque implant for blocking a sector defect.

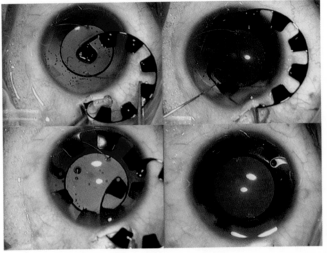

Figure 31-9 Implantation of two multiple-fin segments that are aligned to obtain 360° artificial iris coverage through a small incision.

should be added to the initially calculated IOL, since the optic sits more posteriorly in the more crowded capsular bag.

After implantation, the artificial iris rings remain quite stable and the tension ring component of the aniridia ring can lend support to the capsule by distributing zonular tension evenly around the equator of the capsular bag.

Caution should be exercised when implanting these devices because they are brittle and susceptible to fracture. When planning for surgery with the endocapsular ring type iris implants, it is advisable to order an extra piece in case a ring is fractured during surgical manipulation. Furthermore, the capsular bag can become somewhat crowded after three devices have been inserted. Finally, great care must be taken not to damage the fragile capsule of patients with congenital aniridia.

The Ophtec IPS consists of modular units designed to be implanted in-the-bag (Figure 31-10). This is available in the same variety of colors being offered in its range of Model 311 full-sized aniridia implants. The IPS modular device includes the bilobed elements, which, when assembled, re-establishes an intact diaphragm, a capsular tension ring, and a locking element to secure the implant once the device has been assembled in the bag. The surgeon has to be gentle during the assembly and locking of the device, as it requires a fair amount of manipulation within the capsular bag.

While the black iris devices improve optical function without any improvement in cosmesis, the other colored devices made by Ophtec BV go one step further to achieve a better cosmetic match with the native iris of the fellow eye. Although this is an improvement, the result may still be suboptimal, because only a single shade is available for each color, which when applied evenly to the entire iris surface, leads to a flat, two-dimensional, untextured unnatural iris appearance, even if the color shade were an exact match to the fellow. Morcher now offers multiple shade colored iris prostheses.

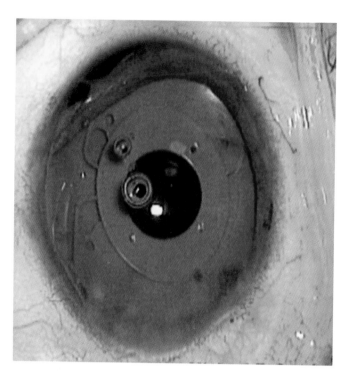

Figure 31-10 The Ophtec IPS multi-piece device is seen here in situ within the capsular bag with the two elements and central locking ring with 3 mm aperture in place. A CTR and PCIOL are also within the capsule.

If the 50C rings are chosen, the foldable optic chosen should have a diameter of 6.5 mm to eliminate edge glare, while a standard 6 mm lens optic is acceptable for models 50D, E, and F. When placing the IOL, the ideal optic position is posterior to both iris rings. An additional 0.5–1.0 diopter of optic power

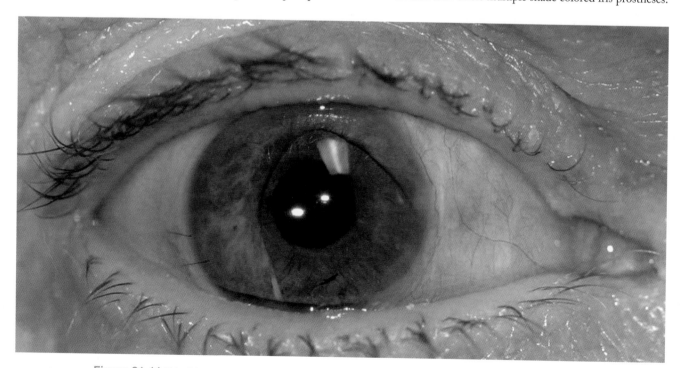

Figure 31-11 This slit lamp photo shows a patient who had an iridociliary melanoma resected, leaving an inferonasal iris defect and profound glare. At the time of cataract surgery, a Humanoptics custom iris device was placed into the capsular bag with a PCIOL and a CTR. Her glare was completely eliminated.

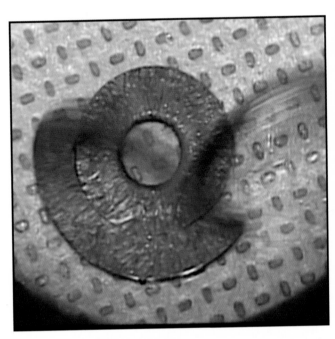 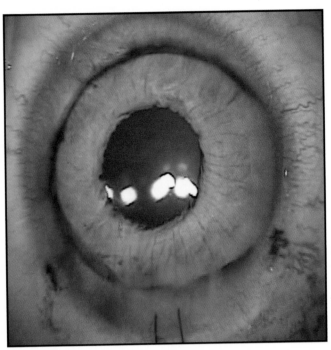

Figure 31-12 This Humanoptics custom iris prosthesis was matched to the vestigial iris stump in this 4-year-old congenital aniric with dense cataract. The device is trephinated to the size of the capsular bag (left), then implanted in-the-bag with a PCIOL. Note the difference in appearance of the device after implantation. The more blue appearance of the residual iris stroma is artifactually altered by trypan blue used during the capsulorrhexis for visualization of the prosthesis during implantation of the device.

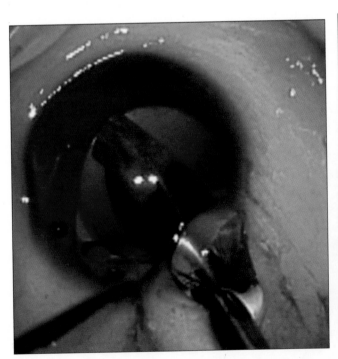 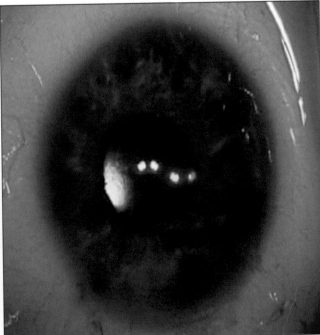

Figure 31-13 This Humanoptics iris device is inserted with forceps. Note the apparent iris detail (right).

A new iris implant has been designed to address this problem. Dr. Schmidt Inraocularlinsen has developed an iris implant made of a flexible material that may be custom tailored to be an exact match with the fellow iris. This extremely flexible device may be rolled up into a cylinder for insertion through a small cataract incision. Each iris device is meticulously crafted to match its fellow in color and shade as well as texture for a remarkably natural appearance. The manufacturer requires an anterior segment photograph to be taken of the fellow eye for this matching to be done.

This device is designed to be attached to the scleral wall with horizontal mattress sutures being passed through the peripheral silicone material itself, in a similar fashion to the method used to repair an iridodialysis. The device is quite flexible in its deployment, as the material may be cut to size with a corneal trephine to match the corneal diameter, or with scissors to the desired shape and size. If only a sector defect needs to be repaired, it is possible to suture the implant after being cut to size, to the remaining normal iris tissue. Further research is being carried out in this area to assess the suitability of this implant for in-the-bag fixation without sutures.

The technology for iris reconstruction will continue to improve as several groups are working on other prosthetic iris devices. In the future we can expect refinements in structure, flexibility, and implantation techniques.

References

[1] Britten MJA. Follow-up of 54 cases of ocular contusion with hyphaema, with special reference to the appearance and function of the filtration angle. Br J Ophthalmol 1965;49:120–127.
[2] Weidenthal DT. Experimental ocular contusion. Arch Ophthalmol 1964;71:77–81.
[3] Wolff SM, Zimmerman I.E. Chronic secondary glaucoma associated with retrodisplacement of iris root and deepening of the anterior chamber angle secondary to contusion. Am J Ophthalmol 1962;54:547–563.
[4] Paton D, Craig J. Management of iridodialysis. Ophthalmic Surg 1973;4:38–39.
[5] Osher RH, Snyder ME, Cionni RJ. Modification of the Siepser slip-knot technique. J Cataract Refract Surg 2005;31:1098–1100.
[6] Reihnhard T, Sundmacher R, Althaus C. Irisblenden-IOL bei traumatischer aniridie. Klin Monatsbl Augenheilkd 1994;205:196–200.
[7] Sundmacher R, Reihnhard T, Althaus C. Black diaphragm intraocular lens for correction of aniridia. Ophthalmic Surg 1994;25:180–185.
[8] Sundmacher R, Reihnhard T, Althaus C. Black diaphragm intraocular lens in congenital aniridia. Ger J Ophthalmol 1994;3:197–201.
[9] Thompson CG, Fawzy K, Bryce IG et al. Implantation of a black diaphragm intraocular lens for traumatic aniridia. J Cataract Refract Surg 1999;25:808–813.
[10] Osher RH, Burk SE. Cataract surgery combined with implantation of an artificial iris. J Cataract Refract Surg 1999;25:1540–1547.

IRIS PROSTHESES

High Myopia

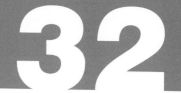

Roger F. Steinert, MD

INTRAOPERATIVE CONSIDERATIONS

CONTENTS

- Preoperative Evaluation
- Intraoperative Considerations
- Postoperative Care

CHAPTER HIGHLIGHTS

>> Surgical challenges of long eye and deep anterior chamber

>> Complications associated with high myopia

>> Special surgical techniques in high myopia

Cataract surgery in the presence of high axial myopia poses a number of challenges for the surgeon. Special consideration must be given to these patients at each stage of the preoperative, operative, and postoperative periods. Table 32-1 summarizes these key considerations in high myopia.

PREOPERATIVE EVALUATION

A comprehensive preoperative evaluation is performed on all cataract patients. In the case of high axial myopia, however, the surgeon must pay particular attention to the fundus exam. High myopia is associated with a higher risk of both peripheral and macular retinal pathologic conditions. Measurement of macular visual potential is important if there is disturbance of the pigment epithelium or evidence of atrophy or neovascularization from the choroid. Preoperative evaluation of potential visual acuity is covered in Chapter 3.

The peripheral retina in high axial myopia is more vulnerable to pathologic conditions that increase the risks of retinal detachment. A careful preoperative peripheral retinal examination is mandatory. However, visualization of the peripheral retina, even with aggressive scleral depression, may not reveal preexisting peripheral retinal pathologic conditions because of impaired visualization caused by the cataract.

The other primary challenge facing the cataract surgeon preoperatively, in the presence of high myopia, is determination of the intraocular lens (IOL) power. First, the accuracy of the A-scan biometry and the subsequent calculation of the IOL power are subject to more variability in high myopia than in patients with a normal-sized eye. If the axial myopia is accompanied by a posterior staphyloma, the precise determination of the axial length at the fovea is often imprecise.

Even with an accurate determination of the axial length, the IOL power formulas have less accuracy in the more extreme ranges. Studies have indicated that the SRK-T formula is more accurate in high axial myopia than other formulas (see Hoffer KJ [1993] and Holladay JT [1998] in Further Reading and Chapter 4). Even then, however, there is considerably more variability in the IOL power accuracy in these cases.

The surgeon must discuss with the patient the intended postoperative IOL power goal. While some myopes value excellent distance uncorrected vision, other myopes have enjoyed the ability to read with spectacles. Determining the desired postoperative refractive goal is a key step in the preoperative surgical planning.

INTRAOPERATIVE CONSIDERATIONS

High axial myopia poses a high risk of complication with retrobulbar or peribulbar anesthesia. The larger and longer globe fills more of the orbit, and the passage of a needle posteriorly is more prone to inadvertently penetrating the sclera. Moreover, the sclera in high axial myopia is thinner, resulting in less resistance to penetration by an anesthetic injection needle (see Chapter 8).

High myopes typically have deeper anterior chambers and less residual formed vitreous than the average patient. Therefore, the surgeon may face excessive anterior chamber deepening on introducing the phacoemulsification tip and irrigation. If so, the height of the infusion bottle should be lowered. There may also be more mobility of the nucleus, related both to zonular laxity and the lack of vitreous support. The vitreous body is frequently more liquefied than in a similar-aged emmetrope. As a result, the surgeon should expect to face a deeper anterior chamber and more anteroposterior movement of the crystalline lens and capsule in the course of the phacoemulsification. Moreover, there is less vitreous support for the posterior capsule, and many

Table 32-1 Special elements in cataract surgery for high myopia

Preoperative
Peripheral retina exam
Macular exam
Potential acuity testing
Biometry, postoperative refractive goal determination, and IOL power calculation
Intraoperative
Risk of retrobulbar/peribulbar anesthetic injection
Increased anterior-chamber depth
Reduced nuclear support
Postoperative
Preservation of a clear posterior capsule/capsulotomy complications minimized
Surveillance for peripheral retinal breaks/early detection of retinal detachments

surgeons have observed that the posterior capsule has the potential for rupturing during surgery at a higher rate in high axial myopia. Furthermore, if the posterior capsule does rupture, the liquefied vitreous will not provide normal resistance to posterior migration of nuclear fragments. The patient is, therefore, at higher risk for loss of nuclear fragments into the deep vitreous and against the retina. Should this complication occur, the anterior-segment surgeon should obtain the assistance of a skilled vitreoretinal surgeon in the safe removal of the nuclear fragments. If a vitreoretinal surgeon is available, this can be done immediately in the course of the cataract surgery. If not, then the cataract surgeon should complete the anterior cleanup and obtain an immediate postoperative consultation to schedule the patient for an expeditious removal of the posterior lens fragments by the vitreoretinal surgeon.

In the presence of this complication, a frequently debated issue is whether the cataract surgeon should place the IOL primarily or whether the patient should be left in an aphakic state. If the nuclear fragments that remain are quite large and dense, a vitreoretinal surgeon may choose to bring the fragments up through the pupil and deliver them through a limbal incision, rather than attempt a posterior ultrasonic fragmentation of a very large and dense nucleus. If the nuclear fragments are reasonably small, however, the vitreoretinal surgeon will usually feel comfortable with posterior ultrasonic fragmentation of the remaining nucleus. In that case, the presence of an IOL will not impede the vitreoretinal surgeon's maneuvers. Ideally, a cataract surgeon should develop a good working relationship with a vitreoretinal surgeon and explore the vitreoretinal surgeon's preferences regarding IOL placement under these circumstances.

High axial myopia presents one other challenge for a surgeon who wishes to perform surgery through a corneal scleral incision rather than a limbal or fully clear corneal incision. In true high axial myopia, the sclera may be markedly thinned. The surgeon needs to anticipate that dissection should be more shallow than usual to avoid inadvertent penetration through the sclera onto the ciliary body while attempting to dissect a scleral tunnel incision.

POSTOPERATIVE CARE

Maintaining the integrity and clarity of the posterior capsule is generally regarded as important in reducing the frequency of vitreoretinal complications. In addition, a broad area of clear posterior capsule and a large optic assist in the examination of the patient's retina postoperatively. A pupil that is not traumatized during surgery and does not have postoperative synechia inhibiting dilation also contributes to good postoperative care. Therefore, the cataract surgeon should use a meticulous technique with a centered capsulorrhexis, thorough cortical cleanup, and great care to maintain the integrity and clarity of the posterior capsule. The choice of IOL should be influenced by these considerations.

A large optic, either 6 or 6.5 mm, is preferable to a smaller optic. Using an IOL optic material that will interfere least with subsequent vitreoretinal surgery, if needed, and an IOL optic edge that is configured to inhibit posterior capsule opacification is recommended. Currently, the lens of choice in this circumstance has a square or modified square edge (see Chapter 37).

Because the high axial myopic patient is at higher risk for retinal detachment, it is advisable to carefully examine the peripheral retina with wide dilation and scleral depression with indirect ophthalmoscopy early postoperatively, such as several weeks, but also to perform such an examination at more frequent intervals. Many postoperative detachments do not occur for many months or years after the surgery. If there is difficulty in visualization of the peripheral retina or a question about the advisability of "prophylactic" laser treatment of suspicious peripheral lesions, consultation with a vitreoretinal surgeon is recommended (see Chapter 56).

If the posterior capsule opacifies to the point of functional visual impairment, then Nd:YAG laser posterior capsulotomy may be indicated. To minimize the disturbance to any residual formed vitreous and to maintain as much integrity of the barrier function of the capsule–IOL complex, the surgeon is advised to use the lowest amount of energy necessary to open the posterior capsule and to keep the size of the capsular opening smaller than the optic (see Chapter 51).

Further Reading

Alldredge CD, Elkins B, Alldredge OC. Retinal detachment following phacoemulsification in highly myopic cataract patients. J Cataract Refract Surg 1988;24:777–780.

Apple DJ, Solomon KD, Tetz MR, et al. Posterior capsular opacification. Surv Ophthalmol 1992;37:73–115.

Buratto L, editor. Phacoemulsification: principles and techniques. Thorofare, NJ: Slack; 1988.

Buratto L, Buratto LE, editors. Cataract surgery in axial myopia. Milano: Ghedini; 1994.

Coonan P, Fung WE, Webster RG, et al. The incidence of retinal detachment following extracapsular cataract extraction: a ten year study. Ophthalmology 1985;92:106.

Curtin BJ. The myopias: basic science and clinical management. Hagerstown: Harper and Row; 1985.

Francois JG, Goes F. Comparative study of ultrasonic biometry of emmetropes and myopes, with special heredity of myopia. Biometrie Oculaire Clinique Parigi Masson, 1976.

Hoffer KJ. The Hoffer Q formula: a comparison of theoretic and regression formulas. J Cataract Refract Surg 1993;19:700–712.

Hoffman P, Pollock A, Oliver M. Limited choroidal hemorrhage associated with intracapsular cataract extraction. Arch Ophthalmol 1984;102:1761–1765.

Holladay JT. IOL power calculation for the unusual eye. In: Gills JP, Fenzyl R, Martin RG, editors. Cataract surgery: the state of the art. Thorofare, NJ: Slack; 1998. p. 197–205.

Hollick EJ, Spalton DJ. The effect of capsulorrhexis size on posterior capsule opacification. Presentation at ASCRS Meeting, Boston, 1997.

Hollick EJ, Spalton DJ, Ursel PG, et al. Lens epithelial cell regression on the posterior capsule with different intraocular lens material. Br J Ophthalmol 1998;82:1182–1188.

Hymans SW, Bialik M, Neumann E. Myopia-aphakia. Br J Ophthalmol 1975;59:480.

Jaffe NS, Clayman HM, Jaffe MS. Retinal detachment in myopic eye after intracapsular and extracapsular cataract extraction. Am J Ophthalmol 1984;97:48–52.

Koch PS. Phacoemulsification in patients with high myopia. In: Phacoemulsification in difficult and challenging cases. New York: Thieme Medical Publishers; 1999.

Osterlin S. Vitreous changes after cataract extraction. In: Freeman HM, Hirose T, Schepens CL, editors. Vitreous surgery and advances in fundus diagnosis and treatment. New York: Appleton-Century Crofts; 1977. p. 15–21.

Percival SPB. Long term complications from extracapsular cataract surgery. Trans Ophthalmol. Soc UK 1985;104:915–918.

Praeger DL. Five years' follow-up in the surgical management of cataracts in high myopia treated with the Kelman phacoemulsification technique. Ophthalmology 1979;86:2024–2033.

Retzlaff J. A new intraocular lens calculation formula. J Am Intraocul Implant Soc 1980;6:148–152.

Retzlaff JA, Sanders DR, Kraff MC. Development of the SRK/T intraocular lens implant power calculation formula. J Cataract Refract Surg 1990;16:333–340.

Rickman-Barger L, Florine CW, Larson RS, et al. Retinal detachment after neodymium YAG laser capsulotomy. Am J Ophthalmol 1989;107:531–536.

Sanders DR, Retzlaff J, Kraff MC. Comparison of empirically derived and theoretical aphakic refraction formulas. Arch Ophthalmol 1983;101:956–967.

Selley LF, Barraquer J. Surgery of the ectopic lens. Ann Ophthalmol 1973;35:1127.

Shah GR, Gills JP, Durham DG, et al. Three thousand YAG laser posterior capsulotomies: an analysis of complications and comparison to polishing and surgical discission. Ophthalmic Surg 1986;17: 473–477.

Ursell PG, Spalton DJ, Pande MV, et al. The relationship between intraocular lens biomaterials and posterior capsule opacification. J Cataract Refract Surg 1998;24:352–360.

POSTOPERATIVE CARE

Nanophthalmos, Relative Anterior Microphthalmos, and Axial Hyperopia

Richard K. Parrish, II, MD, Kendall Donaldson, MD, MS,
Marianne B. Mellem Kairala, MD
and Richard J. Simmons, MD

33

CONTENTS

CHAPTER HIGHLIGHTS

>> Anatomic classification of small eyes

>> Uveal effusion syndrome

>> Angle closure and the lens

>> Surgical techniques

>> Intraocular lens power calculation and piggyback lenses

Understanding the anatomic differences in small eyes gives surgeons a framework for surgical planning in these challenging cases.

CLASSIFICATION AND TERMINOLOGY

Microphthalmos – the result of developmental arrest of ocular growth during gestation – usually occurs sporadically, but can be inherited in an autosomal-dominant or recessive pattern. It is often associated with systemic diseases, including genetic or environmental disorders, or those of unknown causes.[1,2] Evaluation of microphthalmic patients should be interdisciplinary, with special attention given to the history of the disease and examination of other family members.

Because microphthalmos is a heterogeneous condition, with many possible and overlapping presentations, the authors prefer to use an anatomic classification for these eyes, based on anterior chamber depth and total axial length (Tables 33-1 and 33-2).[3,4]

SHORT ANTERIOR CHAMBER DEPTH WITH SHORT AXIAL LENGTH: NANOPHTHALMOS, COLOBOMATOUS, AND COMPLEX MICROPHTHALMOS

Duke-Elder[5] in 1964 described three categories of microphthalmos: simple microphthalmos, or nanophthalmos, which is a short eye with no other associated morphologic anomalies; colobomatous microphthalmos, related to incomplete closure of embryonic fissure; and complex microphthalmos, not related to closure of the fissure, but associated with systemic anomalies and other anterior and posterior malformations of the eye.

Nanophthalmos (Simple Microphthalmos)

Nanophthalmos is a rare condition characterized by a total axial length that is at least two standard deviations below the mean for age or less than 20.5 mm.[6] There are no systemic or other ocular morphologic abnormalities.[5,7] Many authors, including Duke-Elder and Naumann, have synonymously used the terms "simple microphthalmos" and "nanophthalmos."[5,6,8,9]

Although microphthalmos in general is a fairly common ocular malformation found in all races,[1] nanophthalmos is a very rare form. Most cases of nanophthalmos are sporadic, but recently genetic studies of several nanophthalmic pedigrees showed autosomal recessive inheritance.[10] In 1998, the first human gene locus associated with autosomal-dominant nanophthalmos was identified on chromosome 11 and named NNO1.[11] A family history of nanophthalmos is often unknown, but patients sometimes report relatives, without a specific gender predilection, who were blind from unknown cause, consistent with angle-closure glaucoma.

Younger patients usually present for evaluation of poor visual acuity related to a high refractive error, which usually is fully

		Axial length	
		Shorter	Longer
Anterior chamber depth	Shallower ... Deeper	Simple microphthalmos = Nanophthalmos Colobomatous microphthalmos Complex microphthalmos	Relative anterior microphthalmos
		Axial hyperopia	Normal

Modified from Holladay J: Achieving emmetropia in extremely short eyes with two piggyback posterior chamber intraocular lenses, *Ophthalmology* 103:1118-1123, 1996; Auffarth GU, Blum M, Faller U et al: Relative anterior microphthalmos: morphometric analysis and its implications for cataract surgery, *Ophthalmology* 107:1555-1560, 2000.

Table 33-2 Anatomic classification of short eyes

2.1. Short anterior-chamber (AC) depth with short axial length

    2.1.1. Nanophthalmos (simple microphthalmos)

    2.1.2. Colobomatous microphthalmos

    2.1.3. Complex microphthalmos

2.2. Short AC depth with normal axial length

    Relative anterior microphthalmos

2.3. Normal AC depth with short axial length

    Axial hyperopia

correctable with corrective lenses. Consequently, these patients often remain undiagnosed until middle age, when complications most commonly develop. If one or more clinical features are present, the diagnosis of nanophthalmos should be considered. If left untreated, this condition often results in blindness.

Clinical features

The most prominent clinical features seen in nanophthalmos are described here and are summarized in Table 33-3.

Table 33-3 Nanophthalmic clinical features

Short axial length	Moderate to high axial hyperopia
Small cornea	Thick sclera
Shallow anterior chamber	Thickened choroid
Marked iris convexity	Angle closure glaucoma*
Normal or increased lens thickness	Uveal effusions*
High lens/eye volume ratio	Exudative retinal detachment*

*May develop these features in the late course of the disease.

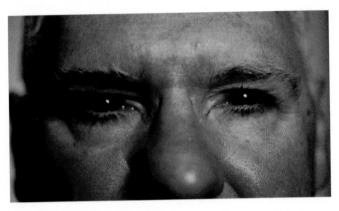

Figure 33-1 Nanophthalmos. Eyes deeply set with narrow palpebral fissures.

Nanophthalmos is a bilateral disease in which the eyes are deeply set with narrow palpebral fissures (Figure 33-1).

The eyes are uniformly small, usually about two-thirds of the normal volume, but have an increased crystalline lens to total eye volume ratio. The crystalline lens can be normal or can have a slightly increased anteroposterior length (Figure 33-2). Nanophthalmos is typically associated with microcornea, with corneal diameters between 9.5 and 11 mm. The central and peripheral anterior chamber depths are also very shallow, from less than 1 mm to 2.7 mm.[6] Pupils usually dilate poorly, and eyes have a wide amplitude of intraocular pulse pressure, the mechanism of which is unknown. The disproportion between lenticular and ocular volume contributes to the shallowing of the central anterior

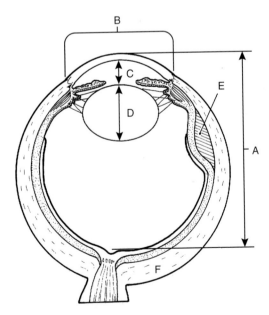

Figure 33-2 Schematic drawing of nanophthalmic eye showing the main ocular findings. A, short axial length; B, reduced corneal diameter; C, shallow anterior chamber; D, normal or increased lens thickness and high lens/eye volume ratio; E, thickened uveal tract with intrachoroidal or suprachoroidal peripheral uveal effusions; F, thickened scleral wall.

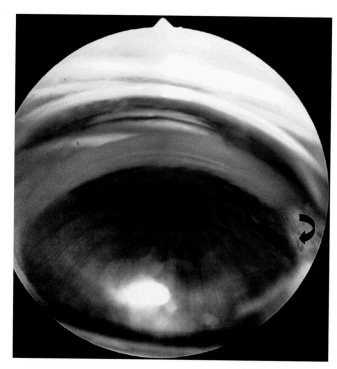

Figure 33-3 Gonioscopic view of a nanophthalmic eye showing marked iris convexity, "Vesuvio iris." Note the patent surgical iridectomy (arrow).

Table 33-4 Scleral abnormalities in nanophthalmic eyes

Collagen fibers
Variations in the size of collagen fibers[23,27,28]
Increased fraying and splitting of collagen fibers[23]
Disordered lamellar arrangement of collagen bundles[22,29]

Extracellular matrix
Glycosaminoglycan deposits[22–24]
Increased fibronectin content[28]

effusions in the late course of the disease and may be associated with exudative retinal detachment (Figure 33-4).

Brockhurst described the association of nanophthalmos and spontaneous uveal effusion in 1974.[8] The pathophysiology of nanophthalmic uveal effusion has been postulated by Brockhurst to be related to the compression of vortex veins and by Gass, to be associated with the reduced scleral permeability to proteins. In both cases, the primary cause is the abnormal sclera found in nanophthalmic eyes.[13,19,27,30–32]

Nanophthalmic uveal effusion (intrachoroidal, suprachoroidal, or both)[33] can occur spontaneously, and usually develops between the fourth and seventh decades, or acutely after intraocular surgery. Uveal effusion can lead to choroidal and exudative retinal detachment spontaneously or after intraocular procedures. The choroidal detachment causes retinal pigment epithelium dysfunction, which may promote leakage of serous fluid into the subretinal space and lead to an exudative retinal detachment. The progressive accumulation of noninflammatory fluid in the choroid leads to an increase in the sclerochoroidal[34] thickness and can be noted by ultrasound or magnetic resonance imaging.

chamber and to the marked peripheral convexity of the iris, and is responsible for the appearance of "Vesuvio iris" (Figure 33-3). Early in life, the angle can remain wide open despite the central shallowing of the anterior chamber, but later the peripheral anterior chamber progressively shallows and closes the filtration angle. High hypermetropia with a range between +7.25 and +20.00[6] typifies this condition. Depending on the corneal and lens refractive power, nanophthalmic patients can have lower degrees of hyperopia or, very rarely, myopia.[2,5–8,12–14]

Nanophthalmic eyes are also characterized by very thick choroid and sclera. In normal eyes the mean combined sclerochoroidal thickness is approximately 1.01 mm, but nanophthalmic patients have values between 0.75 and 4 mm (mean of 2.78 mm), as described in a series of 32 eyes of 16 patients with nanophthalmos.[6]

Retinal findings in nanophthalmic patients include chorioretinal folds, macular hypoplasia, cystic macular degeneration, retinal pigmentary degeneration, retinitis pigmentosa, and disc drusen.[15–18] The distinguishing feature of nanophthalmic eyes is the abnormally thick and inelastic sclera.[8,19,20] Ultrastructural and histochemical studies demonstrate abnormal scleral collagen fibers (Table 33-4) and an alteration in the metabolism of glycosaminoglycans and fibronectin production by scleral cells.[21–28] It has been speculated that the restriction of normal eye growth by the thick sclera is the underlying pathophysiology of nanophthalmos.

Untreated nanophthalmic eyes are likely to develop gradual progressive narrowing of the anterior chamber angle, formation of peripheral synechiae, and elevation of intraocular pressure (IOP). Nanophthalmic eyes characteristically develop spontaneous uveal

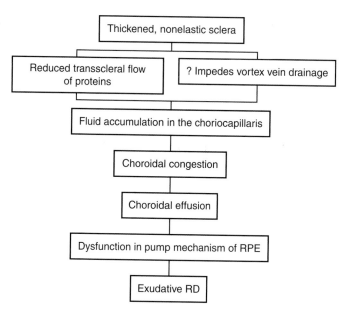

Figure 33-4 Proposed pathogenesis of uveal effusion and retinal detachment in nanophthalmic eyes. RD, Retinal detachment; RPE, retinal pigment epithelium.

Chronic angle-closure glaucoma usually develops painlessly in middle age and is associated with a progressive increase in intraocular pressure. As the crystalline lens enlarges anteroposteriorly with age, relative pupillary block increases, with progressive shallowing of the central and peripheral anterior chamber, narrowing and gradually closing off the angle.[33] Angle closure is usually precipitated by an anteriorly located peripheral annular uveal effusion or exudative retinal detachment, which causes the forward rotation of the ciliary body, forward movement of the peripheral iris, and consequent increase in the relative pupillary block.[9,33] Pupillary block, an early component of this angle closure, is not the sole mechanism of angle closure. Therefore, a patent peripheral iridotomy, which eliminates pupillary block, does not prevent progressive choroidal effusion that may result in further angle closure.

Colobomatous Microphthalmos

Colobomatous microphthalmos results from involution of the primary optic disc or incomplete closure of the embryonic fissure,[5] which is usually closed by the sixth week of gestation. The typical colobomatous defect is located inferonasally and is frequently associated with other ocular anomalies. According to the grade of involvement regarding the ocular and surrounding tissues, these anomalies can vary from a small iris coloboma or choroidal coloboma to clinical orbital cysts, with extrusion of intraocular tissues through the sclera.[1,4] The visual pathways and the occipital cortex may also be hypoplasic.[5]

Complex Microphthalmos

Complex microphthalmos is associated with other syndromes (Table 33-5)[35] and further anatomic malformations of the anterior or posterior segment of the eye, but it is not related to the incomplete closure of the embryonic fissure. This is a heterogeneous group of conditions in which the microphthalmia is secondary to the other ocular abnormalities.[4,5]

Table 33-5 Syndromes associated with microphthalmia

Trisomy 13 (Patau's syndrome)
Chromosome 18 deletion syndrome
Congenital rubella
Hallermann-Streiff syndrome
LSD (lysergic acid diethylamide) embryopathy
Goldenhar's syndrome
Oculodentodigital syndrome
Pierre Robin syndrome
Oculocerebrorenal syndrome
Focal dermal hypoplasia
Francois' syndrome
Ullrich's syndrome

Modified from Ritch R: Glaucoma related to other ocular disorders. In Richt R, Shields M, editors: *The secondary glaucomas*, St Louis, 1982, Mosby, pp 55-57.

Congenital cataracts are common[1] in these patients and are usually associated with poorly developed or defective retinal and optic nerve structures, which further compromise the visual prognosis.

SHORT ANTERIOR CHAMBER DEPTH WITH NORMAL AXIAL LENGTH: RELATIVE ANTERIOR MICROPHTHALMOS

In 1980, Naumann coined the term 'relative anterior microphthalmos' (RAM) to describe smaller than usual eyes that did not fit into any classification. He described eyes with an axial length greater than 20 mm and a horizontal corneal diameter between 9 and 11 mm, but with disproportionately smaller anterior segment volumes.

The terminology and classification used for RAM and microcornea are confusing. Microcornea is a classification based exclusively on the dimension of the cornea (smaller than 10 mm) and can occur as part of the simple, colobomatous, and/or complex microphthalmos.

RAM refers to those eyes with a normal axial length and a disproportionate smaller anterior segment, despite the corneal diameters, which may be in the microcornea or in the lower normal range. These eyes show no other morphologic macroscopic malformations and can easily be overlooked at slit-lamp examination. RAM is more common than nanophthalmos and high hyperopia (Table 33-6).

Like nanophthalmic patients, RAM patients are at high risk of developing chronic angle-closure glaucoma as a result of the crowded anterior segment; however, these eyes do not have scleral abnormalities or uveal effusion. If pupillary block is untreated, then angle-closure glaucoma will progress.

Table 33-6 Anatomic parameters in relative anterior microphthalmos vs. nanophthalmos

Ocular Parameters	Relative Anterior Microphthalmos	Nanophthalmos
Corneal diameter	Average: 10.7 mm Range: 9–11 mm	Average: 10.3 mm Range: 9.5–11 mm
Anterior chamber depth	Average: 2.2 mm Range: 0.98–3.70 mm	Average: 1.46 mm Range: 1–2.7 mm
Anteroposterior lens thickness	Average: 5.05 mm Range: 3.49–6.46 mm	Average: 5.18 mm Range: 4.20–7.26 mm
Total axial length	Average: 21.92 mm Range: 20.29–23.89 mm	Average: 17 mm Range: 14.5–20.5 mm
Refractive error	Average: −0.13 diopters Range: −6.0–+7.5 diopters	Average: +13.60 diopters Range: +7.25–+20.00 diopters

Modified from Auffarth GU, Blum M, Faller U et al: Relative anterior microphthalmos: morphometric analysis and its implications for cataract surgery, *Ophthalmology* 107:1555-1560, 2000.

NORMAL ANTERIOR CHAMBER DEPTH WITH SHORT AXIAL LENGTH: AXIAL HIGH HYPEROPIA

A third group of microphthalmic eyes are characterized by high hyperopia but normal anterior chamber depth, despite the short axial length. These eyes usually do not have the same complications as the two previous groups and the morphology of the anterior chamber is normal. The main issue in this group of patients is the high refractive error.

■ PREOPERATIVE ASSESSMENT ■

The potential hazards of cataract surgery or glaucoma surgery in eyes with nanophthalmos and, to a lesser extent, RAM, demand the identification of patients with these conditions preoperatively to allow for the necessary prophylactic measures to be taken, thus, minimizing the likelihood of serious complications during cataract surgery and in the postoperative period.

NANOPHTHALMOS

Evaluation for Potential Nanophthalmic Glaucoma

Eyes with small corneal diameters and refractive errors of greater than 8 diopters (D) of hypermetropia, and axial lengths of less than 20.5 mm, should be evaluated for other features of nanophthalmos before intraocular surgery is performed, and special attention should be given to evaluation of potential nanophthalmic glaucoma.

Indentation or compression gonioscopy can be performed with a mirrored goniolens, such as Zeiss or Sussman. The extreme iris convexity in microphthalmic eyes and indentation of the small cornea that can produce Descemet's folds, obscures visualization of the angle. A child's 12 mm Koeppe lens, bilaterally inserted, offers a clear view with simultaneous comparison of both eyes and allows for examination by multiple observers without moving the lens;[33] however, this requires special equipment and proficiency with this skill.

Ultrasound biomiscroscopy (UBM) may be used to document the relationship between the anterior chamber structures and the anatomy of the angle to identify peripheral choroidal effusions (Figure 33-5).

B-scan ultrasonography may be used to verify the thickness of the sclera and choroid, as well as the presence of uveal effusions that can be difficult to detect by clinical exam.

In view of the high risk of angle-closure glaucoma, it is important to evaluate and document the optic disc in all eyes, irrespective of the IOP. Optic nerve visualization and photography may not be possible due to poor dilation in nanophthalmic eyes. If the angle is extremely narrow, laser iridotomy should be performed before attempting pharmacologic mydriasis. In these cases, documentation of the disc may be achieved by drawings or imaging techniques that do not require dilation, such as confocal scanning laser ophthalmoscopy and scanning laser polarimetry.

In nanophthalmic patients, the prophylactic and therapeutic approach depends on the status of this condition, which may be divided into five stages (Table 33-7).[33]

Therapy of Nanophthalmos

In 1980, Brockhurst[30] described the successful use of vortex vein decompression by the dissection of a large partial-thickness sclerectomy around the vortex veins for the treatment of nanophthalmic uveal effusions. In 1983, based on his hypothesis that the primary cause of the idiopathic uveal effusion syndrome was the impairment of transscleral outflow of proteins by the abnormal sclera, Gass[19] proposed a new surgical technique: a quadrantic equatorial partial-thickness sclerectomy. The successful use of this scleral-thinning procedure, without vortex-vein decompression, in patients with nanophthalmic uveal effusion, supports the hypothesis that the barrier effect of sclera is more important than the vortex-vein obstructing effect.[31,36–38]

Uveal effusion usually resolves within several months of surgical intervention.[19,31,38] However, recurrence of uveal effusion several months or years after the first scleral thinning procedure has been reported, in which case, repetition of the surgery proved to be successful.[31,36] Recurrence can be explained by the wound healing at the sclerectomy, with the scar tissue blocking the bypass created surgically.[39] Recently, new techniques have been proposed to minimize the scarring of the sclerectomy sites and to promote long-term control of uveal effusion. Akduman, Adelberg, and Del Priore[40] described the successful use of topical mitomycin-C (0.3 mg/mL for $2\frac{1}{2}$ min) over the sclerectomy sites, and Krohn and Seland[41] reported the use of absorbable gelatin film to cover the scleral bed after the procedure in order to maintain a low resistance to transscleral outflow and prevent scarring.

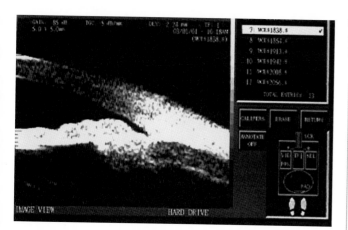

Figure 33-5 Ultrasound biomiscroscope image of nanophthalmic eye showing the anatomy of the angle. Note the thickened choroidal layer.

Table 33-7 Stages of nanophthalmic glaucoma	
Stage 1	Narrow angles; nanophthalmos recognized/no elevation of intraocular pressure
Stage 2	Progressive narrowing of the angle/angle closure threatened but not present
Stage 3	Progressive narrowing of the angle/angle partially closed
Stage 4	Extensive angle closure/increased intraocular pressure controlled with medical therapy
Stage 5	Angle closed by synechiae/intraocular pressure uncontrolled by medical therapy

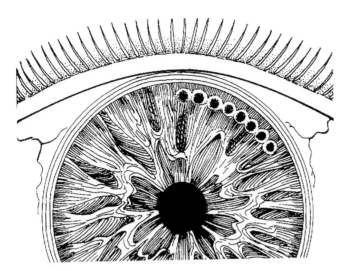

Figure 33-6 Gonioplasty burns from 1 to 2 clock hours.

Table 33-8 Laser settings for gonioplasty in nanophthalmos	
Power	200–500 mW
Spot size	250–500 μm
Time	0.2–0.5 s
Applications	Three to five burns per clock hour
Each session	3–4 clock hours

In stage 1 and 2, nanophthalmic eyes with anterior chamber angles that are judged to be narrow and occludable angles with indentation gonioscopy, prophylactic laser iridotomy is indicated. Uveal effusions after prophylactic laser trabeculoplasty and retinal photocoagulation in nanophthalmic patients have been reported.[36,42]

The thicker than normal iris in nanophthalmic eyes makes penetration of the stroma with neodymium:yttrium-aluminum-garnet (Nd:YAG) laser usually more difficult than in other eyes with chronic narrow angle configuration. To facilitate perforation, argon laser burns should be applied to thin the proposed iridotomy site before final treatment with the Nd:YAG laser.[43]

Although successful iridotomies eliminate pupillary block, the peripheral iris can remain convex and the angle narrow in these eyes. Despite the patent iridotomy, the angle may progressively narrow (stage 3). In this stage, laser gonioplasty, or peripheral

iridoplasty, can be used to flatten the peripheral iris, widen the angle, and prevent the development of peripheral anterior synechiae. Gonioplasty in some cases may cause separation of early peripheral anterior synechiae.

To perform gonioplasty, after miosis is achieved with 2% pilocarpine hydrochloride, a mirrored contact gonioscopic lens is used to visualize the peripheral iris and to apply low-power argon laser burns. With a spot size of 250–500 μm and a laser power of 200 mW, and a duration or 200 ms, the power is slowly increased until a localized iris burn with contraction is observed. Gonioplasty is applied to 3–4 clock hours at a time (Figures 33-6 and 33-7, Table 33-8), and caution is taken not to over-treat, as that could cause injury to the dilator muscle fibers and result in mydriasis. Widening of the angle achieved by gonioplasty may gradually lessen, in which case repeated iridoplasty may be of value. The procedure may be performed multiple times until it is no longer beneficial. In many cases, the anterior chamber angle may be prevented from closing for several years (Figure 33-8).

If gonioplasty fails to maintain a functioning open angle, before IOP is permanently elevated, sclerectomies may be employed to widen the angle by reducing the amount of fluid in the supra-choroidal space. The technique has been used since the 1980s and is illustrated in Figures 33-9A–E.

At stage 4, when angle closure is extensive and the IOP is substantially elevated, the authors opt to treat with topical

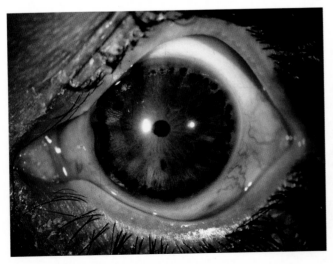

Figure 33-7 Appearance of nanophthalmic eye following successful opening of the entire angle with argon laser gonioplasty, done in multiple sessions.

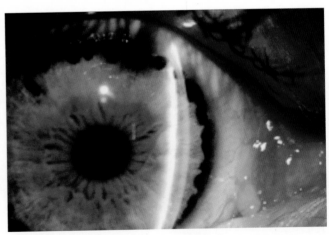

Figure 33-8 Nanophthalmic eye showing the narrow, but open angle maintained with multiple sessions of argon-laser gonioplasty.

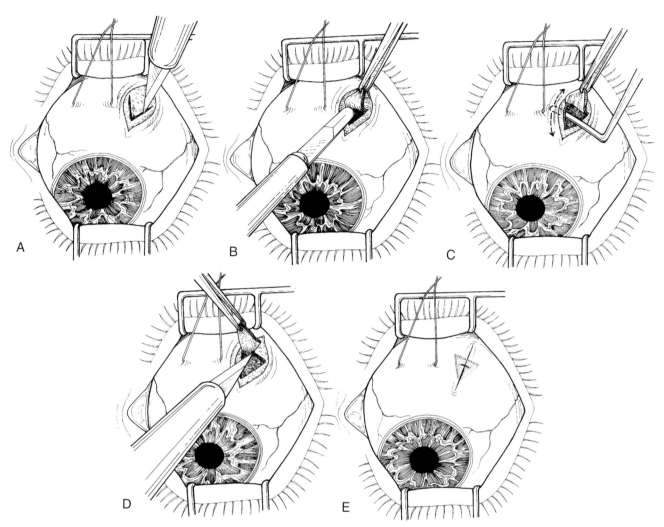

Figure 33-9 **A,** After a radial incision is created in both lower quadrants, a full-thickness triangular scleral flap 4 × 4 × 4 mm is created, with its apex at 3.5 mm from the limbus, over the pars plana. **B,** Flap is dissected posteriorly to expose the underlying choroid. **C,** Cyclodialysis spatula is then advanced to both sides of the sclerectomy, tangentially to the sclera, to drain any existing fluid from the suprachoroidal spaces. **D,** Full-thickness scleral flaps are excised completely, leaving two full-thickness triangular sclerectomies in each lower quadrant. **E,** Conjunctival incisions are closed with one or two 10-0 interrupted nylon sutures.

aqueous humor suppressants, such as beta blockers, carbonic antihydrase inhibitors, and alpha agonists until they become ineffective. Stage 5 is defined by extensive synechial closure of the angle at which time further laser iridotomy, laser gonioplasty, and medical therapy are ineffective. At this point, two IOP-lowering strategies are available: filtering surgery or a cycloablative procedure.

In stage 5, when glaucoma is such that trabeculectomy can be temporarily deferred, the authors prefer to perform prophylactic anterior sclerectomies (as shown in Figures 33-9A–E) in the two lower quadrants, 4 to 6 weeks before the filtering procedure to allow recovery before trabeculectomy. However, if the IOP is so severely elevated that immediate surgery is necessary, anterior sclerectomies may be performed at the time of the trabeculectomy. We modified our trabeculectomy procedure to

minimize hypotony in nanophthalmic eyes, using high-viscosity viscoelastic in the anterior chamber to prevent sudden decompression of the anterior chamber, replacing sutures in the flap to allow rapid closure and making scleral flap closure tighter than usual.

Cyclodestructive procedures are generally used as a last resort when other attempts to control IOP have failed.

Phacoemulsification in nanophthalmic patients may be performed when IOP is well controlled and should be performed after, or simultaneously with, prophylactic sclerectomies. The use of early phacoemulsification as a therapy for narrow angles and as a prophylaxis for angle-closure glaucoma in nanophthalmos is hypothetical and controversial. It can be considered in the face of progressive narrowing of the angle despite other treatments, before extensive synechiae are formed.

COLOBOMATOUS AND COMPLEX MICROPHTHALMOS

Despite different pathophysiologies, colobomatous and complex, microphthalmos can be assessed in the same manner because the common and more important feature is the presence of associated ocular or systemic pathologic conditions. In both cases, the final visual acuity is extremely variable and depends on the grade of disorganization of ocular tissues and integrity of the visual pathway. The presence of congenital cataracts is common in both diseases[1] and is usually associated with poorly developed or defective retinal and optic nerve structures that will further compromise the visual prognosis. For these reasons, cataract surgery is not always indicated in these patients. In children, the health and systemic prognosis of the child should be carefully considered, and the pediatrician should perform a thorough evaluation before the decision to perform cataract surgery is made.

In viable eyes with some expectation of visual acuity improvement, some surgeons[44] recommend using corneal diameter measurements to determine surgical planning as follows:

- Eyes with corneal diameters of less than 5 mm probably should not have cataract surgery unless the cataracts are bilateral. In such cases, surgery without an intraocular lens (IOL) is indicated. Surgery should be performed in the eye with the largest cornea and longest axial length or the one presenting the most normal ocular structures. The correction of aphakia in these cases should be done with spectacles.

- If the corneal diameter is between 6 and 9 mm, a rigid gas-permeable contact lens with a reduced diameter could be adapted.

- In complex microphthalmic eyes with corneal diameters greater than 9 mm, a posterior chamber IOL should be considered.

Patients with choroidal colobomas are at a higher risk for retinal detachment and should be warned of the symptoms.[1] Therefore, any retinal area susceptible to retinal detachment should be treated prophylactically before surgery.

RELATIVE ANTERIOR MICROPHTHALMOS

Indications for cataract extraction in eyes with relative anterior microphthalmos are the same as for normal eyes. Auffarth et al.[4] found that lens removal alone leads to a significant IOP reduction and a decrease in the number of glaucoma medicines in eyes with RAM. The main complication after cataract surgery in these eyes is iridovitreal block. Because of the increased incidence of cornea guttata, transitory or permanent corneal edema can occur following cataract surgery. Another risk factor for cataract surgery in this group is the increased incidence of the pseudoexfoliation syndrome.[4]

AXIAL HYPEROPIA

Phacoemulsification surgery in high hyperopic patients is carried out using the standard surgical technique. In addition to cataract extraction, clear lensectomy for refractive correction in the absence of significant opacity of the lens may be another indication for phacoemulsification. Other techniques for refractive correction in low-to-moderate hyperopic patients include laser in situ keratomileusis (LASIK), photorefractive keratectomy, and laser thermal keratoplasty.[45]

Clear lens extraction in high hyperopic eyes was first described by Lyle and Jin[46] in 1994, in six patients with refractive errors between +4.25 and +7.87, with axial lengths greater than 20.5 mm. No complications were reported during surgery or in the postoperative period. Refractive lensectomy for high hyperopia may have several advantages over other refractive techniques. It has the ability to correct higher refractive errors, offers a higher predictability of refractive outcome, does not cause irregular astigmatism, and it is less likely to result in regression hyperopia.[47] The risks of retinal detachment, loss of accommodation, and of endophthalmitis, in addition to the difficulty in obtaining an optimal IOL selection without using a piggyback IOL implantation, have prevented the widespread acceptance of this treatment for high hyperopia.

Regardless of the indication for phacoemulsification, either cataract extraction or refractive correction, there may be difficulties in the calculation of the implant power[48,49] because of the disproportion between anterior and posterior segments. In addition, extremely high hyperopic eyes require high-power IOLs that are often not available. Piggyback implantation of two IOLs has been used in these eyes with mixed results.

■ INTRAOCULAR LENS ASSESSMENT IN EYES WITH EXTREMELY SHORT AXIAL LENGTH ■

AXIAL LENGTH MEASUREMENT

The measurement of axial length is a critical determinant of the IOL power and a final refractive result in any patient. This is particularly true in extremely short eyes, where a minor error in axial length measurement can lead to a large and unexpected refractive error.[3] An accurate axial length determination can be a challenge in these eyes because most ultrasound biometry devices are calibrated with the average velocities of normal-sized eyes, and some still have limitations of axial length range, not measuring values of less than 21.5 mm.[49] Because of the short axial length, the posterior wall echo can be of great intensity, sometimes making it necessary to reduce the gain to obtain a clear echo (Figure 33-10).[48] Any

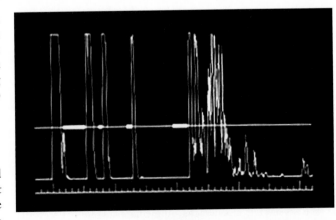

Figure 33-10 Biometry of a nanophthalmic eye. Total axial length is 16.98 mm, lens thickness is 5.05 mm, and anterior chamber depth is 2.77 mm.

flattening of the corneal surface during applanation biometry can also account for significant IOL calculation errors. Immersion biometry and/or optical biometry with partial coherence inferometry (PCI) (IOL Master, Zeiss Humphrey Systems) may be useful in these cases to obtain more accurate results.

LENS POWER CALCULATION

IOL power calculations for extremely short eyes remain a problem for the cataract surgeon. This can be attributed to the poor predictability of the older formulas. Current third-generation formulas (SRK/T, Holladay II, Hoffer Q, and Haigis) that take into account variables such as anterior chamber depth, corneal diameter, and lens thickness, have improved refractive predictability.[3,49–51] Theoretical formulas have been shown to be more accurate than empirical ones in microphthalmic eyes.[52,53] In a study of IOL calculations, Inatomi et al.[52] demonstrated that all of the formulas tested still showed a tendency for residual hypermetropia. A recent study of short eyes (axial length below 22 mm) showed that the Hoffer Q formula was significantly more accurate than the SRK-T in determining the correct IOL power.[54] This study, by Gavin and Hammond, is the largest retrospective and prospective examination of lens power (41 eyes) in this group of patients (axial length range 21.96–20.29 mm with a mean of 21.51 mm).[54] Until newer and more accurate formulas are available, calculations for eyes with an axial length of <22 mm should be made using more than one formula for comparison and should be weighted toward the results of the Hoffer Q formula.

IMPLANT CHOICE

Implant choice is another challenge for the surgeon, because rigid polymethylmethacrylate (PMMA) IOLs with a power greater than +45.0 D and foldable lenses greater than +40.0 D are not available.[54,55] Implanting two PMMA posterior chamber lenses to achieve the desired total lens power was proposed by Gayton[56] in 1993, when +35.0 D was the maximum power available. These piggyback implantations later proved to offer better optical quality and cause less spherical aberration than a single lens with such a high dioptric power.[3] In 1996, Shugar[57] implanted two acrylic foldable lenses in six patients. He combined the advantages of small-incision surgery and the increased biocompatibility of the acrylic material. Acrylic lenses are most suitable for the higher power IOL that is implanted posteriorly in planned piggyback implantation, because the high refractive index of acrylic lenses allows them to be thinner and flatter than PMMA or silicone lenses. To avoid interlenticular membrane formation from the growth of lens epithelial cells between the IOLs, many surgeons advocate that the anterior piggyback IOL should have a silicone optic, be of low power, and be placed in the sulcus.

Gills and Cherchio[58] calculate the lens power by dividing the total power equally between the two lenses, whereas others prefer to place two-thirds of the lens power in the more posterior lens and one-third anteriorly.[49] This last option offers more advantages. By placing the more powerful lens posteriorly within the bag, spherical aberrations can be reduced. Inserting the least powerful lens in the sulcus facilitates access to the lens in case an exchange for a different power lens is necessary at a later date.

MODIFICATIONS IN CATARACT SURGERY TECHNIQUE IN MICROPHTHALMIC EYES

Standard large-incision extracapsular cataract extraction in eyes with increased IOP results in a sudden drop in pressure to atmospheric values, which can lead to dilation of the choroidal vascular bed increasing the risk of intrachoroidal effusion, suprachoroidal or intrachoroidal hemorrhage, or expulsive hemorrhage. This technique is dangerous in eyes with short anterior-chamber depth, and specifically in nanophthalmic eyes, in which the inelasticity of the sclera makes these complications more likely.

Phacoemulsification allows avoidance of intraocular hypotony during surgery. When performing phaco surgery, these eyes should be carefully prepared and the IOP lowered to normal levels preoperatively. If topical medications and mechanical pressure-lowering devices (e.g., Honan's balloon) are not sufficient to lower the pressure to less than 25 mm Hg, 20% mannitol IV, 1–2 mL/kg body weight, should be employed 15–30 min before surgery. In rare cases, the surgery can be performed under general anesthesia with controlled hypotension, resulting in a reduction in arterial pressure, thus decreasing the risks associated with a dramatic pressure drop.[48]

Topical and intracameral anesthesia may have some advantage over peribulbar and retrobulbar anesthesia, as local infiltration causes an increase in orbital volume, which may precipitate an increase in posterior pressure and vortex vein congestion. Clear corneal incisions in eyes with shallow anterior chamber depths offer the surgeon a better anatomic approach to the lens and allow the employment of smaller and safer incisions.[49] A shorter and more anterior corneal tunnel will help to prevent iris prolapse and facilitate manipulation of the nucleus.[48] A temporal approach is especially useful in these microphthalmic eyes which are typically deeply set in a normal-sized orbit.

Maximal control over intraocular fluid dynamics is critical, and the new technology phaco machines offer great advantages over older ones. Paracentesis should be done carefully and gradually, avoiding the iris and anterior capsule. Intraoperative hypotony should be avoided as much as possible.

In severely hyperopic eyes, RAM, and nanophthalmic eyes, the shallow anterior chambers limit the distance between the anterior capsule and the corneal endothelium resulting in limited workspace for phacoemulsification. These eyes often have low endothelial cell counts and risk corneal decompensation following cataract extraction. The Arshinoff soft-shell technique using a cohesive viscoelastic in the center of the anterior chamber and a dispersive viscoelastic above it, may better stabilize the eye, decrease iris prolapse, and protect the endothelium.[49,59]

Posterior synechiae and pupillary membranes, if present, should be dissected off the anterior capsule with an iris spatula. A 30-gauge needle can also be placed on the viscoelastic syringe to perform viscodisection while using the cutting edge of the needle to facilitate this process. If viscoelastic substance and pharmacologic agents (including 10% phenylephrine) fail to increase the pupil size, mechanical dilation of the pupil or sphincterotomies may be needed.

The size of capsulorrhexis should be selected in accordance with the IOL plan. For a single implant 5–6 mm is adequate.

Generous use of viscoelastic is recommended to hyperinflate and maintain the anterior chamber depth, despite the posterior vitreous pressure. This will help depress and flatten the anterior capsule, thus preventing radial extension of the capsulorrhexis. For piggyback implantation, a larger (6.5–7 mm) capsulorrhexis is preferred so that the border of the anterior capsule does not cover the edge of the IOL.[60]

The use of a Kelman–Mackool phaco tip may facilitate surgical manipulation as its tip is bent downward toward the cataract.[49,56] It is important to remember to enter the eye with the phacoemulsification handpiece in the irrigation position. Chilled balanced salt solution (BSS) may help to prevent incision burns in these shallow, anterior chambers.[60]

The anterior epinucleus should be removed before phacoemulsification of the nucleus to allow more space for working in the anterior chamber. During nucleus removal, a chopping technique[48,49,59] with high vacuum and short pulses of ultrasound may be helpful. The surgeon should start with a lower phaco power and increase it, as dictated by nuclear density, up to an efficient rate. Working in the nucleus at the level of the iris plane or in the posterior chamber avoids the endothelium and helps maintain the integrity of the incision.

The risk of a posterior capsular rupture is increased in these eyes because of the frequent presence of significant posterior pressure, weakened zonules, and floppy capsules.[61] To reduce the incidence of this complication, vacuum should be decreased during the removal of the last pieces of nucleus, and a second instrument should be used to protect the posterior capsule.

Automated irrigation–aspiration should be done thoroughly to prevent interlenticular opacification in the case of piggyback implantation.

If a single IOL is planned, there are no changes in the technique. In the case of piggyback implantation, the first lens should be placed in the bag, with the haptics oriented vertically. The second lens should then be inserted into the sulcus vertically with forceps, while maintaining downward pressure on the optic through the side port with the second instrument. The haptics of the two lenses should remain perpendicular to each other, increasing the separation between the optics and perhaps decreasing the incidence of interlenticular opacification.[56] Special attention should be given to viscoelastic removal from behind and between the two lenses.

The incision should be closed with a 10-0 nylon suture to protect against wound leakage and hypotony in the postoperative period, which could lead to a disastrous outcome, especially in nanophthalmic eyes.

POSTOPERATIVE MONITORING

Careful observation is required following any anterior segment surgery in microphthalmic eyes. Some surgeons re-evaluate the patient 4–6 hours after surgery for IOP and anterior-chamber-depth evaluation.

Cataract extraction can dramatically improve the IOP in many cases with narrow angles (e.g., RAM). After surgery, eyes with persistent IOP elevation can be treated with laser trabeculoplasty because their angles are now more accessible.[48]

In patients who undergo piggyback IOL implantation, a dilated exam is recommended every 4–6 months for evaluation of interlenticular opacification.[48]

COMPLICATIONS OF SURGERY

Many complications that arise during and after surgery in microphthalmic eyes are the same as those observed in the routine phacoemulsification of normal-sized eyes. However, they tend to occur with much higher frequency, depending on the disproportion between anterior and posterior chamber depths.[48] Microphthalmic eyes are predisposed to positive vitreous pressure and iris prolapse resulting in technically more challenging cases.[60]

CORNEAL BURNS

Microphthalmic eyes with shallow anterior chambers are at greater risk of corneal burns given the proximity of the endothelium to the phacoemulsification tip. The use of chilled BSS has been shown to reduce the incidence of this complication. Inserting the phaco handpiece in the irrigating position with careful positioning of the tip in the anterior chamber prior to phacoemulsification also reduces this complication.

RUPTURE OR DISINSERTION OF POSTERIOR CAPSULE

The posterior capsule is thin in microphthalmic eyes and very susceptible to ruptures that can extend dramatically because of the positive vitreous pressure present in these small eyes. Surgery may lead to partial or total zonular dialysis. There is no consensus on the best course of action when implantation of a posterior chamber IOL is not feasible due to lack of capsular support. An anterior chamber IOL is difficult to implant in a shallow anterior chamber and, if implanted, carries with it a high risk of subsequent corneal decompensation. Immediate or subsequent scleral fixation of the implant is an extremely risky maneuver associated with uveal effusions and hemorrhage.[48] This is especially true for nanophthalmic eyes, which are most susceptible to these complications.

UVEAL EFFUSIONS/HEMORRHAGES

As emphasized earlier, nanophthalmos is a special group of microphthalmic eyes distinguished by its abnormal sclera. Uveal effusions in this group of patients can occur spontaneously or may be precipitated by cataract extraction, glaucoma surgery, argon laser trabeculoplasty, and even prophylactic laser iridotomy.[42,62] Any eye surgery can precipitate or worsen a previous effusion by inflammatory increase of protein leakage or by reduction of transscleral hydrostatic pressure during intraoperative and/or postoperative hypotony. The effusions can be intrachoroidal, suprachoroidal, or both.

Suprachoroidal hemorrhage is more common in nanophthalmic patients. The sudden decompression of the eye during surgery may lead to choroidal engorgement that cannot be handled because of the inelastic sclera.

In case of sudden uveal effusion or hemorrhage, surgery must be interrupted, and tight closure of wounds must be performed. No further intervention is advised until the problem is resolved.

RETINAL DETACHMENTS

Exudative retinal detachment can occur in isolation after surgery or following postoperative uveal effusion if treatment of the latter is delayed or fails. Treatment of exudative retinal detachment consists of performing multiple sclerectomies, as described previously in this chapter (see Figure 33-9A–E).[37,41,42,62,63]

ANGLE-CLOSURE GLAUCOMA

Many nanophthalmic and RAM eyes have narrow angles with crowded anterior chambers; therefore, the surgeon should be guarded to the possibility that a strong preoperative dilation on the day of surgery may induce a primary angle closure attack in the most susceptible eyes.[60] Secondary angle closure can be caused by sudden peripheral uveal effusion and/or exudative retinal detachment, which causes a forward rotation of the ciliary body, forward movement of the peripheral iris, and pseudophakic pupillary block.[9,33]

If the aqueous is misdirected to the vitreous instead of to the posterior chamber, malignant glaucoma can occur. Cycloplegic and mydriatic therapy should be initiated, together with steroids, and Nd:YAG laser to the anterior hyaloid face through a patent iridectomy may be attempted. If suprachoroidal effusion is also present, surgical drainage of fluid may be required. Posterior vitrectomy should be kept as a last resort for treatment of this complication.[48]

INTERLENTICULAR OPACIFICATION

Also known as interpseudophakos opacification or interpseudophakos Elschnig pearls, this late complication of piggyback IOL implantation recently became the subject of diverse studies and research.[57,64,65] It is characterized by the ingrowth of lens epithelial cells in the space between the two IOLs and results in a hyperopic shift in these patients. It occurs most commonly 1–3 years following the piggyback IOL implantation.

This complication appears to be related to the border apposition of the anterior capsule toward the surface of the anterior lens. To avoid this problem, the authors recommend the use of a larger capsulorrhexis and the insertion of one lens in the bag and the other in the sulcus, instead of inserting both lenses into the bag. Thorough cleaning of epithelial cells from the remaining anterior and posterior capsule should be performed. In patients with microphthalmos and narrow angles, both lenses may be inserted into the bag, as this maximizes the anterior chamber depth and angle dimensions.[57] Some surgeons believe that interlenticular cellular ingrowth is minimized when the optic of the anterior IOL is silicone.

If an interlenticular opacity develops, treatment varies from the use of Nd:YAG in the borders of anterior capsulorrhexis to an IOL exchange. If a lens exchange is necessary due to interlenticular opacification, the surgeon should base the IOL calculation on previous measurements because a hyperopic shift may have occurred.

References

[1] Bateman J. Microphthalmos in development abnormalities of the eye. Int Ophthalmol Clin 1984;24:87–106.
[2] Warburg M. Genetics of microphthalmos. Int Ophthalmol 1981;4:45–65.
[3] Holladay J. Achieving emmetropia in extremely short eyes with two piggyback posterior chamber intraocular lenses. Ophthalmology 1996;103:1118–1123.
[4] Auffarth GU, Blum M, Faller U, et al. Relative anterior microphthalmos: morphometric analysis and its implications for cataract surgery. Ophthalmology 2000;107:1555–1560.
[5] Duke-Elder S. Normal and abnormal development: congenital deformities. In: Duke-Elder S, editor. System of ophthalmology. St Louis: Mosby; 1964. p. 488–495.
[6] Singh O. Nanophthalmos: a perspective on identification and therapy. Ophthalmology 1982;89:1006.
[7] Weiss A. Simple microphthalmos. Arch Ophthalmol 1989;107:1625–1630.
[8] Brockhurst R. Nanophthalmos with uveal effusion: a new clinical entity. Trans Am Ophthalmol Soc 1974;LXXII:371–404.
[9] Ryan E. Nanophthalmos with uveal effusion. Ophthalmology 1982;89:1013–1017.
[10] Altintas A, Acar MA, Yalvac IS, et al. Autosomal recessive nanophthalmos. Acta Ophthalmol Scand 1997;75:325–328.
[11] Othman MI, Sullivan SA, Skuta GL, et al. Autosomal dominant nanophthalmos (NNO1) with high hyperopia and angle-closure glaucoma maps to chromosome 11. Am J Hum Genet 1998;63:1411–1418.
[12] O'Grady R. Nanophthalmos. AJO 1971;71:1251–1253.
[13] Calhoun F. The management of glaucoma in nanophthalmos. Trans Am Ophthalmol Soc 1975;73:97.
[14] Cross H. Familial nanophthalmos. AJO 1976;81:300–306.
[15] Ghose S. Bilateral nanophthalmos, pigmentary retinal dystrophy, and angle-closure glaucoma: a new syndrome? Br J Ophthalmol 1985;69:624.
[16] MacKay C, Shek MS, Carr RE, Yanuzzi LA, Gouras P. Retinal degeneration with nanophthalmos, cystic macular degeneration, and angle-closure glaucoma. Arch Ophthalmol 1987;105:366–371.
[17] Buys YM, Pavlin CJ. Retinitis pigmentosa, nanophthalmos, and optic disc drusen: a case report. Ophthalmology 1999;106:619–622.
[18] Serrano JC, Hodgkins PR, Taylor DS, et al. The nanophthalmic macula. Br J Ophthalmol 1998;82:276–279.
[19] Gass J. Uveal effusion syndrome: a new hypothesis concerning pathogenesis and technique of surgical treatment. Retina 1983;3:159–163.
[20] Gass J. Idiopathic serous detachment of the choroid, ciliary body, and retina (uveal effusion syndrome). Ophthalmology 1982;89:1018–1032.
[21] Yamani A, Wood I, Sugino I, et al. Abnormal collagen fibrils in nanophthalmos: a clinical and histologic study. Am J Ophthalmol 1999;127:106–108, (erratum Am J Ophthalmol 1999;127:635).
[22] Trelstad R. Nanophthalmic sclera: ultrastructural, histochemical, and biochemical observations. Arch Ophthalmol 1982;100:1935.
[23] Stewart D. Abnormal scleral collagen in nanophthalmos. Arch Ophthalmol 1991;109:1017–1025.
[24] Shiono T. Abnormal sclerocytes in nanophthalmos. Graefes Arch Clin Exp Ophthalmol 1992;230:348–351.
[25] Kawamura M. Biochemical studies of glycosaminoglycans in nanophthalmic sclera. Graefes Arch Clin Exp Ophthalmol 1995;233:58–62.
[26] Kawamura M. Immunohistochemical studies of glycosaminoglycans in nanophthalmic sclera. Graefes Arch Clin Exp Ophthalmol 1996;234:19–24.
[27] Yue B. Nanophthalmic sclera: morphologic and tissue culture studies. Ophthalmology 1986;93:534.
[28] Yue B. Nanophthalmic sclera: fibronectin studies. Ophthalmology 1988;95:56–60.
[29] Ward RC, Gragoudas ES, Pon DM, et al. Abnormal scleral findings in uveal effusion syndrome. Am J Ophthalmol 1988;106:139–146.
[30] Brockhurst R. Vortex vein decompression for nanophthalmic uveal effusion. Arch Ophthalmol 1980;98:1987–1990.
[31] Johnson M. Surgical management of the idiopathic uveal effusion syndrome. Ophthalmology 1990;97:778–785.
[32] Shaffer R. Discussion of Calhoun FP Jr: The management of glaucoma in nanophthalmos. Trans Am Ophthalmol Soc 1975;73:119–120.
[33] Simmons R. Nanophthalmos: diagnosis and treatment. In: Epstein D, editor. Chandler and Grant's glaucoma. Philadelphia: Lea & Febiger; 1986. p. 251–259.
[34] Jalkh A. Diffuse choroidal thickening detected by ultrasonography in various ocular disorders. Retina 1983;3:277–283.
[35] Ritch R. Glaucoma related to other ocular disorders. In: Ritch R, Shields M, editors. The secondary glaucomas. St Louis: Mosby; 1982. p. 55–57.
[36] Good W. Recurrent nanophthalmic uveal effusion syndrome following laser trabeculoplasty. Am J Ophthalmol 1988;106:234–235.
[37] Casswell AG, Gregor ZJ, Bird AC. The surgical management of uveal effusion syndrome. Eye 1987;1(pt 1):115–119.
[38] Allen KM, Meyers SM, Zegarra H. Nanophthalmic uveal effusion. Retina 1988;8:145–147.
[39] Morita H. Recurrence of nanophthalmic uveal effusion. Ophthalmologica 1993;207:30–36.
[40] Akduman L, Adelberg DA, Del Priore LV. Nanophthalmic uveal effusion managed with scleral windows and topical mitomycin-C. Ophthalmic Surg Lasers 1997;28:325–327.
[41] Krohn J, Seland JH. Exudative retinal detachment in nanophthalmos. Acta Ophthalmol Scand 1998;76:499–502.
[42] Lesnoni G, Rossi T, Nistri A, et al. Nanophthalmic uveal effusion syndrome after prophylactic laser treatment. Eur J Ophthalmol 1999;9:315–318.
[43] Belcher CD, Greff LJ. Laser therapy of angle-closure glaucoma. In: Albert DM, Jakobiec FA, editors. Principles and practice of ophthalmology. Philadelphia: WB Saunders; 2000.
[44] Biglan AW. Pediatric cataract surgery. In: Albert DM, editor. Ophthalmic surgery: principles and techniques. Cambridge: Blackwell Science; 1999. p. 970–1014.
[45] Fink A. Refractive lensectomy for hyperopia. Ophthalmology 2000;107:1540–1548.
[46] Lyle W, Jin GJ. Clear lens extraction for the correction of high refractive error. J Cataract Refract Surg 1994;20:273–276.
[47] Vicary D. Refractive lensectomy to correct ametropia. J Cataract Refract Surg 1999;25:943–948.
[48] Buratto L, Bellucci R. Cataract surgery and intraocular lens implantation in severe hyperopia. In: Buratto L, Osher RH, Masket S, editors. Cataract surgery in complicated cases. Milano, Italy: Slack Inc; 2000. p. 73–85.
[49] Fine IH, Hoffman RS. Phacoemulsification in high hyperopia. In: Buratto L, Osher RH, Masket S, editors. Cataract surgery in complicated cases. Milano, Italy: 2000. p. 67–72.
[50] Fenzl R. Refractive and visual outcome of hyperopic cataract cases operated on before and after implementation of the Holladay II formula. Ophthalmology 1998;105:1759–1764.
[51] Bartke TU, Auffarth GU, Uhl JC, et al. Reliability of intraocular lens power calculation after cataract surgery in patients with relative anterior microphthalmos. Graefes Arch Clin Exp Ophthalmol 2000;238:138–142.

[52] Inatomi M, Ishii K, Koide R, et al. Intraocular lens power calculation for microphthalmos. J Cataract Refract Surg 1997;3:1208–1212.

[53] Huber C. Effectiveness of intraocular lens calculation in high ametropia. J Cataract Refract Surg 1989;15:667–672.

[54] Gavin EA, Hammond CJ. Intraocular lens power calculations in short eyes. Eye 1–4, Published online, 16 March 2007.

[55] Alcon laboratories, Inc. Intraocular Lenses Product Guide. 2007.

[56] Shugar JK. Cataract surgery in microphthalmos. In: Buratto L, Osher RH, Masket S, editors. Cataract surgery in complicated cases. Milano, Italy: Slack Inc; 2000. p. 90–93.

[57] Gayton J. Implanting two posterior chamber intraocular lenses in a case of microphthalmos. J Cataract Refract Surg 1993;19:776–777.

[58] Shugar J. Implantation of multiple foldable acrylic posterior chamber lenses in the capsular bag for high hyperopia. J Cataract Refract Surg 1996;22:1368–1372.

[59] Gills JP, Cherchio M. Phacoemulsification in high hyperopic cataract patients. In: Lu LW, Fine IH, editors. Phacoemulsification in difficult and challenging cases. New York: Thieme Medical Publishers; 1999. p. 21–31.

[60] Dodick JM, Hsu J. Personal technique for cataract removal in high hyperopia. In: Buratto L, Osher RH, Masket S, editors. Cataract surgery in complicated cases. Milano, Italy: Slack Inc; 2000. p. 86.

[61] Gayton J. Cataract surgery and hyperopia. In: Buratto L, Osher RH, Masket S, editors. Cataract surgery in complicated cases. Milano, Italy: Slack Inc; 2000. p. 87–88.

[62] Buratto L, Osher RH, Masket S. Cataract surgery in complicated cases. Milano, Italy: Slack Inc; 2000. p. 466.

[63] Bellows A. Choroidal effusion during glaucoma surgery in patients with prominent episcleral vessels. Arch Ophthalmol 1979;97:493–497.

[64] Faulborn J, Kolli H. Sclerotomy in uveal effusion syndrome. Retina 1999;19:504–507.

[65] Stasiuk R. Interface Elschnig pearl formation with piggyback implantation. J Cataract Refract Surg 2000;26:157–158.

[66] Gayton J. Interlenticular opacification: clinicopathological correlation of a complication of posterior chamber piggyback intraocular lenses. JCRS 2000;26:330–336.

Cataract Surgery in the Presence of Other Ocular Comorbidities

34

Hiroko Bissen-Miyajima, MD, PhD

CONTENTS

- Ocular Surface Disorders
- Diabetes
- Retinitis Pigmentosa
- Eyelid Abnormalities
- Bleeding disorders

CHAPTER HIGHLIGHTS

>> Surgical impact of ocular surface disease

>> Optimization of patients with diabetes mellitus

>> Altered capsule in retinitis pimentosa

>> Anticoagulation

The new technology of phacoemulsification and aspiration and intraocular lens (IOL) implantation facilitates cataract surgery with smaller incisions and fewer complications. These developments have expanded the indications for cataract surgery for eyes with other ocular pathologies.

◾ OCULAR SURFACE DISORDERS ◾

DRY EYE

Knowledge of the presence of pre-existing dry eye before ocular surgery became an important issue with the increasing worldwide popularity of laser in situ keratomileusis (LASIK). Research on the corneal effects of cataract surgery has focused primarily on the endothelium. However, the effects on the epithelium, such as superficial punctate keratopathy (SPK) and epithelial defects, seem to be more common. Patients often complain postoperatively of ocular discomfort with a dry-eye sensation. Dry eye after cataract surgery can be categorized into two groups: the first is the worsening of pre-existing dry-eye symptoms and the second is surgically induced dry eye. The possible effects of cataract surgery on the ocular surface are shown in Table 34-1.

PREOPERATIVE MANAGEMENT

A Dry Eye Workshop recently determined that "dry eye is a multifactorial disorder of tears and the ocular surface associated with symptoms of discomfort or visual disturbances."[1] If there is any doubt about the presence of dry eye before cataract surgery, the patient should be informed that the dry eye may worsen for a couple of months after cataract surgery. Epithelial defects after cataract surgery often develop in patients with decreased tear production. If dry eye is suspected, fluorescein staining of the corneal epithelium and rose bengal staining should be performed, and tear film break-up time should be determined before surgery. If SPK is present, artificial tears or eye drops containing hyaluronic acid should be prescribed to improve the corneal condition. If SPK is refractory to treatment, intracanalicular plugs should be considered. Eye drops containing a preservative such as benzalkonium chloride should be avoided.[2]

SURGICAL PROCEDURE

The side effects of topical anesthesia on the corneal epithelium are well known, and, therefore, application of anesthetic eye drops should be minimal. Exposure to the light source of the operating microscope also should be minimal. The type of incision (sclerocorneal or corneal) does not seem to be problematic in these patients.

POSTOPERATIVE MANAGEMENT

Eye drops containing a preservative tend to cause epithelial problems. Nonsteroidal anti-inflammatory drugs, such as diclofenac sodium, affect the corneal epithelium in certain cases. For patients already diagnosed with dry eye, only antibiotic and steroid regimens should be prescribed. Additional eye drops, such as artificial tears, increase the stability of the precorneal tear film. If SPK is severe in the early stage, the treatment plan may be adjusted to avoid resistant keratopathy. Severe SPK is sometimes

Table 34-1 Effects of cataract surgery on the ocular surface

Preoperative	Dry eye
During surgery	Corneal and conjunctival dryness due to exposure
	Drying from the light source of the operating microscope
	Topical anesthesia
Incision	Transient ischemia due to the separation of the conjunctival and episcleral vessel
	Corneal denervation
Postoperative	Incomplete lid closure
	Eye drops (steroid, diclofenac natrium, preservative)

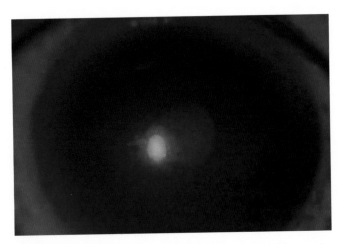

Figure 34-1 Superficial punctate keratopathy. Fluorescein staining over the entire cornea is observed.

seen 1 week after surgery (Figure 34-1). In such cases, all eye drops except artificial tears might have to be stopped. If no improvement is seen, autologous serum eye drops may be prescribed.[3] The procedure for making these eye drops is shown in Table 34-2. Another approach is to use an eye protector or goggles to avoid tear film evaporation.

Table 34-2 Preparation of autologous serum application

40 mL of blood is obtained
↓
Centrifuge for 5 min at 1500 revolutions/minute
↓
Serum is separated
↓
Serum put into a bottle with a coating protective against ultraviolet light
↓
Serum diluted to 20% with physiologic saline

Intracanalicular plugs are useful when the patient still has a dry-eye sensation. Absorbable plugs developed for dry eye after LASIK also can be used.

STEVENS–JOHNSON SYNDROME/OCULAR PEMPHIGOID

Despite refinements to cataract surgery techniques, manipulation inside the eye in the presence of poor conditions on ocular surface remains challenging. The reconstruction of the ocular surface for severe cicatricial keratoconjunctivitis such as Stevens–Johnson syndrome or ocular pemphigoid has changed in the last 10 years. A two-step surgery, ocular surface reconstruction first and cataract surgery second, is advantageous over simultaneous surgeries consisting of cataract extraction and implantation of allograft limbal tissue and amniotic membrane.[4] With the development of tissue engineering, the application of cultivated autologous oral mucosal epithelial tissue seems to result in longer stability of the ocular surface.[5] Micro-incision surgery also is advantageous for these critical cases. The potential problems associated with cataract surgery in eyes with cicatricial kerato-conjunctivitis are shown in Table 34-3.

OCULAR SURFACE RECONSTRUCTION

The patient's oral mucosal tissue is excised and the epithelial cells are cultured. Amniotic membrane is used for the substrate. A cultivated oral mucosal epithelial sheet is handled carefully and spread over the cornea after removing the cicatricial tissue (Figure 34-2). The sheet is sutured with 8-0 Vicryl and a medical-use contact lens is put in place.

CATARACT SURGERY

If the corneal clarity improves after treatment with cultivated oral mucosal epithelium, cataract surgery can then be planned. The pupil should be dilated and the surgical technique with some additional aid considered. Regarding simultaneous surgery, either peribulbar or retrobulbar anesthesia is recommended. However, cataract surgery alone can be performed under routine anesthesia, i.e., under topical anesthesia.

The incision size is small, and both sclero-limbal and clear corneal incisions work well. Creating a capsulorrhexis in the presence of a hazy cornea is difficult. With the combination of capsule staining and an ophthalmic viscosurgical device (OVD), the capsulorrhexis is easier to make (Figure 34-3). Phacoemulsification using a small-diameter sleeve is beneficial for this type of

Table 34-3 Complications in cataract surgery with cicatricial keratoconjunctivitis

Eye lid	Adhesion of palpebral and bulbar conjunctiva
Cornea	Dermal tissue over the cornea
	Irregular surface
	Delayed reepithelization
Wound closure	

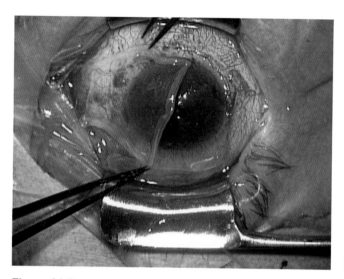

Figure 34-2 Cultivated oral mucosal epithelial transplantation. After removing the cicatricial tissue, the oral mucosal sheet is spread.

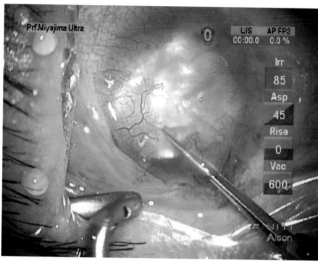

Figure 34-3 Capsulorrhexis. The stained capsule can be observed.

complicated case. The pupil dilation is usually poor, and the small sleeve allows more space in which to manipulate the lens fragments (Figure 34-4). Another pearl for cases with severe corneal opacity is the use of a microkeratome. For these eyes, a penetrating corneal transplantation is critical. The microkeratome can be used to make the flap including the opaque corneal tissue, and then, under the flap, the clear corneal stroma can be confirmed.[6] In such cases, the surface of the corneal bed is rough and a contact lens or irrigating fluid should be applied over the surface to improve the visibility.

Even when the incision size is small, the reepithelization of the incision site may take longer than when performing uncomplicated cataract surgery. The thermal effects from the ultrasound tip can cause thermal burns on the tissue.[7] Since this complication is critical in these cases, recent technology with hyper-pulse phacoemulsification, which reduces the risk of thermal injury, is

highly recommended. The corneal or scleral tissue is usually extremely thin. If the surgeon doubts that the incision will be self-sealing, the incision should be sutured (Figure 34-5).

An OVD is a helpful tool during most procedures that protects the ocular tissue, such as the cornea, iris, and posterior capsule, with appropriate application. In addition, the OVD can be injected in order to separate the cortex and epinucleus from the capsule, and facilitates a safe and efficient phacoemulsification.

The new IOLs and insertion techniques also can be used during these complicated cases.

Postsurgical management is much easier than previous reconstruction with limbal allograft implantation using immunosuppression. In addition to the eye drops used routinely after cataract surgery, preservative-free artificial tears are administered frequently.

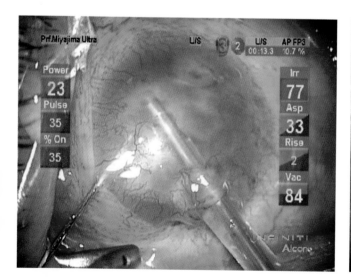

Figure 34-4 Phacoemulsification. Implantation of amniotic membrane. A small sleeve allows more space to manipulate inside the eye.

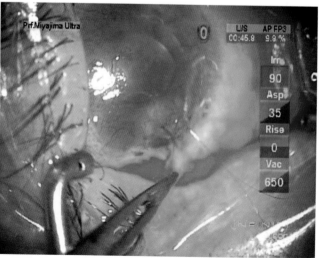

Figure 34-5 Suturing the incision. The corneal tissue is thin and suturing is mandatory.

DIABETES

In patients with diabetes, several complications seem to develop more often compared to normal patients (Table 34-4).

PREOPERATIVE MANAGEMENT

Controlling diabetes is necessary. With the help of primary care doctor or internist, the HbA1c level should be adequately controlled.

SURGICAL PROCEDURE

Minimal invasiveness of the eye should be considered. Surgery sometimes becomes complicated due to poor pupil dilation. A new viscoadaptive OVD, such as Healon 5 (Advanced Medical Optics) is a helpful tool for dilating the pupil during any procedure. Excessive contact with the iris increases postoperative inflammation in the anterior chamber and may cause unexpected bleeding. If vitrectomy for diabetic retinopathy has been performed, the surgeon should be prepared for an unstable anterior chamber and pre-existing rupture of the posterior capsule. If laser coagulation for diabetic retinopathy is planned after cataract surgery, a larger anterior capsulotomy and the diameter of the IOL optic should be considered. There also may be difficulty in controlling intraocular pressure in patients undergoing hemodialysis. For those patients, the OVD in the anterior chamber should be removed completely at the end of surgery.

POSTOPERATIVE MANAGEMENT

Controlling anterior-chamber inflammation should be done more carefully than in uncomplicated cases. Some reports show a higher incidence of cystoid macular edema in patients with diabetes. Synechia is more common, and mydriatic eye drops can be used if posterior synechia may develop. Epithelial problems also are common. Surgeons may prescribe artificial tears for temporary use.

RETINITIS PIGMENTOSA

Anterior subcapsular opacification is common in patients with retinitis pigmentosa. A very small opacity in the center of the lens may diminish the visual acuity, since the visual field is concentric in these patients. Some patients may complain of glare as the first symptom of cataract.

Table 34-4 Possible complications of cataract surgery in patients with diabetes

Bleeding
Poor dilation
Delayed reepithelialization
Iritis
Possible effect on diabetic retinopathy
Insufficient wound closure
Infection
Increased blood sugar level due to topical or general steroid

SURGICAL PROCEDURE

The capsule is thin and handling the capsule is complicated. The capsulorrhexis tends to decrease in size after surgery.[8] If the capsulorrhexis is extremely small, it should be enlarged at the end of surgery. Phacoemulsification is usually not difficult, since the cataract is an anterior subcapsular opacification and the nucleus is not very hard. An IOL with an ultraviolet cut is preferable for implantation.

POSTOPERATIVE MANAGEMENT

If the capsulotomy has become too small and affects the visual acuity, YAG laser capsulotomy is performed. Generally, sunglasses are recommended when patients are in sunlight.

EYELID ABNORMALITIES

PREOPERATIVE MANAGEMENT

The surgical challenge for patients with eyelid abnormalities is obtaining sufficient ocular exposure. For most cases, a lid speculum cannot be used and a suture may be needed to open the upper and lower lids. Especially in cases of symblepharon, planning should include how to open the eyelid and perform cataract surgery with poor ocular exposure.

SURGICAL PROCEDURE

With any difficult case, the routine technique with which the surgeon is most confident should be performed. If the eye can be opened, the entrance of the incision should be well planned. In cases with symblepharon, pannus is also common, and the incision site should be planned to avoid unnecessary hemorrhaging. If phacoemulsification is completed, IOL implantation can be done in the usual manner. Another problem is intraoperative visibility. If the eye is opened with a suture or lid speculum, irrigating water will pool between the upper and lower lids, disturbing the visibility. A cannula that absorbs the water or a lid speculum with an aspiration system is helpful.

BLEEDING DISORDERS

The use of anticoagulant therapy is most often seen for these disorders.[9] With the introduction of topical anesthesia and clear corneal incisions, routine cataract surgery can be performed in patients with bleeding disorders.

PREOPERATIVE MANAGEMENT

If cataract surgery is performed through a clear corneal incision under topical anesthesia, the patient can remain on anticoagulant therapy.[7] If the use of peribulbar or retrobulbar anesthesia is planned during surgery, there is a risk of hemorrhage during the injection. The surgeon should consider the effects on systemic conditions associated with stopping the anticoagulants, such as thrombosis or embolism, and should consult the prescribing doctor if the systemic condition of the patient seems critical.

SURGICAL PROCEDURE

A technique should be chosen that poses less risk of encountering vessels. A clear corneal incision is ideal. Special caution should be taken when the eye is fixed with forceps, because this may cause excessive subconjunctival hemorrhaging.

POSTOPERATIVE MANAGEMENT

If a patient has discontinued the anticoagulant, the medication can be started again after the postoperative visit.

References

[1] No authors listed. The definition and classification of dry eye disease: report of the Definition and Classification Subcommittee of the International Dry Eye Workshop. Ocul Surf, 2007;5:75–92.

[2] Gasset AR. Benzalkonium chloride toxicity to the human cornea. Am J Ophthalmol 1977;84: 169–171.

[3] Tsubota K, Goto E, Shimmura S, Shimazaki J. Treatment of persistent corneal epithelial defect by autologous serum application. Ophthalmology 1999;106:1984–1989.

[4] Bissen-Miyajima H, Monden Y, Shimazaki J, Tsubota K. Cataract surgery combined with ocular surface reconstruction in patients with severe cicatricial keratoconjunctivitis. J Cataract Refract Surg 2002;28:1379–1385.

[5] Nishida K, Yamato M, Hayashida Y, et al. Corneal reconstruction with tissue-engineered cell sheets compose of autologous oral mucosal epithelium. N Engl J Med 2004;351:1187–1196.

[6] Shimmura S, Omoto M, Den S, Bissen-Miyajima H, Tsubota K, Shimazaki J. Microkeratome-assisted phacoemulsification. J Cataract Refract Surg 2005;31:1699–1701.

[7] Bissen-Miyajima H, Shimmura S, Tsubota K. Thermal effect on corneal incisions with different phacoemulsification ultrasonic tips. J Cataract Refract Surg 1999;25:60–64.

[8] Hayashi K, Hayashi H, Matsuo K, Nakao F, et al. Anterior capsule contraction and intraocular lens dislocation after implant surgery in eye with retinitis. Ophthalmology 1998;105:1239–1243.

[9] Shuler JD, Paschal JF, Holland GN. Antiplatelet therapy and cataract surgery. J Cataract Refract Surg 1992;18:567–569.

BLEEDING DISORDERS

part vi

INTRAOCULAR LENSES

The Evolution of the Intraocular Lens

35

Kenneth J. Hoffer, MD, FACS

CONTENTS

CHAPTER HIGHLIGHTS

>> Personal view of the key developments in intraocular lenses (IOLs)

>> The role of Casanova in IOLs

>> Sir Harold Ridley and the RAF pilot

>> The Giants

In a short book chapter, it is impossible to cover every aspect and personality in the history of the intraocular lens (IOL). Therefore, this synopsis is limited by the historical materials at my disposal and my personal recollections.

PREHISTORY

The history of implanting a lens in the human eye to eliminate the "first complication of cataract surgery" – aphakia – dates back to Casanova[1-3] (1725–1798). In his memoirs he related that in 1764 the Italian oculist Tadini had mentioned to him the idea of implanting a lens after cataract surgery. Casanova passed the idea to Casaamata[2] of Dresden in 1795, and he attempted to introduce a glass lens into the eye after removing a cataract and watched it immediately slide back toward the fundus. Choyce[4] stated that in 1939, John Foster of Leeds, England, made a jocular reference to the possibility of artificial lens implantation in an after-dinner speech at the Leeds Medical Society. Strampelli[5] told of the unpublished fruitless attempts of Marchi to fixate quartz lenses with platinum wires in the anterior chambers of animals in 1940.

RIDLEY ERA

In the autumn of 1948, a medical student was observing Harold Ridley extract a cataract at St. Thomas's Hospital in London. The student asked him why he was not going to replace the lens he had just removed. This simple question was the direct stimulus for Ridley to consider implanting an IOL. Ridley was born in Leicestershire, the eldest son of a Navy eye surgeon, and attended Cambridge. He was the head of his surgical division and a well-respected eye surgeon of his time. Fortunately, in August of 1999 (before his death on May 25, 2001), I had the opportunity to visit him and his charming wife Elizabeth at their home (Figure 35-1). I asked him if this story of the medical student was apocryphal, he said that it was absolutely true. In addition, he told me that the medical student was a woman. As it turns out, that was not the case and the student's name was Stephen Perry. Sir Ridley told me that he had asked John Pike of Rayners (Rayner & Keeler, Choleywood, England) to fashion a lens of polymethylmethacrylate (PMMA [from International Chemical Industries]) because he had noted no ill effects from stationary particles of PMMA in the eyes of Royal Air Force pilots (especially Gordon Cleaver, a Battle of Britain pilot) who had sustained injuries from shattered Spitfire canopies during World War II. The lens (Figure 35-2B) that they made was shaped like the human lens with a diameter of 8.35 mm weighing 112 mg, and it was sterilized using 1% cetrimide solution.

History was made on November 29, 1949, when Ridley implanted the first lens in a 42-year-old woman after an extracapsular cataract extraction. The surgery went well, but unfortunately, lens-power calculation became of utmost importance when her

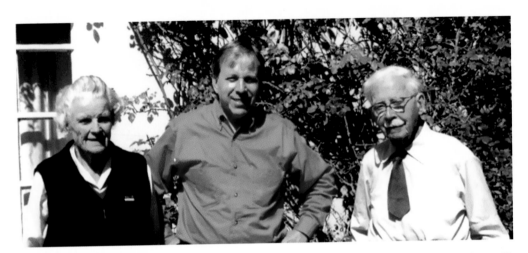

Figure 35-1 Sir Harold and Lady Elizabeth Ridley with the author at their home near Salisbury, England, on August 30, 1999. (Photo by Marcia Hoffer.)

postoperative refractive error was -18.00 to $6.00 \times 120°$ (a -21.0 diopter [D] overcorrection). I had assumed that Sir Harold (see Figure 35-2A) had removed the lens and replaced it with a proper power, but he told me that he was not able to do anything to correct the situation, and that a second lens was implanted 9 months later with the same result. Needless to say, the method of predicting the correct IOL power was changed. After Ridley's first public report at Oxford in 1951, many others followed his example, such as Arruga, Barraquer, Epstein, and Pafique, as well as Warren Reese of Philadelphia (the first American to implant an IOL, on St. Patrick's Day in 1952). The first paper published on IOLs was by Ridley in 1951.[6-7] The major complications were severe hyphema, downward decentration, iris atrophy, glaucoma, and anterior and posterior (6%) dislocation and inflammation. The cetrimide molecule was found to cling to the IOL and later to be released, which caused inflammation. In 1956, Cornelius Binkhorst[8] of Terneuzen, Holland, suggested sterilizing the IOLs using ultraviolet (UV) (253.7 nm) radiation, which was used by some surgeons (Cox-Uphoff) in America in the 1970s. In 1958, Strampelli placed IOLs into the patient's earlobes for 3–4 months to humanize them before implanting them into the eye. Precipitates on the implants did not occur. In 1957, Frederick Ridley[9] of England (no relation) introduced the sodium hydroxide sterilization method (Figure 35-3A) (soak in 10% NaOH for 1 h at 30 °C, store in 0.1% NaOH, neutralize on use with 0.5% $NaHCO_3$, rinse with saline). This method was embraced and used universally until 1978

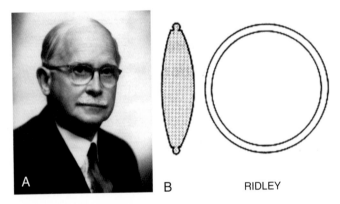

Figure 35-2 A, Sir Harold Ridley. **B**, Original Ridley posterior chamber lens implant circa 1949.

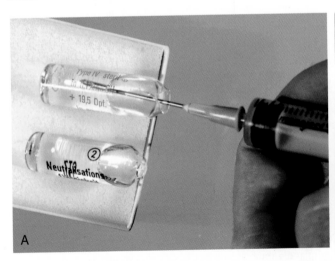

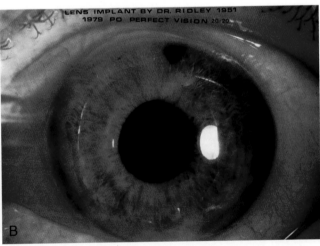

Figure 35-3 A, Sodium hydroxide/bicarbonate sterilization method. **B**, An eye with a Ridley posterior chamber IOL (implanted by Sir Harold Ridley in 1951) with uncorrected 20/20 vision in 1979. (Photo by Kenneth J. Hoffer, in 1979.)

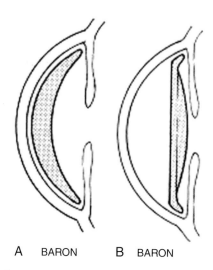

A BARON   B BARON

Figure 35-4 A, Original Baron anterior chamber lens, the very first anterior chamber lens. B, Baron plano-convex anterior chamber lens design.

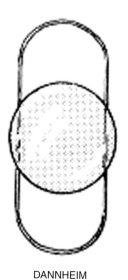

DANNHEIM

Figure 35-6 Original Dannheim closed-loop anterior chamber lens design.

when the U.S. Food and Drug Administration (FDA) mandated ethylene oxide sterilization, which had been introduced by American manufacturers.

Overall, Ridley implanted about a thousand of these lenses. I had the opportunity to examine one of his patients (see Figure 35-3B) in Santa Monica in 1979. The 85-year-old woman had received the implant in 1951 (at age 57) and had an uncorrected visual acuity of 20/20 with a perfectly placed lens for over one-quarter of a century. Although these lenses weren't all bad, because of complications 15% of the Ridley designs were removed, and the implant was beginning to lose favor with those who were using it. Because of this, the pioneers looked for a better place to put Ridley's invention.

For a thorough description of the life of this incredible pioneer, see the book on Ridley's life by David Apple, MD.

■ STRAMPELLI ERA ■

The next site considered for IOL placement was the anterior chamber; the aim being to prevent posterior dislocation and to enable its use in intracapsular and extracapsular surgery. The first to carry out this technique was Baron[10] of France on May 13, 1952. He designed a huge convexo-concave piece of plastic (Figure 35-4A) that was 1 mm thick centrally and rested in (filled) the angle. It came into contact with the corneal endothelium and had the expected results. He, therefore, changed the design to one of plano-convex (Figure 35-4B), but to no avail. Scharf[11] of Germany was next with his quadripodal design, which he first implanted on September 26, 1953. Then 2 days later, Strampelli[12] of Rome implanted the first of his designs (Figure 35-5), which looked like an Iolab Azar lens (B&L, San Dimas, Calif.) but was of solid plastic. Because of his early success and Choyce's later modifications of his original design, Strampelli has been credited with originating the anterior chamber IOL. Many got into the act after this; Schrek and Bietti, and even Sir Harold with his own tripod design. It was Dannheim[13] of Germany who came up with the idea of a closed-loop haptic (Figure 35-6) using elastic-supporting loops made of supramide (similar to the Leiske lens [Surgidev] of the late 1970s and 1980s). Over 650 of these IOLs were implanted. Lieb and Guerry followed with a lens

Figure 35-5 A, Original Strampelli tripod anterior chamber lens design. B, Phakic eye containing an original Strampelli anterior chamber lens.

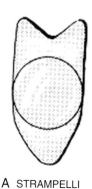

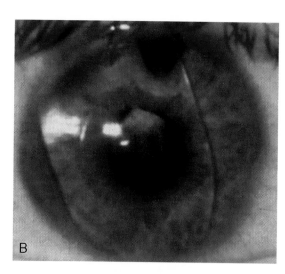

A STRAMPELLI   B

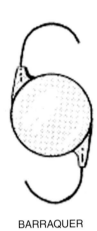

BARRAQUER

Figure 35-7 Original Barraquer open-loop anterior chamber lens design.

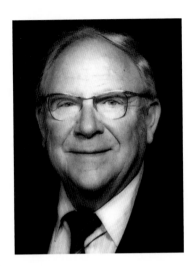

Figure 35-8 Mr. Peter Choyce, MD.

using three closed loops. Barraquer[14] of Barcelona removed half of each loop (Figure 35-7) of the Dannheim lens (giving it an S shape), creating the first open-loop lens, which was later used by Shearing of Las Vegas to create the first flexible-loop, posterior-chamber lens in the late 1970s. However, we're jumping ahead. The primary result of all these early forays into the anterior chamber was bullous keratopathy, dissolving of supramide loops, and chronic inflammation, but the lenses did not dislocate into the vitreous.

■ CHOYCE ERA ■

D. Peter Choyce (Figure 35-8) (died August 8, 2001), who assisted Sir Harold in London, took up the Strampelli concept and implanted his first Choyce Mark I anterior-chamber lens (Rayner) in 1956 (Figure 35-9A). The Mark II–VIII (Figure 35-9B) (including the final Mark IX) (Figure 35-9C) designs modified the optic curvature and the form of the haptic feet and tips. He perfected the Strampelli design such that it became the very first IOL

(Coburn Optical, Ind.) to receive FDA approval in the United States, for which he was justifiably proud. Jerrold Tennant of Dallas, Texas, patented the Choyce Mark VIII design in the United States and helped popularize the lens in America as an alternative to the American-made metal-looped prepupillary lenses (Figure 35-10), which were causing so many problems for intracapsular surgeons. Choyce never benefited financially from the success of his IOL designs and I believe resented the fact that others benefited financially from his design (Tennant). In the early 1980s, Charles Kelman took the Choyce design a step further to the Multiflex designs we use today.

Edward Epstein (Figure 35-11A) of Johannesburg, South Africa, had fairly good success with the original Ridley implant, but because of dislocations, he changed the design to fixate the lens using the pupil. He called this the Collar-Stud lens (see Figure 35-11B) and implanted the first one in June 1953. After noting pigmentary glaucoma in a high percentage of the 40 eyes he had given implants, he switched to some anterior-chamber designs and then developed the Maltese-Cross lens (see Figure 35-11C). This lens had four plates

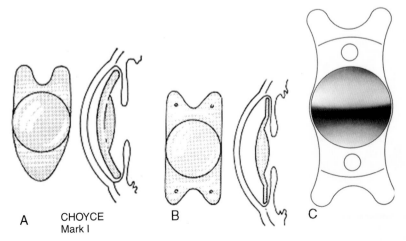

A CHOYCE Mark I   B   C

Figure 35-9 **A,** Choyce Mark I tripod anterior chamber lens design. **B,** Choyce Mark VIII quadripod anterior chamber lens design. **C,** Final Choyce Mark IX anterior chamber lens design.

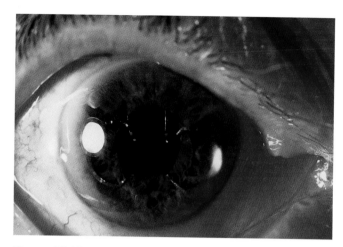

Figure 35-10 First patient ever to receive an American-made (McGhan) metal-loop intracapsular iris clip lens design by Dennis Shepard in 1976. The eye ultimately became blind after several years.

Statements such as "implanting such a foreign body is malpractice," "recklessness," "viciousness" (Derrick Vail, publicly to Ridley on the podium at the American Academy of Ophthalmology (AAO) after Ridley gave his invited lecture [Vail's remarks are published in the Transactions of the American Academy of Ophthalmology and Otolaryngology, January/February 1953]) and "intraocular time bomb" (Richard Troutman) caused many potentially interested surgeons to be wary of joining this merry band. Sir Stewart Duke-Elder of London hated Ridley for what he had done, and he and Vail were very close friends. This public ridicule of his new idea caused Ridley a great deal of psychological pain, and led to his suffering from depression for some time.

It was the integrity, pioneering perseverance, and intellectual and surgical acumen of one man that kept this subject alive to herald in the modern era. Cornelius Binkhorst (Figure 35-12A), of Terneuzen, Holland, had learned about lens implantation from Sir Harold in London, and gradually came to believe that there had to be a better way. He came up with a totally different design that he thought would prevent corneal decompensation, as well as posterior dislocation. He designed the prepupillary iris clip lens (see Figure 35-12B) in 1957 and implanted the first one on August 11, 1958. They were manufactured by both Rayner and Kurt Morcher (Bad Cannstatt, Ebitzweg, Germany). He first presented this lens publicly in Middelburg on the Isle of Walcheren on October 3, 1958. The term "pseudophakia" to indicate the presence of an IOL was inaugurated by Binkhorst at Oxford in 1959. The 5 × 0.6 mm biconvex lens had two pairs of flexible supramide wire loops. The posterior pair was drilled into the posterior surface of the optic and bent at right angles to extend peripherally. They were inserted through the pupil and came to lie against the posterior surface of the iris, but they did not touch the ciliary body. The distance, loop tip to loop tip, was 7 mm, and they prevented the lens from moving forward. After being constricted, the pupil took the shape of a square with a diagonal length of 4 mm. The anterior loops were parallel to the posterior, but 0.75 mm anterior to them. They were mounted on the equator of the optic and were adjacent to the anterior surface of the

(blades) extending from the optic. The anterior two were fenestrated, and the posterior two were solid. The pupil was woven around the plates such that the lens was held in the pupil. In America, at the instigation of Richard Troutman and Cornelius Binkhorst's brother Richard, the same design with four solid plates was produced by an optician named Michael Copeland, becoming known as the Copeland–Binkhorst lens. This lens was used prominently by many American surgeons such as Jaffe, Galin, Osher, and Hamdi. Epstein was never given credit for his design by his American copiers.

■ BINKHORST ERA ■

Things were not looking good for lens implants in the late 1950s and 1960s, and many of the pioneers were abandoning their designs. The bad results led prominent ophthalmologists, especially in America, to deride and ridicule the entire concept.

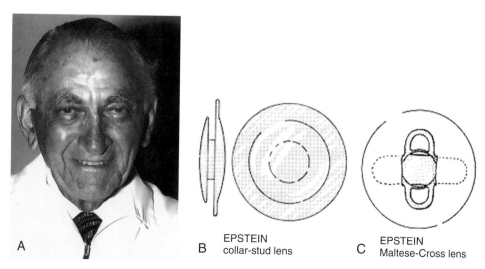

EPSTEIN
collar-stud lens

EPSTEIN
Maltese-Cross lens

Figure 35-11 A, Dr. Edward Epstein. B, Epstein Collar-Stud pupil-fixated lens design. C, Epstein Maltese-Cross pupil-fixated lens design.

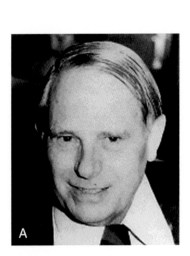

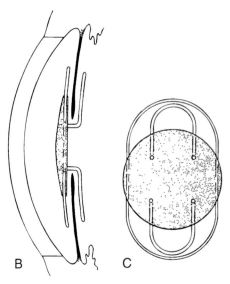

Figure 35-12 **A**, Dr. Cornelius D. Binkhorst. **B**, Binkhorst Iris Clip pupil-fixated lens design (side view). **C**, Iris-clip lens (front view).

iris a safe distance from the anterior chamber angle. The lens weighed 6 mg, compared with the Ridley lens at 112 mg.

In 1963, Syvyateslav Fyodorov[15] (Figure 35-13) of Archangel, Russia, changed the relationship of the anterior and posterior loops from parallel to perpendicular. This was subsequently known as the Binkhorst–Fyodorov lens and it became quite popular in America. He also published the first IOL power formula in 1967.

Few realize that in 1967 the biconvex lens shape for IOLs was changed by Binkhorst to a simple convexo-plano shape at the suggestion of his brother Richard (New York) for the purpose of decreasing obstruction of aqueous flow through the pupil, thus, increasing the accuracy of the IOL power calculation, and, theoretically, lessening spherical aberration. By the 1970s, this became the shape of all IOLs until the American manufacturer Coburn

Optical (later Storz, now Bausch & Lomb) came out with their first PMMA biconvex lens designs in the late 1980s. Although there were really no accounts of optical aberrations with the convexo-plano design, Holladay championed the biconvex design for the company, based on theoretical grounds, and it was soon to become the shape of all IOLs by all manufacturers. Later, several reports (including one by Atchison[16]) establishing that for PMMA lenses the convexo-plano was the best optically, and that biconvex was only superior in lenses made of silicone. Nothing changed however, the die had been cast. In 1968 Fyodorov,[17] working with Zakharov, replaced the anterior loops with three equidistant small prongs (pintles) and changed the posterior loops from two to three. Because of its "antennae" appearance, it was called the Fyodorov Sputnik lens (see Figure 35-13B). With the

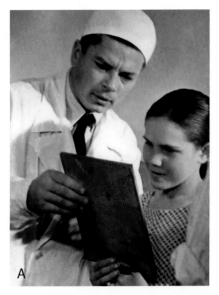

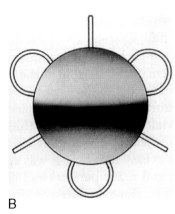

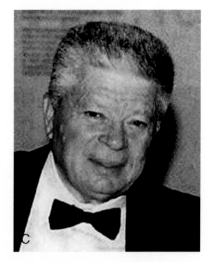

Figure 35-13 **A**, Dr. Syvataslav Fyodorov as a young surgeon in Archangel, Russia. **B**, Fyodorov-Zakharov pupil-fixated Sputnik lens design. **C**, Fyodorov in later life.

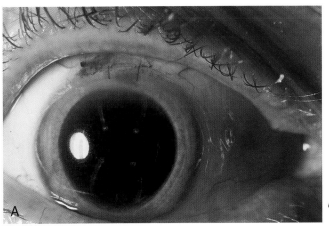

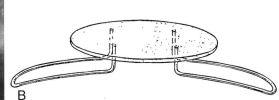

Figure 35-14 A, Eye containing a Binkhorst two-loop iridocapsular lens implant circa 1976. B, Binkhorst two-loop iridocapsular lens design.

increase of posts in the pupil from four to six, the pupil took on a rounder shape when constricted. The lens only weighed 0.9 mg in aqueous and the design was quite successful for intracapsular and extracapsular implantation, but it was difficult to obtain them in America during the Cold War years. To meet the demand, American manufacturers copied it, but they used heavier metal posterior loops and pintles that, because of their weight, caused tearing of the iris sphincter, chronic cystoid macular edema (CME), and dislocation, and the lens fell in popularity.

Various other changes were made in the iris clip lens from 1961 to 1971, but what really created the IOL revolution in the early 1970s was the change made by Binkhorst[18] to his iridocapsular design (Figure 35-14), and the change made by Jan Worst, his Dutch protégé, to his Medallion sutured lens (Figure 35-15A).

Binkhorst originally designed the iridocapsular lens for use in children in 1965, but soon realized that it was the lens of choice for all eyes. The anterior loops of the iris clip lens were removed, and the posterior loops were changed to 0.15 mm platinum–iridium wire because they were to be imbedded in iris and capsule tissue (he feared supramide could biodegrade over time like the Dannheim lenses.) This increased the lens weight to 15.1 mg. He implanted the first style with supramide loops on September 16, 1965, and with metal loops on October 27, 1965. The two-loop lens became his lens of choice for all cataract cases by 1973. What is most interesting in the evolution of IOLs is that as a result of the 1974 American revolution in IOL surgery, Binkhorst advocated extracapsular surgery and the use of the two-loop lens. His successes were the basis for the rapid increase in interest in IOLs in America, but Americans ignored Binkhorst's advice and proceeded with intracapsular designs, such as the iris clip and Copeland lenses. Phacoemulsification was completely ignored by most IOL surgeons because the "incision had to be extended to get the lens in."

Jan Worst, of Groningen, Holland, attempted to eliminate the anterior loops and replaced them with a flat, thin, superior plate extension of the optic with two holes to allow the lens to be sutured to the superior iris. It was called the Worst Medallion lens (Medical Workshop, Groningen, Holland) (see Figure 35-15A), and he implanted the first one on December 18, 1970. His success added to the enthusiasm and excitement in America in 1974. Worst made several other designs with iridectomy clipping devices[19] (see Figure 35-15B) and recommended stainless-steel sutures for fixation. These ideas were not as popular in America.

So far this chapter has liberally relied on the first textbook on IOLs by Marcel Nordlohne[20] (Figure 35-16) in 1975 for many of its historical facts and has subsequently relied on the excellent textbook on IOLs by David Apple.[21]

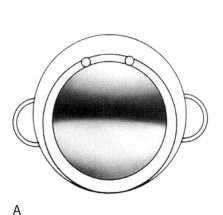

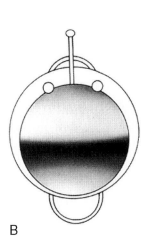

Figure 35-15 A, Worst Medallion sutured pupil-fixated lens design. B, Worst Platina iridectomy clip pupil-fixated lens design.

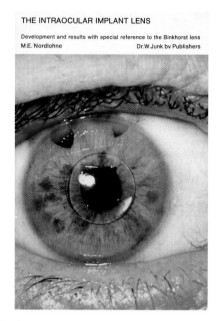

THE INTRAOCULAR IMPLANT LENS

Development and results with special reference to the Binkhorst lens
M.E. Nordlohne   Dr.W.Junk bv Publishers

Figure 35-16 The cover of the first intraocular lens textbook by Nordlohne (Junk Publishers) in 1975.

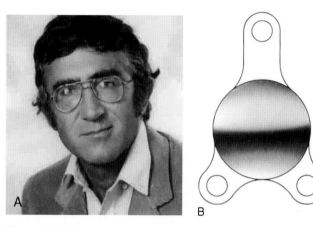

Figure 35-17 A, Mr. John L. Pearce, MD. **B**, Original Pearce tripod posterior chamber lens design.

■ THE REVOLUTION: 1970s ■

The 1970s was a decade of revolution and change in IOL surgery. It began with the use of lenses such as the Copeland, Binkhorst iris clip, Sputnik, iridocapsular, and Choyce Mark VIII, and it ended with the Simcoe and Shearing posterior chamber lenses.

POSTERIOR CHAMBER ERA

Through most of the 1970s, two camps of lens implanters developed: those performing intracapsular surgery and using their favorite IOL design (90%), and those (including myself) using phacoemulsification and implanting the iridocapsular lens (10%). In 1975, John Pearce[22] (Figure 35-17A) of England took the lead back into the posterior chamber with his one-piece PMMA tripod lens (see Figure 35-17B). James Little of Oklahoma City and Eric Arnott of London followed suit with their design and later so did William Harris of Dallas in 1977. Things were rather quiet until 1977, when Shearing[23] of Las Vegas advocated implanting a flexible-loop Barraquer anterior chamber lens into the posterior chamber and called it "ciliary body" (later ciliary sulcus) fixation. Several prominent phacoemulsification trainers in California, such as Richard Kratz and Robert Sinskey, began using the Shearing lens (Model 101, Iolab Corp.) (Figure 35-18A) and teaching it in their courses. The loops were stiff and in the shape of the letter J. Often the lens would become trapped in the pupil, so at the suggestion of Kratz (Iolab ignored

Figure 35-18 Shearing flexible-loop posterior chamber lens designs. **A**, Original Shearing stiff J loop. **B**, "Sinskey" soft J loop. **C**, Kratz–Johnson crimped J loop.

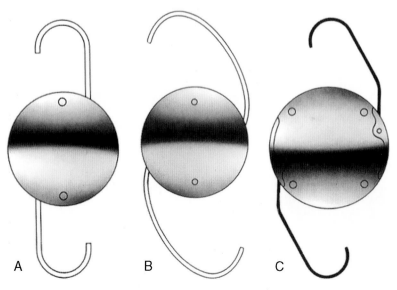

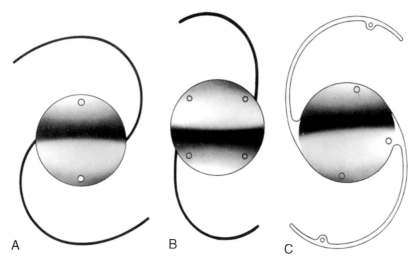

Figure 35-19 Simcoe flexible-loop posterior chamber lens designs. **A,** Original Simcoe wide C loop. **B,** Modified short C loop. **C,** One-piece PMMA C-loop lens.

Shearing's previous request to do this[24]), the loops were angulated 10° anteriorly to keep the optic posterior to the pupil. This was the very first modification of this posterior-chamber IOL and was given the name Model 101K because Kratz refused to attach his name to it. What many will find surprising is that the next modification ever to be made to this posterior-chamber IOL was the addition of the Hoffer[25] ridge to the optic, and for the same reason it was called the Model 101H (see Figure 35-29C).

Through the early and mid-1980s, it became increasing evident that the posterior chamber lens should be implanted completely in the capsular bag to eliminate all contact with uveal tissue. The stiffness of the loops and the jagged "can-opener" capsulotomy made this technically difficult. In the same year as Shearing (1977) (or perhaps earlier), William Simcoe of Tulsa designed long sweeping loops (Figure 35-19A) that came off the lens optic at a very low angle rather than perpendicular, so that they were very flexible and could be "dialed" into the capsular bag. Simcoe and others later recommended shortening the loops so that they took on the shape of the letter C (see Figure 35-19B and C).

Shearing had obtained a method patent for his design and, in attempting to protect his intellectual property, filed legal actions against all the manufacturers making a posterior-chamber lens that was not licensed. In their defense, these manufacturers relied on Simcoe's claim of having really been the first to implant a posterior-chamber lens when he cut off the posterior loops, snipped the anterior loops of an iris clip lens, and implanted them into the capsular bag, which he did before Shearing's patent. These court battles were notorious and contentious, and even led to an Academy meeting podium fistfight, as well as the exhumation of the body of a patient in whom Simcoe claimed to have inserted such an implant (the family was paid to exhume the body).[24] The claimed lens was not found, but Simcoe states that the hospital records were in disarray and that it would be impossible to know which patients had received these initial lenses. Perhaps we will never know who was first.

All posterior-chamber lenses had loops of supramide and latter Prolene. In the mid-1980s, Wayne Callahan* used computer lathes

(Cilco, Huntington, WVa; now Alcon Surgical, Ft. Worth, Tex.) to fashion the first all-PMMA one-piece, posterior-chamber lenses. Early models were stiff and thick, but as development proceeded, they became thin and flexible. The Jaffe, Arnott,[26] and Bechert designs (with Hoffer ridges) became popular throughout the 1980s (Figure 35-20).

In 1980, Kratz asked Iolab to make a crimp in the J loop (to decrease its stiffness), but refused to allow his name to be used on the lens model, so Iolab called it the Sinskey lens[24] (see Figure 35-18B). Later, other manufacturers copied this "soft-J" design, and they were called the Kratz and Kratz–Johnson lenses (see Figure 35-18C). Other posterior-chamber designs, such as the Anis lens (Figure 35-21A) and the Galand disc lens (Figure 35-21B) were defining the future direction of lens design until the foldable lenses caused their demise.

■ THE 1980s ANTERIOR CHAMBER LENS DISASTER ■

The use of anterior chamber lenses continued throughout the 1980s and became extremely popular with intracapsular surgeons, especially when problems with American-manufactured iris-supported lenses (with metal loops [see Figure 35-10]) became an issue. Choyce slimmed down the Mark VIII to the Mark IX in 1978. American manufacturers copied the Mark VIII lens, and most were poorly made and poorly polished, leading to the Ellingson uveitis–glaucoma–hyphema syndrome.[27] In 1977, Robert Azar of New Orleans came out first with a copy of the Strampelli lens with the letters of his last name embossed as molded projections on the surface of the optic, lest someone forget who designed it. He later (1982) changed the design to one with closed loops, called the Azar 91Z (Iolab) (Figure 35-22A), to compete with the Leiske closed-loop lens (Figure 35-22B), both of which became extremely popular in the United States.

Other surgeons designed closed-loop designs (see Figure 35-22) fashioned after the original Dannheim lens. History was repeating

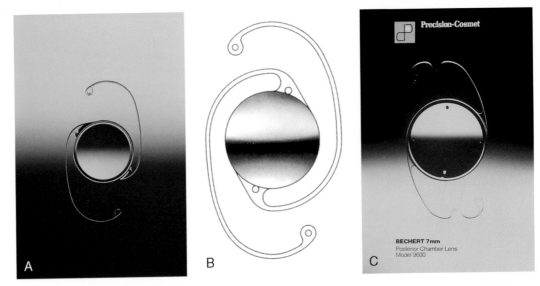

Figure 35-20 **A**, Jaffe short, encircling loop, all-PMMA one-piece lens with Hoffer ridge. **B**, Arnott large, encircling loop, all-PMMA one-piece lens. **C**, Bechert all-PMMA one-piece 7 mm lens design with Hoffer ridge.

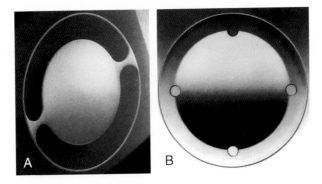

Figure 35-21 Later "Ridleyesque" posterior chamber lens designs. **A**, Anis large closed-circle lens. **B**, Galland disc lens design.

itself by those unfamiliar with it or totally unwilling to learn its lessons. Lens designs such as the Leiske (1978, Surgidev), Shepard (1979), Hessberg (1981, Intermedics), Dubroff (1981), Optiflex (1981), Feaster (1982), Stableflex (1983, Optical Radiation Corp.), and the Copeland anterior-chamber lens (see Figures 35-22B–G) were being implanted in great numbers throughout the United States. Many of these lenses ultimately led to multiple complications and had to be removed, often during a corneal transplantation for bullous keratopathy. These designers were all committed to the concept that a one-size, anterior-chamber lens that could fit eyes of all sizes, which was to the detriment of many patients.

During this period, Charles Kelman[28] of New York (Figure 35-23H), the inventor of phacoemulsification, refrained from implanting IOLs. He finally gave in and designed an anterior-chamber lens tripod (by "cutting the plastic out of it" [similar to the attempt by Boberg-Ans in 1961]). It was made of solid PMMA lathe-cut in the shape of a "pregnant 7," with an optic of 4.5 mm and special foot plates to impinge in the angle that he first implanted in 1978. The first to make this lens was

Precision-Cosmet of Minnesota (Figure 35-23A). A slight modification was later made by Heyer-Schulte (Irvine, Calif. [later AMO]), and they improved it to the Omnifit in 1981 (see Figures 35-23B and C). Collaborating with Wayne Callahan at Cilco, Kelman designed the extremely flexible Quadriflex (1981) quadripodal design, which later was modified to the Multiflex I (1982) (see Figures 35-23D and E). Both had four-point angle fixation with the haptics coming off the same side of the lens optic. The former looked like a "pregnant E," but the haptics of the Multiflex were unique in that their design allowed internal flexion in the same plane as the haptics without forward movement of the optic. This was the answer and is now the basis for all safe anterior-chamber lens implantation used today. When a high incidence of optic entrapment by the pupil was noted, Kelman directed that the haptics should exit the lens optic from opposite sides, and these became the S-flex and the Multiflex II (see Figure 35-23F). The most unique attribute of the Multiflex II was that Cilco originally made the lens in seven different sizes (see Figure 35-23G), from 11.5–14.5 mm (in 0.5 mm steps), so that any size of eye could be fitted safely without making the eye withstand the constant pressure of an oversized lens. This was never repeated by any other company. It has always been my theory that if this had been done with all the closed-loop anterior-chamber lenses, the disasters they caused might have been prevented. The "one-size-fits-all" anterior-chamber lens goal of the surgeons who experimented with it was the cause of untold loss of sight.

Kelman always strongly advocated precise horizontal corneal diameter measurement and intraoperative gonioscopy to ensure proper sizing during the procedure. This advice was ignored by most implanting surgeons to their peril. For intracapsular cataract extraction (ICCE), secondary and backup implantations, I switched from the Rayner Choyce Mark VIII to the Cilco Kelman Multiflex II in 1983 and (following Kelman's teachings) have not had to remove a personally implanted Multiflex II for any reason.

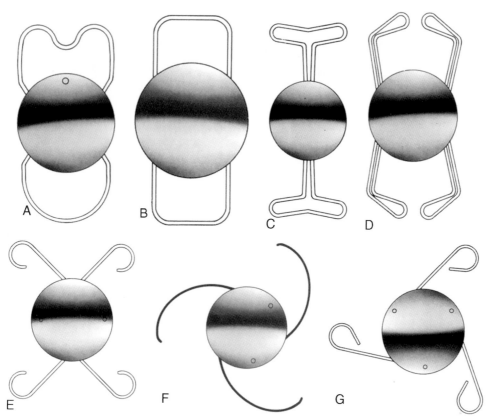

Figure 35-22 The troublesome closed-loop anterior chamber lenses. **A**, Azar 91Z lens (1982). **B**, Leiske lens (1978). **C**, Hessberg lens (1981). **D**, Stableflex lens (1983). **E**, Shepard lens (1979). **F**, Dubroff lens (1981). **G**, Copeland anterior chamber lens (1982).

■ PHAKIC INTRAOCULAR LENSES TO CORRECT AMETROPIA ■

Jan Worst designed his iris plane Lobster Claw lens for aphakia in 1976, which sat on the surface of the iris and was fixated by two haptic claws that imbricated the anterior stroma of the iris in the nondilating midperiphery portion. This lens was used extensively in Europe, India, and Pakistan for aphakia and today is being used in a different version as a phakic IOL for the correction of refractive errors (Artisan Lens, Ophtec, Fla.) This lens has received FDA approval for use in the US and is called the Verisys (AMO, Irvine, CA) (Figure 35-24A). Undeterred by the failures of Strampelli, Barraquer, and many other early pioneers who attempted to use anterior chamber lenses in phakic eyes, Georges Baikoff of Marseilles, France, modified the Multiflex II lens for the same purpose, beginning with the Domilens ZB lens (see Figure 35-24B). This was later changed to the B&L Nuvita lens (see Figure 35-24C) and ultimately the CIBA Vision Vivere lens, which has PMMA haptics but an acrylic foldable optic that is multifocal (see Figure 35-24D). All such ICLs have been removed from the market due to chronic ongoing endothelial cell loss. In the 1980s, Fyodorov and Zuev were working on phakic IOLs for the posterior chamber, starting with the Mushroom pupillary centering lens, which ultimately led to the Staar ICL (Collamer) (see Figure 35-25A), and the Medennium PRL (Silicone) (Figures 35-25B and C), which was developed by

Dimitrii Dementiev, MD (see Figure 35-25D) of Milano, Italy. The Staar lens has received FDA approval, while the US studies of the PRL have been suspended.

■ SMALL INCISION ERA ■

Phacoemulsifiers always disliked enlarging their small, 3.5 mm incision to implant a 6–7 mm solid PMMA optic IOL. What was needed was a lens optic that could be folded and enter the 3.5 mm incision.

In the mid-1970s, Keiki Mehta[29] (Figure 35-26) of Bombay, India, fabricated iris clip lenses using silicone for the optic with no intention of folding them. He told me what he was doing at that time and, 10 years later, how they had all turned yellow over time and that he had, therefore, abandoned their use. In the early 1980s, Edward Epstein started making posterior-chamber IOLs of silicone with the intention of folding them. However, once Thomas Mazzacco (Healdsburg, Calif.) (see Figure 35-26) began folding and implanting plate haptic silicone IOLs (Staar Surgical, Covina, Calif.) through a 3.5 mm phaco incision, the world of lens implantation changed forever. From this point on, the popularity of phacoemulsification went from 40 to 95%. At first, they didn't ensure that the lenses were entirely in the capsular bag, and complications ensued. Around 1981, Calvin Fercho[30] of Fargo, ND (see Figure 35-27A), invented the complete circular capsulorrhexis (later to be popularized by Thomas Neuhann [Munich,

SMALL INCISION ERA

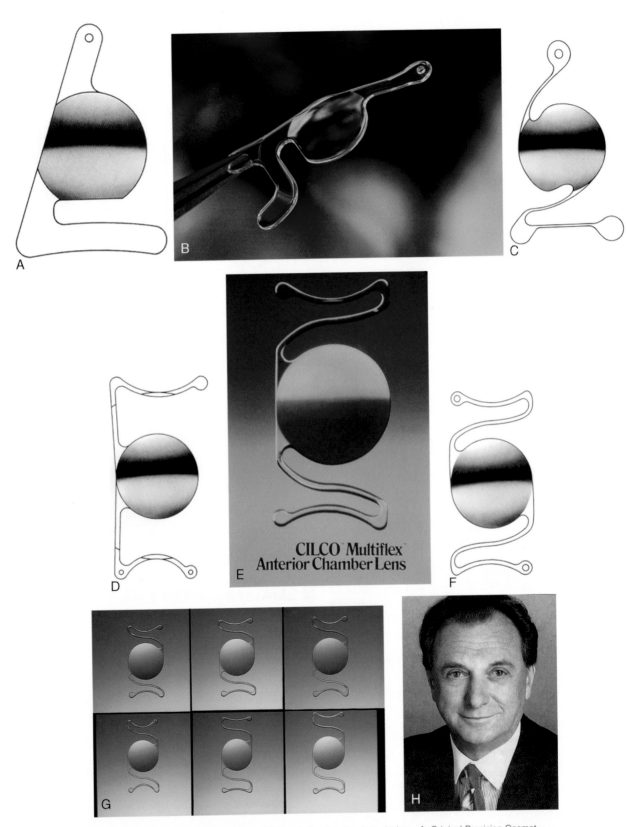

Figure 35-23 The successful Kelman all-PMMA anterior chamber lens designs. **A,** Original Precision-Cosmet "pregnant-7" tripod lens (1978). **B,** Heyer–Schulte tripod design. **C,** AMO Omnifit tripod lens. **D,** Cilco Quadriflex lens (1981). **E,** Cilco Multiflex I lens. **F,** Cilco Multiflex II lens (1982). **G,** Six (of seven) different sizes of the Cilco Multiflex II lens (note difference in design between the shortest and the longest). **H,** Charles D. Kelman, MD.

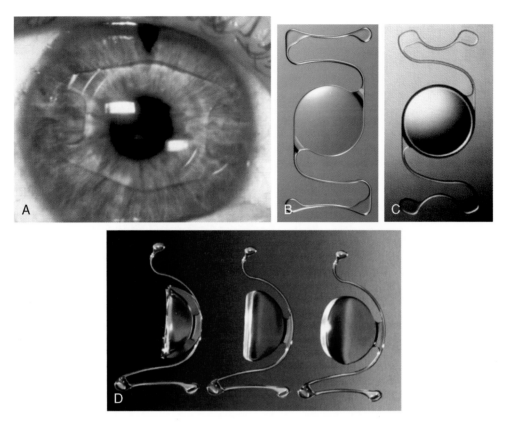

Figure 35-24 Phakic lens implant designs. **A,** Eye containing the Ophtec Artisan Worst "lobster claw" iris-supported lens. **B,** Original Baikoff Domilens ZB anterior chamber lens. **C,** Baikoff B&L Nuvita anterior chamber lens. **D,** Latest Baikoff foldable-optic acrylic/PMMA CIBA Vision Vivere anterior chamber lens.

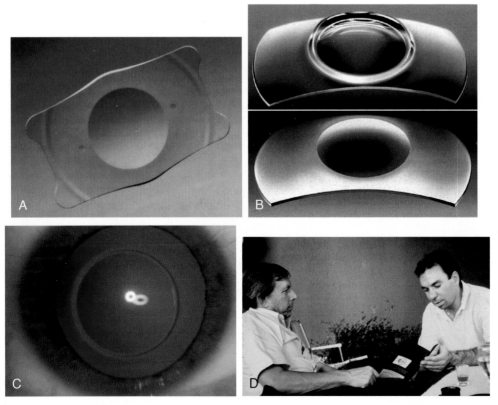

Figure 35-25 Phakic posterior chamber lens implant designs. **A,** Staar ICL. **B,** Medennium myopic (upper) and hyperopic (lower) PRL lenses. **C,** Eye containing myopic Medennium PRL. **D,** The author (Dr. Kenneth Hoffer) with Dr. Dimitrii D. Dementiev (designer of PRL) in Milano, Italy in 1997.

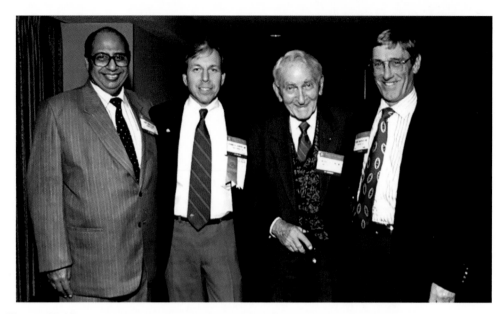

Figure 35-26 The silicone pioneers. Left to right: Drs. Keiki Mehta, Kenneth Hoffer (the author), Edward Epstein, and Thomas Mazzacco.

Germany] and Howard Gimble [Calgary, Canada] while Fercho was undergoing prostate cancer treatment) (see Figure 35-27B). It soon became apparent that the plate haptic silicone lens worked best if placed entirely in the capsular bag with an intact, round central capsulorrhexis of adequate size. The FDA only approved it with this stipulation.

■ VISCOSURGICAL AGENTS ■

Endre Balazs[31] began the research on using hyaluronic acid as a replacement for vitreous. Soon David Miller (Boston) and Roger Stegman (South Africa) began talking about its use for anterior segment surgery. Balazs presented his work at the 1979 AAO meeting in San Francisco. It just so happened that the AAO had asked me to be the discussant for that paper. After giving a presentation, in which the idea was cautiously lauded, I recommended that it be supplied in a preset syringe ready for use in all cataract surgery. I also warned of the potential for antigenicity and intraocular pressure rise. After sitting down, two gentlemen from Pharmacia (of Sweden) approached and asked if I would be interested in doing some research with their new product called Healon. When I agreed, I soon received vials of Healon and performed the first phacoemulsification/IOL viscosurgery in America in November 1979. I was soon using it for every cataract surgery I performed. After 6 months of excellent results (except for temporary

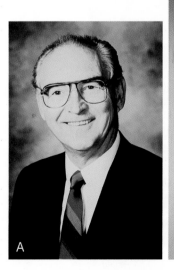

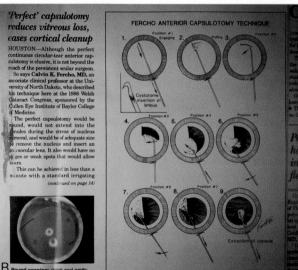

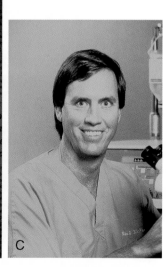

Figure 35-27 Cataract surgery innovators. **A**, Dr. Calvin Fercho. **B**, Ocular Surgery News article (November 15, 1986) first to describe circular capsulotomy. **C**, Dr. Michael McFarland.

rises in intraocular pressure), I warned the company that they had better be well prepared with a huge supply before they bring it to the market because I believed that it would become the standard in cataract surgery immediately. They did not follow my advice, and 6 months after its introduction, they were back-ordered on the product for almost 1 year. In that intervening period, many surgeons looked for ways to bring about the same result without the expense of Healon. Needless to say, everyone is aware of the profound effect Healon and subsequent viscosurgical agents have had on the safety and ease of lens implant surgery.

DEVICE AND MATERIAL DEVELOPMENTS

Probably the most important development in cataract and lens implant surgery was the introduction of the Zeiss motorized zoom microscope in 1965, which allowed surgeons to see the red reflex while operating. The first motorized zoom, focus, and X–Y controls were introduced in 1970. This has had a great effect on the increasing use of extracapsular surgery.

Based on the experience of James Gills of Tarpon Springs, Florida, many surgeons abandoned the routine use of a peripheral iridectomy with posterior-chamber lenses during the 1980s. Michael McFarland (see Figure 35-27C) of Pinebluff, Arkansas, first proposed the concept of self-sealing sutureless incisions, and Howard Fine popularized making the incision in clear corneal surgery. In 1990, John Shepherd[32] of Las Vegas invented the in-the-bag fracturing, hydration, and quartering of the nucleus for phacoemulsification, later popularized by Gimble and others. All these advances made the surgery simpler and safer, as well as shortening the recovery time for the eye dramatically.

One of the most interesting developments was the elimination of retrobulbar injections. R.M. Redmond[33] of Belfast, Northern Ireland, had written a paper in April 1990 about performing extracapsular cataract surgery using local anesthesia without a retrobulbar injection (Figure 35-28A). After reading the paper, I invited him to present his experience at my IOL Course[34] at the AAO Meeting in October 1991 (Figure 35-28B). Many prominent cataract surgeons were also lecturing at, or attending this course, and Redmond's presentation drew excited interest. Soon there followed many surgeons attempting topical anesthetics for IOL surgery, especially with clear corneal incisions. Redmond Smith of London had also eliminated retrobulbar injections since April of 1985. He also eliminated O'Brien lid akinesia in June 1987 and used a locking speculum to prevent the patient from blinking. Gills recommended intraocular xylocaine in addition to the topical anesthetic.

In 1979 Barasch and Poler[35] tried making IOL optics out of glass. This was done by Lynell, Inc., and they used a new polymer, Elastimide, to fashion haptics to hold the glass optic. Because of the increased index of refraction of glass, the lenses were very thin. When the yttrium-aluminum-garnet (YAG) laser caused several of these lenses to crack inside the eye, the FDA recalled them. Staar Surgical used the Elastimide material for the haptics of their three-piece silicone posterior chamber lenses.

Acrylic lenses were the next logical offshoot from research into optical-quality materials that could be folded like silicone. The edge architecture of the original popular models caused persistent haloes (because of acrylic's higher index of refraction) in a sporadic but persistent number of extremely unhappy patients. After many years of ignoring the issue, Alcon finally made changes in the edge design in the newer acrylic lens styles, but there are still reports of this nagging phenomenon.

Extracapsular cataract extraction under local anaesthesia without retrobulbar injection

R M Redmond, N L Dallas

Abstract
Day-case cataract surgery and the need for local anaesthesia are likely to increase. Retrobulbar (and peribulbar) anaesthetic injection is a common technique in cataract surgery, but serious complications are persistently reported. Subconjunctival injection is an alternative that avoids these risks. This retrospective study compares two groups of patients that underwent extracapsular cataract surgery under local anaesthetic. One group (retrobulbar) had uncomplicated retrobulbar injection with bupivicaine and hyaluronidase. The other group (non-retrobulbar) had superior bulbar, subconjunctival infiltration

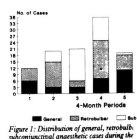

Figure 1: Distribution of general, retrobulbar, subconjunctival anaesthetic cases during the

Patients and methods

A

ACADEMY Instruction Courses — Tue
OCT 15, 1991

Course 261 Room: CTR – B2
Periods 2 through 5 9:45 AM – 4:15 PM
Modern Phaco/ECCE Implant Surgery: 1991 †
Kenneth J Hoffer, MD, Santa Monica, CA; Bradley R Straatsma, MD, Los Angeles, CA; David B Davis II, MD, Hayward, CA; R D Redmond, MD, Belfast, Northern Ireland; William F Maloney, MD, Vista, CA; Thomas V Cravy, MD, Santa Maria, CA; Stephen A Obstbaum, MD, New York, NY; Calvin K Fercho, MD, Fargo, SD; Howard V Gimbel, MD, Calgary, AB, Canada; Thomas Neuhann, MD, Munich, West Germany; David J Apple, MD, Charleston, SC; Aziz Y Anis, MD, Lincoln, NE; R M Redmond, MD, London, England
This course will cover, step-by-step, the latest techniques and options available to achieve 100% in-the-bag IOL placement using either ECCE or Phaco and any size incision and lens style. Due to its rise in popularity, there will be an emphasis on phacoemulsification. Preop and postop considerations will be covered as well as IOL designs, preventing power errors, incision control, and newer ideas in handling vitreous encounters. Practical clinical information will be stressed in areas such as anesthesia, incisions, capsulorrhexis, hydrodissection, nuclear cracking, lens insertion techniques, and incision closure. Novice and experienced phaco surgeons should gain useful tips. (Bas, Int, Adv)

B

Figure 35-28 A, Article by Mr. R.M. Redmond, MD, on topical anesthesia in the British Journal of Ophthalmology in April 1990. B, Academy course where Redmond first presented topical anesthesia in America.

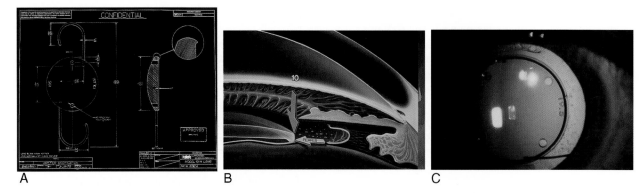

Figure 35-29 **A**, First mechanical drawing by Iolab of the Hoffer ridge lens. **B**, Graphic depiction of the increased pressure caused at the edge of the lens by the ridge. **C**, An eye with an Iolab ridge lens demonstrating the blockage of Elschnig pearls at the edge of the lens optic.

■ YAG LASER AND LENS DESIGN ■

The challenging and sometimes complicated surgical posterior capsulotomy became outdated when Aron-Rosa[36] of Paris, France, and Fankhauser[37] of Switzerland independently introduced the YAG laser in the early 1980s. Aron-Rosa began clinical trials in October 1978 and did 5000 eyes over a period of 4 years. Fankhauser did his first YAG capsulotomy in November 1980. Soon reports of IOL damage from the laser began to appear. Contrary to common belief, the Hoffer laser ridge optic[38] was designed in 1978 for two equally important purposes. The first was to increase the pressure at the edge of the optic to create an increased barrier to the migration of lens epithelial cells onto the posterior capsule (Figures 35-29B and C). The second was to create a space between the back surface of the IOL and the posterior capsule to prevent damage to the IOL during the performance of a posterior capsulotomy. Iolab made the first ridge lenses (Figure 35-29A), but they were soon followed by Cilco, CooperVision (Bellevue, Wash.) and then most other companies. The stimulus for its popularity was the increased use of the YAG laser, which was causing severe pitting in lens optics without the spacing. Other ideas for spacing ensued, such as a meniscus optic (William Myers, CooperVision), Prolene riders (Lawrence Castleman, MD, Ioptex, San Leandro, Calif.), and partial ridges (Kratz-Johnson, AMO). For the Hoffer ridge to block Elschnig pearl formation and prevent posterior capsule opacification (PCO), the haptics had to be angled anteriorly (to increase posterior pressure) and the lens had to be placed entirely in the capsular bag (uniform pressure on entire ridge). Because neither of these rules was adhered to during the lenses' popular period from 1983 to 1989, reports of the effects of the ridge on PCO were conflicting, although several studies showed a definite positive effect.[39] No adverse effects of this lens modification have been reported after 18 years of use. After the disastrous recall of the Azar 91Z, Iolab claimed that it was the Hoffer ridge lenses that kept them afloat. As studies began to show that convex-surface-posterior lenses decreased PCO, and with the increased production of more-accurate lasers, most surgeons turned toward biconvex IOLs without the ridge in the 1990s. The Hoffer ridge optic was successfully made on biconvex PMMA IOLs (Coburn Optical)

and with silicone (AMO), but never brought on the market. Today, many IOLs use a sharp edge design based on this barrier concept.

UV protection was also an issue strongly advocated by Diana Langley in the 1980s and soon it became a standard in IOL fabrication.

■ MULTIFOCAL INTRAOCULAR LENSES ■

In 1982, after seeing a patient referred with severely decentered Shearing lenses bilaterally (Figure 35-30B), I postulated a concept[40] of multifocality for IOLs. The patient had 20/20 vision without correction but was also correctable to 20/20 with an aphakic spectacle correction. I concluded that the only way this could be possible would be if her brain were selecting the clearest image of the two being presented by the pseudophakic and aphakic zones of her pupil. I immediately attempted to patent the concept, but Jack Hartstein had applied for this with contact lens in 1975 (Figure 35-30A). I pressured Iolab into fabricating a 50/50 split bifocal IOL for research purposes. After they made five such lenses (see Figure 35-30C) for me in their research and development division, they lost interest in the idea while they turned their attention to research with partial-depth positioning holes. Frustrated, I was able to get Ioptex to clean, polish, verify the powers, and sterilize these lenses. With thorough informed consent, I implanted them in three patients, uniocularly. They worked, but I had to remove one because of annoying images. Three years later, I learned that John Pearce, working with Iolab, was implanting central bullet bifocal IOLs by Iolab in England. This was soon followed by the diffractive multifocal (3M) and the various other manufacturer designs, including the Array lens by Allergan (AMO). After Alcon purchased the 3M IOL division, they abandoned the multifocal because of the strict FDA testing asked of them. Allergan persisted, and they ultimately received FDA approval. All the other designs gradually faded away. Ironically, I do not implant multifocal IOLs.

Today there a number of approved methods to provide multifocality including so-called "accommodating IOLs." How this all shakes out will be known in the future.

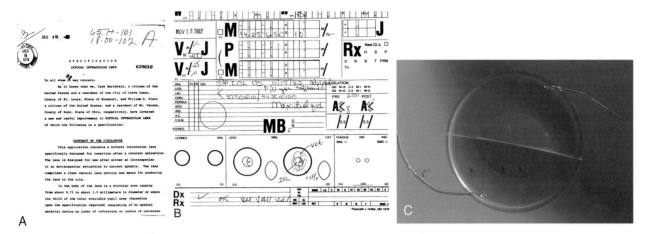

Figure 35-30 **A,** Harstein bifocal intraocular lens patent application, December 8, 1975. **B,** Chart of patient with bilateral dislocated posterior chamber lenses, November 18, 1982. **C,** Original 1983 Hoffer split bifocal intraocular lens.

■ LENS IMPLANT SOCIETIES ■

It is impossible to relate the history of IOLs without touching on the societies that sprang up to deal with them. Choyce[4] came up with the idea of setting up an organization for the study of lens implants in 1964. It took a couple of years for him to convince Ridley, but they did it in 1966 and held their first meeting as the Intraocular Implant Club (IIC) on Wednesday, July 14, 1966, in Oxford, England. Ridley was the first president, followed by Strampelli in 1970. It was the Paris meeting on Saturday, June 1, 1974, at the Meridien Hotel adjoining the Palais des Congres after the close of the Twenty-second International Congress of Ophthalmology, that saw the tremendous surge of interest in IOLs. Forty-four members and 88 nonmembers attended; most were from America. After the formation of the American society and other national implant societies, they changed the name to the International IIC (IIIC).

In March 1974, I conceived of the idea of an American society for lens implantation to bring together the disparate factions then present in the implant world here in the United States. I had not yet heard of the IIC. I wanted the society to hold educational meetings and publish a scientific journal because at that time there was no forum for presenting or publishing reports on the subject. I persuaded three colleagues to help me (Drs. John Darin, Jeremy Levenson, and Stephen Cooperman). Together we organized and incorporated the society as the American Intra-Ocular Implant Society (AIOIS) in August 1974, whose name was changed to the American Society of Cataract & Refractive Surgery (ASCRS) in 1983 (Figure 35-31). After 1 year, Dr. Cooperman went on to other things including a stint in jail for fraudulent art theft in the late 90s.

When I visited Cornelius Binkhorst in Terneuzen, Holland, in November 1974, he was very kind to me, but expressed his great concern about this "American Implant Society" he had heard I

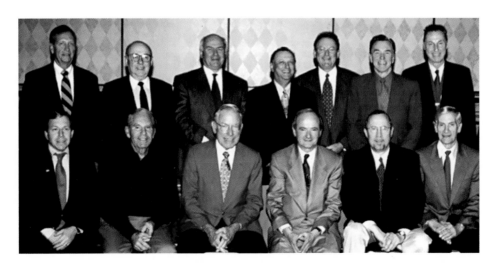

Figure 35-31 Past presidents of the American Society of Cataract & Refractive Surgery (ASCRS) (in chronological order of holding office). Bottom row: Kenneth J. Hoffer (1974–1975), Norman S. Jaffe (1975–1977), Robert C. Drews (1977–1979), Miles A. Galin (1979–1980), Henry M. Clayman (1980–1983), Manuc C. Kraff (1983–1985). Top row: Guy E. Knolle (1989–1991), Jack M. Dodick (1991–1993), John D. Hunkeler (1993–1995), Charles D. Kelman (1995–1997), David Karcher (Executive Vice President 1981–present), Spencer P. Thornton (1997–1999), Robert M. Sinsky (1999–2000).

had founded. I reassured him that we had no intention of overshadowing the IIC, of which he was then president.

I don't think he completely believed me, but he finally dropped the subject. Needless to say I was disconcerted because I never thought of the little society I had started as trying to take over for the IIC, but looking back on it now, he was right; it did. One year later, to quell his continued fears about AIOIS, I urged him to create a European Implant Lens Council, which would be an amalgamation of European national implant societies over which he could preside. As president, he ultimately did just that, and the European Council later became the European Society of Cataract & Refractive Surgery (ESCRS).

■ FIRST INTRAOCULAR LENS POWER CALCULATIONS ■

As proven by Sir Harold's first two cases, correct calculation of the IOL power is essential and a vital part of the history of IOLs. When I learned in 1974 that Jan Worst was using A-scan ultrasound axial length for IOL power calculation, Karl Ossoinig's (Figure 35-32A) (Iowa City) A-scan lectures[41] (1972) were brought to mind prompting me to call him regarding the instrument to be used. Santa Monica Hospital agreed to purchase the recommended Kretz 7200-MA unit from Austria and a keratometer and to provide a facility where I could perform the tests. The new facility was called the "Eye Lab."

Before inserting my first IOL (Medallion ICCE) on April 22, 1974, I performed the first A-scan IOL power calculation in the Western Hemisphere.[42] Dr. Ossoinig was on the telephone from Iowa talking me through the calibration of the Kretz unit and the measurement of the photographs. For his willingness to help me, I will be eternally grateful. It worked!

Before this time, American lens implanters used a standard 18.0-D prepupillary lens for all eyes, expecting the patient to be as myopic or hyperopic as he or she was before surgery. In the mid-1970s, Dennis Shepard (Santa Maria, Calif.) devised a nomogram based on the patient's preoperative refractive error. After the word spread about the Eye Lab, many other ophthalmologists sent their patients to the Eye Lab for IOL power calculation, including Dr. Henry Hirschman, who sent his patients by limousine to Santa Monica from Long Beach. After months of personally performing the exam myself, I finally decided to train a technician. The Eye Lab's photographer, Don Allen, was the closest at hand, and after 2 months he picked it up easily and became the first IOL power-calculation technician in America. Don died several years ago, and I honor him here.

Working with Lou Katz of Sonometrics, I designed the first A-scan ultrasound unit (see Figure 35-32B) specific for IOL power calculation (DBR-100).[42] It ushered in the era of automatic measuring gates and the applanation technique, of which the latter turned out to be less accurate than the Ossoinig immersion technique but became and remains the standard to this day. In 1974, I programmed the Colenbrander and Hoffer IOL formulas on a Hewlitt-Packard programmable calculator. It took hundreds of presentations at the AAO and ASCRS meetings, as well as numbers of "9 diopter surprises" to make A-scan the standard of care nationwide. The efforts of formula developers such as Tom Lloyd, Don Sanders, John Retzlaff, Manus Kraff, Thomas Olsen, Jack Holladay, and Wolfgang Haigis cannot be left unmentioned.

■ CONCLUSION ■

One thread runs clear through this history of IOLs. Since Jaques Daviel[43] (Paris) performed the first intentional intracapsular cataract extraction on April 8, 1747, most, if not all, of the steps of innovation (and mistakes) leading to what we do today were devised and carried out by individual, private, practitioner, cataract surgeons throughout the world without university or government research funding. To all of them, we owe a debt of gratitude.

Ridley lived long enough (94 years) to have his invention implanted into his own eyes, realize the benefit to humanity he

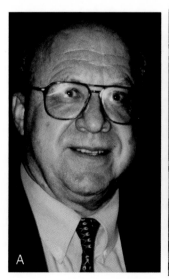
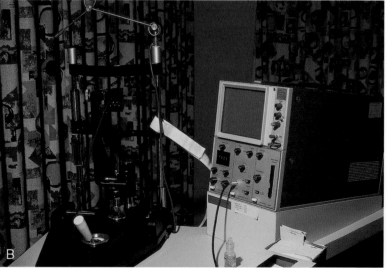

Figure 35-32 A, Karl C. Ossoinig, MD, of Iowa City. B, The first intraocular lens power specific A-scan ultrasound unit in 1975 (Sonometrics DBR-100).

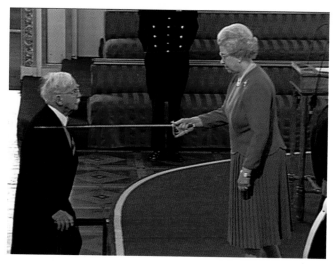

Figure 35-33 Queen Elizabeth II knighting Sir Harold Ridley in London, March 2000.

had provided, and be knighted by his Queen (Figure 35-33). For that we can all be grateful; what a unique and lucky man he was.

With the passing of four giants, Ridley, Choyce, Binkhorst, and Fyodorov, I dedicate this chapter to their memory. I am grateful for having known them.

References

[1] Taieb A. Des mèmoires di Casanova á l'operation di Ridley. Arch Ophtalmol (Paris) 1955;15:501–503.
[2] Münchow W. Zur Geschichte der intraokularen Korrektur der Aphakie. Klin Monatsbl Augenheilkd 1964;145:771–777.
[3] Ascher KW. Prosthetophakia two hundred years ago. Am J Ophthalmol 1965;59:445–446.
[4] Choyce DP. Recollections of the early days of intraocular lens implantation. J Cataract Refract Surg 1990;16:505–508.
[5] Strampelli B. L'évolution des lentilles plastiques de chambre antérieui: derniéres acquisitions techniques. An Inst Barraquer III 1962;4:519–530.
[6] Ridley H. Intra-ocular acrylic lenses. Trans Ophthalmol Soc UK 1951;71:617–621.
[7] Ridley H. Intra-ocular acrylic lenses after cataract surgery. Lancet 1952;I:118–121.
[8] Binkhorst CD, Flu FP. Sterilization of intra-ocular acrylic lens prostheses with ultra-violet rays. Br J Ophthalmol 1956;40:665–668.
[9] Ridley F. Safety requirements for acrylic implants. Br J Ophthalmol 1957;41:359–367.
[10] Baron A. Tolérance di l'oeil à matiére plastique: prosthéses optiques cornéennes. Bull Soc Ophtalmol Paris 1953;9:982–988.
[11] Scharf J. Demonstration eiener neuartigen Kunststofflinse zur Korrecttur der Aphakie, mit Vorstellung operierter Patienten. Klin Monatsbl Augenheilkd 1956;128:233–235.
[12] Strampelli B. Sopportabilità di lenti acriliche in camera anteriore nella afachia e nei vizi di refrazione. Ann Otall 1954;80:75–82.
[13] Dannheim H. Vorderkammerlinse mit elastischen Halteschlingen. Ber Dtsch Ophthal Ges Heidelberg 1956;60:267–268.
[14] Barraquer J. Complicaciones de la inclusion segun los diversos tipos de lentes. An Inst Barraquer 1962;III-4:588–592.
[15] Fyodorov SN. Application of intraocular pupillary lenses for aphakia correction (translation). Vestn Oftal (Mosk) 1965;78:76–83.
[16] Atchison DA. Optical design of poly(methyl methacrylate) intraocular lenses. J Cataract Refract Surg 1990;16:178–188.
[17] Fyodorov SN. Scientific research in behalf of the medical practice (translation). Nauka I Zjiznj (Science Life) 1972;8:93–95.
[18] Binkhorst CD, Gobin MHMA. Pseudophakia after lens injury in children. Ophthalmologica (Basel) 1967;154:81–87.
[19] Platina, 1973
[20] Nordlohne ME. History of intraocular lens implants. In: The intraocular implant lens: development and results with special reference to the Binkhorst lens. The Hague: Dr W Junk BV; 1975. p. 14–36.
[21] Apple DJ, Kincaid MC, Mamalis N, et al. Intraocular lenses: evolution, designs, complications and pathology. Baltimore: Williams & Wilkins; 1989. p. 11–41.
[22] Pearce JL. New lightweight sutured posterior chamber lens implant. Trans Ophthalmol Soc UK 1976;96:6–10.
[23] Shearing SP. Mechanism of fixation of the Shearing posterior chamber intra-ocular lens. Contact Intraocul Lens Med J 1979;5:74–77.
[24] Shearing SP. The genesis of the posterior chamber lens. In: Kwitko ML, Kelman CD, editors. The history of modern cataract surgery. The Hague, Netherlands: Kuglen Publications; 1998. p. 139–146.
[25] Hoffer KJ. Five Year's Experience with the ridged laser lens implant. In: Emery JM, Jacobson AC, editors. Current concepts in cataract surgery (eighth congress). New York: Appleton-Century Crofts; 1983. p. 296–299.
[26] Arnott EJ, Condon R. The totally encircling loop lens-followup of 1,800 cases. Cataract 1985;2:13–18.
[27] Ellingson FT. Complications with the Choyce Mark VIII anterior chamber implant (uveitis-glaucoma-hyphema). J Am Intraocul Implant Soc 1977;3:199–201.
[28] Kelman CD. Anterior chamber lens design concepts. In: Rosen ES, Haining WM, Arnott EJ, editors. Intraocular lens implantation. St Louis: Mosby; 1984. p. 239–245.
[29] Mehta KR, Sathe SN, Karyekar SD. The new soft intraocular lens implant. J Am Intraocul Implant Soc 1978;4:201–205.
[30] Fercho C. "Perfect" capsulotomy reduces vitreous loss, eases cortical cleanup. Ocular Surgery News November 15, 1986.
[31] Pape LG, Balazs EA. The uses of sodium hyaluronate (Healon) in human anterior segment surgery. Ophthalmology 1980;87:699–705.
[32] Shepherd JR. In situ fracture. J Cataract Refract Surg 1990;16:436–438.
[33] Redmond RM, Dallas NL. Extracapsular cataract extraction under local anesthesia without retrobulbar injection. Br J Ophthalmol 1990;74:203–204.
[34] Modern Phaco/ECCE Implant Surgery. 1991 AAO Course #261. Anaheim, Calif; October 1991.
[35] Barasch KR, Poler S. Intraocular lens weights and the vitreous. Ophthalmic Surg 1979;10:65.
[36] Aron-Rosa D, Aron JJ, Griesemann M, et al. Use of the neodymium YAG laser to open the posterior capsule after lens implant surgery: a preliminary report. J Am Intraocul Implant Soc 1980;6:352–354.
[37] Fankhauser F, Roussel P, Steffen J, et al. Clinical studies on the efficacy of high power laser radiation upon some structures of the anterior segment of the eye. Int Ophthalmol 1981;3:129–139.
[38] Hoffer Ridge Patent. US Patent #4,244,060, issued January 13, 1981, US Patent #RE 31,626, reissued July 10, 1984.
[39] Westliing AK, Calissendorff BM. Factors influencing the formation of posterior capsular opacities after extracapsular cataract extraction with posterior chamber lens implant. Acta Ophthalmol 1991;69:315–320.
[40] Hoffer KJ. Personal history in bifocal intraocular lenses. In: Maxwell A, Nordan LT, editors. Current concepts of multifocal intraocular lenses. Thorofare, NJ: Slack, Inc; 1991. p. 127–132.
[41] Ossoinig KC. Standardized echography: basic principles, clinical applications, and results. Int Ophthalmol Clin 1979;19:127.
[42] Hoffer KJ. The history of IOL power calculation in North America. In: Kwitko ML, Kelman CD, editors. The history of modern cataract surgery. The Hague, Netherlands: Kuglen Publications; 1998. p. 193–208.
[43] Daviel J. A new method of curing cataracts by extraction of the lens. Mem Royal Acad Surg (Paris) 1753;2:337.

CONCLUSION

Polymethylmethacrylate Intraocular Lenses

Richard L. Lindstrom, MD

CONTENTS

- Optic Materials
- Loop and Haptic Materials
- Manufacturing Techniques
- Sterilization
- General Design Characteristics, and Optic Size and Shape
- Loop Size, Shape, and Configuration
- Surface Modification of Polymethylmethacrylate Lenses
- Conclusions

CHAPTER HIGHLIGHTS

>> Original material and design considerations

>> Factors in biocompatibility of intraocular lens

>> Lessons learned in manufacturing

This chapter reviews the historical evolution and current status of intraocular lenses (IOLs) with an optic manufactured of polymethylmethacrylate (PMMA). Although a comprehensive review of the literature has been performed and selected references provided, the perspectives presented are those of the author's. In the following chapters, the historical evolution and current status of IOLs with an optic manufactured from foldable materials and of those with a multifocal optic also are reviewed.

The earliest reference to lens implantation is credited to Tadini, an eighteenth-century oculist.[1-3] According to his memoirs, Casanova met him in 1766 in Warsaw, where Tadini showed him a box with small spheres that were well polished and suggested that such globes might be placed under the cornea in the place of the crystalline lens. No confirmation is available that Tadini ever actually did perform such an implant operation.

Approximately 30 years later, in 1795, a Dresden ophthalmologist, Casaamata, performed a cataract operation and implanted an artificial lens.[1-3] Apparently, Casaamata performed the procedure by inserting the glass lens through a wound in the cornea.

He immediately realized the procedure would not be successful as the glass lens fell deeply into the vitreous. Thus the first implantation of an IOL and the first severe complication, total lens dislocation into the vitreous, appear to belong to Casaamata.

The modern era of lens implantation begins with Harold Ridley of London.[4-6] At the end of a cataract operation in the fall of 1949, Ridley reported he was asked by a medical student why he did not replace the cataractous lens he was removing with a new one. Apparently this gave Ridley the impetus to explore the possibility of lens implantation. During World War II, many ophthalmologists had noted that perforating eye injuries from airplane canopies made from acrylic Perspex plastic often resulted in minimal intraocular irritation secondary to the material itself. It, therefore, became accepted that acrylic was relatively inert in the eye. This, and the fact that acrylic has a relatively high refractive index of 1.49 and a low specific gravity of 1.19, prompted Harold Ridley to select this material for his initial investigations into lens implantation.

Ridley originally designed his lens to imitate the natural lens. Its diameter was 8.35 mm, and its weight was 112 mg in air and 70.4 mg in water, as compared with a modern IOL, which weighs less than 4 mg in water. On November 29, 1949, at St. Thomas Hospital in London, Harold Ridley implanted the first posterior-chamber lens into the capsular bag after an extracapsular cataract extraction. It is amazing that his original choice of material, method of cataract extraction, and selection of in-the-bag implantation have been affirmed after more than 40 years of trial-and-error investigation in this field.

The second lens was implanted almost 1 year later, on August 23, 1950. Unfortunately, the initial two patients' postoperative refractive results were significantly myopic, one refracting at −20.0 and one at −15 diopters (D). Ridley then recalculated the basic optics for the lens and began a series of about 750 implants, which extended to approximately 1959. These early lens-implant patients had a significant rate of complications, including severe postoperative inflammation and lens dislocation. Lens dislocation occurred in approximately 13% of the cases, usually into the vitreous. Many patients also developed late secondary glaucoma. Nonetheless, many of these implants performed well for many years (Figure 36-1).

Ridley's work stimulated several other surgeons to become interested in the idea of lens implantation. In an attempt to

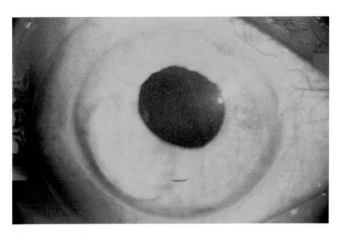

Figure 36-1 Ridley posterior-chamber lens implant in an eye, nearly 40 years after implantation.

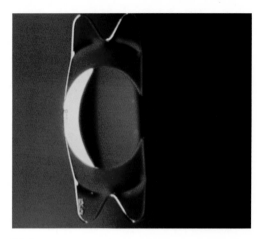

Figure 36-2 Choyce–Tennant, rigid, anterior-chamber intraocular lens.

reduce the high incidence of dislocation, most of these surgeons abandoned the posterior chamber and began to design anterior-chamber, angle-fixated lenses. The first published reports of such lenses came from Strampelli.[7] His lens can be considered the precursor of the rigid, one-piece, anterior-chamber lenses. Of particular interest is the original work by Dahnheim, whose closed-loop, anterior-chamber lens most closely resembles the closed-loop, anterior-chamber lenses that gained great popularity in the United States in the 1980s before being withdrawn from the market for an unexpectedly high incidence of uveitis, glaucoma, hyphema, cystoid macular edema, and corneal decompensation.[8] Of equal interest is the open-loop, anterior-chamber lens of Barraquer, which was later modified successfully as a posterior-chamber lens by Shearing.[9,10] It remains today one of the most popular IOL designs in the world.

Unfortunately, the early anterior-chamber, angle-fixated lenses resulted in a very high incidence of secondary corneal decompensation. Barraquer actually reported a 67% incidence of late corneal decompensation, and he had to remove 50% of his lens implants, many of which were implanted for the correction of myopia in phakic eyes.[9]

These anterior-chamber angle-fixated lenses were the first lenses that suggested to ophthalmologists that long-term follow-up might be required to confirm the level and severity of complications. For example, Strampelli did not notice a high incidence of bullous keratopathy until almost 5 years postoperatively, with most of his patients doing well in the initial postoperative period.

In 1964, Peter Choyce designed a lens, named the Mark VIII, based on his continuing work in anterior-chamber angle fixation (Figure 36-2).[8] This was the first lens implant to perform in a reasonable fashion over an extended period in many surgeons' hands. This lens was implanted without any major change in design between 1964 and 1978. One of the major factors in the improved success of the Mark VIII lens of Choyce was a significant improvement in the quality of manufacturing, which was quite crude in many of the early implant designs.

A continuing significant complication rate with the anterior-chamber angle-fixated lens caused many ophthalmologists to turn to the pupil or iris for fixation of a lens implant. Pioneers of iris-fixated lenses included Epstein of South Africa,[11] Binkhorst[12–14]

and Worst[15] in the Netherlands, and Fyodorov[8] in the Soviet Union.

The original work of Edward Epstein led to a lens shaped like a Maltese cross, with four wings extending from a central optical part. Epstein abandoned this design because of secondary complications, especially inflammation. A similar lens under the name of Copeland was widely used in the United States in the 1970s (Figure 36-3). Unfortunately, a high incidence of chronic iris irritation, secondary cystoid macular edema, and bullous keratopathy caused this lens also to fall into disuse.

A major contributor to the generation of iris support and later iridocapsular lenses was Cornelius Binkhorst, who developed the concept of the iris clip implant. Modifications of this lens, especially the Binkhorst four-loop iris clip lens, gave results superior to those that had been obtained with the early posterior-chamber and anterior-chamber angle-fixated implants.

Jan Worst, also working in Holland, had the concept of improved fixation through the use of a suture or metal clip. This led to a series of lenses called the Medallion lens implants, which also presented improved results over the previous generation of implants.

At the same time, working in the Soviet Union, Syvataslav Fyodorov developed a group of lenses commonly called the Sputnik lenses, which also became popular. However, there continued to be a significant rate of dislocation, cystoid macular edema, and secondary corneal decompensation with these lens implants.

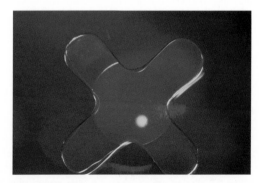

Figure 36-3 Copeland pupil-supported lens.

Unsatisfied with the results himself, Binkhorst recognized the benefits of extracapsular cataract extraction. He went on to develop a series of iridocapsular lenses, which achieved their primary fixation from the capsular bag after extracapsular cataract extraction and a secondary fixation and centration through pupil support.[13] It was soon discovered that the frequency and severity of cystoid macular edema, dislocation, and corneal decompensation were significantly lower with the capsular-fixated lenses.

The concept of iridocapsular fixation gained increasing support and led to a renewed interest in extracapsular cataract extraction. This set the stage for a return to the posterior chamber.

In 1977, John Pearce, working in England, reevaluated the concept of capsular fixation of a posterior chamber lens.[16,17] Beginning with a small, 4 mm optic, tripod-shaped lens, which he sutured to the iris to obtain secondary fixation, he showed that posterior-chamber lenses could be safely and effectively implanted without a high complication rate. The work of Pearce stimulated the imagination of several other ophthalmologists, including Shearing[10] and Simcoe,[18] who modified the Barraquer flexible, open-loop anterior-chamber lens for use in the posterior chamber. Shearing developed the J-loop posterior-chamber lens, with semiflexible loops for implantation either into the ciliary sulcus or the capsular bag[10] (Figure 36-4). This lens proved almost immediately to be successful and demonstrated a relative ease of implantation with a lower complication rate than had been noted with any other implant design. Many brilliant and innovative surgeons then dedicated themselves to improving on the open-loop posterior-chamber lens implant.[19–50] The end result of the evolution is discussed later in this chapter.

At about the same time that one group of pioneers was returning to the posterior chamber with good success, there was a rebirth of interest in the closed-loop anterior-chamber lens (Figure 36-5). The attractiveness of this concept was clear in that most surgeons were accomplished at intracapsular cataract extraction and did not wish to learn the skill of extracapsular extraction required for posterior-chamber lens implantation. The popularity of the closed-loop anterior-chamber lenses peaked in approximately 1982, followed by a total withdrawal from the market by 1988 because of an intolerable incidence of secondary complications, including cystoid macular edema, secondary glaucoma, uveitis, hyphema, and corneal decompensation[51–55] (Figure 36-6).

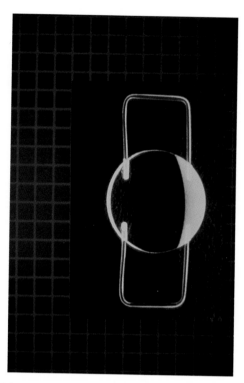

Figure 36-5 The popularity of the Leiske closed-loop anterior-chamber lens peaked between 1982 and 1983.

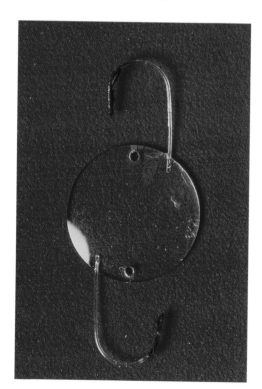

Figure 36-4 Original Shearing J-loop posterior-chamber lens used a 5 mm optic and polypropylene loops.

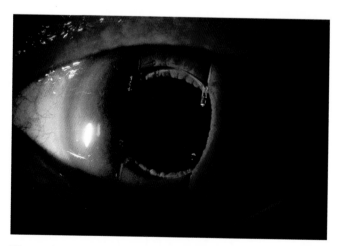

Figure 36-6 Pupil-blocked glaucoma associated with uveitis and recurrent microhyphema in a patient who received a Leiske closed-loop anterior-chamber lens implant.

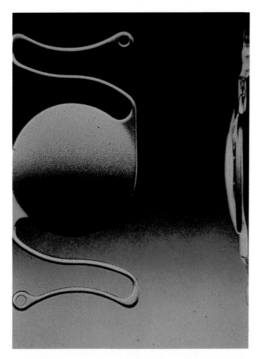

Figure 36-7 Kelman flexible, open-loop, one-piece, anterior-chamber lens.

About the same time, Charles Kelman introduced his flexible, three-point and four-point fixation, one-piece PMMA open-loop anterior chamber lenses, which have continued to perform successfully to this day (Figure 36-7).

■ OPTIC MATERIALS ■

The optic material for an IOL is required to meet several challenges. It must be able to be lathed or molded and polished to a high optical quality, it must be biocompatible and durable with minimal induction of inflammation, it must be nonantigenic and noncarcinogenic, and it must be sterilizable. To meet the requirement for a light weight, it requires a high index of refraction. It is remarkable that Harold Ridley, in his first work, selected a material that has continued to stand the test of time, PMMA.

PMMA is a polymer of methylmethacrylate monomer (Figure 36-8). PMMA is manufactured through the addition polymerization of methylacrylic acid methyl ester, which is itself derived from acrylic acid.[56] Additional agents such as ultraviolet light absorbers may be added to the plastic to enhance its capabilities.[57–59] Various

$$
\left(\begin{array}{ccc} H & & CH_3 \\ | & & | \\ C & - & C \\ | & & | \\ H & & CO \\ & & | \\ & & OCH_3 \end{array}\right)_n
$$

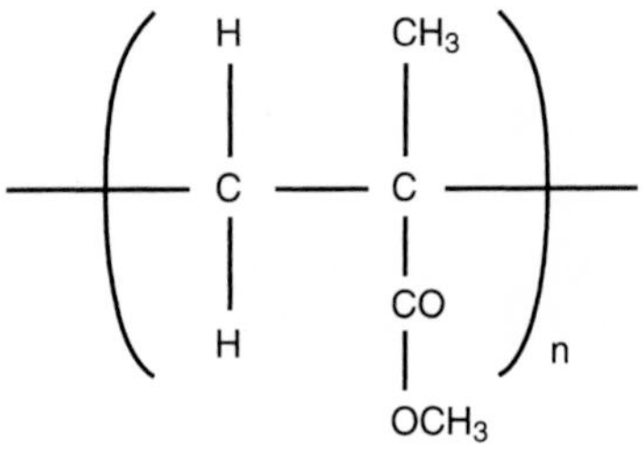

Figure 36-8 Chemical structure of polymethylmethacrylate.

forms of PMMA are available commercially. PMMA used in lathe-cut or compression-molded IOLs is a high-molecular-weight type, such as the Perspex CQ , manufactured by Imperial Chemical Industries. Another form of manufacturing, injection molding, uses a lower-molecular-weight PMMA, such as that manufactured by Rohm & Haas.

PMMA is a light, durable material with a specific gravity of 1.19. It has a refractive index of 1.49. The average molecular weight of Perspex CQ is in the range of 2.5 to 3 million Daltons. At temperatures lower than 100° C it is hard, but the material can melt at temperatures of 140° C or higher.

Although the monomer is toxic, the polymer is inert and is well tolerated in the eye with minimal inflammatory reaction.[60–62] Release of monomer from PMMA was not a concern until the development of the neodymium:yttrium-aluminum-garnet (Nd:YAG) laser for capsulotomy, which has the potential to damage the PMMA optic.[63–67] It has been shown that substances toxic to cultures of various ocular cell lines can be released from PMMA IOLs that are directly hit with Nd:YAG laser bursts of approximately 5 mJ. Fortunately, this has not resulted in significant problems, because much lower energy levels are used, and direct blows to the lens are rare. The higher-molecular-weight, lathe-cut, compression-molded, and cast-molded IOLs are more resistant to Nd:YAG laser damage than the injection molded lenses.

Although PMMA is relatively inert, it is not totally inert in the eye. It does not appear to activate complement or induce chemotaxis of leukocytes, but a cellular reaction does occur on its surface, even in clinically well-tolerated implants.[68–70]

PMMA transmits a broad spectrum of light, including near-ultraviolet light, a possible source of retinal damage.[71] Therefore, ultraviolet-absorbing materials have been added to PMMA optics to reduce this potential toxicity.[57–59] The ultraviolet absorber may be added through covalent bonding or by simply mixing the chromophores with the PMMA. Although it has not been confirmed that ultraviolet absorption has a clinical value, most current PMMA lenses contain ultraviolet light absorbers, usually a benzophenone or benzotriazole.

■ LOOP AND HAPTIC MATERIALS ■

Most PMMA optic lenses are supported by one or more loops or haptic configurations. These may be broadly divided onto one-piece and multipiece IOLs. In the one-piece lenses, the entire lens is manufactured of the same PMMA. In the multipiece lenses, the loop or haptic is composed of a second material. These alternative materials are discussed in the following paragraphs.

An initial material selected for support loops was polyamide, a synthetic material consisting of long molecular chains that contain the amido group at regular intervals. The polyamides include materials such as Nylon 6, Supramid, and Perlon. In the American literature, nylon is basically synonymous with polyamide. These materials retain a high degree of breakage resistance and are quite flexible. They can be manufactured in various diameters, and the manufacturing technology to create various shapes is readily available. Unfortunately, nylon undergoes hydrolysis, resulting in fragmentation over time after implantation into tissue.[15,72] For this reason, polyamide materials were abandoned for use as loops to support optics.

Another suture material, polyethyleneglycolterephthalate, commonly known as Dacron or Mersilene, is also a potential material for IOL loops.[73] Unlike nylon, it is hydrophobic rather than hydrophilic and does not appear to undergo biodegradation. However, it is less elastic and stiffer than the favored polypropylene. Although it is not currently popular for use in IOL loops, Mersilene suture is often used for wound closure and can be used for iris fixation or transscleral fixation of posterior chamber or iris-supported IOLs.

The most popular material for three-piece posterior chamber lenses other than PMMA has been polypropylene (Prolene).[74] Polypropylene has a high tensile strength and, in contrast to nylon, has no hydrolysable binding sites. In a vascular tissue, it is biologically inert and relatively stable, although it is subject to oxidative biodegradation, especially when exposed to light.[72] Elongation of polypropylene is significantly greater than that of Mersilene. It also appears to have a relatively short structural memory, making it possible to implant lenses with compressible polypropylene loops in a space smaller than the diameter of the lens without the loops causing continuous pressure on the tissues.

Polypropylene continues to be a widely employed material for loops of posterior chamber lenses. However, it has two potential problems.

In vitro, polypropylene materials have demonstrated increased levels of complement fragments, which attract circulating inflammatory cells.[70] The clinical importance of this finding is not clear. To date, only one study by Tuberville and Wood[75] has measured complement levels in pseudophakic eyes. This study found that complement levels in posterior chamber IOL pseudophakic eyes were not different than in phakic eyes. The type of haptic material in the patients studied was not differentiated, however.

One in-vitro assay indicated that more bacteria adhere to polypropylene than to PMMA haptics.[76] In a retrospective case-control clinical comparison of endophthalmitis, Menikoff et al.[77] reported that 87% of their cases involved polypropylene-looped lenses. Because of the low incidence of endophthalmitis and the time frame of this study, it is not clear if the more frequent involvement of polypropylene-looped lenses is a function of other confounding factors or represents a clinically significant phenomenon.

Nonetheless, polypropylene has stood the test of time as a support loop in posterior chamber lenses. Yet most surgeons have come to favor PMMA. Metal-looped, iris-supported lenses had a short period of popularity, particularly platinum-iridium and titanium. Today, all metal-looped lenses have been removed from the market because of a high rate of complications.[78]

Another potential haptic material put to use more recently is polyimide. This is a synthetic material of variable construction that contains an imino (NH) group and benzoyl ring. This material is capable of withstanding high temperatures and high-energy radiation, and may be heat sterilized. At this time, polyimide is used as a support loop in some three-piece silicone IOLs, and it is performing in a satisfactory fashion.

In summary, the most popular materials to provide haptic support for a lens implant continue to be PMMA itself, polypropylene, and polyimide. All three appear to perform in a satisfactory fashion, especially if placed inside the capsular bag. The possible oxidative biodegradation of polypropylene and its ability to induce inflammation have reduced its popularity, especially when

sulcus fixation or anterior-chamber angle fixation is selected. The dominant trend is toward one-piece, all-PMMA posterior-chamber lenses.

■ MANUFACTURING TECHNIQUES ■

There are at least five different ways to manufacture IOLs today from PMMA material.[78] Although the exact details of the manufacturing process are often proprietary, a brief review follows.

The most popular method is lathe cutting, in which lenses are cut out of a PMMA blank, usually of a high-molecular-weight acrylic, such as Perspex CQ. Initially, PMMA cast sheets are received as raw material. PMMA cast sheets are preformed and then, using a computer-aided microlathe, lens blanks are cut to the appropriate specific spherical radius for the optic power. The lens blanks are polished. In three-piece lenses, the loops are then formed and attached. In one-piece lenses, the lens optic is lathe cut with a diamond-tip tool to the radius of curvature, and the haptic shape is milled to size and shape. A modern lathe can be programmed to produce a variety of lens shapes and powers. After formation, most lenses are tumble polished, using a drum filled with small spheres that rotate slowly for hours to days. This results in very smooth edges. As an alternative, polishing pads may be used to buff the surface and edges.

In a second manufacturing technique, compression molding is added to the lathe cutting. After creating the lens with a lathe, the implant is placed into a mold, and heat and pressure are applied to shape the lens into its final form. The lens is then carefully polished. This manufacturing technique produces a lens that requires less polishing than a lens produced solely by lathe cutting.

A third method is compression polymerization, in which well-aged and dried base material is poured into a hard stainless-steel mold and slowly warmed under high pressure until polymerization occurs. High pressure is maintained as the material is cooled by blowing.

Fourth, the lenses may be cast molded. Cast molding requires the use of resin in a distilled and purified form. PMMA monomer is crystallized into a pregel or prepolymer residue. The pregel is vacuum processed, filtered, and poured into molds of the desired optical configuration. Lens blanks are cast in a curing cycle similar to that used to prepare cast sheet PMMA.

Finally, lenses may be injection molded. In injection molding, the plastic is heated and then injected into a steel mold. As it softens, it takes the shape of the PMMA mold. After the PMMA cools, the blank is removed from the mold and the edges are polished.

It is clear that manufacture of IOLs by any of these techniques is sophisticated and requires highly skilled technical capability. For an IOL to be suitable for implantation it must be within 0.25 D of stated power; have the proper shape and configuration within 0.25 mm; have a uniform, smooth surface and edges; be chemically pure without any residual monomer, ethylene oxide, or contaminants; be clean of surface debris; and be sterile. Although all manufacturers incorporate careful practices and all IOLs are inspected, it is the surgeon's responsibility to perform a final inspection as well. This may be done under high power with the operating microscope. If the lens shows any imperfection, it should be rejected for implantation and returned to the manufacturer.

■ STERILIZATION ■

PMMA lenses cannot be heat sterilized because the material will melt. Most PMMA lenses are sterilized by ethylene oxide, which is the only technique that is approved by the United States Food and Drug Administration. Ethylene oxide is a cyclic ether that can be toxic to tissue and adheres only to plastic. Although it is an effective sterilizer, all IOLs must be quarantined after sterilization until excess ethylene oxide evaporates and reaches a nontoxic level. Ethylene oxide residual continues to be a concern as a possible cause of postoperative inflammation after implantation of IOLs. The alternative technique of sodium hydroxide sterilization is not used in the United States, but is potentially effective.

■ GENERAL DESIGN CHARACTERISTICS, AND OPTIC SIZE AND SHAPE ■

IOL optics range in size from 4.5 to 7.5 mm. The potential advantage of a larger optic is a lens that is more forgiving of decentration and one that is less likely to produce unwanted optical aberration as a result of light deflecting off the edge of the optic.[79,80] In addition, there is a reduced likelihood of complications such as pupillary capture. An optic size of 6.5–7 mm is appropriately popular with surgeons using planned extracapsular cataract extraction in which a large incision is made (Figure 36-9).

As more surgeons convert to phacoemulsification and use of continuous-tear anterior capsulectomy, smaller optic lenses are becoming more popular.[81–83] In particular, lenses with a round optic of 5–5.5 mm are currently favored by many phacoemulsification

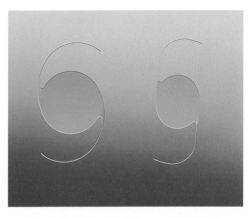

Figure 36-10 A 7 mm round optic, one-piece, all-polymethylmethacrylate, posterior-chamber lens side by side with a 5 × 6 mm oval lens. (Courtesy Storz Corporation, St. Louis, Mo.)

surgeons (Figure 36-10). Because lens implants placed inside the bag after capsulorrhexis show minimal decentration, this optic size seems satisfactory for most older patients.[79] However, these lenses have the potential for increased optical aberration as a result of edge light deflection. Several manufacturers are working on edge treatments to reduce the unwanted visual images created when a lens implant edge is exposed in the pupil.

Oval optics, especially those 5 × 6 mm in diameter, are available and also allow implantation through a relatively small incision. Unfortunately, inside a continuous-tear circular anterior capsulectomy, some lenses decenter in the axis perpendicular to the loops, rendering the extra optical diameter in the opposite meridian less helpful. In addition, the oval lenses appear to induce a higher incidence of unwanted glare or reflection off the edge of the 5 mm portion of the optic, which is usually somewhat thicker. Currently, oval lenses are rarely used as most surgeons favor round optic lenses.

In regard to shape, biconvex lenses appear to be the soundest design. In addition to simulating the natural lens and providing a good optical quality, the posterior convex portion of the optic in close apposition to the posterior capsule appears capable of retarding opacification from Elschnig pearls.[84–86] A biconvex implant design also presents a relatively low profile, which enhances implant-to-iris clearance.

Other design shapes, including meniscus, planoconvex, and those with laser spacing ridges, are still preferred by some surgeons but are significantly less popular. Many lenses have one or more small holes placed in the optic or adjacent to the optic–haptic junction to aid the surgeon in positioning the lens within the eye. Although some surgeons find these useful, with modern flexible-loop capsular bag lenses, positioning holes are probably unnecessary and in some cases can produce unwanted optical aberrations.[37] Use of the optic–haptic junction for manipulation as an alternative to positioning holes in the optic is currently favored by most surgeons because this configuration reduces the chance of postoperative unwanted visual aberrations.

■ LOOP SIZE, SHAPE, AND CONFIGURATION ■

Loop materials currently used in most posterior chamber lenses include PMMA, polypropylene, and polyamide. One-piece and three-piece PMMA lenses, three-piece polypropylene lenses, and

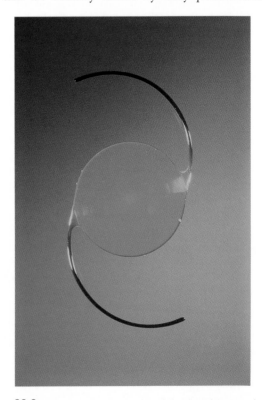

Figure 36-9 Modern one-piece, all-polymethylmethacrylate, open-loop, posterior-chamber lens with a 6.5 mm optic. (Courtesy IOLAB Corporation, Claremont, Calif.)

polyamide haptic lenses have excellent track records with no strong scientific evidence to support one over the other. However, there is an increasing trend toward use of one-piece, all PMMA lenses among experienced surgeons. Theoretically, the absence of a junction between two materials reduces the chance for a discontinuity at which inflammatory cells and debris could accumulate. Several studies have shown that the capsular bag stretches only from approximately 9.5 to approximately 11 mm after cataract extraction and that the diameter of the ciliary sulcus is only 11.5–12.5 mm.[46] This has led to a trend toward shortening the overall tip-to-tip diameter of posterior chamber IOLs. These so-called capsular bag lenses are usually 11.5–12.5 mm from tip to tip. These lenses provide a relative ease of implantation without excess capsular stretch and striae in the postoperative period. Nonetheless, the longer tip-to-tip diameter lenses have achieved an excellent track record over the past 10 years.

Multiple-loop configurations – beginning with the J-loop lens, followed by the Y-loop configurations popularized by Kratz and Sinskey, through the longer and more gradual C-loop, and on to the modified C loop, which is most popular today – are available without any strong scientific proof favoring one over the other. The choice of loop configuration is usually made by the preference of the individual surgeon and influenced by ease of implantation. The majority of surgeons use a modified or short C configuration. Loops are usually angled to a small degree, in the belief that this will reduce pupil capture and iris chafe and place the optic more directly in contact with the posterior capsule.[87] An angulation of 3–10° is usually preferred. Some loops also contain holes or notches for specialized implantation forceps or for use in scleral fixation. Some loops are colored to provide easier visualization during and after implantation into the eye. Increased visibility of the loops can assist in ensuring that the implant is inside the capsular bag (Figure 36-11).

The most popular lenses of today appear to be those manufactured with biconvex optics, which are round and between 5 and 6.5 mm in diameter. In most cases, these lenses are one-piece or three-piece tumble-polished biconvex optics with haptics of PMMA. The preferred overall diameter is 12–12.5 mm, with a modified short C loop and an angulation of approximately 5°. Results with these lenses are superb, and surgeons can use them with confidence.

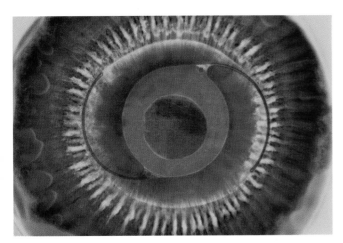

Figure 36-11 A colored-loop, one-piece, all-polymethylmethacrylate, posterior-chamber lens inside the capsular bag, as viewed by a Miyake eye model posterior photograph. (Courtesy IOLAB Corporation, Claremont, Calif.)

Other alternative lens designs continue to attract small but loyal followings, including various closed-loop designs such as those advocated by Sheets and Anis for capsular-bag fixation.[29,88] In addition, disc or plate lenses have been investigated, especially in Europe.[6]

■ SURFACE MODIFICATION OF POLYMETHYLMETHACRYLATE LENSES ■

With improvements in surgical technique and equipment, the incidence of postoperative inflammation following cataract surgery has reduced dramatically. Nevertheless, evidence has shown that a low-grade inflammatory response occurs to the IOL implant.[89–91] Clinical and histologic studies have demonstrated that a foreign-body reaction likely occurs in all eyes following IOL implantation.[92–94] This inflammatory reaction may result in synechiae, cellular and pigmented deposits on the IOL, and uveitis. Certain conditions, such as pre-existing uveitis, diabetes, glaucoma, or a young age may predispose a patient to this event.

Despite PMMA being a relatively inert material in the human eye, its biocompatibility is compromised in one respect, that of surface molecular structure. The ends of the long polymer chains of PMMA, when exposed to the surface of the IOL, can induce inflammatory responses. Knowledge of this interaction potential has stimulated much research into methods of modifying the surface of PMMA lenses such that the exposed polymer ends are either chemically modified or coated with another material.[42,43]

In particular, the use of a heparin coating on the IOL has been investigated and has been shown to reduce early postoperative inflammation in high-risk eyes.[44,45] This IOL is created by inducing electrostatic adsorption of heparin onto the surface of the PMMA IOL. In-vitro experiments have demonstrated a reduced activation of human granulocytes with heparin coating of PMMA. Furthermore, platelet adhesion and growth of human fibroblasts are reduced.[95]

A coating of heparin has been shown to decrease the number and severity of lens deposits. In addition, the likelihood of formation of adhesions to the IOL is decreased.[96–98] Some have found heparin-coated IOLs to be free of cellular deposits and to reduce the incidence of inflammatory complications, compared with unmodified PMMA lenses.[99] In addition, fewer lens deposits lead to a clearer implant and better visual acuity.[100] These benefits have been found not only for high-risk eyes but also for routine cases.[101] Care must be taken in implanting heparin-coated IOLs because the heparin can be mechanically destroyed in the areas where the lens is grasped.[102] The clinical consequences of this occurrence are not currently known.

Another modification of PMMA IOL surfaces has been introduced by Bausch & Lomb Surgical. This innovation, known as fluorine surface modification, is unique in that it produces a permanent, irreversible change in the molecular structure and composition of the IOL surface. Again, this change results in an enhanced biocompatibility with decreased cellular adsorption and adhesions.[103] Fluorine-surface modified lenses have been used in the correction of pediatric aphakia, a procedure in which the postoperative inflammatory response can be significant. These lenses have demonstrated a reduced cicatricial response compared with unmodified PMMA lenses.[104]

CONCLUSIONS

Although IOLs have historically been placed in the anterior-chamber angle, pupillary space, or posterior chamber, the posterior chamber has been confirmed to be the safest and most effective for primary implantation.

Surgeons have the opportunity to select from a large variety of IOL designs. Most of the differences are small modifications based on individual preference, but some design features have been shown to be advantageous through clinical experience and scientific study. PMMA is clearly a superior material for lens implant. Biconvex optics appear to be preferred over other shapes. In addition, a round optic appears to be superior to an oval optic. The trend is, therefore, toward one-piece, biconvex PMMA lenses, which may have a slight advantage over three-piece lenses.

The short modified C-loop haptic appears to be a good compromise between ease of implantation and solid fixation and centration. Reduction in the overall tip-to-tip loop diameter to 12–12.5 mm is consistent with ocular anatomy, and loops that angle forward 3–10° reduce contact between the lens and the iris, and thereby the chance for pupillary capture. In addition, implantation within the capsular bag appears to be superior to sulcus fixation because the lens is sequestered from contact with vascular tissue.

Positioning holes and notches on the lens loops are unnecessary for most surgeons for routine implantation and may result in secondary complications, such as optical aberration or difficulty in IOL removal. Most lenses incorporate an ultraviolet light absorber in spite of the absence of strong evidence in its favor. Loop coloration may ease implantation for the surgeon beginning in this field, but is not required for most experienced surgeons. Surface modification may be useful to reduce the postoperative inflammatory response, particularly in high-risk cases.

The evolution to the current state of the art in posterior chamber lenses over a period of more than 40 years represents a marvel of collaboration between manufacturers, ophthalmic surgeons, and patients throughout the world.

References

[1] Jaffe NS, Clayman HM, Hirschman H, et al. Pseudophakos. St Louis: Mosby; 1978.
[2] Alpar JJ, Fechner PU. Fechner's intraocular lenses. New York: Thieme-Stratton; 1986.
[3] Gorin G. History of ophthalmology. Wilmington, Del: Publish or Perish Inc; 1982.
[4] Ridley H. Intraocular acrylic lenses. Trans Ophthalmol Soc U K 1951;71:617–621.
[5] Ridley H. Intraocular acrylic lenses: 10 years' development. Br J Ophthalmol 1960;44:705–712.
[6] Ridley H. Safety requirements for acrylic implants. Br J Ophthalmol 1957;41:359–367.
[7] Strampelli B. Les lentilles camerules après six annees d'experience. Acta Ophthalmol Belgica 1958;2:1692–1698.
[8] Nordlohne ME. The intraocular implant lens: development and results with special reference to the Binkhorst lens. The Hague: Dr W Junk Publishers; 1975.
[9] Drews RC. The Barraquer experience with intraocular lenses: 20 years later. Ophthalmology 1982;89:386–393.
[10] Shearing S. A practical posterior chamber lens. Contact: IOL Med J 1978;4:114–117.
[11] Epstein E. Modified Ridley lenses. Br J Ophthalmol 1959;43:29–33.
[12] Binkhorst CD, Leonard PAM. Results in 208 iris-clip pseudophakos implantations. Am J Ophthalmol 1967;64:947–956.
[13] Binkhorst CD, Kats A, Leonard PAM. Extracapsular pseudophakia. Am J Ophthalmol 1972;73:625–636.
[14] Binkhorst CD. Iris-clip and irido-capsular lens implants (pseudophakia): personal techniques of pseudophakia. Br J Ophthalmol 1967;51:761–771.
[15] Worst JGF. Iris sutures for artificial lens fixation: perlon vs. stainless steel. Trans Am Acad Ophthalmol Otolaryngol 1976;88:102–104.
[16] Pearce JL. Pearce-style posterior chamber lenses. J Am Intraocul Implant Soc 1980;6:33–36.
[17] Pearce JL. Intraocular lenses. Curr Opin Ophthalmol 1992;3:29–38.
[18] Baikoff F. L'insertion capsulaire des implants de Simcoe. J Fr Ophtalmol 1981;4:14–23.
[19] Clayman HM. Ultraviolet-absorbing intraocular lenses. J Am Intraocul Implant Soc 1984;10:429–432.
[20] Olson RJ, Kolodner H, Kaufman HE. The optical quality of currently manufactured intraocular lenses. Am J Ophthalmol 1979;88:548–555.
[21] Simpson MJ. Optical quality of intraocular lenses. J Cataract Refract Surg 1992;18:86–90.
[22] Drews RC, Smith ME, Okun N. Scanning electron microscopy of intraocular lenses. Ophthalmology 1978;85:415–424.
[23] Yamanaka A, Matsumoto T, Nakama K, et al. Physical and chemical analysis of intraocular materials. J Am Intraocul Implant Soc 1979;5:131–136.
[24] Apple DJ, Mamalis N, Olson RJ, et al. Intraocular lenses: evolution, designs, complications and pathology. Baltimore: Williams & Wilkins; 1989. p. 405–426.
[25] Shepard DD. The dangers of metal-loop intraocular lenses. J Am Intraocul Implant Soc 1977;3:42–45.
[26] Drews RC. Quality control and changing indications for lens implantation. Seventh Binkhorst Medical Lecture, 1982. Ophthalmology 1983;90:301–310.
[27] Clayman HM. Intraocular lenses. In: Duane TD, Jaeger EAD, editors. Clinical ophthalmology. Philadelphia: JB Lippincott; 1991.
[28] Galin MA, Turkish L. Studies of intraocular lens sterilization: the effect of NaOH on B. subtillis spores. J Am Intraocul Implant Soc 1980;6:18–20.
[29] Maida JW, Sheets JH. Intraocular lenses: a review of 1,000 consecutive cases. Contact: IOL Med J 1978;4:95–101.
[30] Olmos EZ, Roy FH. Results of over 1,000 intraocular lens implants in the last five years. Contact: IOL Med J 1980;6:162–170.
[31] Jaffe NS. Results of intraocular lens implant surgery. Am J Ophthalmol 1978;85:13–23.
[32] Kaufman HE, Katz JI. Endothelial damage from intraocular lens insertion. Invest Ophthalmol 1976;15:996–1000.
[33] Miller D, Doane MG. High-speed photographic evaluation of intraocular lens movements. Am J Ophthalmol 1984;97:752–759.
[34] Severin SL. The Severin posterior chamber lens for intracapsular surgery. Contact: IOL Med J 1980;6:291–293.
[35] Kratz RP, Mazzocco TR, Davidson B, et al. A comparative analysis of anterior chamber, iris-supported, capsule-fixated, and posterior chamber intraocular lenses following cataract extraction by phacoemulsification. Ophthalmology 1981;88:56–58.
[36] Stark WJ, Worthen DM, Holladay JT, et al. The FDA report on intraocular lenses. Ophthalmology 1983;90:311–317.
[37] Brems RN, Apple DJ, Pfeffer BR, et al. Posterior chamber intraocular lenses in a series of 75 autopsy eyes. Part III: Correlation of positioning holes and optic edges with the pupillary aperture and visual axis. J Cataract Refract Surg 1986;12:367–371.
[38] Kratz RP. Intraocular lenses: complications associated with intraocular lenses, Ophthalmology 1979;86:659–661.
[39] Crawford JB. A histopathological study of the position of the Shearing intraocular lens in the posterior chamber. Am J Ophthalmol 1981;91:458–461.
[40] Hoffer KJ. Five years' experience with the ridges laser lens implant. In: Emery JM, Jacobson AC, editors. Current concepts in cataract surgery. Norwalk, Conn: Appleton & Lange; 1984. p. 296–299.
[41] Maltzman B, Haupt E, Cucci P. Effect of laser ridge on posterior capsular opacification. J Cataract Refract Surg 1989;15:644–647.
[42] Ratner BD, Mateo NB. Surface modification of intraocular lenses. Ophthalmol Clin North Am 1991;4:277–293.
[43] Hofmeister FM, Yalon MS, Iida S, et al. In vitro evaluation of iris chafe protection afforded by hydrophilic surface modification of polymethylmethacrylate intraocular lenses. J Cataract Refract Surg 1988;14:514–519.
[44] Larson R, Selen G, Bjorklund H, et al. Intraocular PMMA lenses modified with surface-immobilized heparin: evaluation of bio-compatibility in vitro and in vivo. Biomaterials 1989;10:511–516.
[45] Phillipson B, Fagerholm P, Calel B, et al. Heparin surface modified intraocular lenses: three month follow-up of a randomized, double-masked clinical trial. J Cataract Refract Surg 1992;18:71–77.
[46] Assia EI, Legler UFC, Libby CC, et al. Size and configuration of the capsular bag after short and long-term fixation of PC-IOL's in-the-bag. Presented at the American Society of Cataract and Refractive Surgery Annual Meeting, Boston, 1992.
[47] Masket S. Pseudophakic posterior iris chafing syndrome. J Cataract Refract Surg 1986;12:252–256.
[48] Van-Oye R, Budo C, Galand A, et al. Two year postoperative results of Galand lens implantation. J Cataract Refract Surg 1986;12:135–139.
[49] Gunning FP, Greve EL. Intracapsular cataract extraction with implantation of the Galand disc lens: a retrospective analysis in patients with and without glaucoma. Ophthalmic Surg 1991;22:531–538.
[50] Kratz RP. Intracapsular versus extracapsular cataract extraction for intraocular lens implantation. Int Ophthalmol Clin 1979;19:179–194.
[51] Keates RH, Ehrlich DR. "Lenses of chance": complications of anterior chamber implants. Ophthalmology 1978;85:408–414.
[52] Reidy JJ, Apple DJ, Googe JM, et al. An analysis of semi-flexible, closed loop anterior chamber intraocular lenses. J Am Intraocul Implant Soc 1985;11:344–352.
[53] Lim ES, Apple DJ, Tsai JC, et al. An analysis of flexible anterior chamber lenses with special references to the normalized rate of explantation. Ophthalmology 1991;98:243–246.
[54] Beehler CC. A review of 100 cases of flexible anterior chamber lens implantation. J Am Intraocul Implant Soc 1984;10:188–190.
[55] Smith PW, Wong SK, Start WJ, et al. Complications of semi-flexible closed loop anterior chamber intraocular lenses. Arch Ophthalmol 1987;105:52–57.
[56] Saunders JJ. Organic polymer chemistry. New York: Chapman and Hall; 1973.
[57] Mainster MA. Spectral transmittance of intraocular lenses and retinal damage from intense light sources. Am J Ophthalmol 1978;85:167–170.
[58] Gupta A. Long-term aging behavior of ultraviolet absorbing intraocular lenses. J Am Intraocul Implant Soc 1984;10:309–314.
[59] Kraff MC, Sanders DR, Jampol LM, et al. Effect of an ultraviolet filtering intraocular lens on cystoid macular edema. Ophthalmology 1985;92:366–369.
[60] Holyk PR, Eifrig DE. Effects of monomeric methylmethacrylate on ocular tissues. Am J Ophthalmol 1979;88:385–395.
[61] Galin MA, Chowchuvech E, Turkishfd L. Uveitis and intraocular lenses. Trans Ophthalmol Soc UK 1976;96:16–167.
[62] Turkish L, Galin MA. Methylmethacrylate monomer in intraocular lenses of polymethylmethacrylate. Arch Ophthalmol 1980;98:120–121.
[63] Terry AC, Stark WJ, Newsome DA, et al. Tissue toxicity of laser-damaged intraocular lens implants. Ophthalmology 1985;92:414–418.
[64] Mellerio J, Capon MMRC, Docchio F, et al. A new form of damage to PMMA intraocular lenses by Nd:YAG laser photodisruptors. Eye 1988;2:376–381.
[65] Bath PR, Romberger AB, Brown P. A comparison of Nd:YAG laser damage thresholds for PMMA and silicone intraocular lenses. Invest Ophthalmol Vis Sci 1986;27:795–798.
[66] Loertscher H. Laser-induced breakdown for ophthalmic applications. In: Troken SL, editor. YAG Laser ophthalmic microsurgery. Norwalk, Conn: Appleton & Lange; 1983. p. 40–67.
[67] O'Connell RM, Deaton TF, Saito TT. Single and multiple shot laser damage properties of commercial grade PMMA. Appl Optics 1984;23:682–688.
[68] Wolter JR. Foreign body giant cells on intraocular lens implants. Graefes Arch Clin Exp Ophthalmol 1982;1219:103–111.

[69] Sievers H, Von Domarus D. Foreign-body reaction against intraocular lenses. Am J Ophthalmol 1984;97:743–751.

[70] Tuberville AW, Galin MA, Perez HD, et al. Complement activation by nylon and polypropylene-looped prosthetic intraocular lenses. Invest Ophthalmol Vis Sci 1982;22:727–733.

[71] Grossman LW, Knight WB. Resolution testing of intraocular lenses. J Cataract Refract Surg 1991;71:84–90.

[72] Kronenthal FL. Intraocular degradation of non-absorbable sutures. J Am Intraocul Implant Soc 1977;3:222–238.

[73] Jaffe NS. Polyethylene terephthalate (Dacron) in intraocular surgery. Ophthalmology 1981;88:955–958.

[74] Clayman HM. Polypropylene. Ophthalmology 1981;88:959–964.

[75] Tuberville AW, Wood TO. Aqueous humor protein and complement in pseudophakic eyes. Cornea 1990;9:249–253.

[76] Dilly PN, Sellors PJ. Bacterial adhesion to intraocular lenses. J Cataract Refract Surg 1989;15:317–320.

[77] Menikoff JA, Speaker MG, Marmor M, et al. A case-control study of risk factors for postoperative endophthalmitis. Ophthalmology 1991;98:761–1768.

[78] Olson RJ. Intraocular lens quality: update 1979. J Am Intraocul Implant Soc 1980;6:16–17.

[79] Hansen SO, Tetz MR, Solomon KD, et al. Decentration of flexible loop posterior chamber intraocular lenses in a series of 222 postmortem eyes. Ophthalmology 1988;95:344–349.

[80] Assia EI, Castanada VE, Legler UF, et al. Studies on cataract surgery and intraocular lenses at the Center for Intraocular Lens Research. Ophthalmol Clin North Am 1991;4:251–266.

[81] Gimbal HV, Neuhann T. Development, advantages and methods of the continuous tear capsulorhexis technique. J Cataract Refract Surg 1990;16:33–37.

[82] Apple DJ, Assia EI, Wasserman D, et al. Evidence in support of the continuous tear anterior capsulotomy (capsulorhexis technique). In: Cangelosi GC, editor. Advances in cataract surgery: transaction of the New Orleans Academy of Ophthalmology. Thorofare, NJ: Slack; 1991. p. 21–47.

[83] Armstrong TA. Refractive effect of capsular bag lens placement with the capsulorhexis technique. J Cataract Refract Surg 1992;18:121–124.

[84] Hansen SO, Solomon KD, McKnight GT, et al. Posterior capsule opacification and intraocular lens decentration. Part I: Comparison of various posterior chamber lens designs implanted in the rabbit model. J Cataract Refract Surg 1988;14:605–613.

[85] Born CF, Ryan DK. Effect of intraocular lens optic design on posterior capsule opacification. J Cataract Refract Surg 1990;16:188–192.

[86] Setty S, Percival S. Intraocular lens design and inhibition of epithelium. Br J Ophthalmol 1989;73:918–921.

[87] Johnson SH, Kratz RP, Olson PF. Transillumination defect and microhyphema syndrome. J Am Intraocul Implant Soc 1984;10:425–428.

[88] Galand A, Van Oye R, Budo C, et al. Results of implantation in the capsular bag: a short-term review of 1588 cases. Trans Ophthalmol Soc U K 1985;105:562–566.

[89] Jennette JC, Eifrig DE, Paranjape YB. The inflammatory response to secondary methylmethacrylate challenge in lens-implanted rabbits. J Am Intraocul Lens Implant Soc 1982;8:35–37.

[90] Mondino BJ, Nagata S, Glovsky MM. Activation of the alternative complement pathway by intraocular lenses. Invest Ophthalmol Vis Sci 1985;26:905–908.

[91] Mondino BJ, Rao H. Effect of intraocular lenses on complement levels in human serum. Acta Ophthalmol 1983;61:76–84.

[92] Ohara K. Biomicroscopy of surface deposits resembling foreign body giant cells on implanted intraocular lenses. Am J Ophthalmol 1985;11:260–267.

[93] Wolter JR. Cytopathology of intraocular lens implantation. Ophthalmology 1985;92:135–142.

[94] Bryan III JA, Peiffer Jr RL, Brown DT, et al. Morphology of pseudophakic precipitates on intraocular lenses removed from human patients. J Am Intraocul Lens Implant Soc 1985;11:260–267.

[95] Larsson R, Selen G, Bjorklund H, et al. Intraocular PMMA lenses modified with surface-immobilized heparin: evaluation of biocompatibility in vitro and in vivo. Biomaterials 1989;10:511–516.

[96] Ygge J, Wenzel M, Philipson B. Cellular reactions on heparin surface-modified versus regular PMMA lenses during the first postoperative month. Ophthalmology 1990;97:1216–1223.

[97] Miyake K, Maekubo K. Comparison of heparin surface modified and ordinary PCLS: a Japanese study. Eur J Implant Refract Surg 1991;3:95–97.

[98] Borgioli M, Coster DJ, Fan RFT. Effect of heparin surface modification on polymethylmethacrylate intraocular lenses on signs of postoperative inflammation after extracapsular cataract extraction. Ophthalmology 1992;99:1248–1255.

[99] Percival SPB, Pai V. Heparin-modified lenses for eyes at risk for breakdown of the blood–aqueous barrier during cataract surgery. J Cataract Refract Surg 1993;19:760–765.

[100] Jones NP. Extracapsular cataract surgery with and without intraocular lens implantation in Fuchs' heterochromic uveitis. Am J Ophthalmol 1989;108:310–314.

[101] Trocme SD, Hung-ir L. Effect of heparin-surface-modified intraocular lenses on postoperative inflammation after phacoemulsification: a randomized trial in a United States patient population. Ophthalmology 2000;107:1031–1037.

[102] Dick B, Kohnen T, Jacobi KW. Alteration of heparin coating on intraocular lenses caused by implantation instruments. Klin Moatsbl Augenheilkd 1995;206:460–466.

[103] Eloy R, Parrat D, Tran Min Duc CE, et al. In vitro evaluation of inflammatory cell response after CF4 plasma surface modification of poly (methyl methacrylate) intraocular lenses. J Cataract Refract Surg 1993;19:364–370.

[104] Thouvenin D, Arne JL, Lesueur L. Comparison of fluorine-surface-modified and unmodified lenses for implantation in pediatric aphakia. J Cataract Refract Surg 1996;22:1226–1231.

Foldable Intraocular Lenses, Edge Design, and Aspheric Optics

37

Roger F. Steinert, MD

CHAPTER HIGHLIGHTS

>> Materials used in foldable intraocular lenses (IOLs)

>> Impact of foldable IOLs on astigmatism and vision

>> Edge design, posterior capsule opacification, and photic phenomena

>> Impact of aspheric optics

>> Biocompatability of foldable IOLs

>> Anterior IOL cellular ongrowth

FOLDABLE INTRAOCULAR LENSES AND SMALL-INCISION SURGERY

The soft implant material that makes up a foldable intraocular lens (IOL) enables a 6 mm diameter optic intraocular lens (IOL) to be inserted through a 3 mm or smaller incision with minimal trauma. For forceps insertion, the surgeon grasps the IOL, bends it in half with folding forceps, grasps the folded IOL with insertion forceps then maneuvers the lens through the incision until the IOL and haptics are appropriately situated. For insertion with an implantation device, the surgeon grasps the IOL with holding forceps, positions the IOL in the device, inserts the tip of the device through the incision, and implants the IOL. Some implantation injector systems allow for the IOL to be shipped in the unfolded state and then folded into the inserter without manual handling, increasing the ease and reliability of the folding process and reducing the potential for contamination.

As the IOL slides into position inside the capsular bag or within the ciliary sulcus, the optic unfurls to resume its original shape. Visual recovery from the aphakic state is almost immediate. Visual acuity after cataract surgery and IOL implantation is nearly always an improvement over vision through a crystalline lens with a cataract, especially with small foldable IOLs and small-incision surgical techniques. While a major advantage of small-incision cataract surgery is that it minimizes corneal shape changes that induce astigmatism and delay visual recovery,[1-3] the small incision also provides increased surgical and postoperative safety.

SMALL-INCISION SURGERY

EFFECT OF INCISION SIZE ON ASTIGMATISM

Surgically induced changes in the structural stability of the cornea may produce or aggravate corneal astigmatism that may not be amenable to correction postoperatively with a spherocylindrical spectacle lens. Surgically induced astigmatism can adversely affect postoperative refraction and the stability of the patient's vision over time. Incision length, location, shape, orientation, and suture technique and material are factors. Numerous clinical studies have consistently concluded that smaller incisions lead to better early postoperative uncorrected and corrected visual acuity. In addition, rates of induced astigmatism decline as the incisions become progressively smaller, down to near neutrality in incisions between 2.5 and 3 mm.[1-9]

EFFECT OF INTRAOCULAR LENS IMPLANTATION ON INCISION SIZE

Surgically induced astigmatism may correlate with small incision sizes, but forcible insertion of the folded IOL through the wound may widen the wound, and the final incision may not be as small as the initial keratome incision. Steinert and Deacon[10] developed a set of incision-size gauges to study the dimensional stability of incisions during cataract extraction and IOL implantation. Steinert-Deacon gauges (Capital Instruments, Ltd., Wan Chai, Hong Kong) are the equivalent thickness of conventional metal

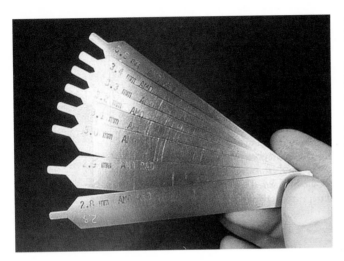

Figure 37-1 Steinert-Deacon incision-size gauges. (From Steinert R, Deacon J: Enlargement of incision width during phacoemulsification and folded intraocular lens implant surgery, *Ophthalmology* 103:220–225, 1996.)

keratomes and are manufactured in 0.2 mm increments (Figure 37-1). The gauges were initially tested in 51 consecutive patients undergoing phacoemulsification.

In the 46 cases of temporal clear corneal incisions performed with diamond keratomes, the initial incision was significantly wider than the keratome blade (0.16 ± 0.08 mm; $P < 0.0001$). After phacoemulsification and irrigation–aspiration, the incision was again significantly wider (0.09 ± 0.06 mm; $P < 0.0001$). If the incision was not widened before insertion of the folded silicone IOL, significant enlargement occurred once more (0.26 ± 0.05 mm; $P < 0.0001$). The final insertion size after forceps insertion of a three-piece silicone foldable IOL was not statistically different than injector insertion of a plate haptic silicone IOL ($P = 0.56$). The investigators concluded that the incision has limited capacity for elastic deformation and may be vulnerable to tearing or irreversible stretching.

IMPLANTATION DEVICES FOR SMALL-INCISION SURGERY

Implantation insertion devices provide uniform folding of the IOL and to allow the IOL to be inserted through smaller incisions than is possible with forceps.[11–12] Unlike forceps, inserters isolate the IOL from the external environment, reducing the risk of introducing surface pathogens into the eye at the time of implantation. For most inserters, the surgeon or technician fills the cartridge with viscoelastic, grasps the IOL with holding forceps, loads the IOL in the cartridge, closes the cartridge, and places it in the handpiece. The surgeon enters the incision with the insertion tip of the handpiece and delivers the IOL into the capsular bag or ciliary sulcus. Not all inserters are appropriate for inserting the IOL into the sulcus.

The next generation of insertion systems eliminates the need for manual loading of the IOL into the inserter. In addition to improved ease of use, an automated loading system brings consistency of loading, thus, reducing the potential complication of

damage to the IOL during insertion, and the potential for the bacterial contamination of the IOL due to handling.

The challenge of automated pre-loaded insertion systems stems from bio-material constraints. Foldable IOL materials cannot be kept in their folded state for extended periods without permanent damage to the material. Therefore, the IOL cannot be shipped in a pre-folded compressed condition. Second, the materials in the injection cartridges typically are chosen, in part, due to inherent lubricity that facilitates the passage of the compressed IOL. These materials may interact with the different material of the IOL optic producing undesirable secondary chemical changes. For these reasons, automated systems have designs that allow the IOL optic to be shipped uncompressed and in contact with a different plastic than the injector itself, yet still allow it to be transferred into the compression chamber and inserter without manual instrumentation.

■ MATERIALS AND OPTICS ■

In the early 1950s, Scales[13] defined an ideal material for implantation into human tissues as chemically inert, stable, not physically modified by contact with tissues, and acceptable to the body, with no inflammation, foreign body response, or tissue chafe. The desired material would be neither carcinogenic nor allergenic, have the capability of being fabricated into the desired form, be able to resist mechanical strains, and be easy to sterilize.

For ophthalmic applications, the material should be optically transparent, and be able to remain so for long periods, be capable of being manufactured into a high resolving power, be able to block ultraviolet (UV) radiation in the 330–400 nm wavelengths, and be implantable through a small incision.

ACRYLIC POLYMERS

The history of acrylic materials used in foldable IOLs begins with polymethylmethacrylate (PMMA), an acrylic material with excellent tissue tolerance that has been used successfully in ophthalmology, oral and dental surgery, orthopedics, and plastic and reconstructive surgery (see Chapter 36). Acrylic materials are polymers synthesized from esters (monomers) of acrylic acid or methacrylic acid. The methyl ester of methacrylic acid, methylmethacrylate, readily polymerizes to PMM. It is a hard, rigid, strong thermoplastic material with excellent optical clarity. It has low water and gas diffusion constants and is highly resistant to the effects of light, oxygen, and hydrolysis. The pure polymer readily transmits UV light but can be manufactured with UV-absorbing chromophores to block ultraviolet energy from reaching the retina.

HYDROPHOBIC ACRYLIC POLYMERS

These polymers are members of the same family as rigid PMMA, but they are tailored for specific optical and mechanical properties by altering the side groups of a standard methacrylate backbone. PMMA and hydrophobic acrylic polymers are similar in their negligible water content and high refractive indices (e.g., 1.55 for AcrySof (Alcon) and 1.47 for Tecnis acrylic (AMO) compared to 1.49 for PMMA). Unlike PMMA, hydrophobic acrylic materials have a relatively long hydrocarbon side chain for increased flexibility at the typical operating room temperatures of 18–22°C. The glass transition temperature (T_g) for PMMA is 105°C, approximately 15.5–21.5°C for AcrySof,[14] and 13°C for Sensar. The T_g is the temperature at which the polymer chains soften from their low-temperature rigid state to their flexible high-temperature form. Thus the lower the T_g, the easier the IOL material is to fold at standard room temperatures.

The AcrySof lens optic is molded from a phenylethyl acrylate and phenylethyl methacrylate polymer (US Patent 5,290,892; 1994). The Sensar lens optic is cut from a sheet of ethyl acrylate, ethyl methacrylate, and trifluoroethyl methacrylate polymer, then cryolathed into its final shape (US Patent 4,834,750; 1989).

HYDROPHILIC ACRYLIC POLYMERS

This class of IOLs is made with hydrophilic acrylic (hydrogel) polymers. Commonly, the IOL optic is lathe cut and polished from a composite material.

A variant is the Collamer IOL (STAAR). Collamer is a hydrogel-collagen copolymer consisting of a HEMA-based acrylic copolymer into which about 0.01% porcine collagen and a UV-absorbing chromophore have been bonded.[18] Because of its high water content, it is wet packed in a glass vial containing the sterile lens in balanced salt solution (BSS) and placed in a pouch for shipping. The lens is removed from the vial with blunt forceps and loaded into a disposable plastic cartridge. The cartridge is inserted into a disposable plastic injector.

In clinical use, early- and late-onset calcification of hydrophilic IOL materials has been a common source of optical degradation.[19–20] The most common reason for explantation of hydrophilic lenses is calcification, sometimes many years after the original implantation surgery.[21] An animal model developed by Buchen illustrates the appearance of calcium deposits on the surface of a hydrophilic IOL[22] (Figure 37-2).

SILICONE ELASTOMERS

Silicone is used in medicine for prosthetic devices, estradiol-releasing vaginal rings, intracoronary stents, subdermal and transdermal implants, intrauterine contraceptive devices, catheters, nasolacrimal intubation tubes, finger joints, and a variety of other clinical situations. In ophthalmology, silicone is used for contact lenses, scleral buckles, keratoprostheses, glaucoma shunts, and IOLs. Silicone is inert, stable at high temperatures, flexible and elastic at a wide range of temperatures, and nonadhesive to tissues. Silicone IOLs are optically clear and have refractive indices ranging from 1.42 to 1.46.

Silicone elastomers are safe, stable, and inert over the long term. Silicone IOLs showed no change in optical performance or surface quality in UV and hydrolytic stress tests designed to mimic 20 years of aging.[23,24] Questions have been raised about the advisability of implanting silicone IOLs in patients at risk for vitreoretinal surgery, because silicone oil used as an intravitreal tamponade may adhere to the solid silicone IOL optic and obstruct the surgeon's view.[25–27] Acrylic IOLs have frequently been the lenses of choice for patients with a history of ocular inflammation, pseudoexfoliation, and diabetic retinopathy or for patients at risk of future vitreoretinal surgery; however, McLoone et al.[28] showed silicone oil adherence to acrylic lenses in vitro. The mean percentage coating of silicone oil on PMMA IOLs was 20.8% and that on foldable hydrophobic acrylic IOLs was from 17.1 to 21.5% ($P = $ NS). One hydrogel IOL (Aqua-Sense, Ophthalmic Innovations International; Ontario, Calif.) had 17.8%, and another (Raysoft, Rayner Intraocular Lenses, UK) had 5.2% coating from silicone oil ($P < 0.001$ vs. the other lenses).

VACUOLES

Vacuoles in foldable IOL materials, particularly hydrophobic acrylics, are ascribed to water vapor that accumulates in microvoids within the material. The number and size of microvoids are affected by the manufacturing process.

Vacuoles within the IOL have been reported in several studies of patients with AcrySof IOL implants.[29–33] Christiansen et al.[30] reported that 42 eyes implanted with AcrySof IOLs all exhibited some degree of vacuole formation that appeared as glistenings under slit-lamp observation. Laboratory studies suggest that temperature elevations increase the level of glistenings[34] as does the addition of serum to AcrySof IOLs in aqueous humor.[35] The presence of vacuoles in the IOL at mild-to-moderate levels does not appear to affect visual function. However, high levels of vacuole formation can decrease visual acuity,[30,32] decrease contrast sensitivity,[29,32,33] and interfere with the ability to target a neodymium:yttrium-aluminum-garnet (Nd:YAG) laser for posterior capsulotomy.[32]

OPTIC EDGE DESIGNS

Initially, most PMMA and foldable IOLs had rounded edges. Manufacturers now design optics with sharp or squared edges to inhibit the growth of lens epithelial cells over the posterior capsule. Nishi, Nishi, and Sakanishi[36] reported that an AcrySof IOL with a sharp optic edge had a significantly greater effect in

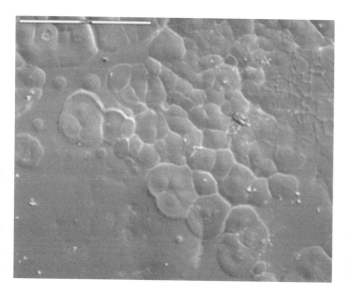

Figure 37-2 Scanning electron micrograph of calcification on the surface of a hydrophilic intraocular lens in an animal model (courtesy Rakhi Jain, Ph.D.)

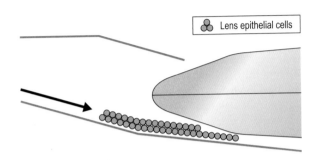

Figure 37-3 Schematic representation of epithelial cell migration under the rounded edge of an intraocular lens.

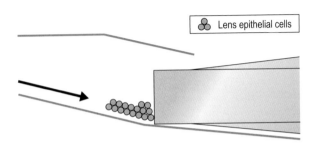

Figure 37-4 Schematic representation of epithelial cell migration inhibited by the sharp posterior edge of an intraocular lens in contact with the posterior capsule.

inhibiting posterior capsule opacification (PCO) than a PMMA IOL with rounded edges. Later, Nishi, Nishi, and Wickstrom[37] looked at the influence of IOL design and materials, implanting an AcrySof acrylic IOL in one eye and a CeeOn silicone IOL in the other eye of seven rabbits. Both IOLs had a sharp, rectangular optic edge. Miyake-Apple views showed that migrating lens epithelial cells were inhibited at the optic edge of five of the six rabbits available for evaluation. Overall, there was no apparent difference in PCO development between the two IOLs for the first 3–4 weeks. The study suggests that IOL design is an important factor in preventing PCO (Figures 37-3 and 37-4).

With the square-edge hydrophobic acrylic IOL, some patients have reported bothersome edge glare and negative dysphotopsias.[38–41] Holladay, Lang, and Portney[42] conducted ray tracings of biconvex IOLs that were identical except that the edge was either round or square. The sharp-edge design formed an arclike pattern of reflected light on the retina, and the round-edge design formed a diffuse image (Figure 37-5).

Rounding the biconvex lens reduced the peak intensity of the reflected glare image by 90%. The authors concluded that the glare images from the sharp edge appeared like a thin crescent or partial ring in the periphery of the retina opposite the image of the glare source and that rounding the edges significantly reduced the peak intensity of the reflected glare image.

An alternative explanation for the photic phenomena reported by patients with the square-edge AcrySof IOL comes from a study comparing equiconvex silicone (LI16U) and PMMA (P359UV) IOLs with an unequal biconvex acrylic (MA60BM) IOL.[43] The refractive indices for the three IOLs were 1.43, 1.49, and 1.55, respectively. This study suggested that the unequal biconvex design produced greater postoperative glare and external reflections than the equiconvex IOLs. Further, an increase in the refractive index from 1.43 to 1.55 increased the amount of reflected light fivefold.

Another approach to edge design was taken by the Sensar (acrylic) and ClariFlex (silicone) lenses. The Sensar IOL has a standard rounded edge. The Sensar with OptiEdge and ClariFlex have a sharp vertical edge on the posterior surface, a sloped edge along the side of the IOL, and a rounded anterior edge (Figure 37-6). The ray tracings of this new design show less reflection off the posterior surface than a conventional square-edge design and dispersion of light rays through the anterior surface (Figure 37-7). These lessons from early improvements in reducing photic phenomena continue to be evolved in new IOL edge designs.[44] Some studies find variations in rates of complaints about dysphotopsia based on IOL design[45] while others report that some patients perceive similar dysphotopsias with two markedly different IOL designs.[46]

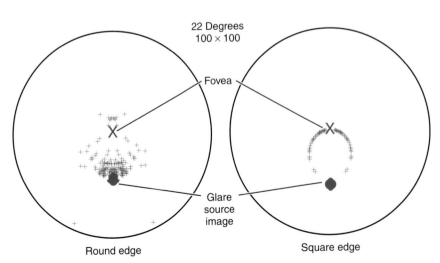

Round edge

Square edge

Figure 37-5 Distribution of internally reflected light on the retina. (From Holladay J, Lang A, Portney V: Analysis of edge glare phenomena in intraocular lens edge designs, *J Cataract Refract Surg* 27:614–621, 2001. Copyright (2001) with permission from Elsevier.)

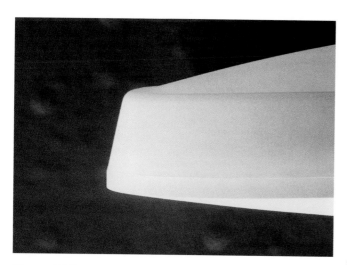

Figure 37-6 Edge design of the Sensar with OptiEdge and ClariFlex IOLs. (Courtesy AMO Surgical.)

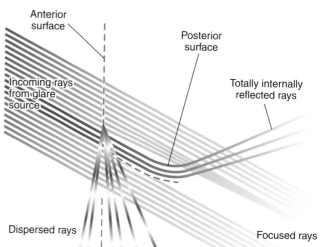

Anterior surface

Posterior surface

Totally internally reflected rays

Incoming rays from glare source

Dispersed rays

Focused rays

Figure 37-7 Ray tracings of the Sensar with OptiEdge. (Courtesy AMO Surgical.)

■ ASPHERIC OPTICS ■

The understanding of sophisticated optics and its relevance to clinical ophthalmology is credited to corneal laser refractive surgery. Vision symptoms that were not consistent with excellent high-contrast visual acuity rapidly led to an understanding of the impact of large-aperture optics and aberrations on the quality of vision. This understanding rapidly found its way into cataract and IOL surgery.

The natural corneal curvature has an asphericity that averages +0.27 μ RMS. In youth, this is balanced by a lenticular asphericity averaging −0.27 μ RMS, leading to minimal total spherical aberration.

The original conventional IOL designs all had optics designed on elementary optics, which resulted in positive spherical aberration in the IOL. This increased the total spherical aberration of the eye after cataract and IOL surgery, with resultant loss of image quality [47–49,53,60,61] and loss of contrast sensitivity.[50]

IOL designs increasingly address the issue of the spherical aberration of the eye. Aspheric optics clinically improve quality of vision and contrast sensitivity compared to spherical optics.[51–54]

The original IOL design with aspheric optics was the lens that is now known as the AMO Tecnis aspheric series of lenses (e.g., Z9000 series). These IOLs are designed with −0.27 μ RMS spherical aberration (Figures 37-8 and 37-9). These IOLs have proved to improve the quality of vision with large pupils, night vision, and night vision with glare.[45,46]

Subsequent aspheric designs have targeted different ranges of spherical aberration. The Bausch & Lomb aspheric design (LI61AO) targets zero asphericity in the IOL, not attempting to alter the corneal asphericity. The Alcon aspheric IOLs (e.g., SN60WF series) are designed for −0.17 μ RMS of asphericity, striking a middle ground. Aspheric IOLs must be centered within 0.4 mm of the pupil center to results in optical benefit.[57] The lower the negative asphericity, the less benefit to a well-centered IOL but, correspondingly, the less degradation from decentration or tilt.[58]

Another factor in the total visual performance of an IOL is chromatic aberration and its balance with spherical aberration. The interaction of these two factors can have an important impact on depth of focus in aspheric IOLs. An analysis of a variety of commercial IOL models showed marked variation in depth of focus, particularly under low-light conditions, with the best depth of focus achieved by the Tecnis aspheric IOL.[59]

One common situation alters corneal asphericity: corneal refractive surgery. Both radial keratotomy and myopic excimer laser refractive surgery generally increase positive spherical aberration. Wavefront-guided and wavefront-optimized corneal myopic refractive surgery also usually increases spherical aberration, but less than in the case of non-"customized" or "guided" treatment. Hyperopic corneal refarctive surgery, on the other hand, tends to decrease positive spherical aberration. As a rule, therefore, a patient with prior myopic corneal refractive surgery will benefit from an IOL with maximal negative aspheicity. A patient with prior hyperopic corneal refractive surgery may do better with one of the original IOL designs that have positive spherical aberration. If possible, patients with prior corneal refractive surgery should have a preoperative measurement of corneal aberrations to guide the optimal IOL selection.

■ BIOCOMPATIBILITY ■

FOREIGN-BODY REACTION

Clinical measures of biocompatibility include cellular deposits on the capsule, capsule opacification, postoperative blood–aqueous barrier breakdown, cellular reaction at the anterior capsule–IOL interface, and postoperative inflammation. Amon[60] calls biocompatibility one of the most important prerequisites of an intraocular implant and raises concerns about the use of the term in the medical literature. He quotes the definition from the International Dictionary of Medicine and Biology, "Biocompatibility is the capability of a prosthesis implanted in the body to exist in harmony with tissue without causing deleterious changes."[61]

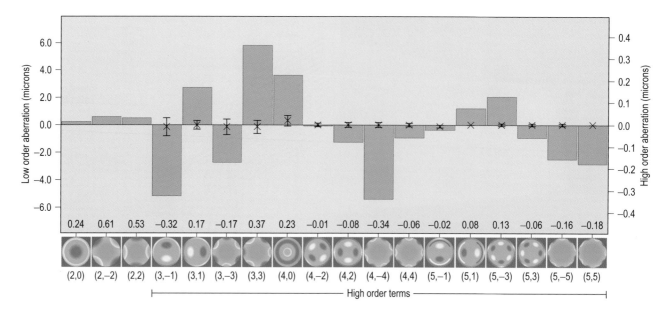

Figure 37-8 Total ocular aberrations measured by the Hartman-Shack method in a patient with a spherical optic intraocular lens. Note the amount of spherical aberration in particular (term 4,0 at 0.23 μ RMS).

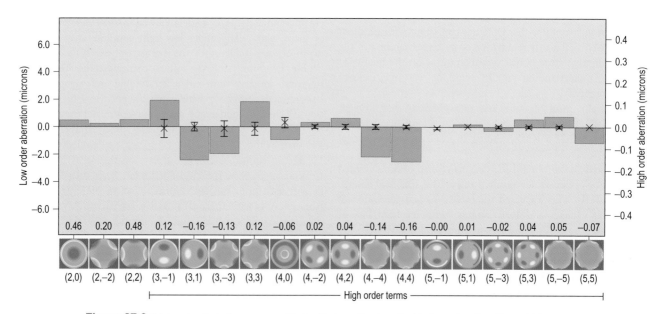

Figure 37-9 Total ocular aberrations measured by the Hartman-Shack method in the patient from Figure 37-8 after exchange of the intraocular lens (IOL) for an aspheric optic IOL with negative asphericity of −0.27 μ RMS. Note the reductions in aberrations, particularly spherical aberration, which is reduced to −0.06 μ RMS, closely matching the theoretical result of 0.23−0.27 = −0.04 μ RMS).

Ideally, the IOL should remain an inert refractive element within the intraocular structures, but it does react with different tissues in the eye, specifically the uvea and the capsular bag. Capsular biocompatibility, according to Amon, occurs when there is minimal or no lens epithelial cell proliferation over the posterior or anterior capsule. Similarly, uveal biocompatibility exists when the IOL causes only a very mild foreign-body reaction despite the close proximity or direct contact between the IOL and uveal tissue.

ANTERIOR CAPSULE OPACIFICATION

Posterior capsule opacification and the role of the IOL are covered in detail in Chapter 51. Less widely recognized and discussed is lens epithelial cell migration onto the anterior surface of the IOL. Hollick, Spalton, and Ursell[62] looked at surface cytologic features of PMMA, silicone, and hydrogel IOLs and their effect on the blood–aqueous barrier as an indicator of biocompatibility. They found that patients who had hydrogel IOLs implanted were significantly more likely to have lens epithelial cells on the anterior surface of the IOL for a longer period than those with PMMA or silicone IOLs ($P < 0.001$). The investigators commented that lens epithelial cells grew over the anterior surface to a much greater extent and in a completely different pattern on the hydrogel IOLs than the PMMA or silicone IOLs.

Müllner-Eidenböck et al.[63] conducted a prospective, randomized clinical study of lens epithelial cell migration onto the anterior capsule in 15 eyes, each implanted with one of four IOLs: the HydroView, MemoryLens, AcrySof, or CeeOn 920. The greatest ongrowth was seen with the hydrophilic acrylic IOLs, HydroView and MemoryLens, which had 86.7 and 73.4%, respectively, at 30 days and 86.7 and 22%, respectively, at 180 days. The lowest rates were seen with the hydrophobic acrylic AcrySof IOL (86.7% at 30 days and 0% at 180 days) and CeeOn 920 silicone IOL (26.7% at 30 days and 19.9% at 180 days).

Lenis and Philipson[64] observed 25 cataract patients with HydroView hydrogel IOL implants for up to 12 months. Lens epithelial cells were detected on the anterior IOL surface in 13 patients (52%). Most of these were within 1 mm of the capsulorrhexis border, with four cases of cell proliferation centrally. Overall, this migration and proliferation did not affect visual acuity.

House et al.[65] evaluated 41 cases of AcrySof IOL implantation in 31 patients. They found granular deposits of what they classified as lens epithelial cell proliferation on the anterior surface of the IOL in 18 cases (44%) at 3 to 5 weeks after surgery. The deposits did not have an effect on visual acuity.

Koch, Kalicharan, and van der Want[66] reported on 62 (of 196; 33.2%) eyes implanted with a HydroView IOL that developed a layer of lens epithelial cells on the anterior surface of the IOL optic between 8 and 98 weeks after surgery. The presence of the lens epithelial cell membrane produced visual symptoms varying from low vision to hazy vision or light scatter. Removal of the membrane by Nd:YAG laser treatment or surgical membranectomy alleviated the visual symptoms.

Schauersberger et al.[67] found significantly higher levels of anterior ongrowth of lens epithelial cells on the round-edge HydroView hydrophilic acrylic IOL than the square-edge AcrySof or round-edge Sensar hydrophobic acrylic IOLs from 30 days to 1 year after surgery ($P = 0.015$). They concluded that, unlike in PCO, IOL material plays a greater role than edge design in anterior lens epithelial cell ongrowth.

INFLAMMATORY REACTION

The trauma of cataract surgery and IOL implantation can trigger a breakdown in the blood–aqueous barrier, with an outpouring of proteins and macrophages to repair tissue and isolate the foreign body from the ocular tissues. The foreign-body reaction depends on the IOL material and the pre-existing status of the ocular tissues, such as diabetic retinopathy. The inflammatory response is measured subjectively by slit-lamp grading of cells and flare, or objectively by a laser flare photometer.

Hollick, Spalton, and Ursell[62] measured the effect of PMMA, silicone (SI30NB), and hydrogel (HydroView) IOL implantation on the blood–aqueous barrier by laser flare and cell meter (Kowa, Osaka, Japan). At 1 month after surgery, small cells were present on 4 of 30 hydrogel, 11 of 30 PMMA, and 15 of 30 silicone

IOLs ($P = 0.01$). The hydrogel lenses showed a significantly shorter duration and lower grades of small cells than the silicone or PMMA IOLs ($P < 0.001$ for both). At the same visit, epithelioid cells were most pronounced on the PMMA (11 of 30), present in only 1 of 30 silicone IOLs, and not present on the hydrogel IOLs ($P < 0.001$). Lens epithelial cells, on the other hand, were present at 1 month on 20 of 30 hydrogel IOLs, 12 of 30 PMMA IOLs, and 0 of 30 silicone IOLs. Lens epithelial cells reached a peak between 1 week and 1 month after surgery and then regressed. The hydrogel IOLs had significantly greater numbers that did not regress, and in half the patients the lens epithelial cells formed a confluent sheet along the entire 360° of the capsulorrhexis rim, probably because of migration from the capsulorrhexis.

In a study by Samuelson, Chu, and Kreiger[68] the levels of postoperative inflammatory giant-cell deposits were measured in patients 6 months after combined cataract and glaucoma surgery. The level of inflammatory giant-cell deposits was slightly higher in patients with an acrylic IOL (AcrySof) than in patients with a silicone IOL (PhacoFlex II); however, the difference was not statistically or clinically significant.

References

[1] Steinert RF, Brint SF, White SM, et al. Astigmatism after small incision cataract surgery: a prospective, randomized, multicenter comparison of 4- and 6.5-mm incisions. Ophthalmology 1991;98:417–423, discussion 423–424.
[2] Hayashi K, Hayashi H, Nakao F, et al. The correlation between incision size and corneal shape changes in sutureless cataract surgery. Ophthalmology 1995;102:550–556 (see comments).
[3] Brint S, Ostrick D, Bryan J. Keratometric cylinder and visual performance following phacoemulsification and implantation with silicone small-incision or poly(methyl methacrylate) intraocular lenses. J Cataract Refract Surg 1991;17:32–36.
[4] Pfleger T, Skorpik C, Menapace R, et al. Long-term course of induced astigmatism after clear corneal incision cataract surgery. J Cataract Refract Surg 1996;22:72–77.
[5] Olson R, Crandall A. Prospective randomized comparison of phacoemulsification cataract surgery with a 3.2-mm vs a 5.5-mm sutureless incision. Am J Ophthalmol 1998;125:612–620.
[6] Oshika T, Nagahara K, Yaguchi S, et al. Three year prospective, randomized evaluation of intraocular lens implantation through 3.2 and 5.5 mm incisions. J Cataract Refract Surg 1998;24:509–514.
[7] Müller-Jensen K, Barlinn B. Corneal refractive changes after AcrySof lens versus PMMA lens implantation. Ophthalmologica 2000;214:320–323.
[8] Hayashi K, Hayashi H, Oshika T, et al. Fourier analysis of irregular astigmatism after implantation of 3 types of intraocular lenses. J Cataract Refract Surg 2000;26:1510–1516.
[9] Shimizu K. Clear-cornea cataract incision: astigmatic consequences. In: Masket S, Crandall AS, editors. Atlas of cataract surgery. London: Martin Dunitz Ltd; 1999. p. 129–139.
[10] Steinert R, Deacon J. Enlargement of incision during phacoemulsification and folded intraocular lens implant surgery. Ophthalmology 1996;103:220–225.
[11] Hagan Jr. Initial experience with the MONARCH IOL delivery system for insertion of the 5.5 mm: ACRYSOF intraocular lens. Mo Med 1999;6:555, 561–562.
[12] Olson R, Cameron R, Hovis T, et al. Clinical evaluation of the Unfolder. J Cataract Refract Surg 1997;23:1384–1389.
[13] Scales J. Discussion on metals and synthetic materials in relation to tissues: tissue reactions to synthetic materials. Proc R Soc Med 1953;46:647–652.
[14] Anderson C, Koch DD, Green G, et al. Alcon AcrySof Acrylic Intraocular Lens. In: Martin RG, Gills JP, Sanders DR, editors. Foldable intraocular lenses. Thorofare, NJ: Slack, Inc; 1993. p. 161–177.
[15] Fernando GT, Crayford BB. Visually significant calcification of hydrogel intraocular lenses necessitating explantation. Clin Experiment Ophthalmol 2000;28:280–286.
[16] Werner L, Apple D, Escobar-Gomez M, et al. Postoperative deposition of calcium on the surfaces of a hydrogel intraocular lens. Ophthalmology 2000;107:2179–2185.
[17] Jiráskova N, Rozsíval P, Lilaková D, et al. Evaluation of 150 MemoryLens implantations. InterNet J Ophthalmol 2000;5:7–11, www.unich.it/injo/200.htm.
[18] Brown D, Grabow H, Martin R, et al. Staar Collamer intraocular lens: clinical results from the phase I FDA core study. J Cataract Refract Surg 1998;24:1032–1038.
[19] Izak AM, Werner L, Pandey SK, Apple DJ. Calcification of modern foldable hydrogel intraocular lens designs. Eye 2003;17:393–406.
[20] Tehrani M, Mamalis N, Wallin T, Dick HB, Stoffelns BM, Olson R, et al. Late postoperative opacification of MemoryLens hydrophilic acrylic intraocular lenses: case series and review. J Cataract Refract Surg 2004;30:115–122. (erratum J Cataract Refract Surg 30:1391, 2004).
[21] Mamalis N, Davis B, Nilson CD, Hickman MS, Leboyer RM. Complications of foldable intraocular lenses requiring explantation or secondary intervention – 2003 survey update. J Cataract Refract Surg 2004;30:2209–2218.
[22] Buchen SY, Cunanan CM, Gwon A, Weinschenk 3rd JI, Gruber L, Knight PM. Assessing intraocular lens calcification in an animal model. J Cataract Refract Surg 2001;27:1473–1484.
[23] Francese JE, Pham L, Christ FR. Accelerated hydrolytic and ultraviolet aging studies on SI-18NB and SI-20NB silicone lenses. J Cataract Refract Surg 1992;18:402–405.
[24] Christ FR, Fencil DA, Van Gent S, et al. Evaluation of the chemical, optical, and mechanical properties of elastomeric intraocular lens materials and their clinical significance. J Cataract Refract Surg 1989;15:176–184.
[25] Khawly J, Lambert R, Jaffe G. Intraocular lens changes after short- and long-term exposure to intraocular silicone oil: an in vivo study. Ophthalmology 1998;105:1227–1233.

[26] Apple D, Federman J, Krolicki T, et al. Irreversible silicone oil adhesion to silicone intraocular lenses: a clinicopathologic analysis. Ophthalmology 1996;103:1555–1561, discussion 1561–1562.

[27] Apple DJ, Isaacs RT, Kent DG, et al. Silicone oil adhesion to intraocular lenses: an experimental study comparing various biomaterials. J Cataract Refract Surg 1997;23:536–544.

[28] McLoone E, Mahon G, Archer D, et al. Silicone oil-intraocular lens interaction: which lens to use? Br J Ophthalmol 2001;85:543–545.

[29] Dhaliwal DK, Mamalis N, Olson RJ, et al. Visual significance of glistenings seen in the AcrySof intraocular lens. J Cataract Refract Surg 1996;22:452–457.

[30] Christiansen G, Durcan FJ, Olson RJ, et al. Glistenings in the AcrySof intraocular lens: pilot study. J Cataract Refract Surg 2001;27:728–733.

[31] Dogru M, Tetsumoto K, Tagami Y. Optical and atomic force microscopy of an explanted AcrySof intraocular lens with glistenings. J Cataract Refract Surg 2000;26:571–575.

[32] Mitooka K, Shiba T, Tsuneoka H, et al. A case of intraocular lens eye with decrease in visual function by glistening. Ganka 1998;40:1501–1504.

[33] Mitooka K, Tsuneoka H. Glistening. Practical Ophthalmol 1999;52:66–67.

[34] Shiba T, Mitooka K, Tsuneoka H. [Study of causal mechanism of glistening occurring in AcrySof intraocular lens]. IOL & RS 2000;14.

[35] Dick HB, Olson RJ, Augustin AJ, et al. Vacuoles in the Acrysof intraocular lens as factor of the presence of serum in aqueous humor. Ophthalmic Res 2001;33:61–67.

[36] Nishi O, Nishi K, Sakanishi K. Inhibition of migrating lens epithelial cells at the capsular bend created by the rectangular optic edge of a posterior chamber intraocular lens. Ophthalmic Surg Lasers 1998;9:587–594.

[37] Nishi O, Nishi K, Wickstrom K. Preventing lens epithelial cell migration using intraocular lenses with sharp rectangular edges. J Cataract Refract Surg 2000;26:1543–1549.

[38] Davison JA. Positive and negative dysphotopsia in patients with acrylic intraocular lenses. J Cataract Refract Surg 2000;26:1346–1355.

[39] Farbowitz MA, Zabriskie NA, Crandall AS, et al. Visual complaints associated with the AcrySof acrylic intraocular lens (1). J Cataract Refract Surg 2000;26:1339–1345.

[40] Mamalis N. Complications of foldable intraocular lenses requiring explanation or secondary intervention: 1998 survey. J Cataract Refract Surg 2000;26:766–772.

[41] Masket S. Truncated edge design, dysphotopsia, and inhibition of posterior capsule opacification. J Cataract Refract Surg 2000;26:145–147.

[42] Holladay J, Lang A, Portney V. Analysis of edge glare phenomena in intraocular lens edge designs. J Cataract Refract Surg 1999;25:748–752.

[43] Erie JC, Bandhauer MH, McLaren JW. Analysis of postoperative glare and intraocular lens design. J Cataract Refract Surg 2001;27:614–621.

[44] Bournas P, Drazinos S, Kanellas D, Arvanitis M, Vaikoussis E. Dysphotopsia after cataract surgery: comparison of four different intraocular lenses. Ophthalmologica 2007;221:378–383.

[45] Shambhu S, Shanmuganathan VA, Charles SJ. The effect of lens design on dysphotopsia in different acrylic IOLs. Eye 2005;19:567–570.

[46] Trattler WB, Whitsett JC, Simone PA. Negative dysphotopsia after intraocular lens implantation irrespective of design and material. J Cataract Refract Surg 2005;31:841–845.

[47] Uchio E, Ohno S, Kusakawa T. Spherical aberration and glare disability with intraocular lenses of different optical design. J Cataract Refract Surg 1995;21:690–696.

[48] Holladay JT, Piers PA, Koranyi G, van der Mooren M, Norrby NE. A new intraocular lens design to reduce spheriacal aberration of pseudophakic eyes. J Refract Surg 2002;18:683–691.

[49] Mester U, Dillinger P, Anterist N. Impact of a modified optic design on visual function: clinical comparatiuve study. J Cataract Refract Surg 2003;29:652–660.

[50] McClellan JS, Marcos S, Burns SA. Age-related changes in monochromatic wave aberrations of the human eye. Invest Ophthalmol Vis Sci 2001;42:1390–1395.

[51] Bellucci R, Scialdone A, Buratto L, Moreselli S, Chierego C, Criscuoli A, et al. Visual acuity and contrast sensitivity comparison between Tecnis and AcrySof SA60AT intraocular lenses: a multicenter randomized study. J Cataract Refract Surg 2005;31:712–717.

[52] Packer M, Fine IH, Hoffmann RS, Piers PA. Prospective randomized trial of an anterior surface modified prolate intraocular lens. J Refract Surg 2002;18:692–696.

[53] Marcos S, Barbero S, Jimenez-Alfaro I. Optical quality and depth-of-field of eyes implanted with spherical and aspheric intraocular lenses. J Refract Surg 2005;21:223–35.

[54] Kershner RM. Retinal image contrast and functional visual performance with aspheric, silicone, and acrylic intraocular lenses. Prospective evaluation. J Cataract Refract Surg 2003;29:1684–1694.

[55] Bellucci R, Morselli S, Piers P. Comparison of wavefront aberrations and optical quality of eyes implanted with five different intraocular lenses. J Refract Surg 2004;20:297–306.

[56] Casprini F, Balestrazzi A, Tosi GM, Miracco F, Martone G, Cevenini G, et al. Glare disability and spherical aberration with five foldable intraocular lenses: a prospective randomized study. Acta Ophthalmol Scand 2005;83:20–25.

[57] Wang L, Koch DD. Effect of decentration of wavefront-corrected intraocular lenses on the higher-order aberrations of the eye. Arch Ophthalmol 2005;123:1226–1230.

[58] Altmann GE, Nichamin LD, Lane SS, Pepose JS. Optical performance of 3 intraocular lenses designs in the presence of decentration. J Cataract Refract Surg 2005;31:574–585.

[59] Franchini A. Compromise between spherical and chromatic aberration and depth of focus in aspheric intraocular lenses. J Cataract Refract Surg 2007;33:497–509.

[60] Amon M. Biocompatibility of intraocular lenses. J Cataract Refract Surg 2001;27:178–179.

[61] International dictionary of medicine and biology. New York: Churchill Livingstone; 1986.

[62] Hollick E, Spalton D, Ursell P. Surface cytologic features on intraocular lenses: can increased biocompatibility have disadvantages? Arch Ophthalmol 1999;117:872–878.

[63] Müllner-Eidenböck A, Schauersberger J, Kruger A, et al. Cellular reactions on anterior surfaces of four different types of foldable lenses. Spektrum der Augenheilkunde 1998;12:218–223.

[64] Lenis K, Philipson B. Lens epithelial growth on the anterior surface of hydrogel IOLs: an in vivo study. Acta Ophthalmol Scand 1998;76:184–187.

[65] House P, Barry C, Morgan W, et al. Postoperative deposits on the AcrySof intraocular lens. Aust N Z J Ophthalmol 1999;27:301–305.

[66] Koch MU, Kalicharan D, van der Want JJ. Lens epithelial cell layer formation related to hydrogel foldable intraocular lenses. J Cataract Refract Surg 1999;25:1637–1640.

[67] Schauersberger J, Amon M, Kruger A, et al. Lens epithelial cell outgrowth on 3 types of intraocular lenses. J Cataract Refract Surg 2001;27:850–854.

[68] Samuelson TW, Chu YR, Krieger RA. Evaluation of giant-cell deposits on foldable intraocular lenses after combined cataract and glaucoma surgery. J Cataract Refract Surg 2000;26:817–823.

[69] Fine I, Hoffman R, Packer M. Clear-lens extraction with multifocal lens implantation. Int Ophthalmol Clin 2001;41:113–121.

[70] Auffarth G, Dick H. Multifocal intraocular lenses: a review. Ophthalmologe 2001;98:127–137.

[71] Ge J, Arellano A, Salz J. Surgical correction of hyperopia: clear lens extraction and laser correction. Ophthalmol Clin North Am 2001;14:301–313.

[72] Steinert RF, Giamporcaro JE, Tasso VA. Clinical assessment of long-term safety and efficacy of a widely implanted silicone intraocular lens material. Am J Ophthalmol 1997;123:17–23.

[73] Menapace R. Evaluation of 35 consecutive SI-30 PhacoFlex lenses with high-refractive silicone optic implanted in the capsulorrhexis bag. J Cataract Refract Surg 1995;21:339–347.

[74] Colin J. Clinical results of implanting a silicone haptic-anchor-plate intraocular lens. J Cataract Refract Surg 1996;22:1286–1290.

[75] Oshika T, Suzuki Y, Kizaki H, et al. Two year clinical study of a soft acrylic intraocular lens. J Cataract Refract Surg 1996;22:104–109.

[76] Mengual E, Garcia J, Elvira JC, et al. Clinical results of AcrySof intraocular lens implantation. J Cataract Refract Surg 1998;24:114–117.

[77] Afsar AJ, Patel S, Woods RL, et al. A comparison of visual performance between a rigid PMMA and a foldable acrylic intraocular lens. Eye 1999;13:329–335.

[78] Kobayashi H, Ikeda H, Imamura S, et al. Clinical assessment of long-term safety and efficacy of a widely implanted polyacrylic intraocular lens material. Am J Ophthalmol 2000;130:310–321.

[79] Oner FH, Gunenc U, Ferliel ST. Posterior capsule opacification after phacoemulsification: foldable acrylic versus poly(methyl methacrylate) intraocular lenses. J Cataract Refract Surg 2000;26:722–726.

[80] Hollick E, Spalton D, Ursell P, et al. The effect of polymethylmethacrylate, silicone, and polyacrylic intraocular lenses on posterior capsular opacification 3 years after cataract surgery. Ophthalmology 1999;106:49–54, discussion 54–55.

[81] Brown D, Ziemba S. Collamer intraocular lens: clinical results from the US FDA core study. J Cataract Refract Surg 2001;27:833–840.

Presbyopia Correcting Intraocular Lenses

Roger F. Steinert, MD, Richard L. Lindstrom, MD
and David F. Chang, MD

38

CONTENTS

CHAPTER HIGHLIGHTS

>> The 10 principles of presbyopia intraocular lens (IOL) practice

>> Monovision, multifocal IOLs, and accommodating IOLs compared

>> Optical principles of multifocality

>> Neuroadaptation

>> Biomechanical concepts of accommodationg IOL designs

>> Managing the disappointing postop outcome

>> Key points and rules for successful presbyopia IOL practice

The normal eye is constructed to allow the various refracting surfaces and ocular media to focus parallel rays of light coming from a distant object onto the retina. The eye can also adjust its refractive power through the accommodative process to bring near objects into focus. The cortex of the young lens is a soft, easily molded material contained in an elastic capsule. The traction of the zonular fibers opposes the natural tendency of the lens to assume a spherical shape. Contraction of the ciliary muscles relaxes the zonular attachment sites inward toward the lens equator, reducing the tension on the zonules and allowing the lens to move anteriorly and the highly elastic capsule to increase the convexity of the lens.[1] The resultant steepening of the anterior and posterior poles and anterior movement of the lens change the focal plane, resulting in accommodation.

For the cataract patient, intraocular lens (IOL) implantation surgery has overcome the loss of visual function associated with the removal of cataracts. However, because most IOLs are monofocal, the loss of accommodation becomes significant with surgery. Although the loss of accommodation is not absolute because increased depth of field secondary to small pupillary diameter[2,3] or mild astigmatism[4-7] provides a degree of apparent accommodation (pseudoaccommodation), the need to correct the resultant loss of accommodation (presbyopia) is clinically apparent.

The most common treatment methods for presbyopia are reading glasses or, in cases of ametropia, bifocal spectacles. The difficulties in adapting to bifocal lenses can be considerable. As the add power is increased in strength, trifocal or multifocal reading segments may be required to enable a greater range of focus.

Three strategies expand the range of functional vision without spectacle aid:

1. Monovision
2. Multifocal IOLs
3. Accommodating IOLs.

MONOVISION

In typical monovision, monofocal IOLs are implanted such that one eye is focused for good uncorrected distance vision, while the other eye of the patient is focused at either intermediate or near distance, depending on the visual requirements and preferences of the patient. The mechanism of monovision is known as *interocular blur suppression*. The image processing system of the visual cortex suppresses the blurred image from one eye so that it does not interfere with the image from the in-focus eye. Successful monovision contact lens wearers have two orders of magnitude greater interocular blur suppression capacity than unsuccessful monovision contact lens wearers.[8] Suppression is less effective in dim illumination.

Monovision results in three inherent visual compromises:

1. Reduced binocular visual acuity
2. Reduced stereopsis
3. Reduced contrast sensitivity.

The impact on binocular visual acuity is modest, averaging 0.04 to 0.08 logMAR units reduction. That impact is increased when the dominant eye has residual oblique astigmatism.[8] The mean decrease in stereopsis is 37 arc sec with monovision contact lenses, but unsuccessful contact lens wearers averaged 50–62 arc sec greater reduction in stereoacuity than successful monovision patients.[9] Monovision reduces contrast sensitivity, especially at higher spatial frequencies (>4 cycles/°).[10] The improvement in a patient's contrast sensitivity under binocular viewing conditions (both eyes corrected for distance) is known as *binocular summation*. This diminishes to monocular levels at about 1.5 diopters (D) of monovision, then further declines (known as *binocular inhibition*) until a low point at about 2.5 D of monovision. With further defocus, the contrast sensitivity returns to the monocular levels.[11]

In refractive surgery, monovision can be simulated preoperatively with a trial frame or a contact lens trial. In a patient with significant visual impairment due to cataract, however, the patient cannot possibly appreciate the visual tolerance of monovision in a preoperative simulation. In refractive surgery, approximately two-thirds of patients have the ability to tolerate at least a modest amount of monovision, while the remainder dislikes experiencing any difference between their two eyes.[9,12,13] Some surgeons will only utilize a monovision strategy in patients who had monovision in contact lenses or with refractive surgery prior to the onset of cataract. Other surgeons have a strategy of creating monovision in most or all of their patients.[14] As is the case with refractive surgery, tolerance of monovision drops considerably when the near-focus eye exceeds −1.5 D. Therefore, these patients must understand that they will gain intermediate vision but not necessarily be able to read fine print without spectacle assistance. Also, as in refractive surgery, a high degree of accuracy is required in the correction of the distance eye, because a patient's ability to function without spectacles will be highly dependent on a single eye.[13]

MULTIFOCAL INTRAOCULAR LENSES

Bifocal and multifocal spectacles and some contact lenses are designed for alternating vision. The individual's gaze is directed through the portion of the lens containing the appropriate dioptric power for the target plane of focus. Usually the majority of the lens provides distance vision, and an inset dioptric add at the bottom of the lens is used for near vision. Such a design is not feasible for a multifocal IOL. An individual cannot "look through" different areas of an IOL.

Multifocal IOLs use the principle of simultaneous vision. Different areas of the IOL are designed with different focal planes, usually for near and distance vision. At any given time, one image is in focus at the retina, and the second image is highly defocused with very little structure. Distant objects are focused by the distance power of the lens and defocused by the near power. For near objects, the reverse is true; near objects are focused by the near power of the lens and defocused by the distance power.

MULTIFOCAL OPTICS

Multifocal IOLs produce simultaneous images using either diffractive or refractive optics. Although the term multifocal is widely used for these IOLs, most designs are actually bifocal.

All diffractive IOLs are inherently bifocal. These IOLs typically consist of an anterior refractive surface with multiple, concentric, microslope rings on the posterior surface (Figure 38-1A). The microslope rings diffract the incoming light, creating a diffraction pattern (Figure 38-1B). Distance and near foci are formed by the combination of the anterior refractive surface with the zero and first orders of diffraction, respectively, created by the posterior surface. In the Alcon ReSTOR design (Figure 38-2), the ratio of distance to near increases as the pupil size increases, due to a modification of the diffractive rings known as *apodization*.[15] Apodization is intended to reduce the problem of halo and glare at night. However, the ability to read in dim light, such as a menu in a restaurant, is also reduced. An alternative diffractive design is the Abbott Medical Optics (AMO) Tecnis multifocal, which has uniform distribution of distance and near focus at all pupil sizes (Figure 38-3). Both the Tecnis and the ReSTOR offer an aspheric refractive optic in an effort to reduce net spherical aberration and thereby reduce that contributing factor to halo and glare. Numerous multifocal IOLs are available internationally but not sold in the US due to FDA restrictions.[16]

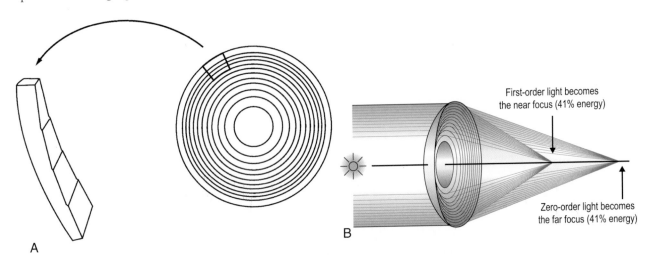

First-order light becomes the near focus (41% energy)

Zero-order light becomes the far focus (41% energy)

A

B

Figure 38-1 **A,** The optical principle of a diffractive intraocular lens, with refractive optics on the anterior surface curvature and diffraction optics on the posterior side of the optic. **B,** Two focal lengths are created by the zero order and first order diffractions.

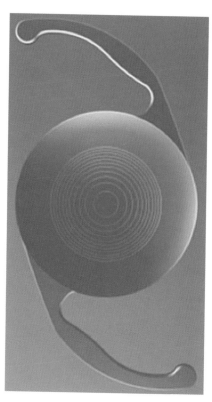

Figure 38-2 Alcon ReSTOR Model SA60D3 (courtesy Alcon Labs).

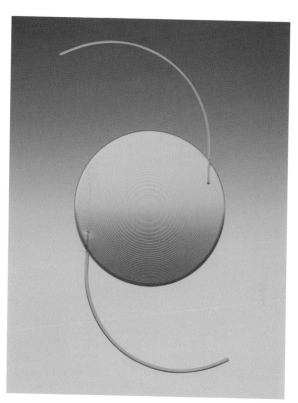

Figure 38-3 AMO Tecnis ZMAOO (courtesy Abbott Medical Optics).

Refractive multifocal IOLs, in contrast, achieve more than one plane of focus by alternating zonular rings of different refracting power.

True multifocality has been attempted with the designs of the AMO Array (Figure 38-4) and ReZoom (Figure 38-5) and the now discontinued Domilens Progress IOLs. The Array and ReZoom are distance-dominant, simultaneous-vision, zonal-progressive lenses. They combine a posterior refractive surface with multiple anterior aspheric refractive zones of continuously varying power. Beginning with the central zone, distance power is placed centrally in each odd ring (1, 3, and 5). The power increases toward the periphery of the odd-numbered rings to form a smooth transition with the even zones (2 and 4) that emphasize near vision with a 3.5 D add in the Array and a weaker, intermediate distance dominated near component in the ReZoom (3.2 D at the IOL plane and 2.6D at the spectacle plane).

The amount of light transmitted to the retina for image formation also differs among IOL designs. With diffractive IOLs, approximately 41% of the transmitted light is allocated to the distance focus and 41% to the near focus. (These ratios vary with aperture size in the apodization modification employed by the Alcon ReSTOR.) The remaining 18% of the transmitted light is lost to higher orders of diffraction that are not focused at the retina.[15,17] In contrast, refractive IOLs transmit all of the available light to the retina. For bifocal refractive IOLs, the transmitted light is divided between near and distance foci. Multifocal IOLs focus the transmitted light for intermediate vision in

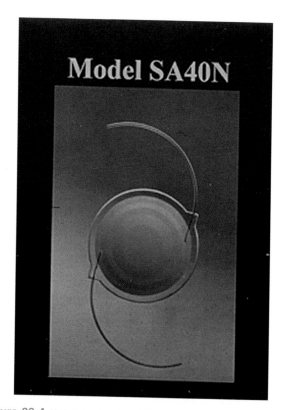

Figure 38-4 AMO Array (courtesy Abbott Medical Optics).

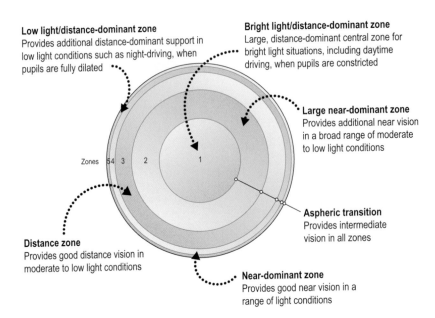

Low light/distance-dominant zone
Provides additional distance-dominant support in low light conditions such as night-driving, when pupils are fully dilated

Bright light/distance-dominant zone
Large, distance-dominant central zone for bright light situations, including daytime driving, when pupils are constricted

Large near-dominant zone
Provides additional near vision in a broad range of moderate to low light conditions

Aspheric transition
Provides intermediate vision in all zones

Distance zone
Provides good distance vision in moderate to low light conditions

Near-dominant zone
Provides good near vision in a range of light conditions

Zones 5 4 3 2 1

Figure 38-5 AMO ReZoom (courtesy Abbott Medical Optics).

addition to near and distance vision. For example, the Array MIOL allocates 50% of transmitted light to distance focus, 37% to near focus, and 13% to intermediate focus (based on a 4 mm pupil). The decrease in the percentage of light transmitted through diffractive bifocal IOLs compared with the Array MIOL may result in decreased contrast acuity for patients' distance and intermediate vision.[18]

OPTICAL ISSUES: CONTRAST SENSITIVITY, HALOS, AND GLARE

Multifocal IOLs distribute the light energy into different focal planes. It is inevitable, therefore, that there will be loss of contrast sensitivity on clinical testing. Atebara and Miller demonstrated the physical basis for the patient's ability to decode the multifocal image presented to the retina as well as the unavoidable loss of contrast sensitivity due to the superimposition of the in focus and out of focus images on the retina (Figures 38-6A and B).[19]

Because vision consists of continuous decoding and image processing by the visual cortex, rather than a pixel-by-pixel translation of the retinal image, patients with normal macular function typically tolerate the multifocal image better than would be expected by the basic physical optics of this lens design. In addition, many observations have concluded that patients experience improvement in the quality of vision over time. This is termed *neuroadaptation*.[20-22] A well-known piece of evidence for this phenomenon is shown in Figure 38-7. A patient of Michael Woodcock, MD, who was an artist received the Array multifocal IOL and painted the same scene immediately after surgery (see Figure 38-7A) and then again at 3 months (see Figure 38-7B). A marked improvement in the amount of glare and halo is evident, even though her eye did not physically change during that interval. Training regimens may be of benefit in encouraging neuroadaptation.[23]

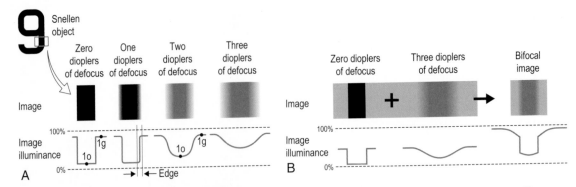

Figure 38-6 **A,** The optical physics of defocusing. The edges become blurred and the black center becomes gray. The illuminance curves under each image quantify these changes. **B,** A bifocal retinal image combines an in-focus and out-of-focus image. The illuminance curve is the sum of the two curves of the two images. Because the edge still has some sharp change from light to dark, the patient can accurately perceive the image and decode the letter being seen. The blunting of the edge of the image and the reduction in the total blackness (elevation of the bottom of the curve) both contribute to loss of contrast sensitivity. (Courtesy of David Miller, MD.)

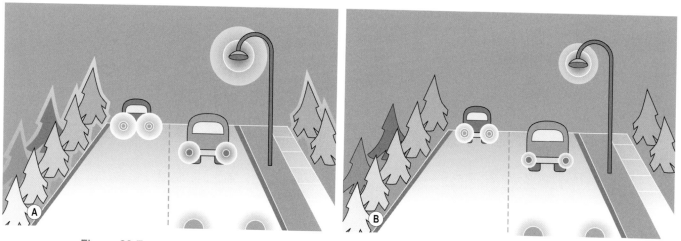

Figure 38-7 A, A patient's perception of night glare immediately after receiving an Array multifocal intraocular lens. B, The patient's perception 3 months later. Note marked reduction in glare around lights and the haze around objects such as trees (courtesy Abbott Medical Optics).

Patients with bifocal/multifocal IOLs gain the ability to see at near but lose some contrast sensitivity. In most studies, the amount of contrast sensitivity loss was within tolerable limits for visual function. For example, using the contrast acuity charts of 96, 50, 25, and 11% thresholds, early studies ($n = 291$ patients total) consistently reported no significant difference in contrast sensitivity at high thresholds (96 and 50%) between the Array MIOL and monofocal IOLs.[26–29] These same studies found that at 11% contrast, contrast sensitivity was significantly lower (approximately 1 line) with the Array MIOL than with a monofocal IOL. However, when comparing binocular vision, contrast sensitivity at 11% did not differ significantly between the Array MIOL and the monofocal IOL.[26–29] The findings at 25% were mixed; some studies found a significant decrease in contrast sensitivity with the Array MIOL ($n = 193$ total patients),[27,28] whereas other studies did not ($n = 98$ total patients).[26,29] The reduction in low-contrast acuity had little effect on everyday visual tasks.[27] Bilateral implantation of the Array MIOL alleviated some of the reduced contrast sensitivity at low contrast levels.[26]

Modification of a monofocal IOL with the creation of an aspheric contour (negative spherical aberration) that compensates for the positive spherical aberration of the cornea has been reported to improve contrast sensitivity compared to a non-aspheric but otherwise equivalent monofocal IOL design for both the AMO Tecnis and Alcon AcrySof IOLs.[30–33] Whether an aspheric multifocal optic will result in the same improvement in contrast sensitivity has not yet been proven but similar improvement with asphericity seems likely.

Driving simulation studies can help define any potential for functional visual performance loss associated with a reduction in low-contrast acuity. At night, car headlights can decrease contrast sensitivity and increase glare. A prospective, masked, parallel-group comparison of 33 bilateral Array MIOL patients and 33 bilateral monofocal IOL patients assessed driving performance during night, night with glare, and fog conditions.[34] There was no significant difference between the groups for 26 of the 30 driving performance measurements. The four measures that were different were in favor of the monofocal subjects. These were the percentage of correctly recognized warning signs at night in clear

weather, sign recognition distances for guide and warning signs in fog, and detection distance for one of four hazards (suitcase). The multifocal patients performed, on average, within safety guidelines (American Association of State Highway and Transportation Officials).[34] Schmitz et al.[35] compared the effect of glare from halogen lights (which are similar to oncoming automobile headlights) on contrast sensitivity in patients with an Array MIOL or a monofocal IOL. There were no significant differences in contrast sensitivity between the two groups in the presence of moderate or strong glare. A significant difference between the two groups was found only at the lowest spatial frequency (3 cpd) without halogen glare. Together, these studies suggest that driving vision with an Array MIOL is similar to that with a monofocal IOL. Nevertheless, patients with multifocal IOLs should exercise caution when driving at night or under poor visibility conditions. While US FDA approval of multifocal IOLs requires some type of driving simulation testing in order to gain approval, only the Array has published results in a peer-review journal.

Photic phenomena such as glare and halos occasionally occur in patients with refractive multifocal,[24,25,36–39] diffractive multifocal,[40,41] and monofocal IOL implants.[36,37,42] As is the case with the inevitable loss of contrast sensitivity with multifocal optics, glare and halo are inevitable with multifocal IOLs due to the fundamental optical physics of this design. As shown in Figure 38-8, when a patient looks at a distant object, the portion of light energy that passes through the reading element in the IOL will come into focus anterior to the retina, and then diverge as a blur circle at the retinal plane. Under diffusely even illumination conditions, the lower light energy of the diffused out of focus image will not be perceived by most patients. The lower energy out of focus blur is masked by the higher light energy of the surrounding peripheral image. At night, those conditions are often different. When a patient looks at a headlight, for example, the headlight has high energy compared to the surrounding periphery, which is dark. The out-of-focus blur circle is, therefore, visible, and the patient perceives this as a halo. Efforts to reduce halos and glare include aspheric optics, aspheric blending and choice of refractive zone size, location, and power in refractive

- When looking at distance, the light rays passing through the near portion of the IOL optics are focused in front of the retina. These light rays then diverge and become a faint blur around the focused image at the retina.

- Under dim illumination, patient sees the out of focus image as a halo.

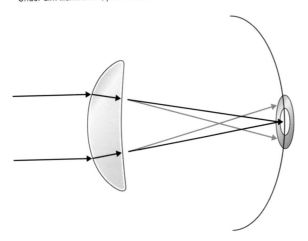

Figure 38-8 Halo occurs due to the distant source light rays passing through the near-focus portion of the optic, coming to focus in front of the retina and then diverging outward as a ring as the light reaches the retina.

multifocal IOLs, and the apodization and ring placements in diffractive multifocal IOLs.

With the original Array SA40N multifocal IOL, for example, one study reported moderate halos and glare in up to 46.2% and severe halos and glare in 14% of eyes.[43] In a multicenter study of the Alcon AcrySof ReSTOR SA30D3 diffractive IOL, severe halos were reported by 4.2% and glare by 8.5% of patients.[40] Measurement of straylight before and after cataract surgery found that straylight declined after cataract surgery more so with a monofocal IOL (Acrysof SA 60AT) than with a diffractive multifocal IOL (AcrySof ReSTOR SA60D3).[44]

Even though some patients experienced halos or glare with the Array multifocal IOL, they would choose to have the Array MIOL implanted again.[24,25,27] Further, overall quality of life and satisfaction were higher in multifocal patients than monofocal patients.[24,25] Similarly, the second generation refractive and diffractive multifocal IOLs result in high levels of patient satisfaction, with excellent uncorrected distance vision. Because of the design of the add power, the Alcon ReSTOR typically gives higher levels of vision at near (effective add is 3.2 D at the spectacle plane), whereas the AMO ReZoom is equal or stronger at intermediate distances (effective add is 2.6 D at the spectacle plane).[45]

■ ACCOMMODATING INTRAOCULAR LENSES ■

Accommodating IOLs have the potential to provide superior image quality compared to multifocal lenses, because competing retinal images are avoided. A lens that moves axially can also be expected to provide a full and continuous range of accommodative shifts. Distance, intermediate, and near focus should all theoretically be attainable with no loss of contrast sensitivity or unwanted nighttime images. The design objective of an accommodating IOL is to use the patient's own natural accommodation mechanism to modify the power of the IOL, in a manner that increases the effective power of the lens due to the action of the ciliary muscle.

The pioneering initial design to meet to this challenge was the CrystaLens AT-45 (eyeonics, Aliso Viejo, CA, now a division of Bausch & Lomb, Rochester NY). The original commercial design of the AT-45 (Figure 38-9A) has been replaced with the AT-50 (Figure 38-9B), featuring a larger optic (5 mm instead of 4.5 mm) and a square configuration to the haptics. These IOLs have two hinges positioned at the edges of the plate portion of the haptic.[46] The hinges are designed to allow the lens to flex anteriorly and posteriorly with contraction of the ciliary muscles. The design goal was to provide up to 2.5 D of accommodation because the anterior movement of the optic would increase its effective power. Clinical experience with these lenses was markedly less powerful, however, and the US FDA labelling for the Crystalens states that 1.0 D of accommodation is provided. A third generation of the Crystalens with an optic modification to provide more depth of focus – the "HD" – was introduced in 2008.

The concept of gaining accommodative benefit by anterior motion of the IOL optic is also the basis of the design of other lenses, including the HumanOptics and the Lenstec TetraFlex models.

Some monofocal IOLs have also been demonstrated to have anterior motion due to accommodative effort.[47]

The Synchrony IOL (Visiogen, Inc., Irvine, California) was the first dual-optic accommodating IOL to be implanted into human eyes. This is a single-piece foldable lens made of advanced generation silicone material. The lens is implanted through a 3.8 mm incision with a pre-loaded disposable injector. The IOL has a 5.5 mm diameter high-powered anterior optic (+32 D) coupled with a 6 mm diameter minus-power posterior optic (Figure 38-10). The amount of minus power is varied in order to correct each individual eye to emmetropia. The two optics are connected and separated by silicone struts that exert a specific amount of spring-like tension against the capsular bag, keeping it open at all times. The uncompressed lens complex is 3.8 mm long axially and 9.8 mm wide. When compressed, the total axial lens thickness decreases to 2.2 mm. The IOL is sized so as to fill the capsular bag, where it should be confined by a centered capsulorrhexis that is smaller in diameter than the anterior optic (Figure 38-11).

The Synchrony IOL is designed to utilize the natural mechanism of phakic accommodation according to the Helmholtz theory – namely zonular restraint and relaxation of the capsular bag shape. Specifically, the resting ciliary body maintains zonular tension, which is transmitted to the bag. This produces outward circumferential movement of the capsular equator, axial shortening of the capsular bag, and compression of the two Synchrony optics. This also generates strain energy that is stored in the connecting springs. With accommodative effort, the zonules relax, releasing their tension on the capsular bag. With relaxation of the bag, the spring-like struts move the anterior optic forward, thereby increasing the overall optical power of the IOL.

For an axially moving optic, the refractive shift achieved for each millimeter of movement is proportional to the dioptric power of the lens. According to ray tracing analysis, 1.5 mm of anterior movement of a +32 D IOL should theoretically produce

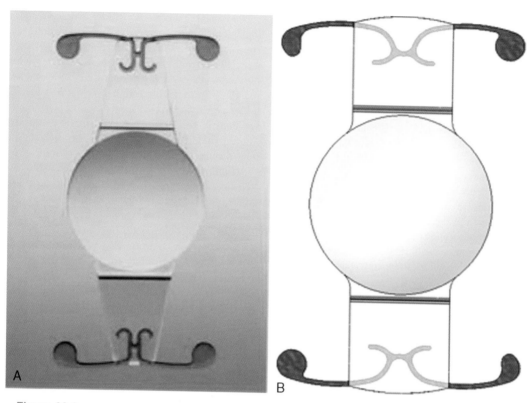

Figure 38-9 A, The CrystaLens AT-45. B, The Crystalens AT-50 (courtesy Eyeonics Division, Bausch & Lomb).

a refractive shift of approximately 3.3 D.[48] In contrast, the same movement of a +19 D lens would only induce a change of 1.2 D. The dual optic strategy seeks to provide every individual eye with a moving +32 D lens, by varying the minus power of the coupled posterior optic. This design maximally leverages the accommodative effect of any axial movement of the front lens.

In late 2007, enrollment for the Synchrony IOL FDA clinical trial was completed and more than 450 eyes were implanted. The lens is now awaiting FDA submission and approval. Because of its mechanism of action, this IOL design dictates certain mandatory surgical objectives. The surgeon must create an astigmatically neutral temporal incision. A preloaded, disposable

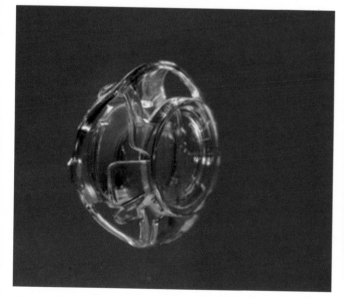

Figure 38-10 The Visiogen Synchrony dual optic accommodating intraocular lens (courtesy Visiogen).

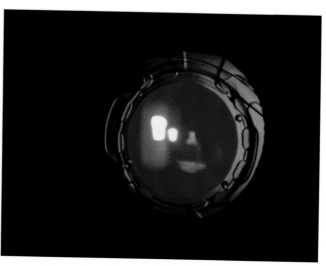

Figure 38-11 The Synchrony IOL implanted inside the capsular bag (courtesy David Chang, MD).

ACCOMMODATING INTRAOCULAR LENSES

injector system is used to implant the IOL through a 3.8 mm clear corneal or scleral pocket incision. The capsulorrhexis must be round, symmetric, intact, and approximately 4.5–5 mm in diameter. With too large an opening, the springs can push the anterior optic partially out of the bag. Thorough cortical clean up is critical in order to maintain capsular flexibility. Polishing or vacuuming the underside of the anterior lens capsule is recommended in order to reduce the tendency for anterior capsule opacification (ACO). Because of the size and design of the lens, removal of viscoelastic is best performed with bimanual irrigation–aspiration, which can access the space in between the two optics.

Some objective evidence of actual lens movement is necessary to prove true ciliary muscle mediated accommodation. The front and back surfaces of each of the paired Synchrony optics are well visualized with high-frequency ultrasound biomicroscopy (UBM). By using a near card to stimulate accommodation in the contralateral phakic eye, separation of the optics can be consistently imaged by UBM (Figure 38-12A and B).

As with all presbyopic lens technologies, proper patient selection, the ability to consistently attain emmetropia, and flawless surgery are important prerequisites for success. In addition, a lens system that requires a pliable and elastic capsular bag must further withstand the test of avoiding capsular fibrosis over time. Rabbit studies were performed by Werner and colleagues to study the rate of capsular fibrosis and capsule contraction with the dual optic bag-filling design of the Synchrony.[49] Bilateral eye implantations were performed with the Synchrony in one eye, and a silicone plate haptic IOL in the second eye as the control. There was no capsular fibrosis or opacification in the Synchrony eye, compared with extensive fibrosis, capsular contraction, and anterior and posterior capsule opacification in the control eye. A similar bilateral rabbit eye study was performed using two piggybacked hydrophobic acrylic IOLs as the control. Inter-pseudophakic opacification readily appeared in the piggyback IOL eyes, but not in the Synchrony eyes.

Many new concepts are under development in pursuit of a highly functioning and reliable accommodating IOL. The NuLens consists of two rigid PMMA plates and a flexible polymer. In principle, vitreous pressure on the back plate during accommodation forces increased anterior optic curvature of a soft optical material. A different approach to harnessing hydraulic fluid pressure is under development by PowerVision. Their "Fluid Vision IOL" has fluid in peripheral chambers that is designed to be pumped into the middle of a flexible fluid-filled optic during accommodation, thereby increasing its radius of curvature.

A different fluid concept is the basis of the "LiquiLens" from Vision Solution Technologies. Inside the optic are two fluids of different specific gravity and refractive index. When the eye rolls down to read something, the higher index of refraction fluid moves into the line of sight, increasing the optical power of the IOL.

The ultimate accommodating IOL would be a flexible polymer that could be injected into the capsular bag after removal of the crystalline lens. Many technical obstacles remain to be solved in order to implement such a lens, including removal of the natural lens leaving much of the capsule intact, prevention of capsular fibrosis and opacification from residual lens epithelial cells, and development of a non-toxic polymer that could be injected and then cured inside the eye while also assuming the correct shape and optical power.

■ OPTIMIZING RESULTS ■

Lens replacement with presbyopia-correcting IOLs is *refractive* surgery more than *cataract* surgery. This has implications for the surgeon's approach and management, and implications for a patient's expectations.

Selection of the "right" patient for a presbyopia IOL is more art than science, but following 10 basic rules will improve the likelihood of a satisfied patient.

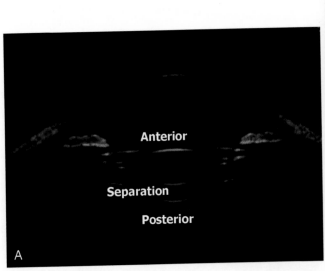

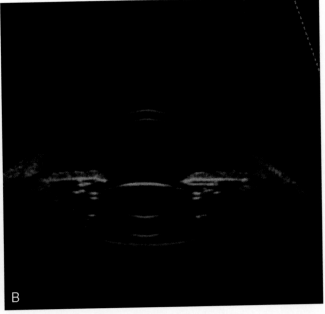

Figure 38-12 A, The position of the Synchrony optics while the fellow eye is focused at distance. **B,** The position of the Synchrony optics with the fellow eye focused at near. Note the greater distance between the posterior optic and the back side of the anterior optic.

THE 10 PRINCIPLES OF PRESBYOPIA INTRAOCULAR LENS PRACTICE

1. The patient must be motivated to increase the range of daily functions that can be performed without spectacle correction. A patient who does not mind using glasses, or perhaps even prefers his or her appearance with glasses, is not likely to appreciate the optical compromise of a multifocal IOL or the extra expense of a premium IOL. The other aspect of this analysis is an assessment of personality. While there is no specific or absolute personality guideline, a patient should have a positive and optimistic personality in order to avoid postoperative disappointment with perceived lack of a perfect outcome.

2. A patient receiving a multifocal IOL must understand and be willing to be patient with the process, recognizing that it may take several months to adapt to the new visual perception system.

3. The surgeon and staff must assess the vision function needs and goals of each patient, differentiating distance, intermediate, and near visual tasks, and the lighting conditions under which those tasks are performed. These answers should then be correlated with objective measures of the pupils under photopic, mesopic, and scotopic lighting levels. These measurements will guide the selection of a specific multifocal IOL design, and also reveal whether the optic size of an accommodating IOL is adequate to avoid edge glare.

4. Because the goal of presbyopia IOL implantation is a wide range of functional vision without glasses, accurate IOL power measurement and calculation is critical.

5. Postoperative astigmatism greater than 0.75 D begins to degrade the quality of uncorrected vision. The surgeon must plan the incision location and know the average astigmatic shift of that incision based on the preoperative corneal cylinder, and be comfortable with performing astigmatic keratotomy (see Chapter 24).

6. Because multifocal IOLs inherently involve optical compromise, they should be avoided in eyes with pre-existing optical impairments, such as maculopathy, amblyopia, glaucoma with central visual field loss, or in patients whose history suggests that those problems have a significant probability of developing.

7. The ocular surface is the dominant optical element in the eye. Careful preoperative assessment of aqueous tear deficiency and meibomian gland disease is important to pre-treat those conditions. If the quality of the surface cannot be improved, a presbyopia IOL may not be the best choice.

8. The surgeon must have a high level of skill so that complications are rare. A well-centered and correctly sized capsulorrhexis, thorough cortical removal, and intact capsular bag are essentials in obtaining a consistently good result with these IOLs. Because complications do occur for all surgeons, however, the patient should be aware that circumstances during surgery might lead to a change in the choice of implants.

9. Staged implantation means allowing enough time between the surgeries on the two eyes so that the visual function of the first eye can be accurately assessed. For many surgeons, that interval averages 2 weeks, but this may need to be longer if there is any uncertainty about the outcome of the first eye. By using the outcome of the first eye to guide the second, the surgeon can optimize the IOL power selection. Moreover, there is an opportunity to select a different IOL for the second eye if the patient feels the first IOL is deficient. This strategy is often called "custom matching" or "mix-and-match." [50]

10. Do not promise, nor allow the patient to think, that glasses will never be needed. Under the best of circumstances this may occur. However, many patients with presbyopia IOLs gain a much wider range of function with unaided vision, but still require spectacles for specific needs. In the business world, this is referred to as "Under-Promise and Over-Deliver." As a corollary, remember to celebrate success. The patient has no way of knowing what vision would have been like had a monofocal IOL been used. In an understated manner, make sure that a postoperative patient is shown the near vision that has been achieved compared to the typical outcome for a monofocal IOL.

APPROACH TO UNEXPECTED POSTOPERATIVE OPTICAL COMPLAINTS

When a postoperative patient presents with complaints about vision with a presbyopia IOL, the surgeon must work methodically to determine the cause if the case was uncomplicated and the anatomical result looks normal. The process begins with taking a good history. The surgeon, not a technician, needs to listen carefully to the patient and ask non-leading questions in order to obtain an accurate picture of what images the patient perceives. For example, "glare" has vastly different meanings to different people.

The pupil is often overlooked as the source of difficulty. Because the staff may have dilated a patient before the surgeon first examines him, the patient may need to return for a second visit. The patient will appreciate that the surgeon and staff sincerely are concerned and are working hard to address the problem.

The optical work-up for complaints about clarity or about glare begins with a careful refraction, guided by corneal topography. Care must be taken to use a defogging technique in the refraction in order to determine the point where the distance vision ceases to improve, as it is easy to be deceived by "over-minusing" the patient and determining a manifest refraction that is not at distance, but rather somewhere within the near portion of the IOL optic. Corneal topographic mapping is important to detect astigmatism, both regular and irregular.

If distance vision is correctable to an acceptable level, but is inadequate in the uncorrected state, a determination can be made about improvement with strategies such as astigmatic keratotomy or corneal laser refractive surgery. On the other hand, if uncorrected distance vision is adequate but intermediate or near vision is inadequate, the strategy of *staged implantation* allows the surgeon to select a different IOL power or IOL model to address the deficiencies of the first implanted eye (Figure 38-13).

A different challenge occurs when a patient perceives that vision is unacceptable at all distances and refractive correction

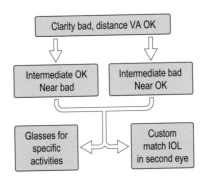

Figure 38-13 Algorithm for managing inadequate intermediate and near vision.

does not improve the outcome. Figure 38-14 shows a decision algorithm for this situation. The ocular surface is the first area that should be carefully examined, as the impact of a poor-quality tear film has been underappreciated, and the findings are subtle. In addition to careful inspection of the lid margins and tear film break-up, the use of vital stains such as lissamine green or rose bengal are important. Ocular surface treatment begins with artificial tears and lid hygiene, but may need to include topical cyclosporine A and non-penetrating corticosteroid drops, punctal plugs, and systemic agents such as doxycycline, flaxseed oil, and omega-3 fatty acids. If the tear film is optimized, the underlying corneal contour is the next suspect. Corneal topography will reveal irregularities or unsuspected astigmatism. Next, attention turns to the deeper structures, with optical coherence tomography (OCT) being the key to detecting maculopathies, and visual field testing and color vision tests helping to detect optic pathway disorders (along with neuro imaging studies, if needed). Only after ruling out all of these issues the posterior capsule can be considered as the source, unless the opacity is unusual and unequivocal. More subtle posterior capsule opacities can most definitely impact the quality of vision in multifocal IOLs compared to monofocal

IOLs because the multifocal optics have already reduced contrast sensitivity. However, once the posterior capsule has been opened by Nd-YAG laser capsulotomy, an IOL exchange becomes higher risk. Therefore, opening the posterior capsule should be an intervention reserved for cases when other sources of vision impairment have been excluded and posterior capsule opacity is the most likely source of the visual difficulty.

A different decision and management algorithm is needed to approach a patient with acceptable acuity but photic phenomenon such as halo and glare (Figure 38-15). The patient must first be asked to determine which eye is the source of the difficulty. Many patients have not thought to check. Have the patient draw the phenomenon. One person's halo is often quite different from another. Try to simulate the glare in the office, typically with light sources such as a muscle light. If the complaint can be duplicated in office, determining whether certain interventions are helpful can be efficiently pursued.

The workup continues with the measurements on the right side of the Figure 38-15 algorithm. Refractive errors and corneal distortions may be treatable sources of halo and glare. Astigmatism may require astigmatic incisions; many optical issues are best addressed with corneal laser refractive procedures.

One maneuver of particular benefit is the use of nighttime driving spectacles to reduce the perception of halos from oncoming headlights in patients with multifocal IOLs. After determining the optimum distance vision correction, added minus power is placed, typically −0.5 to −0.75 D. Figure 38-16A shows that the cause of the halo is the light focused in front of the retina. Figure 38-16B illustrates that with added minus power correction, while the distance focus will be degraded slightly, the benefit is that the halo circle is now closer to the retina and, therefore, smaller. For some patients, this simple step will make the halos at night become tolerable.

The relationship of the IOL to the pupillary aperture is the other main source of remediable glare and halo. This pathway is shown on the left side of Figure 38-15. The IOL may be well-centered in the capsular bag, but the pupil is eccentric to

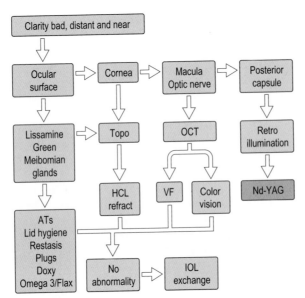

Figure 38-14 Algorithm for diagnosing and managing complaints of poor quality vision with presbyopia intraocular lens.

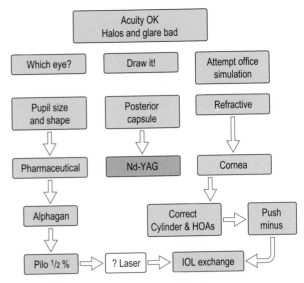

Figure 38-15 Algorithm for diagnosing and managing complaints of halos, glare, and photic phenomena with presbyopia intraocular lens

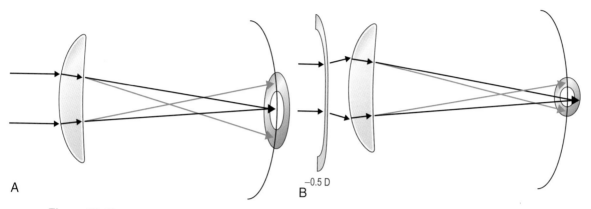

Figure 38-16 A, Halos caused by the defocused light from the near portion of the intraocular lens optic (see also Figure 38-8). B, A low-minus lens used for night driving will reduce the size of the halo by bringing the focal point closer to the retina.

it, or the pupil may be too large or too small. Pharmacologic interventions that may reduce night glare symptoms are brimonidine 0.1% or 0.15% (Alphagan, Allergan), which does not actively constrict the pupil but rather acts to reduce natural mydriasis, and pilocarpine hydrochloride. For most patients, the weakest commercial concentration of 0.5% is adequate, but if the reaction is too intense, a compounding pharmacy can prepare lower concentrations under sterile conditions.

Lasers can be of assistance with pupil issues in several ways. A small pupil can be enlarged with photocoagulation spots applied as a ring outside the sphincter muscle. Alternatively, the Nd-YAG laser can create multiple small sphincterotomies (for details on Nd-YAG sphincterotomy, see Chapter 52). Donnenfeld reported a successful technique to shift the pupil to gain better centration (verbal presentation, *American Academy of Ophthalmology*, 2007). A green photocoagulator is set at 500 μ spot size, 500 milliwats, and 500 ms. Three to five spots are applied in the mid-periphery of the iris in a circumferential arc in the direction toward which the pupil needs to move. Experience indicates that the performance of multifocal IOLs degrades with pupil mis-match greater than 0.3–0.5 mm.

Opacification of the posterior capsule is another source of glare that can be treated. As is the case of suboptimal vision, however, the clinician must be wary of being seduced into attributing glare to the posterior capsule until other sources of glare have been ruled out *and* exchange of the IOL is not under consideration. Once the posterior capsule is open, an IOL exchange carries a much higher risk of complications such as cystoid macuar edema, retinal detachment, and endophthalmitis.

■ SUMMARY ■

Multifocal IOLs have the principal advantage that they function without moving parts, and, therefore, have more predictable visual performance. However, variables remain, especially related to pupil size and variable ability of patients to adapt to processing the multifocal image. Accommodating IOLs offer the potential for higher quality of vision, with absence of glare, halo, and loss of contrast, with optical quality identical to a monofocal IOL with the same optic. The principal challenge is harnessing the action of the ciliary muscle. Reduction in flexibility of the capsular bag as the eye heals can reduce or eliminate any IOL optic movement. As a result, many surgeons are utilizing a modified monovision strategy in conjunction with current accommodating IOLs.

▌ KEY POINTS

- Allow time between 1st and 2nd eye surgery to assess satisfaction
  - Staged implantation
- Listen to the patient
- Convey sincere concerns as a partner with the patient
- Carefully pursue options
- Intraocular lens exchange is the last option
- Posterior capsulotomy limits ability to resolve the problem without further complications

▌ RULES FOR THE PRESBYOPIA INTRAOCULAR LENS SURGEON

1. Only implant a presbyopia intraocular lens (IOL) in a patient who prioritizes functional vision without glasses
2. The patient must both *hear* and *understand* that the goal of the presbyopia IOL is a wider range of functional vision without glasses, and that glasses may still be needed for a few particular activities
3. Do not place a multifocal IOL in an eye that already has compromised visual function from another source
   - Macular disease
   - Optic neuropathy
   - Amblyopia
   - Advanced glaucoma
4. Remember that you are now a *refractive surgeon*
   - Assessment
   - Planning
   - Postoperative management
5. Under promise – Over achieve – Undersell – Celebrate success

References

[1] Duffey RJ, Zabel RW, Lindstrom RL. Multifocal intraocular lenses. J Cataract Refract Surg 1990;16:423–429.

[2] Koch DD, Samuelson SW, Haft EA, et al. Pupillary size and responsiveness: implications for selection of a bifocal intraocular lens. Ophthalmology 1991;98:1030–1035.

[3] Verzella F, Calossi A. Multifocal effect of against-the-rule myopic astigmatism in pseudophakic eyes. Refract Corneal Surg 1993;9:58–61.

[4] Bradbury JA, Hillman JS, Cassells-Brown A. Optimal postoperative refraction for good unaided near and distance vision with monofocal intraocular lenses. Br J Ophthalmol 1992;76:300–302.

[5] Percival P. An update on multifocal lens implants. Doc Ophthalmol 1992;81:285–292.

[6] Sawusch MR, Guyton DL. Optimal astigmatism to enhance depth of focus after cataract surgery. Ophthalmology 1991;98:1025–1029.

[7] Datiles MB, Gancayco T. Low myopia with low astigmatic correction gives cataract surgery patients good depth of focus. Ophthalmology 1990;97:922–926.

[8] Schor C, Landsman L, Erickson P. Ocular dominance and the interocular suppression of blur in monovision. Am J Optom Physiol Opt 1987;64:723–730.

[9] Jain S, Arora I, Azar DT. Success of monovision in presbyopes: review of the literature and potential applications to refractive surgery. Surv Ophthalmol 1996;40:491–499.

[10] Pardhan S, Gilchrist J. The effect of monocular defocus on binocular contrast sensitivity. Ophthalmic Physiol Opt 1990;10:33–36.

[11] Loshin, Loshin. Cornear. Int Cont Lens Clin 1982;9:161–173.

[12] Wright KW, Guemes A, Kapadia MS, Wilson SE. Binocular function and patient satisfaction after monovision induced by myopic photorefractive keratectomy. J Cataract Refract Surg 1999;25:177–182.

[13] Braun EHP, Lee J, Steinert RF. Monovision in LASIK. Ophthalmology 2008;115:1196–202, Epub 2007 Dec 3.

[14] Angelucci DD. Steps to maximize success with pseudophakic monovision. Ophthalmology Management 2008;12:39–41.

[15] Davison JA, Simpson MJ. History and development of the apodized diffractive intraocular lens. J Cataract Refract Surg 2006;32:849–858.

[16] Patel S, Alio J, Feinbaum C. Comparison of Acri.Smart multifocal IOL, Crystalens AT-45 acommodative IOL, and Technovision PresbyLASIK for correcting presbyopia. J Refract Surg 2008;24:294–299.

[17] Akutsu H, Legge GE, Luebker A, Lindstrom RL, et al. Multifocal intraocular lenses and glare. Optom Vis Sci 1993;70:487–495.

[18] Pieh S, Weghaupt H, Skorpik C. Contrast sensitivity and glare disability with diffractive and refractive multifocal intraocular lenses. J Cataract Refract Surg 1998;24:659–662.

[19] Atebara NH, Miller D. An optical model to describe image contrast with bifocal intraocular lenses. Am J Ophthalmol 1990;110:683–687.

[20] Webster MA, Georgeson MA, Webster SM. Neural adjustments to image blur. Nat Neurosci 2002;5:839–849.

[21] Artal P, Chen L, Fernandex EJ, et al. Neural compensation for the eye's optical aberrations. J Vis 2004;4:281–287.

[22] Artal P. Neural adaptation to aberrations. Cataract and Refract Surg Today 2007;7:76–77.

[23] Kaymak H, Fahle M, Ott G, Mester U. Intraindividual comparison of the effect of training on visual performance with ReSTOR and Tecnis diffractive multifocal IOLs. J Refract Surg 2008;24:287–293.

[24] Javitt J, Brauweiler HP, Jacobi KW, et al. Cataract extraction with multifocal intraocular lens implantation: clinical, functional, and quality-of-life outcomes. Multicenter clinical trial in Germany and Austria. J Cataract Refract Surg 2000;26:1356–1366.

[25] Javitt JC, Steinert RF. Cataract extraction with multifocal intraocular lens implantation: a multinational clinical trial evaluating clinical, functional, and quality-of-life outcomes. Ophthalmology 2000;107:2040–2048.

[26] Arens B, Freudenthaler N, Quentin CD. Binocular function after bilateral implantation of monofocal and refractive multifocal intraocular lenses. J Cataract Refract Surg 1999;25:399–404.

[27] Steinert RF, Aker BL, Trentacost DJ, Smith PJ, et al. A prospective comparative study of the AMO ARRAY zonal-progressive multifocal silicone intraocular lens and a monofocal intraocular lens. Ophthalmology 1999;106:1243–1255.

[28] Vaquero M, Encinas JL, Jimenez F. Visual function with monofocal versus multifocal IOLs. J Cataract Refract Surg 1996;22:1222–1225.

[29] Steinert RF, Post Jr CT, Brint SF, et al. A prospective, randomized, double-masked comparison of a zonal-progressive multifocal intraocular lens and a monofocal intraocular lens. Ophthalmology 1992;99:853–860, discussion 860–861.

[30] Mester U, Dillliger P, Anterist N. Impact of a modified optic design on visual function: clinical comparative study. J Cataract Refract Surg 2003;29:652–660.

[31] Bellucci R, Scialdone A, Buratto L, Morselli S, Chierego C, Criscuoli A, et al. Visual acuity and contrast sensitivity comparison between Tecnis and AcrySof SA60AT intraocular lenses: a multicenter randomized study. J Cataract Refract Surg 2005;31:712–717.

[32] Packer M, Fine IH, Hoffmann RS, Piers PA. Improved functional vision with a modified prolate intraocular lens. J Cataract Refract Surg 2004;30:986–992.

[33] Awwad ST, Warmerdam D, Bowman W, Dwarakanathan S, Cavanagh HD, McCulley JP. Contrast sensitivity and higher order aberrations in eyes implanted with AcrySof IQ SN60WF and AcrySof SN60AT intraocular lenses. J Refract Surg 2008;24:619–625.

[34] Featherstone KA, Bloomfield JR, Lang AJ, et al. Driving simulation study: bilateral array multifocal versus bilateral AMO monofocal intraocular lenses. J Cataract Refract Surg 1999;25: 1254–1262.

[35] Schmitz S, Dick HB, Krummenauer F, et al. Contrast sensitivity and glare disability by halogen light after monofocal and multifocal lens implantation. Br J Ophthalmol 2000;84:1109–1112.

[36] Dick HB, Krummenauer F, Schwenn O, et al. Objective and subjective evaluation of photic phenomena after monofocal and multifocal intraocular lens implantation. Ophthalmology 1999;106: 1878–1886.

[37] Haring G, Dick HB, Krummenauer F, et al. Subjective photic phenomena with refractive multifocal and monofocal intraocular lenses: results of a multicenter questionnaire. J Cataract Refract Surg 2001;27:245–249.

[38] Hunkeler JD, Coffman TM, paugh J, Lang A, Smith P, Tarantino N. Characterization of visual phenomena with the array multifocal intraocular lens. J Cataract Refract Surg 2002;28:1195–1204.

[39] Nijkamp MD, Dolders MGT, de Branbander J, van den Borne B, Hendrikse F, Nuijts RMMA. Effectiveness of multifocal intraocular lenses to correct presbyopia after cataract surgery: a randomized controlled trial. Ophthalmology 2004;111:1832–1839.

[40] Kohnen T, Allen D, Boureau C, Dublineau P, Hartman C, Mehdom E, et al. European multicenter study of the AcrySof ReSTOR apodized diffractive intraocular lens. Ophthalmology 2006;113:578–584.

[41] Chiam PJT, Chan JH, Agarwal RK, Kasaby S. ReSTOR intraocular lens implantation in cataract surgery: quality of vision. J Cataract Refract Surg 2006;32:1459–1463.

[42] Franchini A, Zamma Gallarati B, Vaccari E. Analysis of straylight effects related to intraocular lens edge design. J Cataract Refract Surg 30:1531–1536.

[43] Sen HN, Sarikkola A-U, Uusitalo RJ, Laatikainen L. Quality of vision after AMO Array multifocal intraocular lens implantation. J Cataract Refract Surg 2004;30:2483–2493.

[44] de Vries NE, Franssen L, Webers CAB, et al. Intraocular straylight after implantation of the multifocal AcrySof ReSTOR SA60D3 diffractive intraocular lens. J Cataract Refract Surg 2008;34:957–962.

[45] Chang DF. Prospective functional and clinical comparison of bilateral ReZoom and ReSTOR intraocular lenses in patients 70 years or younger. J Cataract Refract Surg 2008;34:934–941.

[46] Cumming JS, Kammann J. Experience with an accommodating IOL. J Cataract Refract Surg 1996;22:1001.

[47] Marchini G, Pedrotti E, Modesti M, Visentin S, Tosi R. Anterior segment changes during accommodation in eyes with a monofocal intraocular lens: high frequency ultrasound study. J Cataract Refract Surg 2008;34:949–956.

[48] McLeod SD, Portney V, Ting A. A dual optic accommodating foldable intraocular lens. Br J Ophthalmol 2003;87:1083–1085.

[49] Werner L, Pandey SK, Izak AM, et al. Capsular bag opacification after experimental implantation of a new accommodating intraocular lens in rabbit eyes. J Cataract Refract Surg 2004;30: 1114–1123.

[50] Gunenc U, Celik L. Long-term experience with mixing and matching refractive Array and diffractive CeeOn multifocal intraocular lenses. J Refract Surg 2008;24:233–242.

The Correction of Astigmatism During Cataract Surgery with Toric Intraocular Lenses

Stephen S. Lane, MD and David F. Chang, MD

39

CHAPTER HIGHLIGHTS

>> Preoperative patient assessment

>> Surgical planning

>> Implantation technique

INTRODUCTION

Astigmatism is caused by refractive aberrations in the cornea or lens that focus light unevenly onto the retina, consequently, distorting images. In recent years there has been increasing interest in correcting astigmatism at the time of cataract surgery or refractive lens exchange to achieve emmetropia. Cataract surgeons and cataract patients, today hope to achieve 20/20, or better, visual acuity with spectacle independence for distance vision. Approximately 15–29% of cataract patients have more than 1.00 diopter (D) of preoperative corneal or refractive astigmatism,[1,2] which can prevent them from achieving the uncorrected 20/20 visual acuity and spectacle freedom that they might desire. Astigmatic treatment options available to cataract surgeons include:

1. spectacles or contact lenses

2. peripheral corneal relaxing incisions (limbal relaxing incisions (LRIs))

3. laser refractive surgery (laser in-situ keratomileusis (LASIK) or photorefractive keratectomy (PRK))

4. toric intraocular lenses (IOLs).

While all are viable options, glasses and contact lenses have the disadvantage of being inconvenient, expensive and quite patient dependent with regard to cosmetic and lifestyle issues. The main drawbacks of LRIs are their limited refractive range and lack of predictability. The unpredictability is a function of the amount of desired correction and the patient's age. Increasing patient age amplifies the relaxing effect of any incisional keratotomy but this relationship unfortunately is not linear. The same length LRI may be ineffective in a 50-year-old patient, yet powerful in a 90-year-old patient. Besides patient age, other variables include the peripheral corneal thickness and corneal diameter. Given these variables, the greater the amount of targeted astigmatism effect, the more inconsistent and unpredictable the results of LRIs are. Finally, although truly accurate incisions should theoretically produce 1:1 "coupling" that does not affect the spherical power, longer LRIs in older patients often result in slight overall corneal flattening.

Laser surgery, while quite predictable, can be accompanied by postoperative pain and discomfort, potential flap complications (LASIK), and glare and haloes. This adds significant expense and requires a second and separate surgical procedure. A toric IOL is designed to minimize image distortion by focusing the light that is otherwise scattered by corneal astigmatism. Toric lenses come in multiple powers and correct for aphakia as well as pre-existing corneal astigmatism. They avoid the variability inherent in a manual corneal incision, do not require new surgical skills, and give highly predictable results when they are properly aligned.

Critical to the success of any toric IOL is rotational stability within the capsular bag. For every degree of misalignment off the desired axis there is a 0.033% loss of cylinder correction. For example, 1.5 D of corneal cylinder would call for a 2.25 D IOL aligned at the proper meridian to fully correct the cylindrical error. As illustrated in Figure 39-1, 15° of misalignment would reduce the correction by half (0.75 D) and 30° of misalignment would result in no correction at all. Proper toric IOL alignment requires accurate and precise positioning at the time of surgery and long-term postoperative rotational stability. Currently, two toric IOLs have been approved by the US Food and Drug Administration (FDA) and are available for implantation in the US.

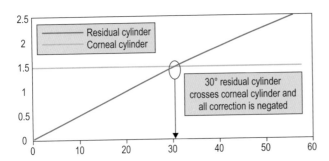

Figure 39-1 Residual cylinder as a function of mis-alignment, assuming 2.25 D Toric intraocular lens and 1.5 D corneal cylinder.

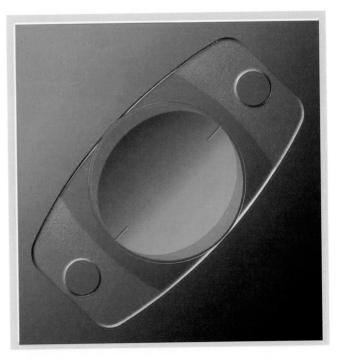

Figure 39-2 Staar Toric intraocular lens (Courtesy of STAAR Surgical, Monrovia, Calif).

■ PREOPERATIVE CONSIDERATIONS FOR TORIC INTRAOCULAR LENS IMPLANTATION ■

In determining the targeted astigmatic correction preoperatively, one must consider the fellow eye refraction and the patient's desire to see without glasses. For example, with +2.50 D of against-the-rule (ATR) astigmatism in a pseudophakic fellow eye, it may not be advisable to eliminate all ATR astigmatism in the surgical eye. Alternatively, surgical astigmatism reduction for +1.00 D of astigmatism should be strongly considered when implanting a multifocal IOL. To avoid "flipping" the axis, it is generally best to err on the side of under-correcting rather than over-correcting pre-existing astigmatism. Irregular or asymmetric astigmatism are not amenable to standard surgical approaches. Corneal topography is helpful in diagnosing and evaluating these situations.

■ STAAR TORIC INTRAOCULAR LENS ■

The Staar model AA4203 silicone plate haptic toric IOL became the first FDA-approved toric lens in November 1998 (Figure 39-2). Several earlier studies had suggested that the plate haptic design might provide better long-term rotational stability compared to traditional three-piece designs with looped haptics. In 1994, Shimizu published a study showing significant late rotation of conventional three-piece IOL with polypropylene haptics by 3 months postoperatively.[3] The three-piece IOLs always rotated in a counter-clockwise direction, with 25% of the 47 lenses rotating >20°, and 21% >30° off axis. In a study using serial digital photographs, Patel reported in 1999 that late, delayed postoperative rotation (>10°) was more frequent with three-piece IOLs (37%) than it was with plate haptic lenses (14%).[4] Like Shimizu, he also found that three-piece IOL designs rotated counter-clockwise.

However, Patel's study also examined early postoperative rotational stability, and found that both lens designs rotated during the immediate postoperative period. By 2 weeks, 41% of three-piece and 38% of plate haptic lenses had rotated >10°. However, severe early rotation (>30°) was much more frequent with the plate haptic design (24% vs. 5%). Presumably, it was not until the capsular bag contracted that the corners of the plate haptic lens were able to resist natural rotational forces. It is important to note

that Patel's study only evaluated a 10.5 mm-long plate haptic IOL, which is shorter than the Staar's two toric IOL sizes (10.8 and 11.2 mm). The plate haptic IOL studied also lacked the large fixation fenestration on the haptic that is used in current designs.

In addition to being available in these two plate haptic sizes, the Staar toric IOL comes in two astigmatic powers. The +2.00 toric lens corrects approximately 1.4 D of keratometric astigmatism, while the +3.50 toric add corrects approximately 2.3 D at the spectacle plane. The "TF" model lens has an overall length of 10.8 mm and was the original FDA-studied design. Subsequently in 1999, Staar introduced a longer 11.2 mm "TL" model that is available for spherical powers of <23.5 D. The TL plate haptics also have a matte finish to make them less slippery and to better resist rotation.

STAAR TORIC INTRAOCULAR LENS CLINICAL RESULTS

Clinical studies of the shorter 10.8 mm Staar AA4203 TF toric IOL have reported a significant rate of early rotation.[5-8] In the US FDA study (using only the shorter TF model), 24% of the IOLs implanted ended up more than 10° off axis. In terms of more severe misalignment, 12% were >20° off, 8% were >30° off, and 5% were >45° off axis) (Figure 39-3).

Three additional published clinical studies evaluated the shorter Staar TF toric IOL. In a series of 130 TF toric IOLs, Sun et al. reported that 25% rotated >20°, 7% rotated >40°, and 9% of the toric IOLs were repositioned.[5] Rumsworth et al. reported a smaller series of 37 eyes with the 10.8 mm TF IOL.[6] They had better rotational stability with only 19% rotated >10° off axis, and only one patient (3%) requiring repositioning. They found that greater IOL

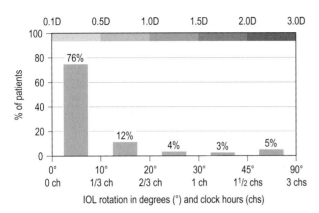

Figure 39-3 Rate of toric intraocular lens misalignment in U.S. FDA study cohort (Courtesy of STAAR Surgical, Monrovia, Calif).

rotation correlated with increasing axial length. Finally, Leyland et al. published a small series of 22 eyes implanted with the TF toric IOL in which 18% rotated >30° and 23% rotated >15°.[7]

In 2002 Till et al. reported a mixed series that included both TF (63%) and TL (37%) toric IOLs.[8] This was the first published report to include data on the TL IOL. Fourteen percent of all of the IOLs (TL and TF) rotated >15° off axis. Nine percent of the IOLs needed to be repositioned, although in some patients it was deemed too late to safely do this. The rotation rates were similar between the TF and TL IOL sub-groups, but the authors did not specify how they selected which IOL to implant.

One of the authors (DFC) published the only study that specifically evaluated the early rotational stability of the longer Staar toric IOL.[9] Results from an expanded series have also been reported, in which excellent rotational stability was achieved in a consecutive series of 80 TL (11.2 mm) toric implants.[10] Seventy-three percent of the IOLs were within 5° of target axis; 89% were within 10° of target axis; 96% were within 15° of target axis (Table 39-1). These results represent a marked improvement over data from the FDA trial (Figure 39-3) and from previous series[5–8] in which the shorter TF IOL was used.

This was also the first study to demonstrate a negligible early rotation rate with any toric IOL, with 2.5% (2/80) of the TL toric IOLs requiring repositioning. Taken together, these studies imply that the length of the plate haptic toric IOL is the most critical factor in early rotational stability of this design. Earlier studies utilizing shorter toric plate haptic IOLs exclusively may have fostered a misperception of higher early rotation rates than would be found with the currently available technology.

Table 39-1 Distribution of alignment relative to desired axis of 80 consecutive cases with longer Staar TL toric IOL

Axis misalignment	≤5 degrees	10 degrees	15 degrees	≥20 degrees
No. of eyes (80)	58	13	6	3
% of eyes	73%	16%	7%	4%

STAAR TORIC INTRAOCULAR LENS SURGICAL TECHNIQUE

For both the Staar and Alcon toric IOLs the spherical power is calculated in the same way as it is for a conventional IOL, and the astigmatic power is selected without having to adjust the spherical power. Hash marks on the Staar optic allow the cylindrical power of the IOL to be surgically aligned with the steeper "plus" axis of astigmatism (Figure 39-4A). In determining the toric power and axis of the IOL, one should use the keratometric reading, rather than the refraction, to avoid any potential influence of lenticular astigmatism. Rigid contact lens wear should be discontinued for several weeks in order to improve the accuracy of keratometry readings. These particular patients should understand that they will not be able to wear rigid contact lenses in the future.

Informed consent should include discussing the potential for unwanted lens rotation – particularly in the early postoperative period. Depending upon the degree of misalignment, the resulting astigmatism might be the same as, or even worse than, the preoperative amount and surgical realignment may be necessary or advisable. Finally, a plate haptic IOL should not be implanted if there is a torn capsulorrhexis, posterior capsule, or zonular dialysis. Some surgeons inform patients about this possibility.

The following guidelines are recommended for implanting the Staar toric IOL:

1. Always use the longer "TL" IOL if available in the desired power (<23.5 D).

2. Proper surgical alignment of the toric IOL is crucial. Notes or diagrams brought to the operating room can help to assure choosing the correct astigmatic axis. Use a felt-tipped pen to mark cardinal positions with the patient sitting upright prior to surgery. This avoids potential cyclotorsion that can occur with squeezing the lids, lying supine, or following a periocular anesthetic injection.

3. Under the operating microscope, use a degree gauge to mark the steep (+) axis of astigmatism on the limbus with the marking pen (Figure 39-4A). Once the toric IOL is implanted, its axis marks can be aligned with these ink marks and double-checked against the preoperative notes or chart.

4. Use an astigmatically neutral, temporal clear corneal incision (Figure 39-4B).

5. Use a cohesive ophthalmic viscosurgical device (OVD), e.g. Healon (AMO), Provisc (Alcon), Amvisc (Bausch & Lomb). Compared to dispersive OVDs, these are less likely to coat and lubricate the IOL surface.

6. Use the irrigation–aspiration handpiece to remove OVD trapped behind the IOL (Figure 39-4C) in order to maximize prompt contact between the IOL and the posterior capsule (Figure 39-4D).

7. Do not overinflate the eye, which tends to maximally inflate the capsular bag. Leaving the eye somewhat "softer" than usual allows a more flaccid capsular bag to collapse around the plate haptic lens more quickly.

8. Plate haptic IOLs should never be implanted in the ciliary sulcus, or in the presence of a torn capsulorrhexis or posterior capsule.

With the Staar toric IOL, proper IOL sizing is critical for initial rotational stability. Until the capsular bag begins to contract within

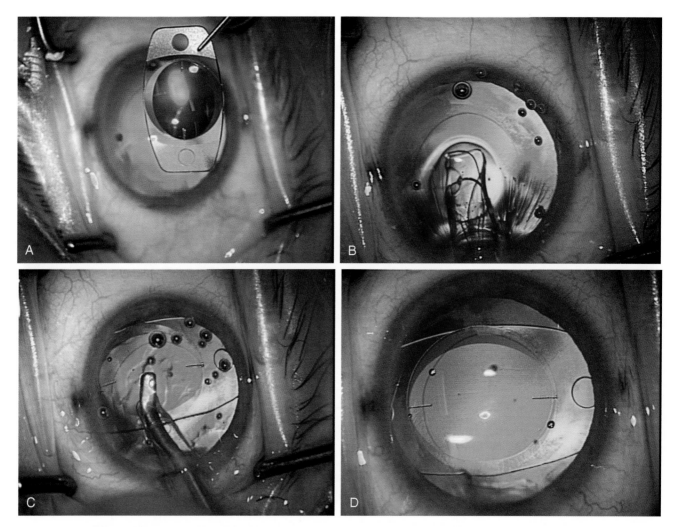

Figure 39-4 Implantation of Staar toric TL intraocular lens (IOL). 90° axis has been marked with felt pen prior to insertion (**A**). IOL is injected through a temporal clear corneal incision (**B**). Irrigation–aspiration handpiece is used to aspirate ophthalmic viscosurgical device (OVD) from behind the IOL optic (**C**). IOL hash marks are aligned with the 90° axis pen marks, coinciding with the (+) axis of astigmatism (**D**).

the first day or so, a plate haptic IOL that is too small for the bag can rotate. A dilated exam should be performed on postoperative day one (POD 1) to check the IOL axis because any significant rotation will usually occur between the time of surgery and the first postoperative morning. If indicated, surgical repositioning should be performed within the first postoperative week, if possible. Under topical anesthesia, the capsular bag can be reopened with BSS or with a small amount of OVD, in order to allow the toric IOL to be dialed into alignment. Greater force is required to rotate the IOL after the capsular bag fully contracts, which in turn increases the chance of tearing the capsular bag or zonules. Fortunately, late rotation has not been a problem reported with the Staar toric IOL either in the literature or in the authors' experience.

■ ACRYSOF TORIC INTRAOCULAR LENS ■

The AcrySof toric lens (Alcon Laboratories, Inc., Fort Worth, TX) is composed of a hydrophobic acrylic polymer that has UV and blue-light absorbers. The lens is built on the same truncated-edged platform as the AcrySof Natural Single-Piece IOL (Alcon Laboratories, Inc.). (Figure 39-5). The toric lens easily folds in half and may be inserted through an incision measuring less than 3 mm using the Monarch II injector (Alcon Laboratories, Inc.).

The AcrySof toric IOL examined in the FDA clinical investigation was provided in three cylinder powers at the IOL plane: 1.50, 2.25, and 3.00 D (Table 39-2). In the future, additional power options will be offered. Initially, the AcrySof toric IOL is available in a spherical range between 16.00 and 25.00 D in 0.50 D increments. The optic design maintains the same thickness for the central optic in all models of the AcrySof toric IOL as with the monofocal models SA60AT and SN60AT. The posterior toric optic design results in slight variations in the edge's thickness around the circumference of the optic due to the different curvature of the principal meridians. This variation between the principal meridians changes as the cylinder power changes from model to model. The importance of this design is that it provides a full 6 mm toric optic with a central optic thickness, IOL volume, IOL delivery characteristics, and A-constant that are consistent among all AcrySof toric IOL models.

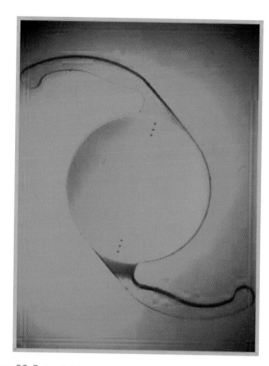

ACRYSOF TORIC INTRAOCULAR LENS

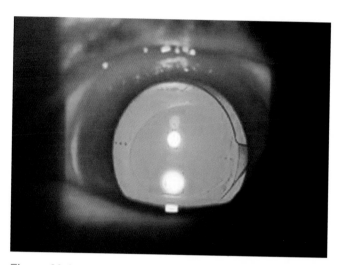

Figure 39-6 AcrySof Toric intraocular lens successfully placed within the capsular bag demonstrating the shrink-wrap effect of the capsular bag around the IOL.

Figure 39-5 AcrySof Toric IOL demonstrating the linear dots that are to be aligned on the steep meridian of the cornea.

Table 39-2 AcrySof Toric IOL Cylinder Powers

Acysof Toric IOL Model	Cylinder Power of IOL (D)	Cylinder Correction @ Corneal Plane* (D)
SN60T3	1.5	1.03
SN60T4	2.25	1.55
SN60T5	3.00	2.06

*Based on an average human eye.

ACRYSOF TORIC INTRAOCULAR LENS CLINICAL RESULTS

The FDA monitored US clinical trial, was a multicenter, prospective comparison of the AcrySof toric IOL (models SA60T3, SA60T4, and SA60T5 – a group referred to as SA60TT in this chapter) and a control spherical IOL (SA60AT). This clinical trial assessed lens rotation, residual astigmatism, uncorrected visual acuity (UCVA), and spectacle freedom for distance vision. Approximately 250 subjects received the SA60TT, and 250 subjects were implanted with the non-toric SA60AT. All subjects were followed for 1 year after lens implantation in their first eye, but only the 6-month data are available. The AcrySof toric IOL demonstrated excellent stability within the capsular bag. The average rotation was less than 4° from the lens' initial placement through 6 months postoperatively (Figure 39-7).

The three toric models (SA60T3, SA60T4, and SA60T5) were used in the clinical study to correct 1.50, 2.25, and 3.00 D of astigmatism, respectively, at the IOL plane. The AcrySof toric IOL significantly reduced or eliminated absolute residual refractive cylinder when compared to the control lens. Specifically, the

The lens design has two major features that limit posterior capsular opacification (PCO). First, its biomaterial adheres to the capsular bag via a single layer of lens epithelial cells. The resulting lack of space through which essential, life-sustaining nutrients can pass ultimately leads to the cells' death. Subsequently, the AcrySof material adheres directly to the lens capsule via common extracellular proteins such as fibronectin and collagen IV.[11] This adhesive property also minimizes the lens' rotation-crucial to success with a toric IOL.

The design of the Acrysof toric IOL's posterior optic edge also increases its ability to maintain a clear posterior capsule and ultimately reduces the need for an Nd:YAG capsulotomy.[11] Apple et al. showed that an IOL's square, truncated optic edge creates a barrier to the migration of lens epithelial cells, thereby leaving the visual axis clear of PCO.[12] The lens' haptic design provides maximum conformance to the capsular bag and thus offers the greatest possible surface area for adherence between the IOL and the capsular tissue. This quality, in turn, enhances the rotational stability of the IOL and leads to a pronounced shrink-wrap effect (Figure 39-6) during the early postoperative period that locks lens into place within the lens capsule.

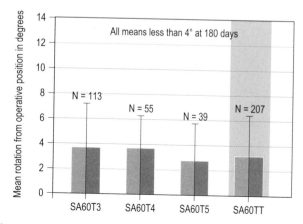

Figure 39-7 AcrySof Toric IOL mean rotation by Model

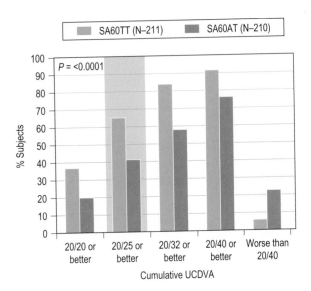

Figure 39-8 Uncorrected visual acuity results from the US clinical trial for the AcrySof Toric intraocular lens.

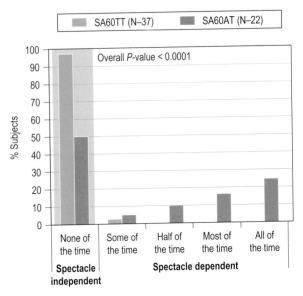

Figure 39-10 Spectacle freedom following bilateral implantation

SA60TT lenses were three times more likely to achieve a residual refractive cylinder of 0.50 D or less compared with the control. At the 6-month visit, approximately 66% of the unilateral toric subjects and 41% of the unilateral control subjects achieved a UCVA of 20/25 or better. For those patients ($n = 37$) who received AcrySof toric IOLs bilaterally, 97% achieved 20/25 or better UCVA compared with 77% of controls ($n = 22$) (Figure 39-8).

Additionally, the AcrySof toric IOL significantly improved subjects' spectacle freedom for distance vision relative to the control lens. In the clinical study, 60% of patients who received the toric lens in one eye achieved spectacle freedom for distance vision. Of the 37 toric subjects and the 22 control subjects who underwent bilateral IOL implantation, 97% of those who received the AcrySof toric IOL achieved spectacle freedom for distance vision compared with 50% of the control subjects (Figures 39-9 and 39-10). In the

FDA trial, the AcrySof toric IOL minimized PCO, provided excellent vision, and allowed maximal conformance to the capsular bag while minimizing the IOL's rotation. All of these characteristics are critical for accurate cylindrical correction. One of the authors compared the Staar and AcrySof toric IOLs in separate consecutive series (90 and 100 cases) and found that the AscrySof demonstrated superior rotational stability.[13] The mean IOL rotation was 5.56 degrees ±8.49 (SD) in the AA4203 group and 3.35±3.41 degrees in the AcrySof SN60T group (P Z.0232). One AcrySof SN60T IOL (1%) and 8 AA4203 IOLs (8.9%) were 15 degrees or more off axis (P Z.01).

ACRYSOF TORIC INTRAOCULAR LENS SURGICAL TECHNIQUE

Implantation of the AcrySof toric IOL implantation follows a similar procedure to that of most modern small-incision cataract surgeries, using phacoemulsification and in-the-bag IOL placement. Extra corneal marking steps are included to ensure proper positioning of the toric correction. To account for cyclorotation, the cornea is marked at the 3 and 9 o'clock limbus while the patient is in an upright position. Once the patient is positioned for surgery, an astigmatism marker is used to mark the axis of the steep corneal meridian using the previously placed 3 and 9 o'clock marks as reference points for the 180° meridian. Following phacoemulsification the IOL is inserted into the capsular bag utilizing a Monarch II injector. Following insertion, the lens begins to naturally unfold within the capsule. The surgeon then carefully aligns axis indication marks on the IOL with the previously placed marks denoting the steep meridian of the cornea. Care must be taken to remove the ophthalmic viscosurgical devise (OVD) from behind the IOL without disrupting the IOL position. A final positioning step following OVD removal may be necessary to reposition the lens on axis.

Two key factors for a successful surgical outcome are the choice of astigmatic power of the IOL and the proper identification of the axis of the steep meridian of the cornea. Both are calculated using software provided by Alcon Laboratories Inc., called the Toric IOL

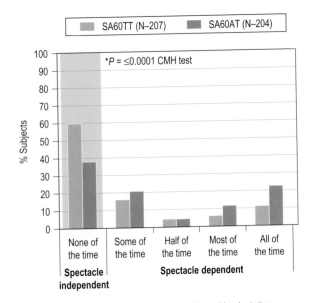

Figure 39-9 Spectacle freedom following unilateral implantation.

Calculator. The A-constant and keratometric analysis are entered into the software, and the Toric IOL Calculator uses this information along with an assumption of the astigmatic effects of the cataract incision (surgically induced astigmatism), to calculate the appropriate astigmatic power correction and position of the steep axis.

The importance of a toric IOL's rotational stability within the capsular bag cannot be overstated with respect to its effectiveness. Because proper axial alignment of a toric IOL maximizes the amount of astigmatism correction, the surgical positioning of the axis must be as accurate as possible. During the early postoperative period, IOLs may rotate within the capsular bag until it contracts, or until they form a bioadhesive bond with the posterior capsule.[14] Compared to the slippery surface of a silicone optic, the tacky surface of the AcrySof material immediately clings to the capsule and allows for this fixation to occur soon after the IOL's implantation.[11,15] Finally, the AcrySof toric IOL is built upon a single-piece hydrophobic acrylic platform that, as a spherical lens, is far more popular than a silicone plate haptic design. As a result, the injector and insertion technique should be very familiar to surgeons already using the spherical AcrySof lens.

■ TORIC INTRAOCULAR LENSES – THE FUTURE ■

The ideal time to correct astigmatism would be 1–2 weeks postoperatively. By this time, an accurate refraction can be performed that will include the net effect of the phaco incision. Furthermore, enough capsular bag shrinkage to prevent IOL rotation or movement will have occurred by this time. A light-adjustable IOL whose spherical and toric power could be modified postoperatively would be the ultimate solution for achieving emmetropia. Calhoun Vision has developed a proprietary lens material consisting of a silicone matrix with diffusible, photo-reactive monomers. Using an external, near UV, non-laser light source, the optic thickness can be altered in order to precisely change the refractive power of the lens postoperatively. Early clinical results have confirmed that both spherical and astigmatic adjustment is possible. This technology could potentially generate a toric IOL that was custom-adjusted and perfectly aligned.

■ CONCLUSION ■

Toric IOLs are an excellent complement or alternative to corneal astigmatic relaxing incisions. They are particularly useful for those patients where limbal relaxing incisions are not powerful or predictable enough. For those patients whose astigmatism exceeds the amount that is correctable with currently available toric IOL powers, these lenses can be combined with corneal astigmatic incisions or laser refractive surgery. The use of toric IOLs is but another example of our ability to merge cataract and refractive surgical objectives for those patients wanting to reduce their spectacle dependence.

References

[1] Hoffer KJ. Biometry of 7,500 cataractous eyes. Am J Opthalmol 1980;90:360–368, correction: 890

[2] Grabow HB. Intraocular correction of refractive errors. In: Kershner RM, editor. Refractive keratotomy for cataract surgery and the correction of astigmatism. Thorofare, NJ: Slack, Inc; 1994. p. 79–115.

[3] Shimizu K, Misawa A, Suzuki Y. Toric intraocular lenses: correcting astigmatism while controlling axis shift. J Cataract Refract Surg 1994;20:523–526.

[4] Patel CK, Ormonde S, Rosen PH, Bron AJ. Postoperative intraocular lens rotation: a randomized comparison of plate and loop haptic implants. Ophthalmology 1999;106:2190–2196.

[5] Sun XY, Vicary D, Montgomery P, Griffiths M. Toric intraocular lenses for correcting astigmatism in 130 eyes. Ophthalmology 2000;107:1776–1781, discussion by RM Kershner, 1781–1782.

[6] Ruhswurm I, Scholz U, Zehetmayer M, et al. Astigmatism correction with foldable toric intraocular lens in cataract patients. J Cataract Refract Surg 2000;26:1022–1027.

[7] Leyland M, Zinicola P, Bloom P, Lee N. Prospective evaluation of a plate haptic toric intraocular lens. Eye 2001;15:202–205.

[8] Till JS, Yoder PR, Wilcox TK, Spielman JL. Toric intraocular lens implantation: 100 consecutive cases. J Cataract Refract Surg 2002;28:295–301.

[9] Chang DF. Early rotational Stability of the Longer Staar Toric IOL – 50 Consecutive (TL) IOLs. J Cataract Refract Surg 2003;29:935–940.

[10] Chang DF. The STAAR Toric intraocular lens: indications and pearls. In: Gills J, editor. A complete surgical guide for correcting astigmatism. Thorofare, NJ: Slack, Inc; 2003.

[11] Linnola RJ, Sund M, Ylonen R, Pihlajaniemi T. Adhesion of soluble fibronectin, laminin, and collagen type IV to intraocular lens materials. J Cataract Refract Surg 1999;25:1486–1491.

[12] Apple DJ, Ram J, Foster A, Peng Q. Elimination of cataract blindness: a global perspective entering the new millennium. Surv Ophthalmol 2000;45(Suppl.):S1–S196.

[13] Chang DF. Comparative rotational stability of single-piece open-loop acrylic and plate-haptic silicone toric intraocular lenses. J Cataract Refract Surg 2008;34:1842–1847.

[14] Vukich JA. Toric intraocular lens. In: Ford JG, Karp CL, editors. Cataract surgery and intraocular lenses: a 21st century perspective. Singapore: Clinical Education Division of the Foundation of the American Academy of Ophthalmology; 2001. p. 144–151.

[15] Linnola RJ, Salonen JI, Happonen RP. Intraocular lens bioactivity tested using rabbit corneal tissue cultures. J Cataract Refract Surg 1999;25:1480–1485.

CONCLUSION

Intraocular Lens Spectral Filtering

Martin A. Mainster, PhD, MD, FRCOphth
and Patricia L. Turner, MD

40

CONTENTS

CHAPTER HIGHLIGHTS

>> Spectral sensitivity and photoreceptors

>> Ganglion cell photoreception and circadian rythms

>> Acute and chronic phototoxicity

>> The science behind the AMD-phototoxicity debate

Intraocular lens (IOL) implantation became standard practice in the mid-1970s.[1] The clear polymethylmethacrylate (PMMA) IOLs in use then were shown in 1978 to transmit potentially harmful ultraviolet (UV) radiation to the retina.[2,3] UV-blocking IOLs were adopted widely in the 1980s.[4] A 1986 recommendation that IOLs block violet light in addition to UV radiation[4] was followed in the 1990s by introduction of IOLs that attenuated both UV and visible light.[5,6]

Retinal phototoxicity from environmental light exposure has been postulated to cause age-related macular degeneration (AMD).[2,7–15] This phototoxicity-AMD hypothesis remains unproven, but it has motivated manufacturers to attach light-absorbing chromophores to constituent monomers in IOL optics. Chromophores can decrease (attenuate, block, filter) IOL transmission of UV and visible optical radiation to the retina. IOLs that block visible radiation impose limits on the light available for vision and circadian photoentrainment,[16–18] thereby balancing pseudophakic photoreception with photoprotection. This chapter explores that balance and its impact on vision and health.

BACKGROUND

A pseudophake's retina is potentially vulnerable to damage from ultraviolet (UV) radiation ($\lambda < 400$ nm), visible light (400–700 nm) and infrared (IR) radiation ($\lambda > 700$ nm). Violet (400–440 nm) and blue (440–500 nm) light are the shortest wavelength regions of the visible spectrum.[17,19] The cornea shelters the eye against UV radiation shorter than 300 nm and IR radiation longer than 1400 nm.[20] The crystalline lens provides intraocular protection, shielding the retina from most UV radiation between 300 and 400 nm.[20–22] IOL chromophores are needed for pseudophakes to have UV protection comparable to that of the crystalline lens.[2,3]

Transmittance spectra describe the percentage of light of different wavelengths that passes through a lens, as shown in Figure 40-1. Phototoxicity action spectra characterize the relative hazardousness of photosensitizers or photopigments at different optical wavelengths, as shown in Figure 40-2.[16,23] Luminous efficiency spectra describe the relative effectiveness of different wavelengths in stimulating photopic, scotopic or circadian responses, as shown in Figure 40-3. Transmittance, phototoxicity and luminous efficiency spectra permit analysis of how IOL chromophores affect photoreception, photoprotection and IOL optical performance.[16]

IOLs can be divided into different classes based on their transmission spectra. UV-transmitting IOLs do not have optical radiation absorbing chromophores bound to their optic monomers.[4,16] Standard UV-blocking IOLs have chromophores that block UV radiation and possibly some additional violet light.[4,16] Blue-blocking IOLs have chromophores that block UV radiation and a substantial amount of violet and blue light.[16,18,24,25]

Intense light can cause acute photochemical retinal damage (photic retinopathy or retinal phototoxicity) at retinal temperature increases far too low for thermal retinal injury (retinal photocoagulation).[23,26] There are two classic types of acute retinal phototoxicity. Blue-green and UV-blue photic retinopathy[10,17,18,26–29] are archetypes of photopigment-mediated and photosensitizer-mediated retinal phototoxicity, respectively.[23] A photosensitizer is a substance that can generate potentially harmful reactive oxygen species when exposed to optical radiation of an appropriate wavelength.[23] UV-blue phototoxicity requires roughly 100 times more retinal irradiance than blue-green phototoxicity.[10,27–29] The two phototoxicities can be differentiated by their action spectra, as shown in Figure 40-2.

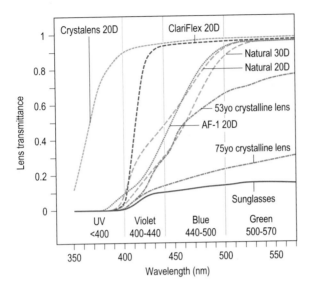

Figure 40-1 The spectral transmittance of UV-transmitting (Eyeonics Crystalens AT-45 20 D), UV-blocking (AMO ClariFlex 20D) and blue-blocking (Alcon AcrySof Natural SN60AT 20 D and 30 D; Hoya AF-1 20 D) intraocular lenses. Spectral transmittances are also shown for (1) neutral gray sunglasses (Sunglasses)[225] and (2) 53- and 75-year-old crystalline lenses.[20]

Blue-green (Noell-type, class 1 or white light) photic retinopathy was discovered in 1966.[30] Its action spectrum and the luminous efficiency spectrum of aphakic scotopic vision are similar because both processes are mediated by the rod photopigment rhodopsin.[30–33] Thus, any spectral filter that reduces acute blue-green phototoxicity produces an equivalent decrease in scotopic sensitivity. Figure 40-2 illustrates that blue-green phototoxicity

peaks at around 500 nm (blue-green) and decreases at shorter (blue) and longer (green) wavelengths. A static IOL spectral filter that substantially reduces the risk of blue-green phototoxicity would produce significant decreases in scotopic, mesopic and photopic photoreception.

UV-blue (Ham-type, class 2 or "blue light hazard") photic retinopathy was discovered 10 years later in 1976.[10,15,28,34–36] One of its primary mediators is lipofuscin, a photosensitizer in the retinal pigment epithelium (RPE).[13,15,23,37] Figure 40-2 shows that the severity of UV-blue phototoxicity increases rapidly with decreasing wavelength, similar to the action spectrum of lipofuscin. Therefore, UV radiation is much more hazardous than violet light, which is much more hazardous than blue light. Figure 40-2 also shows that macular xanthophyll protection is highest in blue light but decreases rapidly in the violet part of the spectrum where all-*trans*-retinal and lipofuscin phototoxicity increase and porphyrin phototoxicity peaks.[38–42] Thus, photosensitizer phototoxicity is maximal in the UV and violet part of the spectrum where intraretinal protection from macular xanthophyll is least effective.[16,23]

There are three classes of retinal photoreceptors:

1. Cone photoreceptors, which are responsible for photopic (bright light) and contribute to mesopic (intermediate light) vision[43–45]

2. Rod photoreceptors, which contribute to mesopic and provide scotopic (dim light) vision[32,33,46]

3. Retinal ganglion photoreceptors, which contribute to pupillary light response, unconscious circadian photoreception and perhaps even to conscious vision.[47–50] There are three types of cone photoreceptors: short-, middle-, and long-wavelength-sensitive cones which have peak spectral sensitivities around 420 nm (S-cone), 530 nm (M-cone) and 560 nm (L-cone), respectively.[43,45,51]

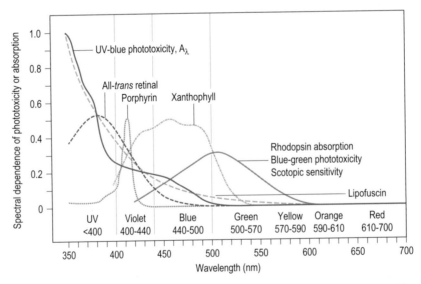

Figure 40-2 Acute UV-blue[34, 35, 53] (A_λ) and lipofuscin[13,15] phototoxicity rise rapidly in the violet part of the spectrum, where all-*trans*-retinal phototoxicity increases,[42] porphyrin phototoxicity peaks[13, 41] and intraretinal protection from macular xanthophyll decreases.[38] The potential hazardousness of acute UV-blue phototoxicity increases with decreasing wavelength, so UV radiation is more hazardous than violet light, which is more hazardous than blue light. Acute blue-green retinal phototoxicity has an action spectrum similar to aphakic scotopic sensitivity because rhodopsin mediates both processes.[30–33] Its action spectrum peaks around 500 nm (blue-green) and decreases at shorter and longer wavelengths, as depicted in this figure by the absorption spectrum of rhodopsin.[226] The curves illustrate spectral dependence but their magnitudes can not be compared directly.

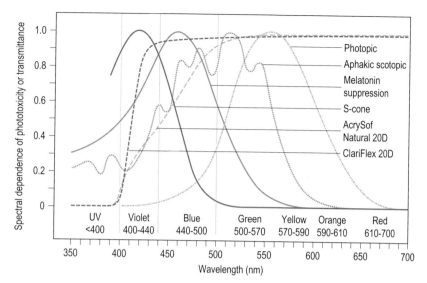

Figure 40-3 S-cone ($\lambda_{max} \sim 420$ nm),[43,45] melatonin suppression ($\lambda_{max} \sim 460$ nm),[47,48,52] aphakic scotopic ($\lambda_{max} \sim 500$ nm)[33] and photopic ($\lambda_{max} \sim 555$ nm)[38] spectral sensitivities. Original rather than curve-fitted aphakic scotopic luminous efficiency data are shown. The curves illustrate spectral dependence but their magnitudes can not be compared directly. The spectral transmittances of UV-blocking (AMO ClariFlex 20D) and blue-blocking (Alcon AcrySof Natural SN60AT 20D) IOLs are also shown.

As shown in Figure 40-3, blue-blocking IOLs affect S-cone, circadian and rod photoreception[16-18] because of their peak spectral sensitivities of roughly 420 nm (violet),[43] 460 nm (blue),[47,48,52] and 500 nm (blue-green),[32,33] respectively.

■ SPECTRAL FILTERING ■

The spectral transmittance of IOLs in air or water can be measured directly with a spectrophotometer. Figure 40-1 presents the transmittances in water of (1) UV-transmitting, (2) UV-blocking, and (3) blue-blocking IOLs.[16] UV-transmitting and UV-blocking IOLs have a clear appearance, whereas blue-blocking IOLs have a yellowish appearance.

The international consensus standard A_λ phototoxicity function[53] shown in Figure 40-2 is used widely to estimate the risk of acute industrial retinal phototoxicity. It is based on acute UV-blue photic retinopathy studies in young dilated monkeys performed with brilliant light exposures from lasers or powerful xenon lamps equivalent to those used in the classical Zeiss photocoagulator.[34,54] UV radiation, violet light and blue light account for 67, 18 and 14% of potential pseudophakic UV-blue phototoxicity, respectively.[16,17]

The effect of different IOLs or crystalline lenses on photoprotection or photoreception can be estimated by multiplying phototoxicity[53] (Figure 40-2), aphakic scotopic sensitivity[33] (Figure 40-3) and circadian photoreception (melatonin suppression sensitivity)[48,52] (Figure 40-3) wavelength-by-wavelength with the spectral transmittance of an IOL or a crystalline lens of a particular age (Figure 40-1).[16] Table 40-1 shows the percentage difference between the performance of each IOL and a standard UV-blocking IOL.[16] If chronic light exposure does

play some role in AMD, its action spectrum is unknown may differ from that of acute UV-blue phototoxicity (A_λ).

■ PHOTOTOXICITY AND AMD ■

AMD is a complex multifactorial process. Smoking and age are the only AMD risk factors documented consistently in different populations.[55-63] Postulated mechanisms for the pathogenesis of AMD include RPE dysfunction with subsequent basal laminar deposits,[56] decreased choroidal perfusion,[64] genetic defects,[65] retinoid deficiency,[66,67] inflammation[68,69] and phototoxicity from environmental light exposure.[2,7-15] The phototoxicity-AMD hypothesis posits that: (1) repeated environmental light exposure causes chronic photochemical retinal damage in the human retina, and (2) this phototoxic damage is a significant risk factor for AMD.[2,7-15,23]

An important failure of the phototoxicity-AMD hypothesis is its lack of supporting epidemiological evidence despite two decades of careful study: 9 of the 11 major epidemiological studies examining the hypothesis failed to support it. Two population-based studies did find an association between AMD and environmental light exposure,[70,71] but five other large population-based investigations did not,[58,72-75] including a study by Taylor[58] who directed the earlier positive Waterman study.[70] Four large case-control studies failed to correlate light exposure with AMD,[76-79] one of which found that sunlight exposure was actually higher in controls than AMD subjects.[78] If there were a strong correlation between environmental light exposure and AMD, these large epidemiological studies should have provided convincing evidence of its existence. Their failure to do so may be due to: (1) the possibility that environmental light exposure is not a significant cause of AMD, (2) an inherent difficulty

Table 40-1 Photoprotection and photoreception relative to the UV-blocking ClariFlex 20D IOL: positive and negative percentages indicate better and worse performance, respectively.[16]

	UV-Blue Photoprotection	Aphakic Scotopic Sensitivity†	Melatonin Suppression
Eyeonics Crystalens AT-45	−150%	+10%	+14%
AMO ClariFlex 20D	–	–	–
Hoya AF-1	+43%	−15%	−27%
Alcon AcrySof Natural 20D	+40%	−14%	−27%
Alcon AcrySof Natural 30D	+57%	−21%	−38%
4.5 year old*	+35%	−24%	−30%
53 year old*	+61%	−37%	−48%
75 year old*	+82%	−76%	−80%
Sunglasses**	+89%	−86%	−100%

†The percentage loss in aphakic scotopic sensitivity is the same as the percentage gain in blue-green phototoxicity protection (the rod photopigment rhodopsin mediates both processes)[16]
*Human crystalline lens spectral transmittance data from Boettner and Wolter[20]
**Sunglasses spectral transmittance data from Marmor[225]

in accurately estimating a subject's cumulative light exposure, or (3) other factors such as variable genetic susceptibility that obfuscate already weak correlations.

There is still no convincing evidence to prove or disprove an association between cataract surgery and AMD.[80] The Beaver Dam and Blue Mountain Eye Studies found that cataract surgery was correlated with late AMD,[81–83] but the Age-Related Eye Disease Study[84] and recent Swiss,[85] Chinese[86] and German studies did not.[87] If there were an association between cataract surgery and AMD, it is probably due to shared risk factors or the physiological effects of intraocular surgery.[16,83,88]

Early interest in the phototoxicity-AMD hypothesis was generated by a 1920 report that the presence of cataract decreases the risk of AMD.[7] Later studies found that AMD risks actually increase with cataract formation.[81,88] Interest in the phototoxicity-AMD hypothesis has been sustained by studies showing that the photosensitizer lipofuscin accumulates with aging in the retinal pigment epithelium (RPE).[89–91] Photic retinopathy and AMD both involve oxidative stress,[13,15,92,93] but that doesn't mean that phototoxicity causes AMD any more than it means that AMD causes retinal phototoxicity.

It is reasonable to use IOL chromophores to prevent UV radiation from reaching the retina because UV radiation is potentially harmful and not useful visually. Nonetheless, there is little evidence to document the clinical value of UV-blocking chromophores, despite their widespread use for more than 2 decades. Indeed, the widely-marketed Eyeonics Crystalens is a UV-transmitting IOL (cf., Figure 40-1). No histopathologic difference in macular aging or degeneration was found in eyes with UV-transmitting or UV-blocking IOLs.[94] One study reported that UV-blocking IOLs reduce postoperative cystoid macular edema,[95] but three later studies refuted that conclusion.[96–98]

UV-blocking IOLs have been reported to reduce the incidence of pseudophakic erythropsia, a transient reddish visual discoloration that can occur after exposure to a bright outdoor environment.[99,100] A vitreous fluorophotometry study showed that blood–retinal barrier disruption is decreased in eyes with UV-only or blue-blocking IOLs in comparison to UV-transmitting IOLs,[101] but the significance of this finding is uncertain because there were no associated retinal abnormalities and IOL chromophores themselves can affect fluorophotometric measurements. Short-wave cone sensitivity was studied in eight bilateral pseudophakes with a UV-blocking IOL in one eye and a UV-transmitting IOL in their contralateral eye.[102] The UV-blocking IOL had better sensitivity in six of the eight subjects, but again no retinal abnormalities were observed,[102] and the finding may represent visual adaptation rather than hypothetical photic injury.

Acute UV-blue and RPE lipofuscin phototoxicities increase with decreasing wavelength,[34,53] so it is not surprising that short wavelength blocking filters decrease the risk of acute phototoxic injury in RPE cell culture and animal experiments.[103,104] Acute retinal phototoxicity experiments and the phototoxicity-AMD hypothesis have been used as a rationale for blue-blocking IOLs, however, despite the fact that AMD is a chronic process, whereas experimental photic retinopathy occurs only when retinal defenses are acutely overwhelmed by abnormally high light exposures. Acute phototoxicity can injure the retina but it can not simulate AMD, just as staring at the sun can scar the fovea but it can not simulate a lifetime of normal environmental light exposure.[16] In the United States, the Centers for Medicare and Medicaid Services concluded in 2005 that "the relationship between blue light and AMD is speculative and not proven by available evidence."[105] In the absence of proven efficacy, use of blue-blocking IOL chromophores does not represent evidence-based medicine.

Pupillary area and crystalline lens transmittance decrease progressively with aging, reducing retinal illuminance and phototoxic risks. If age-related increases in RPE cell phototoxicity[15,37] are taken into consideration in addition to age-related decreases in crystalline lens transmittance[15,106] and pupil area,[107,108] then 20–30 year olds have the highest risk of acute retinal phototoxicity, as shown in Figure 40-4. When phototoxic risks are

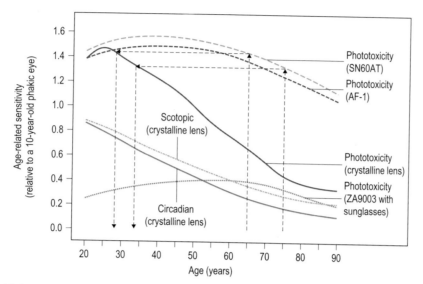

Figure 40-4 Acute UV-blue retinal phototoxicity risk, scotopic sensitivity (rod photoreception) and circadian photoreception (melatonin suppression) for phakic eyes ("crystalline lens") relative to a 10-year-old phakic eye, taking into consideration age-related (1) decreases in crystalline lens transmittance[106] and pupil area[107,108] and (2) increases in RPE cell phototoxicity[37] due to accumulating lipofuscin. Age-related phototoxicity risks are also shown for pseudophakic eyes with (1) 20 D blue-blocking IOLs (Alcon AcrySof Natural SN60AT and Hoya AF-1) and (2) 20 D UV-blocking IOLs (AMO Tecnis ZA9003) combined with sunglasses.[225] The dashed lines show that when acute phototoxic risks are compared for pseudophakic and phakic eyes, 65- and 75-year-old pseudophakes with a 20 D blue-blocking SN60AT IOL have equivalent ocular ages (EOAs) of 28- and 34-year-old phakic adults, respectively. The UV-blocking IOL with sunglasses combination provides better age-matched protection than phakic eyes or blue-blocking IOLs. Important caveats include the facts that (1) nine of the 11 major epidemiological studies found no correlation between environmental light exposure and AMD, (2) acute phototoxicity experiments can not simulate AMD, and (3) if hypothetical chronic retinal phototoxicity does occur, its action spectrum is unknown.

compared for phakic and pseudophakic eyes, 65- and 75-year-old pseudophakes with a 20 D blue-blocking IOL have equivalent ocular ages (EOAs) of 28- and 34-year-old phakic adults, respectively (Figure 40-4).

Blue-blocking IOLs reduce light useful for photoreception, as will be discussed below. In return, as shown in Table 40-1, they provide 50% less acute UV-blue photoprotection than sunglasses and 20% less photoprotection than 53-year-old crystalline lenses. Most AMD occurs in phakic adults over 60 years of age.[63,109] Thus, if light is a risk factor for AMD in some older adults, then sunglasses should be worn in bright environments because blue-blocking IOLs provide less photoprotection than younger crystalline lenses that don't prevent AMD.[16,26] An important difference between sunglasses and blue-blocking IOLs, however, is that people can remove their sunglasses when they choose to do so for optimal scotopic or circadian photoreception. Spectral filtering IOLs and sunglasses alone or in combination do not protect pseudophakes against acute injuries from direct solar or welding arc observation.[110,111]

■ PHOTOTOXICITY AND MELANOMA ■

Exposure to ultraviolet radiation is an important environmental risk factor in the oncogenesis of cutaneous melanoma, but photocarcinogenesis is not retinal phototoxicity. Photocarcinogenesis is caused primarily by DNA damage and mutations due to UV-B ($280 < \lambda < 320$ nm) radiation,[112,113] whereas photic retinopathy is typically caused by apoptosis from longer wavelength UV-A ($320 < \lambda < 400$ nm) radiation and visible light.[23]

The use of blue-blocking IOLs was advocated in a study reporting that decreasing violet and blue light reduces uveal melanoma cell culture proliferation stimulated by intense, 12-h short-wavelength-light exposures.[114] Six other reports in the medical literature found, however, that blue light inhibits the growth of melanoma and leukemia cells in vitro.[115,116] Regardless of these studies' relative merits, there is no evidence that blue-blocking IOLs reduce the risk of choroidal melanoma in human beings. Indeed, the medical literature does not support a significant role for sunlight in the pathogenesis of uveal melanoma.[117,118] Additionally, recent epidemiological evidence shows that the incidence of uveal melanoma actually increases with decreasing solar exposure,[119] consistent with the long reported inverse relationship between solar UV-B and non-skin cancer mortality, which may be mediated by the beneficial effects of vitamin D.[120,121]

■ PHOTOPIC VISION ■

Cone photoreceptors are responsible for photopic vision.[38,122] Normal cone photoreception and subsequent neural processing provide a remarkable constancy in the apparent color of an object despite changes in the circumstances under which it is viewed.[19,123–125] For example, people with normal color vision can properly distinguish traffic signal colors through different sunglass tints in different lighting situations. Additionally, (1) the spectral sensitivity of phakic and aphakic photopic vision is similar despite crystalline lens blockage of shorter wavelength light[126] and (2) the appearance of color returns largely to normal within a few months of implantation of a UV-blocking IOL, despite the IOL's increased transmittance of shorter wavelength light.[127] In general, most people adjust satisfactorily to vision with UV-transmitting, UV-blocking or blue-blocking IOLs.

Clinical D-15 and FM 100-hue tests do not detect color vision abnormalities in pseudophakes with blue-blocking or standard UV-blocking IOLs.[128–134] Nonetheless, (1) color disparity problems required explanation of a blue-blocking IOL in an individual with a UV-blocking IOL in the contralateral eye,[135,136] (2) 20 D and 30 D blue-blocking IOLs reduce light transmittance by 65% and 80%, respectively, at the 420 nm peak sensitivity of S-cones (vs. only a 20% reduction with a UV-blocking IOL), (3) tritan defects with blue-blocking filters can be demonstrated with a Moreland anomaloscope in pseudophakes,[137] (4) blue-blocking IOLs are not recommended for United States Air Force aircrew because of operational color vision requirements,[137] and (5) blue-blocking IOLs reduce photopic luminance contrast.[138]

Blue-blocking IOLs do not improve clinical contrast sensitivity in comparison to UV-blocking IOLs[129–131,133] because the photopic performance of a pseudophakic eye is determined at medium and high spatial frequencies primarily by wavelengths between 500 and 600 nm that are focused better on the retina than shorter or longer wavelengths.[139] Thus, wavelengths shorter than 500 nm contribute little to medium or fine detail modulation transfer, accounting for the failure of blue-blocking chromophores to improve photopic pseudophakic contrast sensitivity significantly.[131,139] There is also no improvement in disability glare because blue-blocking filters reduce target luminance by the same proportion as veiling luminance from the glare source.[140]

MESOPIC AND SCOTOPIC VISION

Spectral filters affect rod photoreception, which is responsible for scotopic (dim light) and contributes to mesopic (intermediate light) vision.[38,122] Rod photoreceptors even influence cone-mediated visual function at photopic (bright light) luminances.[141–144] Blue light (400–440 nm) provides 35% of aphakic scotopic sensitivity and 7% of photopic sensitivity.[16] Thus, blue light is much more important for vision in dim- than bright-light environments. In comparison, potentially more hazardous violet light provides only 10% of scotopic and 1% of aphakic photopic sensitivity.[16]

Rod photoreceptor mediated vision is important in daily life. Cone photoreceptors image headlight illuminated objects during night driving, but rod photoreceptors provide the remaining visual field.[145,146] Driving, mobility and peripheral vision problems are all associated with rod-mediated but not cone-mediated dark adaptation parameters.[147] When you get up in the middle of night and lighting is too dim to see color in objects, you are using rod-mediated vision.

Scotopic sensitivity and other rod-mediated visual functions decline with aging because (1) rod photoreceptor sensitivity and populations decrease,[55,148–152] (2) crystalline lens yellowing reduces transmission of blue light to the retina,[21,106,153] and (3) decreasing pupil size reduces retinal illumination.[108,154] Figure 40-4 shows the age-related decline in rod sensitivity due to optical factors. These optical factors decrease effective scotopic retinal illuminances for 65- and 75-year-old phakic eyes to only 37 and 26% of 10-year-old phakic eyes, respectively. Aarnisalo

demonstrated that filtering out blue and violet light reduces scotopic sensitivity.[155] UV-blocking IOLs provide equivalent ocular ages for rod photoreception roughly 15 years younger than blue-blocking IOLs. A recent study showed that AcrySof Natural IOL pseudophakes have decreased scotopic vision at violet and blue wavelengths;[156] a type of vision loss correlated with night driving difficulties.[157]

Table 40-1 shows that a 20 D UV-blocking IOL provides 37% better scotopic sensitivity than a 53-year-old crystalline lens. In comparison, blue-blocking IOLs offer 14–21% less scotopic sensitivity than a UV-blocking IOL. A 14–21% loss of scotopic sensitivity is difficult to measure clinically and small compared to the broad range of visual sensitivity.[158,159] Nonetheless, (1) it is a decrease in sensitivity, (2) standard static perimetric tests are poor surrogates for tasks performed in dim illumination such as ambulation and driving, (3) scotopic vision deficits are worse in people with AMD and diabetic retinopathy,[160–164] (4) decreased night vision is a significant problem for older adults prompting many to curtail nighttime activities, such as driving,[165–170] and (5) impaired dark adaptation increases older adults' risks of falling.[171] Forty percent of people over 65 years of age fall each year,[172] increasing their risk of debilitating injury, long-term hospitalization and death.[173]

CIRCADIAN PHOTOENTRAINMENT

Spectral filters also affect unconscious circadian photoreception, which is essential for good physical and mental health, because it adjusts (photoentrains) our body to environmental day–night cycles.[16,174] Circadian photoreception is mediated by blue-light sensitive retinal ganglion photoreceptors that were discovered in 2002 and comprise roughly 1% of all human retinal ganglion cells.[47,48,175–177] Axons of retinal ganglion cells controlling conscious vision synapse in the lateral geniculate nuclei of the thalamus. Axons of retinal ganglion photoreceptors synapse primarily in nonvisual nuclei including the paired suprachiasmatic nuclei of the hypothalamus, which constitute the human body's master biological clock.[178–180]

The suprachiasmatic nuclei control melatonin production by the pineal gland, synchronizing hormonal, metabolic and physiologic processes to diurnal and seasonal rhythms. The biological advantage of circadian rhythmicity is that it permits the body to anticipate and prepare for essential daily activities. For example, it takes time to upregulate protein synthesis and increase blood sugar, heart rate and blood pressure before dawn.[16,174] Suprachiasmatic nuclei have their own intrinsic periodicity, so the biological advantages of circadian rhythmicity would be lost without effective photoentrainment of the suprachiasmatic nuclei to external environmental diurnal rhythms.

Melatonin is an important hormone in circadian rhythmicity. It conveys timing information from the suprachiasmatic nuclei, helping synchronize peripheral clocks throughout the human body. Melatonin itself is an important anti-oxidant, anti-cancer and anti-aging hormone.[178–184] It may even help protect the RPE against the oxidative stresses involved in AMD.[185–187] Melatonin is secreted by the pineal gland at a specific time in the daily cycle, facilitating sleepiness, which is accompanied by reduced core body temperature.[178,179,188] Bright-light suppresses melatonin secretion, increasing core temperature, alertness and cognition.[189–192] Nocturnal suppression of melatonin synthesis by light is a widely used proxy for the function of suprachiasmatic nuclei. Effective blue-light exposure is crucial in synchronizing melatonin suppression to environmental day–night cycles. The response of melatonin to light exposure parallels circadian and retinal ganglion photoreception,[176,177,193] and blue light optimally promotes alertness and good cognition in comparison to longer wavelengths.[194]

Circadian photoreception (melatonin suppression) has a characteristic spectral efficiency that peaks in the blue part of the spectrum at 460 nm, as shown in Figure 40-3. This blue-light dependence arises because retinal ganglion photoreceptors utilize the blue-light sensitive photopigment melanopsin.[47,48,178,179,195,196] Blue light provides 55% of melatonin suppression. As shown in Table 40-1, conventional UV-blocking IOLs provide 48% better circadian sensitivity than a 53-year-old lens, but blue-blocking chromophores offer 27–38% less sensitivity than UV-blocking IOLs.[16]

Circadian rhythmicity is often disturbed in older adults and people with insomnia, depression and memory loss.[197–199] Circadian dysfunction occurs in many clinical disorders including coronary artery disease and hypertension,[200–202] diabetes,[203,204] Alzheimer's disease,[205–207] multiple sclerosis,[208,209] and numerous forms of cancer.[210–212] Health-care risks are correlated with both the degree and duration of circadian disruption. Numerous clinical studies have shown the risks of disturbed circadian photoentrainment and the benefits of optimal rhythmicity.[213–216]

Blindness has widespread physiological effects. Light can not suppress melatonin in people without ganglion, rod and cone photoreception. Thus, melatonin levels are higher and cancer risks lower in total photoreceptive blindness because of melatonin's anti-cancer properties.[217–219] Nonetheless, overall life expectancy is decreased, probably due to the adverse effects of chronic cortisol elevation associated with circadian dysfunction. Even mild visual impairment doubles mortality risks.[220] Cataract itself is associated with poorer survival not explained by "traditional" risk factors. Circadian dysfunction may be an important non-traditional risk factor.

Age-related pupillary miosis[107,108] and natural crystalline lens aging[106] limit the blue light needed for retinal ganglion photoreceptors, contributing to circadian dysfunction and its systemic consequences.[221] These optical factors reduce the effective circadian retinal illuminance of 65- and 75-year-old phakic eyes to only 27 and 17% of that of 10-year-old phakic eyes, respectively (cf., Figure 40-4). Age-related losses in retinal ganglion photoreceptor sensitivity may also occur, although pertinent data currently are not available. If circadian photoreception is compared in phakic and pseudophakic eyes, UV-blocking IOLs provide equivalent ocular ages for circadian photoreception 15–20 years younger than blue-blocking IOLs, as shown in Figure 40-5. Less light is the likely cause of decreased melatonin suppression in older adults and some elderly sedentary lifestyles may provide only half the total daily luminance of young adults.[222]

Retinal ganglion cell photoreception is not conscious, so its decline can not be recognized directly. Fortunately, light therapy and cataract surgery can help. Light therapy has been shown to reduce insomnia and return peak nocturnal melatonin levels of older adults to youthful levels.[222] Cataract surgery has also been shown to decrease insomnia and daytime sleepiness.[223,224] Thus, improved retinal ganglion photoreception is an important consideration in cataract surgery, extending its potential benefits beyond better vision to improved systemic and mental health and increased longevity.

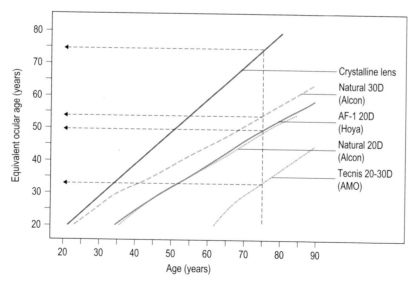

Figure 40-5 Equivalent phakic ocular ages for circadian photoreception in pseudophakic eyes with blue-blocking (Alcon AcrySof Natural SN60AT and Hoya AF-1) or UV-blocking (AMO Tecnis ZA9003) intraocular lenses (IOLs). Results take into consideration age-related decreases in crystalline lens transmittance[106] and pupil area.[107,108] UV-blocking IOLs provide equivalent ocular ages 15–20 years younger than blue-blocking IOLs. For example, the dashed line shows that 75-year-old pseudophakes have equivalent phakic ocular ages of 54, 50, and 33 with 30 D blue-blocking, 20 D blue-blocking, and 20 or 30 D UV-blocking IOLs, respectively.

■ CONCLUSION ■

Most contemporary IOLs utilize UV-blocking chromophores, but UV-transmitting IOLs are still being used, and blue-blocking IOLs have been introduced in recent years. Blue light is needed for good vision in dim environments. Bright, well-timed blue-light exposure is essential for circadian photoreception, which helps assure optimal physical and mental health.[174] Age-related crystalline lens yellowing and pupillary miosis restrict the blue light reaching an older adults' retina.[52] Blue-blocking IOLs permanently limit this short wavelength light needed for scotopic, mesopic, S-cone and circadian photoreception. UV-blocking IOLs provide substantially better rod and circadian photoreceptor function than 53-year-old crystalline lenses.[16]

Current blue-blocking IOLs sacrifice some of the improved photoreception of UV-blocking IOLs to increase protection against acute UV-blue phototoxicity in an effort to reduce the hypothetical risk of AMD. CMS concluded, however, that "the relationship between blue light and AMD is speculative and not proven by available evidence."[105] This conclusion is probably based on the facts that (1) large epidemiological studies have failed repeatedly to provide convincing evidence of a link between environmental light exposure and AMD, and (2) there is no clinical or experimental proof that normal light exposure or repetitive acute phototoxicity causes AMD. Furthermore, current blue-blocking IOLs provide less protection than young crystalline lenses which do not prevent AMD.

After 3.5 billion years of evolution on Earth, life is well adapted to its blue sky. Cataract surgery is a once-in-a-lifetime opportunity for patients to overcome natural aging and obtain better circadian rhythmicity and vision in dim light. Cataract surgery is performed to improve a patient's vision and quality of life. Ophthalmologists improve conscious visual photoreception with cataract surgery. Improving unconscious blue-light dependent circadian photoreception extends the benefits of cataract surgery beyond conscious, image-based vision to improved health and longevity.

REFERENCES

[1] Apple DJ, Sims J. Harold Ridley and the invention of the intraocular lens. Surv Ophthalmol 1996;40:279–292.

[2] Mainster MA. Solar retinitis, photic maculopathy and the pseudophakic eye. J Am Intraocul Implant Soc 1978;4:84–86.

[3] Mainster MA. Spectral transmittance of intraocular lenses and retinal damage from intense light sources. Am J Ophthalmol 1978;85:167–170.

[4] Mainster MA. The spectra, classification, and rationale of ultraviolet-protective intraocular lenses. Am J Ophthalmol 1986;102:727–732.

[5] Ishida M, Yanashima K, Miwa M, Hozumi S, Okisaka S. Influence of the yellow-tinted intraocular lens on spectral sensitivity. Nippon Ganka Gakkai Zasshi 1994;98:192–196.

[6] Yokoyama Y, Iwamoto H, Yamanaka A. Blue light-filtering foldable acrylic intraocular lens. J Artif Organs 2006;9:71–76.

[7] van der Hoeve J. Eye lesions produced by light rich in ultraviolet rays: senile cataract, senile degeneration of the macula. Am J Ophthalmol 1920;3:178–194.

[8] Ts'o MO, La Piana FG, Appleton B. The human fovea after sungazing. Trans Am Acad Ophthalmol Otolaryngol 1974;78:OP–677.

[9] Young RW. A theory of central retinal disease. In: Sears ML, editor. New directions in ophthalmic research. New Haven, Conn: Yale University Press; 1981. p. 237–270.

[10] Mainster MA. Light and macular degeneration: a biophysical and clinical perspective. Eye 1987;1:304–310.

[11] Marshall J. The ageing retina: physiology or pathology. Eye 1987;1:282–295.

[12] Reme C, Reinboth J, Clausen M, Hafezi F. Light damage revisited: converging evidence, diverging views? Graefes Arch Clin Exp Ophthalmol 1996;234:2–11.

[13] Boulton M, Rozanowska M, Rozanowski B. Retinal photodamage. J Photochem Photobiol B 2001;64:144–161.

[14] Burkle A. Mechanisms of ageing. Eye 2001;15:371–375.

[15] Margrain TH, Boulton M, Marshall J, Sliney DH. Do blue light filters confer protection against age-related macular degeneration? Prog Retin Eye Res 2004;23:523–531.

[16] Mainster MA. Violet and blue light blocking intraocular lenses: photoprotection versus photoreception. Br J Ophthalmol 2006;90:784–792.

[17] Mainster MA. Intraocular lenses should block UV radiation and violet but not blue light. Arch Ophthalmol 2005;123:550–555.

[18] Mainster MA, Sparrow JR. How much blue light should an IOL transmit? Br J Ophthalmol 2003;87:1523–1529.

[19] Pokorny J, Smith VC, Verriest G, Pinckers AJLG. Congenital and acquired color vision defects. New York: Grune & Stratton; 1979.

[20] Boettner EA, Wolter JR. Transmission of the ocular media. Invest Ophthalmol 1962;1:776–783.

[21] van Norren D, Vos JJ. Spectral transmission of the human ocular media. Vision Res 1974;14:1237–1244.

[22] Mellerio J. Yellowing of the human lens: nuclear and cortical contributions. Vision Res 1987;27:1581–1587.

[23] Mainster MA, Boulton M. Retinal phototoxicity. In: Albert DM, Miller JW, Blodi BA, Azar DT, editors. Principles and practice of ophthalmology. 3rd ed. London, UK: Elsevier; 2008. p. 2195–2205.

[24] Ernest PH. Light-transmission-spectrum comparison of foldable intraocular lenses. J Cataract Refract Surg 2004;30:1755–1758.

[25] Davison JA, Patel AS. Light normalizing intraocular lenses. Int Ophthalmol Clin 2005;45:55–106.

[26] Mainster MA, Turner PL. Retinal injuries from light: mechanisms, hazards and prevention. In: Ryan SJ, Hinton DR, Schachat AP, Wilkinson P, editors. Retina. 4th ed. London, UK: Elsevier; 2006. p. 1857–1870.

[27] Kremers JJ, van Norren D. Two classes of photochemical damage of the retina. Lasers Light Ophthalmol 1988;2:41–52.

[28] Mellerio J. Light effects on the retina. In: Albert DM, Jakobiec FA, editors. Principles and practice of ophthalmology, 1 vol. Philadelphia: W. B. Saunders Company; 1994. p. 1326–1345.

[29] Gorgels TG, Van Norren D. Two spectral types of retinal light damage occur in albino as well as in pigmented rat: no essential role for melanin. Exp Eye Res 1998;66:155–162.

[30] Noell WK, Walker VS, Kang BS, Berman S. Retinal damage by light in rats. Invest Ophthalmol 1966;5:450–473.

[31] Noell WK. Possible mechanisms of photoreceptor damage by light in mammalian eyes. Vision Res 1980;20:1163–1171.

[32] Wald G. Human vision and the spectrum. Science 1945;101:653–658.

[33] Griswold MS, Stark WS. Scotopic spectral sensitivity of phakic and aphakic observers extending into the near ultraviolet. Vision Res 1992;32:1739–1743.

[34] Ham Jr WT, Mueller HA, Sliney DH. Retinal sensitivity to damage from short wavelength light. Nature 1976;260:153–155.

[35] Ham Jr WT, Ruffolo Jr JJ, Mueller HA, Guerry 3rd D. The nature of retinal radiation damage: dependence on wavelength, power level and exposure time. Vision Res 1980;20:1105–1111.

[36] Reme CE, Grimm C, Hafezi F, Iseli HP, Wenzel A. Why study rod cell death in retinal degenerations and how? Doc Ophthalmol 2003;106:25–29.

[37] Rozanowska M, Jarvis-Evans J, Korytowski W, Boulton ME, Burke JM, Sarna T. Blue light-induced reactivity of retinal age pigment. In vitro generation of oxygen-reactive species. J Biol Chem 1995;270:18825–18830.

[38] Wyszecki G, Stiles WS. Color science. 2nd ed. New York: John Wiley & Sons, Inc; 1982.

[39] Pease PL, Adams AJ, Nuccio E. Optical density of human macular pigment. Vision Res 1987;27:705–710.

[40] Werner JS, Donnelly SK, Kliegl R. Aging and human macular pigment density. Appended with translations from the work of Max Schultze and Ewald Hering. Vision Res 1987;27:257–268.

[41] Anderson HL. Building molecular wires from the colours of life: conjugated porphyrin oligomers. Chem Commun 1999;9:2323–2330.

[42] Rozanowska M, Sarna T. Light-induced damage to the retina: role of rhodopsin chromophore revisited. Photochem Photobiol 2005;81:1305–1330.

[43] Merbs SL, Nathans J. Absorption spectra of human cone pigments. Nature 1992;356:433–435.

[44] Stockman A, Sharpe LT, Fach C. The spectral sensitivity of the human short-wavelength sensitive cones derived from thresholds and color matches. Vision Res 1999;39:2901–2927.

[45] Stockman A, Sharpe LT. The spectral sensitivities of the middle- and long-wavelength-sensitive cones derived from measurements in observers of known genotype. Vision Res 2000;40:1711–1737.

[46] Stockman A, Sharpe LT. Into the twilight zone: the complexities of mesopic vision and luminous efficiency. Ophthalmic Physiol Opt 2006;26:225–239.

[47] Brainard GC, Hanifin JP, Greeson JM, et al. Action spectrum for melatonin regulation in humans: evidence for a novel circadian photoreceptor. J Neurosci 2001;21:6405–6412.

[48] Thapan K, Arendt J, Skene DJ. An action spectrum for melatonin suppression: evidence for a novel non-rod, non-cone photoreceptor system in humans. J Physiol 2001;535:261–267.

[49] Hankins MW, Lucas RJ. The primary visual pathway in humans is regulated according to long-term light exposure through the action of a nonclassical photopigment. Curr Biol 2002;12:191–198.

[50] Dacey DM, Liao HW, Peterson BB, et al. Melanopsin-expressing ganglion cells in primate retina signal colour and irradiance and project to the LGN. Nature 2005;433:749–754.

[51] Stockman A, Sharpe LT, Merbs S, Nathans J. Spectral sensitivities of human cone visual pigments determined in vivo and in vitro. Methods Enzymol 2000;316:626–650.

[52] Charman WN. Age, lens transmittance, and the possible effects of light on melatonin suppression. Ophthalmic Physiol Opt 2003;23:181–187.

[53] ACGIH. Threshold limit values and biological exposure indices. Cincinnati, Ohio: American Conference of Governmental Industrial Hygienists; 2000.

[54] Ham Jr WT, Mueller HA, Ruffolo Jr JJ, Guerry 3rd D, Guerry RK. Action spectrum for retinal injury from near-ultraviolet radiation in the aphakic monkey. Am J Ophthalmol 1982;93:299–306.

[55] Curcio CA, Millican CL, Allen KA, Kalina RE. Aging of the human photoreceptor mosaic: evidence for selective vulnerability of rods in central retina. Invest Ophthalmol Vis Sci 1993;34:3278–3296.

[56] Spraul CW, Lang GE, Grossniklaus HE, Lang GK. Histologic and morphometric analysis of the choroid, Bruch's membrane, and retinal pigment epithelium in postmortem eyes with age-related macular degeneration and histologic examination of surgically excised choroidal neovascular membranes. Surv Ophthalmol 1999;44:S10–S32.

[57] Zarbin MA. Current concepts in the pathogenesis of age-related macular degeneration. Arch Ophthalmol 2004;122:598–614.

[58] McCarty CA, Mukesh BN, Fu CL, Mitchell P, Wang JJ, Taylor HR. Risk factors for age-related maculopathy: the Visual Impairment Project. Arch Ophthalmol 2001;119:1455–1462.

[59] Seddon JM, Ajani UA, Sperduto RD, et al. Dietary carotenoids, vitamins A, C, and E, and advanced age-related macular degeneration. Eye Disease Case-Control Study Group. JAMA 1994;272:1413–1420.

[60] Tso MO. Pathogenetic factors of aging macular degeneration. Ophthalmology 1985;92:628–635.

[61] Smith W, Mitchell P, Leeder SR. Smoking and age-related maculopathy. The Blue Mountains Eye Study. Arch Ophthalmol 1996;114:1518–1523.

[62] van Leeuwen R, Ikram MK, Vingerling JR, Witteman JC, Hofman A, de Jong PT. Blood pressure, atherosclerosis, and the incidence of age-related maculopathy: the Rotterdam Study. Invest Ophthalmol Vis Sci 2003;44:3771–3777.
[63] Evans JR, Fletcher AE, Wormald RP. 28,000 Cases of age related macular degeneration causing visual loss in people aged 75 years and above in the United Kingdom may be attributable to smoking. Br J Ophthalmol 2005;89:550–553.
[64] Friedman E. A hemodynamic model of the pathogenesis of age-related macular degeneration. Am J Ophthalmol 1997;124:677–682.
[65] Fan BJ, Tam PO, Choy KW, Wang DY, Lam DS, Pang CP. Molecular diagnostics of genetic eye diseases. Clin Biochem 2006;39:231–239.
[66] Curcio CA, Owsley C, Jackson GR. Spare the rods, save the cones in aging and age-related maculopathy. Invest Ophthalmol Vis Sci 2000;41:2015–2018.
[67] Curcio CA. Photoreceptor topography in ageing and age-related maculopathy. Eye 2001;15:376–383.
[68] Narayanan R, Butani V, Boyer DS, et al. Complement factor H polymorphism in age-related macular degeneration. Ophthalmology 2007;114:1327–1331.
[69] Schaumberg DA, Christen WG, Kozlowski P, Miller DT, Ridker PM, Zee RY. A prospective assessment of the Y402H variant in complement factor H, genetic variants in C-reactive protein, and risk of age-related macular degeneration. Invest Ophthalmol Vis Sci 2006;47:2336–2340.
[70] Taylor HR, West S, Munoz B, Rosenthal FS, Bressler SB, Bressler NM. The long-term effects of visible light on the eye. Arch Ophthalmol 1992;110:99–104.
[71] Tomany SC, Cruickshanks KJ, Klein R, Klein BE, Knudtson MD. Sunlight and the 10-year incidence of age-related maculopathy: the Beaver Dam Eye Study. Arch Ophthalmol 2004;122:750–757.
[72] Hirvela H, Luukinen H, Laara E, Sc L, Laatikainen L. Risk factors of age-related maculopathy in a population 70 years of age or older. Ophthalmology 1996;103:871–877.
[73] Delcourt C, Carriere I, Ponton-Sanchez A, Fourrey S, Lacroux A, Papoz L. Light exposure and the risk of age-related macular degeneration: the Pathologies Oculaires Liées à l'Age (POLA) study. Arch Ophthalmol 2001;119:1463–1468.
[74] Clemons TE, Milton RC, Klein R, Seddon JM, Ferris 3rd FL. Risk factors for the incidence of Advanced Age-Related Macular Degeneration in the Age-Related Eye Disease Study (AREDS) AREDS report no. 19. Ophthalmology 2005;112:533–539.
[75] Arnarsson A, Sverrisson T, Stefansson E, et al. Risk factors for five-year incident age-related macular degeneration: the Reykjavik Eye Study. Am J Ophthalmol 2006;142:419–428.
[76] Hyman LG, Lilienfeld AM, Ferris 3rd FL, Fine SL. Senile macular degeneration: a case-control study. Am J Epidemiol 1983;118:213–227.
[77] Risk factors for neovascular age-related macular degeneration. The Eye Disease Case-Control Study Group. Arch Ophthalmol 1992;110:1701–1708.
[78] Darzins P, Mitchell P, Heller RF. Sun exposure and age-related macular degeneration. An Australian case-control study. Ophthalmology 1997;104:770–776.
[79] Khan JC, Shahid H, Thurlby DA, et al. Age related macular degeneration and sun exposure, iris colour, and skin sensitivity to sunlight. Br J Ophthalmol 2006;90:29–32.
[80] Smith BT, Belani S, Ho AC. Light energy, cataract surgery, and progression of age-related macular degeneration. Curr Opin Ophthalmol 2005;16:166–169.
[81] Klein R, Klein BE, Wong TY, Tomany SC, Cruickshanks KJ. The association of cataract and cataract surgery with the long-term incidence of age-related maculopathy: the Beaver Dam eye study. Arch Ophthalmol 2002;120:1551–1558.
[82] de Jong PT, Lubsen J. The standard gamble between cataract extraction and AMD. Graefes Arch Clin Exp Ophthalmol 2004;242:103–105.
[83] Cugati S, Mitchell P, Rochtchina E, Tan AG, Smith W, Wang JJ. Cataract surgery and the 10-year incidence of age-related maculopathy: the Blue Mountains Eye Study. Ophthalmology 2006;113:2020–2025.
[84] Ferris 3rd FL. Discussion of a model of spectral filtering to reduce photochemical damage in age-related macular degeneration. Trans Am Ophthalmol Soc 2004;102:95.
[85] Sutter FK, Menghini M, Barthelmes D, et al. Is pseudophakia a risk factor for neovascular age-related macular degeneration? Invest Ophthalmol Vis Sci 2007;48:1472–1475.
[86] Xu L, Li Y, Zheng Y, Jonas JB. Associated factors for age related maculopathy in the adult population in China: the Beijing eye study. Br J Ophthalmol 2006;90:1087–1090.
[87] Baatz H, Darawsha R, Ackermann H, et al. Phacoemulsification does not induce neovascular age-related macular degeneration. Invest Ophthalmol Vis Sci 2008;49:1079–1083.
[88] Freeman EE, Munoz B, West SK, Tielsch JM, Schein OD. Is there an association between cataract surgery and age-related macular degeneration? Data from three population-based studies. Am J Ophthalmol 2003;135:849–856.
[89] Dorey CK, Wu G, Ebenstein D, Garsd A, Weiter JJ. Cell loss in the aging retina. Relationship to lipofuscin accumulation and macular degeneration. Invest Ophthalmol Vis Sci 1989;30:1691–1699.
[90] Delori FC, Goger DG, Dorey CK. Age-related accumulation and spatial distribution of lipofuscin in RPE of normal subjects. Invest Ophthalmol Vis Sci 2001;42:1855–1866.
[91] Sparrow JR, Boulton M. RPE lipofuscin and its role in retinal pathobiology. Exp Eye Res 2005;80:595–606.
[92] Winkler BS, Boulton ME, Gottsch JD, Sternberg P. Oxidative damage and age-related macular degeneration. Mol Vis 1999;5:32.
[93] Beatty S, Koh H, Phil M, Henson D, Boulton M. The role of oxidative stress in the pathogenesis of age-related macular degeneration. Surv Ophthalmol 2000;45:115–134.
[94] van der Schaft TL, Mooy CM, de Bruijn WC, Mulder PG, Pameyer JH, de Jong PT. Increased prevalence of disciform macular degeneration after cataract extraction with implantation of an intraocular lens. Br J Ophthalmol 1994;78:441–445.
[95] Kraff MC, Sanders DR, Jampol LM, Lieberman HL. Effect of an ultraviolet-filtering intraocular lens on cystoid macular edema. Ophthalmology 1985;92:366–369.
[96] Colin J, Ropars YM, Bonissent JF, Mimouni F. Cystoid macular oedema and intraocular lenses with ultraviolet filters. J Eur Implant Soc 1987;4:5–10.
[97] Clarke MP, Yap M, Weatherill JR. Do intraocular lenses with ultraviolet absorbing chromophores protect against macular oedema? Acta Ophthalmol (Copenh) 1989;67:593–596.
[98] Komatsu M, Kanagami S, Shimizu K. Ultraviolet-absorbing intraocular lens versus non-UV-absorbing intraocular lens: comparison of angiographic cystoid macular edema. J Cataract Refract Surg 1989;15:654–657.
[99] Jordan DR, Valberg JD. Dyschromatopsia following cataract surgery. Can J Ophthalmol 1986;21:140–143.
[100] Bennett LW. Pseudophakic erythropsia. J Am Optom Assoc 1994;65:273–276.
[101] Miyake K, Ichihashi S, Shibuya Y, Ota I, Miyake S, Terasaki H. Blood–retinal barrier and autofluorescence of the posterior polar retina in long-standing pseudophakia. J Cataract Refract Surg 1999;25:891–897.
[102] Werner JS, Steele VG, Pfoff DS. Loss of human photoreceptor sensitivity associated with chronic exposure to ultraviolet radiation. Ophthalmology 1989;96:1552–1558.
[103] Sparrow J, Miller AS, Zhou J. Blue light-absorbing intraocular lens and retinal pigment epithelium protection in vitro. J Cataract Refract Surg 2004;30:873–878.
[104] Wenzel ACG, Reme CE. Protective effect of the AcrySof Natural IOL on retinal damage induced by acute blue light in mice. Symposium on Cataract, IOL and Refractive Surgery, Abstract 2004;515:131.
[105] Centers-for-Medicare-&-Medicaid-Services. Medicare program: disapproval of adjustment in payment amounts for new technology intraocular lenses furnished by ambulatory surgical centers. Fed Regist 2005;70:15337–15340.
[106] Barker FM, Brainard GC. The direct spectral transmittance of the excised human lens as a function of age, FDA 785345-6. Washington, DC: US Food and Drug Administration; 1991.
[107] Yang HC, Chung SK, Baek NH. Decentration, tilt, and near vision of the array multifocal intraocular lens. J Cataract Refract Surg 2000;26:586–589.
[108] Loewenfeld IE. Pupillary changes related to age. In: Thompson HS, Daroff R, Frisen L, Glaser JS, Sanders MD, editors. Topics in neuro-ophthalmology. Baltimore, MD: Williams and Wilkins; 1979. p. 124–150.
[109] Seddon JM, Chen CA. Epidemiology of age-related macular degeneration. In: Ryan SJ, Hinton DR, Schachat AP, Wilkinson P, editors. Retina, 4th ed. 2 vol. London, UK: Elsevier Publishers; 2006. p. 1017–1027.
[110] Mainster MA, Ham Jr WT, Delori FC. Potential retinal hazards. Instrument and environmental light sources. Ophthalmology 1983;90:927–932.
[111] Mainster MA. Solar eclipse safety. Ophthalmology 1998;105:9–10.
[112] Gilchrest BA, Eller MS, Geller AC, Yaar M. The pathogenesis of melanoma induced by ultraviolet radiation. N Engl J Med 1999;340:1341–1348.
[113] Singh AD, Rennie IG, Seregard S, Giblin M, McKenzie J. Sunlight exposure and pathogenesis of uveal melanoma. Surv Ophthalmol 2004;49:419–428.
[114] Marshall JC, Gordon KD, McCauley CS, de Souza Filho JP, Burnier MN. The effect of blue light exposure and use of intraocular lenses on human uveal melanoma cell lines. Melanoma Res 2006;16:537–541.
[115] Ohara M, Kawashima Y, Katoh O, Watanabe H. Blue light inhibits the growth of B16 melanoma cells. Jpn J Cancer Res 2002;93:551–558.
[116] Ohara M, Kawashima Y, Watanabe H, Kitajima S. Effects of blue-light-exposure on growth of extracorporeally circulated leukemic cells in rats with leukemia induced by 1-ethyl-1-nitrosourea. Int J Mol Med 2002;10:407–411.
[117] Fernandes BF, Marshall JC, Burnier Jr MN. Blue light exposure and uveal melanoma. Ophthalmology 2006;113:1062, author reply 1062.
[118] Shah CP, Weis E, Lajous M, Shields JA, Shields CL. Intermittent and chronic ultraviolet light exposure and uveal melanoma: a meta-analysis. Ophthalmology 2005;112:1599–1607.
[119] Yu GP, Hu DN, McCormick SA. Latitude and incidence of ocular melanoma. Photochem Photobiol 2006;82:1621–1626.
[120] Boscoe FP, Schymura MJ. Solar ultraviolet-B exposure and cancer incidence and mortality in the United States, 1993–2002. BMC Cancer 2006;6:264.
[121] Grant WB. An ecologic study of cancer mortality rates in Spain with respect to indices of solar UVB irradiance and smoking. Int J Cancer 2007;120:1123–1128.
[122] Rodieck RW. The first steps in seeing. Sunderland, MA, USA: Sinauer Associates, Inc; 1998.
[123] Land EH. The retinex theory of color vision. Sci Am 1977;237:108–128.
[124] Valberg A, Lange-Malecki B. "Colour constancy" in Mondrian patterns: a partial cancellation of physical chromaticity shifts by simultaneous contrast. Vision Res 1990;30:371–380.
[125] Gegenfurtner KR, Sharpe LT. Color vision: from genes to perception. Cambridge, UK: Cambridge University Press; 1999.
[126] Verriest G. The spectral curve of relative luminous efficiency in different age groups of aphakic eyes. 13, Colour Vision Deficiencies II, International Symposium. Edinburgh UK: 1973, Basel, Switzerland: Karger; 1974.
[127] Delahunt PB, Webster MA, Ma L, Werner JS. Long-term renormalization of chromatic mechanisms following cataract surgery. Vis Neurosci 2004;21:301–307.
[128] Cionni RJ, Tsai JH. Color perception with AcrySof natural and AcrySof single-piece intraocular lenses under photopic and mesopic conditions. J Cataract Refract Surg 2006;32:236–242.
[129] Hayashi K, Hayashi H. Visual function in patients with yellow tinted intraocular lenses compared with vision in patients with non-tinted intraocular lenses. Br J Ophthalmol 2006;90:1019–1023.
[130] Leibovitch I, Lai T, Porter N, Pietris G, Newland H, Selva D. Visual outcomes with the yellow intraocular lens. Acta Ophthalmol Scand 2006;84:95–99.
[131] Marshall J, Cionni RJ, Davison J, et al. Clinical results of the blue-light filtering AcrySof Natural foldable acrylic intraocular lens. J Cataract Refract Surg 2005;31:2319–2323.
[132] Raj SM, Vasavada AR, Nanavaty MA. AcrySof Natural SN60AT versus AcrySof SA60AT intraocular lens in patients with color vision defects. J Cataract Refract Surg 2005;31:2324–2328.
[133] Rodriguez-Galietero A, Montes-Mico R, Munoz G, Albarran-Diego C. Comparison of contrast sensitivity and color discrimination after clear and yellow intraocular lens implantation. J Cataract Refract Surg 2005;31:1736–1740.
[134] Vuori ML, Mantyjarvi M. Colour vision and retinal nerve fibre layer photography in patients with an Acrysof Natural intraocular lens. Acta Ophthalmol Scand 2006;84:92–94.
[135] Shah SA, Miller KM. Explantation of an AcrySof Natural intraocular lens because of a color vision disturbance. Am J Ophthalmol 2005;140:941–942.
[136] Mackool RJ. Explantation of an AcrySof natural intraocular lens because of a color vision disturbance. Am J Ophthalmol 2006;142:890, author reply 890–891.
[137] Rubin RM, Ivan DJ, Tsang AC, Edberg M, Gooch J. The impact of blue-blocking intraocular lenses on color vision performance, poster number 423. *American Academy of Ophthalmology, 2006 Annual Meeting*. Las Vegas, NV; 2006.
[138] Pierre A, Wittich W, Faubert J, Overbury O. Luminance contrast with clear and yellow-tinted intraocular lenses. J Cataract Refract Surg 2007;33:1248–1252.
[139] Zhao H, Mainster MA. The effect of chromatic dispersion on pseudophakic optical performance. Br J Ophthalmol 2007;91:1225–1229.
[140] Steen R, Whitaker D, Elliott DB, Wild JM. Effect of filters on disability glare. Ophthalmic Physiol Opt 1993;13:371–376.
[141] Naarendorp F, Frumkes T. The influence of short-term adaptation of human rods and cones on cone-mediated grating visibility. J Physiol 1991;432:521–541.
[142] Mohand-Said S, Hicks D, Leveillard T, Picaud S, Porto F, Sahel JA. Rod-cone interactions: developmental and clinical significance. Prog Retin Eye Res 2001;20:451–467.
[143] Stabell B, Stabell U. Effects of rod activity on color perception with light adaptation. J Opt Soc Am A Opt Image Sci Vis 2002;19:1249–1258.
[144] Buck SL. Rod-cone interactions in human vision. In: Chalupa LM, Werner JS, editors. The visual neurosciences, 1 vol. Cambridge, MA: The MIT Press; 2004. p. 863–878.
[145] Gegenfurtner KR, Mayser H, Sharpe LT. Seeing movement in the dark. Nature 1999;398: 475–476.
[146] Gegenfurtner KR, Mayser HM, Sharpe LT. Motion perception at scotopic light levels. J Opt Soc Am A Opt Image Sci Vis 2000;17:1505–1515.
[147] Owsley C, McGwin Jr G, Scilley K, Kallies K. Development of a questionnaire to assess vision problems under low luminance in age-related maculopathy. Invest Ophthalmol Vis Sci 2006;47:528–535.

[148] Sturr JF, Zhang L, Taub HA, Hannon DJ, Jackowski MM. Psychophysical evidence for losses in rod sensitivity in the aging visual system. Vision Res 1997;37:475–481.
[149] Jackson GR, Owsley C, Cordle EP, Finley CD. Aging and scotopic sensitivity. Vision Res 1998;38:3655–3662.
[150] Jackson GR, Owsley C, McGwin Jr G. Aging and dark adaptation. Vision Res 1999;39:3975–3982.
[151] Schefrin BE, Tregear SJ, Harvey Jr LO, Werner JS. Senescent changes in scotopic contrast sensitivity. Vision Res 1999;39:3728–3736.
[152] Jackson GR, Owsley C. Scotopic sensitivity during adulthood. Vision Res 2000;40:2467–2473.
[153] Pokorny J, Smith VC, Lutze M. Aging of the human lens. Appl Opt 1987;26:1437–1440.
[154] Yang Y, Thompson K, Burns SA. Pupil location under mesopic, photopic, and pharmacologically dilated conditions. Invest Ophthalmol Vis Sci 2002;43:2508–2512.
[155] Aarnisalo EA. Effects of yellow filter glasses on the results of photopic and scotopic photometry. Am J Ophthalmol 1988;105:408–411.
[156] Jackson GR. Pilot study on the effect of a blue-light-blocking IOL on rod-mediated (scotopic) vision. *American Society for Cataract and Refractive Surgery, Washington DC, 2005 Annual Meeting, April 15-20, 2005*. Surgery ASoCaR, Translator. Washington, DC, USA: 2005.
[157] Scilley K, Jackson GR, Cideciyan AV, Maguire MG, Jacobson SG, Owsley C. Early age-related maculopathy and self-reported visual difficulty in daily life. Ophthalmology 2002;109:1235–1242.
[158] Reeves A. Visual adaptation. In: Chalupa LM, Werner JS, editors. The visual neurosciences, 1 vol. Cambridge, MA: The MIT Press; 2004. p. 851–862.
[159] Werner JS. Night vision in the elderly: consequences for seeing through a "blue filtering" intraocular lens. Br J Ophthalmol 2005;89:1518–1521.
[160] Brown B, Brabyn L, Welch L, Haegerstrom-Portnoy G, Colenbrander A. Contribution of vision variables to mobility in age-related maculopathy patients. Am J Optom Physiol Opt 1986;63:733–739.
[161] Sunness JS, Rubin GS, Applegate CA, et al. Visual function abnormalities and prognosis in eyes with age-related geographic atrophy of the macula and good visual acuity. Ophthalmology 1997;104:1677–1691.
[162] Owsley C, Jackson GR, Cideciyan AV, et al. Psychophysical evidence for rod vulnerability in age-related macular degeneration. Invest Ophthalmol Vis Sci 2000;41:267–273.
[163] Owsley C, Jackson GR, White M, Feist R, Edwards D. Delays in rod-mediated dark adaptation in early age-related maculopathy. Ophthalmology 2001;108:1196–1202.
[164] Greenstein VC, Thomas SR, Blaustein H, Koenig K, Carr RE. Effects of early diabetic retinopathy on rod system sensitivity. Optom Vis Sci 1993;70:18–23.
[165] Kline DW. Light, ageing and visual performance. In: Marshall J, editor. The susceptible visual apparatus, 16 vol. London, UK: Macmillan Press; 1991. p. 150–161.
[166] Charman WN. Vision and driving – a literature review and commentary. Ophthalmic Physiol Opt 1997;17:371–391.
[167] Owsley C, McGwin Jr G. Vision impairment and driving. Surv Ophthalmol 1999;43:535–550.
[168] Klein BE, Klein R, Lee KE, Cruickshanks KJ. Associations of performance-based and self-reported measures of visual function. The Beaver Dam Eye Study. Ophthalmic Epidemiol 1999;6:49–60.
[169] Mainster MA, Timberlake GT. Why HID headlights bother older drivers. Br J Ophthalmol 2003;87:113–117.
[170] Owsley C, Stalvey BT, Phillips JM. The efficacy of an educational intervention in promoting self-regulation among high-risk older drivers. Accid Anal Prev 2003;35:393–400.
[171] McMurdo ME, Gaskell A. Dark adaptation and falls in the elderly. Gerontology 1991;37:221–224.
[172] Hausdorff JM, Rios DA, Edelberg HK. Gait variability and fall risk in community-living older adults: a 1-year prospective study. Arch Phys Med Rehabil 2001;82:1050–1056.
[173] Donald IP, Bulpitt CJ. The prognosis of falls in elderly people living at home. Age Ageing 1999;28:121–125.
[174] Turner PL. Circadian photoreception: an important new consideration in cataract surgery. *Australasian Society of Cataract and Refractive Surgeons, 2006 Annual Meeting, July 14–17, 2006*. Hayman Island, Australia: 2006.
[175] Van Gelder RN. Non-visual ocular photoreception. Ophthalmic Genet 2001;22:195–205.
[176] Berson DM, Dunn FA, Takao M. Phototransduction by retinal ganglion cells that set the circadian clock. Science 2002;295:1070–1073.
[177] Brainard GC, Hanifin JP. Photons, clocks, and consciousness. J Biol Rhythms 2005;20:314–325.
[178] Menaker M. Circadian rhythms. Circadian photoreception. Science 2003;299:213–214.
[179] Abbott A. Restless nights, listless days. Nature 2003;425:896–898.
[180] Macchi MM, Bruce JN. Human pineal physiology and functional significance of melatonin. Front Neuroendocrinol 2004;25:177–195.
[181] Reiter RJ, Tan DX, Manchester LC, El-Sawi MR. Melatonin reduces oxidant damage and promotes mitochondrial respiration: implications for aging. Ann N Y Acad Sci 2002;959:238–250.
[182] Reiter RJ. Mechanisms of cancer inhibition by melatonin. J Pineal Res 2004;37:213–214.
[183] Leon-Blanco MM, Guerrero JM, Reiter RJ, Calvo JR, Pozo D. Melatonin inhibits telomerase activity in the MCF-7 tumor cell line both in vivo and in vitro. J Pineal Res 2003;35:204–211.
[184] Leon-Blanco MM, Guerrero JM, Reiter RJ, Pozo D. RNA expression of human telomerase subunits TR and TERT is differentially affected by melatonin receptor agonists in the MCF-7 tumor cell line. Cancer Lett 2004;216:73–80.
[185] Marchiafava PL, Longoni B. Melatonin as an antioxidant in retinal photoreceptors. J Pineal Res 1999;26:184–189.
[186] Liang FQ, Aleman TS, ZaixinYang, Cideciyan AV, Jacobson SG, Bennett J. Melatonin delays photoreceptor degeneration in the rds/rds mouse. Neuroreport 2001;12:1011–1014.
[187] Liang FQ, Green L, Wang C, Alssadi R, Godley BF. Melatonin protects human retinal pigment epithelial (RPE) cells against oxidative stress. Exp Eye Res 2004;78:1069–1075.
[188] Lerchl A. Biological rhythms in the context of light at night (LAN). Neuro Endocrinol Lett 2002;23:23–27.
[189] Lambert GW, Reid C, Kaye DM, Jennings GL, Esler MD. Effect of sunlight and season on serotonin turnover in the brain. Lancet 2002;360:1840–1842.
[190] Yannielli P, Harrington ME. Let there be "more" light: enhancement of light actions on the circadian system through non-photic pathways. Prog Neurobiol 2004;74:59–76.
[191] Espana RA, Scammell TE. Sleep neurobiology for the clinician. Sleep 2004;27:811–820.
[192] Flory JD, Manuck SB, Matthews KA, Muldoon MF. Serotonergic function in the central nervous system is associated with daily ratings of positive mood. Psychiatry Res 2004;129:11–19.
[193] Hattar S, Lucas RJ, Mrosovsky N, et al. Melanopsin and rod-cone photoreceptive systems account for all major accessory visual functions in mice. Nature 2003;424:76–81.
[194] Lehrl S, Gerstmeyer K, Jacob JH, et al. Blue light improves cognitive performance. J Neural Transm 2007;114:457–460, Epub Jan 25 2007.
[195] Skene DJ. Optimization of light and melatonin to phase-shift human circadian rhythms. J Neuroendocrinol 2003;15:438–441.
[196] Foster RG. Neurobiology: bright blue times. Nature 2005;433:698–699.
[197] Haimov I, Laudon M, Zisapel N, et al. Sleep disorders and melatonin rhythms in elderly people. BMJ 1994;309:167.
[198] Terman M, Terman JS. Light therapy for seasonal and nonseasonal depression: efficacy, protocol, safety, and side effects. CNS Spectr 2005;10:647–663, quiz 672.
[199] Jones SH. Circadian rhythms, multilevel models of emotion and bipolar disorder – an initial step towards integration? Clin Psychol Rev 2001;21:1193–1209.
[200] Yaprak M, Altun A, Vardar A, Aktoz M, Ciftci S, Ozbay G. Decreased nocturnal synthesis of melatonin in patients with coronary artery disease. Int J Cardiol 2003;89:103–107.
[201] Scheer FA, Kalsbeek A, Buijs RM. Cardiovascular control by the suprachiasmatic nucleus: neural and neuroendocrine mechanisms in human and rat. Biol Chem 2003;384:697–709.
[202] Dominguez-Rodriguez A, Abreu-Gonzalez P, Garcia M, et al. Light/dark patterns of interleukin-6 in relation to the pineal hormone melatonin in patients with acute myocardial infarction. Cytokine 2004;26:89–93.
[203] Aronson D. Impaired modulation of circadian rhythms in patients with diabetes mellitus: a risk factor for cardiac thrombotic events? Chronobiol Int 2001;18:109–121.
[204] Bughi S, Shaw S, Bessman A. Laser damage to retinal ganglion cells: the effect on circadian rhythms. J Diabetes Complications 2006;20:184–187.
[205] Skene DJ, Swaab DF. Melatonin rhythmicity: effect of age and Alzheimer's disease. Exp Gerontol 2003;38:199–206.
[206] Reiter RJ, Cabrera J, Sainz RM, Mayo JC, Manchester LC, Tan DX. Melatonin as a pharmacological agent against neuronal loss in experimental models of Huntington's disease, Alzheimer's disease and parkinsonism. Ann N Y Acad Sci 1999;890:471–485.
[207] Wu YH, Feenstra MG, Zhou JN, et al. Molecular changes underlying reduced pineal melatonin levels in Alzheimer disease: alterations in preclinical and clinical stages. J Clin Endocrinol Metab 2003;88:5898–5906.
[208] Kanabrocki EL, Ryan MD, Hermida RC, et al. Altered circadian relationship between serum nitric oxide, carbon dioxide, and uric acid in multiple sclerosis. Chronobiol Int 2004;21:739–758.
[209] Kanabrocki EL, Vesely DL, Hermida RC, et al. Circadian distribution of hematology variables in subjects with multiple sclerosis. Clin Ter 2006;157:241–247.
[210] Schernhammer ES, Hankinson SE. Urinary melatonin levels and breast cancer risk. J Natl Cancer Inst 2005;97:1084–1087.
[211] Karasek M, Kowalski AJ, Suzin J, Zylinska K, Swietoslawski J. Serum melatonin circadian profiles in women suffering from cervical cancer. J Pineal Res 2005;39:73–76.
[212] Schernhammer ES, Laden F, Speizer FE, et al. Night-shift work and risk of colorectal cancer in the nurses' health study. J Natl Cancer Inst 2003;95:825–828.
[213] Armstrong SM, Redman JR. Melatonin: a chronobiotic with anti-aging properties? Med Hypotheses 1991;34:300–309.
[214] Erren TC, Reiter RJ, Piekarski C. Light, timing of biological rhythms, and chronodisruption in man. Naturwissenschaften 2003;90:485–494.
[215] Magri F, Sarra S, Cinchetti W, et al. Qualitative and quantitative changes of melatonin levels in physiological and pathological aging and in centenarians. J Pineal Res 2004;36:256–261.
[216] Pauley SM. Lighting for the human circadian clock: recent research indicates that lighting has become a public health issue. Med Hypotheses 2004;63:588–596.
[217] Hahn RA. Profound bilateral blindness and the incidence of breast cancer. Epidemiology 2004;2:208–210.
[218] Bellastella A, Sinisi AA, Criscuolo T, et al. Melatonin and the pituitary-thyroid axis status in blind adults: a possible resetting after puberty. Clin Endocrinol (Oxf) 1995;43:707–711.
[219] Feychting M, Osterlund B, Ahlbom A. Reduced cancer incidence among the blind. Epidemiology 1998;9:490–494.
[220] McCarty CA, Nanjan MB, Taylor HR. Vision impairment predicts 5 year mortality. Br J Ophthalmol 2001;85:322–326.
[221] Herljevic M, Middleton B, Thapan K, Skene DJ. Light-induced melatonin suppression: age-related reduction in response to short wavelength light. Exp Gerontol 2005;40:237–242.
[222] Mishima K, Okawa M, Shimizu T, Hishikawa Y. Diminished melatonin secretion in the elderly caused by insufficient environmental illumination. J Clin Endocrinol Metab 2001;86:129–134.
[223] Asplund R, Lindblad BE. Sleep and sleepiness 1 and 9 months after cataract surgery. Arch Gerontol Geriatr 2004;38:69–75.
[224] Asplund R, Ejdervik Lindblad B. The development of sleep in persons undergoing cataract surgery. Arch Gerontol Geriatr 2002;35:179–187.
[225] Marmor MF. Double fault! Ocular hazards of a tennis sunglass. Arch Ophthalmol 2001;119:1064–1066.
[226] Brown PK, Wald G. Visual pigments. In single rods and cones of the human retina. Direct measurements reveal mechanisms of human night and color vision. Science 1964;144:45–52.

Secondary Intraocular Lens Implantation and Stabilization

Roger F. Steinert, MD and Martin S. Arkin, MD, PhD

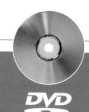

41

CONTENTS

- Surgical Procedure
- Studies of Secondary Intraocular Lenses
- Complications
- Comparison of Sutured Posterior-Chamber Intraocular Lenses with Open-Loop Flexible Anterior-Chamber Intraocular Lenses
- Conclusions

CHAPTER HIGHLIGHTS

>> Pros and cons of different fixation sites

>> Detailed surgical method of iris and scleral suture techniques

>> Results

>> Avoiding complications

The approach to the repair of a subluxating intraocular lens (IOL) or the secondary implantation of an IOL involves similar choices. In both cases, the dominant issue is the desired location of new IOL placement and the method of fixation in that location.

The surgeon has four principal alternatives for fixation of secondary IOLs:

1. Standard capsular bag-fixated or sulcus-fixated posterior-chamber (PC) lenses

2. Transscleral suture-fixated PC lenses

3. Peripheral iris suture-fixated PC IOLs

4. Anterior chamber (AC) lenses.

If capsular support is available standard PC lenses placed in the ciliary sulcus or, preferably, in the capsular bag are the standard of care. If capsular support is absent, the decision is more controversial. Sutured PC IOLs have become increasingly popular over the past decade, but audience surveys in multiple major meetings indicate that many surgeons will select an open-loop flexible AC IOL in the absence of a specific contraindication. Extensive debate persists between these options because of the limited number of studies that are available and the lack of controlled studies with long-term follow-up.

The first suture-fixated IOL was implanted a half century ago by Parry.[1] Worst was a pioneer in the use of iris pupil-fixated lenses in the mid-1970s.[1] McCannel reported the use of mid-peripheral iris fixation sutures to stabilize dislocated pupil-fixated IOLs in 1976.[1] Since then, numerous techniques using sutures to secure PC lenses to the iris or sclera have been described. Although many studies report on relatively small numbers of patients with short-term follow-up and fairly good results, few large prospective controlled studies exist. Most of the studies involve concomitant corneal transplantation to treat pseudophakic bullous keratopathy (PBK). This makes the analysis more difficult because these eyes often have a high degree of existing pathologic conditions, and corneal transplants have their own complications, including astigmatism, glaucoma, cystoid macular edema (CME), and graft rejection.

It is rare to find an aphakic patient with an intact posterior capsule. Most aphakic patients have had a complicated phacoemulsification or extracapsular cataract extraction. Aphakic patients with residual capsule often have synechiae between the anterior capsule and posterior iris or between the anterior capsule and posterior capsule. The surgeon has the option of placing a PC IOL in the ciliary sulcus after lysing iridocapsular adhesions or attempting capsular bag placement after reopening the bag. In the rare case where secondary IOL implantation can be achieved using an intact capsular bag in a healthy eye, stability and complication rates are believed to be similar to those of primary PC IOL placement in the sulcus.

Three primary options exist for IOL fixation in the absence of capsular support: transscleral-sutured PC IOLs, peripheral iris-sutured PC IOLs, and flexible open-loop AC IOLs. If both the posterior capsule and the iris are disrupted or absent, then sutured transscleral PC IOLs are the only IOL option. Tables 41-1 to 41-4 review the advantages and disadvantages of each of these IOL styles and those of nonsutured standard PC IOLs.[2–5]

Table 41-5 lists the principal indications for secondary IOL implantation. Clinical scenarios include rupture of the posterior capsule at the time of cataract surgery or a patient with a threatened expulsive hemorrhage in whom the cataract surgery was aborted without IOL placement. Some patients with closed-loop AC IOLs who have been followed closely and have not yet developed generalized corneal edema have been found to have decreasing

Table 41-1 Theoretical properties—nonsutured standard PC IOLs

Advantages	Disadvantages
Low incidence of CME, pupillary block, UGH, PBK	Requires intact posterior capsule and zonules
Less endothelial loss* Mechanical barrier against vitreous movement or diffusion of vasoactive substances that could lead to CME or retinal detachment Positioned at nodal point of the eye Distant from trabecular meshwork	Increased risk of dislocation

CME, Cystoid macular edema; UGH, uveitis-glaucoma-hyphema; PBK, pseudophakic bullous keratopathy.
*Soong HK, Meyer RF, Sugar A: Techniques of posterior chamber lens implantation without capsular support during penetrating keratoplasty: a review, *J Refract Corneal Surg* 5:249–255, 1989.

Table 41-2 Theoretical properties—scleral-sutured standard PC IOLs

Advantages	Disadvantages
? Share advantages of nonsutured PC IOLs	Technically difficult to insert
Can be used with limbal wound or penetrating keratoplasty	Increased operating time
Not dependent on presence of iris tissue	Often requires extensive vitrectomy
Vitreous supported by lens	Suture-related endophthalmitis
Limited pseudophacodonesis	? Risk of epithelial downgrowth from suture path
Minimizes uveal contact	Risk of retinal detachment from vitrectomy and manipulation near the vitreous base Risk of hemorrhage from suture passage through ciliary body Long-term dependence on fixation of IOL by a suture
Ciliary body erosion from haptics*	

PC IOL, Posterior chamber intraocular lens.
*Duffey RJ, Holland EJ, Agapitos PJ et al: Anatomic study of transsclerally sutured intraocular lens implantation, *Am J Ophthalmol* 108:300–309, 1989.

Table 41-3 Theoretical properties—iris-sutured PC-IOLs

Advantages	Disadvantages
? Share advantages of nonsutured	? CME from uveal irritation
PC IOLs	Pigment dispersion
	Technically difficult to insert
	Technique easier to use with penetrating keratoplasty; challenging in closed chamber
	Limited pupillary dilation*
	Pseudophacodonesis
	Requires sufficient iris tissue

PC IOL, Posterior chamber intraocular lens.
*Spigelman AV, Lindstrom RL, Nichols BD et al: Implantation of a posterior chamber lens without capsular support during penetrating keratoplasty or as a secondary lens implant, *Ophthalmic Surg* 19:396–398, 1988.

Table 41-4 Theoretical properties—flexible open-loop AC IOLs

Advantages	Disadvantages
Easier insertion and sizing	Difficult to insert properly—iris tuck
Less operating time including uveiitis, glaucoma, hyphema, CME, PBK	? Lower but persistent risks of older-style AC IOLs,

AC IOL, Anterior chamber intraocular lens; CME, cystoid macular edema; PBK, pseudophakic bullous keratopathy.

PC IOLs to manage subluxed primary PC IOLs. Price et al.[7] believe that capsulorrhexis should help decrease the incidence of this complication. Finally, cataract surgery complications that can lead to IOL exchange include the uveitis-glaucoma-hyphema (UGH) syndrome or chronic pain from closed-loop AC lenses without corneal edema. Doren, Stern, and Driebe[8] found that the UGH syndrome was usually associated with a relatively poor outcome, even with lens exchange. See Chapters 44, 46, and 49 for further discussion of corneal decompensation and the technique of removing closed-loop AC IOLs.

■ SURGICAL PROCEDURE ■

Few patients have an intact posterior capsule and no IOL present. Occasionally, PC IOLs dislocate without extensive capsular bag disruption, and an IOL exchange or repositioning is necessary. Some patients with an old-style rigid AC IOL and PBK may have some capsular support evident at the time of penetrating keratoplasty and IOL exchange. For the few patients in whom secondary placement of a nonsutured standard PC IOL is possible, the two

endothelial cell counts, increasing corneal thickness, localized peripheral corneal edema, or CME. These patients may be candidates for IOL exchange. AC IOLs and sutured PC IOLs are also used to replace malpositioned lenses that are decentered, subluxated into the vitreous, or dislocated near the endothelium. Panton et al.[6] described the use of iris sutures and IOL exchange for scleral-sutured

Table 41-5 Indications for surgery—secondary IOL or IOL exchange

Corneal edema
PBK (usually with IOL exchange)
Closed-loop AC IOLs
Iris-supported IOLs
Modern open-loop AC IOLs
ABK
Aphakia
Prior intracapsular cataract extraction
Contact lens intolerance
IOL complications
Complications during planned extracapsular cataract extraction
IOL exchange of closed-loop AC IOL
Decreased endothelial cell counts
Cystoid macular edema
Malpositioned IOL
UGH syndrome
Pain
IOL power error

ABK, Aphakic bullous keratopathy; AC IOL, anterior chamber intraocular lens; PBK, pseudophakic bullous keratopathy; UGH; uveitis-glaucoma-hyphema.

Table 41-6 Surgical procedure for AC IOL placement

Correct sizing—length 1 mm greater than horizontal white–white distance (limbal diameter)
If feasible, orient incision on steep meridian to reduce postoperative astigmatism
Orient incision to place haptics away from peripheral iridectomies, or rotate IOL away from iridectomies after insertion
Construct pupil preoperatively (e.g. pilocarpine 2% drops, 30 min before operation)
Use viscoelastic substance to maintain anterior chamber
Vitrectomy to clear anterior chamber and wound of vitreous if necessary
Avoid iris tuck, dialysis; some surgeons prefer the use of a Sheets guide
Haptics should rest securely at level of ciliary body band—perform "bounce" test to evaluate both stable fixation and absence of iris tuck

AC IOL, Anterior chamber intraocular lens.

options are capsular bag or ciliary sulcus placement. In patients with an intact posterior capsule, a significant surgical obstacle is reopening the capsular bag. Nevertheless, in cases without extensive fibrosis, the anterior and posterior capsules can be separated. The key is to locate one area in which the anterior capsule edge is not strongly adherent to the posterior capsule. Using this entry point, viscoelastic agents can be very helpful in the separation of the capsular layers. If adhesions are very dense, blunt dissection with cannulas or other instruments can be attempted. In some cases, the adhesions can be left intact focally by creating an extension of an anterior capsulotomy peripheral to the adhesion, using either capsulorrhexis-like tearing techniques or scissors cutting of the anterior capsule. A final alternative is sharp dissection between the anterior and posterior capsules, but this carries greater risk of penetrating the posterior capsule.

If reopening of the capsular bag is not feasible, ciliary sulcus fixation of the IOL is a reasonable alternative. This requires at least peripheral capsular support and intact zonular support. A frequent situation is a posterior capsular rent with an intact anterior capsulorrhexis. It is often necessary to lyse adhesions between capsular remnants and the posterior iris to reconstruct the ciliary sulcus before IOL placement. It is important to visually confirm that the haptics are not inadvertently directed under the anterior capsule during insertion to ensure proper support and avoid vitreous entanglement. If capsular support is focally uncertain, suturing one of the IOL haptics to the iris or sclera is advisable.

It is commonly stated that AC IOLs are easy to insert but difficult to insert correctly. The three most common mistakes made during insertion are incorrect sizing, not taking sufficient steps to avoid iris tuck, and insufficient attention to location of iridectomies and the capacity of haptics to rotate through them. Table 41-6 lists the most important steps in AC IOL placement.

PERIPHERAL IRIS SUTURE FIXATION

Peripheral iris suture fixation of the haptics of a PC IOL is commonly referred to as "McCannel suturing," which is in recognition of the contribution of Malcom McCannel, who first described the technique for passing sutures through the iris to stabilize an IOL that had dislocated postoperatively. McCannel's description was in the context of a pupil-fixated IOL, an IOL style abandoned long ago. However, the basic maneuvers that McCannel described, using long needles to pass sutures through the iris and around elements of the IOL, remain highly useful for the stabilization or secondary implantation of a PC IOL in the absence of adequate capsular support.

Some surgeons advocate these techniques over transscleral suturing in all cases. Others reserve peripheral iris suture fixation for particular indications. These include glaucoma patients for whom an AC IOL is thought inadvisable or anatomically impossible and patients in whom the conjunctiva needs to be preserved for possible future filtration surgery or where a filtering bleb is already present and must be protected. The technique is also attractive in the setting of phacoemulsification under topical anesthesia when capsular support is inadequate. Most patients can be comfortable with intracameral anesthetic, such as 1% nonpreserved lidocaine, while the surgeon places and sutures the IOL to the peripheral iris, whereas taking down conjunctival flaps and passing sutures through the ciliary sulcus and sclera may be unacceptably painful under topical anesthesia.

The basic technique for peripheral iris suturing of a PC IOL begins with constricting the pupil adequately to temporarily capture the PC IOL optic in the pupil anterior to the iris plane, while the haptics remain in the posterior chamber. The technique is illustrated in Figure 41-1. A key in obtaining a round central pupil is to keep the length of the iris suture pass as short as

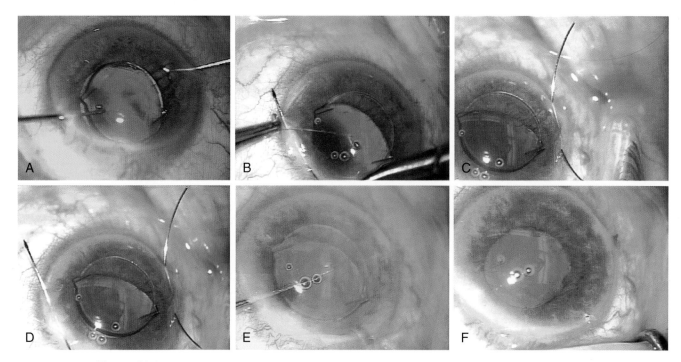

Figure 41-1 McCannel iris suture fixation of a PC IOL. **A,** Kuglen hook in the surgeon's left hand and an Osher Y-hook in the surgeon's right hand are introduced through two paracentesis openings and used to elevate the optic above the iris plane, capturing the optic in the pupil while the haptics remain in the posterior chamber. **B,** A 10-0 polypropylene suture on a fine long needle (Ethicon CTC-6) is passed through the paracentesis, penetrates the iris in the periphery just in front of the haptic, which is indenting the iris stroma, exits the iris as soon as possible after the haptic, and then is driven up through the peripheral clear cornea. **C,** Same maneuver is performed under the opposite haptic. **D,** With both needles remaining in place behind the haptics, the successful capture of the haptics and acceptable location of the IOL in the pupil are verified. **E,** Sutures are tied and cut inside the eye using the "slip knot" technique illustrated for iris suturing in Figure 31-1. Kuglen hook presses the intraocular lens (IOL) optic posteriorly. **F,** Pupil is round, and the IOL is well centered.

possible and as peripheral as possible. Long suture passes bunch up iris tissue. Nonperipheral suture passes inhibit free movement of the pupil. Both errors result in distorted, nonreactive pupils. The repair of a subluxating PC IOL that is not located in the capsular bag is fundamentally the same as a secondary implant with the McCannel technique. The surgeon manipulates the IOL optic anterior to the iris plane while the haptics remain posterior. The pupil is pharmacologically constricted, capturing the optic. The haptics are then suture fixated. In the final step, the optic is then prolapsed posteriorly back into the posterior chamber.

Soong et al.[9] describe both two-point and four-point iris fixation for PC lenses at the time of penetrating keratoplasty.

TRANSSCLERAL SUTURING

Many different alternatives have been presented in the literature for placement of transscleral-sutured PC lenses. Scleral-sutured lenses can be sutured from the inside out (ab interno) or by passing the needles from the outside of the eye inward (ab externo). A combination of scleral and iris sutures has also been described.[10] Transscleral sutures can be oriented vertically, obliquely, or horizontally, except that direct 3 and 9 o'clock horizontal fixation is inadvisable because of the danger of suturing through the long ciliary arteries and nerves in these locations.[11] It is important to do an extensive anterior vitrectomy in most cases before placement of a

sutured PC lens to avoid vitreous incarceration and subsequent retinal traction and detachment.[9,11,12]

Many of the early surgeries performed with scleral-sutured PC IOLs placed the haptics too far posteriorly. The goal is to have the haptics resting in the ciliary sulcus. Anatomic studies have shown that the ciliary sulcus is only 0.83 mm posterior to the limbus in the vertical meridian and only 0.46 mm posterior to the limbus in the horizontal meridian.[4] Duffey et al.[4] passed needles perpendicular to the sclera at 1, 2, and 3 mm posterior to the limbus and found that the needles exited internally at the ciliary sulcus, pars plicata, and pars plana, respectively. These anatomic studies emphasize the importance of keeping transscleral needle penetration sites anteriorly. The surgeon can detect that a needle is being passed too anteriorly by iris movement as the needle penetrates the peripheral iris stroma near the angle. In determining the correct location, the surgeon must be mindful that the anatomic studies are based on a strict perpendicularity of the needle relative to the scleral wall. If the surgeon passes the needle through the scleral wall at an oblique angle (usually tilted toward the iris plane), then the external scleral point will need to be more posterior for the interior scleral point to be at the level of the ciliary sulcus.[13]

The surgeon has the option of creating scleral flaps so that the polypropylene (Prolene) suture knot is buried, avoiding exposed suture ends. Cautery is recommended to retract exposed barbs, should they occur postoperatively, to avoid a possibly entry tract

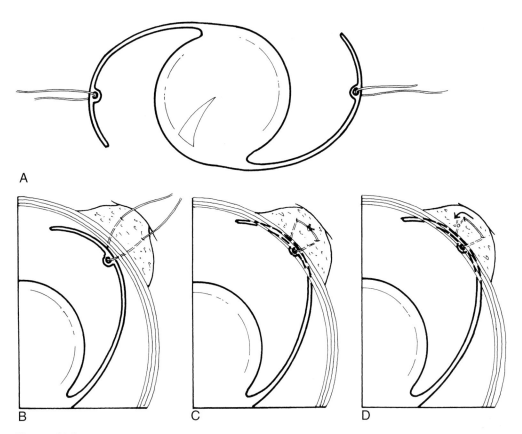

A

B   C   D

Figure 41-2 Lane technique to avoid scleral flaps. **A,** Double-armed polypropylene suture is passed through the haptic positioning hole. **B,** Suture is passed ab interno through the ciliary sulcus, as in Figures 41-3 and 41-4, except that no scleral flap is required. The sutures should be spaced 1.5–2 mm apart. **C,** Suture is tightened and tied with a small 1-1-1-1 knot. **D,** Knot is rotated internally. Conjunctiva is then closed over the smooth suture loop.

for microorganisms or epithelium. If the suture knot is rotated, as in the technique of Stephen Lane shown in Figure 41-2, then no scleral flap is needed.

PC IOLs made specifically for suturing to the sclera have eyelets on the haptic to aid suture fixation and large-diameter optics (7 mm) to compensate for possible decentration. A commonly used model of scleral-sutured IOL is the Alcon CZ70BD.

The ab interno technique for transscleral suture fixation of a PC IOL typically uses polypropylene (Prolene) suture material. A long needle is required for the pass across the anterior chamber: the Ethicon CIF-4 and Ethicon STC-6 and CTC-6 needles are commonly employed[14] (Figures 41-3 and 41-4). The CIF-4 is thicker and affords more control to the surgeon. The needles are passed under the iris, aiming for the ciliary sulcus. A girth hitch can be used to attach the polypropylene suture loop to the IOL haptic (Figure 41-5). Alternatively, sutures can be tied to the haptic, to the haptic eyelets, or proximal to a haptic eyelet.[15] The needles exit the eye under the previously dissected scleral flaps, and the sutures are tied (Figure 41-6). Alternatively, to avoid dissecting scleral flaps and the potential for later erosion of the flap and conjunctiva, with exposure of the suture ends, the suture is passed through the positioning hole in the haptic, and the knot is rotated below the scleral surface (see Figure 41-2). The ab interno technique is adaptable to foldable IOL implantation as well, allowing suture fixation of the IOL while retaining a small incision, which is particularly important if capsule support

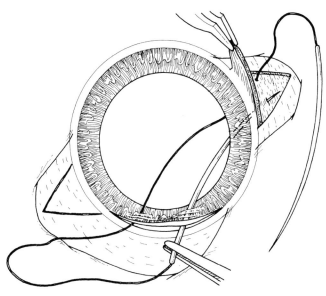

Figure 41-3 Technique for the ab interno approach (also see Figures 41-4 to 41-6). First the long needles are passed under the iris, aiming for the inferior ciliary sulcus. Two needle passes are made for each haptic if four-point fixation is desired. Needles exit under previously dissected scleral flaps.

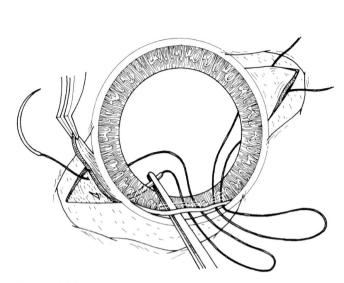

Figure 41-4 A second pair of short needle passes is made under the superior iris for the suture to be tied to the second haptic.

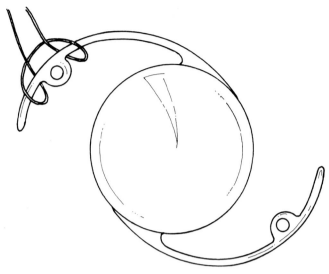

Figure 41-5 Girth hitch can be used to attach the polypropylene suture loop to the intraocular lens (IOL) haptic. This technique is more rapid than tying the suture to the haptic. Alternately, the suture can be attached to the IOL haptics before the transscleral needle passes, but the surgeon must avoid tangling the long sutures.

is lost during primary cataract surgery through a small, clear corneal incision.[16]

The principal advantages of the ab interno (inside-to-outside) approach are that it is more straightforward and possibly faster than the ab externo (outside-to-inside) technique. It is also easier with penetrating keratoplasty. The disadvantages include the fact that the needle is passed under the iris without direct visualization, and the surgeon has to rely on indentation of the iris with the needle from behind to ensure correct placement in the ciliary sulcus.

Lewis[17] first described the ab externo technique of passing the scleral needles from the outside inward. The sutures used for the procedure are 10-0 polypropylene with a long straight needle, such as Ethicon STC-6. Alcon produces Pair Pack Fixation Suture, which is a hybrid combining an SC-5 straight needle on one end and an AUM-5 corneal needle on the other. This is specifically made for the outside-to-inside technique of scleral-sutured PC IOLs. The long straight needle is passed perpendicularly through the sclera (usually under partial-thickness scleral flaps) approximately 0.75 mm posterior to the limbus (Figure 41-7). Inside the

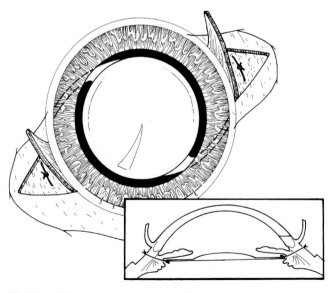

Figure 41-6 After exiting the eye under the previously dissected scleral flaps, the sutures are tied, securing the intraocular lens (IOL) into position. Appropriate suture tension is important to avoid lens decentration. The inset shows the cross-sectional view of the eye with the IOL correctly positioned in the ciliary sulcus.

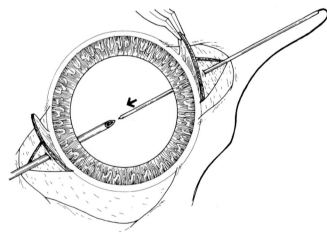

Figure 41-7 Technique for the ab externo approach (also see Figures 41-8 to 41-10). The long, straight solid needle is passed through the sclera (usually under partial-thickness scleral flaps) approximately 0.75 mm posterior to the limbus. Inside the eye, the needle should exit at the ciliary sulcus. A second hollow needle is passed from the opposite side of the eye. A pair of sutures can be used if four-point fixation is desired.

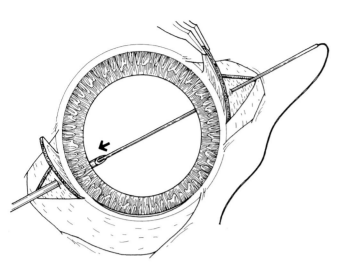

Figure 41-8 Solid needle is "docked" inside the tip of the hollow needle, which has been passed through ciliary sulcus on the opposite side. After docking, the pair of needles are withdrawn together from the eye, with the solid needle inside the hallow needle.

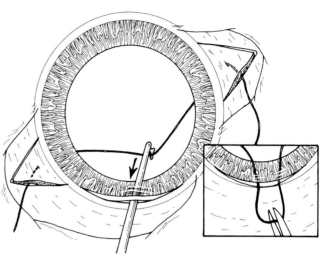

Figure 41-9 A hook is used to pull the suture out through a superior limbal wound so that it can be tied to the intraocular lens.

eye, the needle should penetrate at the ciliary sulcus. The needle is then "docked" inside the tip of a 25-, 27-, or 28-gauge hollow needle, which has been passed through the ciliary sulcus on the opposite side, also with an outside-to-inside technique (Figure 41-8). After the long straight needle with the 10-0 polypropylene is docked within the hollow needle, the hollow needle is withdrawn with the solid needle inside of it. In this way, the polypropylene suture is pulled across the eye. A hook is used to then pull the suture out through a superior limbal wound (Figure 41-9). The suture is cut, and each end is tied to a haptic of the IOL (Figure 41-10). After the IOL is placed into position, the scleral sutures are secured to the sclera.

This procedure can be performed with two sutures per haptic if the surgeon desires four-point fixation to ensure stability (Figure 41-11). The surgeon ties the sutures to the haptics and buries the external knot under a scleral flap (Figure 41-12). The alternative procedure, illustrated in Figure 41-13, allows rotation of the knot to avoid the necessity for scleral flaps and the potential of late exposure of the suture ends, but the antirotational stability of true four-point fixation is not achieved.[15–18]

The advantage of the outside-to-inside approach is greater assurance of the location of internal scleral penetration at the ciliary sulcus. Bleeding may be minimized by using precise measurements and avoiding the highly vascularized pars plicata. In addition, the anterior chamber remains closed during the needle passes, decreasing the duration of ocular hypotony. The disadvantage of the ab externo approach is that it takes longer and it is not applicable with the open-sky situation of penetrating keratoplasty. In addition, if more than one suture pass is performed, it may be hard to keep track of the origin and course of the various suture ends.

If a double-suture technique with knot rotation is selected (see Figures 41-2 and 41-13), the surgeon must be meticulous in achieving a suture orientation that permits easy rotation of the knot (Figures 41-14A and B) and avoiding suture configurations

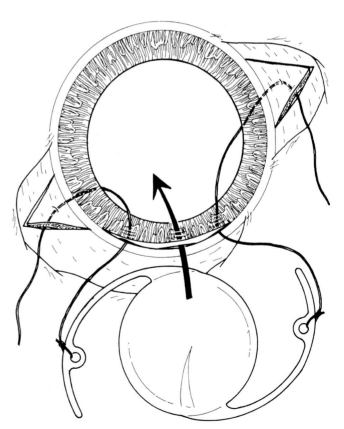

Figure 41-10 Suture is cut, and each end is tied to a haptic of the intraocular lens (IOL). After the IOL is placed into position, the scleral sutures must be anchored to the sclera. Either a "blind pass" in the sclera is made so that the suture is tied to itself, or the transscleral suture is tied to a second suture that has been tied to the sclera with a short partial-thickness pass within the bed of the scleral flap.

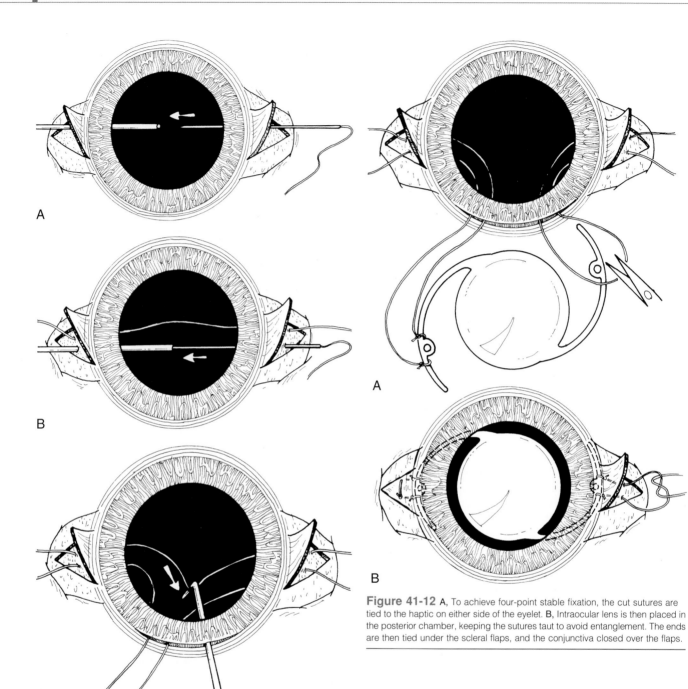

A

B

C

Figure 41-11 A, Double-suture variant of the Lewis ab externo technique begins similar to the single-suture technique, except that the suture entry point under the scleral flap is displaced to one side. **B,** Second suture is passed parallel to the first, with 1–1.5 mm between the two sutures. **C,** Care must be taken to keep the sutures taut to avoid crossing them or confusing which suture originates from each scleral site, while a Kuglen hook or similar instrument withdraws the suture loop through the previously prepared principal incision.

A

B

Figure 41-12 A, To achieve four-point stable fixation, the cut sutures are tied to the haptic on either side of the eyelet. **B,** Intraocular lens is then placed in the posterior chamber, keeping the sutures taut to avoid entanglement. The ends are then tied under the scleral flaps, and the conjunctiva closed over the flaps.

that will resist rotation of the knot (Figures 41-14C–H). Furthermore, the surgeon should orient the suture pass through the opposite haptics in a direction that will resist rotation of the IOL out of the iris plane (Figure 41-14I) rather than allow rotation (Figure 41-14J).

"LASSO" SUTURE FIXATION OF THE CAPSULE/ INTRAOCULAR LENS COMPLEX

A posterior chamber IOL may be properly placed within the capsular bag at the time of initial cataract surgery, and then the entire IOL-capsule complex become unstable and dislocate months or years after surgery. This scenario most commonly occurs after trauma to the globe or in the setting of pseudoexfoliation, where the zonules lose integrity over time. Because the haptics and optic are encapsulated, a standard McCannel suture approach is impossible. To deal with the constraints of this scenario, Steinert devised a technique of trans-scleral "lasso" suture fixation. Trans-scleral sutures are passed through the peripheral capsule so that a loop of suture is created around each haptic.

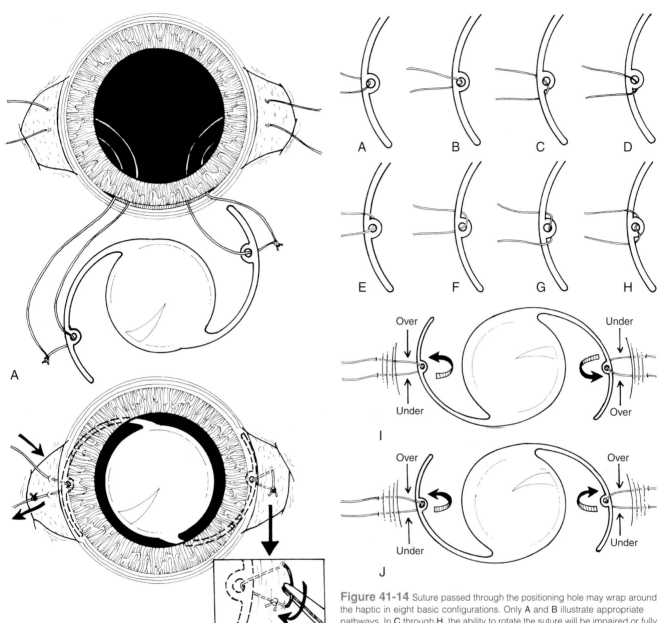

Figure 41-13 In this variant of the double-suture ab externo technique, the goal is to achieve a loop of suture where the knot can be rotated beneath the sclera, avoiding the necessity of a scleral flap and the potential for late erosion of the knot or suture ends. **A,** Cut ends of each suture are passed through the haptic positioning hole and tied. **B,** As the intraocular lens is positioned in the posterior chamber, one end of the suture on each side is pulled so that the knot passes through the sclera to the external eye, where it is cut off. Remaining suture ends are then tied together, and the knot is rotated beneath the sclera (inset), achieving the same end result as illustrated in Figure 41-2.

Figure 41-14 Suture passed through the positioning hole may wrap around the haptic in eight basic configurations. Only **A** and **B** illustrate appropriate pathways. In **C** through **H,** the ability to rotate the suture will be impaired or fully prevented by the circuitous route taken by the suture. Because there are two haptics, a total of 16 configurations are, therefore, possible. **I,** Surgeon should take care to use configuration **A** on one haptic and the opposite configuration **B** on the other haptic. In that manner, torque of the intraocular lens (IOL) is resisted; as one haptic starts to rotate in the direction not resisted by the suture loop, the other haptic meets more resistance (arrows). **J,** When both suture loops have the same configuration, the suture does not resist torque of the IOL (arrows).

STUDIES OF SECONDARY INTRAOCULAR LENSES ■

In studies in conjunction with penetrating keratoplasty, there does not appear to be a major difference in short-term overall results among scleral-sutured PC IOLs, iris-sutured PC IOLs, and modern AC IOLs. Kornmehl et al.[19] reported good results with flexible Kelman Omnifit AC IOLs compared with previous reports of sutured PC IOLs in penetrating keratoplasty. Lindquist et al.,[12] studying scleral-sutured PC IOLs without penetrating keratoplasty, also found results comparable to those in published reports using AC IOLs. Although the difference in complication rate is not striking in any series, some authors have found more complications with the scleral-sutured PC IOLs, compared with either iris-sutured PC IOLs or modern, flexible open-loop AC IOLs. In the setting of penetrating keratoplasty, Schein et al.[20] reported that iris-sutured PC IOLs had the lowest rate of early complications. This may have been a result of the increased complexity of the scleral-suturing techniques, which were relatively new at the time of that study.

Overall results of secondary IOL surgery are better if the initial cataract surgery had been uncomplicated.[8] Eyes with previous cataract surgery complicated by vitreous loss have worse results regardless of the type of IOL used at the second surgery. Vitrectomy at the time of placement of a scleral-sutured IOL does not seem to relate to the final visual acuity.[19,21,22] However, there is at least one report in the literature that contradicts this conclusion; Wong, Koch, and Emery[23] found a 28% incidence of retinal complications if vitrectomy was done at the time of secondary IOL placement.

Visual acuity results with scleral-sutured PC IOLs during penetrating keratoplasty have been similar, for the most part, to those achieved with other modern lens types.

Eighty-two percent of patients had better vision postoperatively compared with the preoperative vision if a combined corneal transplant and scleral-sutured PC IOL was performed.[24] Only 4–10% of patients had worse vision postoperatively, compared with preoperative vision, after scleral-sutured PC IOLs with or without corneal transplantation.[24,25] Several studies agree that approximately 30% of patients have vision of 20/40 or better after penetrating keratoplasty with scleral-sutured PC IOLs.[14,24,26,35] Lass et al.[26] included a control group of patients who had corneal transplants with modern AC IOLs and found that 25% of the AC IOL group had a final vision of 20/40 or better. Thirty-five percent of patients after penetrating keratoplasty with scleral-sutured PC IOLs had a vision of 20/200 or worse.[24] For iris-sutured PC IOLs with corneal transplantation, the final vision was 20/40 or better in approximately 45% of patients.[21] Most authors conclude that modern AC IOLs, scleral-sutured PC IOLs, and iris-sutured PC IOLs all achieve similar short-term results if used with penetrating keratoplasty. There are fewer studies of visual results of sutured lenses alone, without corneal transplantation, and they typically report on smaller numbers of patients. Nonetheless, visual results are reasonable. Patients with good preoperative corrected visual acuity and secondary sutured PC IOL placement usually maintained their preoperative vision.

Wagoner and colleagues reviewed the world literature on IOL implantation in the absence of capsular support, an Ophthalmic Technology Assessment Report on behalf of the American Academy of Ophthalmology, published in 2003, covering the period of 1980 to 2001.[27] Of 189 citations, they found 43 suitable case series or higher level studies, but only six publications suitable for comparative statistical analysis. In a report by Hennig of 2002 cases randomized between an AC IOL and no IOL after intracapsular cataract extraction, the only significant difference was in the rate of glaucoma escalation of treatment, at 1.3% for the AC IOL group vs. 0.2% for the aphakic control group ($P = 0.05$).[28] In the previously cited Schein et al study of 176 patients randomized at PKP, the only significant difference was in the rate of postoperative CME (iris-sutured: 20%; AC IOL: 38%; sclaeral sutured 41%; $P = 0.02$).[20] Note that all of these rates are high, perhaps reflective of many of the PKPs being done

for corneal edema due to closed loop AC IOLs. In a study of PKP patients, Sugar et al found lower endothelial cell loss rates with flexible open loop AC IOLs than iris-sutured or transscleral sutured IOLs, but the difference did not reach statistical significance.[29] Davis found no statistically significant differences between AC IOLs and sutured PC IOLs at PKP.[30] In a nonrandomized case series of secondary implants, Lyle and Jin found minimal differences between AC IOLs and sutured PC IOLs.[31] In the sixth comparative series, Belluci et al compared 35 eyes with AC IOLs to 33 eyes with scleral sutured PC IOLs.[32] No statistically significant differences were found in mean visual acuity, corneal edema, glaucoma escalation, CME, lens tilt or decentration, retinal detachment, or endophthalmitis.

Collins and coworkers looked at the outcomes in Veterans Administration patients after complicated cataract surgery.[33] Four-hundred and thirty-eight eyes had adequate peripheral capsule after anterior vitrectomy and randomly received either an AC IOL or a sulcus fixated PC IOL. A significant difference occurred in visual acuity after 1 year, with 79% of AC IOL vs. 91% of sulcus fixated (unsutured) PC IOL patients achieving 20/40 or better best-corrected visual acuity (BCVA) ($P = 0.003$). In a second arm of that study, looking at 143 eyes with inadequate capsular support for sulcus fixation of a PC IOL, and without randomization, 125 eyes received an AC IOL (87.4%), only two eyes received a sutured PC IOL (1.4%), 11 eyes received no IOL (7.7%), and the implant status was unknown in five eyes (3.5%).[34] Only 66.7% of the inadequate capsule total group achieved BCVA of 20/40 or better, significantly less than either arm of the earlier study ($P = 0.04$). This finding emphasizes that extensive vitrectomy and loss of capsular support is associated with poorer outcomes, independent of the IOL implant.

■ COMPLICATIONS ■

Although overall visual acuity rates are similar among IOL groups, there may be a tendency toward an increased risk of unusual but serious complications with scleral-sutured PC IOLs. These serious complications include retinal detachment, hemorrhagic choroidal detachment, and later lens dislocation.[14] Sundmacher et al.[25] found that there was a 12% rate of severe complications with scleral-sutured PC IOLs. However, they pointed out that many of these eyes had preoperative disease, and half the complications were unrelated to the surgical method. These researchers believed that vascular risk factors predisposed patients to complications from scleral-sutured IOLs. Schein et al.[20] found a greater overall rate of complications with scleral-sutured PC IOLs compared with iris-sutured PC IOLs or modern AC IOLs. However, Heidemann and Dunn[14] reported that the incidences of glaucoma, CME, and graft failure with scleral-sutured PC IOLs were comparable to those with iris-sutured PC IOLs and modern AC IOLs used with penetrating keratoplasty. Table 41-7 compares the relative rates of various complications among the different lens options. This table extrapolates from data derived from initial studies and should be only considered a rough approximation of true relative complication rates.

The most common postoperative complication after scleral-sutured PC IOL implantation is persistent CME.[9] A range of 9–36% of patients with scleral-sutured lenses and penetrating keratoplasty had this complication.[9,36] Schein et al.[20] reported that slightly less macular edema was clinically observed if iris-sutured

Table 41-7 Relative frequency of complications associated with secondary IOLs

Complication	Capsular-Supported PC IOL	AC IOL	Scleral-Sutured PC IOL	Iris-Sutured PC IOL
Acute CME	+	++	++	++
Chronic CME	−	+	+	+
Glaucoma	−	++	+	+
Lens tilt or decentration	−	+	++	++
Polypropylene knot erosion	NA	NA	++	NA
Suture-related endophthalmitis	NA	NA		NA
Endophthalmitis (unrelated to polypropylene suture)	+	+	+	+
Corneal edema	+	++	+	+
Intraoperative bleeding	+	+	++	++
Synechiae	−	++	−	+
Retinal detachment	−	+	++	+
Choroidal detachment	−	+	++	+
Uveitis/iritis	−	++	−	+
Long-term corneal graft failure	−	+	−	−
Risk of polypropylene suture failure	NA	NA	+	+

* −, not associated; +, mild association; ++, strong association; NA, not applicable.
AC, Anterior chamber; CME, cystoid macular edema; IOL, intraocular lens; PC, posterior chamber.

PC IOLs were used, compared with scleral-sutured PC IOLs or flexible open-loop AC IOLs. Although CME was a relatively frequent acute postoperative complication of scleral-sutured lenses, some patients who had a long-standing decrease in vision preoperatively because of CME improved greatly after AC IOL exchange for a scleral-sutured lens.[9,12] Thirty-two percent of patients with preoperative CME had a vision of 20/40 or better postoperatively with penetrating keratoplasty combined with a scleral-sutured PC IOL.[14]

Glaucoma is the second most common complication with scleral-sutured PC IOLs implanted at the same time as a penetrating keratoplasty.[14] It is difficult to determine the cause of this glaucoma because keratoplasty alone is associated with a 5–65% incidence of new onset of glaucoma.[3] Lass et al.[26] found that the mean intraocular pressure was significantly higher with scleral-sutured PC IOLs when compared with penetrating keratoplasty with flexible open-loop AC lenses. However, they recognized that their study may have been somewhat biased by case selection because patients with extensive peripheral synechiae preoperatively did not receive AC IOLs. Holland et al.[35] suspected that scleral-sutured lenses were associated with glaucoma; they found new-onset ocular hypertension in 30.3% of patients after a penetrating keratoplasty with a scleral-sutured PC IOL. Heidemann and Dunn[14] found that 59% of their patients with corneal transplant and scleral-sutured lenses required additional glaucoma medication postoperatively. Therefore, although sutured PC IOLs were not expected on theoretical grounds to be associated with glaucoma, initial studies suggest a possible correlation above that found with corneal transplant alone. Bias resulting from case selection may be responsible for most, or all, of this trend, however.

Lens tilt or decentration is found in 5–10% of patients after scleral-sutured PC lens implantation.[25,36] IOLs with large optics are recommended, so a small degree of decentration is not usually clinically significant. Proper polypropylene suture placement and tension are important in avoiding this complication.

Initially, scleral-sutured lenses were tied under conjunctival flaps alone. However, the high incidence of erosion of the sutures through the conjunctiva prompted surgeons to place these knots under scleral flaps. Solomon et al.[37] found that polypropylene suture erosion was the most common complication of scleral-sutured PC IOLs. Even with scleral flaps, up to 17% of patients have sutures that erode through the conjunctiva.[35,37] This rate greatly exceeds the experience of most surgeons, however. Without scleral flaps, 23.8% of patients have sutures erode through the conjunctiva. Because suture-related endophthalmitis has been reported,[38] it is recommended that all exposed sutures be treated either with cautery or with free scleral grafts.[16] Some have recommended leaving the polypropylene suture ends long so that they lie flatter on the globe, thus avoiding exposure.[12]

PBK has not been a frequently reported complication of scleral-sutured PC IOLs, perhaps partially because of the relatively short follow-up in these early studies of a new technique. If endothelial cell counts are measured after corneal transplantation with scleral-sutured lenses and compared with the results from corneal transplantation with modern AC IOLs, there is no significant difference in endothelial cell loss.[26] Soong et al.[9] found a 19% endothelial cell loss after 1 year with iris-sutured PC IOLs, compared with 28% with closed-loop AC IOLs.

Although bleeding in the form of vitreous hemorrhage or hyphema would be anticipated to be a frequent problem with scleral-sutured lenses because of the proximity of the needle path to the ciliary body, this has not turned out to be the case, and hemorrhages are relatively infrequent.[15]

Heidemann and Dunn[14] reported an 11% incidence of hyphema or vitreous hemorrhage in association with scleral-sutured PC IOLs. Holland et al.,[35] however, reported no hyphemas in 115 cases. The highest reported incidence of bleeding was 22%, reported by Kora, Fukado, and Yaguchi.[39] However, their experience was atypical. Proper passage of the needles through the ciliary sulcus rather than the pars plicata may help prevent this complication. Vitreous hemorrhage, if it occurs, is usually self-limited and spontaneously clears. Massive suprachoroidal hemorrhage is rare.

Although few studies address the question of synechial progression, at least one early report seems to contradict theoretical expectations. Schein et al.[20] found less synechial progression with modern AC IOLs compared with scleral- or iris-sutured PC IOLs. This may, however, result from the fact that AC lenses were oriented in the same meridian as the closed-loop AC lenses that they replaced. New synechiae formation may be limited by the synechiae already present from the older AC lens.

There appears to be a slightly greater risk of retinal detachment with sutured PC IOLs. Soong et al.[9] reported a 2.3% risk of retinal detachment with corneal transplant combined with iris-sutured PC IOL implantation. Three studies with corneal transplantation and scleral-sutured PC lenses reported a 2.7–5.4% risk of retinal detachment after this combined procedure.[14,24,35] Several retinal detachments have been reported with a retinal hole in the meridian of one of the transscleral sutures.[40] Not all studies have identified transscleral suture fixation of PC IOLs as a risk factor for retinal detachment, however.[41] Pathology studies examining eyes that have had sutured PC lenses implanted have found that haptics are usually posterior to the ciliary body adjacent to the pars plana rather than in the ciliary sulcus.[1,4,42] This may increase the risk of retinal detachment. The location of the haptics at the pars plana was found in pathology specimens from both iris- and scleral-sutured PC lenses. The authors explain this finding by the fact that the iris often sags when the globe is fluid filled, making the ciliary sulcus inaccessible internally.[4] They recommend the use of an air bubble to help pull the iris away from the ciliary sulcus. One surgeon used an endoscope to locate the ciliary sulcus intraoperatively.[39] A second explanation for the poor positioning of the haptics with sutured PC lenses is incorrect measurements used in placing the scleral sutures. A surgeon may easily overestimate the distance between the limbus and the ciliary sulcus.

Theoretically, the risk of choroidal detachment ought to increase with the length of operative hypotony. Also, transscleral sutures ought to increase the risk of choroidal hemorrhage or effusion.[14] Early studies seem to bear out this expectation to a small degree. Holland et al.[35] found that choroidal detachments, if they occurred, were often located alongside the site of a transscleral suture. Heidemann and Dunn[24] found that 3.6% of scleral-sutured PC IOLs were associated with a choroidal detachment, although these were nonexpulsive.

Uveitis does not seem to be frequently associated with sutured PC lenses. In a series of 105 penetrating keratoplasties with scleral-sutured PC lenses, there were no reported cases of chronic uveitis.[35] Theoretically, iris-sutured lenses may cause more inflammation as a result of irritation of uveal tissue because of suspension of the relatively heavy IOL from the iris. Pathology specimens

from iris-sutured PC lenses show mild-to-moderate local inflammation, but this has not been shown to be clinically significant.

A disturbing late complication is the report of spontaneous polypropylene suture breakage leading to displaced PC IOLs. Price et al.[43] reported five such cases of late breakage of previously stable iris-supported PC IOLs. It appears that the polypropylene suture was cut by persistent rubbing at the optic hole of the IOL over time. This occurred on average 9 years after the initial surgery. Pathology studies have shown that sutures are the primary fixation point for both iris- and scleral-sutured PC IOLs.[1,42] There is no postoperative fibrosis[14] and no inflammatory reaction around the polypropylene suture.[42]

Accidental cutting of the polypropylene suture is sometimes associated with dislocation of the IOL into the vitreous cavity.[42] This dislocation often is delayed after the cutting of the polypropylene suture, suggesting that the haptic may be embedded into tissue over time, but this fixation is not necessarily adequate to support the IOL long term in the absence of the suture.

Several visual complications are unrelated to the sutured PC IOL procedure. Often age-related macular degeneration was discovered after lens implantation. Vision was found to be limited by this condition in 5.7% of cases after penetrating keratoplasty with scleral-sutured PC IOL.[35] Maculopathy from other causes, such as vascular causes, was found in a minority of cases.

■ COMPARISON OF SUTURED POSTERIOR-CHAMBER INTRAOCULAR LENSES WITH OPEN-LOOP FLEXIBLE ANTERIOR-CHAMBER INTRAOCULAR LENSES ■

In most cases of secondary IOLs, the management decision is between a scleral-sutured PC IOL and AC IOL. There has been no convincing study implicating the modern, flexible open-loop AC IOLs with the many problems associated with the older, rigid closed-loop designs. Modern AC lenses have a greatly decreased incidence of postoperative pain and a decreased incidence of UGH syndrome.[44] Many studies have shown that there is a low rate of overall complications with these newer designs. Apple et al.[1] found that, although 75% of AC IOLs inserted now are of modern, flexible open-loop design, fewer than 15% of complicated AC IOL cases involved flexible open-loop AC IOLs. Mamalis et al.[45] found a favorable outcome in 86% of IOL exchanges to a flexible open-loop design, compared with 90% with exchanges to a standard, nonsutured, in-the-bag PC IOL. The similarity in the results between even standard nonsutured PC IOLs and AC IOLs supports the assertion that both are very stable in the eye. Uveitis is rare with the newer open-loop flexible AC IOLs.[45]

Soong et al.[9] found similar results after penetrating keratoplasty with IOL exchange whether the new lens was an iris-sutured PC lens or a modern AC IOL. Visual results showed that 57–63% of patients after penetrating keratoplasty and modern AC lens placement achieved 20/40 vision or better.[19,46] Endothelial cell counts were also similar with AC and PC lens types. Soong et al.[9] stated that not only were the endothelial cell counts as low with modern AC lenses as with unsutured standard PC IOLs, but they were lower than counts seen with iris-sutured PC lenses:

11.2 vs. 19% loss. The rate of new glaucoma with AC lenses and penetrating keratoplasty is similar to that with penetrating keratoplasty alone.[46] Although persistent CME is a frequent postoperative problem after penetrating keratoplasty and IOL exchange with any lens type, modern AC lenses perform similarly to other lens types in terms of the incidence of CME. Synechiae are usually not formed with the modern AC lenses. Synechiae are commonly seen in the meridian of the haptics with older, rigid AC lens types.

If one accepts the premise that the behavior of an IOL that is retained at penetrating keratoplasty is an indication of the stability of the lens in the eye in general, then the study by Sugar[29] is illuminating. In a study of 469 patients over a 10-year period, he found that vision was best if the older lens was exchanged for a flexible open-loop AC IOL. The results were even better than if iris-sutured PC IOLs were used. Also, corneal transplant failure rates were lowest if flexible open-loop AC lenses were used at the time of penetrating keratoplasty. He found that the corneal transplant failure rate (as opposed to corneal rejection) was highest if closed-loop rigid AC lenses were left in the eye at the time of corneal transplantation and lowest for retained in-the-bag PC IOLs. Retained rigid closed-loop AC lenses were associated with a 33.6% rate of transplant failure. Iris pupillary-supported (not sutured) IOLs were associated with a 28.9% corneal transplant failure rate, and retained primary implanted PC IOLs (standard, unsutured) were associated with only a 6.4% rate of transplant failure. Endothelial cell counts confirmed this data for penetrating keratoplasty and retained IOLs. The rigid closed-loop AC lenses were associated with a 34% drop in endothelial cell counts. Iris pupillary-supported IOLs were associated with a 31% drop in endothelial cell count. However, retained PC IOLs (unsutured) were associated with only a 17% drop in endothelial cell count.

CONCLUSIONS ■

Little debate exists that the placement of a standard PC IOL is the method of choice for a secondary IOL in the presence of sufficient capsular support. In the cases without capsular support, the decision is more difficult. It is impossible to reach firm conclusions regarding sutured PC lenses with present information. It seems clear that modern AC lenses have been disregarded prematurely by some surgeons and that they provide a valuable alternative to sutured PC lenses for many patients. The visual results for most patients with scleral-sutured lenses are comparable to those with other lens types. However, there is some reason to be concerned about the higher risk of some serious complications with scleral-sutured PC IOLs. These complications include a higher risk of retinal detachment, choroidal hemorrhage, lens dislocation, suture exposure and endophthalmitis, glaucoma, and persistent CME. On the other hand, scleral-sutured PC IOLs are an attractive alternative for patients with complications attributable to an AC IOL, such as chronic iritis and CME, and for patients where relative contraindications to an AC IOL are present, such as iris or angle abnormalities.

No large study has yet addressed long-term outcomes in patients randomized between modern, flexible open-loop AC IOLs and scleral-sutured PC IOLs, especially regarding endothelial cell loss.

References

[1] Apple DJ, Price FW, Gwin T, et al. Sutured retropupillary posterior chamber intraocular lenses for exchange or secondary implantation. Ophthalmology 1989;96:1241–1247.
[2] Soong HK, Meyer RF, Sugar A. Techniques of posterior chamber lens implantation without capsular support during penetrating keratoplasty: a review. J Refract Corneal Surg 1989;5:249–255.
[3] Gaster RN, Ong HV. Results of penetrating keratoplasty with posterior chamber intraocular lens implantation in the absence of a lens capsule. Cornea 1991;10:498–506.
[4] Duffey RJ, Holland EJ, Agapitos PJ, et al. Anatomic study of transsclerally sutured intraocular lens implantation. Am J Ophthalmol 1989;108:300–309.
[5] Spigelman AV, Lindstrom RL, Nichols BD, et al. Implantation of a posterior chamber intraocular lens without capsular support during penetrating keratoplasty or as a secondary lens implant. Ophthalmic Surg 1988;19:396–398.
[6] Panton RW, Sulewski ME, Parker JS, et al. Surgical management of subluxed posterior-chamber intraocular lenses. Arch Ophthalmol 1983;111:919–926.
[7] Price FW, Whitson WE, Collins K, et al. Explanation of posterior chamber intraocular lenses. J Cataract Refract Surg 1992;18:475–479.
[8] Doren G, Stern G, Driebe WT. Indications for and results of intraocular lens explantation. J Cataract Refract Surg 1992;18:79–85.
[9] Soong HK, Musch DC, Kowal V, et al. Implantation of posterior chamber intraocular lenses in the absence of lens capsule during penetrating keratoplasty. Arch Ophthalmol 1989;107:660–665.
[10] Stark WJ, Gottsch JD, Goodman DF, et al. Posterior chamber intraocular lens implantation in the absence of capsular support. Arch Ophthalmol 1989;107:1078–1083.
[11] Smiddy WE, Sawusch MR, O'Brien TP, et al. Implantation of scleral-fixated posterior chamber intraocular lenses. J Cataract Refract Surg 1990;16:691–696.
[12] Lindquist TD, Agapitos PJ, Lindstrom RL, et al. Transscleral fixation of posterior chamber intraocular lenses in the absence of capsular support. Ophthalmic Surg 1989;20:769–775.
[13] Yasukawa T, Suga K, Akita J, et al. Comparison of ciliary sulcus fixation techniques for posterior chamber intraocular lenses. J Cataract Refract Surg 1998;24:840–845.
[14] Heidemann DG, Dunn SP. Transsclerally sutured intraocular lenses in penetrating keratoplasty. Am J Ophthalmol 1992;113:619–625.
[15] Hu BV, Shin DH, Gibbs KA, et al. Implantation of posterior chamber intraocular lens in the absence of capsular and zonular support. Arch Ophthalmol 1988;106:416–420.
[16] Oshima Y, Oida H, Emi K. Transscleral fixation of acrylic intraocular lenses in the absence of capsular support through 3.5 mm self-sealing incisions. J Cataract Refract Surg 1998;24:1223–1229.
[17] Lewis JS. Ab externo sulcus fixation. Ophthalmic Surg 1991;22:692–695.
[18] Lewis JS. Sulcus fixation without flaps. Ophthalmology 1993;100:1346–1350.
[19] Kornmehl EW, Steinert RF, Odrich MG, et al. Penetrating keratoplasty for pseudophakic bullous keratopathy associated with closed-loop anterior chamber intraocular lenses. Ophthalmology 1990;97:407–414.
[20] Schein OD, Kenyon KR, Steinert RF, et al. A randomized trial of intraocular lens fixation techniques with penetrating keratoplasty. Invest Ophthalmology 1993;100:1437–1443.
[21] Van Der Schaft TL, Van Rij G, Renardel De Lavalette JGC, et al. Results of penetrating keratoplasty for pseudophakic bullous keratopathy with the exchange of an intraocular lens. Br J Ophthalmol 1989;73:704–708.
[22] Hayward JM, Noble BA, George N. Secondary intraocular lens implantation: eight year experience. Eye 1990;4:548–556.
[23] Wong SK, Koch DD, Emery JM. Secondary intraocular lens implantation. J Cataract Refract Surg 1987;13:17–20.
[24] Heidemann DG, Dunn SP. Visual results and complications of transsclerally-sutured intraocular lenses in penetrating keratoplasty. Ophthalmic Surg 1990;21:609–614.
[25] Sundmacher R, Althaus C, Webster R, et al. Two years experience with transscleral fixation of posterior chamber lenses. Dev Ophthalmol 1991;22:89–93.
[26] Lass JH, DeSantis DM, Reinhart WJ, et al. Clinical and morphometric results of penetrating keratoplasty with one-piece anterior-chamber or suture-fixated posterior-chamber lenses in the absence of lens capsule. Arch Ophthalmol 1990;108:1427–1431.
[27] Wagoner MD, Cox TA, Ariyasu RG, Jacobs DS, Karp CL. Intraocular lens implantation in the absence of capsular support: a report by the American Academy of Ophthalmology. Ophthalmology 2003;110:840–859.
[28] Hennig A, Evans JR, Pradhan D, et al. Randomised controlled trial of anterior-chamber intraocular lenses. Lancet 1997;349:1129–1133.
[29] Sugar A. An analysis of corneal endothelial and graft survival in pseudophakic bullous keratopathy. Trans Am Ophthalmol Soc 1990;87:762–801.
[30] Davis RM, Best D, Gilbert GE. Comparison of intraocular lens fixation techniques performed during penetrating keratoplasty. Am J Ophthalmol 1991;111:743–749.
[31] Lyle WA, Jin JC. Secondary intraocular lens implantation: anterior chamber vs posterior chamber lenses. Ophthalmic Surg 1993;24:375–381.
[32] Bellucci R, Pucci V, Morselli S, Bonomi L. Secondary implantation of angle-supported anterior chamber and scleral-fixated posterior chamber intraocular lenses. J Cataract Refract Surg 1996;22:247–252.
[33] Collins JF, Gaster RN, Krol WF, Colling CL, Kirk GF, Smith TJ. Department of Veterans Affairs Cooperative Cataract Study. A comparison of anterior chamber and posterior chamber intraocular lenses after vitreous presentation during cataract surgery: the Department of Veterans Affairs Cooperative Cataract Study. Am J Ophthalmol 2003;136:1–9.
[34] Collins JF, Gaster RN, Krol WF. Outcomes in patients having vitreous presentation during cataract surgery who lack capsular support for a nonsutured PC IOL. Am J Ophthalmol 2006;141:71–78.
[35] Holland EJ, Daya SM, Evangelista A, et al. Penetrating keratoplasty and transscleral fixation of posterior chamber lens. Am J Ophthalmol 1992;114:182–187.
[36] Hayashi K, Hayashi H, Nakao F, et al. Intraocular lens tilt and decentration, anterior chamber depth, and refractive error after trans-scleral suture fixation surgery. Ophthalmology 1999;106:878–882.
[37] Solomon K, Gussler JR, Gussler C, et al. Incidence and management of complications of transsclerally sutured posterior chamber intraocular lenses. J Cataract Refract Surg 1993;19:488–493.
[38] Schechter RJ. Suture-wick endophthalmitis with sutured posterior chamber intraocular lenses. J Cataract Refract Surg 1990;16:755–756.
[39] Kora Y, Fukado Y, Yaguchi S. Sulcus fixations of posterior chamber intraocular lenses by transscleral sutures. J Cataract Refract Surg 1991;17:636–639.
[40] Rajpal RK, Carney MD, Weinberg RS, et al. Complications of transscleral sutured posterior chamber lenses. Ophthalmology 1991;98:98.
[41] Lee J, Lee J, Chung H. Factors contributing to retinal detachment after transscleral fixation of posterior chamber intraocular lenses. J Cataract Refract Surg 1998;24:697–702.
[42] Lubniewski AJ, Holland EJ, Van Meter WS, et al. Histologic study of eyes with transsclerally sutured posterior chamber intraocular lenses. Am J Ophthalmol 1990;110:237–243.

[43] Price FW, Whitson WE, Collins K, et al. Changing trends in explanting intraocular lenses: a single center study. J Cataract Refract Surg 1992;18:470–474.

[44] Hahn TW, Kim MS, Kim JH. Secondary intraocular lens implantation in aphakia. J Cataract Refract Surg 1992;18:174–179.

[45] Mamalis N, Crandall AS, Pulsipher MV, et al. Intraocular lens explantation and exchange: a review of lens styles, clinical indications, clinical results, and visual outcome. J Cataract Refract Surg 1991;17:811–818.

[46] Hassan TS, Soong HK, Sugar A, et al. Implantation of Kelman-style, open-loop anterior chamber lenses during keratoplasty for aphakic and pseudophakic bullous keratopathy: a comparison with iris-sutured posterior chamber lenses. Ophthalmology 1991;98:875–880.

CONCLUSIONS

Pathology of Cataract Surgery and Intraocular Lenses

**Liliana Werner, MD, PhD, David J. Apple, MD
and Nick Mamalis, MD**

42

CONTENTS

CHAPTER HIGHLIGHTS

>> Interaction of the capsule and the intraocular lens

>> Factors in posterior capsule opacification

>> IOL opacification and discoloration

■ INTRODUCTION ■

Cataract surgery with intraocular lens (IOL) implantation evolved into a highly successful procedure, much of it influenced by technological advances. An estimate 6 million cataract surgeries with intraocular lens (IOL) implantation are performed worldwide each year. The number of surgeries performed in the US was estimated as more than 600,000 in 1982,[1] and approximately 2.4 million in 1996 (*http://www.cignamedicare.com*). In the authors' laboratory at the John A. Moran Eye Center, University of Utah, pathological analyses of pseudophakic human eyes obtained postmortem is performed, as well as of explanted IOLs. These specimens provide great insight into the mechanisms of complications of modern cataract surgery with IOL implantation. In this chapter, the text will focus on two types of postoperative complications: capsular bag opacification,[2–4] and IOL opacification/

Supported in part by a grant from Research to Prevent Blindness, Inc., New York, NY, to the Department of Ophthalmology and Visual Sciences, University of Utah, and by the Research to Prevent Blindness Olga Keith Weiss Scholar Award (to Liliana Werner, MD, PhD).

discoloration leading to explantation.[5] This text is largely, but not exclusively based on the analyses done in the authors' laboratory.

■ CAPSULAR BAG OPACIFICATION ■

Until recently, efforts for the prevention of opacification within the capsular bag were basically concentrated on the prevention of opacification of the posterior capsule. However, research on the prevention of any form of opacification/fibrosis within the capsular bag is increasing in significance, especially now with the advent of specialized IOLs such as accommodative lenses, which are generally designed to enable a forward movement of the optic upon efforts of accommodation. The functionality of such lenses will likely require the long-term transparency and elasticity of the capsular bag. Therefore, prevention of opacification of the anterior capsule, which is essentially a fibrotic entity, and of interlenticular opacification, which is relevant in piggyback implantation but also with dual-optic accommodating lenses, is also very important.

■ HISTOLOGY OF THE CRYSTALLINE LENS ■

The epithelium of the crystalline lens consists of a sheet of anterior epithelial cells ("A" cells) that are a continuity of the cells in the equatorial lens bow ("E" cells) (Figure 42-1). The latter cells comprise the germinal cells that undergo mitosis as they peel off from the equator. They constantly form new lens fibers during normal lens growth. Although both the anterior and equatorial lens epithelial cells stem from a continuous cell line and remain in continuity, it is useful to divide these into two functional groups. They differ in terms of function, growth patterns, and pathologic processes. The anterior or "A" cells, when disturbed, tend to remain in place and not migrate. They are prone to a transformation into fibrous-like tissue (pseudofibrous metaplasia). In sharp contrast, in pathologic states, the "E" cells of the equatorial lens bow tend to migrate posteriorly along the posterior capsule; e.g., in posterior subcapsular cataracts. In general, instead of undergoing a fibrous transformation, they tend to form large,

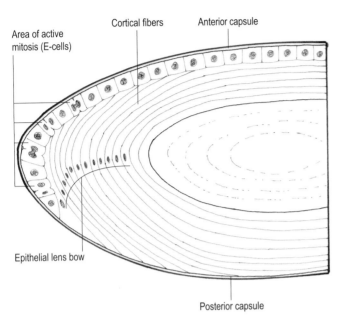

Cortical fibers   Anterior capsule

Area of active mitosis (E-cells)

Epithelial lens bow

Posterior capsule

Figure 42-1 Schematic drawing representing the histology of the crystalline lens.

balloon-like bladder cells (the cells of Wedl). These are the cell types involved in the different forms of capsular bag opacification that may be observed in modern cataract surgery, including posterior capsule opacification, anterior capsule opacification, and interlenticular opacification.[2–4]

■ POSTERIOR CAPSULE OPACIFICATION ■

INTRODUCTION

Secondary cataract or posterior capsule opacification (PCO) is the most common postoperative complication following cataract surgery. Its incidence has decreased over the past few decades as the understanding of its pathogenesis has evolved. Advances in surgical technique, IOL design and materials have all contributed to the gradual decline in PCO incidence. However, it remains a major cause of decreased visual acuity after cataract surgery, occurring at a rate of between 3 and 50% during the first 5 postoperative years.[6]

PATHOGENESIS

PCO results from migration and proliferation of residual lens epithelial cells (LECs) onto the central posterior capsule. When the cells invade the visual axis as pearls, fibrotic plaques, or wrinkles, the patient experiences a decrease in visual function and, ultimately, in visual acuity.[7] As discussed earlier, in pathologic states, the "E" cells of the equatorial lens bow tend to migrate posteriorly along the posterior capsule; e.g., in posterior subcapsular cataracts, and the pearl form of PCO. In general, instead of undergoing a fibrotic transformation, they tend to form large, balloon-like bladder cells (the cells of Wedl). These are the cells that are clinically visible as "pearls" (Elschnig pearls). These equatorial cells are the primary source of classic secondary cataract, especially the pearl form of PCO. In a recent clinical study by Neumayer et al. significant changes in the

morphology of Elschnig pearls were observed within time intervals of only 24 h. Appearance and disappearance of pearls, as well as progression and regression of pearls within these short intervals, illustrate the dynamic behavior of regeneratory PCO.[8]

The "E" cells are also those responsible for formation of a Soemmering's ring, which is a doughnut-shaped lesion composed of retained/regenerated cortex and cells that may form following any type of disruption of the anterior lens capsule. This lesion was initially described in connection with ocular trauma. The basic pathogenic factor of the Soemmering's ring is the anterior capsular break, which may then allow exit of central nuclear and cortical material out of the lens, with subsequent Elschnig pearl formation. A Soemmering's ring forms every time any form of extracapsular cataract extraction (ECCE) is done, whether manually, automated, or with phacoemulsification. For practical purposes it is useful to consider this lesion as the basic precursor of classic PCO, especially the "pearl" form. The LECs have higher proliferative capacity in young compared with old patients; therefore, the incidence of PCO formation is higher in younger patients.

TREATMENT AND PREVENTION

The treatment of PCO is typically neodymium:YAG (Nd:YAG) laser posterior capsulotomy. This is a simple procedure in most cases, but is not without risks. Complications include IOL damage, IOL subluxation or dislocation, retinal detachment, and secondary glaucoma.[9] Therefore, prevention of this complication is important, not only because of the risks associated with its treatment, but also because of the costs involved in the procedure. Extensive research has been performed on the inhibition of LEC proliferation and migration by pharmacologic agents through various delivery systems, or IOL coatings, in vitro and in vivo animal studies. Physical techniques to kill the LECs, as well as immunotherapy, and gene therapy, have also been investigated.[10–12]

While basic research on the effective mechanism for PCO eradication evolves, the practical surgeon can already apply some principles to prevent it. Two major principles that may be applied to prevent PCO are categorized as follows:

1. One should strive to minimize the number of retained/regenerated lens epithelial cells (especially equatorial cells) and cortex following cortical clean up. This is the first line of defense against this complication.

2. If unwanted, proliferative cells remain, one can create a secondary line of defense by erecting a barrier to block growth of cells from the equatorial region (Soemmering's ring) toward the center of the visual axis.

Studies done in the authors' laboratory, as well as clinical studies done in other centers helped in the definition of three surgery-related factors that help in the prevention of PCO (Table 42-1):

1. Hydrodissection-enhanced cortical clean-up

2. In-the-bag IOL fixation

3. Performance of a capsulorrhexis slightly smaller than the diameter of the IOL optic (Figure 42-2).

The same studies helped in the definition of three IOL-related factors for PCO prevention (Table 42-1):

Table 42-1 Surgery- and intraocular-lens (IOL)-related factors for prevention of posterior capsule opacification (PCO)

Six Factors for PCO Prevention	
Surgery-Related Factors	**IOL-Related Factors**
1. Hydrodissection-enhanced cortical clean-up	4. Biocompatible IOL to reduce stimulation of cellular proliferation
2. In-the-bag IOL fixation	5. Contact between the IOL optic and the posterior capsule
3. Capsulorrhexis smaller than the diameter of the IOL optic	6. IOL with a square, truncated optic edge

4. Use of a biocompatible IOL to reduce stimulation of cellular proliferation

5. Enhancement of the contact between the IOL optic and the posterior capsule

6. An IOL with a square, truncated optic edge.

HYDRODISSECTION-ENHANCED CORTICAL CLEAN-UP

Dr. Howard Fine introduced this technique and coined the term cortical cleaving hydrodissection.[13] The edge of the anterior capsule is slightly tented up by the tip of the cannula, while injecting the fluid. The technique is used by many surgeons to facilitate cortex and equatorial lens epithelial cells removal, also enhancing

the safety of the operation. The authors emphasize that complete cortical removal is critical, having a beneficial influence on the prevention of PCO. Following successful cortical cleaving hydrodissection, the operation is also easier and faster.[14] Experimental studies used different solutions during the hydrodissection step of the phacoemulsification procedure, e.g., preservative-free lidocaine 1%, antimitotics, etc.[15,16] Further studies are necessary to establish the safety and utility of these solutions in terms of PCO prevention.

It is especially important to remove all cortical material and "E" cells from the equatorial region of the capsular bag, which contribute to the formation of the Soemmering ring. While a careful cortical clean up and elimination of as many "E" cells as possible is fundamental in reducing the incidence of this complication, the role of anterior capsule polishing and elimination of "A" cells remains to be demonstrated. Indeed, Sacu et al. have recently performed a study to evaluate the effect of anterior capsule polishing on PCO.[17] In this randomized, prospective study, 26 patients received a silicone IOL with a truncated optic in both eyes. The anterior capsule was extensively polished in one eye and was left unpolished in the other eye. Digital slit-lamp photographs taken 1 year postoperatively using a standardized photographic technique showed that anterior capsule polishing caused no significant difference in the outcome of PCO. The same group of authors obtained similar results in another clinical study, with a 3-year follow-up.[18] Some authors actually believe that the postoperative fibrous metaplasia of remaining "A" cells would push the IOL against the posterior capsule, and that would explain the relatively low PCO rates of eyes implanted with silicone lenses having rounded optic edges.[19]

In theory, mechanical devices may also be used with the same objective as the hydrodissection step of the surgery. EpiLoop (PhacoTreat AB, Sweden) is a unique device under investigation, which has been designed to dissect the capsular bag of the crystalline lens from its contents, before their removal by phacoemulsification or extracapsular extraction. It consists of a handle with a cylinder, in which a tip, a movable piston and a flexible filament are placed.

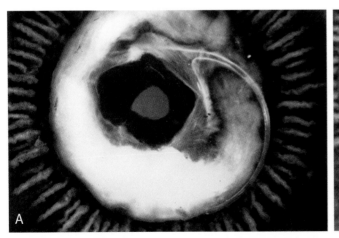 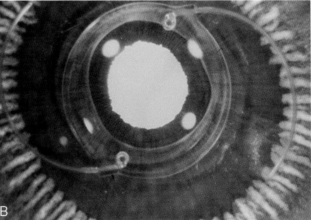

Figure 42-2 Gross photographs of pseudophakic human eyes obtained postmortem, taken from the posterior or Miyake-Apple view. **A**, One of the lens haptics is out of the bag. Extensive Soemmering's ring formation, as well as a posterior capsulotomy due to posterior capsule opacification (PCO) can be observed. **B**, The surgery-related factors for PCO prevention were applied in this case. The intraocular lens (IOL) was symmetrically implanted in the capsular bag, through a capsulorrhexis smaller than the IOL optic diameter, and a thorough cortical clean up was performed.

The filament forms a loop at the end of the tip, which may be expanded or reduced in diameter by moving the piston (Figure 42-3). Generally, two additional corneal incisions are made on each side of the main incision, and the current prototypes of EpiLoop will pass through 1.5 mm wide incisions. After capsulorrhexis, the tip of the device is introduced into the anterior chamber, directing the initial loop between the anterior capsule and the cortex. Then, approximately 3 cm of the filament are introduced, forming a single loop (or multiple loops) that progressively dissects the capsular bag from its contents (Figure 42-4). The procedure is repeated through the three incisions, therefore, covering 360° of the bag. Use of the EpiLoop would eventually reduce time and need of hydrodissection, cortex removal, and capsular polishing by irrigation–aspiration.

IN-THE-BAG INTRAOCULAR LENS FIXATION

The hallmark of modern cataract surgery is the achievement of consistent and secure in-the-bag or endocapsular IOL fixation. The most obvious advantage of in-the-bag fixation is the

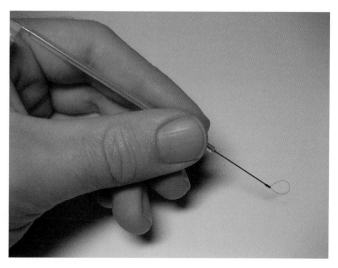

Figure 42-3 Photograph showing the EpiLoop.

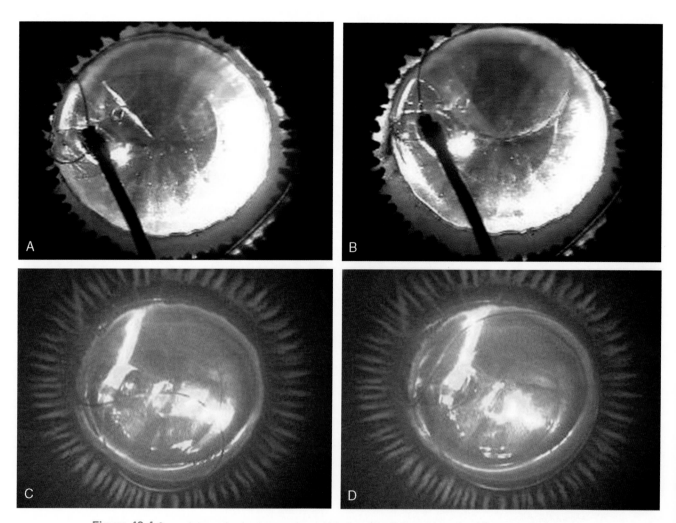

Figure 42-4 Gross photographs showing experimental injection of the EpiLoop blue-colored filament under the capsulorrhexis opening of a human eye obtained postmortem. The loop formed progressively dissected the capsular bag from its contents. **A** and **B**, Anterior or surgeon's view with retroillumination. **C** and **D**, Posterior or Miyake-Apple view.

POSTERIOR CAPSULE OPACIFICATION

accomplishment of good lens centration. However, endocapsular fixation functions primarily to enhance the IOL–optic barrier effect, as it will be discussed later. In a large series of human cadaver eyes implanted with different IOLs analyzed in the authors' laboratory, central PCO and Nd:YAG rates were both influenced by IOL fixation, i.e., less PCO and Nd:YAG capsulotomies in eyes where the IOLs were in the bag.[20]

Dr. Marie-José Tassignon proposed a variation of the in-the-bag IOL fixation concept for PCO prevention, named "bag-in-the-lens" implantation.[21] This involves the use of a twin-capsulorrhexis IOL design, and performance of anterior and posterior capsulorrhexis of the same size. The biconvex lens has a circular equatorial groove in the surrounding haptic, for placement of both capsules after capsulorrhexis. In theory, if the capsules are well stretched around the optic of this lens, the LECs will be captured within the remaining space of the capsular bag and their proliferation will be limited to this space, so the visual axis will remain clear (Figure 42-5). In studies performed in human eyes obtained postmortem, as well as in rabbits, bag-in-the-lens implantation was highly effective in preventing PCO, when the anterior and posterior capsules were properly secured in the IOL groove. More recently, a clinical study was performed comprising 100 eyes of 87 patients who had the bag-in-the-lens IOL implantation between January 2000 and August 2004.[22] The postoperative follow-up ranged between 17 and 72 months. One hundred eyes of 94 patients of the same age and with the same follow-up period were implanted with an IOL of the same biomaterial in the bag. The cumulative Nd:YAG laser frequency rates, defined by Kaplan-Meier survival analysis, showed a zero rate for the bag-in-the-lens implantation. A Nd:YAG laser capsulotomy was performed in 20 eyes having in-the-bag IOL implantation; the cumulative frequency in this group was 2% at 1 year and 20% at 71 months, with a plateau beginning at 42 months.

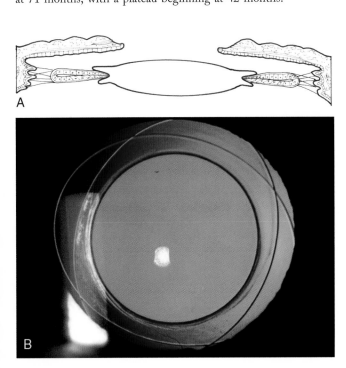

Figure 42-5 Schematic drawing (**A**), and clinical photograph (**B**) showing the bag-in-the-lens concept. (Courtesy of M.J. Tassignon, MD, Belgium.)

CAPSULORRHEXIS SIZE

There is evidence that PCO is reduced if the capsulorrhexis diameter is slightly smaller than that of the lens optic, so that the anterior edge rests on the optic. This helps provide a tight fit of the capsule around the optic analogous to "shrink-wrap," which has beneficial effects in maximizing the contact between the lens optic and the posterior capsule. Another advantage may be the sequestration of the interior compartment of the capsule containing the IOL from the surrounding aqueous humor and any potentially deleterious factors within it, such as inflammatory mediators. In a retrospective clinical study performed at the John A. Moran Eye Center, on patients implanted with different IOLs, including lenses with round or square optic edges, the degree of postoperative PCO was correlated with the degree of anterior capsule overlap.[23] Considering all patients, but also considering the patients distributed in different IOL groups, there was always a significant negative, linear correlation between the degree of overlap and PCO.

BIOCOMPATIBLE INTROCULAR LENS

There are many definitions for the term "biocompatibility." With regards to PCO, materials with ability to inhibit stimulation of cell proliferation are more "biocompatible." The "Sandwich" theory states that a hydrophobic acrylic IOL with bioadhesive surface would allow only a monolayer of lens epithelial cells to attach to the capsule and the lens, preventing further cell proliferation and capsular bag opacification. The authors performed two immunohistochemical studies on the adhesion of proteins to different IOLs that had been implanted in human eyes obtained postmortem.[24,25] Analyses of histological sections demonstrated that fibronectin mediates the adhesion of this hydrophobic acrylic lens (AcrySof, Alcon) to the anterior and posterior capsules. Analyses of explanted lenses confirmed the presence of greater amounts of fibronectin on the surfaces of the same lens (Figure 42-6). However, even though differences among materials exist, in terms of PCO prevention it appears that the geometry of the lens, with a square posterior optic edge is the most important factor (see IOL optic geometry).

BIOMATERIAL PROPERTIES: ANTERIOR CAPSULE OPACIFICATION

The adhesiveness of the material may have a more direct impact on the development of anterior capsule opacification (ACO). This generally occurs much earlier in comparison to PCO, sometimes within 1 month postoperatively. When the continuous curvilinear capsulorrhexis (CCC) is smaller than the IOL optic, the anterior surface of the optic's biomaterial maintains contact with the adjacent posterior aspect of the anterior capsule. Any remaining anterior lens epithelial cells (A cells) in contact with the IOL have the potential to undergo fibrous proliferation; thus, ACO is essentially a fibrotic entity. Studies in the authors' laboratory using pseudophakic human eyes obtained postmortem showed that ACO is more common with silicone IOLs, especially the plate designs, because of the larger area of

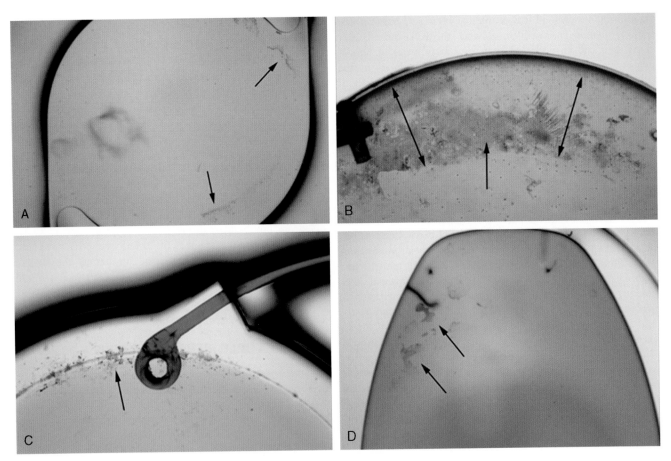

Figure 42-6 Photomicrographs of intraocular lenses explanted from human eyes obtained postmortem. Immunohistochemistry for fibronectin (red; arrows) revealed the presence of significant larger amounts of the protein attached to the surfaces of the hydrophobic acrylic lens in comparison with other biomaterials. This mediates the adhesion of this lens to the capsular bag. (Courtesy of AcrySof, Alcon)

contact between these lenses and the anterior capsule (Figure 42-7).[26,27] However, the same studies showed that the plate design resists contraction forces within the capsular bag better than three-piece silicone lenses with flexible haptics (polypropylene). These latter showed the higher rates of capsulorrhexis

phimosis and IOL decentration as a result of excessive capsular bag fibrosis (Figure 42-8). There is, therefore, a tendency in IOL manufacture favoring haptic materials with higher rigidity, such as poly(methyl methacrylate) (PMMA), polyimide (Elastimide), and poly(vinylidene) fluoride (PVDF).[28] In the same

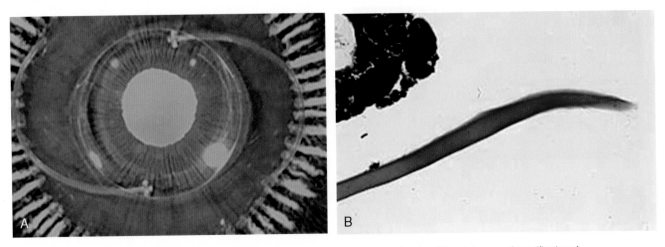

Figure 42-7 Gross photographs from human eyes obtained postmortem showing different degrees of opacification of the anterior capsule (left). **A** and **C,** hydrophobic acrylic intraocular lenses (IOLs).

(Continued)

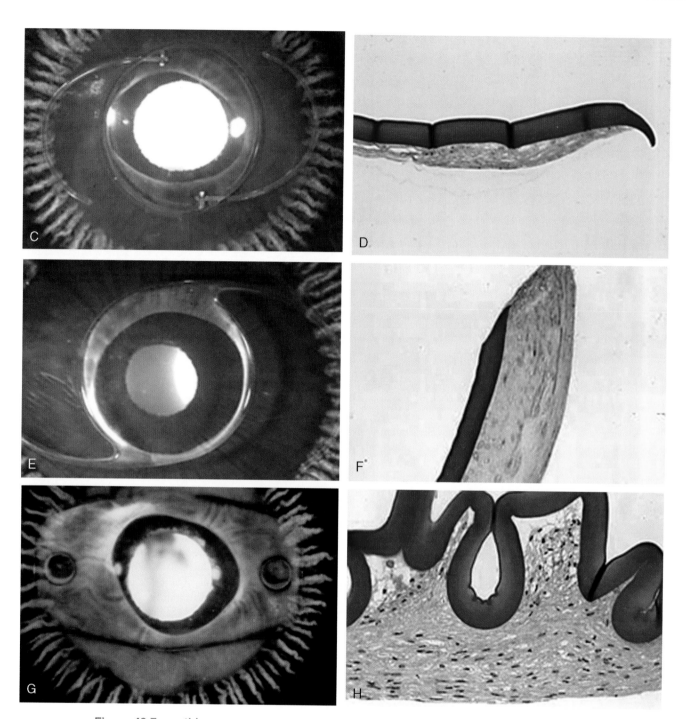

POSTERIOR CAPSULE OPACIFICATION

Figure 42-7, cont'd E, Polymethylmethacrylate IOL. G, Silicone IOL. The corresponding photomicrographs (right; periodic acid Schiff (PAS) stain) were taken at the level of the capsulorrhexis opening. The amount of proliferative fibrocellular tissue opacifying the anterior capsule was found to vary according to the IOL biomaterial keeping contact with the capsule.

studies, ACO was less significant with hydrophobic acrylic lenses having an adhesive surface.

ACO may eventually be prevented by the use of an IOL that does not keep contact with the inner surface of the anterior capsule. The authors evaluated two of such lenses in experimental studies. The first was a dual-optic silicone lens, with lateral expansions of the anterior optic, which are supposed to lift up the anterior capsule minimizing its contact with the anterior optic surface (Synchrony, Visiogen Inc.). No significant ACO was observed in a rabbit model implanted with this lens.[29] The second was a single-piece, hydrophilic acrylic lens, with six haptic components in a 10° angulation in relation to the optic (Concept 360, Corneal, France). The authors observed in human eyes obtained postmortem that this design promotes contact of the optic with the posterior capsule, while the anterior capsule is kept at distance of the anterior optic surface.[30]

ACO has been considered a clinical problem when anterior capsular shrinkage associated with constriction of the anterior

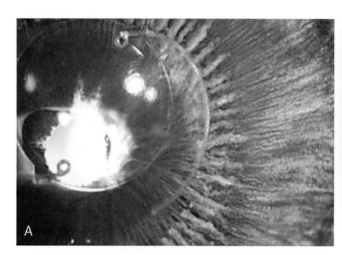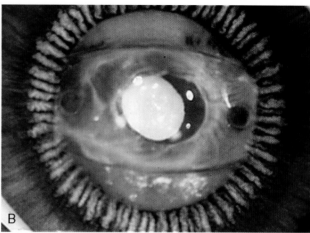

Figure 42-8 Gross photographs from human eyes obtained postmortem (Miyake-Apple view) implanted with a three-piece silicone lens with Prolene haptics (**A**), and a silicone plate lens (**B**). The eyes show capsulorrhexis phimosis due to excessive fibrosis. However, intraocular lens decentration is only observed with the three-piece lens, due to the flexible haptics that are less resistant to contraction forces within the capsular bag.

capsulectomy opening (capsulorrhexis contraction syndrome or capsular phimosis) accompanies excessive anterior capsule fibrosis.[31] This has been especially observed in conditions associated with zonular weakness, e.g., pseudoexfoliation and advanced age, and with chronic intraocular inflammation. Besides phimosis of the CCC opening, excessive zonular traction and its sequelae, IOL dislocation and retinal detachment can also occur because of excessive capsular fibrosis. Excessive opacification of the anterior capsule is problematic in that it hinders visualization of the peripheral fundus during retinal examination. Otherwise, a certain degree of ACO is sometimes considered an advantage, as it can prevent potential dysphotopsia phenomena caused by the square edge of some IOL optic designs. Also, anterior capsule fibrosis with contraction of the capsular bag will push the IOL optic against the posterior capsule, helping in the prevention of PCO according to the "no space, so cells" theory. This mechanism would explain the relatively low PCO rates with some silicone lenses, in the absence of a square optic edge profile, as noted above (see Hydrodissection-enhanced cortical clean-up).[19]

BIOMATERIAL PROPERTIES: INTERLENTICULAR OPACIFICATION

The adhesiveness of the IOL material may also have an influence on interlenticular opacification (ILO) formation. To date, all cases of ILO the authors have analyzed in the laboratory seemed to be related to two hydrophobic acrylic IOLs (AcrySof, Alcon) being implanted in the capsular bag through a small capsulorrhexis, with its margins overlapping the optic edge of the anterior IOL for 360°.[32–34] When these lenses are implanted in the capsular bag through a small capsulorrhexis, the bioadhesion of the anterior surface of the front lens to the anterior capsule edge and of the posterior surface of the back lens to the posterior capsule prevents the migration of the cells from the equatorial bow onto the posterior capsule. This migration may be directed towards the interlenticular space. In this scenario, the two IOLs are sequestered together with aqueous and lens epithelial cells in

a hermetically closed microenvironment. In addition, the adhesive nature of the material seems to render the opacifying material very difficult to remove by any surgical means (Figure 42-9).

Analyses of the above-described cases of ILO in the laboratory allowed the authors to conclude that the opacification within the interlenticular space is derived from retained/regenerative cortex and pearls, which is similar to the pathogenesis of the pearl form of PCO. Based on the common features of different cases of ILO, some surgical methods were proposed for its prevention (Figure 42-10). The first option would be to implant both IOLs in the capsular bag, but with a relatively larger diameter capsulorrhexis. In this scenario, there is a possibility that the cut edge of the rhexis may fuse with the posterior capsule. This should help sequester the retained/proliferated equatorial lens epithelial cells within the equatorial fornix. The other possibility is to implant the anterior IOL in the sulcus and the posterior IOL in the bag with a small rhexis. The rhexis margin will adhere to the anterior surface of the posterior IOL and the cells within the equatorial fornix will also be sequestered.

Re-assessment of factors leading to ILO formation is important because of the development of dual-optic accommodating IOLs to be implanted in the capsular bag (e.g., Synchrony, Visiogen Inc.).[29] Therefore, the authors addressed this issue in the authors' laboratory, by using a rabbit model (Figure 42-11).[35] The authors demonstrated that ILO was significantly associated with pairs of hydrophobic acrylic lenses implanted in the bag, but not with a dual-optic lens. This same study appeared to confirm clinical observations that implantation of two silicone plate lenses in the bag is not associated with ILO. Dr. Joel K. Shugar has been placing a pair of plate-haptic silicone lenses in the capsular bag with the haptics 90° apart and has seen no opacification in this series (Rongé LJ, "Preventing Problems with Piggyback IOLs," EyeNet 2002; 6:21-22). He has recently submitted to the authors' laboratory a pair of postmortem eyes from one of his patients implanted in this manner. Although Nd:YAG laser posterior capsulotomy was necessary because of PCO formation, ILO has not been observed in both eyes

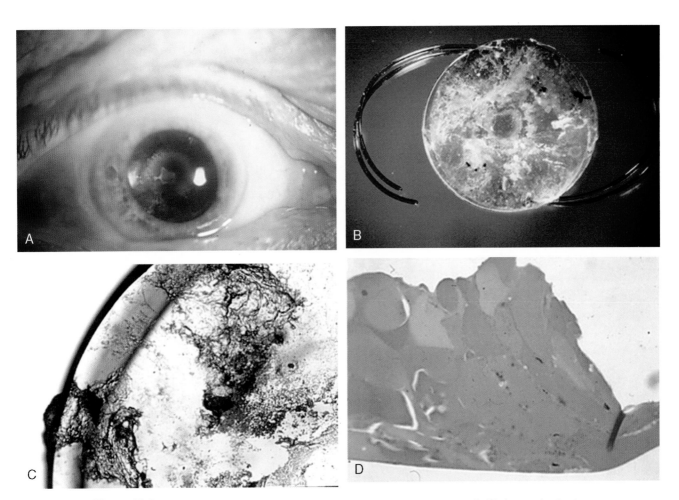

Figure 42-9 Clinical (**A**) (Courtesy of J.L. Gayton, MD, USA), gross (**B**), and light microscopic (**C**) photographs showing cases of interlenticular opacification between piggyback lenses. Histological sections prepared from the specimens (**D**) (periodic acid Schiff (PAS) stain) confirmed that the opacification corresponded to cortical material and pearls, in a pathogenesis similar to that of posterior capsule opacification.

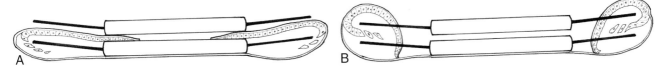

Figure 42-10 Schematic drawings representing surgical methods to prevent interlenticular opacification. **A,** Both intraocular lenses (IOLs) were implanted in the capsular bag via a relatively large capsulorrhexis. **B,** The posterior IOL was implanted in the bag, via a relatively small capsulorrhexis, and the anterior IOL was implanted in the sulcus.

(Figure 42-12). Also, piggyback implantation for correction of residual refractive errors appears to be increasing in popularity, including implantation of a multifocal IOL in pseudophakic patients. However, in these cases the second (anterior) IOL is generally fixated in the ciliary sulcus.

CONTACT BETWEEN THE INRAOCULAR LENS OPTIC AND THE POSTERIOR CAPSULE

Different factors can help maximize the contact between the IOL and the posterior capsule, contributing to the so-called "no space, no cells" concept. The optic/haptic angulation which displaces the optic posteriorly as well as the stickiness of the IOL optic material are the most important lens features in order to obtain a tight fit between lens and capsule. Three-piece lenses manufactured from the different haptic materials currently available today have in general a posterior optic/haptic angulation ranging from 5 to 10°.[28] To keep the advantages of the two above mentioned factors, it is important to achieve endocapsular lens fixation and to create a capsulorrhexis smaller than the diameter of the lens optic.

According to the "no space, no cells" theory, capsular tension rings may also have a role in the prevention of PCO.[36,37] Equatorial capsular tension rings have the ability to maintain the

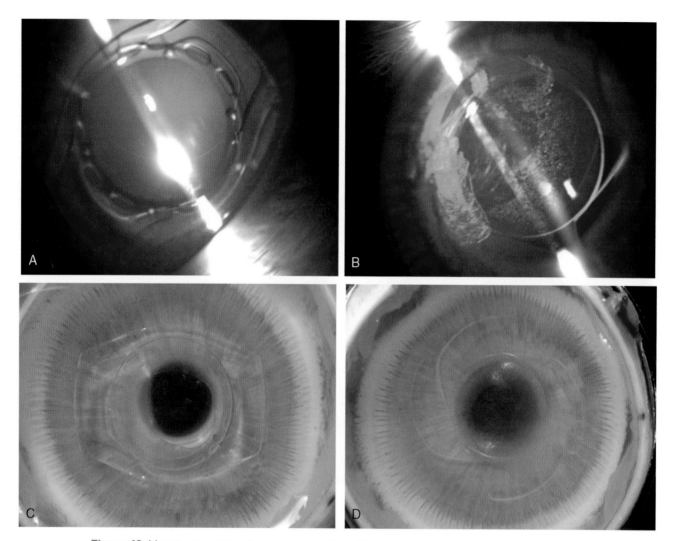

Figure 42-11 Clinical (**A** and **B**), and postmortem gross (**C** and **D**) photographs of rabbit eyes experimentally implanted with a dual-optic silicone lens or a pair of single-piece hydrophobic acrylic lenses. (Courtesy of Synchrony, Visiogen Inc.). Interlenticular opacification was only observed with the pair of hydrophobic acrylic lenses.

contour of the capsular bag and to stretch the posterior capsule. It has been demonstrated by high-resolution laser interferometric studies that there is a space between the IOL and the posterior capsule with different lens designs. With a capsular tension ring in place, this space was found to be smaller or non-existent.[38] Thus, lens epithelial cells would not find a space to migrate and proliferate onto the posterior capsule. Capsular tension rings also produce a circumferential stretch on the capsular bag, with the radial distension forces equally distributed. Formation of traction folds in the posterior capsule, which may be used as an avenue for cell ingrowth is thus avoided.

Capsular tension rings may also have a role in the prevention of opacification of the anterior capsule. The presence of a broad band-shaped capsular ring would keep the anterior capsule leaf away from the anterior optic surface and the posterior capsule. This would ultimately lead to less metaplasia of lens epithelial cells on the inner surface of the anterior capsule with less fibrous tissue formation and, thus, less opacification and contraction of

this structure. A capsular tension ring designed to prevent opacification within the capsular bag was evaluated in two centers, one in Japan (Nishi O, et al.) and the other in Austria (Menapace R, et al.). Both centers reported a significant reduction in PCO and ACO with the rings, in comparison to the contralateral eyes implanted with the same lens design.

INTRAOCULAR LENS OPTIC GEOMETRY

The square, truncated lens optic edge acts as a barrier, preventing migration of proliferative material from the equatorial region onto the posterior capsule (Figure 42-13).[39] The barrier effect is absent with lenses having rounded edges, and proliferative material from the equatorial region has a more free access to the posterior capsule, opacifying the visual axis. The barrier effect of the square optic edge is functional when the lens optic is fully in the bag, in contact with the posterior capsule. When one or both haptics are out of the bag, a potential space exists that allows an avenue

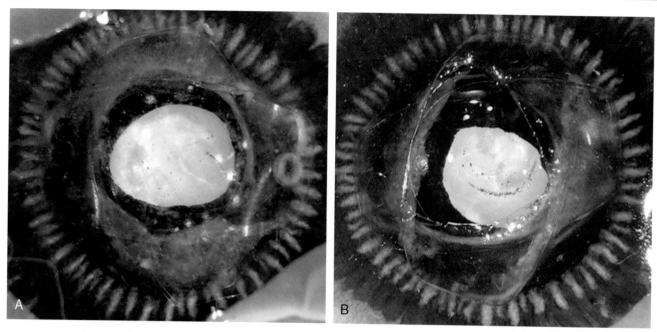

Figure 42-12 Postmortem gross photographs of the left (**A**) and right (**B**) eyes of the same patient, implanted with pairs of silicone plate lenses. Nd:YAG laser was performed for posterior capsule opacification, but there was no interlenticular opacification in these cases. Opacification of the anterior capsule can also be observed.

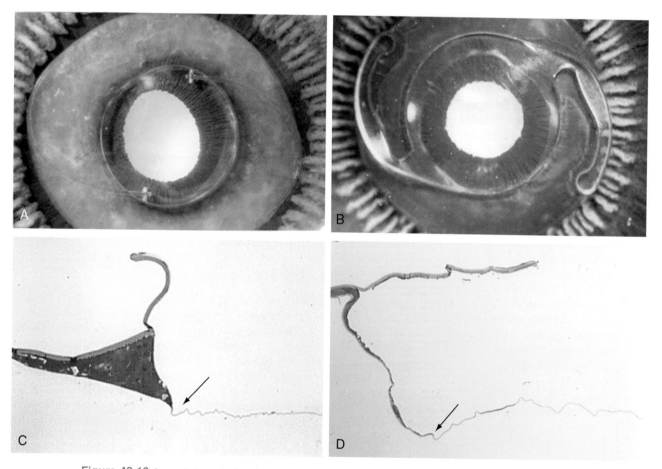

Figure 42-13 Gross photographs from human eyes obtained postmortem, implanted with hydrophobic acrylic lenses with square optic edges (**A** and **B**) (courtesy of AcrySof, Alcon). The corresponding histological sections (**C** and **D**) (Masson's trichrome stain) show the imprint of the square edge onto the posterior capsule (arrows), preventing migration of proliferative/regenerative material (red) from the equatorial region onto the center of the posterior capsule. Note that an extensive Soemmering's ring is present in the eye implanted with the three-piece lens.

for cellular ingrowth towards the visual axis. Different modern lenses manufactured from different materials currently in the market present this important design feature. Some of them have a square edge on the posterior optic surface, while the anterior optic edge remains round in order to prevent disphotopsia (e.g., Sensar, AMO).

Nishi believes that it is not the square optic edge per se that has a preventive effect against PCO, but the capsular bend that is formed in association with this design feature.[40,41] In an earlier rabbit study, Nishi demonstrated that even a silicone IOL with a truncated optic edge of a certain thickness would be able to form a capsular bend, and thus prevent PCO.[41] In a recent rabbit study, the same author compared the outcome of PCO in rabbit eyes implanted with two single-piece AcrySof designs, one with a 5.5 mm optic, and the other with a 7 mm optic. According to his results, adhesion between the anterior and posterior capsules in the periphery of the lens optic would be a fundamental prerequisite for capsular bend formation. He obtained less PCO with the 5.5 mm optic lens and he stated that bulky haptics, such as those of the single-piece AcrySof designs, associated with larger optics would have hampered adhesion between the anterior and posterior capsules, and thus capsular bend formation.[42]

However, in an in vitro study, Bhermi et al.[43] demonstrated that a discontinuous bend in the lens capsule in isolation would be unlikely to be responsible for the observed reduction in PCO formation associated with square edged IOLs. In the authors' experimental and pathological studies on rabbit and human eyes implanted with different IOLs it was observed that there were many instances of a clear barrier effect of the lens square edges preventing cell ingrowth onto the posterior capsule, even in the absence of adhesion between the capsules. This observation was especially valid in human eyes obtained postmortem presenting with important Soemmering's ring formation, likely associated with poor surgical cortical clean up (Figure 42-13C).

Wildeck and Tetz evaluated in an in vitro study the ideal edge sharpness for PCO prevention.[44] Polymethylmethacrylate (PMM) IOLs with 11 different edge designs were especially manufactured for this study. Each lens design was evaluated using the EPCO 2000 system (originally designed for PCO scoring), by calculating the area above the edge from high magnification scanning electron photomicrographs. Also, the ability of the edge to stop cell growth was observed by placing each IOL into cell culture and observing cell growth over 18 days on average. Only three groups of lenses, those with the sharpest edge designs, prevented the growth of lens epithelial cells onto the visual axis of the lens. The edge design that effectively stopped cell growth was characterized by an area above the edge of $13.5\ \mu^2$ at the most.

Evidences from rabbit studies show that the optic-haptic junctions of square-edged single-piece lenses may represent a site for cell ingrowth and PCO formation.[45,46] At the level of those junctions, the barrier effect of the square edge appears to be less effective. The authors obtained better results regarding PCO formation with a hydrophilic acrylic single-piece lens having an "enhanced" square edge, than with the standard model of the same design (Centerflex, Rayner, UK).[45] The enhanced edge provided the lens with a peripheral ridge around the lens optic for 360°. In the standard model, the square edge profile appeared to be absent at the level of the optic-haptic junctions (Figure 42-14). Therefore, the square optic edge is probably the most important IOL design feature for PCO prevention. It appears, however, that it should be present for 360° around the IOL optic in order to provide an effective barrier effect.

■ EXPERIMENTAL DEVICES FOR CAPSULAR BAG TREATMENT ■

SEALED CAPSULE IRRIGATION

As noted above, prevention of PCO relies on removal of lens epithelial cells from the anterior and equatorial regions of the capsular bag after cataract removal. Use of pharmacological and non-pharmacological agents for this purpose in an unsealed system may increase the risk of toxicity to surrounding intraocular structures, especially corneal endothelial cells. Dr. Anthony Maloof has developed a new concept in irrigation of the human lens capsule following lens surgery called sealed capsule irrigation (SCI), which may allow the isolated safe delivery of irrigating solutions containing pharmacological or non-pharmacological agents into the capsular bag following cataract surgery.[47]

Milvella (Sydney, Australia) has recently developed a device called PerfectCapsule™, a sealed delivery system made of biomedical grade soft silicone, which allows the surgeon to reseal the capsular bag. The device consists of a rounded plate containing a suction ring, which abuts the anterior capsule, and an extension arm that passes through a phacoemulsification wound of 2.9 mm. This extension arm carries a vacuum channel, which supplies vacuum to the suction ring, and a combined irrigation–aspiration channel. The irrigation–aspiration channel allows for communication between the sealed capsular bag and the external eye. The overall diameter of the device is 7 mm, with an inner diameter of 5 mm. It was designed to temporarily seal a capsulorrhexis of less than 5 mm, enabling selective and specific irrigation of the internal capsular bag with different solutions (Figure 42-15). Animal and clinical studies demonstrated the effectiveness of PerfectCapsule™ for SCI, without any leakage of the irrigating solutions used into the anterior chamber. Ongoing studies will ascertain the definitive solution(s) to be used in conjunction with this device.

LASER PHOTOLYSIS SYSTEM

A.R.C. Laser (Germany), developed a laser unit for the treatment of the inner compartment of the capsular bag, based on a modification of the Dodick Laser Photolysis system. The unit consists of a q-switched Nd:YAG laser delivering laser pulses with 8 ns pulse length. The energy per pulse can be set at different levels (mJ). The application frequency of the laser pulses is also variable, from 1 to 10 Hz, in 1 Hz increments. The laser light is delivered into the capsular bag via a fiber optic, with a diameter of 0.8 mm connected to an irrigation–aspiration system. After standard phacoemulsification, irrigation and aspiration, the fiber is introduced into the eye, and its tip is directed to the inner compartment of the capsular bag, without touching it. Pulses are then applied to the inner surface of the anterior capsule, and to the equatorial region. Each pulse causes plasma formation, and a shock wave is, therefore, generated, with detachment of the lens epithelial cells from the elastic capsular

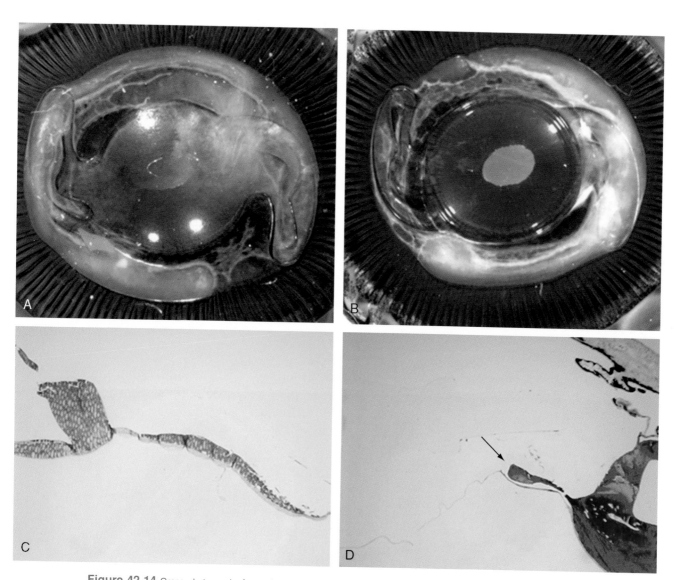

Figure 42-14 Gross photographs from rabbit eyes obtained postmortem, experimentally implanted with hydrophilic acrylic lenses with square optic edges (**A** and **B**) (courtesy of Centerflex, Rayner), and corresponding histological sections (**C** and **D**) (Masson's trichrome stain), cut at the level of the optic–haptic junctions. Posterior capsule opacification started at the level of one optic–haptic junction in **A**. The lens in **B** has a 360 ° enhanced square optic edge. The arrow in **D** shows the barrier provided by the enhanced edge.

bag. Experimental studies in the authors' laboratory with human eyes obtained postmortem demonstrated that use of the probe via two small incisions for bimanual surgery, created 90° apart, allow the treatment of 180° of the capsular bag per incision. The same studies also demonstrated lens epithelial cell removal with energy levels of 5–6 mJ, without disruption of the capsular bag (Figure 42-16).

■ OPACIFICATION/DISCOLORATION OF INTRAOCULAR LENSES ■

The majority of IOLs analyzed at the University of Utah are explants from the US, and a significant number of them are

analyzed because of opacification or discoloration of their optic components.[5] More recently, the Berlin Eye Research Institute in Germany (founded by M. Tetz, MD) was also established as a center for analyses of explanted devices. It is expected that this will expand the scope of independent research on IOL complications, with evaluation of a more significant number of lenses explanted in Europe and Asia. Inability of recognizing a process of IOL opacification or discoloration may prompt surgeons to perform unnecessary surgical procedures, such as Nd:YAG posterior capsulotomies, or vitrectomies, in eyes where the opacification is actually in the IOL itself, and not at the level of the posterior capsule or the vitreous. This may jeopardize subsequent implantation of a new IOL in the capsular bag, among other complications. The causes of IOL opacification and discoloration

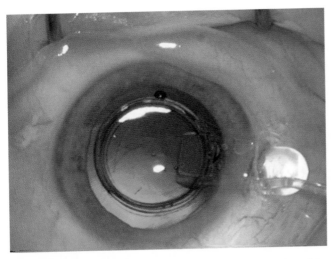

Figure 42-15 Surgical photograph (courtesy of A. Maloof, MD, Australia) showing the PerfectCapsule sealing the capsulorrhexis opening.

reviewed here will be discussed according to their time of presentation: early postoperative (hours or days after surgery), and late postoperative (several months or years after surgery) (Table 42-2).

EARLY POSTOPERATIVE INTRAOCULAR LENS OPACIFICATION/DISCOLORATION

EARLY OPACIFICATION OF SILICONE LENSES BY HYDRATION

Tanaka et al.[48] described early postoperative opacification of a silicone lens (SI40 NB, AMO) in an 83-year-old Japanese patient. In his report, the IOL presented with a "brown haze" on the first postoperative day. The haze did not decrease until day 15 postoperatively, when the IOL was then explanted. Light microscopic evaluation of the explanted lens showed the presence of numerous spheroid structures in the central region of the optic. It was suggested that the haze was secondary to influx of water within the lens, but no analyses to determine possible causative factors were done.

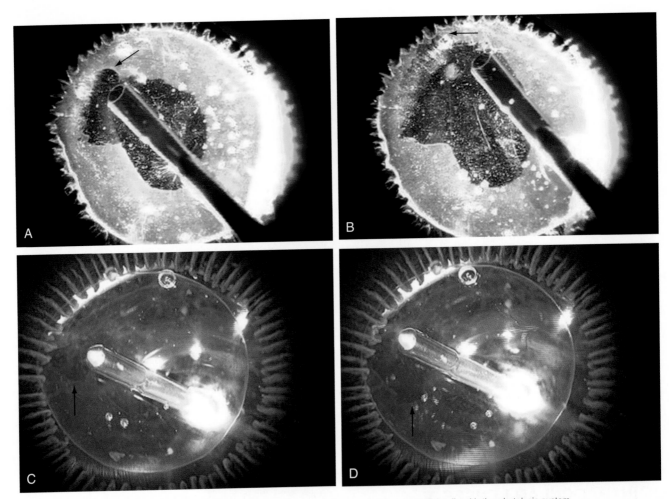

Figure 42-16 Gross photographs showing experimental removal of lens epithelial cells with the photolysis system, from the inner surface of the anterior capsule of a human eye obtained postmortem. The arrows show the progression of the cell removal. **A** and **B**, Anterior or surgeon's view with retroillumination. **C** and **D**, Posterior or Miyake-Apple view.

Table 42-2 Possible causes of clinically significant intraocular-lens (IOL) opacification/discoloration.

IOL Opacification/Discoloration	
Early Postoperative	**Late Postoperative**
Early IOL opacification by water influx	IOL coating with ophthalmic ointment
IOL interaction with capsular dyes	IOL water influx due to incomplete extraction of large polymers during manufacture
IOL coating with ophthalmic ointment	IOL interaction with systemic medications
	IOL coating with silicone oil
	IOL calcification in asteroid hyalosis
	IOL dystrophic calcification
	IOL biomaterial degeneration due to long-term ultraviolet exposure

Later the authors reported similar findings in six patients with three-piece silicone lenses (5 SI40 NB, and 1 SA40 N, AMO), which presented with optic cloudiness as early as a few hours after implantation (Figure 42-17). Two of these cases had been previously reported in collaboration with Hilgert et al., who had a total of four similar cases (Figure 42-3).[49,50] The lenses were implanted in four different locations in Brazil, and in France. A thorough review of the history of the lenses evaluated in this study was done by the manufacturer, according to their serial numbers. Although all the implantations in Brazil were done in different locations, and the lenses were from different manufacturing lots, it was determined that they had been all stored in a same area in Brazil, pre-operatively. Spraying of the storage area with cleaning and insecticide agents was reportedly performed (Internal AMO Materials Research report, March 26, 2004). Gross and microscopic analyses were done in the authors' laboratory in the dry and hydrated states. The lenses actually showed whitish optic

discoloration in the hydrated state, but became transparent upon complete dehydration (Figure 42-18). Suspect exogenous chemical compounds were identified in gas chromatography-mass spectrometry (GC-MS) analyses; general classes included terpenes and ketones, typically found in industrial cleaning agents and fumigants. The authors, therefore, hypothesized that chemical contamination of the lenses might have occurred pre-operatively. This might have caused surface changes, rendering the relatively hydrophobic silicone surfaces more hydrophilic, allowing influx of water and, therefore, opacification of the IOL optic.

Most IOLs are enclosed in semi-permeable packages to allow sterilization by ethylene oxide gas. Storage facilities and operating theaters that are sprayed with aerosolized cleaning solutions, disinfectants, insecticides, or other volatile chemicals may be inadvertently introducing chemicals through vapor-permeable packages and onto the lenses. This may cause surface changes in the IOL promoting opacification by water ingress in the aqueous environment. Cleaning/disinfection procedures of IOL storage areas should be carefully monitored. As a general precautionary measure, all IOLs should be stored in a clean, dry environment, at room temperature, and be protected from potentially harmful fumigant sprays.

In collaboration with Elgohary et al., the authors have recently analyzed two other cases of early postoperative opacification of SA40 N lenses.[51] The two IOLs came from different production batches and were implanted by different surgeons on different lists using two different ophthalmic viscosurgical device (OVD) materials. Moreover, one of the patients had a similar procedure on the other eye but the IOL remained clear. In the two patients, the opacification was noted within 2–8 weeks after surgery, although it is possible that the opacification had developed soon after implantation of the IOLs, i.e., within days or even intraoperatively. The two lenses appeared clinically grayish-white to brownish in color. Only one lens was explanted and it resumed clarity when removed from the balanced salt solution. This, in addition to the absence of deposits on the surface or within the optic substance, suggested that the opacification was related to hydration of the lens optic. Although laboratorial analyses were not done on the second implant, the similarity in clinical features and time of onset suggests a similar mechanism of opacification. A chromatographic peak for lidocaine was detected in the extract prepared from the suspension liquid of the explanted

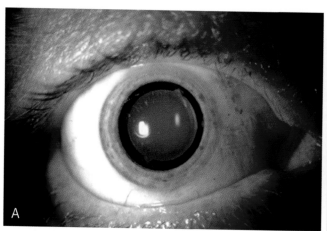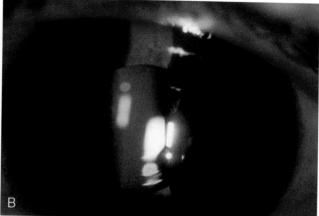

Figure 42-17 Clinical photographs showing optic whitish discoloration of the SI40 NB, AMO (**A**) (courtesy of C.R. Hilgert, MD, Brazil), and of the SA40 N, AMO (**B**) (courtesy of P. Rozot, MD, France).

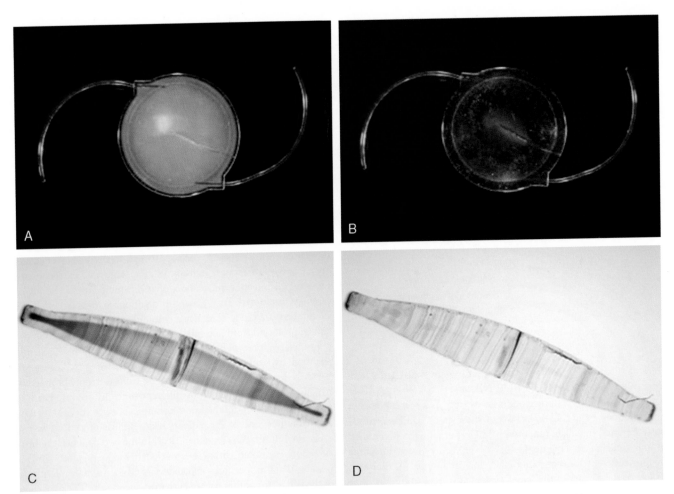

Figure 42-18 Gross (**A** and **B**), and light microscopic (**C** and **D**) photographs of one of the silicone lenses explanted in Brazil because of early opacification. The optic opacity decreases upon dehydration of the lens.

lens but not in the blank water extract, which indicated that it was not an analytical artifact. Cataract surgery had been performed under local subtenon anesthesia (lignocaine 2%) in this case. This does not necessarily suggest a causal relationship to the opacification, and further investigation is necessary to assess the exact cause of the lenses' opacification in these cases.

INTRAOCULAR LENS INTERACTION WITH CAPSULAR DYES

The authors described for the first time the occurrence of blue discoloration of an IOL by a capsular dye.[52] The lens was a hydrophilic acrylic design (Acqua, Mediphacos, Brazil). The patient was a 79-year-old Caucasian male patient, who underwent cataract surgery with implantation of this hydrophilic acrylic design. Trypan blue 0.1% was injected under an air bubble to stain the anterior capsule before capsulorrhexis. Seven days after surgery, the patient presented with "dark and double" vision (monocular diplopia). The IOL was decentered superiorly and appeared dark blue. The lens was explanted 2 months after surgery and submitted for gross and microscopic analyses performed in a dry state and after hydration. Analyses of the lens revealed that the dark-blue staining was denser within the optic component, especially in the optical periphery. The blue discoloration

could not be removed after 24 h of immersion of the lens in balanced salt solution at 37°C. The same analyses were performed on two unused lenses of the same design, which had been immersed in diluted trypan blue solutions (0.01% and 0.001%). Permanent staining of the unused lenses was also obtained after immersion in the experimental solutions (Figure 42-19).

Most of the currently available hydrophilic acrylic lenses have water contents ranging from 18 to 28%. They are packaged in a vial containing distilled water or balanced salt solutions, thus being already implanted in the hydrated state and in its final dimensions. Hydration renders these lenses flexible, enabling the surgeons to fold and insert them through small incisions. To the authors' knowledge, the Acqua lens is manufactured from the hydrophilic acrylic material with the highest water content (73.5%) currently used for the manufacture of IOLs. This lens is implanted in the dry state, its expansion depending on its hydration by the fluids within the capsular bag. It appears that minimal amounts of dye still present in the capsular bag during IOL implantation may be absorbed by this lens. Therefore, capsular dyes should not be used in association with the Acqua lens.

After this report, trypan blue, ICG and fluorescein sodium have been tested in laboratory settings to evaluate their interaction with various IOL materials. These tests showed that only the hydrophilic acrylic lenses could significantly absorb commonly used

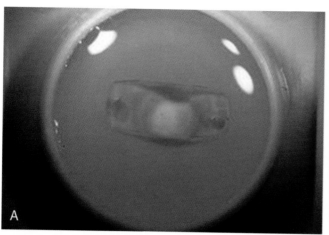
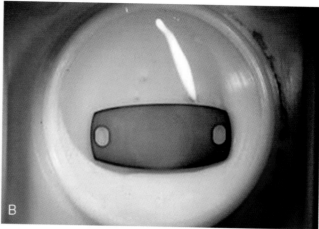

Figure 42-19 Gross photograph taken during experimental immersion of an Acqua lens in a 0.001% trypan blue solution (A). Eight hours later, the dye was completely absorbed by the lens (B).

capsular dyes.[53] Although experimental studies demonstrated that silicone lenses do not significantly interact with commonly used capsular dyes, the authors reported one case of blue discoloration of a silicone IOL.[54] The patient was a 52-year-old man who underwent uneventful phacoemulsification with implantation of a SI40 NB (AMO) in the right eye. A "blue dye" was used to enhance visualization during capsulorrhexis. Postoperatively, the patient presented with corneal edema and a discolored IOL. The lens was, therefore, explanted and exchanged. The corneal edema resolved within 1 month after the initial surgical procedure. After explantation, gross and microscopic analyses of the explanted silicone lens revealed that its surface and internal substance had been permanently stained blue (Figure 42-20). It has then been determined in this case that methylene blue had been inadvertently used instead of trypan blue to stain the anterior capsule. Of course, the most significant problem in this case was not the discoloration of the IOL itself, but the use of a solution that was not appropriate for the intraocular environment, raising concerns about toxic anterior segment syndrome (TASS).

INTRAOCULAR LENS COATING WITH OPHTHALMIC OINTMENT

The authors have recently reported eight cases of TASS related to an oily material within the anterior chamber of the patients' eyes.[55] The eight patients had undergone uneventful phacoemulsification by the same surgeon via clear corneal incisions, with implantation of the same three-piece silicone lens design (SoFlex LI 61U, Bausch & Lomb). Postoperative medications included antibiotic/steroid ointment, and pilocarpine gel; each eye was firmly patched at the end of the procedure. On the first postoperative day, some patients presented with diffuse corneal edema, increased intraocular pressure (IOP), and an oily, film-like material within the anterior chamber, coating the corneal endothelium. The others presented with an oily bubble floating inside the anterior chamber, which was later seen coating the IOL (Figure 42-21). Additional surgical procedures required included penetrating keratoplasty ($n = 4$), IOL explantation ($n = 6$), and trabeculectomy ($n = 1$). Two corneal buttons were analyzed

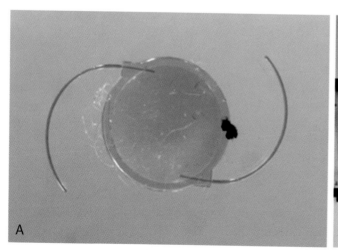
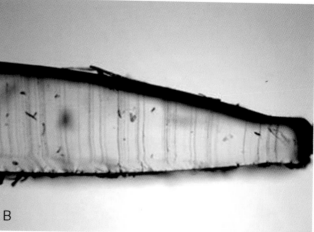

Figure 42-20 Gross (A) and light microscopic (B) photographs of a silicone lens discolored in blue due to inadvertent intraoperative use of methylene blue instead of trypan blue.

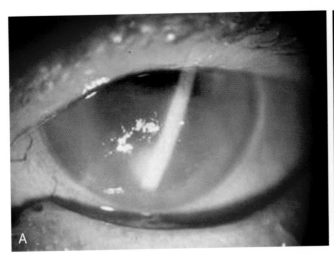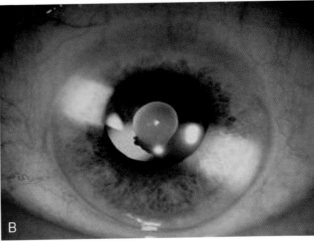

Figure 42-21 Clinical photographs taken during the first week after cataract surgery with intraocular lens implantation, showing corneal edema (**A**), and a large oily bubble floating into the anterior chamber, corresponding to ophthalmic ointment (**B**) (courtesy of W.A. Nash, MD, FRCSC, Canada).

histopathologically, two explanted IOLs underwent gross and light microscopic analyses (as well as surface analyses on one of them), and four other explanted IOLs underwent GC-MS.

Pathological examination of the corneas showed variable thinning of the epithelium, with edema. The stroma was diffusely thickened, and the endothelial cell layer was absent. Evaluation of the explanted IOLs confirmed the presence of an oily substance coating large areas of their anterior and posterior optic surfaces (Figure 42-22). GC-MS of the lens extracts identified a mixed chain hydrocarbon compound, which was also found in the GC-MS analyses of the ointment used postoperatively. Therefore, the results indicated that the ointment gained access to the eye, causing the postoperative complications described. These cases highlight the importance of appropriate wound construction and integrity, as well as the risks of tight eye patching following placement of ointment. McDonnell et al. evaluated the dynamic morphology of clear corneal cataract incisions by creating clear corneal incisions in human and rabbit eyes obtained postmortem.[56]

They found that at low pressures, wound edges tended to gape starting at the internal aspect of the wound. In a retrospective study, Shingleton et al. demonstrated that a significant percentage of eyes having clear corneal phacoemulsification had an IOP of 5 mm Hg or less 30 min after surgery.[57] The possibility of intraocular penetration of any kind of ointment used postoperatively, not only in cataract surgery, but in different types of penetrating procedures should, therefore, be anticipated.

Ophthalmic ointment may also gain intraocular access after surgery, but only coat the IOL implanted later postoperatively. The authors have recently evaluated the case of a patient who underwent uneventful phacoemulsification with implantation of a three-piece silicone IOL (SI30 NB, AMO) via a 3 mm scleral tunnel incision.[58] Postoperative medications included antibiotic/steroid drops and ointments. Eight months postoperatively, the patient started having recurrent episodes of anterior chamber inflammatory reaction. Suspicion of lens instability causing the reactions led to two repositioning procedures, including

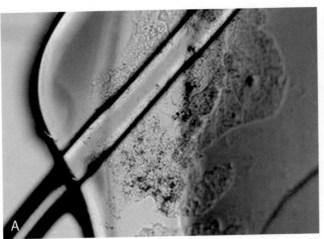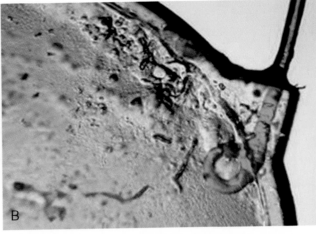

Figure 42-22 Light microscopic photographs showing three-piece silicone lenses explanted because of coating with ophthalmic ointment observed early (**A**) or late (**B**) postoperatively.

performance of McCannel sutures. Finally, 18 months postoperatively, the IOL presented with a "greasy" film and it was later exchanged (Figure 42-22B). GC-MS analysis of the ointment used after each surgical procedure showed several compounds that had mass spectra characteristic of hydrocarbons similar to those detected in the extract prepared from the explanted IOL. In this case, it is possible that the ointment entered the anterior chamber after the IOL repositioning procedures, perhaps through clear corneal paracentesis usually required for the placement of McCannel iris-suture fixation. The first observation of globules on the IOL was only noted 5 months after the last procedure. The reasons for this late onset remain unclear to us. Chen et al. have also recently reported a case where an oily-like material was only observed inside the anterior chamber in the late postoperative period after cataract surgery.[59] The material was identified as ointment by Fourier transform infrared and confocal Raman microspectroscopies.

LATE POSTOPERATIVE INTRAOCULAR LENS OPACIFICATION/DISCOLORATION

LATE POSTOPERATIVE INTRAOCULAR LENS OPACIFICATION/DISCOLORATION OF SILICONE LENSES

There were reports on brownish discoloration and central haze of silicone lenses in the early 1990s.[60–62] In general, this complication was considered clinically insignificant; IOL explantation has rarely been performed. These reports have suggested that the brown haze was due to light scatter from water vapor that may diffuse into the silicone when immersed in an aqueous medium. This may be caused by some anomaly of the curing process during the manufacture of those lenses or by incomplete extraction of large polymers. Ultraviolet blocking agents did not seem to be an issue with lens discoloration since the phenomenon was also observed with silicone IOL models not containing these

agents. Additional filtration steps in the manufacturing process of silicone lenses seemed to solve the problem.

Silicone IOL opacification/discoloration has also been associated with the long-term use of systemic medications. Katai et al. reported on a patient who was treated with amiodarone for 3 years and developed brown discoloration of the silicone lenses in both eyes.[63] Jones and Irwin described the case of a patient who developed a rose discoloration of the silicone lenses in both eyes after receiving rifabutin for 10 months.[64] Recently, there have been reports from South India on green discoloration of silicone IOLs.[65] The phenomenon was noted at 6 months postoperatively, but as the patients were asymptomatic, the lenses were not explanted. To date, careful scrutiny of the medical and surgical history of the patients failed to reveal factors that might have predisposed the IOLs to green discoloration. A previous report from Pakistan had also described a similar complication.[66] Another report from India provided photographic documentation of green discoloration of a silicone IOL in a severely vasculitic, pseudophakic eye. This finding was observed 3 weeks after retinal angiography using intravenous sodium fluorescein 2%.[67]

Opacification/discoloration of silicone lenses in the late postoperative period was also observed in relation to deposition of material on the lens surfaces. The interaction of silicone oil, used in vitreoretinal surgery, with standard silicone IOLs in a given patient is a well-documented clinical complication.[68] Irreversible adherence of silicone oil to the IOL optic may lead to different sequelae, including visual disturbances and visual loss for the patient, as well as obstruction of the vitreoretinal surgeon's view into the eye. This is a complication not generally seen by the implanting cataract surgeon but, rather, at a later stage in a patient's postoperative course, by a vitreoretinal surgeon (Figure 42-23). Experimental studies showed that, although silicone IOLs show maximal adherence to silicone oil, other lens biomaterials are not immune to this complication. Silicone oil coverage was related to the dispersive energy component of the surface charge of the IOL biomaterial. Low dispersive energy materials had less silicone oil coverage, while those

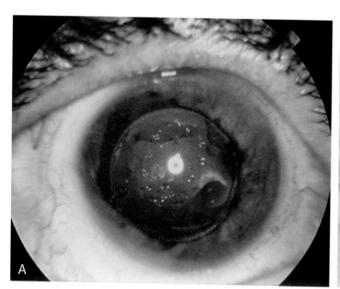
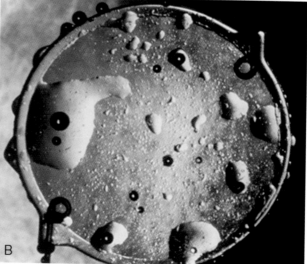

Figure 42-23 Clinical (**A**) and gross (**B**) photographs showing coating of silicone intraocular lenses by silicone oil used in vitreoretinal surgery.

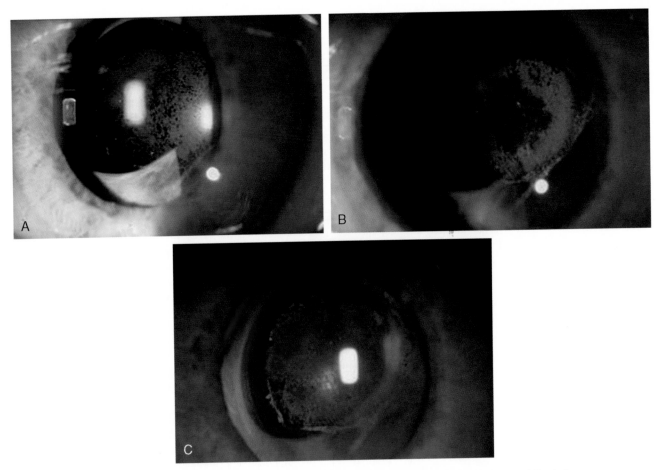

Figure 42-24 Clinical photographs of a patient implanted with a silicone plate lens, in an eye with asteroid hyalosis. The intraocular lens surface deposits could be partially removed with Nd:YAG application (**B**), but re-accumulated after the procedure (**C**) (courtesy of J.P. Gills, MD, USA).

with higher dispersive energy had more oil coverage. Regardless of the degree of oil-induced cloudiness of the IOL, visual loss is often severe by the time most patients develop severe vitreoretinal disease that requires radical treatment with silicone oil. Therefore, the clinical importance of this complication actually relates most significantly to patients who may be deemed to have a high propensity

for severe vitreoretinal disease that may require silicone oil treatment at a later date.

Calcified deposits leading to significant opacification requiring explantation were observed on the surface of silicone IOLs in eyes with asteroid hyalosis (Figures 42-24 and 42-25).[69–71] Four cases were initially reported in the literature, all with silicone plate

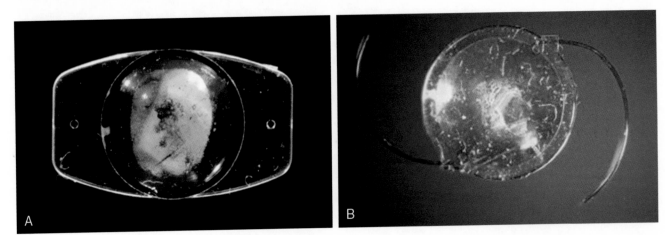

Figure 42-25 Gross photographs of a plate (**A**), and a three-piece (**B**) silicone lens explanted because of surface calcification in association with asteroid hyalosis.

lenses in patients with unilateral asteroid hyalosis.[69,70] Whitish deposits appeared only on the posterior optic surface of the lens late postoperatively. Two out of the four reported patients had diabetes. In two of the cases, the deposits were noted before Nd:YAG laser capsulotomy was performed. Fast re-accumulation of the deposits on the posterior surface of the lenses was described after the procedure. In the other two cases, it is not clear whether or not the deposits were present before the Nd:YAG procedure. While in the three cases reported by us, the deposits were observed mostly within the area of the Nd:YAG capsulotomy,[69] in the case by Wackernagel et al., the deposits also appeared on the periphery of the optic, covered by the posterior capsule.[70]

Later the authors described the first similar case related to a three-piece silicone lens, in a patient with bilateral asteroid hyalosis.[71] The 76-year-old diabetic woman underwent uneventful cataract surgery in 1994 with implantation of a SI30 NB (AMO) IOL in the left eye. A Nd:YAG laser posterior capsulotomy was performed 2 years after cataract surgery, but persistent whitish deposits were observed on the posterior optic surface of the lens. Over the next 3 years, the opacification increased in the region corresponding to the capsulotomy: the IOL was explanted and exchanged. The right eye had cataract surgery in 1995 and the acrylic lens implanted in this eye developed no opacities after 6 years.

There are only few cases in the recent literature describing the association between dystrophic calcification of silicone lenses and asteroid hyalosis. Calcification of silicone lenses in the absence of this vitreous condition has not been reported. Indeed, in the absence of asteroid hyalosis, long-term calcified deposits were previously observed only on the surface or within the substance of some hydrophilic acrylic IOL designs. There is, therefore, increasing evidence that the material opacifying the silicone lenses is derived from the asteroid bodies, or derived from a similar process that results in this vitreous condition, as its composition was found to be similar to that of hydroxyapatite (calcium and phosphate). The latter is more likely the case because the asteroid calcium is already "out of solution." It is, however, still unclear why only a few cases have been observed, while there have probably been many implantations of silicone lenses of various designs in patients with asteroid hyalosis. Careful clinical examination of pseudophakic patients with asteroid hyalosis will confirm if this phenomenon is more widespread, but only significant enough to require IOL explantation in a few cases. This will also confirm if the phenomenon is restricted to silicone lenses. Without such knowledge, it is difficult to proscribe silicone IOL implantation in the presence of asteroid hyalosis.

LATE POSTOPERATIVE INTRAOCULAR LENS OPACIFICATION/DISCOLORATION OF HYDROPHILIC ACRYLIC LENSES

Since 1999, optic opacification of some hydrophilic acrylic IOL designs has been a significant complication leading to IOL explantation. The four major designs manufactured in the US involved in the problem were (Figure 42-12) the Hydroview (Bausch & Lomb),[72,73] the MemoryLens (Ciba Vision),[74,75] the SC60B-OUV (Medical Developmental Research),[76–78] and the Aqua-Sense (Ophthalmic Innovations International).[79,80] The deposits causing the opacification were basically found on the optical surfaces of the Hydroview and the MemoryLens, while they were predominantly found within the substance of the SC60B-OUV and the Aqua-Sense (Figures 42-26 to 42-29). Surface deposits were also significantly observed with this latter design. Histochemical methods, as well as surface analytical analyses demonstrated the composition of the deposits to be at least in part of calcium and phosphate.

In 1997, Bausch & Lomb changed the Hydroview lens packaging system to incorporate the SureFold holder/folder. As of July 2003, the authors' center has received forty explanted Hydroview lenses for pathological analyses. The interval between the cataract procedure and the time the opacification of the lenses in the authors' series was noted ranged from 5 to 48 months (19.75 ± 11.88). Surface chemistry studies of explanted Hydroview lenses performed by Bausch & Lomb identified the lens deposits as a layered mixture of octacalcium phosphate, fatty acids, salts, and small amounts of silicone compounds. As the silicone gasket sealing the new SureFold cap was the only difference in the manufacturing and packaging of the lenses, this gasket came under suspicion early. The manufacturer has since changed the packaging of the Hydroview, which is now sealed with a gasket made from a perfluoroelastomer (Green G, et al. *An issue resolved. The Hydroview intraocular lens: Development, early reports of calcification and subsequent actions.* White paper Bausch & Lomb; July 29, 2003).

As of March 2004, the authors have analyzed 106 Memory-Lens IOLs, explanted because of late postoperative opacification. The mean time interval between the initial cataract surgery and the diagnosis of lens opacification was 25.8 ± 11.9 months (range 3.3–80.7). The manufacturer correlated the opacification of this design with a change in the polishing process in 1999. The modified manufacturing method used a phosphate buffer in the tumbling process, which would attract more protein. The process would then continue to progress with the deposition of minerals, most likely calcium, on top of the protein film. According to the manufacturer, a worldwide recall of this lens in April 2000 (associated with cases of sterile hypopyon) also included all Memory-Lens IOLs manufactured using the modified tumbling process. Ciba Vision then changed the polishing process and re-introduced the MemoryLens in October 2000 with the models U940S and CV232, the latter featuring a square optic-edge design.

The mean time to explantation of the SC60B-OUV and Aqua-Sense lenses because of calcification was found to be 20.22 ± 11.02 months, and 16.27 ± 6.45 months, respectively. Besides calcification demonstrated by the authors and others, the analyses of Frohn et al. of 41 SC60B-OUV IOLs indicated premature aging of the ultraviolet blocking agent within the lenses, the source of the opacification, thus, being a change in the IOL material itself.[78] Medical Developmental Research (now EyeKon Medical) changed their polymer supplier, and currently manufactures different hydrophilic acrylic designs, including the SC25-Fold lens, which has recently received Food and Drug Administration approval for clinical investigation in the United States. The calcification problem with the Aqua-Sense design has also been associated with silicone compounds. Ophthalmic Innovations International stated that researchers, using X-ray photoelectron spectroscopy surface analysis, have found trace siloxane species on the surfaces of the opacified lenses. These siloxane

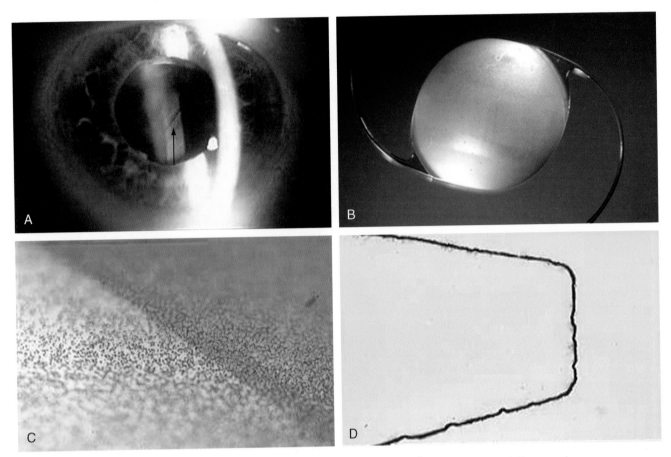

Figure 42-26 Hydroview calcification. **A,** Clinical photograph (courtesy of A. Öhrström, MD, Sweden). The arrow shows forceps marks. **B,** Gross photograph showing a granularity covering the optic surfaces of the explanted lens. **C,** Alizarin red. **D,** Von Kossa method.

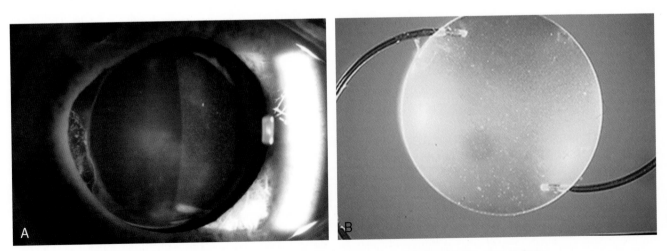

Figure 42-27 MemoryLens calcification. **A,** Clinical photograph (courtesy of A. Crandall, MD, USA). **B,** Gross photograph showing a thin granularity covering the optic surfaces of the explanted lens.

(Continued)

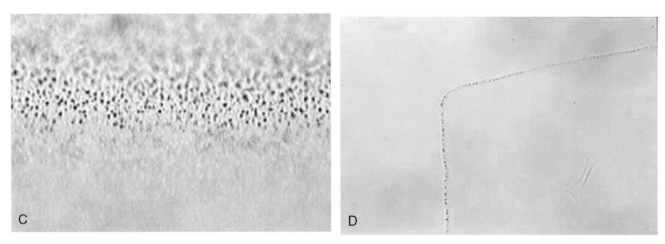

Figure 42-27, cont'd C, Alizarin red. **D,** Von Kossa method.

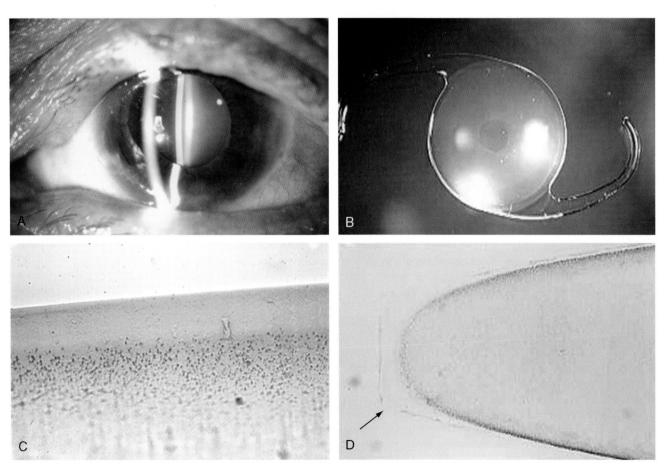

Figure 42-28 SC60B-OUV lens calcification. **A,** Clinical photograph (courtesy of M. Kaskaloglu, MD, Turkey). **B,** Gross photograph showing opacification of the most central optic area of the explanted SC60B-OUV, with a clear optic edge and clear haptics. The calcified nature of the intralenticular deposits was suggested by histochemical methods for calcium, such as alizarin red (**C**), and von Kossa method (**D**). The arrow shows the actual optic edge of the lens.

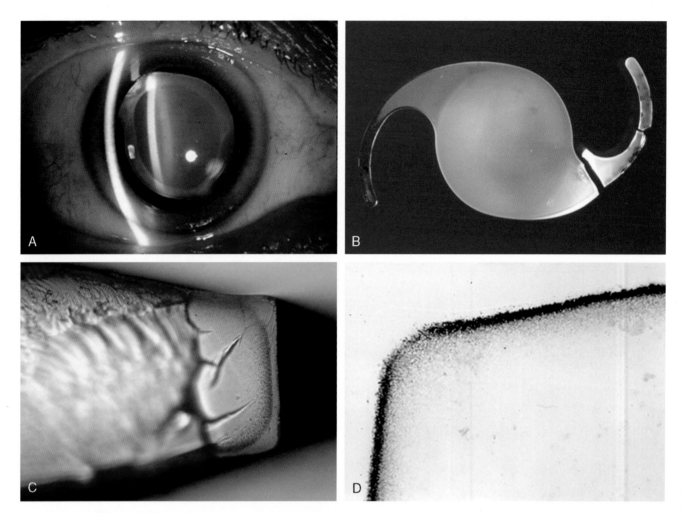

Figure 42-29 Aqua-Sense calcification. **A,** Clinical photograph (courtesy of M. Batterbury, MD, and A. Jacob, MD, UK). **B,** Gross photograph showing opacification of the optic and haptic components of the lens. The calcified nature of the surface and intralenticular deposits was suggested by histochemical methods for calcium, such as alizarin red (**C**), and von Kossa method (**D**).

compounds were hypothesized to have come from the silicone elastomer packaging components used at that time. These packaging components have since been removed and changed to non-silicone materials (Robert Sheehan, Vice President of Regulatory Affairs and Quality Systems, Ophthalmic Innovations International, personal communication, April/2001).

The authors also described dystrophic calcification of hydrophilic acrylic lenses in children (Figure 42-30).[81] Although hydrophilic acrylic lenses are very popular in Europe, the authors analyzed only a handful of IOLs from European manufacturers, which were explanted because of calcification (Figure 42-31).[82,83] By having a center located in Europe, dedicated to analyses of explanted devices, the authors expect to have a better understanding of the different complications leading to explantation of lenses in Europe and Asia, including IOL opacification. Interestingly, there has been a report on calcification of a hydrophilic acrylic lens (model 92S, Morcher, Germany), occurring 2 months after deep sclerectomy with Mitomycin-C for uncontrolled glaucoma. The composition of the calcified deposits was found to be calcium carbonate.[84]

More recently, the authors described for the first time the case of a MemoryLens IOL model CV232 that was explanted 18 months

postoperatively.[85] The patient had decreased visual acuity with the presence of a well-circumscribed, centrally/paracentrally located opacification of the optic. The area had the aspect of a small "lens within the lens" or a regular, round bubble (Figure 42-32). The opacification observed within the CVC232 lens remained well localized, without notable changes in its aspect since it was first noted 1 year after the surgery, until the lens was explanted 6 months later. It was actually difficult to precisely determine the clinical significance of the IOL opacity in that case. The postoperative decrease in visual acuity could eventually be, at least partially, related to posterior capsule opacification (PCO) formation, and eventually to retinal and glaucoma problems. The analyses of the explanted CV232 lens revealed that within the localized round area of opacification there were deposits (large crystals) distributed within an optic "void," seen as a linear breach in sagittal cuts. The authors hypothesized that the precipitation of calcium in this case was a process secondary to the optic defect. The origin of the optic defect remains speculative at this point. The authors are aware of other similar cases with the new CV232 design, including asymptomatic cases where explantation was not necessary and cases where the localized area within the optic has the aspect of a clear

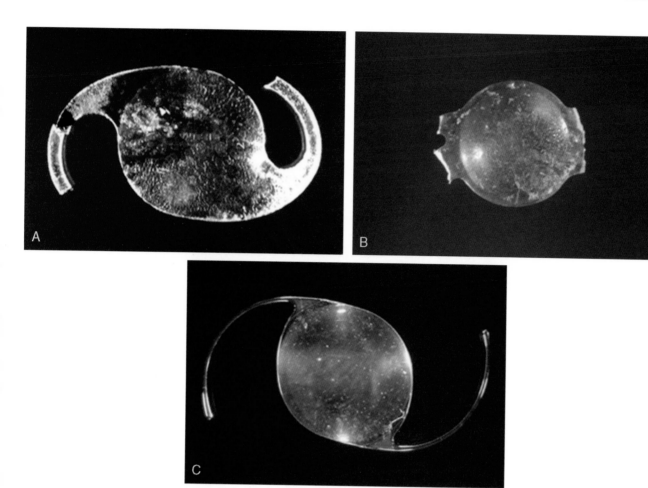

Figure 42-30 Gross photographs showing hydrophilic acrylic lenses explanted from children, because of surface calcification. **A, B**-Lens (courtesy of Hanita, Israel). **B,** Centerflex lens (courtesy of Rayner, UK). **C,** Hydroview (courtesy of Bausch & Lomb, USA).

bubble, without significant opacification. Whether or not secondary calcification will occur within the optic void in these cases at some point in the postoperative period is still unknown.

LATE POSTOPERATIVE INTRAOCULAR LENS OPACIFICATION/DISCOLORATION OF POLYMETHYLMETHACRYLATE LENSES

Snowflake degeneration is a slowly progressive opacification of PMMA IOLs, occurring sometimes 10 years or more after implantation.[3,86] The opacities observed within the IOL optic have the aspect of crystalline deposits. The term "snowflake" relates to the aspect of the individual lesions under high magnification light microscopy. The optic lesions may start as scattered white-brown spots within the substance of the IOL optic and remain stable or slowly progressive (Figure 42-33). Some may gradually increase in intensity and numbers, eventually reaching a point where a visual acuity loss may necessitate removal or exchange of the IOL. The snowflake lesions per se are dry lesions, and should be differentiated from glistenings. These latter are fluid-filled vacuoles, largely described in association with hydrophobic acrylic lenses, but that can also be associated with other materials, including PMMA. Glistenings are generally stated to be clinically insignificant.[87]

It has been suggested that manufacturing variations in some lenses fabricated in the 1980s to early 1990s may be responsible for this problem. It is possible that the late change in the PMMA material process is facilitated by long-term ultraviolet exposure. This is supported by two pathologic observations. First, many opacities have been clustered in the central zone of the optic, extending to mid-peripheral portion but often leaving the distal peripheral rim free of the opacities. This observation would support the hypothesis that lesion formation might relate to the fact that the IOL's central optic is exposed to ultraviolet radiation over an extended period, whereas the peripheral optic may be protected by the iris. Furthermore, the opacities are present most commonly and intensely within the anterior third of the optic's substance.

The authors have recently analyzed a PMMA lens explanted because of snowflake degeneration in the dry and hydrated states (Figure 42-34).[88] The lesions characteristic of the condition were restricted to the central 2 mm of the lens optic in the dry state. This is the smallest area ever observed, and may be related to the fact that the patient's pupils were relatively constricted as noted on the exam before and after dilation. Upon hydration of the explanted lens, an unusual amount of water was collected within the central 4 mm of the lens optic, where multiple linear cracks were present. These cracks were not evident under light microscopy in the dry state. They may

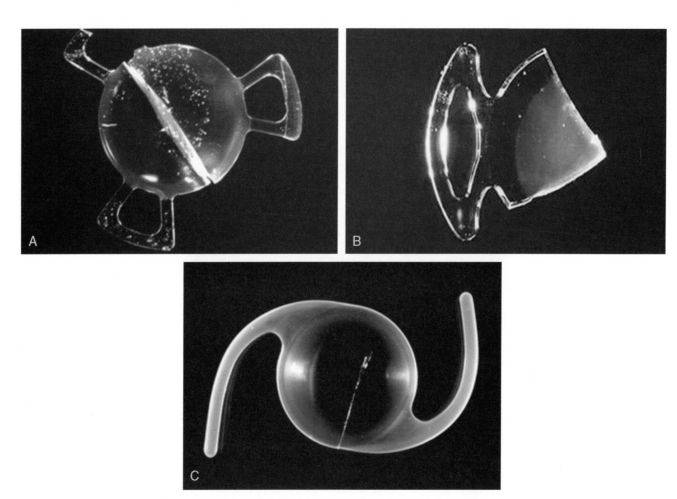

Figure 42-31 Gross photographs showing hydrophilic acrylic lenses manufactured in Europe, explanted because of calcification. **A**, Courtesy of BigBag, IOLtech, France. **B**, Courtesy of StabiBag, IOLtech, France. **C**, Courtesy of 92S, Morcher, Germany.

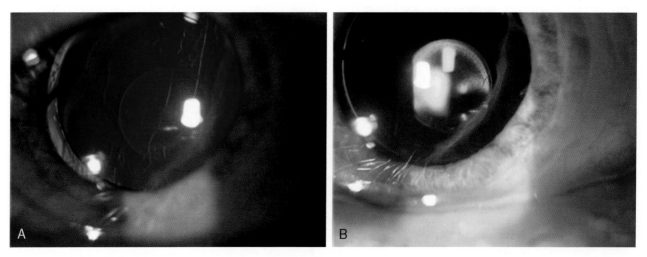

Figure 42-32 Clinical photographs showing a localized optic opacity observed 1 year after MemoryLens implantation (**A** and **B**).

(Continued)

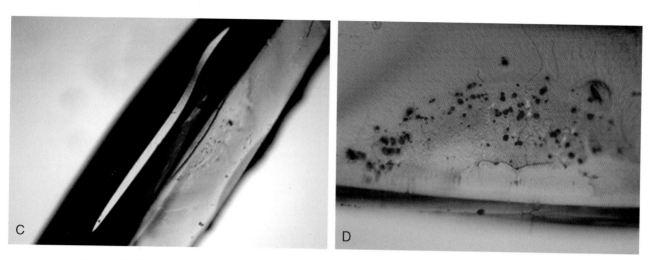

Figure 42-32, cont'd Sagittal analysis of the area involved under light microscopy revealed a linear optic breach (**C**). Alizarin red positive deposits were found within the optic void (**D**).

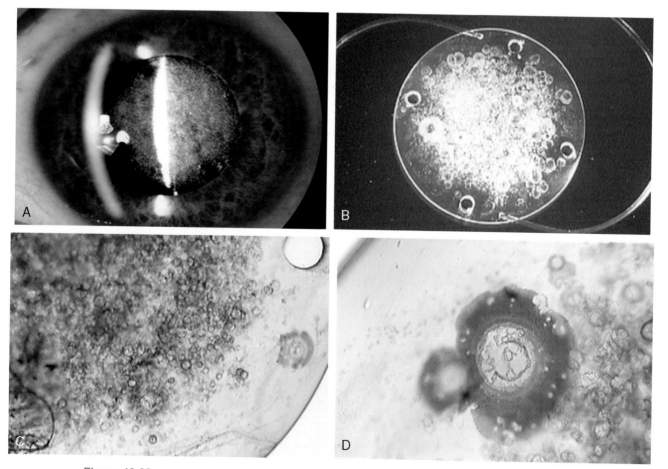

Figure 42-33 Clinical (**A**), gross (**B**), and light microscopic (**C**) photographs showing polymethylmethacrylate lenses, exhibiting snowflake degeneration. The aspect of the individual snowflake lesions can be better observed under high magnification light microscopy (**D**).

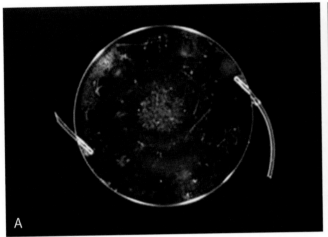
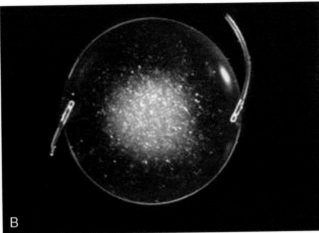

Figure 42-34 Gross photographs of a polymethylmethacrylate lens explanted because of snowflake degeneration, taken at the dry (**A**), and the hydrated (**B**) states. An unusual collection of fluid is observed within and around the area of snowflake lesions.

represent the initial injury before the typical snowflake lesions are seen, or they may be secondary to the initial presence of the more central snowflake lesions. In any case, the clinical significance of snowflake degeneration may depend on the amount of water collected within the area of cracks. The emergence of this complication could have represented a more significant problem, except for the fact that many of the patients implanted with these IOLs are now deceased. However, surgeons must be aware that there are probably still a number of patients living with varying stages of snowflake degeneration.

■ SUMMARY ■

Development of capsular bag opacification is multifactorial, and its eradication depends on the quality of the surgery, as well as on the quality of the IOL implanted. In terms of PCO, each surgery- or IOL-related factor described here does not act in isolation, and it is their interaction that produces the best results. From the authors' analyses it was also observed that factors related to patient's associated conditions, IOL manufacture, IOL storage, surgical techniques and adjuvants, among others, may be involved in a process of IOL opacification or discoloration. The process may involve IOLs manufactured from different biomaterials, and be observed early or late postoperatively. With the increasing numbers of new IOLs in the market every year, constant vigilance is necessary.

References

[1] Stark WJ, Leske MC, Worthen DM, Murray GC. Trends in cataract surgery and intraocular lenses in the United States. Am J Ophthalmol 1983;96:304–310.
[2] Apple DJ, Solomon KD, Tetz MR, et al. Posterior capsular opacification. Major review. Surv Ophthalmol 1992;37:73–116.
[3] Werner L, Apple DJ, editors. Complications of aphakic and refractive intraocular lenses. Philadelphia, PA: Lippincott Williams & Wilkins; International Ophthalmology Clinics, 41(3); 2001.
[4] Apple DJ, Werner L. Complications of cataract and refractive surgery: a clinicopathological documentation. Trans Am Ophthalmol Soc 2001;99:95–109.
[5] Werner L. Causes of intraocular lens opacification or discoloration. J Cataract Refract Surg 2007;33:713–726.
[6] Schaumberg DA, Dana MR, Christen WG, Glynn RJ. A systematic overview of the incidence of posterior capsule opacification. Ophthalmology 1998;105:1213–1221.
[7] Meacock WR, Spalton DJ, Boyce J, Marshall J. The effect of posterior capsule opacification on visual function. Invest Ophthalmol Vis Sci 2003;44:4665–4669.
[8] Neumayer T, Findl O, Buehl W, Georgopoulos M. Daily changes in the morphology of Elschnig pearls. Am J Ophthalmol 2006;141:517–523.
[9] Charles S. Vitreoretinal complications of YAG laser capsulotomy. Ophthalmol Clin North Am 2001;14:705–710.
[10] Fernandez V, Fragoso MA, Billote C, et al. Efficacy of various drugs in the prevention of posterior capsule opacification: experimental study of rabbit eyes. J Cataract Refract Surg 2004;30:2598–605.
[11] Werner L, Legeais JM, Nagel MD, Renard G. Evaluation of Teflon-coated intraocular lenses in an organ culture method. J Biomed Mater Res 1999;46:347–354.
[12] Meacock WR, Spalton DJ, Hollick EJ, et al. Double-masked prospective ocular safety study of a lens epithelial cell antibody to prevent posterior capsule opacification. J Cataract Refract Surg 2000;26:716–721.
[13] Fine IH. Cortical cleaving hydrodissection. J Cataract Refract Surg 1992;18:508–512.
[14] Peng Q, Apple DJ, Visessook N, et al. Surgical prevention of posterior capsule opacification. Part II. Enhancement of cortical clean up by increased emphasis and focus on the hydrodissection procedure. J Cataract Refract Surg 2000;26:188–197.
[15] Vargas LG, Escobar-Gomez M, Apple DJ, et al. Pharmacologic prevention of posterior capsule opacification: in vitro effects of preservative-free lidocaine 1% on lens epithelial cells. J Cataract Refract Surg 2003;29:1585–1592.
[16] Chew J, Werner L, Stevens S, Hunter B, Mamalis N. Evaluation of the effects of hydrodissection with antimitotics using a rabbit model of Soemmering's ring formation. Clin Experiment Ophthalmol 2006;34:449–456.
[17] Sacu S, Menapace R, Findl O, et al. Influence of optic edge design and anterior capsule polishing on posterior capsule fibrosis. J Cataract Refract Surg 2004;30:658–662.
[18] Menapace R, Wirtitsch M, Findl O, Buehl W, Kriechbaum K, Sacu S. Effect of anterior capsule polishing on posterior capsule opacification and neodymium:YAG capsulotomy rates: three-year randomized trial. J Cataract Refract Surg 2005;31:2067–2075.
[19] Spalton DJ. In reply to: Nishi O. Effect of a discontinuous capsule bend. J Cataract Refract Surg 2003;29:1051–1052.
[20] Ram J, Apple DJ, Peng Q, et al. Update on fixation of rigid and foldable posterior chamber intraocular lenses (IOLs). Part II. Choosing the correct IOL designs to help eradicate posterior capsule opacification. Ophthalmology 1999;106:891–900.
[21] Tassignon MJBR, De Groot V, Vrensen GFJM. Bag-in-the-lens implantation of intraocular lenses. J Cataract Refract Surg 2002;28:1182–1188.
[22] Leysen I, Coeckelbergh T, Gobin L, et al. Cumulative neodymium:YAG laser rates after bag-in-the-lens and lens-in-the-bag intraocular lens implantation: comparative study. J Cataract Refract Surg 2006;32:2085–2090.
[23] Smith SR, Daynes T, Hinckley M, Wallin TR, Olson RJ. The effect of lens edge design versus anterior capsule overlap on posterior capsule opacification. Am J Ophthalmol 2004;138:521–526.
[24] Linnola RJ, Werner L, Pandey SK, et al. Adhesion of fibronectin, vitronectin, laminin and collagen type IV to intraocular lens materials in human autopsy eyes. Part I: histological sections. J Cataract Refract Surg 2000;26:1792–806.
[25] Linnola RJ, Werner L, Pandey SK, et al. Adhesion of fibronectin, vitronectin, laminin and collagen type IV to intraocular lens materials in human autopsy eyes. Part II: explanted IOLs. J Cataract Refract Surg 2000;26:1807–1818.
[26] Werner L, Pandey SK, Escobar-Gomez M, et al. Anterior capsule opacification: a histopathological study comparing different IOL styles. Ophthalmology 2000;107:463–471.
[27] Werner L, Pandey SK, Apple DJ, et al. Anterior capsule opacification: correlation of pathological findings with clinical sequelae. Ophthalmology 2001;108:1675–1681.
[28] Izak AM, Werner L, Apple DJ, et al. Loop memory of different haptic materials used in the manufacture of posterior chamber intraocular lenses. J Cataract Refract Surg 2002;28:12292–35.
[29] Werner L, Pandey SK, Izak AM, et al. Capsular bag opacification after experimental implantation of a new accommodating intraocular lens in rabbit eyes. J Cataract Refract Surg 2004;30:11147–11123.
[30] Werner L, Hickman MS, LeBoyer RM, Mamalis N. Experimental evaluation of the Corneal Concept 360 intraocular lens with the Miyake-Apple view. J Cataract Refract Surg 2005;31:1231–1237.
[31] Davison JA. Capsule contraction syndrome. J Cataract Refract Surg 1993;19:582–589.
[32] Gayton JL, Apple DJ, Peng Q, et al. Interlenticular opacification: a clinicopathological correlation of a new complication of piggyback posterior chamber intraocular lenses. J Cataract Refract Surg 2000;26:330–336.
[33] Werner L, Shugar JK, Apple DJ, et al. Opacification of piggyback IOLs associated with an amorphous material attached to interlenticular surfaces. J Cataract Refract Surg 2000;26:1612–1619.

[34] Werner L, Apple DJ, Pandey SK, et al. Analysis of elements of interlenticular opacification. Am J Ophthalmol 2002;133:320–326.

[35] Werner L, Mamalis N, Stevens S, Hunter B, Chew JL, Vargas LG. Interlenticular opacification: Dual-optic versus piggyback intraocular lenses. J Cataract Refract Surg 2006;32:656–662.

[36] Menapace R, Findl O, Georgopoulos M, Rainer G, Vass C, Schmetterer K. The capsular tension ring: designs, applications, and techniques. J Cataract Refract Surg 2000;26:898–912.

[37] Nishi O, Nishi K, Sakanishi K. Inhibition of migrating lens epithelial cells at the capsular bend created by the rectangular optic edge of a posterior chamber intraocular lens. Ophthalmic Surg & Lasers 1998;29:587–594.

[38] Findl O, Drexler W, Menapace R, et al. Accurate determination of effective lens position and lens-capsule distance with 4 intraocular lenses. J Cataract Refract Surg 1998;24:1094–1098.

[39] Peng Q, Visessook N, Apple DJ, et al. Surgical prevention of posterior capsule opacification. Part III. The IOL barrier effect functions as a second line of defense. J Cataract Refract Surg 2000;26:198–213.

[40] Nishi O, Nishi K. Preventing posterior capsule opacification by creating a discontinuous sharp bend in the capsule. J Cataract Refract Surg 1999;25:521–526.

[41] Nishi O, Nishi K. Preventive effect of a second-generation silicone intraocular lens on posterior capsule opacification. J Cataract Refract Surg 2002;28:1236–1240.

[42] Nishi O, Nishi K. Effect of the optic size of a single-piece acrylic intraocular lens on posterior capsule opacification. J Cataract Refract Surg 2003;29:348–353.

[43] Bhermi GS, Spalton DJ, El-Osta AAR, Marshall J. Failure of a discontinuous bend to prevent lens epithelial cell migration in vitro. J Cataract Refract Surg 2002;28:1256–1261.

[44] Tetz M, Wildeck A. Evaluating and defining the sharpness of intraocular lenses: part 1: Influence of optic design on the growth of the lens epithelial cells in vitro. J Cataract Refract Surg 2005;31:2172–2179.

[45] Werner L, Mamalis N, Pandey SK, et al. Posterior capsule opacification in rabbit eyes implanted with hydrophilic acrylic intraocular lenses with enhanced square edge. J Cataract Refract Surg 2004;30:2403–2409.

[46] Werner L, Mamalis N, Izak AM, et al. Posterior capsule opacification in rabbit eyes implanted with single-piece and three-piece hydrophobic acrylic intraocular lenses. J Cataract Refract Surg 2005;31:805–811.

[47] Maloof A, Neilson G, Milverton EJ, Pandey SK. Selective and specific targeting of lens epithelial cells during cataract surgery using sealed capsule irrigation. J Cataract Refract Surg 2003;29:1566–1568.

[48] Tanaka T, Saika S, Hashizume N, Ohnishi Y. Brown haze in an Allergan SI-40NB silicone intraocular lens. J Cataract Refract Surg 2004;30:250–252.

[49] Hilgert CR, Hilgert A, Hofling-Lima AL, Farah ME, Werner L. Early opacification of SI-40NB silicone intraocular lenses. J Cataract Refract Surg 2004;30:2225–2229.

[50] Werner L, Dornelles F, Hilgert CR, et al. Early opacification of silicone intraocular lenses: Laboratory analyses of six explants. J Cataract Refract Surg 2006;32:499–509.

[51] Elgohary M, Zaheer A, Werner L, Ionides A, Sheldrick J, Ahmed N. Opacification of SA40N Array silicone multifocal lens. J Cataract Refract Surg 2007;33:342–347.

[52] Werner L, Apple DJ, Crema AS, et al. Permanent blue discoloration of a hydrogel intraocular lens by intraoperative trypan blue. J Cataract Refract Surg 2002;28:1279–1286.

[53] Ozbek Z, Saatci AO, Durak I, et al. Staining of intraocular lenses with various dyes: a study of digital image analysis. Ophthalmologica 2004;218:243–247.

[54] Stevens S, Werner L, Mamalis N. Corneal edema and permanent blue discoloration of a silicone intraocular lens by methylene blue. Ophthalmic Surg Lasers Imag 2007;38:136–141.

[55] Werner L, Sher JH, Taylor JR, et al. Toxic anterior segment syndrome and possible association with ointment in the anterior chamber following cataract surgery. J Cataract Refract Surg 2006;32:227–235.

[56] McDonnell PJ, Taban M, Sarayba M, et al. Dynamic morphology of clear corneal cataract incisions. Ophthalmology 2003;110:2342–2348.

[57] Shingleton BJ, Wadhwani RA, O'Donoghue MW, et al. Evaluation of intraocular pressure in the immediate period after phacoemulsification. J Cataract Refract Surg 2001;27:524–527.

[58] Chew JJL, Werner L, Mackman G, Mamalis N. Late opacification of a silicone intraocular lens caused by ophthalmic ointment. J Cataract Refract Surg 2006;32:341–346.

[59] Chen KH, Lin SY, Li MJ, Cheng WT. Retained antibiotic ophthalmic ointment on an intraocular lens 34 months after sutureless cataract surgery. Am J Ophthalmol 2005;139:743–745.

[60] Milauskas AT. Silicone intraocular lens implant discoloration in humans. Arch Ophthalmol 1991;109:913–915.

[61] Watt RH. Discoloration of a silicone intraocular lens 6 weeks after surgery. Arch Ophthalmol 1991;109:1494–1495.

[62] Koch DD, Heit LE. Discoloration of silicone intraocular lenses. Arch Ophthalmol 1992;110:319–320.

[63] Katai N, Yokoyama R, Yoshimura N. Progressive brown discoloration of silicone intraocular lenses after vitrectomy in a patient on amiodarone. J Cataract Refract Surg 1999;25:451–452.

[64] Jones DF, Irwin AE. Discoloration of intraocular lens subsequent to rifabutin use. Arch Ophthalmol 2002;120:1211–1212.

[65] Sathyan P, Myint K, Singh G, et al. Late green discoloration of Allergan SI-40NB silicone intraocular lens. J Cataract Refract Surg 2006;32:1584–1585.

[66] Siddique M, Ashraf KM, Qazi ZA. Greenish discoloration of a CeeOn 911A silicone lens. Eye 2005;19:1349–1350.

[67] Grewal SP, Jain R, Grewal D, Gupta R. In vivo fluorescein staining of SI-30NB silicone intraocular lens. J Cataract Refract Surg 2007;33:156–158.

[68] Apple DJ, Isaacs RT, Kent DG, et al. Silicone oil adhesion to intraocular lenses: an experimental study comparing various biomaterials. J Cataract Refract Surg 1997;23:536–544.

[69] Foot L, Werner L, Gills JP, et al. Surface calcification of silicone plate intraocular lenses in patients with asteroid hyalosis. Am J Ophthalmol 2004;137:979–987.

[70] Wackernagel W, Ettinger K, Weitgasser U, et al. Opacification of a silicone intraocular lens caused by calcium deposits on the optic. J Cataract Refract Surg 2004;30:517–520.

[71] Werner L, Kollarits CR, Mamalis N, Olson RJ. Surface calcification of a three-piece silicone intraocular lens in a patient with asteroid hyalosis: a clinicopathologic case report. Ophthalmology 2005;112:447–452.

[72] Werner L, Apple DJ, Escobar-Gomez M, et al. Postoperative deposition of calcium on the surfaces of a hydrogel intraocular lens. Ophthalmology 2000;107:2179–2185.

[73] Pandey SK, Werner L, Apple DJ, Gravel JP. Calcium precipitation on the optical surfaces of a foldable intraocular lens: a clinicopathological correlation. Arch Ophthalmol 2001;120:391–393.

[74] Tehrani M, Mamalis N, Wallin T, et al. Late postoperative opacification of MemoryLens hydrophilic acrylic intraocular lenses: case series and review. J Cataract Refract Surg 2004;30:115–122.

[75] Neuhann IM, Werner L, Izak AM, et al. Late postoperative opacification of a hydrophilic acrylic (hydrogel) intraocular lens: a clinicopathological analysis of 106 explants. Ophthalmology 2004;111:2094–2101.

[76] Werner L, Apple DJ, Kaskaloglu M, Pandey SK. Dense opacification of the optical component of a hydrophilic acrylic intraocular lens: a clinicopathological analysis of 9 explanted lenses. J Cataract Refract Surg 2001;27:1485–1492.

[77] Macky TA, Werner L, Soliman MM, et al. Opacification of two hydrophilic acrylic intraocular lenses 3 months after implantation. Ophthalmic Surg Lasers Imaging 2003;34:197–202.

[78] Frohn A, Dick B, Augustin AJ, Grus FH. Late opacification of the foldable hydrophilic acrylic lens SC60B-OUV. Ophthalmology 2001;108:1999–2004.

[79] Izak AM, Werner L, Pandey SK, Apple DJ. Calcification of modern foldable hydrogel intraocular lens designs. Eye 2003;17:393–406.

[80] Werner L, Hunter B, Stevens S, Chew JJL, Mamalis N. Role of silicon contamination on calcification of hydrophilic acrylic intraocular lenses. Am J Ophthalmol 2006;141:35–43.

[81] Kleinmann G, Apple DJ, Werner L, et al. Postoperative surface deposits on intraocular lenses in children. J Cataract Refract Surg 2006;32:1932–1937.

[82] Neuhann IM, Stodulka P, Werner L, et al. Two opacification patterns of the same hydrophilic acrylic polymer: case reports and clinicopathological correlation. J Cataract Refract Surg 2006;32:879–886.

[83] Kleinmann G, Werner L, Kaskaloglu M, et al. Postoperative opacification of the peripheral optic region and haptics of a hydrophilic acrylic intraocular lens: case report and clinicopathologic correlation. J Cataract Refract Surg 2006;32:158–161.

[84] Moreno-Montanes J, Palop JA, Garcia-Gomez P, et al. Intraocular lens opacification after nonpenetrating glaucoma surgery with mitomycin-C. J Cataract Refract Surg 2007;33:139–141.

[85] Hunter B, Werner L, Memmen JE, Mamalis N. Postoperative localized opacification of the new MemoryLens design: analyses of an explant. J Cataract Refract Surg 2005;31:1836–1840.

[86] Apple DJ, Peng Q, Arthur SN, et al. Snowflake degeneration of polymethylmethacrylate posterior chamber intraocular lens optic material: a newly described clinical condition caused by unexpected late opacification of polymethylmethacrylate. Ophthalmology 2002;109:1666–1675.

[87] Tognetto D, Toto L, Sanguinetti G, Ravalico G. Glistenings in foldable intraocular lenses. J Cataract Refract Surg 2002;28:1211–1216.

[88] Dahle N, Werner L, Fry L, Mamalis N. Localized, central optic snowflake degeneration of a PMMA intraocular lens: clinical report with pathological correlation. Arch Ophthalmol 2006;124:1350–1353.

SUMMARY

part vii

MANAGEMENT OF COMPLICATIONS

Risk Management in Cataract Surgery

Anthony Agadzi, MD, Anne M. Menke, RN, PhD
and Richard L. Abbott, MD

43

CONTENTS

CHAPTER HIGHLIGHTS

>> Legal elements in proving malpractice

>> Informed consent

>> Statistics on malpractice suits and settlements

>> Steps to avoid lawsuits

>> Defense against claims of negligence

■ INTRODUCTION ■

Year after year, cataract surgery accounts for the greatest number of medical malpractice lawsuits against ophthalmologists reported to OMIC, the Ophthalmic Mutual Insurance Company.[1] An analysis of 168 cataract surgery claims over a 10-year span revealed that they represented 33% of the claims, and 24% of the total indemnity paid by OMIC.[2] This chapter will focus on actions surgeons can take before, during, and after surgery to further the two goals of healthcare risk management, namely, promoting the patient's safety and reducing the physician's liability exposure.

■ THE ELEMENTS OF MEDICAL MALPRACTICE ■

In a lawsuit for medical malpractice, or professional negligence, the patient is known as the plaintiff and the physician becomes the defendant. To successfully sue a physician for malpractice,

the plaintiff must prove the existence of four elements: *duty*, a duty of care owed as the result of a physician–patient relationship; *negligence*, a breach in the duty caused by the defendant's negligent act or omission, with negligence defined as a deviation from the standard of care that is determined by expert witness testimony; *causation*, a direct link between the defendant's negligent act or omission and an injury suffered by the plaintiff; and *damages*, pain and suffering, disability and disfigurement, past and future medical bills, lost wages, wrongful death, etc.

During the preoperative-assessment period and informed-consent process for surgery, ophthalmologists weigh up the likely benefit of the procedure for their patients and help them understand the potential risks involved. Despite these educational efforts, patients who experience an unanticipated outcome – a maloccurrence – too often forget that they were forewarned about complications and instead assume that someone was negligent in their care. It is often difficult to persuade patients and other physicians alike that an unanticipated outcome may or may not be the result of error or negligence, and that not all errors are the result of medical malpractice. Indeed, often the investigation of unanticipated outcomes and allegations of negligence reveals that what initially appeared to be malpractice was instead the result of either the disease process itself, or a foreseeable or unpreventable complication of risky, even life- or vision-saving treatment.

An example may help clarify this distinction between malpractice and a maloccurrence. Rupture of the posterior capsule is a well-known complication of cataract surgery. The surgeon is not necessarily negligent if this occurs during the procedure. With this or any other complication, what might be deemed below the standard of care would be the ophthalmologist's failure to:

- explain the potential complication and the likelihood of its occurrence to the patient as part of the informed-consent process

- recognize and address the complication in a timely manner

- inform the patient and document that the complication occurred

- give adequate discharge instructions. These include information about diet, activity, wound care, and the follow-up appointment; how to contact the surgeon; what symptoms to report ("call my office right away if you experience red eye, blurry vision, pain, flashing lights, many floaters, or sensitivity to light"); and the potential consequences of not informing the physician ("these symptoms could indicate a serious infection or a retinal detachment, which if not treated promptly, could lead to vision loss and even blindness")

- refer the patient to a sub-specialist for care in a timely manner if the situation warrants more advanced management.

While a lawsuit may be prompted by a specific event, such as a complication, the entire process of care is scrutized when patients sue physicians for medical malpractice. Experts pore over the medical records in order to evaluate the decision to perform surgery, the preoperative assessment, the choice of anesthesia, surgical approach, intraocular lens (IOL) choice, the quality and timing of the consent, the technical skills of the surgeon, the perioperative monitoring, recognition and management of complications, and postoperative care. Each of these aspects of care will be discussed in turn.

■ PREOPERATIVE CONSIDERATIONS ■

It is hard to defend a cataract surgery lawsuit if the procedure was not indicated in the first place. The plaintiff attorney may allege that the patient's cataract did not interfere with activities of daily living, the cataracts were not the cause of the visual difficulties, or that removal of the cataract would not improve visual acuity in the presence of other ophthalmic conditions, such as diabetic retinopathy or age-related macular degeneration. If both eyes are impacted by cataracts, the plaintiff may allege that the wrong eye was operated on first. Finally, in the case of a (functionally) monocular patient, the plaintiff may claim that the risks of the surgery were simply too great. Depending on source and criteria for selection, rates of inappropriateness of cataract surgery range from 1.7[3] to 37%.[4] These criteria typically include indicators of visual and functional impairment, which may be correctable by glasses or visual aids, situations in which patients cannot undergo surgery because of pre-existing comorbidities, or where underlying ocular conditions imply either a marginal benefit to surgery or clearcut contrandications.

INDICATIONS FOR CATARACT SURGERY

According to the American Academy of Ophthalmology's *Preferred Practice Pattern on Cataract in the Adult Eye*, "the primary indication for surgery is visual function that no longer meets the patient's needs and for which cataract surgery provides a reasonable likelihood of improved vision."[5] Cataract removal is also indicated when the lens opacity inhibits optimal management of posterior segment disease or the lens causes inflammation, angle closure, or medically unmanageable open-angle glaucoma. Notably, preoperative visual acuity is a poor predictor of postoperative functional improvement – and a poor defense of the decision to operate if the cataract does not interfere with the quality of the patient's life. Accordingly, assessment of a patient's near and distance vision under various contrast and lighting situations is highly important.[5] As a risk-management measure, documentation about functional impairment, ideally in the patient's own words or from a visual function questionnaire, should be included in the medical record.[6,7] The same indications extend to (functionally) monocular patients, but because such patients are dependent upon the eye

being considered for cataract surgery, they represent a higher medico-legal risk. Thus, the ophthalmologist should carefully weigh the need for surgery and the type of anesthesia, and is obliged to explicitly inform the patient of the definitive risk of total blindness. Documentation of the decision-making and consent process must be especially complete in such cases.

PREOPERATIVE OPHTHALMIC EVALUATION

In additional to measurements of functional vision, the preoperative ophthalmic evaluation should include assessment and clear documentation of the patient's visual status, acuity and refraction, external and slit-lamp examination including motility and alignment, pupillary function, intraocular pressure and dilated vitreo-retinal exam (or B-scan of posterior segment where poor visualization is present) at the very minimum. Similarly, contrast-sensitivity, glare-testing and potential acuity testing may be other adjunctive parameters on which to gauge and legally justify readiness for cataract surgery. Other tools like specular microscopy may also be useful in predicting poorer outcomes from otherwise routine cataract surgery in eyes with pre-existing endothelial disease. When performed and adequately documented, discussions with a patient about how the results of preoperative ophthalmic testing may influence final outcomes may help mitigate unrealistic patient expectations and prevent undue litigation.

SECOND-EYE SURGERY CONSIDERATIONS

The indications for second-eye surgery are generally along similar lines of first-eye surgery if cataract surgery in the fellow eye is expected to provide similar visual acuities in both eyes.[5] The necessity of second-eye cataract surgery is well established, and rarely challenged in court. In a British study looking at stereoacuity for instance, the number of patients meeting driving standards increased from 52% after first-eye surgery to 86% after second-eye surgery.[8] More recently, the second cross-sectional Blue Mountains Eye Study group demonstrated that a moderate-to-severe unilateral visual impairment caused by eye diseases such as cataract had a measurable impact on health-related quality of life, further underscoring the need for eventual bilateral surgery.[9] This has also been recently corroborated by the Los Angeles Latino Eye cross-sectional population-based study.[10] The importance of visual impairment – of which cataract remains a leading cause – in limiting functional quality of life and the legal ramifications therein should not be underestimated in any discussion of risk management. Visual impairment has been shown to be an important risk factor for falls and hip fractures,[11] and first-eye cataract surgery was shown to independently decrease the rate of falling and fracture over a 12-month period in a randomized controlled trial.[12] Visually significant cataract has also been implicated in a higher likelihood of motor-vehicle accidents.[13,14]

From a medical malpractice perspective, the highest risk for second eye surgery is the interval between procedures. The timing is dictated by several factors, including patient preference and surgical readiness, final visual acuity, medical and refractive stability of the first operated eye, anisometropia and the degree of the need for binocularity, especially as reflected in successful performance of activities of daily living such as driving. The shortest interval between procedures is, of course, simultaneous bilateral cataract surgery. While several reviews of simultaneous bilateral cataract extraction have shown no bilateral complications that resulted in visual loss,[15-18] most ophthalmologists do not operate on both eyes on the same day because of the potential for bilateral visual impairment, and the lost opportunity to adjust surgical plans for the second eye in the event of unanticipated findings or complications in the first. Interest in this scheduling option is growing, nonetheless, particularly in healthcare systems where patients have long waiting times for surgery.[5] At this point in time, at least in the United States, simultaneous bilateral cataract extraction is still considered exceptional, reserved for those patients in whom the risks of anesthesia, co-morbidities, or special travel or other living arrangements preclude the possibility of consecutive surgeries. Even if second-eye surgery is planned from the start, the ophthalmologist must obtain and document informed consent each time. Any additional information about risk gained during the first procedure (e.g., weak zonules or iris instability), must be explained to the patient and documented. The surgeon may either ask the patient to sign a separate consent form, or add the date and signature on a separate line on the first form.

In summary, careful patient selection lies at the forefront of risk management in cataract surgery. The single most important criterion for surgery and outcome measurement is the restoration of vision to meet a patient's functional needs and expectations. Given the potential for improvement in not only visual, but also physical, emotional and mental well-being as a result of cataract surgery, it is important that patient selection involves careful documentation of visual acuity and functional disability as pertains to activities of daily living, as this is the standard against which allegations of malpractice will be measured.

PREOPERATIVE MEDICAL ASSESSMENT

The primary purpose of the preoperative evaluation is to determine if the chosen procedure and anesthesia are safe and appropriate for the patient, and to help anticipate potential complications related to ophthalmic or medical co-morbidities. If a patient experiences an unanticipated outcome, he or she might allege that the assessment was negligent or failed to detect pre-existing medical conditions. While ophthalmologists are medical doctors, as specialists they generally limit their care and treatment to ophthalmic conditions. Accordingly, most ophthalmologists do not perform the preoperative history and physical examination themselves. Instead, they regularly refer the patient to the primary care physician for medical clearance. Ophthalmologists who perform their own preoperative medical assessment should ensure that their history and physical examination skills are up-to-date.

Preoperative assessment for cataract surgery must take into account consideration of past medical, social, family, medication, and allergic history. Extensive medical work-ups with EKG, complete blood counts and serum electrolytes do not appear to decrease perioperative morbidity and mortality, and are thus not routinely performed.[19] Systemic health issues uncovered during the preoperative evaluation may, however, influence an ophthalmologist's decision making regarding anesthetic and surgical technique, thus influencing final visual outcome. Such preoperative concerns should be discussed with the patient as well as primary care physician and anesthesiologist; where indicated, additional testing, such as cardiopulmonary risk assessment,

should be undertaken. The ophthalmologist should clarify with the primary care physician who will be responsible for ordering and reviewing results of preoperative testing, communicating them to the patient and healthcare team, and arranging for any necessary follow-up care.

Particular attention should be paid to patient medication history, especially over-the-counter, anti-coagulant, anti-platelet, and alpha-adrenergic antagonist therapies. Patients should be asked about current and remote use of these medications (especially the latter). There appears to be little evidence favoring the discontinuation of anti-platelet and anti-coagulant medications in the setting of routine cataract surgery.[20] Indeed, cerebrovascular accidents related to inadequate anticoagulation are felt to be the greater threat to patient safety. Surgery on anticoagulated patients must, nonetheless, be carefully managed. First, the surgeon should certainly disclose to the patient the potential for intraoperative bleeding (especially in the setting of retrobulbar anesthesia). Second, careful attention should be paid to the choice of anesthetic route. Finally, the entire surgical team, including the patient, should be instructed to monitor for signs of intra- and postoperative bleeding. From the risk management standpoint, careful documentation of the mutual decision to either continue or temporarily suspend anti-coagulation, as well as choice of alternative anesthetic route employed if any, is imperative.

The use of systemic alpha-adrenergic antagonists for benign prostatic hypertrophy, hypertension, and urinary retention – even years before surgery – has recently been associated with a newly described small-pupil floppy iris syndrome which may increase the risk of complications during cataract surgery.[21,22] During preoperative review and informed consent, a discussion of the possibility of these complications must be documented, equipment to manage them made available, and appropriate surgical technique utilized to minimize risk of a poor outcome.

INFORMED CONSENT

Surgeons are familiar with the duty to obtain the patient's informed consent before invasive and risky procedures. The patient's consent must be both voluntary and informed, and obtained when the patient is able to participate in the decision-making process in a meaningful way, in advance of surgery. Too often equated with the consent form, informed consent is instead a process which begins as an **oral agreement** between the ophthalmologist and the patient that is **reached after a discussion**. The discussion includes the condition, recommended treatment or procedure, and the risks, complications, benefits, and alternatives, as well as the consequences of refusing the recommended treatment or procedure.

Lack of informed consent is rarely the main focus of malpractice lawsuits. Exceptions include when the surgeon performs a procedure that is different from the one planned, or adds one without discussing it with the patient (limbal-relaxing incision during cataract surgery). Jurors readily imagine the difficulty patients feel when trying to make a healthcare decision based upon a layperson's knowledge. This easy identification with patients may explain the attention both plaintiff attorneys and jurors pay to the issue of informed consent. Allegations in lawsuits include failure to warn the patient of a particular complication for which the patient was at increased risk, coerced consent obtained the day of surgery, consent from a patient incapacitated by preoperative medication, or lack of consent for experimental treatment. Lack of documentation of the consent discussion inevitably leads to a credibility battle whose outcome will depend upon subjective factors rather than medical facts.

In general, the duty to obtain informed consent cannot be delegated: the healthcare provider performing the diagnostic procedure or surgery must obtain it. In cases of co-managed care, it is common for the plaintiff attorney and expert to criticize the surgeon for failing to perform his own independent determination of the patient's candidacy and personally conduct the informed consent discussion. Surgeons who co-manage can further decrease the risk of allegations of lack of informed consent by asking the patient to sign a specific consent for the co-management. If the patient has any known risk factors that increase the likelihood of complications, side effects, or poor outcome, the ophthalmologist should discuss these with the patient and document the disclosure discussion. Finally, the informed consent discussion should take place when the patient is awake and aware, free from the effects of any medication that could interfere with the patient's ability to participate in the decision-making process.

The informed consent discussion should always be documented, ideally in two ways. First, the surgeon should include a brief note about the discussion in the medical record. If the discussion took place in a language other than English, document the language used, and the name and relationship of any translator. Specific questions or concerns raised by the patient should be documented, along with the answers. In addition to documenting that the discussion took place, patients should sign a procedure-specific consent form, and be given a copy for review with family or legal guardian. Records and copies of educational materials distributed to patients should be kept readily available.

For elective surgeries, the discussion should take place before the day of the surgery whenever possible. Some patients who had surgery the same day as the informed-consent discussion have later sued for lack of informed consent, arguing that they were coerced into having the procedure and did not have time to weigh the risks and benefits. If the patient cannot be seen until the day of surgery due to time and distance constraints, taking the extra time for discussion will help facilitate patient understanding and ensure that the consent for surgery is not coercive. An extra step for the informed consent includes obtaining information about the patient's medical and ocular health from the referring physician or directly from the patient by telephone or questionnaire. Another strategy is to send the patient an unsigned copy of the procedure-specific form along with other educational information, and to ask the patient to review the materials well in advance of surgery. On the day of surgery, before any medication is administered, the ophthalmologist should conduct the final preoperative assessment and personally obtain the patient's oral consent as well as signature on the consent document.

ANESTHESIA ISSUES

In 2006, OMIC completed a study of its anesthesia claims experience.[23] Out of 2474 claims during this 18-year period, only 78 (or 3%) were related to anesthesia and sedation.[23] While the frequency of anesthesia claims is low, both the percentage of claims resulting in payments (34%) and the severity of the indemnity

awards ($150,000 median payment) were higher than OMIC's overall claims averages (21% and $75,000).[23] Complications of orbital injection anesthesia accounted for the overwhelming majority of anesthesia/sedation-related claims against OMIC insureds (69 claims), while general and topical anesthesia accounted for only five and four claims, respectively.[23] Sedation was an issue in five of the 69 orbital cases.[23] Retrobulbar anesthesia was administered in 49 cases, peribulbar in 16, and O'Brien block in one.[23] Of note is the fact that there were no claims resulting from sub-Tenon's blocks.[23] The injury to the plaintiff was felt to be the result of physician negligence in 13 of the 22 cases that resulted in an indemnity payment.[23] Some incidents of negligence pertained to inadequate control of eye pain, movement, anxiety and level of sedation, as well as negligent administration of orbital injection.

The following guidelines for risk management and anesthesia are critical:

- Document the choice of anesthesia, and decision-making process as discussed with the patient, anesthesia provider, and primary physician, where needed
- Document the patient's informed consent for both the surgical procedure and type of anesthesia, even if administered by an anesthesia provider
- Respect scope of practice, licensure, and competency when providing, delegating, and supervising anesthesia and sedation. Ophthalmologists are usually held vicariously liable for care rendered by their employees, such as nurses and technicians. As a general rule, however, they are not held liable for the negligent acts of anesthesiologists, or certified registered nurse anesthetists even if – for billing and regulatory purposes – they are deemed to be their "supervisors", unless the ophthalmologist directly controls the actions of the anesthesia provider
- Communicate pertinent ocular biometrics or co-morbidity (e.g., long myopic eye, staphyloma, etc.) which may affect the technique of anesthetic administration.

INTRAOCULAR LENS CALCULATION AND SELECTION ISSUES

Following cataract extraction, a patient's final visual acuity expectation depends largely on the type and method of IOL implantation. Any discussion of informed consent, in addition to stating the inability to guarantee a perfect visual outcome, must, therefore, accurately document specific visual goals for both near and distance vision. Issues relevant to lens type include choice of either distance or near acuity with monofocal lenses, dominant eye and depth perception issues in monovision scenarios, or the possibility of unpredictable visual side effects in multifocal lens implants. An additional discussion on the occurrence of temporary anisometropia between the consecutive cataract surgeries, as well as the likelihood of residual refractive error and options for its management, are critical determinants in preventing unnecessary malpractice claims.

According to multiple medico-legal sources, errors related to IOL power miscalculations, size or type, defectiveness, dislocation, or decentration, comprise up to one-third of all cataract-related legal claims.[24,25] Such claims were frequently defensible if there was appropriate documentation and explanation for why a surgeon picked a particular IOL power or type. Further risk-reduction strategies include accurate, repeatable, bilateral ocular biometric measurements derived from precisely calibrated instruments, and performed by well-trained technicians. The use of appropriate lens formulae, as well as appropriate labeling and intraoperative verification of IOL types is critical.

In recent years, in addition to regular monofocal lenses for either distance or near vision, several new "multifocal" intraocular lenses with the ability to provide an expanded range of near-to-distance vision have been developed to more adequately simulate the pre-presbyopic eye. These lenses may not be appropriate for patients with unrealistic personal expectations or strict professional visual acuity requirements (e.g., pilots) as even the most accurate biometry and uncomplicated surgery in the hands of the most adept surgeon, may not guarantee a perfect visual outcome. Since patients often pay more for multifocal lens options, such inflexible expectations can lead to dissatisfaction and ultimately litigation in the event of a suboptimal visual outcome. This may especially be the case in the setting of misleading advertising on the part of the ophthalmologist who "guarantees" spectacle-free near, intermediate and distance acuity. The following points should be documented as part of the informed consent pertaining to patient selection for multifocal lens implantation:

- Discuss presbyopia and alternatives for near vision following cataract surgery with every patient, whether or not you offer "multifocal" IOLs. If you do not offer these IOLs, the discussion can be brief. If patients desire an IOL you do not offer, encourage them to seek care elsewhere.

- Elicit and document information about professional and leisure activities that may influence IOL choice (e.g., accountants and knitters may prefer near vision).

- Discuss side effects associated with multifocal IOLs such as nighttime glare, haloes, or imperfect near or intermediate acuity results and their potential effect on activities of daily living, night driving, or other low-light situations.

- Discuss the possibility of placing a monofocal lens in the event that a multifocal lens cannot be implanted because of an intraoperative complication.

- Discuss the possibility for subsequent IOL exchange in the event of extreme side effects, or symptom intolerance which persists after a reasonable "neuro-adaptive" period.

- Discuss management options and financial implications for both the IOL and any residual refractive error.

- Inform patients having refractive lens exchange of the "off-label" status of IOLs, which are only approved for implantation during cataract surgery.

■ INTRAOPERATIVE CONSIDERATIONS ■

IDENTIFICATION OF THE PATIENT AND SURGICAL SITE

Perhaps no other type of medical error has received more attention than instances where the wrong procedure has been performed. OMIC has had a total of 42 of these "wrong" allegations, which are usually considered by plaintiff attorneys and juries to be completely preventable.[1] The vast majority (26) involved claims of wrong power IOLs, followed by surgery on the wrong eye (10), block on the wrong eye (2), wrong procedure (2), and wrong patient (2).[1] Fully 36% of these cases resulted in indemnity payments totaling $573,515.[1] Surprisingly, in many instances, the patient never filed a lawsuit. Patients who are promptly told the truth, offered an apology, and granted a waiver of the fees associated with the procedure tend to be more forgiving.

Recommendations for preventing site errors include a preoperative verification process, marking the operative site and a "time out" immediately before starting the procedure. The "time out" involves the patient and the entire surgical team and frequently includes a checklist to verify the identity of the patient, correct site and side, procedure, patient position, and any implants, or special equipment. The verification process should be enforced prior to administration of anesthesia as well as before the operative procedure.

SURGICAL STERILE PREPARATION

Once in the operating suite, appropriate sterile instrumentation, preparation and draping of the patient, operating surfaces and equipment is imperative to reducing the risk of intraoperative complications and for facilitating a proper surgical outcome. In a recent review of risk issues in endophthalmitis by OMIC, at least nine out of 32 systems-related errors pertained to failure to sterilize, contaminated ultrasonic baths and equipment malfunction.[26] Appropriate labeling of all medications, injections and liquids used during surgery and on the sterile field is also essential to avoid any complications or intraocular toxicities.

INTRAOPERATIVE COMMUNICATION

Due to the ambulatory nature of most cataract surgery performed today, of utmost importance to risk management is communication between surgeon, anesthesiologist, patient and any ancillary staff members present in the operating room during an encountered complication. Since the cataract patient is frequently awake and relatively lucid during surgery, anxiety management on the part of the surgeon is a key element to patient cooperation during a difficult case, and tactful verbalization of operating room directives to counter a complicated situation can help prevent patient misunderstanding and undue litigation. At times, it may be necessary to conduct a post-procedure "debriefing" to collect necessary information and ensure adequate documentation.

■ POSTOPERATIVE CONSIDERATIONS ■

DOCUMENTATION

Accurate and immediate documentation of the operative report is an imperative risk reduction strategy following routine and complicated cataract surgery, both in the form of a dictated report and a brief entry in the medical record conveying information needed for care in the post-anesthesia care unit. A careful and detailed, customized operative report may be more easily defensible than that created by a standardized template which may omit critical information. Any information gained after the report is dictated should be entered into the record as a correctly labeled and dated addendum. A complete cataract operative report should include indications for surgery, informed consent documentation, record of infection prophylaxis, anesthesia method, surgical technique, recognition of and response to complications or unusual occurrences, as well as the rationale for and type and serial number of IOL used. Unusual occurrences, such as equipment malfunction, should be noted in the medical record in a factual manner without speculation or blame. In addition, the physician should notify the facility risk manager and follow the established protocol for completing an incident report which may contain information that should not be included in the medical record. Incident reports should not be referred to or included in the medical record, and should not be photocopied.

SURGICAL COMPLICATIONS

Corneal complications such as phacoemulsification burns, Descemet's detachments, endothelial decompensation or epithelial erosions, are recognized complications of cataract surgery. Legal claims associated with these complications may be reduced by appropriate informed consent, careful documentation of pre-existing pathology such as endothelial guttae, and precautionary phacoemulsification technique. The latter includes maintenance of adequate irrigation and flow around instrument tips, nuclear-chop techniques to minimize ultrasonic power and time, and appropriate use of ophthalmic visco-dispersive materials.

Despite the common opinion that the iris is merely an obstruction to anterior segment surgery, many claims result from the cosmetic effect of post-surgical iris trauma and distortion;[2] this possibility should be mentioned in any informed consent discussion. Preoperative conditions such as alpha-adrenergic antagonist use or poor dilation are often predisposing factors to iris trauma and need to be taken into account so that appropriate techniques can be anticipated and employed to minimize such scenarios.

Vitreoretinal complications are not only the second most common legal claim, but also the second highest in amount of indemnity paid.[2] Specific issues include those related to retinal detachment, choroidal effusion, exacerbations of age-related macular degeneration, as well as ruptured posterior capsule with dropped or retained lens fragments. Anterior segment surgeons not experienced or trained to perform deep vitrectomy should abstain from retrieving nuclear fragments in the vitreous as such heroic efforts may paradoxically lead to further complications. Instead such patients should promptly be referred to vitreoretinal specialists for follow-up care.

Other miscellaneous complications including intraocular pressure exacerbations in the context of glaucoma emphasize the need for meticulous management of ocular comorbidities, including early referral for sub-specialty care where indicated. Large settlements have resulted from failure to perform and document examinations of the optic nerve, to obtain informed consent for prolonged courses of steroids, and to monitor for steroid-induced side effects.[1]

ENDOPHTHALMITIS AND TOXIC ANTERIOR SEGMENT SYNDROME

Infectious endophthalmitis is one of the most feared complications of ophthalmic surgery. Recently, a type of inflammatory response known as TASS, or toxic anterior segment syndrome,

has also garnered attention. Since OMIC's inception in 1987, endophthalmitis has accounted for 0.6% of claims frequency (150 claims out of 2559 total) and 5% of claims severity ($3,345,964 paid indemnity out of $63,191,199 total).[1,26] Of the 150 endophthalmitis cases, more than three-quarters (78%) of OMIC's endophthalmitis cases have closed without an indemnity payment.[26] The percentage of cases that have settled (22%) and the median settlement amount ($75,000) are comparable to OMIC's overall data.[26] Despite the severity of the outcome for the patient, endophthalmitis settlements have ranged from $9000 to $735,000 compared to a low of $500 and a high of $1.8 million for all settlements. Reflecting the relative novelty of TASS, allegations in all but three of the 150 claims involve an infectious rather than an inflammatory process.[26]

Given the estimated 2 million cataract procedures performed annually in the United States, it is hardly surprising that cataract surgery would account for 61% of all endophthalmitis cases.[26] Less expected, however, is that only 23% of cataract-related endophthalmitis cases resulted in an indemnity payment.[26] During the informed consent process for cataract surgery, ophthalmologists routinely disclose this rare complication, and most actively try to prevent its occurrence by treating pre-existing conditions such as blepharitis, preparing the eye with povidone iodine, and administering antibiotics. Indeed, assuming cataract surgery was indicated in the first place and the endophthalmitis was promptly recognized and treated, expert witnesses view this complication as a tragic maloccurrence rather than malpractice.

Amid ongoing debate of evidence-based guidelines for prevention of endophthalmitis, it is noteworthy that antibiotic administration was not a key issue in any case; nor was patient noncompliance a significant factor.[26] Instead, systems issues and physician-driven processes predominate.[26] While not all adverse events can be prevented, there is much ophthalmologists can do to reduce the incidence of endophthalmitis and TASS. The two primary issues in OMIC's endophthalmitis cases – telephone care and the diagnostic process – indicate the need to carefully screen patients who present with ophthalmic complaints, especially postoperatively, and to educate them about which symptoms to report. Failure to rule out endophthalmitis has resulted in harm to patients and significant liability exposure. Emerging research indicates that the ophthalmologist should also include inflammatory reactions such as TASS and postoperative uveitis in the differential diagnosis. Indeed, mistaking one for the other could lead not only to a delay in treatment but may worsen the outcome. Finally, the prompt use of retinal consultants with early suspicion of endophthalmitis can prevent liability associated with delay in diagnosis and treatment of this dreaded complication.

In the event of an endophthalmitis or TASS outbreak at a surgical facility, an effective response depends upon careful coordination and cooperation among the facility, surgeon, and patient. The facility should contact all affected surgeons, and document the notification efforts. Ophthalmologists in turn need to call all patients operated on that day or during that period, and notify them of the events, screen for symptoms, and educate them about when and why to contact the physician. As in any disclosure discussion, the physician should avoid speculation or blame. Documentation of outreach efforts must be made in the affected patient's medical records. Close follow-up and patient reassurance during such at-risk periods is critical. Particular attention must be given to patients whose surgery falls right before weekends or holidays as provision must be made for on-call coverage.

Given an outbreak, a surgical facility needs to sequester all involved materials, interview staff, and evaluate equipment, devices, solutions, medications, and the sterilization process. All aspects of the investigation should be carefully documented. The investigation will help locate the responsible organism or toxic agent, ascertain liability, and determine what steps to take to remedy any identified problems. Faced with a cluster of either endophthalmitis or TASS cases, both the surgical facility and the individual surgeon will need to decide whether or not it is safe to proceed with other scheduled ophthalmic cases at that location. Ophthalmologists who have an ownership interest in an ambulatory surgical facility may also be involved in these deliberations, and should act as patient advocates promoting quality care. Patient safety should be the driving factor, and all parties must feel confident that the causative factors have been identified and addressed.

DISCLOSURE DISCUSSION

After a detailed informed consent discussion, most patients can understand and accept a single complication, if they have a good working relationship with the surgeon. For this reason, surgeons who co-manage would be well-advised to perform the postoperative care of all patients who experience significant problems. Certain complications, moreover, predispose patients to subsequent ones. If patients are not promptly informed of complications as they occur, and warned that they are also at higher risk of experiencing other problems, they may lose faith in the ophthalmologist and seek out second opinions and legal advice. The best course of action is to invite the patient to be a member of the healthcare team assigned the responsibility of monitoring for, and reporting, symptoms suggestive of complications. Telephone screening protocols that prompt staff members and physicians alike to ask for past surgical history can also reduce the risk of a malpractice suit.[27]

DISCHARGE INSTRUCTIONS, PATIENT FOLLOW-UP AND COMPLIANCE

After cataract surgery, clear, written instruction for appropriate postoperative care must be reviewed with the patient and accompanying family members or surrogates, and appropriate follow-up arranged. While a wide range of postoperative follow-up intervals exists, practitioners should ensure adequate timing to allow for diagnosis of common postoperative complications, such as endophthalmitis, especially within the first postoperative week. In the event of a complicated cataract surgery, more frequent follow-up may be necessary, along with appropriate documentation in the chart of any unusual findings, and the use of outside consultants.

While patient compliance with postoperative antibiotic regimens and follow-up appointments is critical in facilitating improved outcomes, it is not always possible. Where non-compliance and patient attrition become an issue, it is the practitioner's responsibility to document such behavior as well as any attempts made to resolve this problem, such as records of correspondence. When

the practitioner is unable to continue providing care, a documentation of referral or transfer of care is essential to reduce the risk of liability resulting from a poor outcome.

■ CONCLUSION ■

The ultimate goal of risk management in cataract surgery is to maximize safety and satisfactory visual outcome for the patient, while minimizing the ophthalmologist's liability exposure. This can be achieved by implementing current treatment recommendations (e.g., Preferred Practice Patterns), and careful documentation at each stage of the preoperative, intraoperative and postoperative care of the ophthalmic patient as detailed in this chapter. Finally, clear, consistent, and accurate communication with the patient about the treatment plan, risks, expectations, and complications helps foster an effective physician–patient relationship. Taken together, these risk reduction measures may prevent even the worst outcome from translating into a medical malpractice lawsuit.

References

[1] OMIC unpublished data.

[2] Brick DC. Risk management lessons from a review of 168 cataract surgery claims. OMIC Digest Summer, 1997.

[3] Tobacman JK, Lee P, Zimmerman B, et al. Assessment of appropriateness of cataract surgery at ten academic medical centers in 1990. Ophthalmology 1996;103:207–215.

[4] Quintana JM, Escobar A, Arostequi I, et al. Development of appropriateness explicit criteria for cataract extraction by phacoemulsification. BMC Health Serv Res 2006;6:23.

[5] American Academy of Ophthalmology, Prefered Practice Pattern® Guideline. Cataract in the Adult Eye. San Francisco, CA: American Academy of Ophthalmology, 2006. Available at www.aao.org.

[6] Schein OD, Steinberg EP, Cassard SD, et al. Predictors of outcome in patients who underwent cataract surgery. Ophthalmology 1995;102:817–823.

[7] Steinberg EP, Tielsch JM, Schein OD, et al. The VF-14. An index of functional impairment in patients with cataract. Arch Ophthalmol 1994;112:630–638.

[8] Talbot EM, Perkins A. The benefit of second eye cataract surgery. Eye 1998;12:983–989.

[9] Chia EM, Mitchell P, Rochtchina E, et al. Unilateral visual impairment and health-related quality of life: The Blue Mountains Eye Study. Br J Ophthalmol 2003;87:392–395.

[10] Varma R, Wu S, Chong K, et al. Impact of severity and bilaterality of visual impairment on health-related quality of life. Ophthalmology 2006;113:1846–1853.

[11] Tinetti ME, Speechley M, Ginter SF. Risk factors for falls among elderly persons living in the community. N Engl J Med 1988;319:1701–1707.

[12] Harwood RH, Foss AJ, Osborn F, et al. Falls and health status in elderly women following first eye cataract surgery: a randomized controlled trial. Br J Ophthalmol 2005;89:53–59.

[13] Owsley C, Stalvey B, Wells J, et al. Older drivers and cataract: driving habits and crash risk. J Gerontol A Biol Sci Med Sci 1999;54:M203–M211.

[14] Owsley C, McGwin Jr G, Sloane M, et al. Impact of cataract surgery on motor vehicle crash involvement by older adults. JAMA 2002;288:841–849.

[15] Sharma TK, Worstmann T. Simultaneous bilateral cataract extraction. J Cataract Refract Surg 2001;27:741–744.

[16] Chang DF. Simultaneous bilateral cataract extraction. Editorial. Br J Ophthalmol 2003;87: 253–254.

[17] Ramsay AL, Diaper CJ, Saba SN, et al. Simultaneous bilateral cataract extraction. J Cataract Refract Surg 1999;25:753–762.

[18] Beatty S, Aggrawal RK, David DB, et al. Simultaneous bilateral cataract extraction in the UK. Br J Ophthalmol 1995;79:1111–1114.

[19] Schein OD, Katz J, Bass EB, et al. The value of routine preoperative medical testing before cataract surgery. Study of Medical Testing for Cataract Surgery. N Engl J Med 2000;342:168–175.

[20] American Academy of Ophthalmology, Prefered Practice Pattern® Guideline. Cataract in the Adult Eye. San Francisco, CA: American Academy of Ophthalmology, 2006. Available at www.aao.org.

[21] Chang DF, Campbell JR. Intraoperative floppy iris syndrome associated with tamsulosin. J Cataract Refract Surg 2005;31:664–673.

[22] Menke AM. Intraoperative floppy iris syndrome from administration of tamsulosin. http://www.omic.com/resources/risk_man/forms/patient/Flomax-Induced%20Intraoperative%20Floppy%20Iris%20Syndrome.rtf, 2005.

[23] Menke AM. Ocular anesthesia claims: causes and outcomes. OMIC Digest 2006;16:http://www.omic.com/new/digest/Digest_spring06.pdf.

[24] Smith HE. The incidence of liability claims in ophthalmology as compared with other specialties. Ophthalmology 1990;97:1376–1378.

[25] Brick DC. Risk management lessons from a review of 168 cataract surgery claims. Surv Ophthalmol 1999;43:356–360.

[26] Menke AM. Endophthalmitis and TASS: claims results and lessons. OMIC Digest 2006;16:1–7, http://www.omic.com/new/digest/Digest_spring06.pdf.

[27] Menke AM. Responding to unanticipated outcomes for more detailed instructions on disclosure discussions, http://www.omic.com/resources/risk_man/forms/medical_office/UnanticipatedOutcomes.rtf.

CONCLUSION

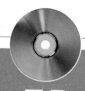

DVD

Intraoperative Complications of Phacoemulsification Surgery

Robert H. Osher, MD, Robert J. Cionni, MD,
Scott E. Burk, MD, PhD and David F. Chang, MD

44

CONTENTS

CHAPTER HIGHLIGHTS

>> Anesthesia issues

>> Controlling capsular defects

>> Managing nuclear fragments

>> Uses of ophthalmic viscosurgical devices

>> Vitrectomy maneuvers

Recognizing and managing intraoperative complications comprises the ultimate test of a cataract surgeon's knowledge, skill, and judgment. Because the intense stress of the moment may impair clear and rapid thinking, the better one has mentally prepared oneself for a complication, the less likely one is to panic.

Taking the time to ponder in advance on how to handle an emergency prepares us to respond correctly almost automatically. This chapter focuses on a constellation of intraoperative complications. Because the majority of these complications will be encountered by every cataract surgeon, a well-prepared and knowledgeable response can maximize the chances for a successful visual outcome.

PATIENT MOVEMENT

One primary drawback of local anesthesia is that the patient is still able to move during surgery. Although movement most often occurs from the patient talking, coughing, or simply fidgeting, occasionally a patient will abruptly sit up and try to leave the operating room while the surgeon is still working.

PREVENTION

As always, the best solution to a problem is to prevent it from occurring. Taping the forehead to the operating table helps to stabilize patients with a head tremor or who are otherwise unable to lie still. This is difficult to do once surgery begins, so assess the patient's level of cooperation and involuntary movement before starting the operation. If a significant head tremor or movement disorder is noted during the preoperative examination, it may be wise to consider general anesthesia.

Allowing the patient to become overly sedated or to fall asleep is also dangerous. The patient may suddenly awaken in a disoriented state and violently thrust the head, resulting in severe intraocular damage. A periodic reminder may aid the somnolent patient in staying awake. Coughing can also cause sudden head movement, as well as significant positive pressure. We ask the patient to warn us if he or she feels a cough coming. A box of cough drops located at the microscope has been helpful on numerous occasions.

To minimize restlessness, be certain that the patient is comfortable before surgery begins. Besides providing ample ventilation beneath the drapes, carefully position the operating table and any supporting pillows so as to minimize neck and back strain.

MANAGEMENT

The anesthesiologist can be invaluable in decreasing excessive patient movement by the administering of the appropriate medications as needed during the procedure. It may occasionally become necessary for the surgeon to be stern with the patient for the sake of surgical safety. With a small, self-sealing incision the surgeon always has the luxury of briefly halting surgery to address a problem with excessive patient movement. Although rarely necessary, small self-sealing incisions can even permit the surgeon to suspend surgery and correct a serious problem before returning to the operating room at a later time or even on another day.

■ RETROBULBAR HEMORRHAGE ■

Severe retrobulbar hemorrhage should necessitate cancellation of intraocular surgery.[1,2] High orbital or intraocular pressure significantly increases the likelihood of complications, such as iris prolapse, posterior capsule rupture, and vitreous loss. Anticoagulant therapy increases the risk of a serious retrobulbar hemorrhage, and we routinely ask our patients to check with their internist regarding the safety of discontinuing anticoagulant use before surgery if a local anesthetic injection anesthetic is planned. For anticoagulated patients topical anesthesia avoids the possibility of retrobulbar hemorrhage.

Proceeding with surgery in the setting of a limited retrobulbar hemorrhage is controversial, and will depend upon many factors, including the surgeon's experience. We have found that phacoemulsification with posterior chamber intraocular lens (IOL) implantation can be performed safely, provided that several criteria are met. First, all bleeding must be stopped by immediate and direct orbital pressure. This not only expedites clotting but also limits the volume of blood accumulation behind the globe. The surgeon should next evaluate the extent of the hemorrhage. Surgery can proceed if the globe is soft and easily retropulsed, the lids are loose and mobile, and proptosis is not excessive. If any of these criteria are not met, either digital massage or placement of a mercury bag against the orbit for 5–10 min may adequately reduce the orbital and intraocular pressure enough so that these parameters are fulfilled. It may also be advisable to perform a lateral canthotomy to reduce lid tightness. If after 30 min the surgeon remains uncertain about the safety of proceeding, it is best to reschedule the surgery rather than risk severe positive pressure intraoperatively.

In rare cases, the accumulation of orbital blood may elevate the intraocular pressure enough to threaten vision. Although the intraocular pressure can be measured quickly using a Schiotz tonometer or tonopen, it is more important to confirm retinal perfusion rather than the exact intraocular pressure. For this reason the authors keep a special lens (Osher panfundus lens, manufactured by Ocular Instruments) readily available, that can be used to quickly view the fundus through the operating microscope. If the central retinal artery is pulsating, its diastolic pressure has been exceeded and there is risk of infarction.

The combination of progressive proptosis, a tight orbit, central retinal artery pulsation, progressive corneal epithelial edema, and high intraocular pressure is an ominous emergency. The surgeon must quickly dissect into the periocular space with a scissors to release an expanding hematoma. If this fails to decompress the globe, the lower and upper lids should be disinserted by an emergency lateral canthotomy and cantholysis. It does not take much time to develop an ischemic optic neuropathy.

In a series of 60 cases of retrobulbar hemorrhage related to the anesthetic injection, only three cases required cancellation because they failed to satisfy the previously mentioned criteria for proceeding with surgery.[3] With few exceptions, the eyes undergoing surgery did not develop intraocular complications, and the postoperative visual results were similar to a control group of patients in whom retrobulbar hemorrhage had not developed.

Although small-incision surgery allows one to deal more easily with the complications associated with a retrobulbar hemorrhage, it does not eliminate them completely. The surgeon who proceeds with surgery in the face of a limited retrobulbar hemorrhage should be comfortable managing an eye with significant positive pressure.

■ COMPLICATIONS OF TOPICAL ANESTHESIA ■

Although this topic is covered elsewhere in this book, several important points should be emphasized. Optimal anesthesia requires appropriate preoperative counseling so that the patient's natural fear of eye surgery is minimized. Confirming adequate topical anesthesia before beginning the operation and then reassuring the patient in a gentle, caring voice are worth the time and effort. The authors instruct the patient to inform them if he or she feels anything uncomfortable, emphasizing that any discomfort can be promptly "numbed" by a few extra eye drops.

While some surgeons find supplemental intracameral anesthesia to be helpful, the most important factor when using topical anesthesia is appropriate patient selection. To prevent unexpected eye movements, the globe should be "stabilized" with a fixation ring, or by a second instrument holding or entering the paracentesis with a second instrument during delicate intraocular maneuvers. Finally, repeated verbal reassurance – "vocal local" – contributes to the safety and comfort of the patient.

■ INCISION ■

Surgeons today have many choices in the design and construction of their phaco incision. The options include scleral tunnel, near-clear, or clear corneal placement with steep axis or temporal location and frown, straight, smile, or even radial incision configurations.[4–6] Although each has its own advantages and disadvantages, which are covered elsewhere in this book, the common goal is to achieve a well-sealed incision that is either astigmatically neutral or in some cases designed to reduce pre-existing astigmatism. A poorly constructed incision will make a routine case difficult. Likewise, a carefully planned and precise incision is an important first step toward achieving success with an extremely difficult case. The following generalities about the incision are discussed to help avoid complications.

PLACEMENT

The foremost determinant of axis placement is ease of surgical access to the globe so that a prominent superior orbital rim will not interfere with the process. This often necessitates a superotemporal or temporal approach. The other considerations for axis placement are astigmatism and, occasionally, special anatomy such as prominent blood vessels, peripheral anterior synechiae, corneal opacities, or a pre-existing filter or ocular tumor.

Another important consideration is the distance from the incision to the central cornea. For any given incision size, the closer the incision is to the central cornea, the greater its tendency will be to alter cylinder along that axis.[7,8] Closer central corneal proximity also increases endothelial cell loss. Incision placement dictates the tunnel length as well. Clear corneal incisions require a shorter tunnel to avoid working too close to the central cornea, whereas scleral tunnel incisions must have a greater length to avoid premature entry. An incision with too short a tunnel length may not be watertight and self-sealing without sutures because there is less flap surface for appositional closure. Short clear corneal incisions might initially be watertight when the globe is repressurized, but may readily leak with any external pressure to the cornea or incision area.[9] To maximize the allowable tunnel length, a clear corneal incision should be started as posteriorly as possible. However, a tunnel that is too long can hinder motion of the phaco tip, causing excessive globe movement during phacoemulsification and undesirable corneal distortion. When creating a scleral pocket incision the surgeon must be careful to avoid excessive bleeding and premature entry. A posterior scleral pocket incision also creates a more difficult, "uphill" approach for the instruments. Mimicking scleral depression, any excessive instrument pressure on the incision can produce significant positive pressure.

Young or highly myopic patients with reduced scleral rigidity are more likely to experience molding or scleral shrinkage around the shaft of the phacoemulsification needle. Therefore, a slightly wider incision may occasionally be desirable in these eyes and will seal better if it hasn't been overly stretched. This is especially true if the surgeon is also attempting to reduce plus cylinder in the axis of the incision.

DEPTH

When a scleral tunnel approach is too deep, the keratome may prematurely enter the chamber angle or even the suprachoroidal space. The former may be associated with iris prolapse, whereas the latter is associated with bleeding and hypotony. If the suprachoroidal space is inadvertently entered, placement of deep sutures may prevent prolonged postoperative hypotony (Figure 44-1). A guarded blade for performing the initial scleral or near-clear corneal groove is helpful, and the incision need not exceed the depth of one half of the scleral thickness.

ANTERIOR CHAMBER ENTRANCE

The width of the entrance into the anterior chamber must be precise in its dimensions. It must allow easy entry of the phacoemulsification needle. Too large an entrance may result in a leaky incision with constant chamber shallowing throughout the operation and may require a temporary suture (Figure 44-2). Too tight an incision will restrict sliding of the phacoemulsification needle shaft, causing eye rotation during phacoemulsification. A tight opening may also constrict irrigation flow around the needle, increasing the chance of thermal injury with resulting incision gape. Finally, trauma to Descemet's membrane is more likely if instruments must be forced through a tight incision. While a certain amount of "snugness" is desirable, the incision should be extended if it is excessively tight.

The entrance through Descemets membrane must be anterior enough to create a self-sealing watertight incision. However, too anterior an entry increases endothelial cell loss and impairs visualization due to corneal striae developing during phacoemulsification. Moreover, too anterior an entry makes manipulation of the proximal pole of the nucleus and subincisional cortex more difficult. Too posterior an entrance invites iris prolapse.

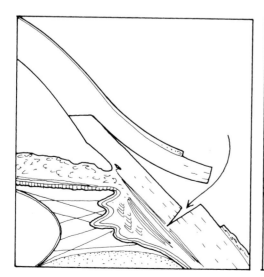 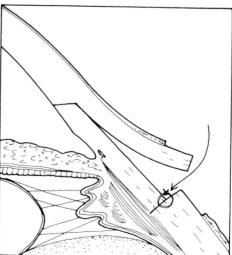

Figure 44-1 Placement of deep sutures when the scleral groove is too deep.

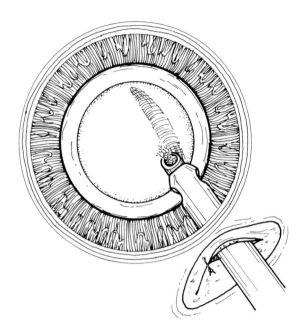

Figure 44-2 Placement of a temporary radial suture for an oversized phacoemulsification incision.

■ INCISION LEAK ■

If the incision is not watertight at the conclusion of the operation, the surgeon has several options to choose from. First, a 30-gauge cannula may be used to inject balanced salt solution (BSS) perpendicularly into the lateral borders of the incision. Hydrating the lateral stroma in this way forces the roof and floor of the tunnel together. If the incision still leaks, it is easy to place an interrupted 10-0 nylon suture that can be either tied and cut or looped for subsequent removal in the office.

Finally, if the incision leak is secondary to gaping from thermal injury, special suturing techniques described by Osher may be required. A radial 10-0 nylon suture is passed from the corneal tissue through the floor and tied, without incorporating the distal margin (the external lip) of the incision. Alternatively, a horizontal 10-0-nylon suture can be passed, bringing the posterior roof to the anterior floor. Each of these techniques helps to compensate for tissue shrinkage and minimize induced cylinder.[10,11]

■ TEAR OF DESCEMET'S MEMBRANE ■

A tear of Descemet's membrane at the anterior chamber entry site can be caused by improper insertion of an instrument through the incision. To avoid this occurrence, the leading tip should be directed posteriorly whenever inserting an instrument. This is difficult in eyes with shallow chambers in which a posteriorly directed instrument would immediately engage the iris. Deepening the anterior chamber with an ophthalmic viscosurgical device (OVD) prior to entry with the keratome or phaco tip will help to prevent this complication. As mentioned earlier, a Descemet's tear is less likely with an incision that is properly sized and constructed.

It is crucial to recognize an early tear in Descemet's membrane so that it is not extended with continuing instrument forces. Inadvertent injection of an OVD into the separation can also extend the detachment. Once recognized, the Descemet's membrane flap can usually be reattached by one of several simple maneuvers. Placing pressure on the posterior lip of the incision at the site of the tear will generate an egress of fluid, which will reposition a small Descemet's membrane flap in most instances. Alternatively, a small air bubble or bolus of OVD can be used to tamponade a torn Descemet's membrane flap back into position where it can be sutured if necessary.

A larger tear may require more extensive suturing. The needle should pass through clear cornea central to the "hinge" of the tear and then be directed peripherally to splint the Descemet's membrane flap into position. The authors have not needed to use gas or tissue glue, although others have reported success with these modalities.[12–15]

■ IRIS PROLAPSE ■

A prolapse of the iris may damage the stroma or sphincter enough to cause postoperative pupil irregularities, iris transillumination defects, peripheral anterior synechiae, or uveal incarceration into the incision. Intraoperatively, acute prostaglandin release may cause constriction of the pupil, whereas rupture of vessels from the minor iris circle may result in intraocular bleeding further complicating the operative procedure. In recent years the use of alpha blockers such as tamsulosin (Flomax), have markedly increased the incidence and severity of iris prolapse.[16]

The cardinal features of this syndrome termed intraoperative floppy iris syndrome (IFIS) include iris billowing, suboptimal dilation, progressive constriction of the pupil, and a tendency toward iris prolapse. It appears that the effect on the smooth muscle of the iris dilator is semi-permanent so that discontinuing the drug does not prevent IFIS. Moreover, the time of onset and the severity of IFIS is highly variable.[17]

Management options include viscomydriasis and mechanical iris retraction with highly retentive OVDs, iris retractors, pupil expansion devices, and adjunctive pharmacologic agents. These include preoperative atropine, intraoperative epinephrine, or intracameral phenylephrine.[18] Trying to enlarge the pupil by using the Fry stretch technique is ineffective and seems to worsen the tendency for iris prolapse.

PREVENTION

A well-constructed incision that extends "uphill" into the clear cornea will help to prevent iris prolapse, whereas too posterior an entry or too large an opening will ensure its occurrence (Figure 44-3). Efforts to both minimize iris trauma and reduce positive pressure will decrease the likelihood of iris prolapse. Any event that acutely raises the intraocular pressure may also cause iris prolapse. Care should be taken to avoid excessive injection of fluid or OVD into the capsular bag or behind the iris.

MANAGEMENT

The surgeon must identify the cause of the iris prolapse in order to manage the underlying problem properly. Excessive external pressure on the globe can be caused by improper speculum

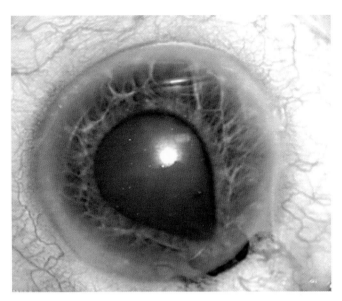

Figure 44-3 Iris prolapse through a posteriorly placed entrance into the anterior chamber.

positioning or a taut bridle suture. A tense and overfilled globe can be softened by aspirating fluid or OVD through a second incision site which reduces the intraocular pressure. If iris prolapse occurs during hydrodissection or viscodissection, neutralizing the pressure gradient between the anterior and posterior chamber can be accomplished by depressing the nucleus within the capsular bag. The iris can be gently repositioned in most cases with the OVD syringe cannula placed through the stab incision, leaving some OVD on the iris surface. If these attempts fail, the surgeon can next perform a small peripheral iridectomy at the site of prolapse to further neutralize the pressure gradient between the anterior and posterior chambers. Excessive manipulation causes the iris to become increasingly more frayed and flaccid, and this must be avoided. At the end of the case the injection of an intracameral miotic agent, judicious use of an OVD, a peripheral iridotomy, and deeply placed sutures help reduce the possibility of iris incarceration in the incision. In cases of IFIS, hydrating the incision before removing irrigating instruments and injecting a miotic agent through the side port incision will decrease the risk of iris prolapse at the end of the procedure.

■ INTRAOCULAR HEMORRHAGE FROM THE INCISION ■

Hemorrhage from the incision may compromise surgical visibility. Blood may also accumulate behind an IOL or dissect through the zonules into the vitreous cavity. Although intraocular hemorrhage will invariably be reabsorbed, it may acutely reduce vision, stimulate inflammation, and accelerate capsular opacification. Clot formation may cause posterior synechiae. For certain complicated cases, some surgeons consider discontinuing anticoagulant therapy before surgery under the direction of the patient's internist. If anticoagulant therapy cannot be discontinued, a clear corneal approach with topical anesthesia is indicated.

Because of the location of larger scleral blood vessels, intraocular hemorrhage is more likely to occur when the incision is temporal, deeper and more posterior than usual. The prompt injection of OVD may limit intraocular hemorrhage by the use of a tamponade at the bleeding site. In addition, elevating the intraocular pressure by overfilling the chamber with adrenalized BSS can often stop bleeding. Occasionally a visible feeder vessel may be amenable to point cautery, as long as it is not within the incision. After the bleeding has stopped, the surgeon should evacuate any intraocular blood before clot formation occurs.

The evacuation of blood from the anterior chamber can be achieved by simply depressing the posterior lip of the incision with a cannula. However, to prevent additional bleeding, it is probably best to aspirate the blood while infusing BSS in a "closed" system, thereby maintaining the intraocular pressure. This can be done through the main incision with an irrigating–aspiration tip or through two side port incisions using separate irrigation and aspiration. The likelihood of postoperative hyphema can be reduced in sutureless procedures by hydrating the incision then firming the globe with BSS at the end of the procedure to attain a high normal intraocular pressure. This maneuver will seal the anterior lip of the incision more tightly, preventing entrance of blood into the anterior chamber.

■ CAPSULORRHEXIS ■

The continuous curvilinear capsulotomy, or capsulorrhexis (see Chapter 14), is arguably the most important step in modern phacoemulsification surgery. The capsulorrhexis is strong enough to be stretched, and resists being torn during nucleus manipulation, cortical removal, and IOL implantation.[19–21] Capsulorrhexis has not only reduced the incidence of anterior capsular tears, but also the incidence of posterior capsule tears (0.2%). Moreover, if a tear in the posterior capsule should occur, an intact capsulorrhexis permits ciliary sulcus placement of a posterior chamber IOL, either with or without optic capture. Alternatively, endocapsular fixation with capture of the optic anterior to the rhexis edge may be possible.

Osher developed the concept of the "safety rhexis" which provides surgeons with a "second chance" if the primary capsulorrhexis is faulty.[22] A 22-gauge needle slash results in an anterior capsular tear with two arms. The lower arm is redirected opposite the orientation of the upper arm, which prevents it from running with the primary tear. The upper arm of the tear is then directed clockwise around the anterior capsule, until the capsulorrhexis is completed peripheral to the original starting point.[23] If a problem occurs with the upper arm, the surgeon may resume the capsulorrhexis by tearing the second edge counterclockwise until it connects with the first arm. There are several different variations of this theme, but the important concept is that if the primary capsulorrhexis flap becomes too difficult to see or control, a second contingency flap has can be created (Figure 44-4).

PERIPHERAL EXTENSION

The frequency with which a radial tear in the capsulorrhexis occurs is usually related to the surgeon's experience. However, certain conditions predispose to this event. Anterior bowing of the lens-iris diaphragm will encourage peripheral extension. This condition is more common in patients with shallow anterior

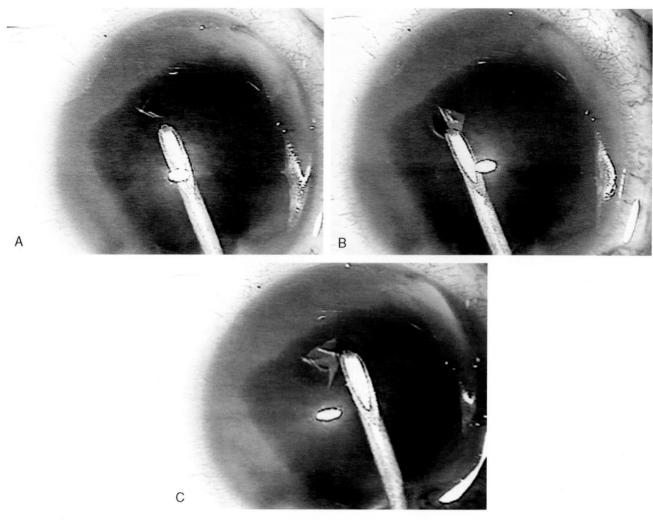

A

B

C

Figure 44-4 Operating microscope view of an eye with aniridia. Trypan blue has been applied to the anterior capsule. **A,** Capsulorrhexis is initiated with a bent 22-gauge needle. **B,** The 22-gauge needle is used to reverse the direction of the lower arm of the capsular tear. **C,** Using the upper arm, the remainder of the capsulorrhexis proceeds normally. However, should the surgeon encounter a problem with the capsulorrhexis, it can be restarted easily in the opposite direction.

chambers and in those with positive intralenticular pressure, such as with a white intumescent cataract. Extension can be caused by excessive convex curvature of the anterior lens capsule that can be conceptualized as a "hill." If the capsular tear runs over the "edge of the hill," it will continue to pursue a "downhill" course, despite attempts to redirect it (Figure 44-5).

In young patients, the leading edge of the anterior capsular tear also has a tendency to run peripherally. This may be due to the elastic forces of the zonulocapsular apparatus, a higher endolenticular pressure, and anterior chamber shallowing associated with lower scleral rigidity. The widely dilated pupil of a young patient may also lend itself to a larger capsulectomy, and if the zonular insertions are encountered, the tear will have a strong tendency to follow the radial course of the zonule, rather than the desired circumferential course. This can also happen when the capsular tear encounters proximal zonules.[24]

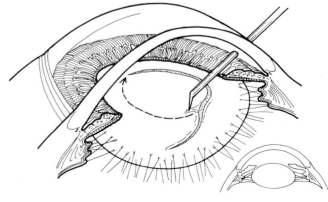

Figure 44-5 Shallowing of the anterior chamber causes the capsule tear to run peripherally "downhill," instead of following the intended course (broken line).

The capsular flap is also more difficult to control in the presence of weak zonules, such as in patients with pseudoexfoliation. As one pulls on the capsular flap, the peripheral capsule is normally immobilized by the zonules. However, with weakened zonules, the peripheral capsule moves along with the flap, until it suddenly wants to slingshot radially outward. Chang has called this phenomenon "pseudoelasticity," in that the loss of flap control is similar to that encountered when tearing an elastic material, such as latex.[25]

This behavior is also seen with elastic capsules in pediatric eyes, but in the case of weakened zonules, it is due to excessive mobility of the peripheral capsule, rather than true capsular elasticity.

Finally, the capsular flap will tend to veer radially with hyperexpansion of the anterior chamber, as can occur in vitrectomized eyes, and in eyes with extreme axial myopia. With severe retropulsion of the entire lens-iris diaphragm, there is significant zonular traction exerted on the peripheral anterior capsule. These forces are directed anteriorly and peripherally, and will tend to pull the flap radially. In these situations, some OVD should be removed so that the anterior chamber is not overinflated, and the lens-iris diaphragm is not displaced posteriorly.

Whenever there is difficulty in controlling the advancing capsulorrhexis flap, a conscious effort is made to create a slightly smaller diameter opening. This both improves control of the flap, and affords enough space to redirect the flap if necessary. The capsulorrhexis diameter should not be so small as to compromise nuclear manipulation or subincisional cortical aspiration. Moreover, it is helpful to flatten the anterior capsular convexity with a generous amount of OVD in eyes with shallow anterior chambers, or whenever difficulty in controlling the capsulorrhexis tear is encountered. If the OVD is extruded, refilling the chamber may be required; alternatively, selecting a more retentive OVD, such as Healon 5, may be tried. It may be helpful to attach a bent needle or cystotome to the OVD syringe to direct the tear, thereby reducing the tendency for the OVD to escape when capsule forceps are manipulated through the incision. Once the chamber deepens, the capsulorrhexis will be easier to guide in the desired direction (Figure 44-6).

When redirecting the tear, it is helpful to "unfold" the anterior capsule back to its original position and then pull the tear towards the center of the pupil, with some mild posteriorly directed force.[22]

Once the tear begins to move more centrally, one can flip the capsule back onto itself in order to proceed.

Occasionally, even in experienced hands, the anterior capsular tear will extend too far peripherally to allow redirection. Persistent heroic attempts to pull the flap centrally may extend the tear around the equator and into the posterior capsule. An experienced surgeon may recognize when the tear is too peripheral by the "feel" of resistance to his or her efforts to redirect the tear. The surgeon should return to the starting point and proceed with a second continuous tear using the "safety" capsulorrhexis strategy or switch to a can-opener technique until the capsulectomy is completed (Figure 44-7).

If the anterior capsule tear has extended too far peripherally to be salvaged, phacoemulsification should be performed with extreme care to minimize any forces directed toward the capsular bag. As a technique, phaco chop is preferable to divide and conquer for this reason. If possible, one should avoid rotating the nucleus, as this typically requires lateral displacement of the nucleus and imparts the greatest force to the torn capsulorrhexis rim. Reducing the irrigation–aspiration flow parameters slows the pace of phacoemulsification in order to avoid sudden fluctuations in chamber depth and excessive fluid movement through compromised zonules. Careful aspiration of cortex from the affected quadrant is performed only after the rest of the cortex has been removed. With a single radial capsulorrhexis tear, a single-piece hydrophobic acrylic IOL with soft haptics would exert the least amount of capsular force during implantation. If a three-piece IOL with stiff haptics is used, consider unfolding the lead haptic in the anterior chamber. This allows one to dial the two haptics into the bag in such a way that the optic is never displaced toward the weakened capsulorrhexis tear. The haptics should be left oriented 90° away from the area of the capsulorrhexis tear. Alternatively, a posterior chamber IOL can be placed in the ciliary sulcus, with or without suture fixation. Iris fixation or an anterior chamber angle-supported IOL are also alternative options.

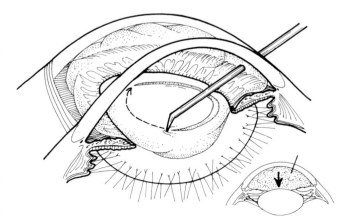

Figure 44-6 Deepening the anterior chamber with viscoelastic allows the capsule to tear along the desired course (broken line).

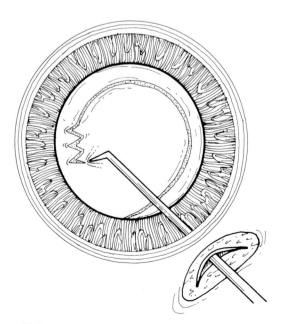

Figure 44-7 Conversion of a capsulorrhexis that ran peripherally into a can-opener capsulotomy.

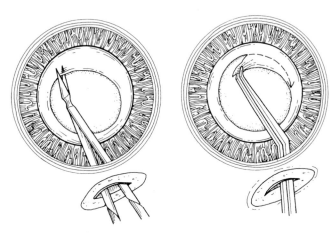

Figure 44-8 Enlargement of the capsulorrhexis. **A**, Capsular edge is incised with intraocular scissors to create a small flap. **B**, Flap is grasped with forceps, and the new tear is directed to rejoin the capsulorrhexis (broken line). This technique may be used to enlarge the capsular opening or to excise a capsular notch and provide a new continuous capsular edge.

In cases in which the capsulorrhexis edge finishes inside the starting point creating a "notch" in the anterior capsule, the surgeon should have a management plan. A fine intraocular scissors can be used to make an angulated cut lateral to the notch. Intraocular forceps are used to grasp the resulting flap and enlarge the capsulorrhexis to create a smooth, continuous tear peripheral to the notch (Figure 44-8A depicts a similar maneuver for enlarging the capsular opening). If the notch is proximal, the surgeon may either use a reverse cutting scissors (Figure 44-9) to create a flap or a micro-incision blade to button-hole the capsule. After creating the button hole, one blade of a long Vannas scissors is introduced into the hole and a snip is made, creating a flap as the button hole is connected to the edge of the capsulorrhexis. The flap is grasped, and the capsulorrhexis is enlarged, thereby excising the notch and replacing it with a continuous edge.

SMALL CAPSULECTOMY

Although too large a capsulorrhexis may lead to peripheral extension, too small a diameter makes the removal of the nucleus and cortex more difficult. A small anterior capsular opening will particularly frustrate surgeons who favor a nucleus tipping or prolapsing technique. Either grooving and then dividing the nucleus within the capsular bag or simply chopping the nucleus into fragments will achieve nuclear disassembly in the face of a small-diameter capsulorrhexis.

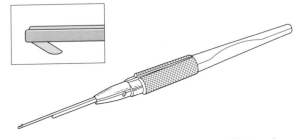

Figure 44-9 Osher reverse cutting scissors, courtesy of Duckworth & Kent: #1-620

A small capsulectomy also complicates sub-incisional cortical aspiration. In some cases it may be necessary to orient the irrigation–aspiration tip so that it is nearly vertical while rotating the eye to reach the subincisional cortex. We believe that it is easier and safer to initiate cortex removal in the subincisional quadrant because the capsular bag will be held partially open by the remainder of the cortex. Surgeons should be prepared to use alternative instrumentation, such as an angled coaxial irrigation–aspiration tip, bimanual irrigation–aspiration handpieces, or a curved aspirating cannula introduced through either the main incision or a side port incision. A small capsulectomy also increases the risk of "capsular block syndrome."[26,27]

In this intraoperative or postoperative syndrome, the capsulorrhexis forms a tight seal against the anterior IOL surface. In the intraoperative form, fluid may become trapped behind the nucleus raising the pressure enough to blow out the posterior capsule. In the postoperative form, OVD is trapped behind the optic and an osmotic gradient can further expand this retrolenticular space. The anterior displacement of the optic will cause an unintended myopic shift, and can result in shallowing of the anterior chamber. A laser capsulotomy, preferably in the anterior capsule peripheral to the edge of the optic, will break the capsulo-lenticular block, allowing this trapped material to escape.

An excessively small capsulorrhexis also predisposes an eye with weakened zonules to the capsulophimosis syndrome. This is characterized by marked contraction of the anterior capsular opening with a severely fibrotic thickening of the capsulorrhexis edge. In severe cases, capsulophimosis syndrome can result in progressive zonular disinsertion and a decentered IOL requiring surgical intervention.[28–31]

To enlarge a small diameter capsulectomy, an intraocular scissors can be used to create an oblique tear in the edge that is angled away from the surgeon, which can be grasped and re-torn with the capsule forceps (Figure 44-8).

This maneuver is safest when performed under the protection of a viscoelastic agent and after the IOL has been implanted. The sub-incisional edge of the anterior capsule is the most difficult to enlarge and requires a reverse cutting scissors or a button-hole slit as described above.

■ THE WHITE CATARACT ■

Historically, the white cataract has been a leading cause of torn capsulorrhexes. While the hard white cataract in the fluid-filled Morgagnian cataract can be challenging, it is the intumescent lens with "swollen" cortex that is most dangerous. Besides the fact that it results in the surgeon's inability to visualize the capsulorrhexis edge because of the absence of a red reflex, elevated endocapsular pressure due to cortical liquefaction also tends to extend the tear radially. Horiguchi and co-workers pioneered the concept of anterior capsular staining, which has become invaluable in visualizing the rhexis edge.[32–39] Osher developed the following three-step method to avoid using an air bubble in the anterior chamber as advocated by other groups.[40]

After Healon 5 is injected into the anterior chamber, a gentle stream of BSS is instilled along the surface of the anterior capsule. This creates a wafer-thin fluid layer separating the anterior capsule from the elevated mass of Healon 5. Finally, indocyanine green (ICG) or trypan blue dye is injected directly into this space, "painting" the intended rhexis size onto the anterior capsule. A special

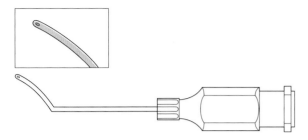

Figure 44-10 Osher Capsular Dye Cannula, Courtesy of Duckworth & Kent: #MMP203.

cannula (Figure 44-10) with the hole directed posteriorly has been designed to minimize the risk of the injected stream going peripherally through the zonules. This technique protects the corneal endothelium, avoids accumulation of dye within the viscoelastic material, and results in superior staining and visualization of the anterior capsule. Other surgeons inject Trypan blue directly into the anterior chamber for about 20 s before lavaging it out with BSS. Trypan blue results in a more intense and persistent staining of the capsule than ICG. With an intumescent white lens, the high intralenticular pressure may violently expand the initial anterior capsular puncture or tear out to the periphery in both directions. Because the resulting large capsular gap appears as a white stripe separating the two trypan blue-stained halves of the anterior capsule, this clinical picture has been called the Argentenian Flag Sign.[41] A tip-off to this possibility is the presence of a swollen anterior cortex and an anterior–posterior measurement of >6 mm by ultrasound biomicroscopy.[42] The judicious use of retentive OVD, capsular staining, central decompression of the lens, a small capsulorrhexis (which can be enlarged), and posterior voiding (balloting) to release posterior cortical pressure will allow the surgeon to minimise risks in these challenging cataracts.

■ CONGENITAL ANIRIDIA ■

The surgeon should be aware of the extreme fragility of the anterior capsule in some patients with congenital aniridia, as initially identified by Osher.[43] Histopathologic analysis with scanning electron microscopy has demonstrated that the fragile anterior capsules are remarkably thin (Figure 44-11).

■ PHACOEMULSIFICATION ■

A variety of complications can occur during phacoemulsification, many of which are discussed in the following paragraphs.

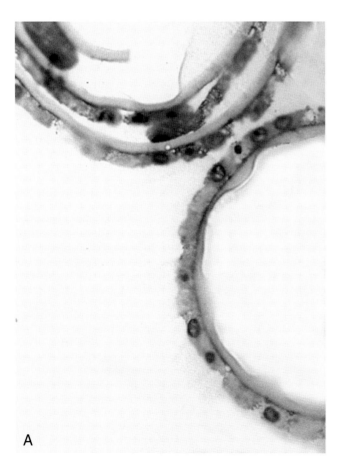

A

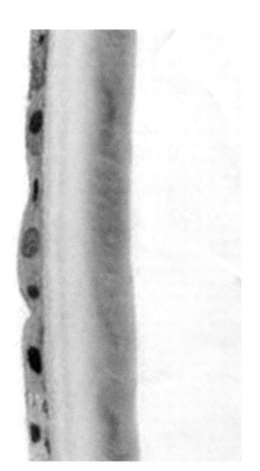

B

Figure 44-11 A, Anterior capsule from a patient with congenital aniridia. Note the thin anterior capsule and curling nature, as compared to **B,** the anterior capsule from a patient without aniridia.

PROBLEMATIC INSERTION OF THE PHACOEMULSIFICATION TIP

Careless insertion of the phacoemulsification tip can tear Descemet's membrane, chafe the iris stroma, and even cause an iridodialysis. These complications are more likely to occur in eyes with shallow chambers in which there is less space between the iris and the cornea. If the incision is constructed properly and the instruments are carefully angled toward the pupil, these complications can be avoided. To better avoid impaling the iris, introduce the phacoemulsification tip bevel down and then rotate the bevel after the tip is safely through the incision.

If iris has prolapsed through the incision before or during insertion of the phaco tip, it should be repositioned using the techniques described earlier. Injecting some OVD over the reposited iris will restrain it, unless the OVD is washed out as soon as the irrigating phaco tip is re-inserted. In such a case, insert the phaco tip dry, and commence irrigation only after the tip and irrigation openings are well inside the anterior chamber.

EXCESSIVE GLOBE MOVEMENT

Improper manipulation of the phacoemulsification handpiece can lead to excessive globe movement. An incision that is too tight or has a longer tunnel makes unwanted globe movement more likely and, occasionally, the incision may need to be slightly enlarged. Flaring the blade inside the incision to create a slightly wider internal opening may suffice. The incision site must always act as a fulcrum for the handpiece. Better instrument access to the incision is one significant advantage of locating it temporally instead of superiorly.

CROWDED ANTERIOR CHAMBER

The presence of a shallow anterior chamber makes phacoemulsification extremely difficult. Descemet's membrane detachments and difficulty reaching the subincisional cortex are more likely to occur as the surgeon tends to direct the incision more anteriorly to avoid the iris. As described earlier, whenever the lens-iris diaphragm is relatively forward, peripheral extensions are more likely to occur during the capsulorrhexis. In addition, iris prolapse and damage to both the iris and corneal endothelium may occur during insertion of the phacoemulsification needle. Spontaneous prolapse of the nucleus can be minimized by carefully sizing the capsulorrhexis and avoiding excessive hydrodissection in these cases. The use of a higher-viscosity OVD will often help to maintain a deeper anterior chamber. The risk of endothelial cell loss is greater during phacoemulsification in these eyes because the turbulence at the phaco tip is occurring at a much closer proximity to the cornea. Fortunately, the anterior chamber will usually deepen significantly on completion of the emulsification.

HYPER-DEEP ANTERIOR CHAMBER

During the phacoemulsification or irrigation–aspiration steps, an unusual deepening of the chamber with pupil widening and posterior displacement of the iris border can occur as a sign of lens iris diaphragm retropulsion syndrome (LIDRS). LIDRS occurs as a result of reverse pupillary block where contact between the iris and the residual anterior capsular rim seals the anterior chamber from the posterior chamber and allows hydrostatic pressure to markedly deepen the anterior segment. LIDRS is managed by either elevating the iris or depressing the anterior capsule with any instrument.[44]

CHAMBER SHALLOWING DURING PHACOEMULSIFICATION

When sudden chamber collapse occurs, there is a risk of damage to the cornea, iris or posterior capsule. Repeated episodes with corneal folding alone may damage corneal endothelial cells and lead to increased postoperative corneal edema. There are several potential causes of anterior chamber collapse.

INSUFFICIENT INFLOW

The amount of irrigation inflow must be enough to maintain the depth of the anterior chamber when an occlusion is cleared. Although excessive irrigation can be traumatic to the corneal endothelium, insufficient infusion that results in chamber instability is more dangerous. Chamber collapse from inadvertent disconnection of the inflow line from the phaco handpiece is particularly hazardous. Besides inadequate bottle height, other causes of insufficient inflow include air block, clogged or kinked irrigation tubing, too tight an incision, or withdrawing the irrigation sleeve port within the incision. Finally, the anterior chamber may shallow if the surgeon is so preoccupied with intraocular maneuvering that he or she accidentally comes off of the foot switch. Continuous irrigation, an idea separately introduced by Osher and Crozafon, may be helpful in preventing chamber collapse.

EXCESSIVE OUTFLOW

Poor chamber stability due to excessive fluid egress will occur if the incision is too large, or is gaped by instrumentation. For example, there is a tendency to lift the phaco tip with deep set eyes or a prominent brow, if one is operating from the superior approach. Tightening a large incision with a suture, or switching to a new incision site should be considered.

The most common cause of chamber shallowing is improper balancing of phaco machine fluidic parameters. Post-occlusion surge describes a momentary chamber shallowing that occurs as soon as an occluded phaco tip clears. Because vacuum levels build within the aspirating line following tip occlusion, fluid will rush in through the phaco tip opening to equalize the vacuum gradient as soon as the occlusion clears. Higher aspiration flow and vacuum rates increase the rate and amount of this unwanted fluid surge. Osher has advocated a slow-motion phacoemulsification technique using a lower aspiration rate, vacuum, and bottle height, which results in a more stable chamber.[45,46]

To allow surgeons the option of safely using higher aspiration flow and vacuum settings, a number of phacodynamic strategies have been designed by the equipment manufacturers. These include the use of smaller lumen phaco tips and stiffer walled aspiration tubing to reduce the compliance, coiled aspiration tubing, and flow restrictors, such as Staar Surgical's Cruise Control. Some manufacturers have added auxiliary irrigation bottles to the machine, or increased the irrigation tubing diameter. Finally, smart pumps with on-board computer sensing can decelerate or reverse speed as the maximum vacuum preset level is approached.

Once the equipment has been optimized, the options for reducing post-occlusion surge are to either raise the irrigation bottle, or decrease the aspiration flow rate or vacuum limit. These measures should be considered during those parts of the procedure where the posterior capsule is directly exposed to the phaco tip or for certain higher risk cases, such as with weak zonules where a lax posterior capsule is more likely to trampoline forward.

INTERNAL CONDITIONS

Any increase in fluid volume within the vitreous cavity may shallow the chamber. Expansion of the blood volume in the choroidal space could be due to a coughing episode or a hemorrhage. A choroidal effusion or zonular compromise leading to fluid misdirection syndrome will also shallow the chamber. These conditions will be covered in more detail later in this chapter.

POSITIVE PRESSURE

The presence of positive pressure increases the difficulty and risk of phacoemulsification. The chamber will tend to become shallow, and iris prolapse and progressive miosis are more likely. The nucleus may spontaneously prolapse forward, and it may be difficult to reposition, forcing the surgeon to perform the emulsification in the anterior chamber. The posterior capsule may bulge forward, which makes it more prone to rupture. Moreover, the capsular bag cannot fully expand, making cortical aspiration and IOL placement more challenging. If positive pressure is encountered, the surgeon must take all steps necessary to identify the cause and, if possible, to correct it.[47]

CAUSES OF POSITIVE PRESSURE

External compression of the globe is a common cause of positive pressure that is often preventable or easily resolved. An excessive volume of retrobulbar or peribulbar anesthetic injection, particularly in a small orbit, can cause globe compression. A poorly designed lid speculum, or one that is improperly placed, can result in positive pressure. However, one that is designed to lift the lids off the globe may not only avoid positive pressure in routine cases but also prevent it in patients with tight lids.

Tight lids associated with narrow palpebral fissures act to tether the globe, leading to positive pressure. Several clues indicate excessive lid pressure. When the eyelids are opened for insertion of the speculum, the surgeon may observe narrowed fissures with little visible sclera, or a blunted lateral canthal angle may be restricting the width of the fissure. Taut lids will also tend to snap closed when opened. Another sign of potential lid pressure is indentation of the conjunctiva by either the lid margin or the speculum. Blepharospasm can cause positive pressure, and can even expel the lid speculum.

After the speculum has been inserted and adequate anesthesia has been obtained, it may occasionally be necessary to perform a lateral canthotomy. A hemostat is used to clamp a few millimeters of the lateral canthal angle for 1 or 2 min. After releasing the hemostat, a horizontal incision is made with scissors through the canthus, and little if any bleeding results.

With temporal incisions, traction sutures are rarely needed any more. Excessive traction from a fixation suture may increase the intraocular pressure by either excessive downward rotation of the globe or actually lifting the globe from the orbit. Therefore, if a traction suture is used, the minimal force required to maintain the globe in its primary position is desirable. One should loosen the suture prior to phacoemulsification when it is not needed to position the globe.

Several specific circumstances that originate within the eye may cause positive pressure. If the posterior capsule has been ruptured or there is a defect in the zonules, posterior misdirection of irrigation fluid may expand the vitreous gel, resulting in anterior displacement of the capsule and iris. Although difficult to recognize, infusion inflow must be reduced to avoid worsening the situation. Air may also shallow the anterior chamber if it gets behind the iris and produces pupillary block. Scleral collapse and indentation can result in chamber shallowing, especially in eyes of young patients with poor scleral rigidity, in eyes that have undergone previous vitrectomy, or in eyes that have been "oversoftened." Choroidal hemorrhage or effusion can cause positive pressure and will often shallow or flatten the anterior chamber. The nanophthalmic eye with a thickened sclera often has positive pressure and may be associated with choroidal effusions.

Another cause of positive pressure is body habitus. When lying flat, obese patients have increased venous stasis in their head, and an increase in orbital venous volume will cause external pressure on their globes. Elevating the head and chest of the patient with slight reverse Trendelenburg positioning can significantly lessen the orbital venous pressure in these patients.

Any condition leading to a Valsalva maneuver may obstruct venous return, elevating orbital and intraocular pressure. Straining with a full bladder, coughing, discomfort, or anxiety must be recognized and managed appropriately before continuing with surgery.

If one must continue with phacoemulsification in the presence of positive pressure, several maneuvers may decrease the risks of complications. Techniques for performing the capsulorrhexis and phacoemulsification in the face of a shallow chamber have already been described.[48]

Entering through a chamber filled with OVD and without infusion may avoid iris trauma. Excessive hydrodissection that might spontaneously prolapse the nucleus should be avoided. The aspiration fluidic parameters should be reduced, and it may be necessary to elevate the bottle. Briefer application of ultrasound pulses may increase safety. It may also be necessary to use a dull second instrument to either hold the nucleus posteriorly or to restrain a bulging posterior capsule while performing the emulsification in the safe zone immediately above it. Adjusting the handpiece angle within the incision may decrease a tendency toward scleral depression, gaping, or torquing of the incision. Although counterintuitive, intravenous hypertonic solutions may actually worsen scleral collapse, causing further chamber shallowing. The use of a more highly retentive OVD such as Healon 5 should aid in maintaining a deeper chamber. Excessive chamber collapse may occasionally require that the cortex be removed using a "dry" manual technique, during which the bag is inflated by OVD rather than irrigation fluid. Intraoperative hydration of the incision may tighten it enough to reduce any incisional leakage.

Rarely, IOL implantation will be prevented by persistent positive pressure despite the use of a retentive OVD. Under these circumstances, the surgeon should be familiar with several emergency maneuvers. First, if the IOL can be introduced into the anterior chamber under viscoelastic protection with adequate corneal clearance, then it can be rotated into the capsular bag within a "closed" system by working through the side port incision(s). This better avoids egress of the OVD, which must eventually be removed and exchanged for BSS or miotic in small aliquots through the side port incision.

If the chamber shallowing is progressive and the surgeon suspects a suprachoroidal hemorrhage, rapid closure of the eye is followed by either indirect ophthalmoscopy or viewing the posterior segment by an Osher pan fundus surgical lens (Ocular Instruments). The management of this severe complication is discussed later in this chapter. However, the incision should be carefully sutured and the procedure should be aborted.

If there is no evidence of a choroidal hemorrhage or effusion, the surgeon can consider either aspirating fluid vitreous using a 25-gauge needle or performing a vitreous tap under direct visualization. This should be done by inserting a vitrectomy tip without any infusion sleeve through a pars plana sclerotomy that is located 3.5 mm behind the limbus. The vitrectomy tip (cutting tip aimed posteriorly) is visualized through the pupil, and as soon as a small amount of vitreous is removed, additional OVD is injected into the AC through a paracentesis.[49] The chamber should deepen to allow the procedure to continue under safer conditions. Because vitreous aspiration increases the risk of hemorrhage, as well as retinal tear or detachment, this maneuver should be used only when clearly necessary.

THERMAL BURN

Regardless of whether a piezoelectric crystal or a magnetostrictive design is operative, the phacoemulsification transducer converts energy into acoustic waves, moving the hollow titanium tip longitudinally back and forth at excursions of approximately 100 μm at a specified frequency. Controversy exists as to whether emulsification of the nucleus occurs because of cavitation or the jackhammer effect of the tip.[50] Friction within the incision causes heat, which is conducted along the titanium phaco needle. The internal and external flow of irrigation–aspiration fluid cools the needle and protects the incision from heat damage. More recently, an oscillatory tip which produces less heat and repulsion of nuclear material has been introduced by Alcon and adds safety to the temperature profile. All current machines allow modifications of the duty cycle permitting "off time" for tip cooling.

If for any reason this internal and external flow of cooling fluid stops, thermal damage can occur within 1–3 s.[51] Loss of inflow of fluid will occur if the tubing becomes kinked or disconnected. Fluid outflow will halt if the tubing becomes occluded. The latter is more likely with a dispersive OVD and a brunescent nucleus, which when admixed together may result in a thicker emulsate. A highly retentive OVD in a low vacuum setting may also result in an obstruction. If there is suddenly no fluid outflow and the incision is snug, gravity fed inflow will also cease. A thermal incision burn will result as soon as continuous mode ultrasound commences. There are several warning signs of clogged aspiration tubing. Partial occlusion might cause reduced followability, resulting in the need to chase nuclear fragments within the anterior chamber. Seeing whitish "smoke" or lens "milk" in front of the tip indicates total tip occlusion. Recognizing this, ultrasound must immediately stop, and the cause must be rectified after the phaco tip is removed.

Several routine safeguards help to prevent thermal burns. As part of the phaco machine priming cycle, adequate irrigation inflow and aspiration outflow within the test chamber are checked. If the anterior chamber has been filled with OVD, one should habitually aspirate a small amount just above the central anterior nuclear surface prior to commencing phacoemulsification. This is particularly important with a brunescent cataract and with a highly retentive OVD. Alternatively, space can be created by initially sculpting a divot in the anterior cortex using bevel-down higher vacuum to prevent occlusion while leaving OVD undisturbed in the anterior chamber. The incision width and tunnel length must not be such that the irrigation tubing is pinched off. Although cooling the BSS and using pulsed ultrasound have been advocated by some surgeons, others prefer an ultrasound needle designed to maintain fluid either through an inner metal sleeve (MacKool), through metallic grooves (Barrett), or using an aspiration bypass hole (Alcon). Finally, power modulation with variable duty cycle results in a hyperpulse mode that significantly reduces heat generation during the ultrasound function. Bimanual microincisional phaco using a bare phaco needle through tight incisions is made possible because of this technology.[52–54]

Should a thermal burn occur, the surgeon must select a suturing technique to properly close the incision, while minimizing iatrogenic astigmatism. A radial suture (gape stitch) passed through the anterior lip and then through the floor, but avoiding the distal lip or a horizontal suture (Osher stitch), bringing together the posterior roof and the anterior floor can serve this purpose.[10,11,16] A typical thermal burn is illustrated in Figure 44-12.

IRIS TRAUMA

Damage to the iris during phacoemulsification can be caused by either iris prolapse or direct injury from the phaco tip or other instruments. Iris prolapse or injury may cause intraoperative miosis, iris depigmentation, bleeding, tissue loss, and an atonic or distorted pupil. Any trauma to the iris whether by contact with

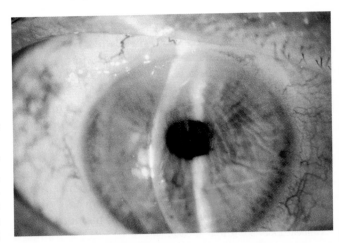

Figure 44-12 Slit-lamp photograph of a thermal burn from phacoemulsification. Note the marked edema and opacification of the superior stroma. Striae extend from the burn in a radial pattern because of heat-induced contraction of the collagen. (Courtesy of Roger F. Steinert, MD.)

instruments, sharp nuclear fragments, or even the IOL will increase prostaglandin release, leading to intraoperative miosis, and postoperative inflammation with cystoid macular edema (CME). Intraoperative miosis is also stimulated by sudden and dramatic fluctuations in the pupil diameter such as with repeated chamber collapse or the abrupt onset and reversal of pupillary block that characterizes LIDRS. Preoperative topical nonsteroidal anti-inflammatory agents, adequate topical cycloplegia, and intracameral alpha agonists such as phenylephrine, or epinephrine will help to maintain pupillary dilation.[55] Bisulfite-free 1:1000 epinephrine can be added to the BSS bottle, or can be directly injected into the anterior chamber. However, because of its acidic pH epinephrine should be diluted 1:3 or 1:4 with BSS or BSS Plus prior to direct intracameral injection.[56] Epi Shugarcaine is a more concentrated combination of epinephrine, lidocaine and BSS which can be used as an intracameral injection in IFIS.[56A]

Direct trauma to the iris from the phacoemulsification tip can be prevented in most cases. Iris trauma is more likely with crowded anterior chambers, with small pupils, and with IFIS. Techniques for inserting the handpiece using an OVD to decrease iris chafing have already been presented. Working centrally in the deepest part of the anterior chamber is preferable. By using low aspiration flow rates during phacoemulsification, events occur more slowly, and inadvertent aspiration of the iris is much less likely. Several small pupil phacoemulsification techniques are very effective,[57] and the surgeon should be experienced in using these techniques. Healon 5 is also effective in achieving viscomydriasis. Radial iridotomy, multiple sphincterotomies, Frye sphincter stretching, the use of iris retracting hooks, and mechanical pupil expansion devices such as the Malyugin ring are all options for managing the small or constricting pupil.[58–67]

Once the iris has been injured, it will often become frayed and flaccid. It may be necessary to use a second instrument as a retractor to prevent repeated prolapse or aspiration of the iris in this situation. Often overlooked is the damage to the iris caused by contact with the exposed metal of the titanium tip that extends beyond the silicone sleeve. For this reason, it is best to minimize the metal exposure when performing phacoemulsification in an eye with a small pupil.

POSTERIOR CAPSULE TEARS

The torn posterior capsule is probably the most frequent of the significant complications encountered by the surgeon learning phacoemulsification, and it continues to occur, albeit rarely, in even the expert's hands. Posterior capsule rupture with vitreous loss increases the risk of endophthalmitis, IOL malposition, cystoid macular edema and retinal detachment.[68] In many instances, posterior capsule rupture can be prevented. However, if a tear does occur, proper management will usually allow a successful procedure with secure placement of a posterior chamber IOL.[69]

PREVENTION

Fortunately, the incidence of posterior capsule rupture decreases with increasing surgical experience. The most challenging posterior capsule tears occur during phacoemulsification because of the presence of residual nucleus and cortex. Several general surgical principles are important for reducing the frequency of this complication.

Besides its advantages for IOL fixation, the continuous curvilinear capsulorrhexis has been a significant advance in the prevention of posterior capsular rupture. The smooth, continuous edge acts like an elastic waistband, by stretching rather than tearing, and this allows the capsular bag to better withstand certain stretching and deforming forces. Proper fluidic settings and stability of the anterior chamber depth are also important in lowering the risk of this complication. Inflow and outflow must be appropriately balanced so as to avoid post-occlusion surge and forward trampolining of the posterior capsule.

Special instrument modifications have also been introduced with the goal of reducing the incidence of this complication. The Dewey radius tip (MST) rounds off the sharp edge of the phaco needle tip. Without any significant impact upon cutting ability, this tip modification provides a safety margin of error should the capsule be aspirated or hit with the phaco needle. The Alcon soft silicone irrigation–aspiration tip provides superior capsular protection compared to traditional metallic tip designs which may have irregular, sharp burrs within the lumen of the aspiration hole capable of snagging and tearing the capsule.

A variety of phaco techniques have been conceived with the universal goal of maximizing capsular safety. Slow-motion phacoemulsification,[70] the use of low-vacuum and low-aspiration parameters, will reduce the tendency toward surge and the chance of the phaco needle piercing through the nucleus and rupturing the posterior capsule.[46] Supracapsular techniques such as phaco flip eliminate the need to perform nuclear emulsification in the proximity of the posterior capsule. Nucleofractis techniques, such as divide and conquer and phaco chop, fragment the nucleus so that manageable pieces can be elevated and then emulsified in the safe supracapsular zone.[69] Phaco chop utilizes mechanical forces to divide the nucleus so that less force is applied to the zonules and capsular bag, as compared to sculpting.[71]

The posterior capsule is most vulnerable as the last remaining nuclear fragments are removed. Without the bulk of nucleus material there to restrain it, the exposed posterior capsule can vault toward the phaco needle with either positive pressure or the slightest bit of post-occlusion surge. In addition to reducing the vacuum and flow settings for this stage of the case, a second instrument may be placed behind the remaining nucleus to guard the posterior capsule. This should keep the capsule from trampolining toward the phaco tip as the occlusion is broken. We recommend dull-fingered instruments, which function as a nucleus manipulator or chopper for this purpose, since any sharp tip can inadvertently puncture the capsule.[72]

Certain types of cataracts increase the risk for posterior capsule rupture. The brunescent nucleus is not only firmer, but also larger in its horizontal and vertical dimensions. Because of this, instrument forces and maneuvers, such as sculpting, cracking, and rotation, are directly transmitted to the capsular bag. In addition, the soft epinucleus is often absent, which brings the phaco tip potentially into much closer proximity to the capsule. In the routine cataract, the epinucleus not only acts as a soft cushion-like shock absorber during sculpting, but also fills the capsular bag enough to prevent collapse (with trampolining of the posterior capsule) as the final mobile fragments are removed. The surgeon should avoid vigorous hydrodissection initially to prevent excessive nuclear mobility during sculpting. Too much fluid injected around the lens may push the nucleus forward against the anterior capsular rim creating an intraoperative capsular block syndrome with a blown-out posterior capsule.[27]

After the central nucleus is debulked and a very deep groove is made, additional hydrodissection either under the anterior capsule or through a nuclear crack loosens the remaining peripheral shell from the capsule, which can be emulsified as it is rotated and chopped. Posterior connecting lamellae can be lifted with a second instrument, or with an injection of dispersive OVD, away from the posterior capsule, where the emulsification can be completed safely.

The young patient with a very soft cataract is also at greater risk for a torn posterior capsule because the second instrument or phacoemulsification tip may more abruptly penetrate the peripheral nucleus to strike or aspirate the capsule. Moreover, poor scleral rigidity results in more fluidic fluctuation of the anterior chamber depth, so lower phaco power, and more conservative fluidic parameters are recommended.

The posterior polar cataract and the cataract associated with posterior lenticonus or lentiglobus may be associated with a weakened or defective central posterior capsule.[73,74] Hydrodissection alone can rupture a thinned posterior capsule or widen any congenital capsular opening. Hydrodissection should, therefore, be partial or avoided in favor of careful hydrodelineation, and fluidic parameters should be reduced appropriately. It is best to assume that the posterior capsule is already open. Minimal nuclear manipulation in a closed system and the skillful use of viscoelastic material for dry cortical removal and tamponade of the tear, as well as converting a tear to a posterior capsulorrhexis, are helpful principles in managing the posterior polar cataract.[75-79]

Patients with congenital aniridia have anterior capsules that are extremely thin and fragile, and are much more likely to tear either into the zonule or around the equator through the posterior capsule.[80] Patients who have had a prior vitrectomy or iridocyclectomy are also at greater risk.

A morgagnian cataract is associated with a dramatic escape of liquefied cortex from the capsular bag when the initial puncture is made into the proximal anterior lens capsule. Careful aspiration of the liquefied cortex will prevent it from obstructing the surgeon's view for the rest of the procedure. As the intumescence is decompressed and the liquid cortex released, the capsular bag will collapse, bringing the anterior and posterior capsule leaflets closer to each other and placing the posterior capsule at risk for being torn during the anterior capsulectomy. Therefore, a viscoelastic agent should be injected through the initial puncture site to refill the capsular bag before proceeding with this challenging capsulorrhexis. The use of a capsular dye such as trypan blue or ICG is recommended for improved capsular visualization in any white cataract[32,33,36-39] (Figure 44-13).

MANAGEMENT

Knowledgeable and skillful management of a posterior capsule tear is essential to the successful outcome of the procedure. At whatever stage the tear is discovered, establishment of a semiclosed pressurized system is necessary. Allowing the anterior chamber to decompress and shallow will cause forward movement of the vitreous, rupture of the anterior hyaloid face, and likely extension of the tear.

If a tear is discovered during phacoemulsification, residual nuclear material may be removed by either continuing phacoemulsification or converting to a larger incision, manual,

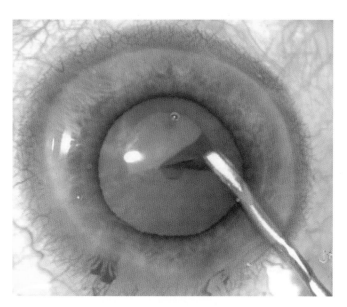

Figure 44-13 Operating microscope view of a Trypan Blue-assisted continuous capsulorrhexis in an eye with an opalescent cataract.

extracapsular technique. If most of the nucleus has already been emulsified and there is no vitreous in the anterior chamber, the surgeon may use the second instrument to maneuver the remaining nucleus away from the tear in order to complete the emulsification. Avoid excessive infusion pressure that could propel the nucleus posteriorly into the vitreous cavity, but do not lower the infusion bottle so much that the chamber is not kept inflated. The second instrument may be placed behind the nuclear fragment to prevent it from descending through a small rent. Use as little longitudinal ultrasound as possible to avoid repelling fragments away, therefore torsional ultrasound may be advantageous (see Chapter 20). Reduced irrigation and aspiration flow rates will effectively slow down surgical events within the eye. Whether or not the nucleus has been removed, the phacoemulsification handpiece should not be removed without simultaneously injecting OVD through the second stab site to prevent chamber shallowing and vitreous prolapse into the AC or to the incision. This is a critical maneuver and may be the deciding factor as to whether or not a vitrectomy must be performed. Because vitreous prolapse will expand any posterior capsular defect, this may also determine whether or not an IOL can be implanted into the capsular bag.

Adherence to several surgical principles should facilitate removal of the cortex without expanding the capsular tear. Consider using lower irrigation and aspiration flow rates to slow the surgical pace. Start by removing cortex in those quadrants that are furthest away from the tear. Cortex should be stripped toward the rent because any force directed away from it will cause its extension. Depending upon the location, it may be necessary to leave some cortex behind, rather than risk extending the tear. The anterior chamber must be kept expanded by an air or OVD injection prior to withdrawing the irrigation-aspiration handpiece. Bimanual irrigation–aspiration instrumentation allows the irrigation and aspiration currents to be dissociated. This permits the irrigation currents to be directed away from the capsular defect, even as nearby cortex is aspirated.

An alternative method of cortical removal is manual aspiration using both a bent cannula and a J-shaped cannula while maintaining the anterior chamber depth with repeated OVD injections. This manual technique of "dry" aspiration of cortex is more time consuming but decreases the risk of extending the tear and precipitating vitreous loss.

If vitreous is aspirated at any point during the procedure, a low-flow bimanual vitrectomy should be performed. This is best accomplished by using an infusion cannula through a second stab site in combination with a separate automated vitrector, which is passed through the capsular tear to perform the anterior vitrectomy. The infusion must not be directed into the vitreous cavity because removing just the prolapsed anterior vitreous is preferable to a massive vitrectomy. An alternative technique is a "dry" (no infusion) vitrectomy that uses repeated OVD injections to maintain the anterior chamber while the vitrectomy is performed.[81] Recently, there has been a trend toward using a pars plana incision for the vitrectomy cutter. Although it carries the theoretical risk of vitreous hemorrhage, this technique avoids drawing more and more vitreous anteriorly into the AC. A new technique for staining the vitreous has been introduced by Burk and colleagues using Kenalog (triamcinolone acetonide), which results in a dramatically improved visibility of the vitreous.[82] A non preserved steroid preparation, Triesence (Alcon) has been approved for visualizing the vitreous.

FOUR SPECIAL MANEUVERS

There are several special techniques that can be utilized in order to continue surgery in the face of a posterior capsular tear (see Chapter 46).

If the nucleus has partially descended through a capsular defect onto the anterior hyaloid face, one must not chase it with the phaco tip. The posterior assisted levitation (PAL) technique popularized by Charles Kelman can be used to rescue the descending nucleus.[83–86] A pars plana sclerotomy is made 3.5 mm behind the limbus, and a spatula is used to maneuver behind the nucleus prior to levitating it forward. Alternatively, an OVD cannula can be used for this purpose. An advantage of the Viscoat PAL technique is that a dispersive OVD can be immediately injected behind the nucleus to buoy and support it prior to further manipulation.[87]

If a vitrectomy must be performed with lens material still present in the anterior chamber, Chang has described the Viscoat Trap technique for preventing posterior descent of the residual nucleus and cortex.[88] Any free floating lens material is elevated toward the cornea with dispersive OVD, which is then used to fill the anterior chamber. The bimanual anterior vitrectomy is then performed using a pars plana sclerotomy for the vitreous cutter. By keeping the cutter tip behind the pupillary plane, any prolapsing vitreous bands will be transsected, without aspirating the Viscoat layer. With the Viscoat Trap, the residual lens material remains supported by the OVD layer, rather than by the vitreous which is being removed.

Mark Michelson has described creating an artificial posterior capsule in order to continue phacoemulsification in the presence of a posterior capsular tear. After the residual nucleus is brought forward into the anterior chamber, a trimmed Sheets glide can be inserted behind it and over the capsular defect.[89] This supports

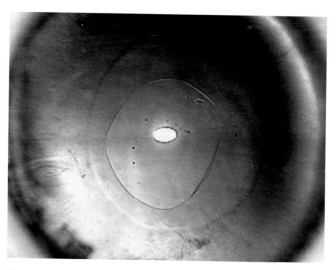

Figure 44-14 Operating microscope view of an ICG-assisted posterior capsulorrhexis in a cadaver eye. Note the light green staining of the capsular bag and the intact anterior capsular rim in the foreground.

the nucleus, and prevents vitreous from being aspirated by the phaco tip.[90]

Finally, the surgeon may be able to convert a small, central linear tear into a posterior capsulorrhexis, as popularized by Howard Gimbel.[91] In this maneuver the anterior hyaloid face is retroplaced with OVD, and a fine forceps is used to grasp and redirect the edge of the tear until a continuous edge is achieved.[92] If this is successfully accomplished, the capsular defect will not expand during IOL implantation into the bag (Figure 44-14).

INTRAOCULAR LENS PLACEMENT IN THE PRESENCE OF A CAPSULAR TEAR

The key to successful placement of an IOL in the presence of a posterior capsule tear is clear visualization and understanding of the compromised capsulozonular anatomy. After OVD placement, the iris is gently retracted with a collar-button instrument (Figure 44-15) to properly inspect the peripheral capsule. Based upon the amount and location of the residual capsule, the surgeon must decide upon the IOL design, and its optimal location and orientation.

A capsulorrhexis with a single radial anterior tear may permit the placement of a single-piece acrylic IOL. This IOL has a very small mass when injected and its haptics open slowly and gently so it is least likely to extend the tear posteriorly, especially when the capsular bag is filled with Healon 5. Furthermore, the lens can be rotated without placing excessive force on the equatorial capsule. Even when the lens has unfolded, the haptic is uniquely soft. Moreover, there is a rapid postoperative bioadhesive effect caused by fibronectin, which seals the IOL to the capsule. The IOL should be positioned so that the haptics are oriented 90° from the axis of the capsulorrhexis tear.

A posterior capsular tear – if converted into a posterior capsulorrhexis – will permit implantation of virtually any PC IOL into the capsular bag. However, in the absence of a posterior capsulorrhexis, placing any IOL into a capsular bag with a small PC rent risks the extension of the defect. This is particularly so for IOLs with stiff haptics because of the need to decenter the

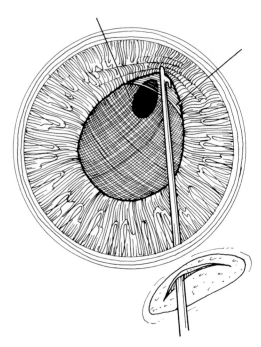

Figure 44-15 Retraction of the iris to visualize the extent of a posterior capsular tear.

optic when dialing it into place. If the posterior capsule tears when the lens is in the bag, the optic may be prolapsed and captured through either the anterior or a posterior capsular opening. It may also be possible to carefully implant a single-piece acrylic IOL into the bag despite the presence of a posterior capsule defect. The capsular bag must be well expanded with OVD if this is to be attempted, and decentering forces must be avoided during implantation. Beware, however, that single-piece acrylic IOLs are unsuitable for ciliary sulcus fixation; thus, if the capsular tear extends, the IOL cannot be moved into the ciliary sulcus and must instead be either captured or explanted.

Instead of using a single-piece acrylic IOL, if the capsulorrhexis is intact, placement of a three-piece IOL with C-loop haptics into the ciliary sulcus should be considered. A single-piece acrylic IOL should not be implanted into the ciliary sulcus because of the thicker haptics, the unfinished sharper edge to the haptics, and the shorter overall length. Most foldable IOLs have an overall length of 13 mm. The exception is the Staar silicone AQ2010 model, which is 13.5 mm in length. A longer overall diameter is more secure when ciliary sulcus fixation is intended. Particularly if the anterior segment is large, capsulorrhexis capture of the optic will prevent a sunset/sunrise postoperative subluxation due to insufficient overall IOL length. Because of the different effective lens position, the power of a posterior chamber IOL must be reduced by approximately 0.5 diopter, depending upon the power of the IOL when the optic is placed in the sulcus.[93–95]

Once the lens is centered within the ciliary sulcus, its fixation should be evaluated by slightly decentering the lens toward each haptic and releasing it to observe for spontaneous recentering (Osher Bounce Test). If it does not recenter itself, the haptic should be rotated to a different meridian.

In the absence of sufficient capsular support, the surgeon has the option to either implant an angle-supported anterior chamber

IOL, or to suture fixate a posterior chamber IOL. Therefore, if an IOL placed within the sulcus still shows signs of poor fixation and will not center itself, and the optic cannot be captured, it should be sutured to the iris or sclera. Alternately, the IOL can be removed and exchanged for an anterior chamber IOL, provided there are no relative contraindications, such as poorly controlled glaucoma, significant peripheral anterior synechiae, or iris tissue loss. If an anterior chamber lens is used, each haptic should always be flexed, lifted, and allowed to reseat itself in the angle to prevent inadvertent iris entrapment. Outside of the USA, a "claw" lens is another useful option that allows for IOL fixation to either the anterior or posterior surface of the iris stroma.[96] Recently, Agarwal has published the use of glue for fixation of a posterior chamber lens without capsular support.

Either air or OVD will establish a formed, pressurized chamber for precise incision closure and prevention of vitreous prolapse. Once the IOL is well centered and its stability has been confirmed, acetylcholine may be used to constrict the pupil. This makes it easier to identify vitreous prolapse and incarceration, while helping to prevent vitreous aspiration as the OVD is removed. OVD can be removed manually or with an irrigation–aspiration handpiece with low infusion. However, if the chamber collapses, there is a risk for further vitreous prolapse or loss of an optic capture. Therefore, the irrigation–aspiration tip should not simply be withdrawn from the incision. Air or BSS should be injected through the stab incision simultaneously with tip withdrawal to prevent momentary chamber collapse and late vitreous prolapse. Air can then be removed in small aliquots and exchanged for a BSS so that the anterior chamber depth is maintained.

Sweeping the pupil with a microhook is always recommended to ensure that there is no prolapsed vitreous remaining. If the posterior capsule was torn but a vitrectomy was not performed, a peripheral iridectomy should be considered as a prophylactic measure against vitreous-induced pupillary block.[97] Intracameral air has the advantage of allowing any vitreous to fall back while delineating transcameral vitreous strands by their interruption of the smooth round bubble observed in the anterior chamber. However, Kenalog staining is the best way to vizualize vitreous strands.[82]

Successful management of posterior capsule rupture and vitreous loss depends upon the surgeon's familiarity and experience with the various management techniques discussed in this chapter. One must mentally be prepared to make these decisions and perform these maneuvers, so that they become automatic amidst the stressful environment of an unplanned complication.

DROPPED NUCLEUS

Posterior dislocation of a partially emulsified nucleus into the vitreous cavity is a complication which is dreaded by every phacoemulsification surgeon. Excessive infusion, gross manipulation, ultrasound repulsion, vitreous syneresis, or forward displacement of the anterior vitreous will cause the nucleus to fall posteriorly.[98A]

As previously discussed, if the nucleus falls back into the mid-to-anterior vitreous, the Viscoat PAL technique may be performed as long as the nucleus can be visualized. If a nuclear piece can be brought forward, there are two options. It can be trapped by either a Sheets Glide, intracameral miotic or OVD followed by phacoemulsification in the anterior chamber, or it can be manually removed with a lens loop through an enlarged incision.[83-90] If the entire nucleus is intact, the surgeon may experience difficulty bringing it forward through the intact capsulorrhexis. The nucleus may require sectioning while the surgeon attempts to maintain the intact capsulorrhexis.

If the nucleus reaches the posterior vitreous or the retinal surface, it should be left alone. The surgeon should remove as much cortex as possible, performing an anterior vitrectomy through the phaco incision or through the pars plana as needed. The patient should be referred to a vitreoretinal specialist for a subsequent three-port pars plana lensectomy and vitrectomy. Heroic attempts to retrieve the nucleus should be avoided because excessive intravitreal maneuvers by an anterior segment surgeon carry a greater risk of retinal tear or detachment. Whether the cataract surgeon elects to implant an IOL before closing the eye or leaves this task to the vitreoretinal specialist must be considered on an individual basis. Optic capture has proven to be very helpful in this critical setting. Traditionally, if the nucleus was very brunescent, the IOL was not implanted initially because the nucleus had to be brought forward in the event that intravitreal fragmentation was not possible. However, newer vitrectomy machines are capable of emulsifying even the densest nucleus.

■ ZONULAR DIALYSIS ■

A preoperative zonular dialysis may be the result of pre-existing trauma or in association with specific disorders (i.e., Marfan syndrome, Weill-Marchesani syndrome). Warning signs include phacodonesis, iridodonesis, vitreous in the anterior chamber, or a visible defect in the zonular region. A slit view of the nucleus that appears off center or a "gap" between the iris border and the lens may provide subtle but important clues to this diagnosis.[98] Pseudoexfoliation is another condition that has a propensity for weakened zonules.

Surgical management of these challenging cases is beyond the scope of this chapter and is reviewed elsewhere.[99-110]

An intraoperative zonular dialysis may result from forceful maneuvers that disinsert the zonules in one region. The causes include a traumatic capsulectomy, excessive maneuvering of the nucleus, or aspiration of either the anterior, equatorial, or posterior capsule with the irrigation–aspiration tip. Prompt recognition and the avoidance of further zonular trauma are the best response. A highly retentive OVD such as Viscoat should be placed over the area of dialysis to restrain the vitreous from prolapsing. Similar principles for managing the torn posterior capsule apply in that all instrument forces should be directed toward rather than away from the quadrant of weakened zonules in order to avoid "unzipping" the adjacent intact zonules. Implantation of a capsule tension ring should be considered upon recognition of a zonular dialysis.

Capsulorrhexis, nuclear removal, and cortical removal may be very difficult when a loose capsular bag cannot provide countertraction. Stabilizing the capsular bag with Prolene iris or capsule retractors and even a capsular tension ring may be necessary for removing the nucleus and cortex in some patients. Cortical stripping may require frequent foot pedal reflux as the lax capsule is easily aspirated. Alternatively, dry cortical removal can be performed by expanding the capsular bag with either Healon5 or a dispersive OVD and then using a straight and a J-shaped cannula (Duckworth & Kent MMP220 MG). The cortex in the area of the zonular dialysis should be removed as the final step. It should not be stripped radially but rather tangential to the region of the dialysis (Figure 44-16). If cortex

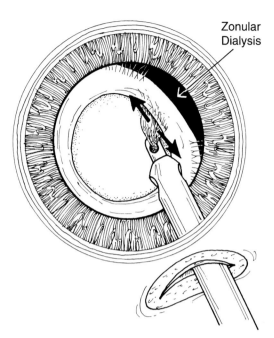

Figure 44-16 Cortical stripping in the presence of a zonular dialysis should always be done using gentle tangential movements (black arrows). Radial forces should be avoided to prevent enlarging the zonular dialysis.

adheres tightly to the capsule, viscodissection may facilitate separation. Excessive attempts to remove every last bit of cortex may not be worth the risk of disinserting more zonules. To prevent vitreous from prolapsing, the capsular bag should be expanded with OVD and chamber shallowing should be avoided.

If vitreous prolapses through the dialysis, either a low-infusion or dry bimanual anterior vitrectomy should be performed. A pars plana approach avoids continuously pulling more and more vitreous forward. Once the anterior segment is free of vitreous, an IOL can be implanted into the capsular bag as long as the anterior capsule ring is intact and the extent of the zonular dialysis is not greater than 4 clock hours. There is some debate regarding the optimal orientation of the IOL. We have placed it both parallel and perpendicular to the zonular dialysis (Figure 44-17A). Perpendicular haptic orientation (Figure 17B) may help resist postoperative capsular contracture that may cause the IOL to decenter. A larger, optic may be helpful if available because a slight decentration may occur as postoperative forces generated by the remaining intact zonules come into play. Silicone plate IOLs are not recommended.

If the zonular dialysis is severe, a posterior chamber IOL may be suture fixated to the sclera or iris as with other eyes without adequate capsular support. An excellent option with a severe zonular dialysis would be a CTR that is suture fixated in the area of the dialysis, as supported by numerous publications since 1993.[100-110] Cionni designed a modification with an eyelet on a hook that allows permanent suture fixation through the ciliary sulcus while the attached capsular tension ring is within the capsular bag (Figures 44-18).[110]

Ahmed has designed a capsule tension segment (CTS) while Assia has recently introduced a capsular anchor.[111,112] Only by reexpanding the loose bag, refixating it to the sclera, and implanting an IOL in the capsular bag is the patient with severe zonular dialysis optimally managed (Figure 44-19).

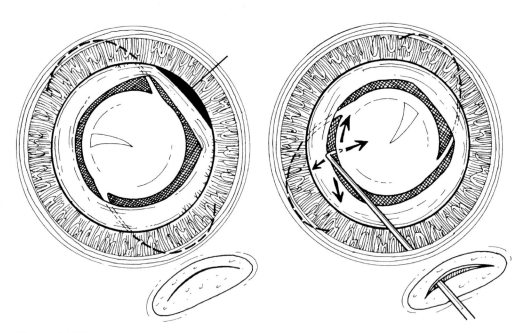

Figure 44-17 Orientation of the intraocular lens (IOL) parallel to (**A**) or perpendicular to (**B**) the zonular dialysis. The "bounce" test is performed with an IOL hook to determine stability (arrows).

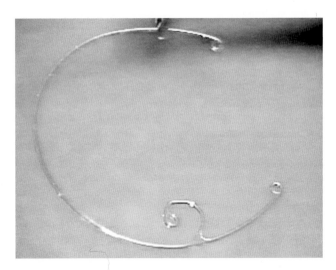

Figure 44-18 The Cionni modified endocapsular tension ring. The ring expands the capsular bag and has an eyelet for permanent fixation to the sclera.

VITREOUS LOSS

Whether related to a zonular dialysis or capsular tear, all anterior segment surgeons will occasionally encounter vitreous. While virtually invisible with the operating microscope, vitreous in the anterior segment makes surgery more difficult and is associated with many serious intraoperative and postoperative complications. Fortunately, meticulous vitreous clean-up can reduce the incidence of vision-threatening complications associated with vitreous loss.[113] Highlighting the difficulty of visualizing vitreous, a recent survey found that over 80% of ophthalmologists have completed surgery only to discover vitreous incarceration postoperatively.[114] Until recently surgeons were forced to use indirect clues to look for vitreous gel in the anterior chamber. Kenalog suspension (triamcinolone acetonide (TA)) solves this problem[82] (Figure 44-20 and video clips 1-3).

INDICATIONS FOR TRIAMCINOLONE USE

Kenalog may be used in the anterior chamber to highlight vitreous known to be present, to check for suspected vitreous, or to confirm that all the vitreous has been cleared from the anterior chamber.

PREPARATION OF TRIAMCINOLONE SUSPENSION

In the original description of TA use, the preservative was removed by a sterile capture-wash technique. Briefly, 0.2 mL of Kenalog-40 is drawn up into a tuberculin syringe and expressed into a 5 μm filter that captures the TA particles. The authors then rinse and resuspend the TA with BSS. The final resuspension volume is 2 mL, giving an approximate concentration of 4 mg/mL. While our TA washing technique removes the benzyl alcohol preservative, it can be tedious, particularly when the encounter with vitreous is unexpected or the operating room staff is unfamiliar with the technique.

Alternatively, some surgeons simply dilute 40 mg/mL TA 1:10 with BSS. However, the final product will contain 0.01% benzyl alcohol preservative. Other surgeons prefer a sedimentation-resuspension-dilution technique. The most conceptually simple version of this technique involves leaving a Kenalog-40 vial sitting undisturbed in the operating room. When TA is needed, the supernatant is drawn off and replaced with an equal volume of BSS. The TA is typically then diluted 1:10 in BSS. Assuming supernatant removal of 90% or greater, the final product will contain

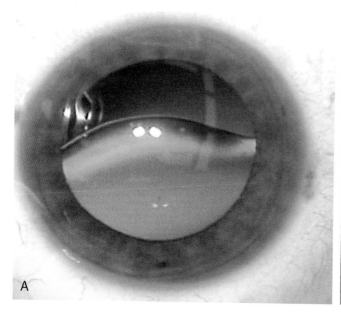

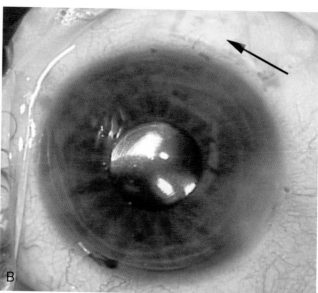

Figure 44-19 A, Operating microscope view of severe zonular laxity in a patient with Marfan syndrome. B, Operating microscope view following phacoemulsification and intraocular lens implantation. Note the fixation loop with eyelet of the Cionni modified endocapsular tension ring (black arrow).

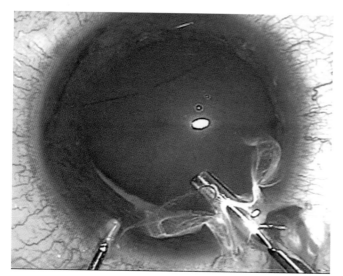

Figure 44-20 Vitreous gel made clearly visible by the injection of Kenalog particles seen streaming into the vitrectomy port.

0.001% benzyl alcohol or less. Finally, preservative-free TA has been recently introduced by Alcon and although expensive, it can be quickly prepared by simple 1:10 dilution.

TECHNIQUE

Kenalog injected directly into the substance of the vitreous provides maximum visualization; dusting the surface of the gel also works, but only until the dusted surface has been removed by vitrectomy at which point reinjection may be performed. A preferred option is to swirl a little Kenalog gently in the anterior chamber to get an overview of the situation, and then bury the cannula tip within the gel and make a very controlled injection. You can watch the vitreous anatomy gradually appear as the particles become entrapped. It is very important to remember that vitreous follows the pressure gradient, and if vitreous is near the wound when fluid comes out, so will vitreous. Inserting the cannula through a paracentesis rather than the phaco incision tends to reduce such reflux.

The vitrectomy should be performed in Cut-I/A mode using a high cut rate (800+), a low aspiration rate (~20), and separate irrigation. Although not always needed, a pars plana approach (3 mm behind the limbus) can be quite helpful. Indeed, in eyes with a large zonular dialysis, we often make a paracentesis, instill Kenalog, and perform the vitrectomy through the pars plana before making the phaco incision.

Finally, all eyes that undergo a vitrectomy require a dilated peripheral fundus examination in the early postoperative period to look for retinal tears.

ALTERNATIVES

Visualization of the vitreous using biostaining ophthalmic dyes has been described.[115,116] While it is true that dye is held in the vitreous briefly, dye in solution is comprised of relatively small molecules that rapidly diffuse away, unless it becomes bound to protein. The capsular dyes are great for binding to basement membrane proteins, but there is very little protein in the vitreous. Thus, the rapid diffusion of dye and the paucity of protein to bind to in the vitreous (compared to elsewhere in the eye) result in an unacceptably low signal-to-noise ratio. After a short time, the consequence is poorly highlighted vitreous and diffuse ocular staining.

If you imagine the vitreous as a three-dimensional microscopic spider web, it becomes more conceptually obvious why the vitreous gel will capture and hold nearly any particulate matter (think of asteroid hyalosis). Certainly, there are alternative particulate suspensions that have been evaluated for vitreous identification.[4] The most notable of these is 11-deoxycortisol, a steroid precursor without glucocorticoid effects.[117] As expected, the suspension of 11-deoxycortisol becomes trapped in vitreous just like TA.

Nonetheless, the authors prefer Kenalog because it is a Food and Drug Administration (FDA) approved medication. It is readily available, nontoxic, and has been used for intraocular injections since 1980.[118–122] In addition, the steroid effect stabilizes the blood–aqueous barrier and minimizes postoperative inflammation in these complicated anterior segment cases. Furthermore, the risk of steroid-induced glaucoma seems to be minimal because only a small amount of TA is used and the majority of it is removed along with the vitreous gel.

VITREOUS PRESENTING POSTOPERATIVELY

Kenalog staining has revealed that vitreous prolapse through the wound or paracentesis occurs in most cases of vitreous loss. Fortunately, vitreous stained with Kenalog is much easier to visualize and remove.

When vitreous incarceration in an incision is discovered postoperatively, the first and most important task is to determine if any vitreous is exposed to the tear film. Vitreous wicking is an open invitation for infection, and unrecognized vitreous wicking undoubtedly accounts for many cases of endophthalmitis associated with vitreous loss. If externalized vitreous is not readily apparent, try staining it with fluorescein sodium because it temporarily highlights the gel bright green. If any externalized vitreous is detected, the patient should be taken back to the operating room for additional vitrectomy using Kenalog as needed.

If there is a peaked pupil, indicating vitreous incarceration, but no evidence for externalized vitreous, YAG laser vitreolysis may be considered. Small strands of vitreous may be broken, but the surgeon must take care to use the minimum energy required to disrupt the strand. Thick vitreous strands will typically necessitate a return trip to the operating room for additional vitrectomy where Kenalog may be used to enhance visualization. In either case, it is important not to leave the eye with vitreous traction. To do so only invites cystoid macular edema and retinal tears.

ACUTE CORNEAL CLOUDING

There is always the remote possibility that the surgeon can inject either the wrong concentration of a drug or even the wrong solution into the eye. The toxic effect upon the corneal endothelium can cause immediate or delayed clouding of the cornea. The authors have seen the cornea become opaque when an inappropriate mixture of Miochol was instilled, and are aware of a case where distilled water was accidentally substituted for BSS.

Prompt recognition followed by immediate intracameral lavage with BSS is indicated. Proper labeling and communication between members of the surgical team should minimize the risk of this potentially disastrous complication.

INADVERTENT CANNULA INJECTION

The accidental injection of a cannula has been reported to cause scleral penetration, iris damage, posterior capsule tear, zonular dialysis, vitreous hemorrhage, and retinal tear.[123] Detachment of the cannula hub from the syringe tip during forceful injection of a solution or OVD creates a sharp projectile capable of penetrating intraocular tissues. Luer lock systems are still no guarantee that a mishap will not occur and vigilance is required to minimize the risk of this complication. Proper set up must be insured by reviewing the potential risk with the surgical staff. Scrub technicians should routinely confirm the security of the connection between the cannula and the filter of the syringe by a forceful "practice injection" prior to handing the surgeon the syringe. If the incision is being hydrated, the cannula tip should be directed into the tissue at right angles to the incision in order to prevent the inadvertent launching of the cannula into the eye should it detach. The surgeon should always inject with the dominant hand while the thumb and index finger of the fellow hand are pinching the hub of the cannula, although discharge of the cannula may still be difficult to prevent. This creates instantaneous tactile feedback the moment the cannula ejects, at which point the surgeon will cease the injection and the index finger will blunt the forward movement of the cannula.

EXPULSIVE SUPRACHOROIDAL HEMORRHAGE

The catastrophic complication of suprachoroidal expulsive hemorrhage is more likely to occur in older patients with brunescent lenses, pre-existing uveitis, glaucoma with elevated intraocular pressure, high myopia, and systemic hypertension. Anticoagulation therapy is another risk factor.[124,125] Early recognition is the key to successful management. Chamber shallowing with positive pressure may be the first sign of a suprachoroidal choroidal hemorrhage. The surgeon may notice a loss of the red reflex, and the patient may complain of pain despite adequate anesthesia. If the surgeon suspects this diagnosis, ophthalmoscopy should be performed to determine whether a suprachoroidal choroidal hemorrhage is developing. Although the indirect ophthalmoscope should be readily available, a lens has been developed by Ocular Instruments (Osher Panfundus lens) that can be kept sterile in "peel aparts" which will allow a quick view of the fundus through the operating microscope. If severe positive pressure is present, a special lens (Osher Gonio-Posterior Pole lens by Ocular Instruments) allows a more magnified view of the optic nerve to confirm perfusion of the central retinal artery.

The globe that suddenly becomes firm demands immediate closure of the eye. If the surgeon is unable to close the incision because of severe pressure, he or she should tamponade the incision with a finger while mannitol is being given.[126] Once the incision has been closed, uveal tissue that has prolapsed can be reposited (or rarely excised), and the anterior chamber can be deepened with air, BSS, or OVD injection. If the anterior chamber fails to deepen or if the incision cannot be safely secured, the surgeon should attempt to drain the suprachoroidal hemorrhage via a posterior sclerotomy 3.5–4 mm posterior to the limbus avoiding the larger vessels that are present at 3 and 9 o'clock. An emergency telephone call to a vitreoretinal surgeon may be advisable.

Once the incision is secure, only a highly experienced surgeon might succeed in removing cortex with a cannula through the stab incision then injecting the IOL through the unenlarged primary incision. As a general rule, the surgeon should avoid the temptation to continue surgery, because any decompression of the anterior chamber will likely induce further hemorrhage. It is far safer to complete the procedure at a later date. Fortunately, this complication is extraordinarily rare with small incision phacoemulsification surgery and the self-sealing incision provides a significant advantage in this sight-threatening situation.

A suprachoroidal effusion or a posterior scleral invagination will often mimic a hemorrhage in its clinical presentation.[127] Again, the main surgical imperative is to close and secure the incision to avoid extrusion of intraocular tissue. Although it may be impossible to distinguish between a suprachoroidal hemorrhage and effusion using ophthalmoscopy, effusions may be circumferential and low-lying. If the incision is secure, one should pull away the operating microscope and simply wait for 5 minutes. Alternatively, the patient can be transported to the holding area and re-examined after 1 hour or so. With repressurization of the globe, a suprachoroidal effusion may resolve after only a few minutes, as evidenced by spontaneous and dramatic softening of the previously firm globe. In this instance, cautiously resuming the procedure is a consideration. However, with self-sealing small incisions, there is literally no point in the procedure where surgery cannot be aborted with the plan of completing the case at a later and safer time.

CONCLUSIONS

Phacoemulsification is an elegant and safe procedure that is rewarding to both the patient and surgeon. Complications will be encountered by every cataract surgeon, and successful management will depend upon the ophthalmologist's experience, skill, and sound judgment. We have reviewed a spectrum of intraoperative complications and offered our perspective in preventing and managing these situations.

As phacoemulsification techniques change, so also will the types and frequency of complications. We encourage surgeons to master and adhere to these basic principles which will still be applicable to new techniques in the future.

References

[1] Feibel RM. Current concepts in retrobulbar anesthesia. Surv Ophthalmol 1985;30:102–110.

[2] Ellis P. Retrobulbar injection. Surv Ophthalmol 1974;18:425–430.

[3] Cionni R, Osher R. Retrobulbar hemorrhage. Ophthalmology 1991;98:1153–1155.

[4] Koch D. Standard analysis of cataract incision construction. J Cataract Refract Surg 1999;17:661–667.

[5] Ernest P, Kiesslue L, Lowery K. Relative strength of cataract incisions in cadaver eyes. J Cataract Refract Surg 1991;17:668–671.

[6] Singer J. Frown incisions for minimizing individual astigmatism after small incision cataract surgery with rigid optic intraocular lens implantation. J Cataract Refract Surg 1991;17:677–688.

[7] Jaffe N, Claymann H. The pathophysiology of corneal astigmatism after cataract extraction. Trans Am Acad Ophthalmol Otolaryngol 1975;79:615–630.

[8] Masket S. Nonkeratometric control of post-operative astigmatism. Am Intraocular Implant Soc J 1985;11:134–147.

[9] Ernest P. Cadaver eye study of the relative stability of clear corneal incisions and scleral corneal incisions used in small incision cataract surgery. Presented at the American Society of Cataract and Refractive Surgery Meeting, Seattle, Wash, May 1993.

[10] Osher RH. Thermal injuries. In: Chang DF, editor. Curbside consultation in cataract surgery. Thorofare, NJ: Slack, Inc; 2007.

[11] Osher R. New suturing techniques. Audiovisual J Cataract Implant Surg 1990; 6.

[12] Kremer I, Stiebel H, Yassur Y, et al. Sulfur hexafluoride injection for Descemet's membrane detachment in cataract surgery. J Cataract Refract Surg 1997;23:1449–1453.

[13] Morinelli EN, Najac RD, Speaker MG, et al. Repair of Descemet's membrane detachment with the assistance of intraoperative ultrasound biomicroscopy. Am J Ophthalmol 1996;121:718–720.

[14] Booth FM, Kurdian P, Liu H. Repositioning of Descemet's membrane: a case report. Aust J Ophthalmol 1984;12:341–343.

[15] Vastine DW, Weinberg RS, Sugar J, et al. Stripping of Descemet's membrane associated with intraocular lens implantation. Arch Ophthalmol 1983;101:1042–1045.

[16] Chang D, Campbell J. Intraoperative floppy iris syndrome associated with tamsulosin. J Cataract Refract Surg 2005;4:664–773.

[17] Osher RH. Association between IFIS and Flomax. J Cataract Refract Surg 2006;32:547.

[18] Gurbaxani A, Packard R. Intracameral phenylephrine to prevent floppy iris syndrome during cataract surgery in patients on tamsulosin. Eye 2007;21:331–332, Epub 2005 Nov 11.

[19] Thim K, Grag S, Corydon L. Stretching capacity of capsulorhexis and nucleus delivery. J Cataract Refract Surg 1991;17:27–31.

[20] Wasserman D, Apple D, Castaneda V, et al. Anterior capsular tears and loop fixation of posterior chamber intraocular lenses. Ophthalmology 1991;98:425–432.

[21] Assia E, Apple D, Tsai J, et al. The elastic properties of the lens capsule in capsulorhexis. Am J Ophthalmol 1991;3:628–632.

[22] Marques FF, Marques DM, Osher RH, Osher JM. Fate of anterior capsule tears during cataract surgery. J Cataract Refract Surg 2006;32:1638–1642.

[23] Osher RH, Falzoni W, Osher JM. Our phacoemulsification technique. In: Buratto L, Werner L, Zanini M, et al., editors. Phacoemulsification principles and techniques. 2nd ed. Thorofare, NJ: Slack Inc; 2003.

[24] Little BC, Smith JH, Packer M. Little capsulorhexis tear-out rescue. J Cataract Refract Surg 2006;32:1420–1422.

[25] Chang DF. Phacoemulsification in high risk cases. In: Wallace RB, editor. Refractive cataract surgery and multifocal IOLs. Thorofare, NJ: Slack Inc; 2001.

[26] Masket S. Postoperative complications of capsulorhexis. J Cataract Refract Surg 1993;19: 721–724.

[27] Miyake K, Ota I, Ichihashi S, et al. New classification of capsular block syndrome. J Cataract Refract Surg 1998;24:1230–1234.

[28] Deokule SP, Mukherjee SS, Chew CK. Neodymium:YAG laser anterior capsulotomy for capsular contraction syndrome. Ophthalmic Surg Lasers Imaging 2006;37:99–105.

[29] Edrich CL, Ghanchi F, Calvert R. Anterior capsular phimosis with complete occlusion of the capsulorhexis opening. Eye 2005;19:1229–1232.

[30] Hohn S, Spraul CW. Complete occlusion of the frontal capsule after cataract-operation in a patient with pseudoexfoliation syndrome – a case report and review of literature. Klin Monatsbl Augenheilkd 2004;221:495–497.

[31] Waheed K, Eleftheriadis H, Liu C. Anterior capsular phimosis in eyes with a capsular tension ring. J Cataract Refract Surg 2001;27:1688–1690.

[32] Horiguchi M, Miyake K, Ohta I, Ito Y. Staining of the lens capsule for circular continuous capsulorhexis in eyes with white cataract. Arch Ophthalmol 1998;116:535–537.

[33] Pandey SK, Werner L, Escobar-Gomez M, et al. Dye-enhanced cataract surgery. Part I. Anterior capsule staining for capsulorhexis in advanced/white cataract. J Cataract Refract Surg 2000;26:1052–1059.

[34] Werner L, Pandey SK, Escobar-Gomez M, et al. Dye-enhanced cataract surgery. Part II. Learning critical steps of phacoemulsification. J Cataract Refract Surg 2000;26:1060–1065.

[35] Pandey SK, Werner L, Escobar-Gomez M, et al. Dye-enhanced cataract surgery. Part III. Posterior capsule staining to learn posterior continuous curvilinear capsulorhexis. J Cataract Refract Surg 2000;26:1066–1071.

[36] Newsom TH, Oetting TA. Indocyanine green staining in traumatic cataract. J Cataract Refract Surg 2000;26:1691–1693.

[37] Pandey SK, Werner L, Apple DJ. Staining the anterior capsule. J Cataract Refract Surg 2001;27:647–648.

[38] Sturmer J. Cataract surgery and the "Blue Miracle." Klin Monatsbl Augenheilkd 2002;219: 191–195.

[39] de Waard PW, Budo CJ, Melles GR. Trypan blue capsular staining to "find" the leading edge of a "lost" capsulorhexis. Am J Ophthalmol 2002;134:271–272.

[40] Marques DM, Marques FF, Osher RH. Three-step technique for staining the anterior lens capsule with indocyanine green or trypan blue. J Cataract Refract Surg 2004;30:13–16.

[41] Perrrone D. Argentina flag sign. Video J Cataract Refract Surg 2001;17.

[42] Centurian V. Intumescent cataract. Video J Cataract Refract Surg 2006;22.

[43] Schneider S, Osher RH, Burk SE, et al. Thinning of the anterior capsule associated with congenital aniridia. J Cataract Refract Surg 2003;29:523–525.

[44] Cionni RJ, Barros MG, Osher RH. Management of lens-iris diaphragm retropulsion syndrome during phacoemulsification. J Cataract Refract Surg 2004;30:953–956.

[45] Wilbrandt H, Wilbrandt T. Evaluation of intraocular pressure fluctuations with differing phacoemulsification approaches. J Cataract Refract Surg 1993;19:223–231.

[46] Osher R. Slow motion phacoemulsification approach. J Cataract Refract Surg 1993;19:667.

[47] Cionni R. Review of positive pressure. Audiovisual J Cataract Implant Surg 1992;8.

[48] Khng C, Osher RH. Surgical options in the face of positive pressure. J Cataract Refract Surg 2006;32:1423–1425.

[49] Chang DF. Pars plana vitreous tap for phaco in the crowded eye. J Cataract Refract Surg 2001;27:1911–1914.

[50] Davis P. Phaco transducers: basic principles and corneal thermal injury. Eur J Implant Ref Surg 1993;5:109.

[51] Osher RH, Injev VP. Thermal study of bare tips with various system parameters and incision sizes. J Cataract Refract Surg 2006;32:867–872.

[52] Soscia W, Howard JG, Olson RJ. Bimanual phacoemulsification through 2 stab incisions. A wound-temperature study. J Cataract Refract Surg 2002;28:1039–1043.

[53] Soscia W, Howard JG, Olson RJ. Microphacoemulsification with WhiteStar. A wound-temperature study. J Cataract Refract Surg 2002;28:1044–1046.

[54] Donnenfeld ED, Olson RJ, Solomon R, et al. Efficacy and wound-temperature gradient of WhiteStar phacoemulsification through a 1.2 mm incision. J Cataract Refract Surg 2003;29: 1097–1100.

[55] Keates R, McGowan K. Clinical trial of flurbiprofen to maintain pupillary dilation during cataract surgery. Ann Ophthalmol 1984;16:919–921.

[56] Shugar JK. Use of epinephrine for IFIS prophylaxis. J Cataract Refract Surg 2006;32:1074–1075.

[56A] Review of Ophthalmology March Vol XVI, 2006 of CRST 2006 September pages 72–74.

[57] Osher R, Gimbel B, Galand A, et al. Small pupil phacoemulsification. Audiovisual J Cataract Implant Surg 1991;7.

[58] Mackool RJ. Small pupil enlargement during cataract extraction: a new method. J Cataract Refract Surg 1992;18:523–526.

[59] Nichamin LD. Enlarging the pupil for cataract extraction using flexible nylon iris retractors. J Cataract Refract Surg 1993;19:793–796.

[60] Shepherd DM. The pupil stretch technique for miotic pupils in cataract surgery. Ophthalmic Surg 1993;24:851–852.

[61] Koch PS. Techniques and instruments for cataract surgery. Curr Opin Ophthalmol 1994;5:33–39.

[62] Fry L. Pupil stretching. Video J Cataract Refractive Surg 1995;9.

[63] Masket S. Avoiding complications associated with iris retractor use in small pupil cataract extraction. J Cataract Refract Surg 1996;22:168–171.

[64] Dinsmore SC. Modified stretch technique for small pupil phacoemulsification with topical anesthesia. J Cataract Refract Surg 1996;22:27–30.

[65] Novak J. Flexible iris hooks for phacoemulsification. J Cataract Refract Surg 1997;23:828–831.

[66] Barboni P, Zanini M, Rossi A, Savini G. Monomanual pupil stretcher. Ophthalmic Surg Lasers 1998;29:772–773.

[67] Oetting TA, Omphroy LC. Modified technique using flexible iris retractors in clear corneal cataract surgery. J Cataract Refract Surg 2002;28:596–598.

[68] Jaffe H. Cataract surgery and its complications. 3rd ed. St Louis: Mosby; 1981. p. 368,9.

[69] Gimble H. Divide and conquer nucleofractis phacoemulsification: development and variations. J Cataract Refract Surg 1991;17:281–291.

[70] Osher RH, Marques DM, Marques FF, Osher JM. Slow-motion phacoemulsification technique. Techniques in Opthal 2003;1:73–79.

[71] Chang DF. Converting to phaco chop: why and how. Ophthalmic Practice 1999;17:4.

[72] Temel M, Osher RH. Posterior capsule tear resulting from faulty instrumentation. J Cataract Refract Surg 2003;29:619–620.

[73] Osher RH, Yu BC, Koch DD. Posterior polar cataracts: a predisposition to intraoperative posterior capsular rupture. J Cataract Refract Surg 1990;16:157–162.

[74] Vasavada A, Singh R. Phacoemulsification in eyes with posterior polar cataract. J Cataract Refract Surg 1999;25:238–245.

[75] Cheng KP, Hiles DA, Biglan AW, Pettapiece MC. Management of posterior lenticonus. J Pediatr Ophthalmol Strabismus 1991;28:143–149.

[76] Vasavada A, Singh R. Phacoemulsification in eyes with posterior polar cataract. J Cataract Refract Surg 1999;25:238–245.

[77] Allen D, Wood C. Minimizing risk to the capsule during surgery for posterior polar cataract. J Cataract Refract Surg 2002;28:742–744.

[78] Fine IH, Packer M, Hoffman RS. Management of posterior polar cataract. J Cataract Refract Surg 2003;29:16–19.

[79] Hayashi K, Hayashi H, Nakao F, Hayashi F. Outcomes of surgery for posterior polar cataract. J Cataract Refract Surg 2003;29:45–49.

[80] Schneider S, Osher RH, Burk SE, et al. Thinning of the anterior capsule associated with congenital aniridia. J Cataract Refract Surg 2003;29:523–525.

[81] Osher R. Dry vitrectomy. Audiovisual J Cataract Refract Surg 1992;8.

[82] Burk SE, Da Mata AP, Snyder ME, et al. Visualizing vitreous using Kenalog suspension. J Cataract Refract Surg 2003;29:645–651.

[83] Kelman C. PALTechnique. Video J Cataract Refractive Surg 1996;12.

[84] Por YM, Chee SP. Posterior-assisted levitation: outcomes in the retrieval of nuclear fragments and subluxated intraocular lenses. J Cataract Refract Surg 2006;32:2060–2063.

[85] Lifshitz T, Levy J. Posterior assisted levitation: long-term follow-up data. J Cataract Refract Surg 2005;31:499–502.

[86] Teichmann KD. Posterior assisted levitation. Surv Ophthalmol 2002;47:78.

[87] Chang DF, Packard RB. Posterior assisted levitation for nucleus retrieval using viscoat after posterior capsule rupture. J Cataract Refract Surg 2003;29:1860–1865.

[88] Chang DF. Viscoelastic levitation of posteriorly dislocated intraocular lenses from the anterior vitreous. J Cataract Refract Surg 2002;28:1515–1519.

[89] Michelson M. The Sheets glide. Video J Cataract Refract Surg 1991;7.

[90] Chang DF. Conquering capsule complications: a video primer, AAO course 629. 2002.

[91] Gimbel HV, DeBroff BM. Intraocular lens optic capture. J Cataract Refract Surg 2004;30: 200–206.

[92] Castaneda V, Tegler U, Tsai J, et al. Posterior continuous curvilinear capsulorhexis. Ophthalmology 1992;99:45.

[93] Osher RH. Adjusting intraocular lens power for sulcus fixation. JCRS 2004;30:20–31.

[94] Suto C, Hori S, Fukuyama E, Akura J. Adjusting intraocular lens power for sulcus fixation. J Cataract Refract Surg 2003;29:1913–1917.

[95] Bayramlar H, Hepsen IF, Yilmaz H. Myopic shift from the predicted refraction after sulcus fixation of PMMA posterior chamber intraocular lenses. Can J Ophthalmol 2006;41:78–82.

[96] Menezo JL, Martinez MC, Cisneros AL. Iris-fixated Worst claw versus sulcus-fixated posterior chamber lenses in the absence of capsular support. J Cataract Refract Surg 1996;22:1476–1484.

[97] Samples JR, Bellows AR, Rosenquist RC. Pupillary block with posterior chamber intraocular lenses. Arch Ophthalmol 1987;105:335–337.

[98] Marques DM, Marques FF, Osher RH. Subtle signs of zonular damage. J Cataract Refract Surg 2004;30:1295–1299.

[98A] Osher RH, Osher JM, Injev V. "Understanding the dropped nucleus." Grand prize winner in the 2008 film festival of the European Society of Cataract and Refractive Surgery.

[99] Osher R. Surgical approach to the traumatic cataract. Audiovisual J Cataract Implant Surg 1987;3.

[100] Osher R, Cionni R, Gimbel H, et al. Cataract surgery in patients with pseudoexfoliation: cataract surgery in patients with pseudoexfoliation syndrome. Eur J Implant Refract Surg 1993;5:46–50.

[101] Cionni RJ, Osher RH. Endocapsular ring approach to the subluxed cataractous lens. J Cataract Refract Surg 1995;21:245–249.

[102] Fine IH, Hoffman RS. Phacoemulsification in the presence of pseudoexfoliation: challenges and options. J Cataract Refract Surg 1997;23:160–165.

[103] Gimbel HV, Sun R, Heston JP. Management of zonular dialysis in phacoemulsification and IOL implantation using the capsular tension ring. Ophthalmic Surg Lasers 1997;28:273–281.

[104] Cionni RJ, Osher RH. Management of profound zonular dialysis or weakness with a new endocapsular ring designed for scleral fixation. J Cataract Refract Surg 1998;24:1299–1306.

[105] Menapace R, Findl O, Georgopoulos M, et al. The capsular tension ring: designs, applications, and techniques. J Cataract Refract Surg 2000;26:898–912.

[106] Menkhaus S, Motschmann M, Kuchenbecker J, Behrens-Baumann W. Pseudoexfoliation (PEX) syndrome and intraoperative complications in cataract surgery. Klin Monatsbl Augenheilkd 2000;216:388–392.

[107] Ahmed II, Crandall AS. Ab externo scleral fixation of the Cionni modified capsular tension ring. J Cataract Refract Surg 2001;27:977–981.

[108] Bayraktar S, Altan T, Kucuksumer Y, Yilmaz OF. Capsular tension ring implantation after capsulorhexis in phacoemulsification of cataracts associated with pseudoexfoliation syndrome: intraoperative complications and early postoperative findings. J Cataract Refract Surg 2001;27:1620–1628.

[109] Gimbel HV, Sun R. Clinical applications of capsular tension rings in cataract surgery. Ophthalmic Surg Lasers 2002;18.

[110] Cionni RJ, Osher RH, Snyder ME. Five years experience with the Cionni modified capsular tension ring. Video J Cataract Refractive Surg 2002;18.

[111] Ahmed II, Chen SH, Kranemann C, Wong DT. Surgical repositioning of dislocated capsular tension rings. Ophthalmology 2005;112:1725–1733.

[112] Michaeli A, Assia EI. Scleral and iris fixation of posterior chamber lenses in the absence of capsular support. Curr Opin Ophthalmol 2005;16:57–60.

[113] Spigelman AV, Lindstrom RL, Nichols BD, Lindquist TD. Visual results following vitreous loss and primary lens implantation. J Cataract Refract Surg 1989;15:201–204.

[114] AAO Spotlight on Cataract 2006 Audience Response questions.

[115] Burk SE, Da Mata AP, Snyder ME. Indocyanine green-assisted peeling of the retinal internal limiting membrane. Ophthalmology 2000;107:2010–2014.

[116] Cacciatori M, Chadha V, Bennett HG, Singh J. Trypan blue to aid visualization of the vitreous during anterior segment surgery. J Cataract Refract Surg 2006;32:389–391.

[117] Kaji Y, Hiraoka T, Okamoto F. Visualizing the vitreous body in the anterior chamber using 11-deoxycortisol after posterior capsule rupture in an animal model. Ophthalmology 2004;111: 1334–1339.

[118] McCuen 2nd BW, Bessler M, Tano Y. The lack of toxicity of intravitreally administered triamcinolone acetonide. Am J Ophthalmol 1981;91:785–788.

[119] Hida T, Chandler D, Arena JE, Machemer R. Experimental and clinical observations of the intraocular toxicity of commercial corticosteroid preparations. Am J Ophthalmol 1986;101: 190–195.

[120] Young S, Larkin G, Branley M, Lightman S. Safety and efficacy of intravitreal triamcinolone for cystoid macular edema in uveitis. Clin Experiment Ophthalmol 2001;29:2–6.

[121] Tano Y, Chandler D, Machemer R. Treatment of intraocular proliferation with intravitreal injection of triamcinolone acetonide. Am J Ophthalmol 1980;90:810–816.

[122] Oh JY, Wee WR, Lee JH, Kim MK. Short-term effect of intracameral triamcinolone acetonide on corneal endothelium using the rabbit model. Eye 2007;21:812–818. Epub 2006 Jun 2.

[123] Osher RH. Iris damage by inadvertent cannula injection. J Cataract Refract Surg 2007;33: 341.

[124] Riderman J, Harbin T, Campbell D. Post-operative suprachoroidal hemorrhage following filtrating procedures. Arch Ophthalmol 1986;194:201–205.

[125] Speaker M, Guerleio P, Riet J, et al. A case control study of risk factors for intraoperative suprachoroidal expulsive hemorrhage. Ophthalmology 1991;98:202–210.

[126] Osher M. Emergency treatment of vitreous bulge and incision gaping complicating cataract surgery. Am J Ophthalmol 1957;44:409–411.

[127] Kirsch RE, Singer JA. Ocular fundus immediately after cataract extraction. Arch Ophthalmol 1973;90:460–463.

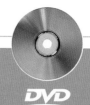

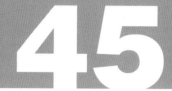

Anterior Vitrectomy Techniques for the Cataract Surgeon

45

*David F. Chang, MD

CONTENTS

CHAPTER HIGHLIGHTS

>> Posterior assisted levitation (PAL) technique

>> Pars plana anterior vitrectomy

>> "Visco trap"

>> The "contingency kit"

Every cataract surgeon must have a game plan for when and how to perform an anterior vitrectomy following posterior capsule rupture. This chapter will review the indications, the goals, and the techniques for managing vitreous loss in this setting. Understanding and mentally rehearsing these strategies in advance will better prepare anterior segment surgeons to properly manage vitreous loss amidst the stress of a surgical complication.

PREVENTING VITREOUS LOSS FOLLOWING POSTERIOR CAPSULAR RUPTURE

Despite a torn posterior capsule, it is frequently possible to avoid rupturing the anterior hyaloid face. The cataract surgeon must

*David F. Chang MD is clinical professor at the University of California, San Francisco, and in private practice in Los Altos, CA. He has no financial interest in any product or instrument mentioned.

avoid the natural reflex to immediately withdraw the phaco tip upon recognizing a posterior capsular tear. Abruptly unplugging the incision causes the anterior chamber to empty and shallow. The resulting posterior pressure gradient will rupture an intact hyaloid face, and vitreous will prolapse anteriorly toward the incision, expanding the capsular defect in the process.

To prevent this undesirable cascade of events the surgeon must fill and stabilize the anterior chamber with an ophthalmic viscosurgical device (OVD) prior to removing the phaco tip. Upon recognizing a capsular tear during phaco or cortical irrigation–aspiration (I–A), the surgeon should keep the anterior chamber pressurized with continuous irrigation while deciding what to do next. Continuing to phaco may be an option with a small zonular dialysis or capsular defect. Before removing the phaco or I–A tip, the surgeon injects OVD through the side port incision while changing from foot pedal position 1 to 0. Once the anterior chamber is filled with OVD, the posterior capsule and anterior hyaloid cannot bulge forward as the incision is unplugged. If phacoemulsification or cortical cleanup is resumed, these same maneuvers must be repeated whenever the instruments are removed.

MANAGING THE NUCLEUS FOLLOWING POSTERIOR CAPSULE RUPTURE

Early recognition of posterior capsule rupture is often the key to avoiding a dropped nucleus. This is because it is much easier to remove the nucleus while it remains anterior to the posterior capsule defect. Because the nucleus is approached from above, continuing instrument and fluidic forces will eventually expand an unrecognized capsular defect enough to allow the nucleus to fall posteriorly.

One must often rely upon indirect clues to recognize a posterior capsular defect because the iris and the nucleus obscure the zonular and posterior capsular anatomy. The first sign of zonular or capsular rupture might be sudden deepening of the chamber with momentary expansion of the pupil, the transitory appearance of a clear red reflex peripherally, or the inability to rotate a previously mobile nucleus. More obvious and alarming signs would be excessive tilting or lateral mobility of the nucleus, or partial descent of the nucleus. Continuing to phaco a large dense lens in the presence of a capsular tear or zonular defect carries a high risk of a dropped nucleus. Recognizing these early warning signs alerts one to manually remove the nucleus through a large incision before it is too late.

If the residual nucleus is small and soft enough, continuing phaco within the anterior chamber over a trimmed Sheet's glide is a consideration. As described by Marc Michelson, the glide serves as an artificial posterior capsule to keep lens material from dropping posteriorly and to shield the phaco tip from aspirating vitreous from below.[1] The incision should be widened slightly to accommodate inserting the phaco tip alongside the glide. Movements of the phaco tip should be minimized to avoid simultaneously displacing the glide. Using bimanual microincisional phaco instrumentation through separate 1.2 mm side ports avoids this problem if the surgeon is adept at this technique.

■ RESCUING A PARTIALLY DESCENDED NUCLEUS – THE VISCOAT POSTERIOR ASSISTED LEVITATION ■

How far the nucleus initially descends will depend upon the vitreous anatomy and the size of the capsular tear. If the defect is large and the vitreous is liquefied, the nucleus will rapidly sink to the retina before the cataract surgeon has any chance to react. Alternatively, the nucleus may partially descend when there is enough remaining capsular support and an intact hyaloid face (Figure 45-1). Such slight posterior displacement can be very subtle. Finally, if the hyaloid face is ruptured with some remaining capsule, the nucleus may tip or partially descend until it is suspended and supported by formed vitreous. In this situation, a rescue technique may be possible.

Attempting to chase and spear a partially descended nucleus with the phaco tip is fraught with risk. Lacking the normal capsular barrier, the posteriorly directed irrigation flow will hydrate and flush more vitreous forward, expanding the rent. The fluid stream will then propel nuclear fragments posteriorly. Attempts to emulsify or aspirate the nucleus may ensnare vitreous into the large diameter phaco tip. The tractional forces from employing suction and ultrasound in the presence of vitreous incarceration can produce a giant retinal tear.

A safer alternative is to elevate the nucleus into the pupillary plane or anterior chamber by manually lifting it from below, but accomplishing this may be difficult for several reasons. First, posterior capsule rupture occurs more frequently when the pupil is small. A small-diameter pupil hampers visibility and together with a small capsulorrhexis will impede levitation of a large nucleus. If the phaco incision is used, the angle of approach may be too steep for an OVD cannula to successfully maneuver behind the nucleus. It is especially difficult to inject OVD beneath the nucleus if there is a small pupil, a small capsulorrhexis, or any prolapsed vitreous. As more and more vitreous exits the eye through the manipulated incision, the nucleus will drop further posteriorly.

Charles Kelman popularized the posterior assisted levitation (PAL) technique by which a cyclodialysis spatula, inserted through a pars plana sclerotomy, is used to lift the nucleus into the anterior chamber from below ("New PAL method may save difficult cataract cases." *Ophthalmology Times* 1994; 19:51).[2] Compared to the phaco incision, a pars plana sclerotomy provides a much better instrument angle for getting behind the nucleus. Richard Packard and the author subsequently published the results of using the dispersive OVD Viscoat (Alcon Laboratories) and the Viscoat cannula to support and levitate the nucleus – the so-called Viscoat PAL technique.[3] An equally effective dispersive agent is Healon D (AMO).

After opening the conjunctiva and applying light cautery, a disposable micro-vitreoretinal (MVR) blade (Alcon, Katena) is used to make a pars plana sclerotomy 3.5 mm behind the limbus. An oblique quadrant should be selected to avoid the long ciliary vessels. The Viscoat cannula tip is then advanced and aimed behind the nucleus under direct visualization. The first step is to inject a bolus of dispersive OVD behind the nucleus to prevent any further descent (Figure 45-2).[3–5] Periodic palpation of the globe confirms that over-inflation has not occurred.

If the nucleus has subluxated laterally, directing dispersive OVD toward the area beneath it will often buoy the nucleus toward a more central position. This is preferable to blindly probing behind the iris with a metal spatula. The cannula tip is then used to mechanically maneuver and elevate the nucleus into the anterior chamber (Figure 45-3). A small capsulorrhexis or pupil will stretch to accommodate the levitation of a greater diameter nucleus. Small aliquots of additional OVD can be injected as

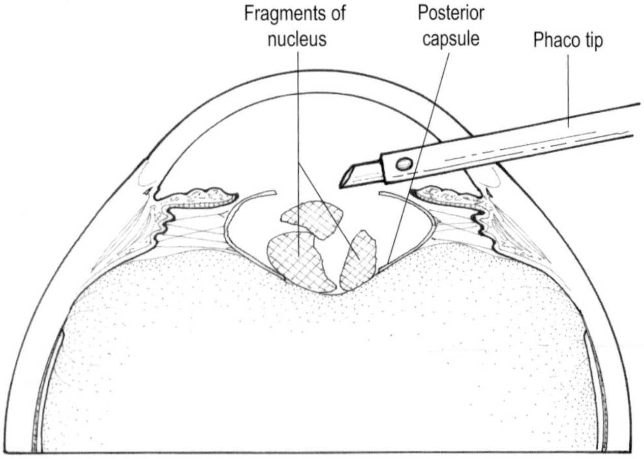

Figure 45-1 Partial descent of nuclear fragments following posterior capsule rupture. (Courtesy of David F. Chang.)

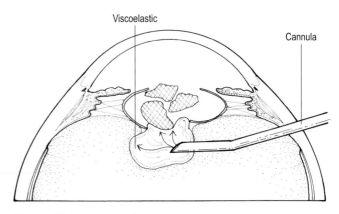

Figure 45-2 Dispersive ophthalmic viscosurgical device (Viscoat) is injected through a pars plana sclerotomy behind the descending nuclear fragments to provide immediate supplemental support. (Courtesy of David F. Chang.)

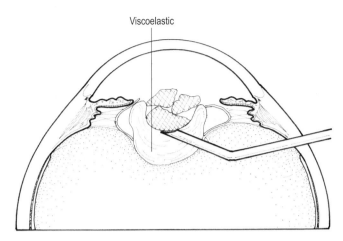

Viscoelastic

Figure 45-3 The Viscoat cannula is used to carefully levitate the nuclear fragments into the anterior chamber. (Courtesy of David F. Chang.)

needed to maneuver and prop up the nucleus. One should never attempt to float the nucleus into the anterior chamber using a massive infusion of dispersive OVD alone. Unlike using liquid perfluorocarbon in a vitrectomized eye, an excessive injection of OVD in this setting will over-inflate the globe and cause vitreous expulsion through the sclerotomy or phaco incision.

Using dispersive OVD to first support and reposition the nucleus prior to definitive manual levitation is the major advantage of the Viscoat PAL variation.[3–5] Because there is no aspiration involved, these PAL maneuvers should minimize iatrogenic vitreous traction and reduce the chance of accidentally touching the retina with a metal spatula tip. However, it is important to keep the cannula tip under direct visualization by focusing the microscope slightly posteriorly.

Once a fragment descends into the mid or posterior vitreous cavity and beyond the microscope's range of focus (without a special viewing lens), it is dangerous to blindly fish for it with any instrument. One should abandon the dropped nucleus and concentrate on removing the residual epinucleus and cortex, while preserving as much capsular support as possible. A thorough anterior vitrectomy must be performed prior to inserting the IOL. Depending upon the capsular anatomy, either an anterior or a posterior chamber IOL can be selected.[5–8] In the absence of capsular support, sutured posterior chamber IOLs are more time consuming to implant and superiority over anterior chamber IOLs has not been demonstrated.[9,10] Since the vitreoretinal surgeon will later use a three-port pars plana fragmatome and vitrectomy technique to remove any retained nucleus, it is preferable to insert an IOL during the initial surgery if possible.

MANAGING VITREOUS LOSS AND RESIDUAL LENS MATERIAL

CONVERTING TO MANUAL EXTRACAPSULAR CATARACT EXTRACTION

Any residual nucleus retrieved with the Viscoat PAL technique can be removed using either of two different approaches. As described earlier, one can resume phaco over a Sheet's glide if there is no vitreous prolapse and the nucleus is soft and of limited size. However, a larger dense nucleus would be more safely removed by converting to a large incision manual extracapsular

cataract extraction (ECCE) approach. This is best done by abandoning the self-sealing temporal phaco incision, and repositioning the surgeon and microscope for a superior incision location.

For patients under topical anesthesia, a posterior sub-Tenon's block can be administered with 2 mL of 2% lidocaine. A small conjunctival-Tenon's buttonhole is made in the inferior conjunctival fornix, avoiding the inferior rectus muscle insertion. Through this, a curved blunt Simcoe sub-Tenon's cannula is threaded alongside and behind the globe. The anesthetic is injected until conjunctival ballooning occurs. After making an adequately large superior ECCE incision, the nucleus should be surrounded and sandwiched by OVD. An irrigating lens loops should be used to extract the nucleus being careful not to lift it against the endothelium as it is withdrawn. Bimanual nuclear expression is contraindicated with an open posterior capsule.

THE VISCO TRAP

As residual nucleus and cortex are removed, the phaco or I–A tip may at some point ensnare prolapsing vitreous. To avoid vitreous traction, the surgeon must immediately stop to perform an anterior vitrectomy before extraction of the remaining lens material can be resumed. Instead of using a coaxial infusion sleeve, a separate self-retaining irrigating cannula should be inserted though an obliquely directed limbal paracentesis. The objective is to keep the irrigation circulating within the anterior chamber where it cannot expand the capsular defect or hydrate the vitreous.

Most cataract surgeons insert the vitrectomy probe through the phaco incision. However, there are multiple drawbacks to this approach. First, the phaco incision is too wide for the sleeveless vitrectomy instrument and will leak. This results in poor chamber stability and allows both irrigation fluid and vitreous to prolapse externally alongside the vitrector shaft. Second, performing the vitrectomy in the anterior chamber will tend to draw more vitreous from the posterior segment forward into the anterior segment. Finally, as more and more vitreous exits the eye through either the vitrectomy instrument or the incision, the residual lens material that it was supporting will sink posteriorly toward the retina. It bears repeating that if the posterior capsule is open, it is the formed vitreous that is preventing the remaining nucleus and epinucleus from descending.

The author has proposed a strategy called the Visco Trap which, when combined with a pars plana anterior vitrectomy, can prevent the posterior loss of residual lens material in this situation.[4,5] The first step is to use a dispersive OVD such as Viscoat or Healon D to corral and lift any mobile lens fragments up toward the cornea. Next, the anterior chamber is completely filled with dispersive OVD in order to support and trap the residual lens material anteriorly as the vitreous is excised from below (Figure 45-4). Even though vitreous has already prolapsed forward, injecting OVD should not exert traction on the retina.

The Visco Trap is so named because of the need to employ a dispersive OVD. To effectively trap lens material the OVD should be maximally retentive so that it is less easily burped out of the eye by incisional manipulation. In addition, dispersive agents such as Viscoat and Healon D better resist aspiration by the I–A or vitrectomy instruments. Finally, small amounts of

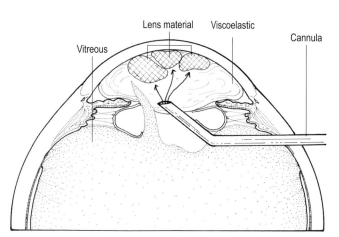

Figure 45-4 Following anterior vitreous prolapse, the residual lens fragments are elevated toward the cornea, where they are trapped by filling the anterior chamber with Viscoat. (Courtesy of David F. Chang.)

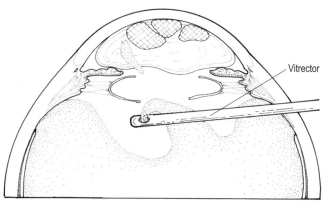

Figure 45-5 The sleeveless vitrectomy cutter is introduced via a pars plana sclerotomy, and kept behind the plane of the capsulorrhexis and pupil. This severs the transpupillary bands, but keeps Viscoat–filled anterior chamber isolated from the vitrectomized posterior chamber. The self–retaining infusion cannula (not shown) is placed through a limbal paracentesis incision. (Courtesy of David F. Chang.)

retained dispersive OVD are less likely to cause a prolonged or severe pressure spike because of the smaller molecular weight of these agents.[11,12]

■ BIMANUAL PARS PLANA ANTERIOR VITRECTOMY ■

As with the Viscoat PAL, the pars plana sclerotomy is made 3.5 mm posterior to the limbus in an oblique quadrant with a disposable MVR blade. The appropriate sized MVR blade is selected (19-gauge for most cutters) so as to avoid too tight an opening. The blade tip is oriented so as to produce a 1.2 mm slit incision that is parallel rather than radial to the limbus. The blade is aimed toward the plane of the posterior capsule and advanced until it is visualized through the pupil. It is possible to perform this step under topical anesthesia alone. As mentioned earlier, a self-retaining irrigating cannula is placed through a limbal paracentesis, and angled toward the pupil. As described by Scott Burk, staining prolapsed vitreous with a triamcinalone suspension to improve visibility is an option.[13] The sleeveless vitrectomy shaft is inserted through the pars plana sclerotomy until the tip can be visualized in the retro-pupillary space. If it does not easily pass through the incision, slightly enlarge the opening rather than force the entry.

METHOD OF PREPARING INTRACAMERAL TRIAMCINOLONE (IF NON-PRESERVED TRIAMCINOLONE IS NOT AVAILABLE)

Triamcinolone is supplied in a sterile vial containing 40 mg in 1 mL of preserved diluent. Burk has recommended a technique of removing the preserved diluent. However, this method of preparation is time-consuming and cumbersome, particularly given the stressful circumstances of a surgical complication. An alternative technique is to store the triamcinolone vial upright so that the precipitated drug settles to the bottom of the vial. Immediately prior to use, the one ml of diluent can easily be drawn off with a 25-gauge needle leaving the precipitated layer of white triamcinolone flakes at the bottom. The triamcinolone is then re-suspended with 3–4 mL of sterile balanced salt solution (BSS) for off label use as a vitreous staining agent.

A thorough bimanual anterior vitrectomy is performed, being careful to focus posteriorly enough to keep the vitrectomy tip under direct visualization at all times. Vitreous traction is minimized by using low aspiration flow and vacuum settings, and maximizing the vitrectomy cutting rate (e.g. >400 cpm). The vitrectomy tip should be moved very slowly and should never aspirate without simultaneous cutting vitreous. With the Viscoat Trap technique, the vitrectomy tip should be kept behind the pupil if possible. This will sever any trans-pupillary bands of vitreous without removing the dispersive OVD that fills the anterior chamber (Figure 45-5). When properly performed, one will see that the anteriorly trapped lens fragments remain immobilized as the vitrectomy is being carried out from below. This is because the OVD-filled anterior chamber has been isolated and partitioned from the vitrectomized posterior chamber.

Using a pars plana sclerotomy is an excellent but underutilized option for performing an anterior vitrectomy. The surgical objectives and principles are the same. One must not aspirate vitreous without cutting it, one should keep the vitrectomy tip under direct microscopic visualization, and one should not attempt to retrieve lens material that is in the posterior vitreous cavity. The main advantage is that using a properly sized pars plana sclerotomy will decrease incisional leak and vitreous prolapse by providing a better fluidic seal. Unlike with a limbal incision, the vitrector will not draw more vitreous forward into the anterior chamber and it will not aspirate the Viscoat partition. Performing the vitrectomy posterior to the pupil and the plane of the capsulorrhexis also decreases the chance of inadvertently cutting either structure. If the capsulorrhexis is preserved, an appropriate foldable posterior chamber IOL may be implanted in the ciliary sulcus with or without optic capture. The sclerotomy can be closed with an interrupted 8-0 Vicryl suture.

Some ophthalmologists would question whether a cataract surgeon has enough training to perform a pars plana anterior vitrectomy. The important distinction is that this is still an anterior vitrectomy performed under direct coaxial microscopic visualization. Posterior vitrectomy requires a special viewing lens, indirect light pipe illumination, and three watertight sclerotomy sites to permit high pressure forced infusion. Anterior vitrectomy following capsular rupture utilizes low-flow, gravity-fed infusion through a limbal cannula, and the sclerotomy need not and should not be tight. Making a 1.2 mm wide pars plana incision is, therefore, the only new skill required of the cataract surgeon. All eyes are at greater risk of retinal tear and detachment following posterior capsule rupture and vitreous loss.[14] Regardless of which vitrectomy incision was used, a careful peripheral retinal exam should be performed postoperatively for this reason. Some anterior segment surgeons may choose to refer these patients to a vitreoretinal sub-specialist.

■ CORTICAL REMOVAL FOLLOWING POSTERIOR CAPSULE RUPTURE ■

Following the retro-pupillary anterior vitrectomy, one can resume aspiration of the remaining cortex or epinucleus that was securely trapped within the Viscoat-filled anterior chamber. One should attempt to work in "slow motion" by lowering the irrigation bottle, and decreasing the aspiration flow and vacuum settings. There are several advantages to using bimanual I–A instrumentation for epinuclear and cortical extraction once the capsule or zonules have ruptured (Figure 45-6). The snug paracentesis incisions provide excellent chamber stability and reduce exiting fluid streams that might further induce vitreous prolapse. This also decreases the total volume of irrigation fluid circulating through the eye.

Without the constraining silicone irrigating sleeve, the aspirating tip can extend further peripherally into the capsular fornices. Burying the aspirating port within the peripheral-most cortex helps to block vitreous from becoming ensnared. Finally, the surgeon can direct the infusion away from the aspirating tip because the irrigation and aspiration currents are dissociated. This avoids further hydrating the vitreous cavity or flushing loose lens material posteriorly. If the aspirating port becomes entangled with vitreous again, one can repeat the Viscoat Trap maneuver followed by additional pars plana anterior vitrectomy. Bimanual cortical I–A can then be resumed.

■ EMERGENCY PREPAREDNESS ■

Posterior capsule rupture and vitreous loss necessitates an unsettling and stressful departure from the surgical routine for both surgeons and their operating room (OR) staff. Anticipating these difficulties, one can prepare for this contingency in several ways. First, one can assign and pre-program a phaco machine memory setting for "emergency" parameters. These might include a decreased bottle height, and reduced aspiration flow rate (20–24 cc/min) and vacuum limit (100–125 mm Hg). This should avoid the need for nursing personnel to hurriedly and manually adjust the settings in the face of posterior capsule rupture.

Second, the OR staff can pre-package special instruments in a "contingency" kit that is kept in a separate sterile peel pack. This avoids the need to urgently search for a seldom-used instrument amidst the stress of an unexpectedly complicated procedure. Based upon the scenarios discussed in this chapter for converting to a large incision ECCE or performing a vitrectomy, one might choose to include a Simcoe sub-Tenon's cannula, corneal scissors, an irrigating lens loop, a self-retaining limbal infusion cannula, and a bimanual I–A handpiece set. Such a contingency set is commercially available (Chang Contingency Kit, Katena) (Figure 45-7), but can be easily assembled and customized using any surgeon's preferred instruments. Vitrectomy instrumentation, disposable MVR blades, Sheet's glides, and a dispersive OVD such as Viscoat should also be available in the operating room.

In summary, cautious adherence to these principles may help surgeons to reduce the risk of dropping the nucleus following posterior capsular rupture. However, there is a fine line dividing maneuvers that are reasonable and safe from those that are overly aggressive or dangerous. Cataract surgeons must be honest in assessing their own level of comfort and expertise. Timely surgical management of a dropped nucleus by a vitreoretinal surgeon at a later date is always preferable to overstepping this fine line.[14]

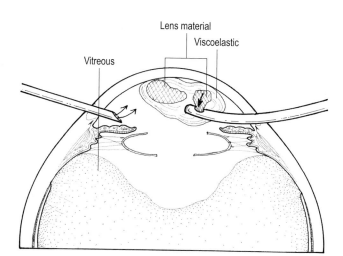

Figure 45–6 The bimanual irrigation–aspiration handpieces allow dissociation of the irrigation and aspiration currents. (Courtesy of David F. Chang.)

Vitreous

Lens material

Viscoelastic

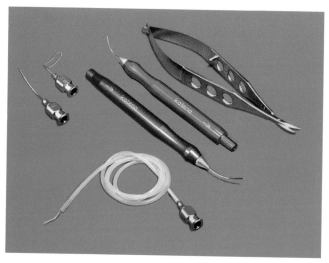

Figure 45-7 Chang Contingency Kit, Katena (author has no financial interest). (Courtesy of David F. Chang.)

References

[1] Michelson MA. Use of a Sheets' glide as a pseudoposterior capsule in phacoemulsification complicated by posterior capsule rupture. Eur J Implant Surg 1993;570–572.

[2] Lifshitz T, Levy J. Posterior assisted levitation: long-term follow-up data. J Cataract Refract Surg 2005;31:499–502.

[3] Chang DF, Packard RB. Posterior assisted levitation for nucleus retrieval using Viscoat after posterior capsule rupture. J Cataract Refract Surg 2003;29:1860–1865.

[4] Chang DF. Managing residual lens material after posterior capsule rupture. Techniques in Ophthalmology 2003;1:201–206.

[5] Chang DF. Strategies for managing posterior capsular rupture. In: Phaco chop: mastering techniques, optimizing technology, and avoiding complications. Thorofare, NJ: Slack Inc; 2004.

[6] Vajpayee RB, Sharma N, Dada T, et al. Management of posterior capsule tears. Surv Ophthalmol 2001;45:473–488 [review].

[7] Gimbel HV, Sun R, Ferensowicz M, et al. Intraoperative management of posterior capsule tears in phacoemulsification and intraocular lens implantation. Ophthalmology 2001;108:2186–2189. discussion 2190–2192.

[8] Arbisser LB, Charles S, Howcroft M, Werner L. Management of vitreous loss and dropped nucleus during cataract surgery. Ophthalmol Clin North Am 2006;19:495–506 [review].

[9] Pokroy R, Pollack A, Bukelman A. Retinal detachment in eyes with vitreous loss and an anterior chamber or a posterior chamber intraocular lens: comparison of the incidence. J Cataract Refract Surg 2002;28:1997–2000.

[10] Kwong YY, Yuen HK, Lam RF, et al. Comparison of outcomes of primary scleral-fixated versus primary anterior chamber intraocular lens implantation in complicated cataract surgeries. Ophthalmology 2007;114:80–85.

[11] Burke S, Sugar J, Farber MD. Comparison of the effects of two viscoelastic agents, Healon and Viscoat, on postoperative intraocular pressure after penetrating keratoplasty. Ophthalmic Surg 1990;21:821–826.

[12] Probst LE, Hakim OJ, Nichols BD. Phacoemulsification with aspirated or retained Viscoat. J Cataract Refract Surg 1994;20:145–149.

[13] Burk SE, Da Mata AP, Snyder ME, et al. Visualizing vitreous using Kenalog suspension. J Cataract Refract Surg 2003;29:645–651.

[14] Scott IU, Flynn Jr HW, Smiddy WE, et al. Clinical features and outcomes of pars plana vitrectomy in patients with retained lens fragments. Ophthalmology 2003;110:1567–1572.

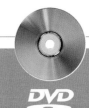

DVD

Surgical Repositioning and Explantation of the Intraocular Lens

Robert H. Osher, MD, Robert J. Cionni, MD,
Michael E. Snyder, MD, Christopher D. Riemann, MD
and Andrea P. Da Mata, MD

46

CONTENTS

- General Methods
- Surgical Techniques
- Conclusions

CHAPTER HIGHLIGHTS

>> Anterior-chamber intraocular lenses (IOL) incarcerated in peripheral anterior synechiae

>> Lasso suture stabilization of posterior-chamber IOLs

>> Techniques for IOL exchange

Although most eyes that undergo cataract extraction and intraocular lens (IOL) implantation are rapidly rehabilitated from an anatomic and visual standpoint, a small percentage of them develop complications that require repositioning, removal, or exchange of the pseudophakos. In the past lens dislocation and chronic intraocular inflammation were the most frequent indications for lens exchange.[1] Occasionally, the cause is faulty lens design, which results in chronic inflammation or opacification of the optic with a reduction of vision justifying an IOL exchange. In other cases, a material interaction creates a problem such as the hydrophillic optic absorbing trypan blue stain and the symptom of blue dyschromatopsia leads to IOL exchange.[2] A lens of an inappropriate size leads to unacceptable lens mobility and an uveitis glaucoma hyphema (UGH) syndrome. Incorrect dioptric power may result in anisometropia, asthenopia, or other refractive symptoms. Improper intraoperative positioning of an anterior chamber lens may cause iris tuck, uveal irritation and a UGH syndrome. A posterior chamber lens may decenter because of any number of reasons, including asymmetric haptic placement, inadequate capsular or zonular support, disproportionate IOL/bag size, progressive posterior synechiogenesis with pupillary capture, endocapsular fibrosis, late zonular dehiscence, enlargement of the neodymium:yttrium-aluminum-garnet laser posterior capsulotomy, or postoperative trauma to the eye.[3,4]

Complications of malpositioned and dislocated anterior chamber lenses include uveitis, glaucoma, hyphema, cystoid macular edema (CME), and corneal decompensation. While a full-blown UGH syndrome is also possible,[5] complications of dislocated posterior-chamber IOLs (PC IOLs) tend to be less severe and are primarily optical in character. For example, PC IOLs can induce diplopia from several causes including binocular symptoms of anisokonia or, by prismatic image displacement. Monocular symptoms are numerous, including blurred vision and monocular diplopia from a refracted image through the edge of the IOL competing with an image through the aphakic portion of the pupil. Decentration and glare may occur as a result of refractive or diffractive effects on the lens edge or, in older IOLs, positioning holes. Rarely, a well-centered IOL with the correct power may mysteriously cause a permanent positive or negative dysphotopsia severe enough to warrant IOL exchange. Similarly, undesired halos or glare may result from multifocal or accommodating IOLs. Patient whim can also lead to a lens explantation, for example, when a request is made to exchange a monofocal IOL for a presbyopic/correcting IOL.

Although surgical intervention is definitive, it is not the only approach available in the management of difficult IOL cases. Conservative observation and pharmacologic therapy should always be considered.[3,4] Many eyes with IOLs that dislocated into the vitreous cavity during the earlier days of implant surgery have maintained excellent aphakic-corrected vision with no surgical intervention. The course of action must reflect the type and location of the lens, the age and health of the patient, the symptoms, the visual acuity, the corneal endothelial health, the presence and severity of intraocular inflammation, and the status of the fellow eye. Conservative therapy such as observation may be appropriate for an eye with an anterior chamber lens that is associated with a peaked or oval pupil, as long as signs and symptoms of intraocular inflammation are absent. Pharmacologic management consisting of topical steroids may be indicated in the case of mild cell and flare that is unassociated with symptoms or with reduced vision. A trial with a nonsteroidal anti-inflammatory agent in combination with a steroid is justified as a first step in symptomatic pseudophakic CME. Edge-related reflections, diplopia, or glare may, in some cases, be managed successfully by topical apraclonidine or pilocarpine. Topical sodium chloride might be preferable to surgery in treating peripheral corneal edema associated with incipient corneal decompensation in an elderly, frail patient who has a low endothelial cell count.[6] The malpositioned iris-supported lens associated with refractive or inflammatory symptoms is less successfully managed by conservative measures because of our recognition that this design is inferior when compared with both open-loop anterior chamber and most other styles of posterior chamber lenses. However, the posterior dislocation of a single haptic of the Copeland lens or the loop of a Binkhorst or Medallion lens may be associated with posterior synechiae or a fixed pupil that acts to prevent dislocation of the optic. Sequential pharmacologic manipulation of the pupil can result in successful repositioning of these older lenses in selected instances.[6–8]

Decentered and dislocated PC IOLs have become more prevalent because these designs account for more than 98% of all lenses implanted in the United States today. The most common presenting complaint with decentration is unwanted optical images caused by the edge of the optic within the pupil. If the symptoms are infrequent and limited to the evening when the pupil is more dilated, the surgeon may elect to manage these patients conservatively by using a topical miotic. More severe or disabling symptoms can be managed by repositioning, explanting, or exchanging the IOL. When complete dislocation of a posterior chamber lens has occurred, historical options include:

1. observation and correction of monocular aphakia by external means
2. IOL repositioning
3. IOL exchange.[8–10]

Effective suturing techniques both for secondary placement of posterior chamber lenses and for repositioning of dislocated lenses have further increased the available options.[11,12]

In this chapter the authors discuss a technical approach to the management of IOL problems that requires surgical intervention.

GENERAL METHODS

PREOPERATIVE EVALUATION

All patients being considered for surgical correction of IOL problems require thorough preoperative evaluation, which includes the determination of a bilateral best-corrected visual acuity, slit-lamp biomicroscopy, gonioscopy, and dilated fundus ophthalmoscopy. Keratometry, topography, A-scan ultrasonography, specular microscopy with endothelial cell count, and, in some instances, potential acuity meter testing should be performed. Ultrasound biomicroscopy can offer valuable insights into the anatomic pathophysiology.[13,14] A review of the original operative report and knowledge of the lens power, style, A-constant, and location which it was originally placed, as well as the postoperative refraction may be useful in achieving a more emmetropic pseudophakic refractive error. IOL master axial length measurements have markedly improved our ability to choose an IOL power for an exchange in the already pseudophakic eye, especially when access to old records no longer exists.

On reviewing all information available, a surgical strategy with a preliminary plan can be made to reposition, remove, and/or exchange the IOL. When surgical intervention is under consideration, a decision must be made with regard to the timing of surgery, the approach (anterior versus posterior), the composition of the surgical team (cataract surgeon, vitreoretinal surgeon, or both)

and how to achieve the disposition of the pseudophakos (repositioning, replacement, or removal). If the pupil fails to dilate in the office, the procedure chosen to correct a malpositioned posterior chamber lens cannot always be finalized at the time of the preoperative examination and should be reassessed during surgery when the pupil is maximally dilated to allow direct visualization of the anatomic relationships. Poor visualization can be managed by either a Fry stretch technique,[17] the use of iris retractors, or a Malyugin ring.[17A] Occasionally, ocular endoscopy can be very helpful in gathering useful anatomic information. Adequate visualization is essential for understanding the pathophysiology of the malpositioned posterior chamber lens and for correcting the underlying problem.

In addition to correcting the IOL problem, the surgeon should take advantage of the opportunity and also correct residual refractive error. Moderate or high astigmatism can be reduced by incision placement, astigmatic keratotomy, limbal relaxing incisions, or even an exchange for a toric IOL. In addition to improving the refractive error, surgical intervention may accomplish other objectives. Synechiae can be separated, the capsular bag can be reopened, Soemmerring's material can be removed, and the posterior capsule can be vacuumed or polished. An iris defect may be repaired by an imbricating suture or even a prosthetic iris device. A pupil can be enlarged, made smaller, or translocated. Zonular weakness can be addressed with a capsular tension ring (CTR).

SURGICAL TECHNIQUES

ANTERIOR CHAMBER INTRAOCULAR LENS

Repositioning of an anterior chamber lens should be performed when a haptic incarcerates iris tissue, when iris has acutely prolapsed into the incision, when the anterior-chamber intraocular lens (AC IOL) haptic migrates through the iridectomy causing decentration, or when the haptic migrates anteriorly contacting the corneal endothelial surface. If diagnosed early, iris incarceration and haptic malposition can be corrected by flexing, lifting, and repositioning the offending haptic. Intolerable optical images might occasionally be corrected by the repositioning of the iris and AC IOL; however, explantation may be required to eliminate unacceptable symptoms.

Although repositioning might suffice in selected cases, IOL explantation is necessary when the lens size is wrong. Lens movement or "propellering" indicates that the lens is too small, while severe tenderness, pupil ovalization, and indentation of the ciliary body suggest that the lens is too large and rigid. Explantation of an AC IOL is also necessary when the lens is associated with chronic UGH syndrome that is resistant to medical therapy.[8,11]

Exchange of an AC IOL depends on the style of the implant and whether any of the haptics are encased in synechiae. The closed-loop anterior chamber lenses, most notably the Azar (91Z), the Leiske, and the Stableflex, have loop haptics that may become enveloped by peripheral anterior synechiae. When synechiae are present, the explantation technique involves severing the haptics from the optic to remove the lens in pieces, thereby avoiding bleeding, iridodialysis, and severe damage to the angle. This can be achieved with an intraocular scissors or by using the YAG laser preoperatively.[16] The optic should be manipulated carefully because the severed haptics are sharp and

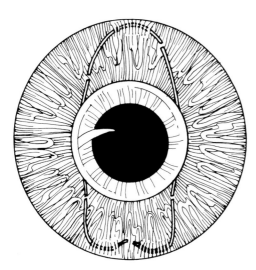

Figure 46-1 Anterior chamber lens with filamentous haptics encased by peripheral anterior synechiae. Scissors are used to sever the haptic from the optic.

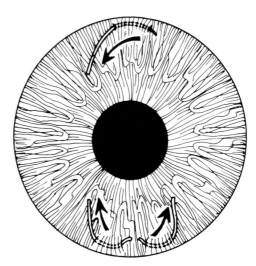

Figure 46-2 After removal of the optic, the severed haptics are backthreaded into the anterior chamber and removed.

potentially hazardous. With viscoelastic material filling the anterior chamber, a spatula placed under the optic serves as a ramp to prevent snagging of the posterior lip of the incision during removal. Since almost all AC IOLs are made of polymethylmethacrylate (PMMA), the incision will need to accommodate the size of the rigid optic, which must be removed in one piece. Once the optic has been explanted, the remaining haptics are threaded back through the synechial tunnels until they are free in the anterior chamber where they can be easily and safely removed (Figures 46-1 and 46-2).

If a posterior capsular remnant is present and offers adequate peripheral support, the AC IOL may be exchanged for a PC IOL. Suture fixation of a posterior chamber lens to either the iris or ciliary sulcus is an excellent option, especially in a patient with glaucoma or with an abnormal anterior segment (e.g., extensive synechiae, angle recession).[17–22] If the posterior capsule is intact and the capsular membranes are fused, sulcus fixation may suffice. Posterior optic capture also provides an elegant alternative by creating a primary posterior capsulorrhexis with capture of the PC IOL optic through the opening.[23]

IRIS-SUPPORTED LENSES

These IOLs are rarely seen today. As a general rule, a dislocated or malpositioned iris-supported lens should be either explanted or exchanged for an anterior or posterior chamber lens. Surgical repositioning of these lenses can be considered in situations where a more extensive explantation-exchange procedure may be risky, such as in an elderly patient with a dangerously low endothelial cell count. In such an instance, the main surgical principle in these eyes (which have invariably undergone previous intracapsular surgery) is to perform minimal manipulation. Before repositioning the IOL an air bubble may be injected through a paracentesis incision to avoid having to deal with the exposed vitreous face. Alternatively, a dispersive ophthalmic viscosurgical device (OVD) can be used since the chance of IOP rise postoperatively will be less than with other agents. If vitreous gel is present and entangled around the IOL, a vitrectomy should be

performed first to prevent traction on the vitreous base and possible retinal detachment. Two microhooks introduced through strategically placed limbal stab incisions are effective for haptic manipulation. These incisions are made just anterior to the corneoscleral junction to avoid bleeding into the eye. One hook is used to retract and depress the iris, while the other elevates and decenters the optic in the opposite direction. The haptics are repositioned, and the pupil is pharmacologically constricted to ensure IOL fixation.

When an iris-fixated IOL is associated with chronic irritation or progressive endothelial cell loss, explantation is the procedure of choice. Separation of posterior synechiae, often in conjunction with an anterior vitrectomy, aids in achieving atraumatic explantation. Retrieval of the lens dislocated into the anterior vitreous can be accomplished using a two-stab anterior approach by ensnaring the visible haptic with a C-shaped hook and ushering the lens back through the pupil and into the anterior chamber. A second hook is then placed under the lens, which reduces the possibility of "losing" the lens. Once the lens is forward, the pupil is constricted with an intracameral miotic trapping the lens in the anterior chamber. At this point, it is safe to open the eye and to remove the lens using a second instrument as a ramp and removing all vitreous adhesions with a mechanical cutter. Significant vitreous entanglement or more posteriorly dislocated iris supported IOLs are best managed with primary vitrectomy techniques as described for dislocated posterior chamber lenses in a subsequent section. Following removal of a dislocated iris-supported lens, either anterior chamber lens implantation or posterior chamber lens implantation with scleral or iris suture support can be performed at the surgeon's discretion (Figure 46-3).

POSTERIOR-CHAMBER INTRAOCULAR LENSES

REPOSITIONING

Repositioning a lens should always be considered as an alternative to an exchange procedure. Repositioning a PC IOL that is decentered secondary to asymmetric haptic fixation may be

SURGICAL TECHNIQUES

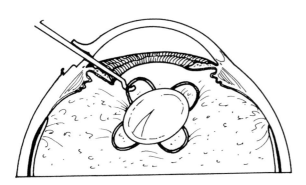

Figure 46-3 Removal of the dislocated iris-fixated lens from the anterior vitreous cavity by a limbal approach using a C-hook.

accomplished by several different methods. If the capsular bag is intact, it is usually possible to inject a less retentive OVD into the bag just beneath the anterior capsule. Unless there is a tear in the capsule, or a previous can-opener capsulotomy, the capsular bag can generally be re-opened. The IOL can be either rotated into the bag or into the sulcus where symmetric haptic fixation will result in centration of the lens. A useful trick is to engage the displaced haptic in the crotch of an Osher curved Y-hook (Bausch & Lomb Y hook STORZ E577), (Duckworth & Kent Y hook, P2443A6-471) while the right hand dials the lens clockwise. The curved Y-hook compresses and lowers the haptic, repositioning it into the bag. Alternatively, the IOL haptics can be rotated into the sulcus (Figure 46-4) with an option of capturing the optic within the anterior capsulorrhexis.

There are many situations where the IOL can be repositioned. The single-piece acrylic IOL that has been inadvertently placed into the ciliary sulcus can be repositioned by reopening the bag with OVD then manipulating the soft, highly flexible haptics. Any IOL captured by the pupil can also be repositioned. An IOL inadvertently inserted backwards can be "summersaulted" using the protection of a retentive OVD to fill the chamber and bag. A small IOL that has decentered in a gigantic capsular bag

can be repositioned by creating either an anterior or posterior optic capture. A slight power shift will occur when prolapsing an optic backwards into the bag or forward, creating an anterior capture through the capsulorrhexis.

If the posterior capsule is open, the capsular bag cannot be reopened since injected OVD will enter the vitreous cavity. Still it is often possible to reposition an IOL. For example, if a single-piece lens is decentered within the torn capsular bag, the optic may be prolapsed forward and captured within an intact capsulorrhexis. An acute central tear may in some cases be converted to a primary posterior capsulorrhexis and the optic may be captured posteriorly. Even when the tear has extended peripherally, it is sometimes possible to snag the optic between two flaps of capsule or a three-piece lens can be repositioned into the ciliary sulcus. A single-piece AcrySof lens should not be placed into the ciliary sulcus because of its thick, square-edged haptics and small overall diameter. A long-standing capsular tear may allow a new capsulotomy to be created in the fused anterior and posterior capsules, presenting another opportunity for optic capture.

Repositioning a decentered PC IOL can also be accomplished by a Lasso Suture, first described by Osher in a Video Symposium on Malpositioned IOLs at the annual meeting of the AAO in 1997.[24] A double-armed 10-0 prolene suture is passed through a stab incision, the first needle going behind the optic and exiting through the ciliary sulcus out through the sclera. The second needle is passed through the same stab incision but the needle is directed above the haptic before exiting through the ciliary sulcus adjacent to the first pass. The externalized arms of the sutures are cinched up ensnaring the haptic, which is tied to the scleral wall. This knot is trimmed and rotated into the sclera. Alternatively, the sutures can be passed beneath a scleral flap.

Subsequently, Steinert modified the lasso suture for the specific case of suture stabilizing a fully in-the-bag IOL. This scenario can occur after trauma, but is most common in the presence of pseudoexfoliation. The IOL-capsule complex may dislocate many years after uncomplicated surgery. In the Steinert technique, a 10-0 polypropylene suture on a long, gently curved needle is

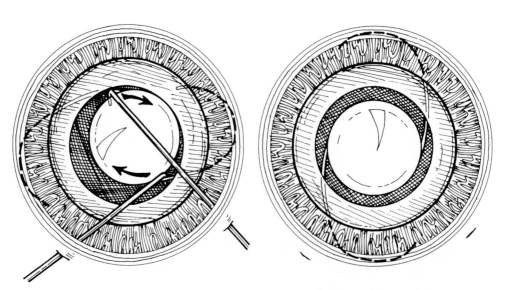

Figure 46-4 Two-hook rotation of a malpositioned posterior-chamber intraocular lens in the ciliary sulcus.

inserted *ab externo* through the ciliary sulcus and directed behind the haptic, up through the capsule between haptic and optic, and then exits through a paracentesis. The needle is then reversed and passed back *ab interno* through the ciliary sulcus approximately 1.5 mm lateral to the first pass. The suture is tied with four square single throws and then rotated beneath the sclera, so that only a conjunctival flap is needed to cover the suture securely. This maneuver is repeated for the second haptic.

There are many other variations of suturing the loop or plate haptics of a decentered PC IOL through the ciliary sulcus to the scleral wall.[25-31] A haptic can be externalized through a stab incision where a knot can secure the haptic to the sclera before repositioning the lens. Other elegant suturing techniques for repositioning a subluxed IOL within the capsular bag secondary to pseudoexfoliation syndrome have been described by Steinert and others.[32-34] A clever technique avoiding conjunctival dissection has been described by Hoffman,[34A] while Agarwal has published a technique of fixating a PC IOL beneath scleral flaps with fibrin glue.[34B] Osher described using a CTR to stabilize an IOL by creating artificial zonules[35] and Fine has described repositioning a subluxed IOL/bag/CTR complex by suturing the ring back to the scleral wall.[34]

The technique of repositioning a PC IOL by fixating the haptics to iris first described by Stark has become very popular.[36-38] The optic of the PC IOL is captured through the pupil and a retentive OVD like Healon 5 is injected into the anterior chamber. The haptics behind the iris become visibile as the OVD deepens the chamber compressing the iris against the haptics. Using a modification of the Siepser suture technique each haptic is secured to the mid peripheral iris (too proximal a pass will result in a "cat's eye" pupil).[39] Finally, the optic is dunked through the pupil and centered in the posterior chamber while the iris provides suture support.

A final word of caution is necessary when the surgeon is attempting to use the ciliary sulcus when the capsular bag has been torn. Most contemporary posterior chamber IOLs have a shorter overall length than the older style lenses which were often 13.5 mm or 14 mm. To ensure that the lens is centered and well supported, the Osher "bounce test" (Figure 46-5) is performed by gently and deliberately decentering the optic toward each haptic which should result in spontaneous recentration. Failure to recenter indicates either a serious problem with the capsular support, permanent deformation of the lens haptic, or inadequate sizing, each of which may indicate the need for suture fixation, explantation, or exchange depending on the nature of the problem. Alternatively, optic capture can be considered.

EXPLANTATION/EXCHANGE

In many instances, repositioning a dislocated PC IOL may not be possible or desirable. This may be related either to structural abnormalities of the implant or to co-existing ocular conditions that necessitate removal and/or exchange. The dislocated lens may have pre-existing structural damage to the haptic, as a result of haptic distortion or breakage precluding adequate refixation. When repositioning is not possible, exchange of the PCIOL for another posterior chamber lens is our strong preference when adequate residual peripheral capsulozonular support is present. This can best be determined when the pupil is widely dilated and after all posterior synechiae between iris and capsule are separated intraoperatively to reconstruct a full-sized posterior chamber. Direct inspection of the peripheral retroiridal anatomy indicates the best axis for implantation and where best fixation of the IOL may be achieved. Provided there is sufficient residual capsular support, three-piece acrylic foldable or a single-piece all-PMMA IOL with a large optic (6–6.5 mm) with a large diameter (12.5–13.5 mm) is preferable to either an anterior chamber lens or a sutured posterior chamber lens. However, there is recent evidence to support the safety of using anterior chamber lenses in these challenging cases.[40] Today it would be rare to explant a lens without also performing an exchange.

EXCHANGE OF THE POSTERIOR-CHAMBER INTRAOCULAR LENS WHEN THE BAG IS INTACT

The most common reason necessitating exchange is inadvertent IOL power miscalculation with either anisometropia or patient

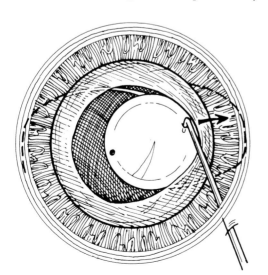
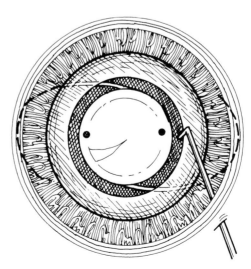

Figure 46-5 The "bounce" test used to ensure that a repositioned posterior-chamber intraocular lens spontaneously recenters.

dissatisfaction. Although some surgeons prefer implanting a piggy back IOL to compensate for the power error this may lead to interface opacification, and undesired optical phenomena especially with a multifocal IOL (MIOL). Sometimes, a monofocal in-the-bag PCIOL will be exchanged for an MIOL based upon a patient's strong desire for presbyopic IOL correction. Preservation of the capsular bag integrity is of utmost importance. Reopening the capsular bag can be performed by pressurizing the anterior chamber with an OVD, then viscodissecting the capsular bag open. A variety of OVDs will perform this task suitably and it may be left to surgeon's discretion. Occasionally, the anterior capsulorrhexis is difficult to elevate from the anterior optic surface of an acrylic PCIOL. Slipping a thin spatula under the edge can achieve a separation. When the adherence seems too tight for this, the capsulorrhexis margin can be gently lifted off the optic using the non-beveled side of the end of a 25- or 30-gauge needle. The OVD cannula can then be slipped under the capsular edge and the bag is expanded. Viscodissection is frequently required in all quadrants and may be accessed by multiple paracenteses or by using different cannula configurations.

Once the capsular bag has been opened, the method of removing the optic depends on whether it is foldable or not. The PMMA optic requires an incision of similar size as the diameter of the optic. Several options exist for the removal of the foldable optics through a smaller incision. Transection with either a scissors or a snare can be achieved under viscoelastic protection before removing each half. Jack Dodick popularized the Hinge technique in which the optic is partially transected leaving the distal fifth intact. When one half of the optic is grasped and ushered into the incision, the other half hinges open and follows.[41]

Paul Ernest developed a clever method for intraocular folding of the IOL.[42] Using OVD protection the lens is maneuvered into the anterior chamber where the superior haptic is prolapsed out of the incision. Next, a spatula is passed under the optic from a side port incision placed across from the primary incision, and a lens insertion forceps is introduced through the main incision over the optic. Upward force of the spatula combined with the downward force of the forceps results in re-folding of the optic, which can then be rotated 90° and explanted.

Another innovative technique was developed by Shuichiro Eguchi. After prolapsing the proximal haptic into the anterior chamber, a radial scissors cut is made in the optic. The lens is then rotated, and a second radial cut is made in the optic 90° away. One-quarter of the lens is explanted and the remaining three-quarters of the lens is rotated out through the small incision.[43]

Crisscross lensectomy is a technique for explanting a silicone plate lens through a small incision developed by Robert Osher utilizing the Eguchi principle.[44] The surgeon makes a radial incision along the longitudinal axis of the lens, rotates the lens 90°, and makes a second radial incision which intersects with the first, freeing a rectangle of the IOL which can be removed. The lens is rotated another 90° and a third radial incision is made along the longitudinal axis. A final 90° rotation allows the last radial incision to intersect and a second rectangle is explanted. The remaining segment of the lens can be maneuvered out through the small incision. The authors have found that the Osher IOL serrated cutting scissors (Duckworth & Kent P1870B) is very effective in cutting either silicone or acrylic material. The serrated blade reduces the tendency of the lens to tilt during the cut.

EXCHANGE OF THE POSTERIOR-CHAMBER INTRAOCULAR LENS WHEN THE BAG IS TORN

The intraoperative findings and the behavior of the IOL will determine whether it can be repositioned or must be explanted. If a lens with a known C or J-loop haptic fails to easily rotate, it is likely that the haptic is either snagged within the zonules or protruding through a tear in the zonules or the capsular bag. Reverse rotation followed by decentration toward the ensnared haptic and then re-rotation can sometimes free it. The lens can then be rotated 90° and a "bounce test" can be performed to confirm centration and fixation. If the haptic has an eyelet or bulbous tip, removal may be more difficult. Continued resistance to rotation indicates that haptic amputation is necessary and the piecemeal removal of the lens may be required. When the severed haptic is stuck within an intact bag, an attempt should be made to inject viscoelastic material under an edge, which often opens the bag, allowing retrieval. Gentle perseverance under the protection of an OVD may enable successful removal, although leaving the amputated haptic behind is preferable to causing additional damage to the capsular bag.[44A]

Regardless of how the IOL is going to be removed, the surgeon must be prepared to deal with vitreous. If minimal vitreous prolapse is present, a dry vitrectomy using a limbal approach can be performed by filling the chamber with an OVD, through which the vitrectomy handpiece is inserted. This vitrectomy technique produces a more limited vitrectomy, with less of a tendency toward collapse of the globe. If vitreous fills the anterior chamber, a limbal bimanual vitrectomy with low-flow irrigation through a second stab incision can be performed.[45] Alternatively, the surgeon may perform the vitrectomy through the pars plana 3.5 mm posterior to the limbus. The surgeon should set the automated vitrector on "cut/IA" and utilize a high cutting rate with moderate vacuum settings. If the posterior capsule is open and vitreous has been removed, maintaining a pressurized anterior chamber is crucial to preventing further vitreous prolapse at the end of the case. OVD can be removed manually in small aliquots and exchanged for BSS or by bimanual irrigation and aspiration through paracenteses after the primary incision has been closed. Instillation of intraocular carbachol and topical medications can provide prophylaxis against an IOP spike following surgery.

Recently, Burk and colleagues described the use of Kenalog suspension (triamcinolone acetonide) to highlight vitreous present in the anterior chamber.[46] (See Chapter 45 for detailed discussion.)

MANAGEMENT OF THE POSTERIORLY LUXATED INTRAOCULAR LENS

Previous sections of this chapter have described many elegant and efficient techniques for the management of the malpositioned IOL when this subluxation is in the realm of the anterior segment – the anterior chamber, the iris plane, the ciliary sulcus, the level of the capsular bag, or at the level of the very anterior vitreous. In these instances, an anterior segment surgeon is well within her/his scope of practice when applying the principles and techniques described earlier in this chapter. When the pseudophakos is completely luxed posteriorly, is entangled in the vitreous, and/or is in contact with the retina, surgical techniques are required which fall into the scope of practice of the subspecialty trained vitreoretinal surgeon – alone or in combination with an anterior segment surgeon. Prior to proceeding with a brief description of these techniques, we will offer some of the considerations involved in deciding on how to manage the more posteriorly dislocated but not yet completely luxed lens implant. Today, a vast majority of the implants in this scenario are PC IOLs.

The individual attending surgeon bears the sole responsibility for deciding which surgical techniques to employ and which surgical cases to attempt. Each patient presents with his/her own unique fact pattern and requires an individualized approach for management. Each surgeon has their own surgical skill set and their own level of comfort with each of the surgical techniques which make up that skill set. Certainly a luxed PC IOL lying on the surface of the macula is best managed by prompt referral to a vitreoretinal surgeon. On the other hand, some anterior segment surgeons would (and should) feel confident managing a severely subluxed PC IOL dangling into the mid-vitreous cavity by one haptic in a patient in whom a previous complete PPVx had been performed and in whom both IOL haptics are easily visualized as not being engaged in vitreous (or residual vitreous skirt). The issue becomes more muddled when surgical management requires vitrectomy techniques. The key question is to determine how much vitrectomy needs to be performed.

The two predominant vitrectomy techniques available for the anterior segment surgeon are the limbal anterior vitrectomy and the limited pars plana anterior vitrectomy. With limbal anterior vitrectomy, the vitreous cutter is inserted into the anterior segment through a limbal incision, most often with the infusion "split", supplied via a separate limbal incision or paracentesis. With limited pars plana anterior vitrectomy, the vitreous cutter enters the eye through a single pars plana sclerotomy or trocar created 3 mm posterior to the surgical limbus. Irrigation is achieved with a cannula inserted into the anterior segment through a separate anterior segment wound. We suggest that purely anterior vitrectomy techniques be limited to the most basic anterior maneuvers and that strong consideration be given to using the limited pars plana anterior vitrectomy techniques in any case requiring manipulation of the anterior vitreous within the vitreous cavity. It is important to stress that neither of these two surgical techniques allow for a complete vitrectomy or for ANY amount of peripheral or posterior vitreous dissection. These limitations relate to the fluidics and the limited visualization inherent to these surgical techniques.

The most important consideration here is the position of the IOL and haptics relative to the vitreous. Careful attention should be paid to identifying if either of the IOL haptics is entangled in the vitreous base with meticulous scleral depressed peripheral retinal examination. If so, freeing the optic from vitreous with a limited anterior vitrectomy is not sufficient and manipulating the IOL without a more complete peripheral vitreous dissection can have disastrous consequences, including retinal detachment with giant retinal tear. Prompt referral to a vitreoretinal surgeon is appropriate.

The decision to proceed with anterior surgical techniques vs. involving a retinal surgeon rests on having the observational skills to accurately and reproducibly identify these and other important anatomical relationships preoperatively, intraoperatively and postoperatively. A simple mental experiment is useful in deciding how to proceed. Imagine a 65-year-old loved one who presents with a mild-to-moderate vitreous hemorrhage in the setting of an acute PVD. You examine the patient and find no retinal tears. How do you feel about this scenario? If you lose sleep and seriously think about a referral to a retinal surgeon, serious consideration should be given to deferring any pars plana vitrectomy in the setting of a subluxed IOL to that same retinal surgeon. If, on the other hand, you feel comfortable discussing the signs and symptoms of a retinal detachment and seeing your loved one back again in a few weeks, and are confident in your negative exam (even when you know that published series have long documented a 50–82% incidence of retinal tear in this scenario),[47-51] then considering limited pars plana anterior vitrectomy techniques may not be so unreasonable.

Special mention should be made of the recent development of 25- and 23-gauge pars plana vitrectomy techniques.[52-57] These technologies allow for transconjunctival trocar placement and allow for microincisional sutureless vitrectomy techniques and have already been employed for limited anterior pars plana vitrectomy.[58,59] The advantages and disadvantages of these new microincisional techniques remain to be elucidated.

If a luxed IOL is to be addressed using three port pars plana vitrectomy techniques, the first step is of course, a complete and meticulous core and peripheral vitrectomy. This, by definition includes peeling of the posterior hyaloid. A very careful peripheral dissection is then performed trimming the vitreous base and carefully disengaging the IOL optic and both IOL haptics from all vitreous attachments. The IOL is then mobilized anteriorly by the placement of a bubble of perfuoro-n-octane, allowing the bubble to float the IOL anteriorly[62] (Figure 46-6), or with a combination of aspiration from the vitreous cutter, or with an extrusion cannula and manipulation with forceps. Once the IOL has been retrieved, it is either repositioned (with or without suture fixation), or explanted and exchanged for a primarily sutured PCIOL or ACIOL.

Whether IOL repositioning or replacement is initially planned, the preoperative planning should include appropriate measurements and calculations for a replacement IOL, in the event that repositioning cannot be successfully achieved. The precise lens type and

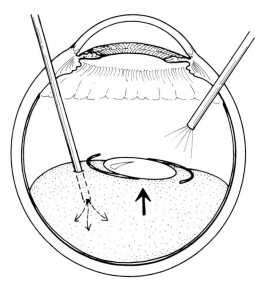

Figure 46-6 Perfluorocarbon liquid flotation of dislocated posterior-chamber intraocular lens into anterior vitreous cavity.

dioptric power of the luxed IOL should also be ascertained. Considerations in the decision to reposition or replace a lens include the structural stability of the lens, the size, and the haptic design. For example, foldable silicone lenses are less amenable to repositioning than all-PMMA lenses because of their greater inherent structural instability. Lenses with smaller optical zones and interhaptic distances are more likely to produce optical edge effects and to be less stable when suspended by scleral sutures than other styles. Similarly, very thin or shortened haptics, particularly older-style J-loops, as well as single piece acrylic lenses are less amenable to primary suture fixation than other styles.

A variety of techniques have been described for repositioning lenses that are displaced into the vitreous.[60–73] Fixation options have been described previously in this chapter including; iris fixation, scleral suture fixation or residual capsular fixation.

In cases of progressive zonulopathy, such as pseudoexfoliation syndrome, a subluxation of the implant lens contained within the capsular bag complex may occur. This can occur, even when the capsular bag contains a capsular tension ring. If the subluxation is mild, a suture can be passed through the capsular bag periphery around the apex of the haptic or around any point of the CTR, then passed transclerally. The other end of the double-armed suture is passed through the sclera and then tied externally. A number of differing suture-passing techniques through the bag and around the haptic/CTR can be equally effective, including some ab externo approaches and suture-docking procedures. When the zonular damage is profound, it is sometimes more facile to remove the entire IOL/bag complex, either in toto or in pieces and exchange the IOL/bag complex for a sutured PC IOL.

The results of several published surgical series on primary positioning by a pars plana route are summarized in Table 46-1. Of 282 eyes with dislocated IOLs, treated by either exchange or repositioning with either scleral or iris fixation to supplement sulcus repositioning, 165 (58%) achieved 20/40 or better final vision. Fifty-seven of 282 (20%) developed CME, which was usually transient and responsive to medical therapy, and 19 (6.7%) developed a retinal detachment postoperatively. Postoperative retinal detachments developed between 10 days and 2 years after surgery, although most occurred within the 2 months of IOL repositioning or exchange. Other reported complications of ciliary sulcus repositioning by a pars plana route with scleral fixation sutures include lens tilt, redislocation, suture erosion, retinal phototoxicity, persistent intraocular pressure elevation, corneal opacification, iris capture, epiretinal membrane formation, suture exposure, persistent uveitis, wound leak with hypotony, choroidal effusions, and vitreous hemorrhage.

DISCUSSION

Surgical treatment of malpositioned and dislocated IOLs remains an important and challenging clinical problem. Several previous publications have summarized the reasons for IOL removal. Although there are many common themes the details are notably affected by the date of the study, and the type of IOL used.

Solomon et al. evaluated 2500 explant cases at the Center for Intraocular Lens Research between 1982 and 1988. Anterior chamber lenses accounted for 59% and were usually explanted because of pseudophakic bullous keratopathy or inflammatory complications. Iris-fixated lenses represented 21%, whereas

Table 46-1 Results of vitrectomy and repositioning for posteriorly dislocated IOLs

Authors	Patients (*n*)	Method	VA ≥20/40	Comments
Sternberg and Michels (1986)	5	Iris/haptic fixation	5/5	
Smiddy and Flynn (1991)	4	Sclera/haptic fixation	3/4	
Maguire et al (1991)	6	Sclera/haptic fixation	4/6	Prior retinal damage in 2/6 eyes
Chan (1992)	12	Sclera/haptic fixation	11/12	CME in 3/12 eyes
Lewis and Sanchez (1993)	8	Sclera/positioning hole fixation; temporary perfluorocarbon	6/8	
Mello et al. (2000)	110 (72 in posterior segment)	Sclera or capsule/haptic fixation	63/110	Postoperative RD in 7/110 eyes CME 19/110 eyes
Thach et al. (2000)	78	Sclera/haptic fixation after temporary externalization of haptic		Postoperative RD in 5/78 eyes CME in 20/78 eyes
Sarrafizadeh et al. (2001)	59	Repositioned with (16) or without (13) sutures with scleral or capsule/haptic fixation Exchanged for sutured PC IOL (13) or AC IOL (17)	12/29 repositioned 19/30 exchanged	Nonrandomized case series comparing repositioning versus exchange of dislocated PC IOL; similar complication rates

CME, Cystoid macular edema; RD, retinal detachment; VA, visual acuity.

posterior-chamber lenses accounted for 20%. The latter were most frequently explanted because of decentration, malposition, or inflammation.[74]

Apple et al. showed that many anterior chamber lenses were explanted because of poor manufacturing, characterized by rough optic and haptic edges, which resulted in chronic iris chafing.[75]

Kraff et al. reported their results of explantation surgery in 1986, at which time anterior chamber lenses were most often removed as a result of corneal decompensation and chronic inflammation. Posterior chamber lenses, which represented only 20% of those explanted in the survey by Kraff et al., were removed because of dislocation, decentration, or incorrect power.[76]

Mamalis et al. reviewed 102 explanted lenses between 1982 and 1989. Anterior chamber lenses, which represented 66.7% of the series, were removed because of pseudophakic bullous keratopathy, UGH syndrome, and CME. Iris-supported lenses made up 17.6%, with pseudophakic bullous keratopathy representing the most frequent reason for removal. PC IOLs represented 15.7% of the explanted lenses, and the underlying cause was most often lens dislocation or decentration. Although approximately 70% of these patients underwent IOL exchange, the overall visual outcome showed that 39% experienced improvement, 46% were unchanged, and 15% showed a worsening of vision following surgery. The most common cause of further visual deterioration was corneal decompensation followed by glaucoma and CME. It was noteworthy that 90% of patients who underwent exchange with a PC IOL had a successful clinical outcome.[77]

In a series of 1400 implant cases published in 1980, Kline and Yang found a 1.7% incidence of lens removal. Corneal edema, CME, uveitis, and iris erosion were the most common causes for explantation.[78]

Smiddy and Flynn reviewed 32 cases of posterior dislocation of posterior chamber lenses. Management consisted of conservative observation without surgery in two eyes, repositioning in 19 eyes, exchange in eight eyes, and explantation without exchange in three eyes. The visual acuity of 20/40 or better was achieved in 69% of eyes in their study.[79]

Doren, Stern, and Driebe reviewed 101 consecutive explantations performed between 1983 and 1987. The majority of lenses removed were anterior chamber styles (53.9%) and iris-fixated lenses (33.7%). Pseudophakic bullous keratopathy was the main reason for explantation (69%) followed by UGH syndrome (9%) and IOL instability (7%). The best visual outcome was attained in eyes with an unstable IOL, half of which attained visual acuity of 20/40 or better. The poorest visual outcome was seen in eyes with UGH syndrome. Although 83% of the eyes in the latter group failed to attain acuity better than 20/200, even these patients benefited by the resolution of pain and better control of the intraocular pressure.[80]

Sinskey, Amin, and Stoppel conducted a retrospective review of 79 patients who underwent IOL exchange. Sixty-one percent were posterior chamber lenses, and 39% were anterior chamber lenses; these were replaced by posterior chamber (76%) and anterior chamber (24%) lenses. Indications for lens exchange included eccentric or displaced IOL (42%), endothelial decompensation (28%), incorrect IOL power (13%), and UGH syndrome (10%). The postoperative visual acuity was better than or equal to 20/30 in 72%, whereas 8% had a loss of one or more lines of visual acuity. Complications encountered following lens exchange included retinal detachment in four eyes, glaucoma in 14 eyes, corneal decompensation in three eyes, and anisometropia in one eye.[81]

Lyle and Jin published a series of eyes undergoing IOL exchange with and without penetrating keratoplasty in 1992. Of the 56 eyes that underwent IOL exchange without penetrating keratoplasty, the type of lens explanted was an AC IOL in 41%, an iris-supported IOL in 14%, and a PC IOL in 45%. The most frequent indications were dislocation of the lens in 20 eyes (36%), incorrect power in 14 eyes (25%), and CME in 11 eyes (20%). The geometric mean visual acuity improved from 20/61 preoperatively to 20/43 postoperatively. A visual acuity of 20/40 or better was attained in 69%, and 46% of eyes gained two or more lines. The main reason for a visual acuity of less than 20/200 was CME (four eyes). The authors noted a better prognosis if either the original lens was a PC IOL or if the original lens was exchanged for a PC IOL. The most frequent complications following explantation included hyphema (23%), CME (18%), posterior capsule opacification (13%), and glaucoma (9%). Isolated cases of choroidal detachment, endophthalmitis, retinal detachment, and lens dislocation also occurred.[82]

Marques et al. studied 49 eyes which had had IOL exchange between 1986 and 2002 performed by the same surgeon. The mean interval between surgeries was 53.8 months and the mean follow-up, 35.6 months. There were 15 eyes with an AC IOL and 34 eyes with a PC IOL originally. The mean interval between the primary surgery and IOL explantation was 82.3 months in the AC IOL group and 37.9 months in the PC IOL group. The main reason for IOL exchange was inflammation (53.3%) in the AC IOL group, and dislocation/decentration (85.3%) in the PC IOL group. The preoperative best corrected visual acuity was similar in both groups, and visual acuity was maintained or improved in 80%. Vitreous prolapse was the main intraoperative complication. The primary indication for IOL exchange was intraocular inflammation in patients with an AC IOL and IOL malposition in patients with a PC IOL.[83]

Dislocation of an IOL with the capsular bag is a late complication of cataract surgery, reported with increasing frequency in recent years. Gimbel et al. reported an identified predisposing condition in 90% of reviewed cases. Pseudoexfoliation was the most common cause, accounting for more than 50% of cases. Other common conditions were uveitis, myopia, and other diseases associated with progressive zonular weakening and capsular contraction. Capsular tension rings probably help but do not prevent this complication. An AC IOL was implanted in 48% of the cases and sutured PC IOL in 26% of the eyes included in this review.[84]

Gross et al. carried out a multicenter analysis of 25 eyes of 22 patients with dislocation of the PC-IOL encased within the capsular bag, secondary to dehiscence of the zonules supporting the capsular bag. They concluded that in-the-bag PC-IOL dislocations are an unusual, sometimes bilateral, late complication of cataract surgery and the most common associated condition was pseudoexfoliation. The dislocated in-the-bag PC-IOL was replaced with an anterior chamber intraocular lens in 60% or repositioned/exchanged and scleral fixated in 40% of eyes. Associated conditions included pseudoexfoliation syndrome 44%, uveitis 16%, and trauma 16%. There was no identifiable cause in 24% of eyes.[85]

Dick et al. reported on a survey of the German Society of Ophthalmic Surgeons which determined that the most common

CONCLUSIONS

reasons for the exchange of foldable monofocal IOLs were lens opacification in 2000, and incorrect IOL power in 2001. In addition to incorrect IOL power and decentration, IOL opacification of hydrophilic IOLs accounted for a very high percentage of the explantations (46%).[86]

The results of a 2001 and a 2003 survey of the American Society of Cataract and Refractive Surgery members and the European Society of Cataract and Refractive Surgeons were reported by Mamalis. The most common complications associated with foldable IOLs that required explantation or secondary intervention were residual ametropia followed by malpositioning and lens opacification.[87,88]

This increased importance of incorrect refractive error as a reason for IOL exchange was corroborated by Jin et al. who evaluated 51 eyes that underwent IOL exchange between January 1998 and December 2004. The overall rate of IOL exchange was 0.77% for all cataract surgeries. Incorrect IOL power (41.2%), decentration/dislocation (37.3%), and glare (7.8%) were the most common indications for IOL exchange. An AC-IOL was used in 14 eyes (27.5%) and a PC-IOL in 37 eyes (72.5%) for IOL exchange. None of the PC-IOLs were sutured to the sclera or iris. Overall, 90.2% of patients obtained a best-spectacle corrected visual acuity (BSCVA) of 20/40 or better. All eyes in the AC-IOL group and 94.6% of eyes in PC-IOL group achieved a visual acuity of between −1 and +5 lines of the pre-exchange vision. The authors suggest that an open-loop flexible AC-IOL poses no greater risk than PC-IOL with respect to visual outcome and safety for IOL exchange.[89]

More recently, Jin et al. evaluated patients who underwent IOL exchange for unexpected postoperative refractive errors. Of 22 cases, the identifiable reasons included: keratometry errors in 5 (23%) and incorrect axial length (AL) determination in 3 (14%). Three other postoperative refractive surprises occurred because the wrong IOL was implanted. After IOL exchange, 82% (18/22) of eyes were within ±0.50 diopters (D) and 86% (19/22) within ±1.00 D of emmetropia. Uncorrected visual acuity was 20/40 or better in 82% of eyes, and BSCVA was 20/40 or better in 95% (21/22) of eyes.[90]

CONCLUSIONS

As ophthalmic surgical practice continues to evolve, a gradual shift has been seen in the frequency and reasons for repositioning or exchanging IOLs. Fortunately, the incidence of pseudophakic bullous keratopathy, UGH syndrome, chronic CME, and even "incorrect" IOL power continues to decline. That said, patient expectations are higher than ever, especially with the advent of presbyopic correcting IOLs. Patients expect excellent uncorrected visual acuity, and in the absence of pathology other than cataract, we are better equipped than ever to fulfill those expectations. Given this, it is incumbent upon surgeons to recognize the etiologies that may require IOL exchange, and make every possible effort to prevent its necessity. Furthermore, surgeons must rectify IOL problems, that are symptomatic, or that may create the potential for other ophthalmic pathology. Explantation of an IOL is always challenging, yet armed with knowledgeable preparation and meticulous ooperative technique the results are generally satisfying to both the patient and the surgeon.

References

[1] Brown DC, Swead JW. Intraocular lens implant exchanges. J Am Intraocul Implant Soc 1985;11:376–379.

[2] Werner L, Apple DJ, Crema AS, et al. Permanent blue discoloration of a hydrogel intraocular lens by intraoperative trypan blue. J Cataract Refract Surg 2002;28:1279–1286.

[3] Flynn Jr HW. Management and repositioning of posteriorly dislocated intraocular lenses. In: Stark WJ, Terry AC, Maumenee AE, editors. Anterior segment surgery: oils, lasers, and refractive keratoplasty. Baltimore: William & Wilkins; 1987. p. 321–329.

[4] Blumenkranz M, Maguire A. Modern management considerations in dislocation of crystalline and intraocular lenses. In: Stirpe M, editor. Advances in vitreoretinal surgery. Rome: Fondazione GB Bietti/Ophthalmic Communications Society; 1992. p. 39–46.

[5] Percival SP, Das SKJ. UGH syndrome after posterior chamber lens implantation. Am Intraocul Implant Soc 1983;9:200–201.

[6] Insler M, Benefield D, Ross V. Topical hyperosmolar solution in the reduction of corneal edema. LAO J 1987;13:149.

[7] Osher RH. Surgical management of the malpositioned posterior chamber lens. Audiovisual J Cataract Implant Surg 1991;VII.

[8] Ellington FR. The uveitis-glaucoma-hyphema syndrome associated with the Mark VIII anterior chamber lens implant. Am Intracellular Implant Soc J 1978;4:50.

[9] Keates RH, Ehrlich DR. "Lenses of change": complications of anterior chamber implants. Ophthalmology 1978;85:408.

[10] Percival SPK, Das SK. UGH syndrome after posterior chamber lens implantation. J Am Intraocul Implant Soc 1983;9:200.

[11] Koch DD. Scleral fixation of posterior chamber implants. Audiovisual J Cataract Implant Surg 1990;VI.

[12] Lubniewski AJ, Holland EJ, Van Meter WS, et al. Histologic study of eyes with transsclerally sutured posterior chamber intraocular lens. Am J Ophthalmol 1990;110:237–243.

[13] Ozdal PC, Mansour M, Deschenes J. Ultrasound biomicroscopy of pseudophakic eyes with chronic postoperative inflammation. J Cataract Refract Surg 2003;29:1185–1191.

[14] Loya N, Lichter H, Barash D, et al. Posterior chamber intraocular lens implantation after capsular tear: ultrasound biomicroscopy evaluation. J Cataract Refract Surg 2001;27:1423–1427.

[15] Fry L. Capsular stretching. VJCRS 1995;XI.

[16] Marques FF, Marques DM, Smith CM, Osher RH. Intraocular lens exchange assisted by preoperative neodymium:YAG laser haptic fracture. J Cataract Refract Surg 2004;30:247–249.

[17] Koch DD. Scleral fixation of posterior chamber implants. Audiovisual J Cataract Implant Surg 1990;VI.

[17A] Chang DF. Use of Malyugin pupil expansion device for intraoperative floppy-iris syndrome: results in 30 consecutive cases. J Cataract Refract Surg 2008;34:835–841.

[18] Price FW. Iris fixation of posterior chamber implants. Audiovisual J Cataract Implant Surg 1990;VI.

[19] Moretsky SL. Suture fixation technique for subluxated posterior chamber IOL through stab wound incision. J Am Intraocul Implant Soc 1984;10:455–480.

[20] Girard LJ, Nino N, Wesson M, et al. Scleral fixation of subluxed posterior chamber intraocular lens. J Cataract Refract Surg 1986;14:326–337.

[21] Anand R, Bowman RW. Simplified technique for suturing dislocated posterior chamber intraocular lens to the ciliary sulcus. Arch Ophthalmol 1990;108:1205–1206. [letter].

[22] Lubniewski AJ, Holland EJ, Van Meter WS, et al. Histologic study of eyes with transsclerally sutured posterior chamber intraocular lens. Am J Ophthalmol 1990;110:237–243.

[23] Gimbel HC, DeBroff BM. Intraocular lens optic capture. J Cataract Refract Surg 2004;30:200–206.

[24] Osher RH. Sewing through the capsular bag: a brief history. Cataract & Refract Surgery Today 2004;4:72–73.

[25] Hoffman RS, Fine IH, Packer M, Rozenberg I. Scleral fixation using suture retrieval through a scleral tunnel. J Cataract Refract Surg 2006;32:1259–1263.

[26] Hoffman RS, Fine IH, Packer M. Scleral fixation without conjunctival dissection. J Cataract Refract Surg 2006;32:1907–1912.

[27] Epley KD, Levine ES, Katz HR. A simplified technique for stable transscleral suture fixation of posterior chamber intraocular lenses. Ophthalmic Surg Lasers 1999;30:398–402.

[28] Chan CK, Agarwal A, Agarwal S, Agarwal A. Management of dislocated intraocular implants. Ophthalmol Clin North Am 2001;14:681–693.

[29] Hannush SB. Sutured posterior chamber intraocular lenses: indications and procedure. Curr Opin Ophthalmol 2000;11:233–240.

[30] Kulkarni K, Zarbin M, Del Priore LV, Tezel TH. Ab externo technique for accurate haptic placement of transscleral sutured posterior chamber intraocular lenses. Ophthalmic Surg Lasers Imaging 2007;38:72–75.

[31] Leon JA, Leon CS, Aron-Rosa D. Endoscopic technique for suturing posterior chamber intraocular lenses. J Cataract Refract Surg 2000;26:644–649.

[32] Arkin MS, Steinert RF. Sutured posterior chamber intraocular lenses. Int Ophthalmol Clin 1994;34:67–85.

[33] Gimbel HV, Condon GP, Kohnen T. Late in-the-bag intraocular lens dislocation: incidence, prevention, and management. J Cataract Refract Surg 2005;31:2193–2204.

[34] Fine IH, Hoffman RS. Phacoemulsification in the presence of pseudoexfoliation: challenges and options. J Cataract Refract Surg 1997;23:160–165.

[34A] Hoffman RS, Fine IH, Packer M. Scleral fixation without conjunctival dissection. J Cataract Refract Surg 2006;32:1907–1912.

[34B] Agarwal A, Kumar DA, Jacob S, et al. Fibrin glue-assisted sutureless posterior chamber intraocualr lens implantation in eyes with deficient posterior capsules. J Cataract Refract Surg 2008;34:1433–1438.

[35] Osher RH. Synthetic zonules. Ophthalmology Times 1997;15.

[36] Stark WJ, Goodman G, Goodman D, Gottsch J. Posterior chamber intraocular lens implantation in the absence of posterior capsular support. Ophthalmic Surg 1988;19:240–243.

[37] Stark WJ, Goodman G, Goodman D, Gottsch J. Posterior chamber intraocular lens implantation in the absence of posterior capsular support. Yan Ke Xue Bao 1989;5:19–23.

[38] Stark WJ, Gottsch JD, Goodman DF. Posterior chamber intraocular lens implantation in the absence of capsular support. Arch Ophthalmol 1989;107:1078–1083.

[39] Osher RH, Snyder ME, Cionni RJ. Modification of the Siepser slip-knot technique. J Cataract Refract Surg 2005;31:1098–1100.

[40] Kwong YY, Yuen HK, Lam RF, et al. Comparison of outcomes of primary scleral-fixated versus primary anterior chamber intraocular lens implantation in complicated cataract surgeries. Ophthalmology 2007;114:80–85, E Pub 2006, Oct 27.

[41] Batlan SJ, Dodick JM. Explantation of foldable silicone intraocular lens. Am J Ophthalmol 1996;122:270–272.

[42] Ernst P. Intraocular refolding. Video J Cataract Refractive Surg 1996;XII.

[43] Eguchi S. Quadrantotomy. VJCRS 2000;XVI.

[44] Osher RH. Criss-cross lensectomy. VJCRS 2005;XXI.

[44A] Trindade FC. Haptic-induced recurrent vitreous hemorrhage and increased intraocular pressure with a hydrophobic acrylic intraocular lens. J Cataract Refract Surg 2009;35:399–402.

[45] Snyder ME, Foster RE. Anterior vitrectomy. Comp Ophthalmol Update 2001;2:149–158.
[46] Burk SE, Da Mata AP, Snyder ME. Visualizing vitreous using Kenalog suspension. J Cataract Refract Surg 2003;29:645–651.
[47] Winslow RL, Taylor BC. Spontaneous vitreous hemorrhage: etiology and management. South Med J 1980;73:1450–1452.
[48] Butner RW, McPherson AR. Spontaneous vitreous hemorrhage. Ann Ophthalmol 1982;14:268–270.
[49] Dana MR, Werner MS, Viana MA, Shapiro MJ. Spontaneous and traumatic vitreous hemorrhage. Ophthalmology 1993;100:1377–1383.
[50] Lindgren G, Sjodell L, Lindblom B. A prospective study of dense spontaneous vitreous hemorrhage. Am J Ophthalmol 1995;119:458–465.
[51] Hasenfratz G. Acute vitreous hemorrhage – possibilities for differential diagnostic, echographic assessment. Fortschr Ophthalmol 1990;87:641–645.
[52] De Juan Jr E, Hickingbotham D. Refinements in microinstrumentation for vitreous surgery. Am J Ophthalmol 1990;109:218–220.
[53] Fujii GY, De Juan Jr E, Humayun MS, Chang TS, Pieramici DJ, Barnes A, et al. Initial experience using the transconjunctival sutureless vitrectomy system for vitreoretinal surgery. Ophthalmology 2002;109:1814–1820.
[54] Fujii GY, De Juan Jr E, Humayun MS, et al. A new 25-gauge instrument system for transconjunctival sutureless vitrectomy surgery. Ophthalmology 2002;109:1807–1812.
[55] Lakhanpal RR, Humayun MS, de Juan Jr E, et al. Outcomes of 140 consecutive cases of 25-gauge transconjunctival surgery for posterior segment disease. Ophthalmology 2005;112:817–824.
[56] Ibarra MS, Hermel M, Prenner JL, Hassan TS. Longer-term outcomes of transconjunctival sutureless 25-gauge vitrectomy. Am J Ophthalmol 2005;139:831–836.
[57] Eckardt C. Transconjunctival sutureless 23-gauge vitrectomy. Retina 2005;25:208–211.
[58] Chalam KV, Shah VA. Successful management of cataract surgery associated vitreous loss with sutureless small-gauge pars plana vitrectomy. Am J Ophthalmol 2004;138:79–84.
[59] Shah VA, Gupta SK, Chalam KV. Management of vitreous loss during cataract surgery under topical anesthesia with transconjunctival vitrectomy system. Eur J Ophthalmol 2003;13:693–696.
[60] Lewis H, Sanchez G. The use of liquid perfluorocarbon in the repositioning of posteriorly dislocated intraocular lenses. Ophthalmology 1993;100:1055–1059.
[61] Sternberg P, Michels RG. Treatment of dislocated posterior chamber intraocular lenses. Arch Ophthalmol 1986;104:1391–1393.
[62] Flynn HW, Buus D, Culbertson WW. Management of subluxated and dislocated intraocular lenses using pars plana vitrectomy instrumentation. Cataract Refract Surg 1990;16:51–56.
[63] Smiddy WE, Flynn HW. Needle assisted scleral fixation technique for relocating posteriorly dislocated IOLs. Arch Ophthalmol 1993;111:161–162.
[64] Smiddy W, Flynn H. Management of dislocated posterior chamber intraocular lenses. Ophthalmology 1991;98:889–894.
[65] Maguire AM, Blumenkranz MS, Ward TG, et al. Scleral loop fixation for posteriorly dislocated intraocular lenses. Arch Ophthalmol 1991;109:1754–1758.
[66] Chan CK. An improved technique for management of dislocated posterior chamber implants. Ophthalmology 1992;99:51–57.
[67] Smiddy WE, Ibanez GV, Alfonso E, et al. Surgical management of dislocated intraocular lenses. J Cataract Refract Surg 1995;21:64–69.
[68] Mello MO, Scott IU, Smiddy WE, et al. Surgical management and outcomes of dislocated intraocular lenses. Ophthalmology 2000;107:62–67.
[69] Thach AB, Dugel PU, Sipperley JO, et al. Outcome of sulcus fixation of dislocated posterior chamber intraocular lenses using temporary externalization of the haptics. Ophthalmology 2000;107:480–484.

[70] Sarrafizadeh R, Ruby AJ, Hassan TS, et al. A comparison of visual results and complications in eyes with posterior chamber intraocular lens dislocation treated with pars plana vitrectomy and lens repositioning or lens exchange. Ophthalmology 2001;108:82–89.
[71] Wong KL, Grabow HB. Simplified technique to remove posteriorly dislocated lens implants. Arch Ophthalmol 2001;119:273–274.
[72] Kokame GT, Atebara NH, Bennett MD. Modified technique of haptic externalization for scleral fixation of dislocated posterior chamber lens implants. Am J Ophthalmol 2001;131:129–131.
[73] Johnson MW, Schneiderman TE. Surgical management of posteriorly dislocated silicone plate intraocular lenses. Curr Opin Ophthalmol 1998;9:11–15.
[74] Solomon K, Apple D, Mamalis N, et al. Complications of intraocular lenses with special reference to an analysis of 2500 explanted intraocular lenses (IOLs). Eur J Implant Ref Surg 1991;3: 195–200.
[75] Apple DJ, Brems RN, Park RD, et al. Anterior chamber lenses. Part I. Complications and pathology and a review of designs. J Cataract Refract Surg 1987;13:157–173.
[76] Kraff M, Sanders DR, Lieberman HL, et al. Secondary intraocular lens implantation. Ophthalmology 1983;90:324–326.
[77] Mamalis N, Crandall A, Pulsipher M, et al. Intraocular lens explantation and exchange: a review of lens styles, clinical indications, clinical results, and visual outcome. J Cataract Refract Surg 1991;17:810–818.
[78] Kline OR, Yang HK. A review of 1400 intraocular lens implant cases. Contact Lens 1981;7: 262–278.
[79] Smiddy W, Flynn H. Management of dislocated posterior chamber intraocular lenses. Ophthalmology 1991;98:889–894.
[80] Doren G, Stern G, Driebe W. Indications for and results of intraocular lens exchanges. J Cataract Refract Surg 1992;18:79–85.
[81] Sinskey RM, Amin P, Stoppel JO. Indications for and results of a large series of intraocular lens exchanges. J Cataract Refract Surg 1993;19:68–71.
[82] Lyle W, Jin JC. An analysis of intraocular lens exchange. Ophthalmic Surg 1992;23:453–458.
[83] Marques FF, Marques DM, Osher RH, et al. Longitudinal study of intraocular lens exchange. J Cataract Refract Surg 2007;33:254–257.
[84] Gimbel HV, Condon GP, Kohnen T, et al. Late in-the-bag intraocular lens dislocation: incidence, prevention, and management. J Cataract Refract Surg 2005;31:2193–2204.
[85] Gross JG, Kokame GT, Weinberg DV. In-the-bag intraocular lens dislocation. Am J Ophthalmol 2004;137:630–635.
[86] Dick HB, Tehrani M, Brauweiler P, et al. Complications of foldable intraocular lenses requiring explantation. Results of the 2000 and 2001 survey in Germany. Ophthalmologe 2003;100: 465–470.
[87] Mamalis N. Complications of foldable intraocular lenses requiring explantation or secondary intervention – 2001 survey update. J Cataract Refract Surg 2002;28:2193–2201.
[88] Mamalis N, David B, Nislon CD, et al. Complications of foldable intraocular lenses requiring explantation or secondary intervention – 2003 survey update. J Cataract Refract Surg 2004; 30:2209–2218.
[89] Jin GJ, Crandall AS, Jones JJ. Changing indications for and improving outcomes of intraocular lens exchange. Am J Ophthalmol 2005;140:688–694.
[90] Jin GJ, Crandall AS, Jones JJ. Intraocular lens exchange due to incorrect lens power. Ophthalmology 2007;114:417–424, Epub 2006 Nov 21.

Issues in Wound Management

Douglas D. Koch, MD, Randall E. Nacke, MD, Li Wang, MD, PhD and Kenneth D. Novak, MD

47

CONTENTS

CHAPTER HIGHLIGHTS

>> Wound construction and endophthalmitis

>> Causes and prevention of wound leakage

>> Complications from dehiscence and their management

The cataract incision serves as more than just the port of access to the anterior segment. It affects ocular integrity and corneal stability. Wound construction is the critical determinant of wound integrity, and the two key elements of the wound are its size and architecture. Wound management following cataract surgery is required in cases of wound leakage, burns or dehiscence.

This chapter will review wound construction, mechanisms of wound healing, factors that can predispose to wound compromise, and the management of wound leakage, burns and dehiscence.

WOUND CONSTRUCTION

The traditional limbal or anterior scleral incision was designed for ready access to the anterior chamber and simple closure with radially oriented sutures. Two or three planes were incorporated into the incision, but the intrascleral (or intralimbal) portion was short (1 mm or less), and the site of entry into the anterior chamber was located near the iris root. In contrast, key elements of the self-sealing scleral tunnel incision include a long (>2 mm) intrascleral component and an anterior entry into the chamber.[1,2] The latter creates an internal corneal valve that is closed by intraocular pressure.

Stimulated in part by the advances in foldable lens design, the small incision (3.5 mm or less) has largely supplanted the traditional 6 to 7 mm incision. Initially, these incisions were simply small scleral tunnels, but the scleral tunnel has in turn largely been supplanted by clear-corneal incisions. Advantages of the clear-corneal incision include avoidance of the conjunctiva and sclera, allowing virtually bloodless surgery; easier access to the eye; safer surgery; and reduced operating time.

The principles of clear-corneal wound construction remain the same: create adequate tunnel length with an internal corneal valve to create a self-sealing wound. Several corneal incision constructions have been used: paracentesis incision, two-plane or grooved incision, hinged incision, and three-plane incision. Ernest et al.[3] showed that clear-corneal incisions demonstrated resistance to leakage comparable to similarly constructed scleral tunnel incisions.[4] In an animal model, Ernest el al.[3] evaluated the role of the site of external opening of the incision on incision healing and stability. They found that starting incisions in the vascular region (limbus) resulted in a fibroblastic response that enhanced incision stability and allowed rapid incision healing within 7 days postoperatively, compared with the 60 days of healing time required for incisions started in the avascular region (cornea). Their findings are compelling, but clinical studies have not yet been performed on the effect of the incision site on factors such as wound integrity and induced astigmatism.

WOUND HEALING

A scleral, limbal, or corneal incision creates a tissue gape that initiates a process of repair by tissue-addition. For scleral and limbal incisions, active wound healing begins within 48 h of surgery; the initial phase is the ingrowth of episcleral vascular tissue.[5,6] Over the next several weeks, this tissue fills the entire incision, creating a fibrovascular plug. Over the ensuing 2 or more years, remodeling occurs, resulting in reorientation of the wound healing collagen so that it becomes parallel to existing scleral collagen. Concurrently, vascularization and cellularity diminish.

At 1 week postoperatively, wound strength is approximately 10% of that found in normal nonincised tissue.[7–9] By 8 weeks postoperatively, this value is roughly 40%, and, by 2 years postoperatively, the wound has regained approximately 75 to 80% of its original strength. Therefore, although the wound is most vulnerable to dehiscence early in the postoperative period, depending

COMPROMISE OF WOUND INTEGRITY

on its size and construction, the cataract incision retains a permanent susceptibility to traumatic dehiscence.[10–12]

Corneal incisions heal by ingrowth of keratocytes,[3] which initially are oriented parallel to the incision and, therefore, perpendicular to lamellae of the cornea stroma. These keratocytes then undergo fibroblastic transformation and, over months, reorient themselves to become parallel to the corneal lamellae. Compared with scleral and limbal wound healing, the wound-healing process of the corneal incision is much slower and ultimately produces a weaker incision, as attested by the relative fragility of corneal graft wounds.

The clinical impact of this slower healing for cataract corneal wounds is not fully understood. For standard 2.5–3.5 mm corneal tunnel incisions, the small incision size and wound construction appear to largely or even fully compensate for the deficiencies in the corneal wound-healing process. However, it is probable that the slower healing of corneal incisions may predispose to problems with dehiscence in poorly constructed small incisions and in incisions longer than 4 mm. It is possible (but unproven to date) that there is greater against-the-wound astigmatic shift with corneal incisions compared with limbal or scleral wounds of the same size.

COMPROMISE OF WOUND INTEGRITY

WOUND LEAKAGE

A wound leak that occurs in the first few days postoperatively is usually due to an inadequate suture closure for that particular wound configuration.

The clinical signs of wound leak include poor vision, ocular hypotony, broad corneal folds, shallow anterior chamber, hyphema, choroidal effusions, choroidal folds, and optic nerve edema. The intraocular pressure is typically less than 5 mm Hg, but occasionally can be higher. The definitive diagnosis is made by instilling concentrated fluorescein, using either fluorescein strips or 2% fluorescein solution. Although both methods are equally effective, use of the solution avoids the sometimes cumbersome act of "painting" the incision with the fluorescein strip. One sign that we find particularly helpful is evaluation of the internal corneal valve: in the presence of a wound leak, the valve can be seen to be gaping with posterior displacement of the posterior portion of the wound. Gimbel, Sun, and DeBroff[13] recommended the use of gonioscopy to recognize internal wound gape during and after surgery.

The seal of the internal corneal valve is intraocular pressure dependent, and an apparently watertight wound can leak as a result of postoperative hypotony. The latter, in turn, can be caused by insufficient chamber inflation at the conclusion of the surgery, sluggish ciliary body function (itself often caused by hypotony), or accidental wound lip compression (e.g., eye rubbing) that leads to aqueous egress. Ultrasound biomicroscopy has been reported to be helpful in detecting a subtle wound leak as a cause of chronic hypotony in a patient 1 year after cataract surgery by phacoemulsification.[14] Using ocular coherence tomography (OCT), Taban et al. examined various self-sealing incisions over various intraocular pressures and found that higher IOP was associated with more tightly sealed wounds in general. Furthermore, larger angle (more perpendicular) incisions sealed better at lower IOP while, conversely, smaller angle (less perpendicular) incisions sealed better at higher IOP.[15]

At multiple junctures during cataract surgery, the corneal or scleral tunnel incision may be subject to compromise that can predispose to later leakage. Excessive episcleral cautery may devitalize the flap, delaying the tissue ingrowth that is essential to wound healing and, in extreme cases, precipitating flap necrosis. Tearing or buttonholing of the roof of the tunnel can make closure difficult, and a groove or dissection into the ciliary body, if sufficiently anterior, can create a deep channel into the anterior chamber. False passages in the tunnel itself with multiple levels of anterior chamber entry may also arise and escape detection and closure. Incorrect suture placement and tying also may distort wound architecture and predispose to leakage. Finally, at the close of surgery, a seton may be left in the tunnel, creating a wound fistula.[16] This may occur with capsular or cortical remnants, vitreous, or prolapsed iris.

Management of wound leak depends on several factors, including etiology, timing, severity, and the structural appearance of the incision. Wound leaks that are noted in the first or second day postoperatively often seal themselves as a result of the postoperative inflammatory process. Wound leaks that occur after the first few days can sometimes be managed medically, particularly if wound apposition is generally good and the integrity of the eye is unaffected. Unfortunately, in the authors' experience this is not often the case, and these cases generally fit into the category of wound rupture requiring surgical repair (discussed later in the chapter). Adjunctive medical management can include the following:

1. *Decreasing or stopping corticosteroid therapy.* This is a logical, if unproven, maneuver to eliminate pharmacologic inhibition of wound healing.

2. *Prophylactic administration of topical antibiotics.* Our preference is one with a broad spectrum of coverage, such as a fourth-generation fluoroquinolone.

3. *Cycloplegia, preferably with a long-acting agent such as atropine or scopolamine.* This may improve ciliary body function by minimizing hypotony-induced ciliary body detachment.

4. *Full-time patching.* This is usually reserved for persistent (>5 days) or severe (<2 mm Hg intraocular pressure and/or shallow anterior chamber) cases.

5. *Use of a 48- or 72-h collagen shield or disposable soft contact lens.* The indications for this are similar to those for patching, and selection is sometimes based on the patient's preferences. It is important to select a lens that covers the incision.

6. *Topical administration of aqueous inhibitors (e.g., beta-blockers).* Theoretically, this will diminish the flow of aqueous through the incision, hastening wound closure.

Resuturing of an early postoperative wound leak may be indicated in several circumstances:

1. If the anterior chamber is flat

2. If intraocular pressure remains low for several days, particularly in the presence of a shallow anterior chamber

3. If iris prolapse occurs

4. If there is extensive external wound gape, particularly if excessive flattening along the meridian of the incision has developed. Alternatively, use of tissue adhesives, such as cyanoacrylate, appears to be well tolerated and may have future applicability.[17]

Recently, interest has increased as to whether clear-corneal incisions and their potential for wound leakage may be associated with an increased incidence of endophthalmitis. Some studies have shown an increase in the incidence of endophthalmitis beginning with the time period of transition to clear-corneal incisions,[18–20] particularly in the setting of observed wound leak.[21] This is further supported by cadaveric and in-vivo studies showing that fluctuation in IOP (simulating eye rubbing and blinking) can compromise wound integrity and cause entry of surface fluids.[22–24] Other studies, however, have not conclusively borne out this trend in incidence.[25–28] No sufficiently large randomized study has yet compared clear-corneal incisions with other types of incisions. However, it is apparent that any incision (corneal, limbal, or scleral) should be sutured if it is not self-sealing at the conclusion of surgery.[29]

WOUND THERMAL BURNS

A wound burn is a thermal injury of the incisional tissue and is characterized by whitening of the overlying corneal tissue, contraction and striae of wound tissue, and wound gape. Wound burns are caused by inadequate cooling of the phacoemulsification tip, which in turn is caused by one or more factors, including occlusion of the phaco tip by nuclear material or dispersive ophthalmic viscosurgical devices (OVD), compression of the irrigation sleeve from an excessively tight incision or poor angulation of the phacoemulsification handpiece, and absence of irrigation fluid. Its incidence may have been increased by advances in small incision surgery and small-caliper phacoemulsification needles.

Bradley et al. in a survey of practicing ophthalmologists found an incidence of wound burn of approximately 0.1% with the majority occurring during fragment removal. Divide-and-conquer and carousel techniques showed a higher incidence than chop techniques,[30] possibly because of the greater tendency to impale larger nuclear pieces with the former approaches.

Prevention of wound burn is of utmost importance. Careful vigilance to the following factors may limit this complication:

1. Matching of wound size to the size and design of the phacoemulsification tip. In addition, it is vital to test fluid flow prior to handpiece insertion. Non-compressible tips such as the Mackool tip with an inner polyimide sleeve and the Microflow fluted tip may also prevent obstruction of irrigation inflow.

2. Clearing of dispersive viscoelastic prior to commencing ultrasound.

3. Setting appropriate vacuum and power settings for a given nucleus density to minimize the risk of tip blockage by nuclear material.

4. Careful nuclear sculpting, avoiding occlusion, and prompt recognition of auditory signals from the phacoemulsification device indicating tip obstruction.

5. Being alert to visible signs of decreased fluid flow ("lens milk") and early wound tissue whitening.

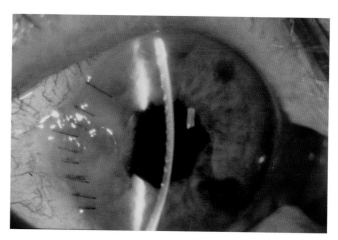

Figure 47-1 Severe wound burn requiring multiple interrupted sutures to achieve a watertight closure. Note the induced corneal striae. The cause was undetected obstruction of the phacoemulsification tip by a dispersive ophthalmic viscosurgical device due to low flow and vacuum settings.

Advances in phacoemulsification machine engineering, perhaps with thermal coupling, may further limit this potentially devastating complication.

If a burn occurs, meticulous suturing of the wound with multiple radial sutures is often needed (Figure 47-1). Another approach is to use a vertical mattress suture to avoid excessive traction on the tissue; however, this can be technically difficult to insert when there is marked tissue contracture. In severe cases, it may be difficult to achieve watertight closure with sutures alone and, occasionally, a scleral patch graft may be necessary. In less severe cases, a bandage contact lens may assist with wound closure, and we have found fibrinogen glue to be an effective adjunct and use it whenever wound integrity is uncertain despite careful suturing.

Wound healing tends to be slow, and sutures typically should be removed only after several weeks elapse. Our preference with severe burns is to begin suture removal only at 3 months postoperatively, when we can be assured that endothelial cells covering the incision have deposited new Descemet's membrane.

Wound burns create astigmatism along the meridian due to both tissue contracture and the sutures. One immediate step to reduce the amount of induced astigmatism is to place a scleral relaxing incision just posterior to the sutures. The depth should be approximately 50%, and the length should match that of the incision.

The tissue contracture often largely regresses over the ensuing year, but some or, rarely, large amounts of astigmatism can persist. The latter can be addressed with relaxing incisions that are made in the peripheral cornea in the area of the burn; these should be conservative in length to prevent overcorrection and can be lengthened if the initial response is inadequate.

WOUND DEHISCENCE

Wound dehiscence typically occurs later postoperatively after the wound has been documented as being closed at one or more postoperative visits. Causes of wound dehiscence are direct ocular trauma or, less commonly, spontaneous loosening or breakage of a suture or tissue melting or necrosis.

Although the actual incidence of wound dehiscence is likely to vary moderately depending on multiple factors, the shift to small-incision surgery and the evolution in techniques of wound design have reduced the incidence markedly, with reports indicating a range of 0.02–1.5%.[31–36] For example, Quraishy and Casswell[34] reported an incidence of traumatic wound dehiscence of 0.4% (21/5600) following extracapsular cataract extraction (ECCE) from 1986 to 1993. From the same hospital, only one case of traumatic wound dehiscence (0.02%) was identified in 4200 phacoemulsification procedures from 1996 to 1998.[35]

FACTORS PREDISPOSING TO WOUND DEHISCENCE

The surgical incision and its closure are only as reliable as the corneoscleral tissue substrate (Figure 47-2). Particularly for larger incisions, wound healing may be delayed or incomplete in the setting of profound systemic illness[33] and malnutrition (particularly vitamin C deficiency).

An unusual example of the role of systemic factors in wound healing occurs with Werner's syndrome, which is an autosomal recessive condition of premature aging associated with cataract formation by the age of 20–40 years. Jonas et al.[37] reported that wound dehiscence occurred in 10 out of 18 cataract wounds at 2.5 to 21 weeks postoperatively. The cause is a presumed deficiency in fibroblast growth potential.

Peripheral ulcerative keratitis and scleritis associated with underlying collagen vascular disease can produce marked scleral and/or corneal thinning, rendering wound closure extremely difficult. These entities also may flare after surgery, leading to melting of the tunnel incision.

Perioperative systemic steroid exposure may predispose to dehiscence of large incisions. Fechner and Wichmann[38] reported a 10% incidence of wound dehiscence in 100 phakic myopic eyes treated with high-dose systemic steroids directly before and after

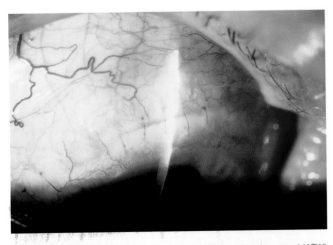

Figure 47-2 Scleral "melting" and 6 diopter (D) of against-the-wound (ATW) astigmatism developed in a 68-year-old white female 3 weeks following uncomplicated planned extracapsular cataract extraction. The wound was resutured, but within 4 weeks there was spontaneous loosening of all sutures and recurrence of 4 D of against-the-wound astigmatism. Note wound gape, scleral edema, and loose sutures. Because of poor scleral integrity, no further wound revision was attempted.

implantation of iris-fixated lenses. The intended suppression of postoperative inflammation apparently interfered with the initial stages of wound healing. Not surprisingly, there is also some evidence that topical corticosteroids may also delay wound healing. Barba et al.[39] reported that corneas treated with topical corticosteroids had less wound healing at 7 days after surgery than untreated corneas or corneas treated with nonsteroidal anti-inflammatory drugs. However, the relevance of these findings to small-incision surgery is unclear, and we are unaware of cases of actual wound dehiscence precipitated by topical corticosteroid use.

MANIFESTATIONS AND MANAGEMENT OF WOUND DEHISCENCE

Manifestations of wound dehiscence include wound leakage (discussed previously), inadvertent filtering bleb, wound rupture, epithelial downgrowth and fibrous ingrowth, and against-the-wound astigmatism.

Inadvertent Filtering Bleb

A wound leak under sealed conjunctiva results in formation of a filtering bleb. The management is again highly dependent on the timing and severity. Filtering blebs noted in the first few days postoperatively typically resolve. This process can be hastened using the medical measures discussed earlier for management of a wound leak.

Filtering blebs that develop after the first several postoperative days usually reflect the breakdown of an initially well-apposed wound, which can occur from trauma, suture breakage or loosening, or scleral melting. Spontaneous resolution of blebs with this cause is less likely because there is insufficient inflammation to promote closure of the incisional gaping.

Regardless of the time of onset and the cause, blebs that persist beyond several days can undergo epithelialization of the fistulous tract. This channel is resistant to medical treatment and many forms of surgical intervention.

Treatment of persistent filtering blebs depends on the level of the intraocular pressure, the overall integrity of the wound, and patient comfort. Surgical repair is indicated in eyes with poorly tolerated hypotony, ocular discomfort due to the size of the bleb, or reduction in vision due to encroachment of the flap over the cornea. Large, thin-walled blebs that "weep" aqueous may predispose to the development of endophthalmitis, and surgical closure should be considered. Filtering blebs accompanied by poor wound apposition typically induce against-the-wound astigmatism, and, if this is excessive for the patient's need, it is a relative indication for surgical repair. Dellen can form adjacent to large blebs, and these can be resistant to standard therapy with topical lubricants.[40] Some patients are uncomfortable because of lid contact with the filtering bleb or may have cosmetic concerns when the bleb is large and cystic; in these situations, bleb repair may be indicated (Figure 47-3).

Closure of a long-standing filtering bleb is complicated by epithelialization of the fistula.[41] Relatively noninvasive methods to close or shrink chronic blebs include cryotherapy, chemical cauterization with trichloroacetic acid, argon laser treatment following application of methylene blue or rose bengal bye (Steinert RF,

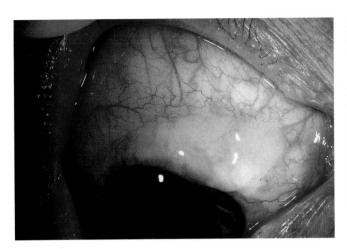

Figure 47-3 Persistent inadvertent filtering bleb 2 years following cataract surgery. The intraocular pressure was 11 mm Hg in this eye and 19 mm Hg in the fellow eye. Patient complained of progressive, severe eye irritation and tearing. Surgical repair consisted of excision of cystic conjunctiva, scraping of fistulous track, closure of the track with interrupted 9-0 nylon sutures, and coverage of the track with a half-thickness scleral flap. The bleb recurred, but at less than 50% of original size, and the intraocular pressure was 14 mm Hg.

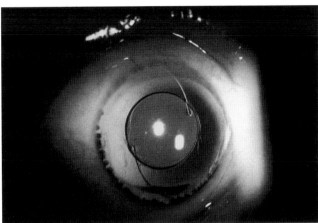

Figure 47-4 Total absence of iris following expulsion that occurred 10 weeks after routine phacoemulsification and intraocular lens implantation through a 3.2 mm clear corneal incision. (From Walker NJ, Foster A, Apel AJ. Traumatic explusive iridodialysis after small incision sutureless cataract surgery. *J Cataract Refract Surg* 30:2223–4. Copyright 2004, with permission from Elsevier.)

personal communication, 1994), neodymium:yttrium-aluminum-garnet (Nd:YAG) laser,[42] and diathermy.[43,44]

Surgical closure of the fistula requires either its excision or sufficient compression and inflammation to foster cicatricial closure. We recommend excision of the conjunctiva that was involved in the filtering bleb to eliminate these channels. The wound must be carefully explored and the fistula identified. The fistulous tract is covered by a layer of endothelial cells, and it should, therefore, be scraped or excised, and, if necessary, the remaining hole covered or filled with a scleral graft or a folded half-thickness scleral flap.[45,46] The wound is then meticulously resutured. If the sutures appear to induce excessive astigmatism, this can be minimized by placing a scleral relaxing incision just posterior to the sutures. This incision is placed at a depth of around 300 μm and should extend the length of the sutured region. Finally, the conjunctiva and Tenon's capsule are advanced and meticulously sutured. Postoperative anti-inflammatory treatment is kept to a minimum. Even with these steps, complete closure of a bleb is not always successful. However, a large bleb can sometimes be dramatically reduced in size and low pressure ameliorated, thereby achieving partial surgical success.

Patients with persistent filtering blebs should be warned of the risk of development of bleb-induced endophthalmitis. The incidence and severity of postcataract endophthalmitis are increased in patients with filtering blebs,[47–49] and early detection is desirable.

WOUND RUPTURE

One of the most severe sight-threatening presentations of wound dehiscence is frank wound rupture,[50–53] which is the traumatic reopening of a wound that had previously been sealed, usually accompanied by extrusion of intraocular contents. Susceptibility to traumatic wound rupture is presumably highly dependent on the size and architecture of the incision, with a possible contribution of the patient's predisposing factors. Indeed, wound failure can occur without apparent precipitating trauma in patients with abnormal sclera or poor healing. Conversely, in patients with small self-sealing incisions, a traumatic rupture of the globe without compromise of the incision is even possible. Case reports of traumatic expulsion of anterior segment structures with resealing of the wounds have been reported, testifying to the unique integrity of these wounds compared to traditional extracapsular wounds[54,55] (Figure 47-4).

Most traumatically induced wound ruptures have extensive structural disruption of the incision with poor wound edge apposition and iris prolapse (Figure 47-5). The amount of damage to the wound is almost always much more widespread than is evident preoperatively. The initial steps of surgical repair consist of dissecting free the conjunctival flap, exploring the incision, reopening of the wound beyond the margin of dehiscence, and freshening of the wound edges by scraping them with a sharp blade.

Iris prolapse occurs in the majority of eyes that sustain late postoperative wound rupture. This may in part be due to the

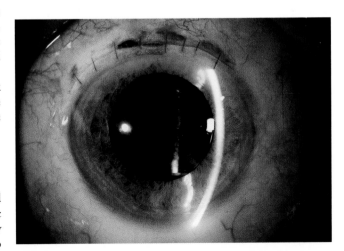

Figure 47-5 Presumably traumatic wound dehiscence that was detected 3 weeks following uncomplicated extracapsular cataract extraction. The patient indicated that he had rubbed the eye. Note iris prolapse; no wound leak occurred.

infrequent use of peripheral iridectomy, which predisposes to a large disparity in pressure between the posterior and anterior chambers at the moment of traumatic wound opening. Iris that is frankly necrotic should be excised and cultured. Viable iris can usually be reposited after it is meticulously scraped to remove any adherent epithelial cells. There is some controversy over the management of iris that has been prolapsed over 24 h because of concern about the introduction of epithelium or microorganisms.[56,57] Epithelial downgrowth has been reported after repositioning an iris that was prolapsed for 7 days. As a general rule, it may be preferable to excise iris that has been prolapsed over 24 h. It is often easiest to reposit iris tissue through a separate stab incision. The surgeon should be cautious to avoid exerting excessive traction on the iris root, which could create an iridodialysis, hemorrhage, or both.

Vitrectomy is performed as needed, and the intraocular lens is repositioned or exchanged as necessary. The wound is then meticulously resutured; our preference is interrupted 10-0 or 9-0 nylon sutures. With limbal and scleral incisions, the conjunctiva is pulled centrally over the peripheral cornea and meticulously sutured at each end to ensure good wound coverage. Topical and broad-spectrum intravenous or oral antibiotics are usually recommended for 2 to 5 days following wound repair.

EPITHELIAL DOWNGROWTH AND FIBROUS INGROWTH

One of the rarest but most insidious manifestations of wound dehiscence is epithelial downgrowth.[58,59] This is a rare complication of cataract surgery and has multiple presentations, including corneal decompensation, severe glaucoma with or without obvious angle closure, chronic anterior uveitis, and the presence of a retrocorneal membrane with a demarcated leading edge[59] (Figure 47-6). The presence of epithelial downgrowth can sometimes be confirmed by irradiating the affected iris with an argon laser. Using laser settings of 300–700 mW and 500 μm spot size, a white blanching is seen at the site of laser treatment, as opposed to a standard burn or brown color change of the normal iris surface. Epithelial downgrowth can sometimes be

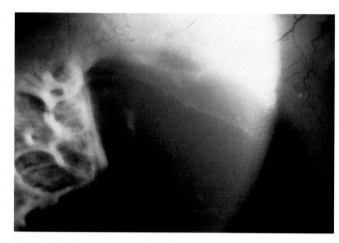

Figure 47-6 Epithelial downgrowth with membrane on corneal endothelial surface 21 months following traumatic wound rupture; note prominent leading edge. Diagnosis was confirmed by frozen section obtained at the time of iridocyclectomy.

diagnosed with specular endothelial microscopy; a demarcation line can be seen separating endothelial cells (which are often abnormal is size and configuration) from dark, poorly defined cells representing the epithelium.[60,61] Definitive diagnosis depends on histopathologic confirmation of the presence of epithelial tissue in the eye.

Another manifestation of epithelial downgrowth is the presence of an intraocular cyst (Figure 47-7).[62] This usually involves the iris and is often adherent to the posterior surface of the cornea. The cyst is slowly expansile and readily transilluminates. An epithelial implantation cyst can readily be transformed into true epithelial downgrowth if the cyst is inadvertently lysed.[63]

The time of onset of epithelial downgrowth is highly variable, but it typically presents within months of the surgery. It appears to be more common in patients who have undergone multiple procedures or in patients who have experienced postoperative complications with wound closure.

Definitive treatment of epithelial downgrowth consists of complete destruction or excision of all intraocular epithelial

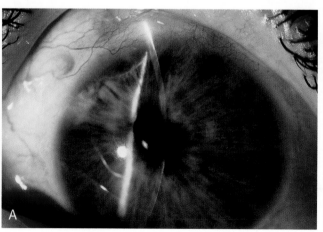
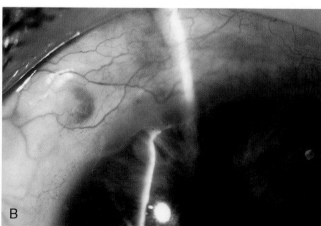

Figure 47-7 A, Iris epithelial cyst that was noted 18 months following intraocular lens exchange and scleral flap recession. **B,** High-magnification detail of the cyst. Patient has done well with 20/40 vision 18 months following iridocyclectomy and suture-fixation of a posterior chamber lens.

tissue. Surgical techniques include some combination of cryotherapy of the involved cornea with the anterior chamber filled with air; iridocyclectomy with excision of the internal corneal flap in the affected region; and pars plana vitrectomy with removal of all involved iris, ciliary body, and lens with endolaser of any suspected involved areas.[16] Unfortunately, the prognosis is poor.[64]

Fibrous ingrowth is the abnormal invasion of the anterior chamber by connective tissue from the incision.[65–67] This condition is uncommonly diagnosed clinically, and it occurs in eyes with deficient wound closure, possibly in the presence of abnormal endothelium. By slit-lamp biomicroscopy it appears as a thick, opaque membrane on the posterior surface of the cornea. Vascularization is sometimes evident. It tends to be slower growing and more clearly demarcated than epithelial downgrowth. It is typically detected histopathologically in tissue from eyes that have undergone incisional repair or in enucleated specimens.

AGAINST-THE-WOUND ASTIGMATISM

For incisions 4 mm and longer, one of the most subtle, but perhaps most common, manifestations of wound dehiscence is excessive flattening along the meridian of the incision.[68] This condition can begin at any time in the first 2 years postoperatively and can progress for years thereafter. A precise definition of this condition is difficult to formulate, in part because the determination of excessive flattening along the meridian of the incision depends on incision size. Shifts of unusual magnitude would include flattening of greater than or equal to 1.5 diopters (D) for a 5 mm or smaller incision, greater than or equal to 2 D for 6–7 mm incisions, and ≥3 D for extracapsular incisions. This process is usually detected first by keratometry, refraction, or computerized videokeratography (Figure 47-8). With computer videokeratography, characteristic asymmetric flattening can often be seen in the semimeridian adjacent to the incision.

Excessive against-the-wound astigmatism is fostered by the tissue addition that occurs as part of the natural wound-healing process, but additional elements are required. Wound construction is

important. A predisposition to excessive flattening along the meridian of the incision becomes more prominent with longer wounds and shorter tunnels. This problem certainly is more common in superior incisions and, indeed, is rarely seen with temporal incisions. Intrinsic patient factors, perhaps labeled "poor healing" for want of a better term, often seem to play a major role (see Figure 47-2).

Treatment in most instances is directed at reducing the induced astigmatism. Although the cause is incisional weakness or dehiscence, surgical repair of the incision is fraught with difficulties and is generally reserved for selected cases detected in the first 2–4 weeks postoperatively. Wound resuturing can induce excessive with-the-wound astigmatism, requires reentry of the eye, and provides no certainty that the process will not recur. For most patients, it is reasonable first to attempt conservative management with glasses or, less commonly, contact lenses. Astigmatic keratotomy or peripheral corneal relaxing incisions are offered to patients who poorly tolerate the strong refractive correction required or who keenly desire improved uncorrected vision. Excimer laser photorefractive keratectomy or laser in situ keratomileusis can be used to address both residual cylindrical and spherical errors.

■ CONCLUSIONS ■

The compromise of wound integrity is a relatively uncommon but potentially devastating complication of cataract surgery. It has multiple manifestations and causes, requiring a wide spectrum of therapeutic responses. It is an evolving area due to advances in wound-construction techniques, particularly the conversion to clear-corneal incisions of diminishing size. Advances in multiple areas, including techniques of wound construction, phacoemulsification machine design, and small-incision IOLs, will further reduce the prevalence and complications of wound compromise.

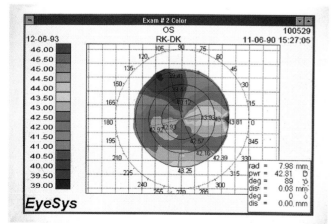

Figure 47-8 Computerized videokeratographic map showing against-the-wound astigmatism (2.75 diopter (D) by keratometry) 4 years following secondary intraocular lens implantation through a superior 7 mm incision. Note asymmetric flattening greater in the semimeridian adjacent to the incision.

References

[1] Ernest PH, Lavery KT, Kiessling LA. Relative strength of scleral corneal and clear corneal incisions constructed in cadaver eyes. J Cataract Refract Surg 1994;20:626–629.

[2] Koch PS. Structural analysis of cataract incision construction. J Cataract Refract Surg 1991;17 (Suppl.):661–667.

[3] Ernest P, Tipperman R, Eagle R, Kardasis C, Lavery K, Sensoli A, et al. Is there a difference in incision healing based on location? J Cataract Refract Surg 1998;24:482–486.

[4] Mackool RJ, Russell RS. Strength of clear corneal incisions in cadaver eyes. J Cataract Refract Surg 1996;22:721–725.

[5] Flaxel JT, Swan KC. Limbal wound healing after cataract extraction. Arch Ophthalmol 1969;81:653–659.

[6] Flaxel JT. Histology of cataract extractions. Arch Ophthalmol 1970;83:436–444.

[7] Gliedman ML, Karlson KE. Wound healing and wound strength of sutured limbal wounds. Am J Ophthalmol 1955;39:859–865.

[8] Masuda K. Tensile strength of corneoscleral wounds repaired with absorbable sutures. Ophthalmic Surg 1981;12:110–114.

[9] Koch DD, Smith SH, Whiteside SB. Limbal and scleral wound healing. In: Healing processes in the cornea. Portfolio Publishing Co, The WoodlandsTexas, USA 1989. p. 165–181.

[10] Hurvitz LM. Late clear corneal wound failure after trivial trauma. J Cataract Refract Surg 1999;25:283–284.

[11] Pham DT, Anders N, Wollensak J. Wound rupture 1 year after cataract operation with 7 mm scleral tunnel incision (no-stitch technique). Klin Monatsbl Augenheilkd 1996;208:124–126.

[12] Routsis P, Garston B. Late traumatic wound dehiscence after phacoemulsification. J Cataract Refract Surg 2000;26:1092–1093.

[13] Gimbel HV, Sun R, DeBroff BM. Recognition and management of internal wound gape. J Cataract Refract Surg 1995;21:121–124.

[14] Machemer HF, Roters S. Ultrasound biomicroscopy of chronic hypotony after cataract extraction. J Cataract Refract Surg 2001;27:327–329.

[15] Taban M, Rao B, Reznik J, Zhang J, Chen Z, McDonnell PJ. Dynamic morphology of sutureless cataract wounds – effect of incision angle and location. Surv Ophthalmol 2004;49(Suppl. 2): S62–S72.

[16] Schaeffer AR, Nalbandian RM, Brigham DW, O'Donnell FE. Epithelial downgrowth following wound dehiscence after extracapsular cataract extraction and posterior chamber lens implantation: surgical management. J Cataract Refract Surg 1989;15:437–441.

[17] Meskin SW, Ritterband DC, Shapiro DE, Kusmierczyk J, Schneider SS, Seedor JA, et al. Liquid bandage (2-octyl cyanoacrylate) as a temporary wound barrier in clear corneal cataract surgery. Ophthalmol 2005;112:2015–2021.

[18] West ES, Behrens A, McDonnell PJ, Tielsch JM, Schein OD. The incidence of endophthalmitis after cataract surgery among the US medicare population increased between 1994 and 2001. Ophthalmol 2005;112:1388–1394.

[19] Cooper BA, Holekamp NM, Bohigian G, Thompson PA. Case-control study of endophthalmitis after cataract surgery comparing scleral tunnel and clear corneal wounds. Am J Ophthalmol 2003;136:300–305.

[20] Nagaki Y, Hayasaka S, Kadoi C, et al. Bacterial endophthalmitis after small-incision cataract surgery. J Cataract Refract Surg 2003;29:20–26.

[21] Wallin T, Parker J, Jin Y, Kefalopoulos G, Olson RJ. Cohort study of 27 cases of endophthalmitis at a single institution. J Cataract Refract Surg 2005;31:735–741.

[22] Sarayba MA, Taban M, Ignacio TS, Behrens A, McDonnell PJ. Inflow of ocular surface fluid through clear corneal cataract incisions: a laboratory model. Am J of Ophthalmol 2004;138:206–210.

[23] Taban M, Sarayba MA, Ignacio TS, Behrens A, McDonnell PJ. Ingress of india ink into the anterior chamber through sutureless clear corneal cataract wounds. Arch Ophthalmol 2005;123:643–648.

[24] McDonnell PJ, Taban M, Sarayba M, Rao B, Zhang J, Schiffman R, et al. Dynamic morphology of clear corneal cataract incisions. Ophthalmol 2003;110:2342–2348.

[25] Ng JQ, Morlet N, Pearman JW, et al. Management and outcomes of postoperative endophthalmitis since the endophthalmitis vitrectomy study. Ophthalmol 2005;112:1199–1206.

[26] Haapala TT, Nelimarkka L, Saari JM, Ahola V, Saari KM. Endophthalmitis following cataract surgery in Southwest Finland from 1987 to 2000. Graefe's Arch Clin Exp Ophthalmol 2005;243:1010–1017.

[27] Monica ML, Long DA. Nine-year safety with self-sealing corneal tunnel incision in clear cornea cataract surgery. Ophthalmol 2005;112:985–986.

[28] Miller JJ, Scott IU, Flynn HW, Smiddy WE, Newton J, Miller D. Acute-onset endophthalmitis after cataract surgery (2000–2004): incidence, clinical settings, and visual acuity outcomes after treatment. Am J of Ophthalmol 2005;139:983–987.

[29] McCulley JP. Low acute endophthalmitis rate: possible explanations. J Cataract Refract Sur 2005;31:1074–1075.

[30] Bradley MJ, Olson RJ. A survey about phacoemulsification incision thermal contraction incidence and causal relationships. Am J of Ophthalmol 2006;141:222–224.

[31] Swan KC, Campbell L. Unintentional filtration following cataract surgery. Arch Ophthalmol 1964;71:77–83.

[32] Lambrou FH, Kozarsky A. Wound dehiscence following cataract surgery. Ophthalmic Surg 1987;18:738–740.

[33] Arango JL, Margo CE. Wound complications following cataract surgery. A case-control study. Arch Ophthalmol 1998;116:1021–1024.

[34] Quraishy MM, Casswell AG. May I bend down after my cataract operation, doctor? Eye 1996;10 (Pt 1):92–94.

[35] Ball JL, McLeod BK. Traumatic wound dehiscence following cataract surgery: a thing of the past? Eye 2001;15(Pt 1):42–44.

[36] Anders N, Pham DT, Wollensak J. Etiology of insufficient wound sealing in cataract operation with the no-stitch technique. Ophthalmologe 1995;92:270–273.

[37] Jonas JB, Ruprecht KW, Schmitz-Valckenberg P, et al. Ophthalmic surgical complications in Werner's syndrome: report on 18 eyes of nine patients. Ophthalmic Surg 1987;18:760–764.

[38] Fechner PU, Wichmann W. Retarded corneoscleral wound healing associated with high preoperative doses of systemic steroids in glaucoma surgery. Refract Corneal Surg 1991;7:174–176.

[39] Barba KR, Samy A, Lai C, Perlman JI, Bouchard CS. Effect of topical anti-inflammatory drugs on corneal and limbal wound healing. J Cataract Refract Surg 2000;26:893–897.

[40] Soong HK, Quigley HA. Dellen associated with filtering blebs. Arch Ophthalmol 1983;101:385–387.

[41] Soong HK, Meyer RF, Wolter JR. Fistula excision and peripheral grafts in the treatment of persistent limbal wound leaks. Ophthalmol 1988;95:31–36.

[42] Geyer O. Management of large, leaking, and inadvertent filtering blebs with the neodymium: YAG laser. Ophthalmol 1998;105:983–987.

[43] Cleasby GW, Fung WE, Webster RG. Cryosurgical closure of filtering blebs. Arch Ophthalmol 1972;87:319–323.

[44] Yannuzzi LA, Theodore FH. Cryotherapy of post-cataract blebs. Am J Ophthalmol 1973;76:217–222.

[45] Clinch TE, Kaufman H. Repair of inadvertent conjunctival filtering blebs with a scleral flap. Arch Ophthalmol 1992;110:1652–1653.

[46] Rao SK, Padmanaban P. An unusual complication of a postcataract filtering bleb. Ophthalmic Surg Lasers 1997;28:601–602.

[47] Mandelbaum S, Forster RK. Endophthalmitis associated with filtering blebs. Intl Ophthalmol Clinics 1987;27:107–111.

[48] Dickens A, Greven CM. Posttraumatic endophthalmitis caused by lactobacillus. Arch Ophthalmol 1993;111:1169.

[49] Phillips 2nd WB, Wong TP, Bergren RL, Friedberg MA, Benson WE. Late onset endophthalmitis associated with filtering blebs. Ophthalmic Surg 1994;25:88–91.

[50] Pham DT, Anders N, Wollensak J. Wound rupture 1 year after cataract operation with 7 mm scleral tunnel incision (no-stitch technique). Klin Monatsbl Augenheilkd 1996;208:124–126.

[51] Routsis P, Garston B. Late traumatic wound dehiscence after phacoemulsification. J Cataract Refract Surg 2000;26:1092–1093.

[52] Kass MA, LaHav M, Albert DM. Traumatic rupture of healed cataract wounds. Am J Ophthalmol 1976;81:722–724.

[53] Blomquist PH, Parrish CM, Elliott JH, O'Day DM. Traumatic wound dehiscence in pseudophakia. Am J Ophthalmol 1989;108:535–539.

[54] Blomquist PH. Expulsion of an intraocular lens through a clear corneal wound. J Cataract Refract Surg 2004;29:592–594.

[55] Walker NJ, Foster A, Apel AJG. Traumatic expulsive iridodialysis after small-incision sutureless cataract surgery. J Cataract Refract Surg 2004;30:2223–2224.

[56] Orlin SE, Farber MG, Brucker AJ, Frayer WC. The unexpected guest: problem of iris reposition. Surv Ophthalmol 1990;35:59–66.

[57] Menapace R. Delayed iris prolapse with unsutured 5.1 mm clear corneal incisions. J Cataract Refract Surg 1995;21:353–357.

[58] Maumenee AE. Treatment of epithelial downgrowth and intraocular fistula following cataract extraction. Tr Am Ophth Soc 1964;62:153–162.

[59] Kuchle M, Green WR. Epithelial ingrowth: a study of 207 histopathologically proven cases. Ger J Ophthalmol 1996;5:211–223.

[60] Smith RE, Parrett C. Specular microscopy of epithelial downgrowth. Arch Ophthalmol 1978;96:1222–1224.

[61] Liang RA, Sandstrom, Leibowitz HM, Berrospi AR. Epithelialization of the anterior chamber. Clinical investigation with the specular microscope. Arch Ophthalmol 1979;97:1870–4.

[62] Knauf HP, Rowsey JJ, Margo CE. Cystic epithelial downgrowth following clear-corneal cataract extraction. Arch Ophthalmol 1997;115:668–669.

[63] Orlin SE, Raber IM, Laibson PR, Shields CL, Brucker AJ. Epithelial downgrowth following the removal of iris inclusion cysts. Ophthalmic Surg 1991;22:330–335.

[64] Stark WJ, Michels RG, Maumenee AE, Cupples H. Surgical management of epithelial ingrowth. Am J Ophthalmol 1978;85:772–780.

[65] Bloomfield SE, Jakobiec FA, Iwamoto T. Fibrous ingrowth with retrocorneal membrane. Ophthalmol 1981;88:459–65.

[66] McDonnell PJ, de la Cruz Z, Green WR. Vitreous incarceration complicating cataract surgery. A light and electron microscopic study. Ophthalmol 1986;93:247–253.

[67] Kremer 1, Zandbank J, Barash D, Ben-David E, Yassur Y. Extensive fibrous downgrowth after traumatic corneoscleral wound dehiscence. Ann Ophthalmol 1991;23:465–468.

[68] Gelender H. Management of corneal astigmatism after cataract surgery. Refract Corneal Surg 1991;7:99–102.

Toxic Anterior Segment Syndrome

48

Nick Mamalis, MD

CONTENTS

CHAPTER HIGHLIGHTS

>> Clinical recognition of toxic anterior segment syndrome (TASS)

>> Causes

>> Treatment

>> Protocol for managing a TASS outbreak

Toxic anterior segment syndrome (TASS) is an acute, sterile postoperative anterior segment inflammation following any anterior segment surgery. This entity is by definition sterile or noninfectious. This condition was initially described as sterile postoperative endophthalmitis, but in 1992, Monson et al.[1] coined the term toxic anterior segment syndrome (TASS). In addition, cases of TASS which are characterized by localized corneal endothelial damage have been termed toxic endothelial cell destruction syndrome (TECDS).[2-6] A recent review/update on TASS as well as its accompanying editorial has provided a detailed, in-depth discussion of this entity.[7,8]

TASS occurs most commonly following cataract surgery, but may occur following anterior-segment surgeries of any kind including glaucoma or cornea transplant surgeries. While TASS is most commonly noted to occur acutely following anterior segment surgery, in rare instances it can have a delayed onset. This postoperative inflammation is sterile or noninfectious and is felt to be caused by a substance that enters the anterior segment either during or immediately after surgery, resulting in toxic damage to intraocular tissues.

CLINICAL SIGNS AND SYMPTOMS

The most common complaint that patients with TASS have is blurred vision. Pain is usually absent which is distinct from cases of postoperative infectious endophthalmitis. The patients may have signs of ocular inflammation and injection. The clinical hallmark of TASS is the fact that the inflammation presents with a relatively immediate onset, usually within 12–48 h of surgery. This inflammation is sterile and Gram-stain and cultures are negative.

The most common clinical finding in TASS is diffuse corneal edema which has been described as "limbus-to-limbus" corneal edema (Figure 48-1). This diffuse corneal edema is due to widespread damage of the corneal endothelial cells. This finding is very different from the focal areas of corneal edema which may occur after routine cataract surgery. A second common finding associated with this entity is marked anterior segment inflammation. This is characterized by diffuse breakdown of blood–aqueous barrier with a marked increase in inflammatory cells in the anterior chamber. These cells may settle to the lower part of the anterior chamber forming a hypopyon (Figure 48-2). In addition, significant breakdown of the blood–aqueous barrier may lead to fibrin formation in the anterior chamber which may extend across the pupil from the iris onto the surface of the intraocular lens and toward the incisions. Finally, TASS may result in damage to the iris which can cause a permanently dilated or irregular pupil with thinning of the iris stroma (Figure 48-3). There may be associated trabecular meshwork damage which can lead to secondary glaucoma which may be difficult to control.

It is important to differentiate the sterile inflammation seen in TASS from an infectious postoperative endophthalmitis. One of the signs that are most helpful in differentiating these two entities is the fact that TASS occurs acutely in the vast majority of cases with signs appearing within the first 12–48 h. In bacterial endophthalmitis, the typical signs do not often appear until 4–7 days postoperatively. The symptoms in these entities are different in that greater than 75% of patients who have an infectious endophthalmitis will have pain. The majority of cases of TASS are pain free. The anterior segment inflammatory changes in both of these entities are often very similar with significant inflammation and hypopyon formation. However, the diffuse corneal edema

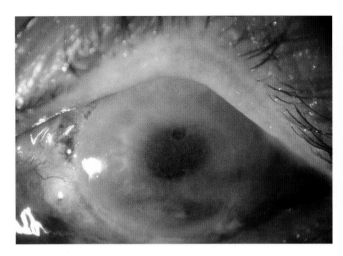

Figure 48-1 Diffuse limbus-to-limbus corneal edema. (From Mamalis N, Edelhauser HF, Dawson DG, Chew J, LeBoyer RM, Werner L: Toxic anterior segment syndrome, *J Cataract Refract Surg* 32:324–333, 2006 (review/update). Copyright 2006, with permission from Elsevier.

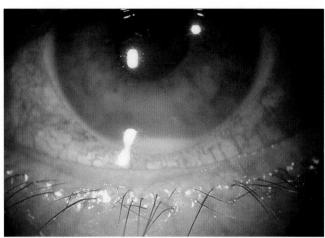

Figure 48-2 Anterior segment inflammation with hypopyon formation. (From Mamalis N, Edelhauser HF, Dawson DG, Chew J, LeBoyer RM, Werner L: Toxic anterior segment syndrome, *J Cataract Refract Surg* 32:324–333, 2006 (review/update). Copyright 2006, with permission from Elsevier.

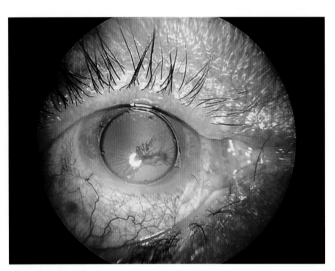

Figure 48-3 Atrophic iris with dilated, slightly irregular pupil. (From Mamalis N, Edelhauser HF, Dawson DG, Chew J, LeBoyer RM, Werner L: Toxic anterior segment syndrome, *J Cataract Refract Surg* 32:324–333, 2006 (review/update). Copyright 2006, with permission from Elsevier.

seen in TASS is often not noted in infectious endophthalmitis. It is important if there is any question of an infectious etiology that anterior chamber and vitreous samples be taken for staining and culture.

■ ETIOLOGY OF TOXIC ANTERIOR SEGMENT SYNDROME ■

Any substance that is used during or immediately after cataract surgery which can access the anterior segment of the eye can cause TASS. The corneal endothelium is especially sensitive to any form of toxic insult as are many of the structures in the anterior segment of the eye in general. The etiology of TASS is relatively broad and may include problems involving irrigating solutions such as balanced saline solution (BSS) and any additives included.[9-13] In addition, any other ophthalmic solutions used during surgery, especially those which contain preservatives or

stabilizing agents may cause toxicity to corneal endothelium and precipitate TASS.[13-15] Medications such as antibiotics and anesthetics which are injected into the eye may also be associated with TASS. Additionally, residues of ophthalmic viscosurgical devices (OVDs) may cause significant postoperative inflammation.[16] Lastly, it is important to remember that any enzymes or detergents that are used in the cleaning of instruments used in anterior-segment surgery may leave behind a residue which could cause TASS.[17-19]

INTRAOCULAR IRRIGATING SOLUTIONS

Intraocular irrigating solutions such as BSS have the potential for causing problems with TASS if there are problems with the composition of the BSS such as incorrect ionic composition, osmolarity, or pH.[9-13]

It is also important to remember that any medication or solutions that are added to the BSS may be associated with potential problems with inflammation. Examples of these include agents to dilate the pupil, such as epinephrine, and antibiotics which are placed into the irrigating solution.

Furthermore, it is important to ensure that there is no contamination in the BSS secondary to materials such as endotoxin. There was an outbreak of TASS in the fall of 2005 which was found to be secondary to endotoxin contamination of BSS. Multiple patients throughout the United States were found to have signs and symptoms of TASS, but cultures of the anterior chamber and vitreous showed no signs of infectious endophthalmitis. These patients tended to occur in clusters and responded well to intense topical corticosteroid treatments. This outbreak was evaluated by investigators from the Intermountain Ocular Research Center at the University of Utah, as well as investigators from the United States Centers for Disease Control (CDC). A thorough investigation of 112 cases from this outbreak by the CDC found that the vast majority of patients were exposed to one particular brand of BSS that was used during cataract surgery. Samples were taken from many different lots of BSS and tested for endotoxin. Several lots of BSS were found to have levels of endotoxin exceeding the allowable limit of 0.5 EU/mL. It was found that this BSS was manufactured by Cytosol Laboratories and distributed by AMO as Endosol. This BSS was withdrawn from the market which resulted in termination of the outbreak (U.S. Food and Drug Administration FDA – Reported Recall – Cytosol Laboratories, Inc. Product Contains Dangerous Levels of Endotoxin. February 13, 2006).

PRESERVATIVES

Ophthalmic solutions which contain preservatives or stabilizing agents may be toxic to the corneal endothelium and result in TASS.[13–15] The corneal endothelium is exquisitely sensitive to preservatives which are used in many topical ophthalmic drops or solutions. One of the most commonly used preservatives is benzalkonium chloride (BAK). There have been multiple reports of patients with significant corneal edema or endothelial cell damage resulting from solutions which are preserved with BAK.[5] In addition, BAK has been found to cause significant corneal edema when used as a preservative with an OVD.[6] Low levels of BAK are safe to use on the surface of the eye, but should be avoided in medications which gain access to the eye during anterior segment surgery.

In addition to preservatives, agents which are used to stabilize intraocular medications have been found to be associated with TASS. The most commonly used stabilizing agents are bisulphites or metabisulphites, which are often used as a stabilizing agent for epinephrine (to maintain the epinephrine in the reduced state) which is added to the BSS to help maintain pupil dilation during cataract surgery. While these stabilizing agents are not considered to be traditional preservatives, they can be toxic to the corneal endothelium, as well as other cells within the anterior segment of the eye and can lead to TASS.[20] It is imperative that any medications placed into the eye during surgery are not only preservative free but free of stabilizing agents.[21]

INTRAOCULAR ANESTHETICS

Intracameral anesthetics are often used in routine cataract surgery to help supplement topical anesthetics. Preservative-free anesthetics which are in a relatively low concentration have not been found to be toxic to the endothelium. However, doses of lidocaine which is preservative free (methylparaben free-MPF) at a level of 2% or higher have been known to cause significant corneal thickening and opacification postoperatively.[22] Although these agents are preservative free, intracameral use of anesthetics can potentially cause corneal endothelial cell damage at a high enough dose.[22–24] Therefore, it is very important that any anesthetics used in anterior-segment surgery are not only of the proper dose but are free of preservatives.

INTRAOCULAR ANTIBIOTICS

Antibiotic agents are an additional source of toxicity when either they are used in irrigating solutions or are injected into the anterior segment of the eye at the conclusion of surgery. These agents are often used to help prevent endophthalmitis. Surgeons had initially advocated the use of either gentamicin sulfate or vancomycin in the irrigating solution (BSS) to help prevent endophthalmitis.[25] However, concerns were raised about the possibility of toxicity, especially with intraocular gentamicin, which has a relatively narrow range of therapeutic versus toxic doses and has been found to cause macular toxicity.[26,27] These agents have been mostly discontinued for use in the BSS for prevention of infection.

There has been recent work done mainly in Europe on the use of intracameral antibiotics which are injected at the conclusion of the surgery to help prevent endophthalmitis. Initial studies in Sweden regarding the use of intracameral cefuroxime for endophthalmitis prophylaxis showed no signs of toxicity with a 1 mg/0.1 cc dose of intracameral cefuroxime.[28] The European endophthalmitis study which has recently been published showed a significant reduction of endophthalmitis following the intracameral injection of cefuroxime at the conclusion of the case.[29] The issue of the use of intracameral antibiotics to prevent endophthalmitis is an important topic that will need to be addressed by surgeons in the United States in the near future. The American Society of Cataract and Refractive Surgery (ASCRS) has established a subcommittee to evaluate the various treatments of endophthalmitis, including intracameral antibiotics. Careful measures need to be taken to ensure that the proper mixing and dosing of the antibiotic is done in the pharmacy in order to prevent the possibility of TASS outbreaks due to improperly dosed or mixed intracameral antibiotics.

In addition to topical drops which may gain access to the eye during cataract surgery, there have been recent reports regarding a relatively delayed-onset TASS secondary to topical ophthalmic ointments gaining access to the anterior chamber of the eye following surgery and causing inflammation.[30] A series of patients were found to have delayed-onset TASS-like symptoms with film or oil-like substance in the anterior chamber, coating the endothelium or on the intraocular lens (IOL). Analysis of this material using chromatography – mass spectral analysis revealed that this material contained a mixed chain hydrocarbon which was also found in the analysis of the steroid-antibiotic ointment that was placed on the patient's eyes following the conclusion of the surgery. Such cases raised the possibility that ointment placed on the surface of the patient's eye at the conclusion of the case followed by tight patching in the setting of a clear cornea wound may lead to ointment gaining access into the anterior chamber of the eye and causing inflammation.

OPHTHALMIC VISCOSURGICAL DEVICES

An additional potential source of TASS are commonly used OVDs (previously referred to as viscoelastics). A large amount of remnant OVD in the anterior chamber of the eye can cause an increase in intraocular pressure (IOP) as well as increased inflammation postoperatively.

An additional problem is the possibility of denatured residual OVD left in either reusable cannulas, tips or handpieces which have not been properly flushed following surgery. This residual OVD may be broken down during sterilization and can cause toxic inflammation following flushing of this material into the eye in subsequent cases.[16] In addition, this OVD may actually retain other materials such as detergents or enzymes which are used during cleaning and processing of instruments that could conceivably lead to inflammation in the anterior segment of the eye or TASS. It is critically important that any reusable cannulas or instruments be thoroughly flushed at the conclusion of a case in order to not allow the OVD to dry on the instruments which can occur when cannulas are exposed to the air, making cleaning very difficult. It is recommended that all cannulas, handpieces or phacoemulsification tips that are exposed to OVD be thoroughly flushed using sterile, deionized, or distilled water to ensure that there is no residue left on the instruments between cases.

CLEANING AND STERILIZATION OF OPHTHALMIC INSTRUMENTS

The cleaning and sterilization of instruments for use in anterior segment surgery has become an important factor in many recent cases of TASS. Beginning in February of 2006, the number of TASS cases reported to the Intermountain Ocular Research Center of the University of Utah, as well as to the TASS center at Emory University and to industry representatives began to increase markedly. Multiple clusters of cases of TASS were found in surgical centers throughout the United States and Canada. The Ad Hoc TASS Task Force was established with funding from the ASCRS to help investigate this outbreak. Two questionnaires regarding instrument reprocessing as well as the use of products in anterior segment surgery were developed and a database was established to investigate the causes of the TASS outbreak

Approximately 130 different centers reporting TASS were evaluated. The Ad Hoc TASS Task Force issued its final report on September 22, 2006 regarding the analysis of this TASS outbreak (Toxic Anterior Segment Syndrome (TASS) Outbreak: Task Force Final Report - *www.ascrs.org* and *www.aao.org*).

There was no conclusive epidemiologic evidence to suggest any one product was responsible for the increase in the TASS cases reported. Also, analysis of the information did not reveal a single cause or point source related to this particular TASS outbreak. However, there were multiple potential etiologic factors which were found to be related to the cases of TASS. The issue of cleaning and sterilization of instruments for cataract surgery was found to be the most important factor involved in many of the cases of TASS. Specifically, the taskforce found that the short time available between cases to properly clean and reprocess instruments was an area of concern. The use of reusable cannulated instruments of any kind was found to be a potential source of TASS because they normally have small internal diameters and openings as small as 0.3 mm. This includes ultrasound and irrigation–aspiration (I–A) handpieces for use during surgery. It is critically important that all reusable handpieces and cannulas are flushed thoroughly at the conclusion of each case. Inadequate flushing may allow a buildup of residual cortex and OVD which could lead to toxic anterior segment inflammation.

Another important area when evaluating the cleaning and sterilization of instruments that was also evaluated by the task force was the use of enzymes or detergents in the cleaning of the instruments. Enzymes or detergents that are used in the cleaning of instruments for anterior-segment surgery may leave a residue which could cause TASS.[18,19]

If any of this residual enzyme or detergent is not properly rinsed from the instruments, it has the potential to cause TASS. Detergents have been found to accumulate on the inner surfaces of reusable instruments, especially when there is dried or residual OVD. It should be noted that the enzymes and detergents are not completely inactivated when exposed to high temperatures used in the autoclaving of instruments. There is a possibility that the residue of detergents and enzymes left in cannulas or phaco or I–A handpieces

may cause potential inflammation. There have been reports of an increase in corneal thickness secondary to endothelial damage in both rabbits and humans due to enzymatic detergents.[13,19]

Initial evaluations of the toxicity of detergents to the corneal endothelium were referred to as the toxic endothelial cell destruction (TECD) syndrome. Reports of severe TECD following cataract surgery have been found to occur from detergent residues on reusable cannulas.[2]

Furthermore, the use of ultrasound baths to clean ophthalmic instruments between cases is a potential source of TASS. The ultrasound baths may become contaminated by Gram-negative bacteria which can produce a heat-stable endotoxin that can survive autoclaving and cause TASS. Even though the bacteria are incapacitated by heat from the autoclave, the endotoxin remains viable. Deposits of the heat-stable lipopolysaccharide endotoxins can remain attached to the instruments or cannulas and can cause significant inflammation in the anterior segment of the eye if they are injected into the eye.[31] Endotoxin is difficult to remove from ophthalmic instruments and may require an alcohol rinse. Consideration should be given to eliminating the use of ultrasound baths in the cleaning of ophthalmic instruments. Ultrasound baths are often necessary to remove bulk contamination on instruments which is important in areas such as general surgery, but is not a factor in most anterior segment ophthalmic surgeries.

TREATMENT OF TOXIC ANTERIOR SEGMENT SYNDROME

Once again, it is important to ensure that an infectious etiology has been adequately ruled out of cases of suspected TASS. Once the toxic agent enters the eye and causes inflammation and damage which leads to TASS, the mainstay of treatment is the suppression of the secondary inflammatory response. The primary treatment for patients with TASS is the use of intense topical corticosteroids to help calm the inflammation and limit the damage not only from the initial toxic insult but also from the secondary immune response. Patient's should be started on topical prednisolone acetate 1% drops every 1–2 h and be carefully followed in the first several days following the onset of TASS. In addition, the IOP should be closely monitored in patients with TASS. Although the pressure may initially be low, recovery of aqueous production by the ciliary body may cause a rapid increase in IOP as the inflammatory reaction decreases. The initial toxic insult causing TASS not only may injure the cornea and iris, but also can cause significant damage to the trabecular meshwork. Lastly, the inflammation can lead to formation of peripheral anterior synechia, which may also contribute to a rise in IOP.

Patients should be followed closely to ensure that the inflammation is not worsening and that the pressure remains stable. Careful slit-lamp examinations of the anterior segment of the eye should be performed regularly to document the resolution of the anterior segment inflammation and corneal edema if it is present.

CLINICAL COURSE

The clinical outcome of a patient with TASS is directly related to the degree of toxic insult to the anterior segment of the eye occurring during or immediately following the surgical procedure. Patients who have a relatively mild case of TASS tend to undergo

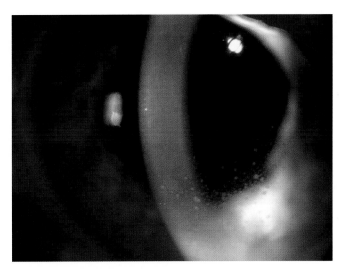

Figure 48-4 Resolving toxic anterior segment syndrome with clearing cornea, rapidly clearing anterior segment inflammation with small residual keratic precipitates.

rapid clearing of the corneal edema over the course of several days to weeks. In addition, the inflammation will clear relatively rapidly with minimal associated sequelae and no permanent damage (Figure 48-4). Patients who have suffered a more moderate insult causing TASS may have a more prolonged course lasting weeks to months with eventual clearing of the cornea and possibility of small residual corneal edema. These patients may also have increased IOP. Patients who have a more severe initial insult often suffer permanent damage to the anterior segment of the eye. This can include diffuse corneal edema which is non-clearing and may require cornea transplantation for treatment (Figure 48-5). In addition, the patient's may suffer other inflammatory sequelae, such as chronic cystoid macular edema. The significant damage to the trabecular meshwork, as well as possible peripheral synechia,

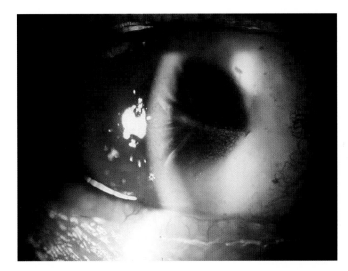

Figure 48-5 Severe toxic anterior segment syndrome with permanent damage showing marked corneal edema and residual chronic anterior segment inflammation.

may lead to a very difficult to control glaucoma, which is often resistant to treatment. Damage to the iris may also lead to a fixed, dilated pupil with significant iris thinning.

■ ANALYSIS OF TOXIC ANTERIOR SEGMENT SYNDROME OUTBREAKS ■

The issue of cleaning and sterilization of instruments has been found to be increasingly related to outbreaks of TASS. Therefore, it is important to analyze how instruments are not only sterilized but also, just as importantly, cleaned prior to actual sterilization. The first step in the proper cleaning of instruments involves flushing or cleaning off any reusable instruments or cannulas at the conclusion of the previous case prior to final sterilization. It is important that any reusable cannulas, handpieces, or tips from phacoemulsification or I–A handpieces be thoroughly flushed at the conclusion of each case. It is important that any residual cortex or OVDs be removed prior to allowing them to dry on the instruments. Many manufacturers recommend that at least 120 cc of sterile, deionized, or distilled water be used to thoroughly flush through all handpieces. It is also important that all instruments which have received any other treatments prior to sterilization undergo a thorough final rinse, once again with sterile deionized water prior to autoclaving or final sterilization.

Processes used for the cleaning of instruments prior to sterilization should also be carefully evaluated. The use of enzymes or detergents for the cleaning of instruments should be re-evaluated, as the use of these materials have the potential to cause TASS. It is unclear whether it is necessary to use either enzymes or detergents following routine ophthalmic surgery, as ophthalmic instruments do not normally have a large bioburden or large amounts of tissue attached to them following surgery. If possible, consideration should be given to the elimination of the use of enzymes or detergents for the cleaning of ophthalmic instruments. Similarly, the use of ultrasound water baths may not be necessary because once again, ophthalmic instruments do not tend to have large bioburdens on them. If ultrasound water baths are used, they should be drained and thoroughly cleaned on a regular basis to prevent the buildup of Gram-negative bacteria and possible endotoxin contamination.

Care should be taken to completely review all of the medications that are used in the cataract surgery and its aftermath. It is important that confirmation be obtained that the anesthetics used intracamerally are preservative free and of the proper dose. In addition, any additives to the BSS, such as epinephrine, should not only be preservative free but should also be bisulphite free. If any intracameral antibiotics or antibiotics in the BSS are used, the proper dosing and dilution of these medications should also be confirmed. Both are off label uses in cataract surgery.

■ PREVENTION OF TOXIC ANTERIOR SEGMENT SYNDROME ■

Since TASS has the possibility of causing significant ocular morbidity, major effort should be focused on the prevention of TASS. It is imperative that surgical centers and hospitals have protocols in place regarding the cleaning and sterilization of instruments and that the entire surgical staff involved in this process is aware of the protocols. It is crucial that the entire surgical team including nurses, operating room technicians, physicians, and pharmacists are aware of what is appropriate for use in ophthalmic surgery and that they be educated about protocols that are in place. The TASS task force investigations of outbreaks of TASS at various surgical centers found that often there were not adequately established protocols in place for the cleaning, processing, and sterilization of instruments. The level and intensity of cleaning of instruments often depended on who was doing the cleaning of the instruments on a particular day and it was often obvious that there were not well-established guidelines in place for the surgical staff.

To help increase the awareness of TASS and to help guide in the prevention of this complication, the Ad Hoc TASS Task Force has taken several steps to create educational materials for surgeons and surgical staff. A video symposium discussing the findings of TASS, etiological factors, and possible ways to prevent TASS comprised of members of the Task Force, as well as representatives from ophthalmic nurse's organizations is available at *www.TASSFacts.com*.

In addition, the members of the Ad Hoc TASS Task Force were involved in a symposium held at Emory University in the fall of 2006 with representatives from the major ophthalmic nurses associations, as well as other personnel with expertise in the cleaning and sterilization of ophthalmic instruments. Input was also obtained from other organizations such as the Centers for Disease Control (CDC) and the Food and Drug Administration (FDA) regarding the development of proper guidelines for the cleaning, sterilization, and processing of ophthalmic instruments. These guidelines are now available to surgeons and their staff on the ASCRS website (*www.ASCRS.org*), as well as the ASORN website and were disseminated with the March 2007 issue of the *Journal of Cataract and Refractive Surgery*. These guidelines should help the surgeons and their staff in the critical process of cleaning and sterilization of instruments with the goal of preventing further TASS outbreaks.

References

[1] Monson MC, Mamalis N, Olson RJ. Toxic anterior segment inflammation following cataract surgery. J Cataract Refract Surg 1992;18:184–189.

[2] Breebaart AC, Nuyts RMMA, Pels E, et al. Toxic endothelial cell destruction of the cornea after routine extracapsular cataract surgery. Arch Ophthalmol 1990;108:1121–1125.

[3] Grimmett MR, Williams KK, Broocker G, Edelhauser HF. Corneal edema after Miochol. Am J Ophthal 1993;116:236–238.

[4] Duffy RE, Brown SE, Caldwell KL, et al. An epidemic of corneal destruction caused by plasma gas sterilization – the toxic cell destruction syndrome investigation team. Arch Ophthalmol 2000;118:1167–1176.

[5] Liu H, Routley I, Teichmann K. Toxic endothelial cell destruction from intraocular benzalkonium chloride. J Cataract Refract Surg 2001;27:1746–1750.

[6] Eleftheriadis H, Cheong N, Sandman S, et al. Corneal toxicity secondary to inadvertent use of benzalkonium chloride preserved viscoelastic material in cataract surgery. Br J Ophthalmol 2002;86:299–305.

[7] Mamalis N, Edelhauser HF, Dawson DG et al. Toxic anterior segment syndrome. J Cataract Refract Surg 2006;32:324–333. [review/update].

[8] Mamalis N. Toxic anterior segment syndrome. J Cataract Refract Surg 2006;32:181–182. [editorial].

[9] Swan KC. Reactivity of ocular tissues to wetting agents. Am J Ophthalmol 1944;27:1118–1122.

[10] Edelhauser HF, Van Horn DL, Schultz RO, et al. Comparative toxicity of intraocular irrigating solutions on corneal endothelium. Am J Ophthal 1976;81:473–481.

[11] Gonnering R, Edelhauser HF, Van Horn DL, et al. The pH tolerance of rabbit in human corneal endothelium. Inv Ophthalmol Vis Sci 1979;18:373–390.

[12] Edelhauser HF, Hanneken AM, Pederson HJ, et al. Osmotic tolerance of rabbit in human corneal endothelium. Arch Ophthalmol 1981;99:1281–1287.

[13] Parikh CH, Edelhauser HF. Ocular surgical pharmacology: corneal endothelial safety and toxicity. Curr Opin Ophthalmol 2003;14:178–185.

[14] Britton B, Hervey R, Kasten K, et al. Intraocular irritation evaluation benzalkonium chloride in rabbits. Ophthalmic Surg 1976;7:46–55.

[15] Green K, Hull DS, Vaughn ED, et al. Rabbit endothelial response to ophthalmic preservatives. Arch Ophthalmol 1977;95:2218–2221.

[16] Kim JH. Intraocular inflammation of denatured viscoelastic substance in cases of cataract extraction and lens implantation. J Cataract Refract Surg 1987;13:537–542.

[17] Richburg F, Reidy J, Apple DJ, Olson RJ. Sterile hypopyon secondary to ultrasonic cleaning solution. J Cataract Refract Surg 1986;12:248–251.

[18] Carter LM, Duncan G, Rennie GK. Effects of detergents on the ionic balance and permeability of isolated bovine cornea. Exp Eye Res 1973;17:409–416.

[19] Parikh C, Sippy BD, Martin DF, Edelhauser HF. Effects of enzymatic sterilization detergents on the corneal endothelium. Arch Ophthalmol 2002;120:165–172.

[20] Edelhauser HF, Hyndivk RA, Zeeb A, Schultz RO. Corneal edema and the intraocular use of epinephrine. Am J Ophthal 1982;93:327–333.

[21] Slack JW, Edelhauser HF, Helenek MJ. A bisulfite-free intraocular epinephrine solution. Am J Ophthal 1990;110:77–82.

[22] Kadonosono K, Ito N, Yazama F, et al. Effect of intracameral anesthesia on the corneal endothelium. J Cataract Refract Surg 1998;24:1377–1381.

[23] Anderson NJ, Nath R, Anderson CJ, Edelhauser HF. Comparison of preservative-free Bupivacaine vs lidocaine for intracameral anesthesia: a randomized clinical trial and in vitro analysis. Am J Ophthal 1999;127:393–402.

[24] Guzey M, Satici A, Dogan Z, et al. The effects of Bupivacaine and lidocaine on the corneal endothelium when applied into the anterior chamber at the concentration supplied commercially. Ophthalmologica 2002;216:113–117.

[25] Gills JP. Filters and antibiotics in irrigating solution for cataract surgery. J Cataract Refract Surg 1991;17:385.

[26] Judson PH. Aminoglycoside macular toxicity after subconjunctival injection. Arch Ophthalmol 1989;107:1282–1283.

[27] Campochiaro PA, Conway BP. Aminoglycoside toxicity – a survey of retinal specialists; implication for ocular use. Arch Ophthalmol 1991;109:946–950.

[28] Montan PG, Wejde G, Setterquist H, et al. Prophylactic intracameral cefuroxime: Evaluation of safety and kinetics in cataract surgery. J Cataract Refract Surg 2002;28:977–981.

[29] Barry P, Seal DV, Gettinby G, et al. ESCRS study of prophylaxis of postoperative endophthalmitis after cataract surgery: Preliminary report of principal results from a European multicenter study. J Cataract Refract Surg 2006;32:407–410.

[30] Werner L, Shear JH, Taylor JR, et al. Toxic anterior segment syndrome and possible association with ointment in the anterior chamber following cataract surgery. J Cataract Refract Surg 2006;32:227–235.

[31] Kriesler KR, Martin SS, Young CW, et al. Postoperative inflammation following cataract extraction caused by bacterial contamination of the cleaning bath detergent. J Cataract Surg 1992;18:106–110.

Corneal Edema after Cataract Surgery

Roger F. Steinert, MD

49

CONTENTS

CHAPTER HIGHLIGHTS

>> Causes of unexpected postop edema

>> Repair of Descemet membrane detachment

>> Is the intraocular lens to blame?

>> When to consider keratoplasty

Corneal endothelial decompensation after cataract extraction is a well-known, although rare complication of all types of cataract surgery. The overall incidence is less than 1%. This chapter reviews the differential diagnosis and treatment of corneal edema after cataract surgery. Chapter 21 addresses combined penetrating keratoplasty and cataract surgery in patients with preoperatively compromised corneas.

PATHOPHYSIOLOGY

The final common pathway for corneal stromal edema occurring after cataract surgery is inadequate endothelial pump function used to keep the corneal stroma and epithelium in their relatively dehydrated and clear state.[1] Elevated intraocular pressure can overwhelm the corneal endothelial pump. Reduction in intraocular pressure (IOP) will reverse the edema in such cases. In a marginally compensated endothelium, lowering of IOP with antiglaucomatous medications from a high-normal to a low-normal reading can make a critical difference in corneal clarity.

The corneal endothelium acts to dehydrate the cornea both actively through an adenosine triphosphate-driven bicarbonate ion pump[2–4] and passively through the integrity of the cellular membrane barrier.[5,6] The adult human corneal endothelium has little ability to replicate in order to replace damaged cells.[7–10]

Endothelial cells do migrate, enlarge, and undergo fibroblastic metaplasia in an effort to cover denuded areas of Descemet's membrane and reestablish the intercellular junctions.[10–12] An adaptive increase in the number of pump sites per cell may occur in diseased corneas.[1] Therefore, some cases of corneal edema will improve over several weeks to months. Inflammation may also transiently reduce endothelial pump function.[13] Elimination of the inflammation may be accompanied by restoration of corneal clarity.

DIFFERENTIAL DIAGNOSIS OF POSTOPERATIVE CORNEAL EDEMA

Table 49-1 lists the principal causes of postoperative corneal edema after cataract surgery.

Surgical trauma is often the culprit in unexpected postoperative corneal endothelial decompensation. Direct local injury to the endothelium with an instrument or a portion of the intraocular lens (IOL) implant will result in a discrete patch of edema. Over time, the migration of adjacent endothelial cells can restore corneal clarity if the area of injury is not overly large. Diffuse edema may result from difficulty in delivering the nucleus in extracapsular cataract extraction or prolonged ultrasound in phacoemulsification, particularly if all or part of the nucleus is fragmented in the anterior chamber. A high volume of balanced salt solution (BSS) infusion alone is generally well tolerated by the corneal endothelium, but prolonged infusion studies have demonstrated increased endothelial injury with regular BSS compared to the enhanced BSS formula use.[14–18]

Toxicity from a variety of chemical contaminants may result in diffuse endothelial decompensation. It is frequently, but not always, accompanied by other evidence of intraocular toxicity, most notably a fixed and dilated pupil and elevated IOP.[19,20] This syndrome is often called toxic anterior segment syndrome (TASS) (see Chapter 48). In more extreme cases, toxicity will result in an excessive inflammatory reaction, ciliary body shutdown and hypotony, or acute retinal inflammation or retinal necrosis (or both).

When toxicity is suspected, all intraocular solutions and medications are suspect and should be reviewed. More commonly, toxicity results from agents not intended for use inside the eye or agents used in excessive concentration. Examples include

Table 49-1 Principal causes of corneal edema after cataract surgery

Surgical trauma
Instruments
IOL
Irrigating solutions
Ultrasonic vibrations
Nuclear fragments
Prior surgery
Primary corneal endothelial disease
Fuchs' dystrophy
Low enthothelial cell density without guttae
Chemical injury
Preservations in solutions
Residual toxic chemicals on instruments (e.g., detergents, dried solutions)
Improper concentrations of solutions (e.g., antibiotics)
Osmotic damage
Direct toxicity
Mistakenly used toxic chemicals, expired agents, or incorrect solutions (e.g., normal saline instead of balanced salt solution)
IOL syndromes
Direct endothelial touch
Long-term toxicity (? inflammatory)
Contact with other ocular tissues
Flat chamber
Iris bombé
Suprachoroidal effusion-hemorrhage
Detachment of Descemet's membrane
Trauma from retained foreign material
Nuclear chips
Particulate matter
Postoperative glaucoma
Inflammation
Membranous ingrowth or downgrowth
Epithelial downgrowth
Fibrous ingrowth
Endothelial proliferation
Vitreous touch-adherence
Absence of IOL and capsule
Brown-McLean syndrome

IOL: Intraocular lens

detergents used in cleaning reusable instruments, incorrect concentrations of additives, use of preserved instead of nonpreserved additives in infusions, or confusing an intended intraocular medication with some other substance that is toxic. Antibiotics particularly can be suspect. Errors in dilution medications may occur. External antibiotics may also inadvertently enter the anterior chamber, particularly through an unsutured wound. A subconjunctival bolus superiorly overlying a superior corneal scleral tunnel may be expressed into the anterior chamber through lid pressure, for example. Aminoglycoside antibiotics, in particular, have profound retinal toxicity at all but the extremely low concentrations.

Detachment of the Descemet's membrane is usually recognized intraoperatively. If not, slit-lamp examination postoperatively is diagnostic.[12,21–24] A glassy membrane similar to the lens capsule will be seen separated from the posterior stroma. If extensive, the exact configuration of the detached membrane can be difficult to interpret. Localized detachments are often in close proximity to their proper anatomic location. If the Descemet's membrane can be brought back into proper anatomic apposition with the posterior stroma, and the endothelium itself has not been irreversibly damaged, the endothelial pump function will itself reattach the Descemet's membrane because of the relative vacuum created by the endothelial pump. This is best accomplished surgically by introduction of an air bubble through a paracentesis wound inferiorly. This can be performed intraoperatively or post-operatively in the operating room or at the slit-lamp microscope in favorable cases. Only when the Descemet's membrane is held away from the stroma by traction is a suture needed. A full-thickness through-and-through 10-0 nylon suture can forcefully reappose an area of intractable detachment (Figure 49-1). Instrumentation of the membrane itself should be avoided if possible because of the local injury to the endothelium that will occur. Use of viscoelastic agents should be avoided in an effort to reappose the Descemet's membrane. If the viscoelastic agent enters between the posterior corneal stroma and the Descemet's membrane, it will prevent reattachment of the membrane and may remain as a barrier indefinitely. Finally, although reattachment of the Descemet's membrane and restoration of corneal clarity is urgent, it is not a true emergency. The endothelium is bathed in aqueous, even in the detached form. The endothelium will remain viable while an orderly reintervention is planned. Abnormal endothelial proliferation will occur with prolonged detachment or improper adhesion.[12,25,26]

UNSUSPECTED LOW PREOPERATIVE ENDOTHELIAL CELL DENSITY

A small portion of the population has a low endothelial cell density not heralded by the presence of corneal guttae.[27,28] To detect these patients preoperatively, some cataract surgeons perform routine preoperative specular microscopy with endothelial cell counts. Other surgeons argue against this routine testing in view of its expense and the fact that a low cell count should not alter the surgical technique; in all cases, the surgeon presumably employs the best available technique to minimize endothelial cell injury. Careful inspection with a broad oblique beam at high magnification under the slit-lamp biomicroscope can, in fact, disclose the endothelial cell pattern. With practice, the surgeon can make a good estimate of the endothelial cell density and pattern. Formal specular microscopy with endothelial cell photography can then be reserved for cases of probable abnormality rather than used as a screening tool.

An occasional patient will experience unexpected corneal edema after apparently atraumatic surgery. In the absence of preoperative specular microscopy, the status of the endothelium in the fellow eye should be examined. A case of naturally low cell density will almost always be bilateral. Examination of the fellow eye will, therefore, help in the differential diagnosis of unexpected postoperative corneal edema.

IOL syndromes are a leading cause of corneal decompensation many years after the surgery. A loose anterior-chamber IOL or a large or loose pupillary-supported iris plane IOL will directly traumatize the corneal endothelium, cause a progressive attrition of endothelial cells, and ultimately lead to clinically evident corneal edema. The edema will characteristically begin in a localized zone over the area of trauma but will progress as the remaining endothelial cells migrate into the area of damage.

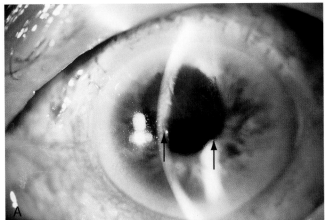
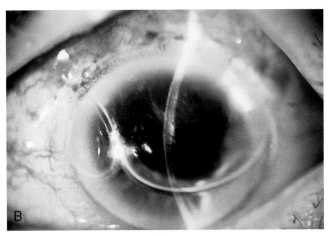
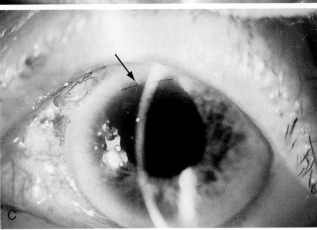

Figure 49-1 A, Detached Descemet's membrane is seen as a glassy membrane in the anterior chamber behind an area of corneal edema. The detachment may be extensive with curling of the Descemet's membrane in on itself well away from the area of edema, or it may be a shallow detachment only seen with a thin slit beam. Often a small amount of blood is trapped at the edge of the inferior detachment (arrows). B, Most Descemet's membrane detachments can be reapposed by placing a large air bubble in the anterior chamber through an inferior paracentesis. C, Particularly where extensive detachment or traction on the membrane exists that cannot be fully relieved, a through-and-through 10-0 nylon suture is needed to forcefully reappose the Descemet's membrane and prevent aqueous access into the space between the posterior corneal stroma and the separated membrane (arrow). After several weeks, the suture may be removed in most cases.

Corneal edema beginning many years after IOL implantation may be due to excessive loss of endothelium at the time of surgery, followed by ongoing normal or accelerated attrition of the remaining endothelium. So-called, closed-loop anterior-chamber IOLs are no longer marketed (Azar 91Z from IOLAB, Leiske Surgidev Style 10, Stableflex from Optical Radiation Corporation, Hesburg from IntraOptics) and have a much higher rate of late corneal decompensation than any other anterior-chamber lenses, especially the Kelman three-foot (Omnifit) and four-foot (Multiflex) styles.[29–31] Many surgeons suspect that all anterior-chamber lenses have a higher rate of long-term complications than do posterior-chamber lenses, whereas other surgeons believe that this perception arises because anterior-chamber lenses are typically employed in complicated cases in which posterior capsule support has been compromised. Adequate data to prove or disprove these viewpoints may never be available.

Late-onset corneal edema associated with anterior-chamber lenses is often preceded by or accompanied by cystoid macular edema, a phenomenon that has been termed the cornea-retina syndrome. A generally accepted explanation for this syndrome is that the anterior-chamber IOL causes chronic subclinical inflammation. Prostaglandins are the inflammatory mediators most often suspected as being capable of causing both cystoid macular edema and corneal endothelial cell loss.

The anterior-chamber IOLs in these cases of cornea-retina syndrome are typically not loose. In fact, gonioscopy reveals peripheral iris synechiae around the closed-loop haptics (Figure 49-2). Special techniques are required to explant these closed-loop anterior-chamber IOLs, as detailed in Figures 49-3 and 49-4 (see also Chapter 46). Simple traction on incarcerated haptic will cause iridodialysis and severe bleeding.

A loose IOL causing corneal edema can be differentiated from the cornea-retina syndrome in two ways. Clinical examination with gonioscopy usually is diagnostic. Specular microscopy also is often diagnostic when the corneal edema is localized to a peripheral area. If the localized edema is due to trauma from a loose IOL, the endothelial cell density increases with increasing distance from the area of edema. In contrast, in the cornea-retina syndrome, the corneal endothelial density will be very low and borderline to maintain compensation throughout the remaining clear cornea.

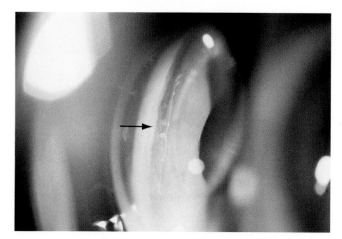

Figure 49-2 Gonioscopic examination of a Stableflex anterior chamber lens shows typical peripheral anterior synechia formation around the distal haptic loop (arrow).

If the cornea decompensates centrally and penetrating keratoplasty is performed, most surgeons will exchange a closed-loop anterior-chamber IOL for either an open-loop anterior-chamber IOL or a suture-fixated posterior-chamber IOL.[32–38] The best type of replacement IOL remains undetermined in regard to both short-term complications and long-term graft survival and recovery of vision.

Management of a patient with late-onset cystoid macular edema or localized corneal edema in the presence of an anterior-chamber IOL is problematic. In most cases of late-onset cystoid macular edema and essentially all cases of localized corneal edema, the endothelium will be severely depleted even when the cornea remains clinically clear. Nevertheless, the longer cystoid macular edema persists, the more likely that it will cause irreversible macular damage even if acute leakage resolves. The author's approach to new late-onset cystoid macular edema is an intense course of topical steroids and nonsteroidal anti-inflammatory agents (e.g., dexamethasone, 0.1%, or prednisolone acetate, 1%, combined with ketorolac, 0.5% [Acular], or diclofenac, 0.1% [Voltaren], both four times daily). If the cystoid macular edema does not improve over 1 month, or resolves but then recurs, exchange of the closed-loop anterior-chamber IOL is strongly indicated. Improvement may occur with a replacement Kelman-style anterior chamber IOL, but the author favors moving to another fixation site, either peripheral iris suture fixation or trans-scleral suture fixation of a posterior-chamber IOL, for the best long-term results. The surgeon must perform atraumatic surgery if the fragile cornea is to remain compensated. Explantation must use the techniques outlined in Figures 49-3 and 49-4. Secondary IOL implantation is reviewed in Chapter 41. Cystoid macular edema is covered in detail in Chapter 54, and management of intraocular inflammation is discussed in Chapter 57.

Table 49-2 outlines the decision-making steps for managing complications of closed-loop anterior-chamber IOLs.

PERIPHERAL CORNEAL EDEMA

Perhaps the rarest and most benign form of corneal edema is the syndrome described by Brown and McLean.[39,40] In the classic syndrome, an aphakic patient experiences peripheral corneal stromal and epithelial edema that spares the superior cornea. Pigment deposits are present on the underlying endothelium. A central zone of 5–7 mm remains clear and compact indefinitely despite the peripheral edema. The peripheral iris may show transillumination, but the trabecular meshwork is not necessarily hyperpigmented. If the patient is bilaterally aphakic, the syndrome is usually present in both eyes. There is no clinical inflammation, and the cause is unknown. Although the classic presentation is following intracapsular cataract extraction, it may occur after extracapsular cataract extraction.[41] Moreover, although the syndrome is said to occur only 6 years or more postoperatively, the author has seen the syndrome appear 3 months after sulcus suturing of a posterior chamber lens in a 40-year-old patient with prior extracapsular extraction of a traumatic cataract (Figure 49-5).

■ TREATMENT OF POSTOPERATIVE CORNEAL EDEMA ■

HYPERTONIC SOLUTIONS

Hypertonic solutions, typically 5% sodium chloride ophthalmic preparations, can improve the visual function of a patient with

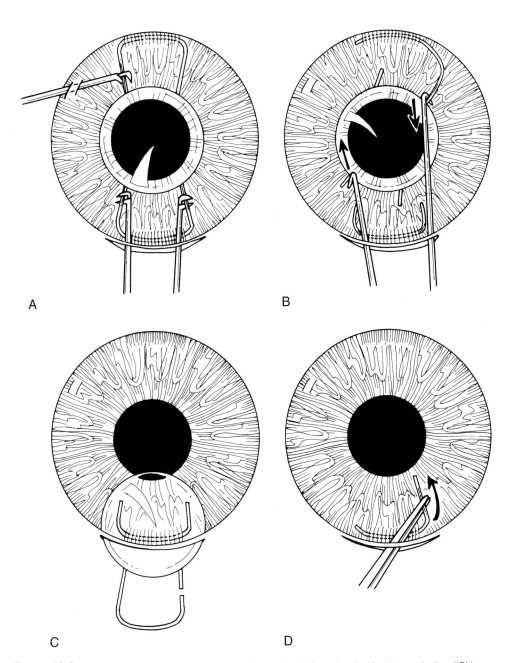

Figure 49-3 Technique for explantation of a Surgidev Style 10 (Leiske) anterior chamber intraocular lens (IOL). **A,** Through an inferotemporal paracentesis, a haptic cutting instrument (Rapazzo haptic cutter, Storz Instruments) is introduced to cut one arm of the inferior haptic. Through the superior wound, with the anterior chamber maintained by viscoelastic solution, both arms of the superior haptic are cut. **B,** Using two IOL manipulating hooks, the IOL is then rotated gently. The inferior haptic uncurls and is drawn through the inferior peripheral anterior synechia without tearing the synechia, which would result in bleeding and an iridodialysis. **C,** The rotated IOL is then delivered through the superior wound, taking care not to snag the iris or the wound on the transected haptic. **D,** The remaining superior haptic is then grasped with a forceps and rotated out of the superior peripheral anterior synechia.

mild, predominantly microcystic epithelial edema. This will be particularly beneficial to the patient on awakening in the morning, when edema is maximal because of lack of evaporation during the night when the eyelids are closed. Use of a 5% sodium chloride ointment at bedtime will also help reduce the accumulation of edema while the eyelids are closed during sleep. However, the use of hypertonic solutions is only palliative. It does not improve or restore endothelial pump function or the integrity of the cell barrier.

ANTI-INFLAMMATORY THERAPY

Reduction of intraocular inflammation may be of benefit in some cases of postoperative edema. Inflammation can cause transient dysfunction of the endothelial pump. Moreover, inflammation may cause some degree of endothelial cell death. By extrapolation, pharmacologic treatment of inflammation with topical steroids and perhaps nonsteroidal anti-inflammatory drugs may help to maximize the surviving endothelium, thus improving the chances that corneal clarity will ultimately return

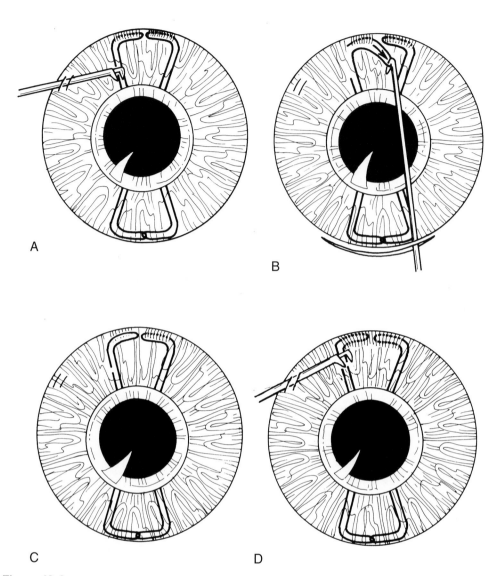

Figure 49-4 Technique for explantation of a Stableflex-style anterior chamber intraocular lens (IOL). **A,** Through an inferotemporal paracentesis, a haptic cutter transects the lateral arm of the haptic. **B,** Sinskey-style hook engages the "toe" of the haptic by direct visualization if possible or by carefully passing it within the two haptic struts. With gentle traction on the "toe," the haptic unfolds and is drawn through the inferior peripheral anterior synechia, avoiding bleeding or iridodialysis. **C,** Freed from the peripheral anterior synechia, the haptic is now loose within the anterior chamber. The same maneuver is now performed on the remaining haptics that are entrapped in peripheral anterior synechia. This should be determined by preoperative gonioscopic inspection and confirmed directly at surgery. Not all four haptics are necessarily engaged in peripheral anterior synechia. Sometimes the "toes" cross, as illustrated in the superior haptics (6 o'clock position in the figure). The IOL hook must engage only the desired haptic and avoid engaging the wrong haptic or both haptics simultaneously. After freeing all of the haptics, the IOL is delivered through the wound. **D,** In occasional cases of extreme inflammatory reaction, the peripheral anterior synechia entirely covers the "toe" of the haptic or both arms of the haptic. In this case, it is best to simply transect the two arms of the haptic as distal as possible and leave the remaining haptic in the angle. The acute angle of the "toe" does not allow a haptic to "uncurl" out of the synechia with traction on the "heel" or upper "leg" of the haptic.

postoperatively. This supposition has not been rigorously proved, but most clinicians will treat patients with strong topical steroids, such as prednisolone acetate (1%) or dexamethasone (0.1%) as often as every 1–2 h in cases of acute postoperative corneal edema. Steroid therapy may be of no benefit in non-inflammation-related corneal edema, however. Topical dexamethasone did not differ from placebo in the rate of occurrence of corneal edema in a controlled study of patients with Fuchs' dystrophy.[42]

CORNEAL TRANSPLANTATION

Restoration of vision in an eye with irreversible corneal edema requires either a posterior lamellar endothelial transplant (Descemet-stripping endothelial keratoplasty (DSEK), Descemet-stripping automated endothelial keratoplasty (DSAEK), deep lamellar endothelial keratoplasty (DLEK), and Descemet membrane endothelial keratoplasty (DMEK)) or full-thickness

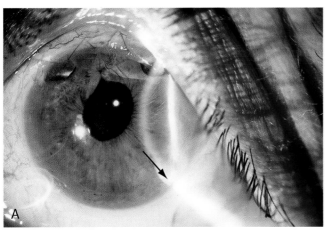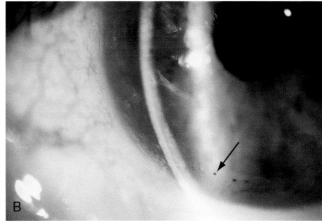

Figure 49-5 A, Slit-lamp photomicrograph of a patient with Brown-McLean syndrome of peripheral corneal edema (arrow). B, High magnification reveals classic pigment deposits on the endothelium underlying the area of edema (arrow).

Table 49-2 Treatment of corneal edema

Eliminate cause
  Treat inflammation
  Lower intraocular pressure
  Remove tissue-IOL contact
  Re-attach Descemet's membrane

Enhance surface dehydration
  Evaporate
  Hypertonic agents

Treat pain
  Lubricants
  Soft contact lenses
  Cautery of the Bowman's layer
  Conjunctival flap

Restore anatomy
  DSEK
  DSAEK
  DLEK
  DMEK
  Penetrating keratoplasty

IOL: Intraocular lens; DSEK: Descemet-stripping endothelial keratoplasty; DSAEK: Descemet-stripping automated endothelial keratoplasty; DLEK: deep lamellar endothelial keratoplasty; DMEK: Descemet membrane endothelial keratoplasty

stromal and epithelial edema, the situation may be so clearly irreversible that it is in the patient's best interest to proceed with penetrating keratoplasty earlier than 3 months after the original cataract extraction.

The treatment options for corneal edema are listed in Table 49-2.

References

[1] Waring GO, Bourne WM, Edelhauser HF, et al. The corneal endothelium: normal and pathologic structure and function. Ophthalmology 1982;89:531.
[2] Maurice DM, Riley MV. The cornea. In: Graymore CN, editor. Biochemistry of the eye. New York: Academic Press; 1970.
[3] Kaye GI, Tice LW. Studies on the cornea. V. Electron microscopic localization of adenosine trisphosphatase activity in the rabbit cornea in relation to transport. Invest Ophthalmol 1966;5:22.
[4] Barfort P, Maurice D. Electrical potential and fluid transport across the corneal endothelium. Exp Eye Res 1974;19:11.
[5] Maurice DM. Cornea and sclera. In: Davson H, editor. The eye. 3rd ed. New York: Academic Press; 1984.
[6] Kreutziger GO. Lateral membrane morphology and gap junction structure in rabbit corneal endothelium. Exp Eye Res 1976;23:285.
[7] Flaxel JT, Swan KC. Limbal wound healing after cataract extraction: a histological study. Arch Ophthalmol 1969;81:653–659.
[8] Kloucek F. The corneal endothelium. Acta Univ Carol [Med] (Praha) 1967;123:321–373.
[9] Van Horn DL, Edelhauser HF, Aaberg TM, et al. In vivo effects of air and sulfur hexafluoride gas on rabbit corneal endothelium. Invest Ophthalmol 1972;11:1036–1038.
[10] Capella JA. Regeneration of endothelium in diseased and injured corneas. Am J Ophthalmol 1972;74:810–817.
[11] Iwamoto T, DeVoe AG. Electron microscopic studies on Fuchs' combined dystrophy. I. Posterior portion of the cornea. Invest Ophthalmol 1971;10:9–28.
[12] Waring GO, Laibson PR, Rodrigues M. Clinical and pathologic alterations of Descemet's membrane: with emphasis on endothelial metaplasia. Surv Ophthalmol 1973–1974;18:325–368.
[13] Dohlman CH, Hyndiuk RA. Subclinical and manifest corneal edema after cataract extraction. In: Transactions of the New Orleans Academy of Ophthalmology, Symposium on the Cornea. St Louis: Mosby; 1972. p. 214.
[14] Edelhauser HF, Van Horn DL, Hyndiuk RA, et al. Intraocular irrigating solutions: their effect on corneal endothelium. Arch Ophthalmol 1975;93:657–658.
[15] Dikstein S, Maurice DM. The metabolic bases to the fluid pump in the cornea. J Physiol 1972;221:29–41.
[16] Dikstein S. Efficiency and survival of the corneal endothelial pump. Exp Eye Res 1973;15:639–644.
[17] Anderson EI, Fischbarg J, Spector A. Fluid transport, ATP level, and ATPase activities in isolated rabbit endothelium. Biochem Biophys Acta 1973;307:557–562.
[18] Anderson EI, Fischbarg J, Spector A. Disulfide stimulation of fluid transport and effect on ATP level in rabbit endothelium. Exp Eye Res 1974;19:1–10.
[19] Breebaart AC, Nuyts RMMA, Pels E, et al. Toxic endothelial cell destruction of the cornea after routine extracapsular cataract surgery. Arch Ophthalmol 1990;108:1121–1125.
[20] Nuyts RMMA, Edelhauser HF, Pels EII, et al. Toxic effects of detergents on the corneal endothelium. Arch Ophthalmol 1990;108:1158–1162.
[21] Samuels B. Detachment of Descemet's membrane. Trans Am Ophthalmol Soc 1928;26:427–437.
[22] Scheie HG. Stripping of Descemet's membrane in cataract extraction. Trans Am Ophthalmol Soc 1964;62:140–152.
[23] Sparks GM. Descemetopexy: surgical reattachment of stripped Descemet's membrane. Arch Ophthalmol 1967;78:31–34.
[24] Zeiter HJ, Zeiter JT. Descemet's membrane separation during five hundred forty-four intraocular lens implantations. J Am Intraocul Implant Soc 1983;9:36–39.
[25] Donaldson DD, Smith TR. Descemet's membrane tubes. Trans Am Ophthalmol Soc 1966;64:89–109.

penetrating keratoplasty. A final decision about proceeding with keratoplasty should usually be deferred 2–3 months postoperatively in case of acute decompensation after cataract surgery. In some cases of marginal corneal endothelial function, clarity is regained within this time frame. If there is active ongoing inflammation, the decision to proceed with keratoplasty should be deferred while intense anti-inflammatory therapy continues, to enhance the probability of transplant survival and restoration of the patient's own corneal clarity. In occasional cases of severe striae with both

[26] Kroll AJ. Proliferation of Descemet's membrane. Arch Ophthalmol 1969;82:339–343.

[27] Kayes J, Holmberg A. The fine structure of the cornea in Fuchs' endothelial dystrophy. Invest Ophthalmol 1964;3:47–67.

[28] Stocker FW. The endothelium of the cornea and its clinical implications. 2nd ed. Springfield, Ill: Charles C. Thomas; 1971.

[29] Solomon KD, Apple DJ, Mamalis N, et al. Complications of intraocular lenses with special reference to an analysis of 2500 explanted intraocular lenses (IOLs). Eur J Implant Refract Surg 1991;3:195.

[30] Lim ES, Apple DJ, Tsai JC, et al. An analysis of flexible anterior chamber lenses with special reference to the normalized rate of lens explantation. Ophthalmology 1991;98:243.

[31] Price Jr FW. Factors contributing to corneal decompensation with the Stableflex lens. J Cataract Refract Surg 1988;14:53–57.

[32] Kozarsky M, Stopak S, Waring GO, et al. Results of penetrating keratoplasty for pseudophakic corneal edema with retention of intraocular lens. Ophthalmology 1984;91:1141.

[33] Speaker MG, Lugo M, Laibson PR, et al. Penetrating keratoplasty for pseudophakic bullous keratopathy. Ophthalmology 1988;95:1260.

[34] Kornmehl EW, Steinert RF, Odrich MG, et al. Penetrating keratoplasty for pseudophakic bullous keratopathy edema associated with closed-loop anterior chamber intraocular lenses. Ophthalmology 1990;97:407–414.

[35] Schein OD, Kenyon KR, Steinert RF, et al. A randomized trial of intraocular lens fixation techniques with penetrating keratoplasty. Ophthalmology 1993;100:1437–1443.

[36] Price Jr FW, Whitson WE. Visual results of suture-fixated posterior chamber lenses during penetrating keratoplasty. Ophthalmology 1989;96:1234–1240.

[37] Soong HK, Meyer RF, Sugar A. Posterior chamber IOL implantation during keratoplasty for aphakic or pseudophakic corneal edema. Cornea 1987;6:306–312.

[38] Soong HK, Musch DC, Kowal V, et al. Implantation of posterior chamber intraocular lenses in the absence of lens capsule during penetrating keratoplasty. Arch Ophthalmol 1989;107:660–665.

[39] Brown SI, McLean JM. Peripheral corneal edema after cataract extraction: a new clinical entity. Trans Am Acad Ophthalmol Otolaryngol 1969;73:465–470.

[40] Brown SI. Peripheral corneal edema after cataract extraction. Am J Ophthalmol 1970;70:326–329.

[41] Flaxel JT, Swan KC. Limbal wound healing after cataract extraction: a histological study. Am J Ophthalmol 1969;81:653–659.

[42] Wilson SE, Bourne WM, Brubaker RF. Effect of dexamethasone on corneal endothelial Fuchs' dystrophy, Invest Ophthalmol Vis Sci 1988;29:357.

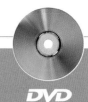

Glaucoma after Cataract Surgery

James W. Hung, MD and Bradford J. Shingleton, MD

50

CHAPTER HIGHLIGHTS

>> Open angle etiologies
>> Causes and treatment of angle closure
>> Medical therapy options
>> Surgical interventions

Advances in instrumentation and cataract surgical techniques have resulted in shorter operating time, smaller incisions, and earlier visual rehabilitation. However, glaucoma following cataract surgery can still be a problem. Elevation in intraocular pressure (IOP) may occur early or late in the postoperative course and can be associated with either an open or closed angle. Many causes exist for IOP elevation after cataract surgery, and it is inappropriate to categorize them all under the terms aphakic or pseudophakic glaucoma.

As cataract surgery has evolved, so have the types of postoperative glaucoma. With the decline in intracapsular cataract surgery and rigid anterior chamber lenses, enzyme glaucoma and the uveitis-glaucoma-hyphema (UGH) syndrome are rarely seen. Planned extracapsular cataract surgery and posterior chamber lens implants brought a rise in pigmentary glaucoma as a result of pigment release from the ciliary sulcus and posterior iris. The widespread use of viscosurgical agents with cataract surgery plays a significant role in early postoperative IOP elevation. Phacoemulsification and clear corneal incisions have lessened glaucoma from wound compression caused by tight suture closure. Clear corneal phacoemulsification also allows cataract surgery to be done in normal and glaucomatous eyes with less risk of postoperative IOP worsening and, indeed, IOP is often reduced after

phacoemulsification. The use of topical anesthesia allows glaucoma patients to continue using their antiglaucoma medications without interruption. At the same time, new types of postoperative anterior segment complications, such as capsular block, are being seen.

Surgeons must also realize that glaucoma after cataract surgery does not always result directly from the surgery itself but may occur after postoperative interventions, such as neodymium: yttrium-aluminum-garnet (Nd:YAG) posterior capsulotomy.

This chapter reviews the wide-ranging differential diagnosis of glaucoma after cataract surgery (Table 50-1) and presents the therapeutic options for the ophthalmologist.

OPEN-ANGLE GLAUCOMAS

PRIMARY OPEN-ANGLE GLAUCOMA

Primary open-angle glaucoma may first become apparent following cataract surgery secondary to anatomic alterations, the natural evolution of the disease, or both. In the early era of cataract surgery, incomplete wound closure with aqueous leakage and low pressure (hypotony) were relatively common. Today, the incidence of inadvertent aqueous leakage is low because of improved incision architecture, finer suture material and more advanced closure techniques. Particularly in planned extracapsular surgery, tight-closure techniques,[1,2] suture compression,[3] and edema[4] may mechanically distort the filtration angle and further compromise aqueous outflow, leading to elevated IOP. Scleral tunnel and clear cornea phacoemulsification techniques reduce but do not eliminate this problem.[2] Even if preoperative IOP control is satisfactory, the risk of an acute pressure rise following uncomplicated intracapsular or extracapsular cataract surgery is greater in eyes with pre-existing glaucoma than in healthy eyes.[5,6]

Besides alterations in angle configuration, early open-angle postoperative IOP increase after cataract surgery may be the result of retained viscosurgical, postoperative inflammation, bleeding, or pigment dispersion.[7]

The long-term effect of cataract surgery on glaucoma control varies depending on the method of cataract extraction. Following intracapsular and extracapsular surgery, several studies have

Table 50-1 Glaucoma after cataract surgery

Open-angle glaucomas

- Primary open-angle glaucoma
- Blood-induced glaucomas
- Hyphema
- Ghost cell glaucoma
- Uveitis
- UGH syndrome
- Lens particle
- Dislocated nuclear fragments
- Corticosteroids
- Viscosurgical agents
- Nd:YAG laser capsulotomy
- Vitreous in anterior chamber
- Cyclodialysis cleft closure
- Alpha-chymotrypsin

Closed-angle glaucomas

- Pre-existing angle-closure glaucoma
- Pupillary block
- Malignant glaucoma
- Neovascular glaucoma
- Epithelial/fibrovascular ingrowth

UGH, Uveitis-glaucoma-hyphema.

reported IOP reduction for weeks to months.[8,9] Other groups have found no long-term pressure reduction.[5,6,10] With clear corneal phacoemulsification, several authors have shown an associated reduction in IOP in normal and glaucoma suspect eyes.[11–16] Patients with glaucoma were shown to have a reduction in IOP plus a lowering in the number of medications necessary to control postoperative IOP.[11] The need for medications tends to slowly increase with time. However, clear-corneal phacoemulsification should not be performed with the intent of achieving better IOP control, but for the secondary benefit of the IOP likely remaining stable or slightly reduced for up to 5 years.[17]

Cataract surgery in eyes with preexisting filtration blebs may result in IOP elevation and decrease in bleb size, but IOP may still remain acceptable for long-term control.[6,18,19]

The presence of a properly positioned posterior-chamber intraocular lens (IOL) implant does not affect IOP. Although closed-loop, anterior chamber IOLs occasionally produce significant IOP elevation, the current semiflexible, one-piece, open-loop style lenses are associated with fewer problems.[20]

An early postoperative rise in IOP may be minimized with topical beta-blockers,[21] topical apraclonidine,[22] systemic carbonic anhydrase inhibitors,[23] topical prostaglandin analogues,[24] and intracameral carbachol.[23] In addition, judicious use and removal of viscosurgical substances are recommended (see Viscosurgical agents). Nonsteroidal anti-inflammatory drugs are ineffective in preventing or decreasing the magnitude of the pressure elevation.[25] Sterile anterior-chamber decompression with the release of aqueous via the paracentesis incision may provide temporary relief of IOP elevation. It is important to check the IOP 30–60 min after decompression because recurrence of IOP elevation may occur.[26]

Persistent postoperative IOP elevation resulting from primary open-angle glaucoma mandates standard treatment protocols. Earlier and more aggressive management is indicated in patients with significant pre-existing glaucomatous optic nerve damage.

BLOOD-INDUCED GLAUCOMAS

HYPHEMA

Blood in the anterior chamber during the early postoperative period typically originates from the scleral cataract incision, an iridectomy, or pupillary sphincter tears.

Patients with postoperative hyphemas may be asymptomatic or have decreased vision. Circulating or layered red blood cells, or both, are seen in the anterior chamber with an open angle. An endocapsular location is an unusual type of postoperative hemorrhage.[27] Pupillary block is uncommon but may develop if bleeding extends into the posterior chamber, occludes an iridectomy, or both. If the anterior hyaloid face is not intact, blood may be seen in the vitreous cavity.

Open-angle glaucoma occurs from trabecular meshwork obstruction by red blood cells, platelets, fibrin, and hemosiderin-filled macrophages. Secondary angle-closure glaucoma results from peripheral anterior synechiae that may develop in the setting of persistent large hyphemas and inflammation.

Any amount of intraocular bleeding may elevate IOP, but larger hyphemas usually cause higher IOPs.[28] Postoperative hyphemas, and glaucoma resulting from them, are generally self-limited and resolve without complications. Management depends on the degree of IOP elevation, the status of the optic nerve, and the presence or absence of sickle cell anemia. A healthy optic nerve can withstand a moderate IOP rise without damage and does not require antiglaucoma therapy. Medical treatment is favored if the IOP is acutely elevated to >40 mm Hg or persistently elevated to >30 mm Hg for 2 weeks.[28] In the presence of pre-existing glaucomatous optic-nerve damage or sickle cell disease, earlier and more aggressive management is required.[28] Aqueous suppressants, especially topical beta-blockers and topical or oral carbonic anhydrase inhibitors (avoided in sickle cell patients), are the preferred medical approach. Hyperosmotic agents may be helpful (e.g., oral isosorbide, 2 mL/kg, or intravenous mannitol, 20% solution, 2 mL/kg over 30 min). It is best to avoid using miotics and prostaglandin analogues, which may exacerbate intraocular inflammation, as well as adrenergic agents, which cause vasoconstriction. Additional therapeutic measures include frequent administration of topical corticosteroids (every 1–2 h) to decrease inflammation; elevating the head of the bed to minimize posterior blood layering; and, if medically possible, avoiding aspirin, aspirin-containing products, sodium warfarin (Coumadin), and nonsteroidal anti-inflammatory agents. Cycloplegics, systemic steroids, and aminocaproic acid are not commonly used for postsurgical hyphemas.

Despite medical therapy, surgical intervention may be required in situations of uncontrolled IOP, corneal blood staining, or a clot of prolonged duration.[28] Traditional IOP criteria for surgical intervention to avoid optic nerve damage in hyphemas are an IOP of >50 mm Hg for 5 days or >35 mm Hg for 7 days. Pre-existing optic nerve damage or sickle cell disease warrants earlier interventions;[27,29] an IOP of <25 mm Hg is desirable in these circumstances. Any sign of corneal blood staining warrants surgical intervention.[28] Patients with compromised endothelial cell function may require earlier intervention. Large clots that persist longer than 10 days or total hyphemas lasting more than 5 days are often evacuated to avoid peripheral anterior synechiae and corneal blood staining.

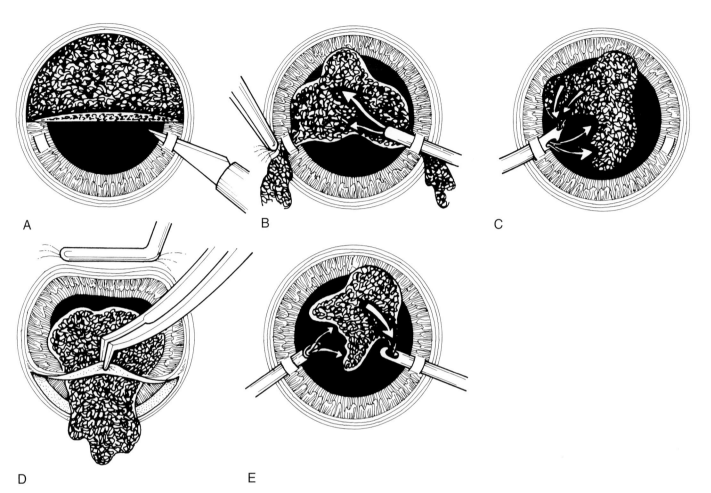

Figure 50-1 Surgical techniques for evacuation of postsurgical hyphemas. **A,** Anterior chamber washout. **B,** Irrigation and aspiration of blood. **C,** Coaxial automated cutting and aspiration of clot. **D,** Clot expression. **E,** Bimanual irrigation and automated cutting.

Surgical techniques for hyphema evacuation include anterior-chamber washout, with or without coaxial irrigation–aspiration, automated cutting-aspiration of clot material, or clot expression (Figure 50-1). Simple removal of circulating red blood cells and debris often suffices for IOP control, but visual rehabilitation is hastened by clot removal. If vitreous is admixed with blood in the anterior chamber, automated cutting-aspiration equipment is required for surgical removal.

LATE HYPHEMAS (SWAN SYNDROME)

Anterior segment hemorrhage months to years after cataract surgery may arise from neovascularization at the surgical incision site,[30–35] vascular iris tufts in contact with anterior chamber IOL haptics in the ciliary sulcus, or blood vessels in contact with posterior chamber IOL haptics in the ciliary sulcus (see also Uveitis-glaucoma-hyphema syndrome and neovascular glaucoma). Patients typically have painless, transient blurring of vision. Visual acuity and IOP depend on the amount of bleeding and trabecular meshwork function. Diagnosis of anterior-chamber bleeding sites is made by gonioscopic identification of neovascularization at the previous wound site or in areas of peripheral

anterior synechia formation. It is uncommon to see bleeding directly from these vessels, but red blood cell "dusting" on the corneal endothelium may be present.

Treatment is often limited to topical medications as needed to control inflammation and IOP. Many eyes have only a single, isolated incident. Recurrent hemorrhages are best managed by laser goniophotocoagulation to the offending vessel when visible, although success with limbal cryopexy has also been reported.[31,36] Long-term acuity deficits or intractable glaucoma are uncommon.[31]

Recurrent bleeding that is related to the haptic placement of an anterior-chamber lens typically requires an IOL exchange. Posterior-chamber lenses without haptic notches or bulbs can often be rotated 90° to position the haptics away from vessels. Haptic cutting and IOL exchange may also be required.

GHOST CELL GLAUCOMA

Erythrocytes begin degenerating within a few days after a vitreous hemorrhage.[37] After 1–3 weeks, they are tan and khaki colored, less pliable, spherical, devoid of intracellular hemoglobin, and freely mobile.[37] These cells are called "ghost cells." After cataract surgery, an intact anterior hyaloid face largely prevents movement

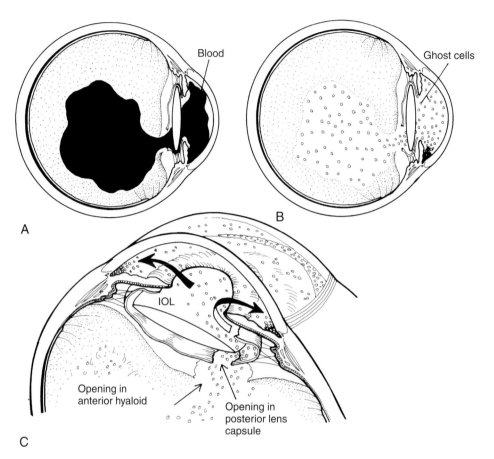

Figure 50-2 Mechanism of ghost cell glaucoma. **A,** Clotted blood in the anterior and posterior chamber. **B,** Erythrocytes degrade to ghost cells. **C,** Rigid khaki-colored ghost cells enter the anterior chamber from the reservoir in vitreous humor through disrupted posterior capsule and anterior hyaloid face. Obstruction of the trabecular meshwork leads to glaucoma.

of cells into the anterior chamber, but any disruption allows easy access (Figure 50-2). Secondary open-angle glaucoma is produced from obstruction of the trabecular meshwork by the ghost cells. IOP may be normal or may rise rapidly to high levels if large numbers of cells are present.[37] Elevated pressure can persist for several months. A fine dusting of ghost cells may be seen on the corneal endothelium, and a layering of cells in the anterior chamber has the appearance of a tan hypopyon (Figure 50-3). The angle is normal or shows a slight khaki discoloration to the trabecular meshwork.

Standard medications are often ineffective in lowering IOP until the number of ghost cells in the anterior chamber has decreased. If the IOP remains persistently elevated despite maximally tolerated medical therapy, an anterior-chamber washout should be considered. Recurrent IOP elevation is common even with repeated anterior-chamber washouts, and a vitrectomy to remove the reservoir of posterior segment ghost cells may be required.[38]

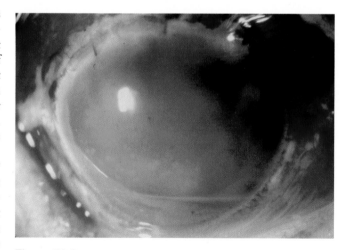

Figure 50-3 Tan "hypopyon" characteristic of ghost cell glaucoma.

UVEITIS

Glaucoma rarely results from the mild postoperative inflammation that is routinely seen after cataract surgery. More commonly, glaucoma occurs in eyes with pre-existing uveitis or in eyes with a more severe inflammatory response. Uveitic glaucoma can be open angle, closed angle, or a combination of both. Open-angle glaucoma results from inflammation-related alterations in the trabecular meshwork. Changes include swelling of the trabecular matrix, endothelial cell dysfunction, or accumulation of inflammatory cells and debris.[39] Corticosteroid treatment and endogenous prostaglandins may also contribute.[40] Angle-closure glaucoma can occur from peripheral anterior synechiae, posterior synechiae, or rubeosis iridis.

Cataract surgery in patients with heterochromic iridocyclitis may be associated with secondary open-angle glaucoma.[41] In these eyes, gonioscopy typically discloses an open angle with fine, iris blood vessels that differ from the coarse, arborizing vessels associated with neovascular angle closure.[42] On entering the anterior chamber, bleeding may occur from these vessels. A secondary, open-angle glaucoma has also been reported in conjunction with episcleritis in a patient with a transscleral-fixated posterior-chamber implant.[43]

Clinical symptoms of uveitis include pain, photophobia, and decreased vision. Any findings on examination may include miosis, perilimbal injection, keratic precipitates, cells and flare in the anterior chamber, and, occasionally, fibrin.

Postoperative uveitic glaucoma is managed medically by controlling inflammation with frequent corticosteroid use. Cycloplegic and sympathomimetic agents are given to prevent or break posterior synechiae. For severe intraocular inflammation, periocular or systemic anti-inflammatory medication may be needed. Elevated IOP is treated with topical beta-blockers, topical or systemic carbonic anhydrase inhibitors, and hyperosmotic agents. Miotic agents and prostaglandin analogues are avoided. Iridectomies should be created to relieve pupillary block when indicated. Laser trabeculoplasty is largely ineffective. If medical therapy fails, filtration surgery with adjunctive antifibrotic treatment or seton placement is indicated.

Rarely, noninflammatory pigment cells circulating in the anterior chamber after posterior chamber IOL implant surgery may be associated with glaucoma.[44] This typically arises with sulcus-fixated IOLs and resultant haptic erosion of pigment from the ciliary body or posterior iris. Iris transillumination may be seen in the area of iris-haptic contact. On gonioscopy, the trabecular meshwork demonstrates dense pigmentation similar to pigment dispersion syndrome. Standard antiglaucoma therapy is instituted, but rarely IOL rotation, removal, or exchange is required.

UVEITIS-GLAUCOMA-HYPHEMA SYNDROME

Uveitis combined with glaucoma and hyphema results from an IOL implant rubbing against the iris. It was a more frequent problem with early versions of iris-fixated and anterior-chamber IOLs[18,45–50] but is also reported with posterior chamber implants.[44,51–53] Causes include imperfections in implant construction, improperly sized lenses, or imperfectly positioned lenses. Initially, patients are treated conservatively with ocular anti-inflammatory and antiglaucoma medications. Patients with persistent glaucoma, recurrent hemorrhage, or endothelial decompensation require the removal of the implant. If the trabecular meshwork has not been irreversibly damaged, the glaucoma will subside.[45,47,50]

LENS PARTICLE GLAUCOMA

Residual cortical material after cataract extraction can cause significant IOP elevation by either open- or closed-angle mechanism.[54] This glaucoma typically occurs early in the postoperative period, although it can occur years later if a Soemmering's ring cataract suddenly opens. Nd:YAG laser rupture of

an epithelial pearl may be the precipitating factor. The patient presents with a red, painful eye. Keratic precipitates, anterior chamber inflammation, and retained lens material are seen.

Lens material causes severe obstruction of trabecular outflow channels,[55] but unlike phacolytic glaucoma, high-molecular-weight proteins are lacking. Obstruction to outflow may also result from macrophages filled with lens material, inflammatory cells, or persistent inflammation. Treatment with topical corticosteroids and antiglaucoma medications, excluding miotic and prostaglandin agents, is usually sufficient until IOP normalizes. Severe inflammation or persistent pressure elevation, or both, may require surgical removal of the residual lens material.

DISLOCATED NUCLEAR FRAGMENTS

With the rise in popularity of phacoemulsification as the preferred method for cataract surgery, the incidence of inadvertent posterior capsule tear and loss of nuclear fragments into the vitreous cavity also increased (Figure 50-4).[56–61] Lens dislocation into the vitreous most often occurs during lens emulsification or cortical cleanup.[57,61–64] It tends to be inversely correlated with the experience of the surgeon performing the phacoemulsification. Other risk factors include inadequate zonular support (pseudoexfoliation, trauma, previous vitrectomy), very hard nuclei, deep-set eyes, poorly dilated pupils, or patient movement during surgery.[57,61,62,65–67]

Lens fragments in the vitreous are a serious problem. Lens particles left in the eye during cataract surgery seem to induce an inflammatory reaction that is somewhat proportional to the size of the displaced fragment.[58] Patients may develop significant visual loss, chronic uveitis, secondary glaucoma, corneal edema, and retinal detachment.[58,68–72] One study reported a 52% incidence of glaucoma in eyes with retained lens fragments.[58]

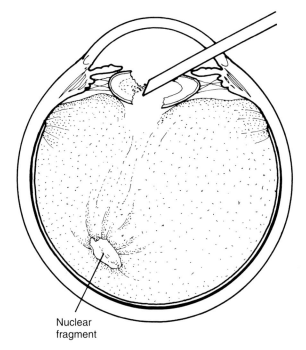

Nuclear fragment

Figure 50-4 Dislocated nucleus fragment in vitreous humor.

Small pieces of lens cortex or a small chip of nucleus without significant corneal edema or glaucoma may only require medical management with topical corticosteroids.[73] However, larger lens fragments are best managed by consultation with a vitreoretinal surgeon. Removal of large lens fragments in the vitreous by an anterior segment approach is not recommended. Aggressive attempts at lens-fragment removal with lens loops, forceps, anterior vitrectomy, or phacoemulsification handpiece should not be done. These maneuvers typically result in vitreoretinal traction and carry a higher risk of retinal tears, retinal detachment, and potential corneal edema or decompensation. The best approach by the cataract surgeon is to perform a thorough cleanup of the vitreous and cortex using appropriate automated vitrectomy cutting instrumentation. An IOL, either anterior or posterior depending on the available capsular support, may be placed. The presence of an IOL does not interfere with the vitrectomy or removal of lens fragments.[58,70,71] The cataract incision should then be tightly closed with sutures. The patient should be referred in a timely fashion to a vitreoretinal surgeon for a three-port pars plana vitectomy-fragmentectomy.[58,72]

Studies on the timing of vitrectomy for removal of retained lens fragments allow some general conclusions to be drawn. Vitrectomy need not be performed the same day. A reasonable time frame for vitrectomy is within 1–2 weeks. Visual acuity is generally improved with vitrectomy within this time frame.[58,61,68–76] There may be a lower chance of elevated IOP in eyes undergoing early vitrectomy.[66,72,74,76] However, a delay in vitrectomy allows time for corneal edema to clear, elevated IOP to be treated, and the patient to be prepared for further surgery.[77,78] Although retinal detachment is the major source of poor visual outcome, excellent visual results are typically achieved. Elevated IOP is managed with standard antiglaucoma medications. Several studies have shown that removal of lens fragments has a beneficial effect on the secondary glaucoma.[70–72,76,79]

See Chapter 44, Intraoperative complications of phacoemulsification surgery, for further discussion of displaced lens fragments after cataract surgery.

CORTICOSTEROIDS

Intraoperative or postoperative administration of topical, periocular, or systemic corticosteroids may produce secondary open-angle glaucoma.[80–88] Topical corticosteroids, a mainstay of postoperative cataract care, are most commonly implicated. Although a less frequent cause of IOP elevation, administration of periocular repository corticosteroids can result in a significant IOP rise that is often delayed.[80,85–88] These depot preparations are used in the treatment of cystoid macular edema or uveitis to increase intraocular drug concentrations and reduce the need for frequent instillation of drops.[80,85–88]

Corticosteroid-induced glaucoma is related to the drug preparation, potency, frequency of administration, and duration of application. With depot preparations, drug release is primarily regulated by the biochemical composition of the corticosteroid. Highly water-soluble compounds diffuse rapidly and are short acting, whereas water-insoluble preparations persist longer.

Individuals with primary open-angle glaucoma,[89] their first-degree relatives,[90] diabetics,[91] and patients with high myopia[92] seem to be at higher risk for steroid-related IOP elevation. In patients without these predisposing factors, the clinician cannot predict which patients will have a pressure rise. Patients of any age may be affected. IOP elevation can occur in the presence of a functioning filter or seton device.[93,94]

Corticosteroids raise IOP by reducing aqueous outflow[95] through effects on glycosaminoglycan metabolism.[96] The release of enzymes that depolymerize glycosaminoglycans is inhibited, and glycosaminoglycans accumulate within the trabecular meshwork.

Diagnosis requires a high index of suspicion and careful questioning. The predominant clinical finding is IOP elevation. The onset of IOP elevation is variable and can be significantly delayed. It may rise within the first week after the start of corticosteroid treatment or not until months or years later. Patients are usually asymptomatic. Eyes generally are not inflamed despite an increased IOP. Depending on the degree and duration of IOP elevation, optic nerve head cupping and visual field loss may or may not be present.

The first step in the management of corticosteroid glaucoma is to stop topical steroid therapy. Clinically significant IOP elevation is treated with the standard antiglaucoma medications. Careful follow-up and monitoring are required. In most cases, IOP returns to normal within days to weeks, although persistent elevation can occur. If corticosteroid medications must be continued, decreasing the strength and frequency or changing the type of corticosteroid and mode of administration may be useful.[97] If periocular corticosteroids have been given, excision of residual steroid material should be considered if IOP cannot be controlled medically.[84,85,87,88] Biochemical analysis of excised depots has shown that significant amounts of periocular corticosteroids can remain for long periods. Laser trabeculoplasty is generally not helpful. If IOP is medically uncontrolled or progressive optic nerve damage occurs, patients require filtering, non-penetrating deep sclerectomy, or tube shunt surgery.

VISCOSURGICAL AGENTS

Viscosurgical agents were introduced into ophthalmic surgery in the early 1970s[98] and have expanded the options available to ophthalmic surgeons greatly by protecting tissue surfaces from mechanical damage, maintaining anterior chamber depth, and assisting in hemostasis. Since then, many materials with varying physical and biochemical properties have become commercially available. Some of these agents include Healon (1% sodium hyaluronate), Healon GV (1.4% sodium hyaluronate), Healon 5 (2.3% sodium hyaluronate), Viscoat (3% sodium hyaluronate/ 4% chondroitin sulfate), Amvisc (1.6% sodium hyaluronate), Vitrax (3% sodium hyaluronate), and OcuCoat (2% hydroxypropylmethylcellulose). Orcolon, a polyacrylamide polymer, was removed from the market because of severe uveitis and secondary glaucoma[99] resulting from contamination with microspheres that obstructed outflow.

The most common complication from use of viscosurgical agents in cataract surgery is a significant, and potentially dangerous, IOP elevation in the early postoperative period.[100–104] The IOP rise peaks between 4 and 7 h postoperatively, and returns to normal within 24–72 h.[105–108] Ocular pain and blurred vision are common presenting symptoms. Corneal edema and stagnation of circulating cells in the anterior chamber may be seen on the slit-lamp examination. The angle is open.

Viscosurgical substances leave the eye through the trabecular meshwork as relatively unchanged large molecules. Even in the presence of intraocular inflammation, little degradation of the viscosurgical substance occurs.[109] Studies demonstrate that these molecules elevate IOP by impairing aqueous humor outflow.[109] Eyes with insufficient trabecular meshwork function before surgery are more likely to have a significant elevation of IOP.[110]

IOP changes after viscosurgical use in cataract surgery have been studied by numerous clinicians. Lane et al.[111] compared early postoperative IOP after use of Healon, Viscoat, and Ocu-Coat. All three agents produced significant IOP elevation at 4 h postoperatively. Holzer et al.[108] found a moderate increase in IOP postoperatively for Healon 5, Viscoat, OcuCoat, and Healon GV. The highest mean IOP was at 4 h, with the highest to lowest IOP by agent being Healon 5, Viscoat, OcuCoat, and Healon GV. At 24 h postoperatively, all groups had a mean IOP of <20 mm Hg.

To reduce the incidence of postoperative IOP elevation, ophthalmic surgeons evacuate the viscosurgical agent at the completion of the procedure. However, its removal only lessens, not eliminates, the incidence of IOP elevation.[102,103,105] Rates of removal vary from agent to agent. Highly viscous agents, such as Healon, Healon GV, and Healon 5, can cause significant IOP increases but require significantly less time to remove from the eye. Conflicting reports exist on the effectiveness of prophylactic treatment with topical beta-adrenergic agents and systemic carbonic anhydrase inhibitors.[112,113]

In the early postoperative period after cataract surgery, IOP should be monitored closely. A clinically significant IOP rise should be treated with either simple release of aqueous via the paracentesis site[114] or antiglaucoma medications. If IOP elevation persists, surgical evacuation of the viscosurgical agent or filtration/seton surgery may be necessary to prevent visual loss.

See Chapter 6 for a detailed discussion of viscosurgical agents.

CAPSULAR BLOCK SYNDROME (OR CAPSULAR BAG DISTENTION SYNDROME)

Capsular block syndrome occurs in patients who have had cataract removal with implantation of a posterior-chamber IOL in the capsular bag after an anterior continuous curvilinear capsulorrhexis.[115–119] Most cases occur immediately postoperatively, but capsular block has been observed as long as 5 years after surgery.[118]

Clinical features of this syndrome include an unexpected myopic overrefraction, anterior displacement of the optic and iris diaphragm, shallowing of the anterior chamber, increased space between the optic and posterior capsule, adherence of the anterior capsule to the IOL, and occasionally a persistent uveitis. Early postoperatively, the IOP may be normal or elevated. If untreated, eyes with capsular block syndrome develop glaucoma, posterior synechiae, and/or posterior capsule opacification with debris within the capsular bag.

To develop this problem, the anterior capsulorrhexis must be smaller than the IOL optic and a viscosurgical agent used. The condition results from a blockage of the egress of fluid contents within the capsular bag. Lens particulates and viscosurgical material are prevented from passing between the IOL optic and the anterior capsule. It is not exactly clear what mechanism draws fluid into the capsular bag and results in its distention.

Postoperatively, capsular block is relieved by performing an Nd-YAG laser anterior capsulotomy peripheral to the edge of the IOL, if observable directly or by first creating a peripheral iridectomy, or by a posterior capsulotomy if anterior capsule cannot be visualized.[119] Although it is uncommon, persistent IOP elevation is treated with standard antiglaucoma medications.

NEODYMIUM:YTTRIUM-ALUMINUM-GARNET (ND:YAG) LASER CAPSULOTOMY

Short-term increases in IOP after an Nd:YAG capsulotomy are well documented[120–123] and they can result in significant and vision-threatening IOP elevation in both aphakic and pseudophakic patients.[124,125] IOP elevation commonly occurs in the first 2 h after the procedure, but may occur later. The rise is typically transient, but may persist.[126] The new onset of glaucoma or the worsening of pre-existing glaucoma can occur.[127] Patients with pre-existing glaucoma appear to be more susceptible to a rise in IOP[128] and should be monitored with extra caution and over the long term after the procedure.[129]

Intermediate and long-term changes in IOP following Nd:YAG capsulotomy also occur.[129–132] Long-term IOP problems after Nd:YAG capsulotomy appear to be correlated with the IOP measurement 1 h following the procedure. Therefore, any patient who has a short-term rise in IOP should be checked regularly thereafter for the possibility of developing long-term IOP problems.[129]

The IOP elevation is caused by reduced facility of outflow from plugging of the trabecular meshwork with capsular particles, inflammatory cells, and protein, as well as from prostaglandin-mediated effects.[133] The number of laser pulses and total energy delivered do not appear to be contributing factors.[127]

Patients undergoing Nd:YAG capsulotomy require close medical observation to detect and treat postoperative pressure elevation. Although varying results have been reported, prophylactic use of timolol,[134] pilocarpine, topical dorzolamide,[135] acetazolamide,[136,137] and topical apraclonidine[138] has been shown to be highly effective in preventing acute pressure spikes following laser treatment. Persistent IOP elevation is managed with standard antiglaucoma medications.

See Chapter 51 for an extensive discussion of Nd:YAG laser capsulotomy.

VITREOUS IN THE ANTERIOR CHAMBER

Secondary open-angle glaucoma from vitreous in the anterior chamber is uncommon. It may occur (1) after intracapsular surgery with iatrogenic or spontaneous breakage of the anterior hyaloid face, (2) after extracapsular surgery with iatrogenic capsular rupture and incomplete vitrectomy, or (3) after posterior capsulotomy.[139,140]

Vitreous within the anterior chambers of enucleated eyes results in trabecular meshwork obstruction and secondarily a decrease in

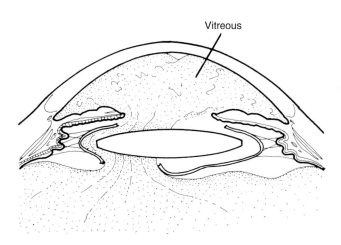

Vitreous

Figure 50-5 Vitreous humor filling the anterior chamber through the posterior capsule opening, leading to obstruction of trabecular meshwork.

aqueous outflow[139] (Figure 50-5). In human eyes, uncertainty exists as to whether vitreous alone, inflammation, or a combination of factors actually causes glaucoma.

IOP elevation is seen a few weeks or months after surgery. Anterior segment inflammation is often minimal. Pressure elevation is treated with standard antiglaucoma therapy. Hyperosmotic and mydriatic agents may help by retracting vitreous from the angle. The effect of miotic agents is variable. Anterior vitrectomy may be successful for medically uncontrolled glaucoma.[139] However, even total removal of vitreous from the anterior chamber and angle does not ensure resolution of the glaucoma.

CYCLODIALYSIS CLEFT CLOSURE

A cyclodialysis cleft is a separation between the scleral spur and ciliary body that produces a direct communication between the anterior chamber and the suprachoroidal space. Cleft formation may occur as an inadvertent complication of cataract surgery. It is, fortunately, an uncommon problem.

Clefts vary in size, and small ones are especially difficult to see with gonioscopy. The size of the cleft is not related to the degree of hypotony.[141]

Postoperative ocular hypotony is the initial typical clinical presentation. Other clinical features include: reduced visual acuity, anterior chamber shallowing, choroidal effusions, optic nerve edema, and macular edema.

Treatment is directed at partial or complete closure of the cyclodialysis cleft. Conservative medical management involves atropine 1% drops twice daily. Cycloplegia helps to promote contact between the sclera and choroid. Miotics and topical steroids are avoided. If medical therapy fails, cyclodialysis clefts can be closed with argon laser, cryotherapy, or placement of sutures.[141,142]

IOP may acutely rise to high levels from either spontaneous or therapeutic closure of the cleft.[143,144] The pressure rise is usually rapid and severe, but generally transient. Management of IOP elevation includes topical beta-adrenergic blockers, topical alpha-2 agonists, topical or systemic carbonic anhydrase inhibitors, and hyperosmotic agents. Miotics should be avoided.

ALPHA-CHYMOTRYPSIN (ENZYME) GLAUCOMA

Although rarely seen today, alpha-chymotrypsin glaucoma was very common following enzyme zonulolysis in intracapsular cataract extraction.[145] In 1964, Kirsch[146] first reported glaucoma from the use of alpha-chymotrypsin in human cataract extraction.

This condition results from acute obstruction of the trabecular meshwork outflow channels by zonular fragments. Scanning electron microscopy of animal eyes demonstrates particulate material blocking the trabecular meshwork near Schlemm's canal and within the uveal meshwork; saline-perfused control eyes show no material.[147] Particles vary in size and shape. Transmission electron microscopy identifies them as zonular fragments and not alpha-chymotrypsin or its by-products. Zonular fragments have also been documented in human eyes.[148] Tonography studies document an impaired facility to outflow. Pilocarpine lowers pressure and improves outflow except during peak pressure rise.[145]

The onset of the IOP rise occurs during the first several days after cataract surgery and may last days to weeks.[50] Clinical findings include mild-to-severe elevation in IOP, corneal edema, normal anterior-chamber depth, and an open angle. IOP elevation is dose dependent. Patients with pre-existing glaucoma have a slightly greater or no greater incidence of this glaucoma. Tonography shows no long-term alteration in trabecular meshwork outflow between 2 and 6 months postoperatively in patients who had previously demonstrated a postoperative pressure increase.[149]

The pressure rise may be prevented or minimized by using a 1:10,000 enzyme dilution instead of 1:5000, limiting the volume used, and irrigating the anterior chamber. Prophylactic use of timolol and acetazolamide may also be of benefit.[36,150] Any postoperative pressure rise should be managed conservatively with antiglaucoma medications until spontaneous resolution occurs, which is usually within 1 week.

■ CLOSED-ANGLE GLAUCOMAS ■

PRE-EXISTING ANGLE CLOSURE

Patients with a previous history of angle-closure glaucoma have an increased risk of glaucoma following cataract surgery, especially if significant angle closure is present preoperatively. However, the degree of preoperative synechial closure is not proportional to the potential severity of postoperative glaucoma. Intense postoperative inflammation and/or prolonged flattening of the anterior chamber can result in permanent peripheral anterior synechiae. A shallow or flat anterior chamber following cataract extraction is commonly associated with a wound leak, choroidal detachment, or both. Medical therapy is initiated, but early surgical intervention may be required to prevent, reduce, or avoid synechial closure, as well as other complications.

PUPILLARY BLOCK

A pupillary block represents a blockage of aqueous humor flow from the posterior chamber to the anterior chamber. It develops when the pupillary space and iridectomies are occluded with vitreous,[151–155] gas,[156] blood,[28] inflammatory materials,[40] capsule,[157] lens cortical material, IOL,[158] or silicone oil.[159] This entity is the most common cause of angle-closure glaucoma following cataract surgery with or without IOL implantation and may complicate both intracapsular[160] and extracapsular cataract extraction.[158,161–163] Anterior-chamber, iris-plane, and posterior-chamber IOL implants have been reported with pupillary block. In addition, pupillary block may occur in the presence of peripheral and sector iridectomies.[158,161–164]

Aphakic pupillary block glaucoma presents days to weeks following surgery with a shallow or flat anterior chamber, elevated IOP, and occlusion of the pupillary space, iridectomies, or both. Pseudophakic block with an anterior chamber implant presents the same way except that (1) the central anterior chamber is deep (the optic holds the iris under it posteriorly), and the peripheral chamber is shallow or flat with an iris bombé configuration (Figure 50-6) or (2) the chamber is uniformly shallow. Although dependent on the stage of glaucoma development, gonioscopy usually shows the filtration angle to be closed.

Medical and laser therapies are used to break pupillary block, deepen the anterior chamber, and prevent chronic angle-closure glaucoma. Iris dilation with cycloplegic-mydriatic agents often eliminates pupillary block. Pupillary block from air can be treated with patient positioning and mydriasis. Elevated IOP is treated with topical beta-adrenergic blockers, topical or systemic carbonic anhydrase inhibitors, and hyperosmotic agents, as needed. Prostaglandin analogues are typically not recommended for angle-closure glaucoma. A laser iridectomy is recommended in conjunction with medical therapy to prevent recurrence. The laser iridectomy is often easier to create before pupillary dilation. Gonioscopy should be performed soon after elimination of pupillary block to assess for residual angle closure. If peripheral anterior synechiae persist, argon laser gonioplasty may be helpful to reduce synechiae and should be performed promptly to maximize success.[165] Surgical goniosynechialysis,[166] filtration surgery, or seton placement may be required for cases of extensive synechiae and high IOP (Table 50-2). The role of routine surgical iridectomy with posterior chamber implants is controversial. Because the risk of pupillary block is low, the general tendency with phacoemulsification and self-sealing incisions (corneal or scleral) is to not perform an iridectomy.[162,167,168]

Table 50-2 Treatment sequence for pupillary block

- Laser iridectomy
- Pupillary dilation
- Reduce IOP medically
- Argon laser gonioplasty—reduce synechiae
- Surgical goniosynechialysis—synechiae with IOP
- Filtration/seton surgery

Reverse pupillary block or "sticky pupil" syndrome may be noted intraoperatively. This blockage of communication between the anterior chamber and the posterior chamber is due to a seal of viscosurgical agent between the iris and the IOL. Any chamber deepening results in an exaggerated concave configuration. Blockage is relieved by the removal of the viscosurgical agent.

MALIGNANT GLAUCOMA (POSTERIOR AQUEOUS DIVERSION)

The term malignant glaucoma conveys the message of a serious form of glaucoma that responds poorly to conventional glaucoma therapy and may result in serious vision loss. The terms ciliary-block glaucoma and posterior aqueous diversion are also used to describe this condition. Both of these terms better describe the pathophysiology, which is blockage of anterior movement of aqueous humor near the junction of the ciliary processes, lens equator, and anterior vitreous face. Aqueous humor is then diverted posteriorly into and behind the vitreous cavity with resultant forward movement of the vitreous and shallowing of the anterior chamber (Figure 50-7). Impermeability of the anterior hyaloid membrane and vitreous body to the anterior flow of

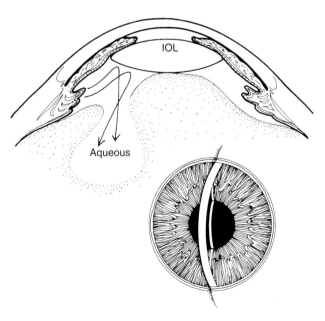

Figure 50-7 Malignant glaucoma with posterior aqueous diversion and shallowing of anterior chamber.

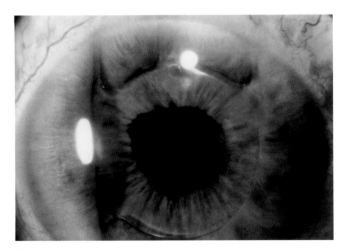

Figure 50-6 Iris bombé with pupillary block.

aqueous humor has been found as perfusion pressure is elevated.[169] Impermeability may be increased by hyaloid to ciliary body apposition. The sequence of events in malignant glaucoma is thought to be initiated by the increased pressure behind a posteriorly detached vitreous, by compaction of the vitreous and, further, decreased fluid movement through it.

Malignant glaucoma may occur following cataract surgery with or without associated trabeculectomy.[170,171] Phakic eyes with a history of angle-closure glaucoma and a degree of closed angle at the time of surgery are at highest risk.[172] Onset may occur intraoperatively or months after surgery.

Clinical characteristics and response to medical therapy, surgery, or both, distinguish malignant glaucoma from choroidal detachment, pupillary block, and suprachoroidal hemorrhage (Table 50-3; see Figure 50-7). In malignant glaucoma, both the central and peripheral anterior chambers are shallow or flat. IOP may be normal or elevated. Choroidal detachment is not seen. Unlike pupillary block glaucoma, clinical findings persist despite having a patent iridectomy. If patency of the iridectomy is questioned, an additional iridectomy should be made to definitively rule out pupillary block. Serous and hemorrhagic choroidal detachments have a characteristic fundus appearance, and a choroidal tap confirms the presence of fluid or blood in the suprachoroidal space.

Medical therapy for malignant glaucoma includes mydriatic-cycloplegic agents (1% atropine, 0.25% scopolamine, 10% phenylephrine),[173] topical or systemic carbonic anhydrase inhibitors, hyperosmotic agents, and topical beta-blockers.[174] Mydriatic-cycloplegic agents presumably act by tightening the lens-iris diaphragm and pulling the lens back against the vitreous, thus stopping the cycle of posterior fluid migration. Miotic or prostaglandin therapy is ineffective and may precipitate or aggravate malignant glaucoma. Medical therapy is continued until the IOP is satisfactorily reduced and the anterior chamber deepens. If treatment is successful, all medications, except cycloplegic agents, are gradually discontinued. Indefinite continuation of cycloplegia is essential to prevent relapse. If medical treatment is unsuccessful after a few days, further therapy with laser or surgery is indicated. In cases of aphakia or pseudophakia, the Nd:YAG laser may be used to disrupt the anterior hyaloid face.[165,171,175] Surgical intervention involves pars plana aspiration of liquid vitreous and restoration of the anterior chamber depth with or without goniosynechialysis.[176,177] (See also Chapter 45.)

NEOVASCULAR GLAUCOMA

Neovascular glaucoma is a secondary angle-closure glaucoma that results from the growth of new blood vessels on the anterior surface of the iris and across the anterior-chamber angle. These vessels grow rapidly and may lead to complete synechial closure of the angle. Iris neovascularization results from retinal hypoxia, typically seen in diabetes mellitus, central retinal vein occlusion, and carotid occlusive disease.[178] Hypoxia leads to the production of a soluble angiogenic factor that causes the proliferation of new blood vessels.[179] The presence of an intact posterior capsule or anterior hyaloid appears to prevent anterior movement of this factor.[180-182] Disruption of the capsule is associated with an increased incidence of rubeosis. The preoperative presence of proliferative diabetic retinopathy also carries a significantly greater risk of the development of neovascular glaucoma following cataract surgery.[180,183]

Several stages exist in the development of rubeosis and neovascular glaucoma. Neovascularization typically begins at the pupillary margin and progresses toward the root of the iris. Interestingly, new vessels may first form around peripheral iridectomies.[184] Patients may have few early symptoms. With advanced disease, the eye becomes very painful with poor vision, conjunctival injection, corneal edema, and very high IOPs. Gonioscopy in early cases shows a normal and open angle, but as the condition progresses, abnormal vessels and areas of synechial closure are seen across the angle. Blood vessels that cross the scleral spur and arborize onto the trabecular meshwork are definitely abnormal.[178] Rubeotic glaucoma can progress to total angle closure within days. Distinguishing between an open and closed angle

Table 50-3 Distinguishing characteristics of shallow or flat anterior chamber

	Malignant Glaucoma	Serous Choroidal Detachment	Pupillary Block	Suprachoroidal Hemorrhage	Wound Leak
Onset	Intraoperatively or any time thereafter	Within the first postoperative week	Early or late postoperatively	Intraoperatively or within the first week	Within the first postoperative week
Anterior chamber	Shallow or flat	Shallow or flat	Shallow or flat	Shallow or flat	Shallow or flat
Intraocular pressure	Normal or elevated	Low	Normal or elevated	Normal or elevated	Low
Fundus	No choroidal detachment	Smooth, light brown choroidal elevations	Normal	Dark brown or red choroidal elevation	Choroidal detachment may or may not be present
Patent iridectomy present	Yes	Yes	No	Yes	Yes
Relief by iridectomy	No	No	Yes	No	No
Relief by suprachoroidal fluid drainage and anterior chamber reformation	No	Yes	No	Yes	No

is important because an open angle signifies an opportunity for achieving vessel regression with panretinal photocoagulation. Panretinal photocoagulation should be performed in rubeotic eyes with retinal ischemic disorders.[184]

Elevated IOP is treated with topical and systemic aqueous suppressants. Because of the presence of inflammation, miotic and prostaglandin agents are avoided. Cycloplegics and topical corticosteroids are used to reduce inflammation. In the early stages of disease, panretinal photocoagulation is performed with the hope of causing vessel regression and preservation of an open angle. It may be possible to avoid glaucoma surgery. Laser goniophotocoagulation appears to be of little value. Intravitreal anti-angiogenic drugs such as bevacizumab (Avastin) have shown promise in reducing anterior segment neovascularization. If the IOP is significantly elevated despite medical treatment, and vision is endangered, urgent filtering surgery with antimetabolite supplementation is required. If this surgery is unsuccessful, seton devices or cyclodestructive procedures have shown some success. The rate of phthisis following cyclodestructive procedures may approximate 10%. Eyes with neovascular glaucoma and no vision are not candidates for surgical therapy. Comfort is best achieved with chronic use of cycloplegic agents and topical steroids.

EPITHELIAL AND FIBROVASCULAR INGROWTH

Epithelial and fibrovascular ingrowth results from either epithelial growth or connective tissue growth into the anterior chamber and across the trabecular meshwork. Both conditions were more common with intracapsular cataract extraction and early surgical techniques. The incidence has significantly decreased over the past decade.[185,186] Associated risk factors include complicated or difficult surgery and poor wound construction or closure with leakage.

The diagnosis of epithelial downgrowth is often delayed. Symptoms may be vague and include tearing, dull pain, redness, photophobia, and blurred vision.[187] Examination may show wound gape, a filtering bleb, and a fistulous tract with positive Seidel testing. Retroillumination of the cornea shows a translucent membrane that is demarcated by a gray line. The leading edge of this line often has a thickened and scalloped appearance (Figure 50-8). Unlike corneal graft rejection, keratic precipitates

are not associated with this line. Corneal edema and deep corneal vascularization may be present. Anterior segment cells and flare are seen. Iris involvement is often extensive and can be delineated with the argon laser. Gonioscopy also helps to assess the extent of epithelialization. Membranes may also grow over the pupil, vitreous face, or IOL implants.

The clinical picture for fibrous ingrowth differs slightly, with membranes appearing gray or white and demonstrating more irregular leading edges. Vascularization is more commonly present.

Histopathologic studies and electron microscopy show that nonkeratinized, stratified squamous epithelium grows over the posterior cornea, angle, iris, ciliary body, vitreous, and retina.[188] Epithelium is also usually seen along the surgical wound, which may or may not have incarcerated tissue. A chronic inflammatory cell infiltrate is frequently present within the tissues.

Glaucoma almost invariably occurs with downgrowth[186] and may result from synechial closure of the angle, pupillary block, and inflammation-related changes. Hypotony may also occur, secondary to a fistula and wound leak.

No medical therapy exists to stop progression from either epithelial or fibrovascular ingrowth.[189] Surgery is the mainstay of treatment. Before surgery is performed, the extent of ingrowth on the iris is delineated with the argon laser. White burns indicate the presence of epithelium. Surgical therapy requires removal of the involved iris, vitreous, and implant. Cryotherapy is applied to the cornea, angle, and ciliary body to devitalize remaining epithelium. Salvage of the globe is the prime consideration. Filtration with antifibrotic agents or seton devices may be needed for pressure control.

See Chapter 53 for a detailed discussion of epithelial and fibrous ingrowth.

TREATMENT OF GLAUCOMA AFTER CATARACT SURGERY: GENERAL PRINCIPLES

As noted previously, all efforts are made to determine the cause of the IOP elevation that develops after cataract surgery. Therapy is directed toward elimination or treatment of the specific cause (Table 50-4). In general, mainstays of therapy include topical and systemic aqueous suppressants. Miotic and prostaglandin agents may be helpful in open-angle glaucomas when there is

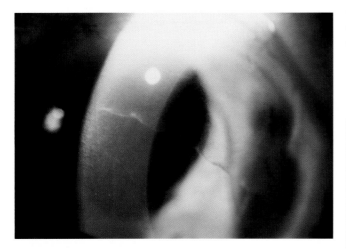

Figure 50-8 Epithelial downgrowth with retrocorneal membrane.

Table 50-4 Glaucoma after cataract surgery: treatment sequence

- Identify and treat specific cause
- Add standard glaucoma medications
- Laser therapy
- Filtration surgery with antimetabolite
- Seton (tube/shunt)
- Cycloablation

no inflammation or chamber shallowing. However, disruption of the blood–aqueous barrier[184] and cystoid macular edema in the early postoperative period have been reported after cataract surgery in patients receiving topical latanoprost.[190–199] Adrenergic agents are generally avoided because of the possibility, albeit small, of cystoid macular edema that may develop after cataract surgery. Apraclonidine and brimonidine are helpful adjuncts for acute therapy of high IOP spikes and are beneficial for short-term IOP treatment from days to weeks. Oral and intravenous osmotic agents are occasionally needed for profound IOP elevations. Eye surgeons should always be alert to the possibility of corticosteroid- or cycloplegic-induced glaucoma that may require cessation of steroid and cycloplegic therapy.

Conventional laser treatment for glaucoma after cataract surgery generally involves laser iridectomy for pupillary block and laser trabeculoplasty for open-angle glaucoma. Argon laser trabeculoplasty and selective laser trabeculoplasty may not be as effective in the pseudophakic patient as in the phakic patient, but still may be helpful treatment modalities for many patients. Laser gonioplasty may be able to reduce synechiae in recently closed angles. Laser therapy is also indicated for malignant glaucoma and neovascular glaucoma, as noted earlier.

Surgery for glaucoma is occasionally required in aphakic and pseudophakic patients. Decisions concerning surgical technique and location of surgery depend largely on the status of the conjunctiva, vitreous, and IOL. Most surgeons prefer to operate in areas of conjunctiva that have not been disrupted by previous surgery.[19] At the same time, it is generally preferable to perform surgery superiorly rather than inferiorly to avoid exposing filtration blebs to a greater risk of infection. Filtration surgical techniques may be either partial thickness or full thickness. Vitreous must be removed if it is present in the area of the sclerectomy. The position of the IOL may direct the surgeon's choice of operative location. In eyes without significant limbal scarring, non-penetrating deep sclerectomy procedures, including viscocanalostomy and canaloplasty may be indicated.

If surgery is required for IOP control, a filtration procedure with intraoperative antifibrotics may be preferred. A limbal-based conjunctival flap is preferred to reduce leaks, but a fornix-based conjunctival flap may be used if necessary. Tight scleral flap closure is favored to minimize the risk of suprachoroidal hemorrhage. Selective laser suture lysis or releasable sutures are used postoperatively to facilitate aqueous egress. Supplemental use of 5-fluorouracil is also added postoperatively if necessary.

If standard filtration surgery with mitomycin-C fails, a tube-shunt seton device is often the next option. Deep sclerectomy procedures (viscocanalostomy and others) may be effective, particularly in eyes with minimal limbal scarring from previous procedures. Aphakic and pseudophakic eyes undergoing laser and surgical procedures more commonly require supplemental glaucoma medications for IOP control postoperatively than do phakic eyes. Because of the risk of visual loss and phthisis, cyclodestructive procedures are reserved for patients in which filtration or tube-shunt procedures fail. Transscleral cyclophotocoagulation is our preferred ciliary body destructive procedure of choice. Endocyclophotocoagulation is not associated with as great an IOP reduction as the transscleral route, but produces much less inflammation.

References

[1] Rich WJ. Further studies on early postoperative ocular hypertension following cataract extraction. Trans Ophthalmol Soc U K 1969;89:639–645.
[2] Rothkoff L, Beidner B, Glumenthal M. The effect of corneal section on early increased intraocular pressure after cataract extraction. Am J Ophthalmol 1978;85:337–338.
[3] Kirsch RE, Levine O, Singer JA. Further studies on the ridge at the internal edge of the cataract incision. Trans Am Acad Ophthalmol Otolaryngol 1977;83:224–231.
[4] Lee PF, Trotter RR. Tonographic and gonioscopic studies before and after cataract extraction. Arch Ophthalmol 1957;58:407–416.
[5] McGuigan LJB, Gottsch J, Stark WJ, et al. Extracapsular cataract extraction and posterior chamber lens implantation in eyes with preexisting glaucoma. Arch Ophthalmol 1986;104:1301–1308.
[6] Savage JA, Thomas JV, Belcher CD, et al. Extracapsular cataract extraction and posterior chamber intraocular lens implantation in glaucomatous eyes. Ophthalmology 1985;92:1506–1516.
[7] Fang EN, Kass MA. Increased intraocular pressure after cataract surgery. Semin Ophthalmol 1994;9:235–242.
[8] Bigger JF, Becker B. Cataracts and primary open angle glaucoma: the effect of uncomplicated cataract extraction on glaucoma control. Trans Am Acad Ophthalmol Otolaryngol 1971;75:260–272.
[9] Linn JG. Cataract extraction in management of glaucoma. Trans Am Acad Ophthalmol Otolaryngol 1971;75:273–280.
[10] Kaufman IH. Intraocular pressure after lens extraction. Am J Ophthalmol 1965;59:722–723.
[11] Shingleton BJ, Gamell LS, O'Donoghue MW, et al. Long-term changes in intraocular pressure after clear corneal phacoemulsification: normal patients versus glaucoma suspect and glaucoma patients. J Cataract Refract Surg 1999;25:885–876.
[12] Tong JT, Miller KM. Intraocular pressure change after sutureless phacoemulsification and foldable posterior chamber lens implantation. J Cataract Refract Surg 1998;24:256–262.
[13] Kim DD, Doyle JW, Smith MF. Intraocular pressure reduction following phacoemulsification cataract extraction with posterior chamber lens implantation in glaucoma patients. Ophthalmic Surg Lasers 1999;30:37–40.
[14] Schwenn O, Dick B, Krummenauer F, et al. Intraocular pressure after small incision cataract surgery: temporal sclerocorneal versus clear corneal incision. J Cataract Refract Surg 2001;27:421–425.
[15] Tennen DG, Masket S. Short- and long-term effect of clear corneal incisions on intraocular pressure. Ophthalmology 1995;102:863–867.
[16] Pohjalainen T, Vesti E, Uusitalo RJ, et al. Intraocular pressure after phacoemulsification and intraocular lens implantation in nonglaucomatous eyes with and without exfoliation. J Cataract Refract Surg 2001;27:26–431.
[17] Shingleton BJ, Pasternack JJ, Hung JW. Three and five year changes in intraocular pressures after clear corneal phacoemulsification in open angle glaucoma patients, glaucoma suspects, and normal patients. J Glaucoma 2006;15:494–498.
[18] Lamping KA, Bellows AH, Hutchinson BT, et al. Long-term evaluation of initial filtration surgery. Ophthalmology 1986;93:91–101.
[19] Shingleton BJ, Alfano C, O'Donoghue MW, Riviera J. The efficacy of glaucoma filtration surgery in pseudophakic patients with or without conjunctival scarring. J Cataract Refract Surg 2004;30:2504–2509.
[20] Berger RO. Fox shield treatment of the UGH syndrome. J Cataract Refract Surg 1986;12:419–421.
[21] Haimann MH, Phelps CD. Prophylactic timolol for prevention of high intraocular pressure after cataract extraction: a randomized, prospective, double-blind trial. Ophthalmology 1981;88:233–238.
[22] Prata Jr JA, Rehder JR, Mello PA. Apraclonidine and early postoperative intraocular hypertension after cataract extraction. Acta Ophthalmol 1992;70:434–439.
[23] Fry LL. Comparison of the postoperative intraocular pressure with Betagan, Betoptic, Timoptic, Iopidine, Diamox, Pilopine Gel, and Miostat. J Cataract Refract Surg 1992;18:14–19.
[24] Scherer WJ, Mielke DL, Tidwell PF et al. Efficacy of latanoprost on intraocular pressure following cataract extraction. J Cataract Refract Surg 1999;25:304.
[25] Strelow SA, Sherwood MB, Broncato LJ, et al. The effect of diclofenac sodium ophthalmic solution on intraocular pressure following cataract extraction. Ophthalmic Surg 1992;23:170–175.
[26] Hildebrand GD, Wickremasinghe SS, Tranos PG, Harris ML, Little BC. Efficacy of anterior chamber decompression in controlling early intraocular pressure spikes after uneventful phacoemulsification. J Cataract Refract Surg 2003;29:1087–1092.
[27] Hagen III JC, Gaasterland DE. Endocapsular hematoma: description and treatment of a unique form of postoperative hemorrhage. Arch Ophthalmol 1991;109:514–518.
[28] Shingleton BJ, Hersh PJ. Traumatic hyphema. In: Shingleton BJ, Hersh PJ, Kenyon KR, editors. Eye trauma. St Louis: Mosby; 1991.
[29] Deutsch TA, Weinreb RN, Goldberg MF. Indications for surgical management of hyphema in patients with sickle cell disease. Arch Ophthalmol 1984;102:566–569.
[30] Benson WE, Karp LA, Nichols CW, et al. Late hyphema due to vascularization of the cataract wound. Ann Ophthalmol 1978;10:1109–1111.
[31] Jarstad JS, Hardwig PW. Intraocular hemorrhage from wound neovascularization years after anterior segment surgery (Swan syndrome). Can J Ophthalmol 1987;22:271–275.
[32] Speakman JS. Recurrent hyphema after surgery. Can J Ophthalmol 1975;10:299–304.
[33] Swan KC. Hyphema due to wound vascularization after cataract extraction. Arch Ophthalmol 1973;89:87–90.
[34] Swan KC. Late hyphema due to wound vascularization. Trans Am Acad Ophthalmol Otolaryngol 1976;81:138–144.
[35] Watzke RC. Intraocular hemorrhage from wound vascularization following cataract surgery. Trans Am Ophthalmol Soc 1974;72:242–248.
[36] Barraquer J, Rutlan J. Enzymatic zonulysis and postoperative ocular hypertension. Am J Ophthalmol 1967;63:159.
[37] Campbell DG, Simmons RJ, Grant WM. Ghost cells as a cause of glaucoma. Am J Ophthalmol 1976;81:441–450.
[38] Summers CG, Lindstrom RI. Ghost cell glaucoma following lens implantation. J Am Intraocul Implant Soc 1983;9:428–433.
[39] Kass MA, Podos SM, Moses RA, et al. Prostaglandin E1 and aqueous humor dynamics. Invest Ophthalmol Vis Sci 1992;2:1022–1027.
[40] Kass MA, Johnson T. Corticosteroid-induced glaucoma. In: Ritch R, Shields MB, Krupin T, editors. The glaucomas. St Louis: Mosby; 1989. p. 1161–1168.
[41] Hart CT, Wrad DM. Intra-ocular pressure in Fuchs' heterochromic uveitis. Br J Ophthalmol 1967;51:739–743.
[42] Lerman S, Levy C. Heterochromic iritis and secondary neovascular glaucoma. Am J Ophthalmol 1964;57:479–481.
[43] Leo RJ, Palmer DJ. Episcleritis and secondary glaucoma after transscleral fixation of a posterior chamber intraocular lens. Arch Ophthalmol 1991;109:617.
[44] Masket S. Pseudophakic posterior iris chafing syndrome. J Cataract Refract Surg 1986;12:252–256.

[45] Alpar JJ. Glaucoma after intraocular lens implantation: survey and recommendations. Glaucoma 1985;7:241–245.
[46] Choyce DP. Complications of the anterior chamber implants of the early 1950s and the UGH syndrome or Ellingson syndrome of the late 1970s. J Am Intraocul Implant Soc 1978;4:22–29.
[47] Ellingson FT. The uveitis-glaucoma-hyphema syndrome associated with the Mark VIII anterior chamber lens implant. J Am Intraocul Implant Soc 1978;4:50–53.
[48] Moses L. Complications of rigid anterior chamber implants. Ophthalmology 1984;91:819–825.
[49] Nicholson DH. Occult iris erosion: a treatable cause of recurrent hyphema in iris-supported intraocular lenses. Ophthalmology 1982;89:113–120.
[50] Obstbaum SA. Management of glaucoma in the implanted patient. J Am Intraocul Implant Soc 1981;7:252–259.
[51] Apple DJ, Mamalis N, Loftfield K, et al. Complications of intraocular lenses: a historical and histopathological review. Surv Ophthalmol 1984;29:1–54.
[52] Pazandak B, Johnson S, Kratz R. Recurrent intraocular hemorrhage associated with posterior chamber lens implantation. J Am Intraocul Implant Soc 1983;9:327–329.
[53] Percival SPB, Das SK. UGH syndrome after posterior chamber lens implantation. J Am Intraocul Implant Soc 1983;9:200–201.
[54] Epstein DL. Diagnosis and management of lens-induced glaucoma. Ophthalmology 1982;89:227–230.
[55] Epstein DL, Jedziniak JA, Grant WM. Obstruction of aqueous outflow by lens particles and by heavy-molecular-weight soluble lens proteins. Invest Ophthalmol Vis Sci 1978;17:272–277.
[56] Emery JM, Wilhelmus KA, Rosenberg S. Complications of phacoemulsification. Ophthalmology 1978;85:141–150.
[57] Monshizadeh R, Samiy N, Haimovici R. Management of retained intravitreal lens fragments after cataract surgery. Surv Ophthalmol 1999;43:397–404.
[58] Gilliland GD, Hutton WL, Fuller DG. Retained intravitreal lens fragments after cataract surgery. Ophthalmology 1992;99:1263–1269.
[59] Irvine WD, Flynn HW, Murray TG. Retained lens fragments after phacoemulsification manifesting as marked intraocular inflammation with hypopyon. Am J Ophthalmol 1992;114: 610–614.
[60] Pande M, Dabbs TR. Incidence of lens matter dislocation during phacoemulsification. J Cataract Refract Surg 1996;22:737–742.
[61] Tommila P, Immonen I. Dislocated nuclear fragments after cataract surgery. Eye 1995;9: 437–441.
[62] Allinson RW, Metrikin DC, Fante RG. Incidence of vitreous loss among third-year residents performing phacoemulsification. Ophthalmology 1992;99:726–730.
[63] Gonvers M. New approach to managing vitreous loss and dislocated lens fragments during phacoemulsification. J Cataract Refract Surg 1994;20:346–349.
[64] Leaming DV. Practice styles and preferences of ASCRS members: 1994 survey. J Cataract Refract Surg 1995;21:378–385.
[65] Guzek JP, Holm M, Cotter JB, et al. Risk factors for intraoperative complications in 1000 extracapsular cataract cases. Ophthalmology 1987;94:461–466.
[66] Margherio RR, Margherio AR, Pendergast SD, et al. Vitrectomy for retained lens fragments after phacoemulsification. Ophthalmology 1997;104:1426–1432.
[67] Streeten BW. Pathology of the lens. In: Albert DM, Jakobiec FA, editors. Principles and practices of ophthalmology: clinical practice. Philadelphia: WB Saunders; 1994. p. 2180–2239.
[68] Hutton WL, Snyder WB, Vaiser A. Management of surgically dislocated intravitreal lens fragments by pars plana vitrectomy. Ophthalmology 1978;85:176–189.
[69] Fastenberg DM, Schwartz PL, Shakin JL, et al. Management of dislocated nuclear fragments after phacoemulsification. Am J Ophthalmol 1991;112:535–539.
[70] Lambrou Jr FH, Steward MW. Management of dislocated lens fragments after cataract surgery. Ophthalmology 1992; 1260–1262.
[71] Kim JE, Flynn Jr HW, Smiddy WE, et al. Retained lens fragments after phacoemulsification. Ophthalmology 1994;101:1827–1832.
[72] Blodi BA, Flynn Jr HW, Blodi CF, et al. Retained nuclei after cataract surgery. Ophthalmology 1992;99:41–44.
[73] Wong D, Briggs MC, Hickey-Dwyer MU et al. Removal of lens fragments from the vitreous cavity. Eye 1997;11:37–42.
[74] Yeo LMW, Charteris DG, Bunce C, et al. Retained intravitreal lens fragments after phacoemulsification: a clinicopathological correlation. Br J Ophthalmol 1999;83:1135–1138.
[75] Watts P, Hunter J, Bunce C. Vitrectomy and lensectomy in the management of posterior dislocation of lens fragments. J Cataract Refract Surg 2000;26:832–837.
[76] Vilar NF, Flynn Jr HW, Smiddy WE, et al. Removal of retained lens fragments after phacoemulsification reverses secondary glaucoma and restores visual acuity. Ophthalmology 1997;104:787–792.
[77] Stilma JS, van der Sluijs FA, van Meurs JC, et al. Occurrence of retained lens fragments after phacoemulsification in the Netherlands. J Cataract Refract Surg 1997;23:1177–1182.
[78] Topping TM. Discussion of paper by Gilliland GD, Hutton WL, Fuller DG. Ophthalmology 1992;99:1268–1269.
[79] Borne MJ, Tasman W, Regillo C, et al. Outcomes of vitrectomy for retained lens fragments. Ophthalmology 1996;103:971–976.
[80] Brubaker RF, Halpin JA. Open-angle glaucoma associated with topical administration of flurandrenolide to the eye. Mayo Clin Proc 1975;50:322–326.
[81] Eisenlohr JE. Glaucoma following the prolonged use of topical steroid medication to the eyelids. J Am Acad Dermatol 1983;8:878–881.
[82] Covell LL. Glaucoma induced by systemic steroid therapy. Am J Ophthalmol 1958;45:108–109.
[83] McDonnell PJ, Kerr Muir MG. Glaucoma associated with systemic corticosteroid therapy. Lancet 1985;2:386–387.
[84] Herschler J. Intractable intraocular hypertension induced by repository triamcinolone acetonide. Am J Ophthalmol 1972;74:501–504.
[85] Herschler J. Increased intraocular pressure induced by repository corticosteroids. Am J Ophthalmol 1976;82:90–93.
[86] Kalina R. Increased intraocular pressure following subconjunctival corticosteroid administration. Arch Ophthalmol 1969;81:788–790.
[87] Mills DW, Siebert LF, Climenhaga DB. Depot triamcinolone-induced glaucoma. Can J Ophthalmol 1986;21:150–152.
[88] Kalina PH, Erie JC, Rosenbaum L. Biochemical quantification of triamcinolone in subconjunctival depots. Arch Ophthalmol 1995;113:867–869.
[89] Armaly MF. Effect of corticosteroids on intraocular pressure and fluid dynamics. II. The effect of dexamethasone in the glaucomatous eye. Arch Ophthalmol 1963;70:492–499.
[90] Becker B, Hahn KA. Topical corticosteroids and heredity in primary open-angle glaucoma. Am J Ophthalmol 1964;57:543–551.
[91] Becker B. Diabetes mellitus and primary open angle glaucoma: the XXVII Edward Jackson memorial lecture. Am J Ophthalmol 1971;71:1–16.
[92] Podos SM, Becker B, Morton WR. High myopia and primary open-angle glaucoma. Am J Ophthalmol 1966;62:1039–1043.
[93] Mermoud A, Salmon JF. Corticosteroid-induced ocular hypertension in draining Molteno single-plate implants. J Glaucoma 1993;2:32–36.
[94] Wilensky JT, Snyder D, Gieser D. Steroid-induced ocular hypertension in patients with filtering blebs. Ophthalmology 1980;87:240–244.
[95] Armaly MF. Effects of corticosteroids on intraocular pressure and fluid dynamics. I. The effect of dexamethasone in the normal eye. Arch Ophthalmol 1963;70:482–491.
[96] Spaeth GL, Rodrigues MM, Weinreb S. Steroid-induced glaucoma. A. Persistent elevation of intraocular pressure. B. Histopathologic aspects. Trans Am Ophthalmol Soc 1977;75:353–381.
[97] Mindel JS, Goldberg J, Tavitian HO. Similarity of the intraocular pressure response to different corticosteroid esters when compliance is controlled. Ophthalmology 1979;86:99–107.
[98] Balazs EA, Freeman MI, Kloti R, et al. Hyaluronic acid and replacement of vitreous and aqueous humor. Mod Prob Ophthalmol 1972;10:3–21.
[99] Seigel MJ, Spiro HJ, Miller JA, et al. Secondary glaucoma and uveitis associated with Orcolon. Arch Ophthalmol 1991;109:1496–1497.
[100] Binkhorst CD. Inflammation and intraocular pressure after the use of Healon in intraocular lens surgery. J Am Intraocul Implant Soc 1980;6:340–341.
[101] Genstler DE, Keates RH. Amvisc in extracapsular cataract extraction. J Am Intraocul Implant Soc 1983;9:317–320.
[102] Glasser DB, Matsuda M, Edelhauser HF. A comparison of the efficacy and toxicity of and intraocular pressure response to viscous solutions in the anterior chamber. Arch Ophthalmol 1986;104:1819–1824.
[103] Obstbaum SA. Glaucoma and intraocular lens implantation. J Cataract Refract Surg 1986;12:257–261.
[104] Olivius E, Thorburn W. Intraocular pressure after surgery with Healon. J Am Intraocul Implant Soc J 1985;11:480–482.
[105] Cherfan GM, Rich WJ, Wright G. Raised intraocular pressure and other problems with sodium hyaluronate and cataract surgery. Trans Ophthalmol Soc UK 1983;103:277–279.
[106] Henry JC, Olander K. Comparison of the effect of four viscoelastic agents on early postoperative intraocular pressure. J Cataract Refract Surg 1996;22:960–966.
[107] Kohnen T, von Her M, Schutte E, et al. Evaluation of intraocular pressure with Healon and Healon GV in sutureless cataract surgery with foldable lens implantation. J Cataract Refract Surg 1996;22:227–237.
[108] Holzer MP, Tetz MR, Auffarth GU, et al. Effect of Healon 5 and 4 other viscoelastic substances on intraocular pressure and endothelium after cataract surgery. J Cataract Refract Surg 2001;27:213–218.
[109] Berson FG, Patterson MM, Epstein DL. Obstruction of aqueous outflow by sodium hyaluronate in enucleated human eyes. Am J Ophthalmol 1983;68:1037–1050.
[110] Handa J, Henry JC, Krupin T, et al. Extracapsular cataract extraction with posterior chamber lens implantation in patients with glaucoma. Arch Ophthalmol 1987;105:765–769.
[111] Lane SS, Naylor DW, Kullerstrand LJ, et al. Prospective comparison of the effects of Occucoat, Viscoat, and Healon on intraocular pressure and endothelial cell loss. J Cataract Refract Surg 1991;17:21–26.
[112] Anmarkrud N, Bergaust B, Bulie T. The effect of Healon and timolol on early postoperative intraocular pressure after extracapsular cataract extraction with implantation of a posterior chamber lens. Acta Ophthalmol 1992;70:96–100.
[113] Paper LG, Balasz EA. The use of sodium hyaluronate (Healon) in human anterior segment surgery. Ophthalmology 1980;87:699–705.
[114] Calhoun Jr FR. The clinical recognition and treatment of epithelialization of the anterior chamber following cataract extraction. Trans Am Ophthalmol Soc 1949;47:498–553.
[115] Davison JA. Capsular bag distension after endophacoemulsification and posterior chamber intraocular lens implantation. J Cataract Refract Surg 1990;16:99–108.
[116] Holtz SJ. Postoperative capsular bag distension. J Cataract Ref Surg 1992;18:310–317.
[117] Miyake K, Ota I, Ichihashi S, et al. New classification of capsular block syndrome. J Cataract Refract Surg 1998;24:1230–1234.
[118] Nishi O, Nishi K, Takahasi E. Capsular bag distension syndrome noted 5 years after intraocular lens implantation. Am J Ophthalmol 1998;125:545–547.
[119] Theng JTS, Jap A, Chee SP. Capsular block syndrome: a case series. J Cataract Refract Surg 2000;26:462–467.
[120] Stark WJ, Worthen D, Holladay JT, et al. Neodymium:YAG lasers: an FDA report. Ophthalmology 1985;92:209–212.
[121] Channell MM, Beckman H. Intraocular pressure changes after neodymium-YAG laser posterior capsulotomy. Arch Ophthalmol 1984;102:1024–1026.
[122] Flohr MJ, Robin AJ, Kelley JS. Early complications following Q-switched neodymium:YAG laser posterior capsulotomy. Ophthalmology 1985;92:360–363.
[123] Slomovic AR, Parrish RK. Acute elevations of intraocular pressure following Nd:YAG laser posterior capsulotomy. Ophthalmology 1985;92:973–976.
[124] Vine AK. Ocular hypertension following Nd:YAG laser capsulotomy: a potentially blinding complication. Ophthalmic Surg 1984;15:283–284.
[125] Richter CU, Arzeno G, Pappas H et al. Intraocular pressure elevation following Nd:YAG laser posterior capsulotomy, Ophthalmology 1985;92:636.
[126] Demer JL, Koch DD, Smith JA, et al. Persistent elevation in intraocular pressure after Nd:YAG laser treatment. Ophthalmic Surg 1986;17:465–466.
[127] Steinert RF, Puliafito CA, Kumar SR, et al. Cystoid macular edema, retinal detachment, and glaucoma after Nd:YAG laser posterior capsulotomy. Am J Ophthalmol 1991;112:373–380.
[128] Keates RH, Steinert RF, Puliafito CA, et al. Long-term follow-up of Nd:YAG laser posterior capsulotomy. J Am Intraocul Implant Soc 1984;10:164–168.
[129] Ge J, Wand M, Chiang R, et al. Long-term effect of Nd:YAG laser posterior capsulotomy on intraocular pressure. Arch Ophthalmol 2000;118:1334–1337.
[130] Leys M, Pameijer JH, deJong P. Intermediate-term changes in intraocular pressure after neodymium-YAG laser posterior capsulotomy. Am J Ophthlamol 1985;100:332–333.
[131] Fourman S, Apisson J. Late-onset elevation of intraocular pressure after neodymium-YAG laser posterior capsulotomy. Arch Ophthalmol 1991;109:511–513.
[132] Jahn C, Emke M. Long-term elevation of intraocular pressure after Nd:YAG laser posterior capsulotomy. Ophthalmologica 1996;210:85–89.
[133] Altamirano D, Mermoud A, Pittet N, et al. Aqueous humor analysis after Nd:YAG laser capsulotomy with the laser flare-cell meter. J Cataract Refract Surg 1992;18:544–558.
[134] Rakofsky S, Koch D, Faulkner, et al. Levobunolol 0.5% and timolol 0.5% to prevent intraocular pressure elevation after neodymium:YAG laser posterior capsulotomy. J Cataract Refract Surg 1997;23:1975–1080.
[135] Hartenbaum D, Wilson H, Maloney S, et al. the Dorzolamide Laser Study Group. A randomized study of Dorzolamide in the prevention of elevated intraocular pressure after anterior segment laser surgery. J Glaucoma 1999;8:273–275.
[136] Parker WT, Clorfeine GS, Stocklin RD. Marked intraocular pressure rise following Nd:YAG laser capsulotomy. Ophthalmic Surg 1984;15:103–104.
[137] Richter CU, Arzeno G, Pappas HR, et al. Prevention of intraocular pressure elevation following neodymium-YAG laser posterior capsulotomy, Arch Ophthalmol 1985;103:912.

[138] Pollack IP, Brown RH, Crandall AS, et al. Prevention of the rise in intraocular pressure following neodymium-YAG posterior capsulotomy using topical 1% apraclonidine. Arch Ophthalmol 1988;106:754–757.

[139] Grant WM. Open-angle glaucoma with vitreous filling the anterior chamber following cataract extraction. Trans Am Ophthalmol Soc 1963;61:196–218.

[140] Samples JR, Van Buskirk EM. Open-angle glaucoma associated with vitreous humor filling the anterior chamber. Am J Ophthalmol 1986;102:759–761.

[141] Epstein DL. Cyclodialysis. In: Epstein DL, Allingham RR, Schuman JS, editors. Chandler and grant's glaucoma. 4th ed. Baltimore: Williams & Wilkins; 1997. p. 573–379.

[142] Reyer EB, Aquino NM. Cyclodialysis cleft in anterior chamber area. In: Hampton Roy F, editor. Master techniques in ophthalmic surgery. Baltimore: Williams & Wilkins; 1995. p. 3–8.

[143] Harbin Jr TS. Treatment of cyclodialysis clefts with argon laser photocoagulation. Ophthalmology 1982;89:1082–1083.

[144] Ormerod LD, Baerveldt G, Green RL. Cyclodialysis clefts: natural history, assessment and management. In: Weinstein GW, editor. Open angle glaucoma. New York: Churchill Livingstone; 1986. p. 201–205.

[145] Kirsch RE. Further studies on glaucoma following cataract extraction associated with the use of alpha-chymotrypsin. Trans Am Acad Ophthalmol Otolaryngol 1965;69:1011–1023.

[146] Kirsch RE. Glaucoma following cataract extraction associated with use of alpha chymotrypsin. Arch Ophthalmol 1964;72:612–620.

[147] Anderson DR. Experimental alpha chymotrypsin glaucoma studied by scanning electron microscopy. Am J Ophthalmol 1971;71:470–476.

[148] Worthen DM. Scanning electron microscopy after alpha chymotrypsin perfusion in man. Am J Ophthalmol 1972;73:637–642.

[149] Jocson VL. Tonography and gonioscopy: before and after cataract extraction with alpha chymotrypsin. Am J Ophthalmol 1965;60:318–322.

[150] Packer AJ, Fraioli AJ, Epstein DL. The effect of timolol and acetazolamide on transient intraocular pressure elevation following cataract extraction with alpha-chymotrypsin. Ophthalmology 1981;88:239–243.

[151] Allen JC. Surgical treatment pupillary block. Ann Ophthalmol 1977;9:661–664.

[152] Anderson DR, Forster RK, Lewis ML. Laser iridotomy for aphakic pupillary block. Arch Ophthalmol 1975;93:343–346.

[153] Chandler PA. Glaucoma from pupillary block in aphakia. Arch Ophthalmol 1962;67:14–17.

[154] Hitchings RA. Aphakic glaucoma: prophylaxis and management. Trans Ophthalmol Soc UK 1978;98:118–123.

[155] Reese AB. Herniation of the anterior hyaloid membrane following uncomplicated intracapsular cataract extraction. Trans Am Ophthalmol Soc 1948;46:73–96.

[156] Chang S, Lincoff HA, Coleman DJ, et al. Perfluorocarbon gases in vitreous surgery. Ophthalmology 1985;92:651–656.

[157] Tomey KF, Traverso CE. Neodymium-YAG posterior capsulotomy for the treatment of aphakic and pseudophakic pupillary block. Am J Ophthalmol 1987;104:502–507.

[158] Samples JR, Bellows AR, Rosenquist RC, et al. Pupillary block with posterior chamber intraocular lenses. Arch Ophthalmol 1987;105:335–337.

[159] Burk LL, Shields MB, Proia AD, et al. Intraocular pressure following intravitreal silicone oil injection. Invest Ophthalmol Vis Sci 1985;26(Suppl.):159.

[160] Sheie HG, Ewing MQ. Aphakic glaucoma. Trans Ophthalmol Soc UK 1978;98:111–117.

[161] Bellows AR, Johnstone MA. Surgical management of chronic glaucoma in aphakia. Ophthalmology 1983;90:807–813.

[162] Cohen JS, Osher RH, Weber P, et al. Complications of extracapsular cataract surgery: the indications and risks of peripheral iridectomy. Ophthalmology 1984;91:826–829.

[163] Van Buskirk EM. Pupillary block after intraocular lens implantation. Am J Ophthalmol 1983;95:55–59.

[164] Forman JS, Ritch R, Dunn MW, et al. Pupillary block following posterior chamber lens implantation. Ophthalmic Laser Ther 1987;2:85–97.

[165] Halkias A, Magauran DM, Joyce M. Ciliary block (malignant) glaucoma after cataract extraction with lens implant treated with YAG laser capsulotomy and anterior hyaloidotomy. Br J Ophthalmol 1992;76:569–570.

[166] Shingleton BJ, Chang MA, Bellows AR, et al. Surgical goniosynechialysis for angle-closure glaucoma. Ophthalmology 1990;97:551–556.

[167] Schulze RR, Copeland JR. Posterior chamber intraocular lens implantation without peripheral iridectomy: a preliminary report. Ophthalmic Surg 1982;13:567.

[168] Simel PF. Posterior chamber implants without iridectomy. J Am Intraocul Implant Soc 1982;8:141–143.

[169] Epstein DL, Hashimoto JM, Anderson PJ, et al. Experimental perfusions through the anterior and vitreous chambers with possible relationships to malignant glaucoma. Am J Ophthalmol 1979;88:1078–1086.

[170] Duy TP, Wollensak J. Ciliary block (malignant) glaucoma following posterior chamber lens implantation. Ophthalmic Surg 1987;18:741–744.

[171] Tomey KF, Senft SH, Antonios SR, et al. Aqueous misdirection and flat chamber after posterior chamber implants with and without trabeculectomy. Arch Ophthalmol 1987;105:770–773.

[172] Simmons RJ, Thomas JV, Yaqub MK. Malignant glaucoma. In: Ritch R, Shields MB, Krupin T, editors. The glaucomas. St Louis: Mosby; 1989. p. 1251–1263.

[173] Chandler PA, Grant WM. Mydriatic-cycloplegic treatment in malignant glaucoma. Arch Ophthalmol 1962;68:353–359.

[174] Dickens CJ, Shaffer RN. The medical treatment of ciliary block glaucoma after extracapsular cataract extraction. Am J Ophthalmol 1987;103:237.

[175] Epstein DL, Steinert RF, Puliafito CA. Neodymium-YAG laser therapy to the anterior hyaloid in aphakic malignant (cilio-vitreal block) glaucoma. Am J Ophthalmol 1984;98:137–143.

[176] Chandler PA, Simmons RJ, Grant WM. Malignant glaucoma: medical and surgical treatment. Am J Ophthalmol 1968;66:496–502.

[177] Lynch MG, Brown RH, Michels RG, et al. Surgical vitrectomy for pseudophakic malignant glaucoma. Am J Ophthalmol 1986;102:149–153.

[178] Wand M. Neovascular glaucoma. In: Ritch R, Shield MB, Krupin T, editors. The glaucomas. St Louis: Mosby; 1989. p. 1063–1110.

[179] Gu QX, Fry GL, Lata GF, et al. Ocular neovascularization. Arch Ophthalmol 1985;103:111–117.

[180] Poliner LS, Christianson DJ, Escoffery RF, et al. Neovascular glaucoma after intracapsular and extracapsular cataract extraction in diabetic patients. Am J Ophthalmol 1985;100:637–643.

[181] Wand M. Hyaloid membrane vs. posterior capsule as a protective barrier. Arch Ophthalmol 1985;103:1112.

[182] Weinreb RN, Wasserstrom JP, Parker W. Neovascular glaucoma following neodymium-YAG laser posterior capsulotomy. Arch Ophthalmol 1986;104:730–731.

[183] Aiello LM, Wand M, Liang G. Neovascular glaucoma and vitreous hemorrhage following cataract surgery in patients with diabetes mellitus. Ophthalmology 1983;90:814–819.

[184] Wand M, Dueker DK, Aiello LM, et al. Effects of panretinal photocoagulation on rubeosis iridis, angle neovascularization, and neovascular glaucoma. Am J Ophthalmol 1978;86:332–339.

[185] Bernardino VB, Kim JC, Smith TR. Epithelialization of the anterior chamber after cataract extraction. Arch Ophthalmol 1969;82:742–750.

[186] Weiner MJ, Trentacoste J, Pon DM, et al. Epithelial downgrowth: a 30-year clinicopathological review. Br J Ophthalmol 1989;73:6–11.

[187] Smith MF, Doyle JW. Glaucoma secondary to epithelial and fibrous downgrowth. Semin Ophthalmol 1994;9:248–253.

[188] Zavala EY, Binder PS. The pathologic findings of epithelial ingrowth. Arch Ophthalmol 1980;98:2007–2014.

[189] Stark WJ, Michels RG, Maumenee AE, et al. Surgical management of epithelial downgrowth. Am J Ophthalmol 1978;85:772–780.

[190] Miyake K, Ota I, Maekubo K, et al. Latanoprost accelerates disruption of the blood–aqueous barrier and the incidence of angiographic cystoid macular edema in early postoperative pseudophakias. Arch Ophthalmol 1999;117:34–40.

[191] Lima MC, Paranhos Jr A, Salim S, et al. Visually significant cystoid macular edema in pseudophakic and aphakic patients with glaucoma receiving latanoprost. J Glaucoma 2000;9:317–321.

[192] Rowe JA, Hattenhauer MG, Herman DC. Adverse side effects associated with latanoprost. Am J Ophthalmol 1997;124:683–685.

[193] Heier JS, Steinert RF, Frederick AR. Cystoid macular edema associated with latanoprost use. Arch Ophthalmol 1998;116:680–682.

[194] Avakian A, Renier SA, Butler PJ. Adverse effects of latanoprost on patients with medically resistant glaucoma. Arch Ophthalmol 1998;116:679–680.

[195] Ayyala RS, Cruz DA, Margo CE, et al. Cystoid macular edema associated with latanoprost in aphakic and pseudophakic eyes. Am J Ophthalmol 1998;126:602–604.

[196] Callanan D, Fellman RL, Savage JA. Latanoprost-associated cystoid macular edema. Am J Ophthalmol 1998;126:134–135.

[197] Thorne JE, Maguire AM, Lanciano R. CME and anterior uveitis with latanoprost use. Ophthalmology 1998;105:1981–1983.

[198] Warwar RE, Bullock JD, Ballal D. Cystoid macular edema and anterior uveitis associated with latanoprost use: experience and incidence in a retrospective review of 94 patients. Ophthalmology 1998;105:263–268.

[199] Moroi SE, Gottfredsdottir MS, Schteingart MT, et al. Cystoid macular edema associated with latanoprost therapy in a case of patients with glaucoma and ocular hypertension. Ophthalmology 1999;106:1024–1029.

Neodymium: Yttrium-Aluminum-Garnet Laser Posterior Capsulotomy

Roger F. Steinert, MD

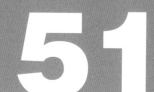

51

CAPSULAR OPACIFICATION

CONTENTS

- Capsular Opacification
- Posterior Capsulotomy

CHAPTER HIGHLIGHTS

>> Factors influencing posterior capsule opacification

>> Preoperative decision making

>> Technique

>> Complications

The neodymium:yttrium-aluminum-garnet (Nd:YAG) laser is a solid-state laser with a wavelength of 1064 mm that can disrupt ocular tissues by achieving optical breakdown with a short, high-power pulse. Optical breakdown results in ionization, or plasma formation, in the ocular tissue. This plasma formation then causes acoustic and shock waves that disrupt tissue.[1,2]

The development of the Nd:YAG laser as an ophthalmic instrument and its application in discussion of the posterior capsule coincided with the conversion from intracapsular to extracapsular surgical techniques in cataract surgery. Before the introduction of the Nd:YAG laser, only surgical cutting or polishing of the posterior capsule could manage opacification of the posterior capsule following extracapsular cataract extraction. Nd:YAG laser posterior capsulotomy introduced a technique for closed-eye, effective, and relatively safe opening of the opacified posterior capsule, and laser capsulotomy rapidly became the standard of care.[3]

CAPSULAR OPACIFICATION

Postoperative opacification of initially clear posterior capsules occurs frequently in patients after they have undergone extracapsular extraction of senile cataracts, although the time to opacification is highly variable. In adults, the time from surgery to visually significant opacification varies from months to years,[4,5] and the rate of opacification declines with increasing age.[6,7] In younger age groups, almost 100% opacification occurs within 2 years after surgery.

The incidence of posterior capsule opacification varies with different studies. Sinskey and Cain[8] reported that 43% of their patients required discussion, with an average follow-up of 26 months and a range from 3 months to 4 years. Emery, Wilhelmus, and Rosenberg[6] found opacification in 28% of their patients with 2 to 3 years of follow-up. Late opacification of the posterior capsule after 3 to 5 years has been reported to be approximately 50%.[9,10] Several studies have reported that the incidence of posterior capsule opacification is lower if a posterior chamber intraocular lens (IOL) is inserted with a convex posterior configuration in close apposition to the posterior capsule.[11-14] Phacoemulsification is associated with lower rates of posterior-capsule opacification than extracapsular cataract extraction.[15]

A study of posterior capsule opacification in 5416 postmortem pseudophakic eyes by Apple et al.[16,17] and Peng et al.[18,19] identified six factors associated with reduced posterior capsule opacification:

1. Hydrodissection-associated cortical cleanup

2. In-the-bag IOL fixation

3. Continuous circular capsulorrhexis diameter slightly smaller than the IOL optic

4. IOL material associated with reduced cellular proliferation. Hydrogel IOLs are associated with the highest rate of posterior capsule opacification; polymethylmethacrylate (PMMA) is intermediate; and silicone and acrylic optic material, the lowest[20,21]

5. Maximal IOL optic to posterior capsule opacification

6. IOL optic geometry with a square, truncated edge[22,23]

Diabetes mellitus may reduce the rate of posterior capsule opacification compared with nondiabetic patients.[24]

Experimental and pathologic studies indicated that posterior capsule opacification occurs as a result of the formation of opaque secondary membranes by active lens epithelial proliferation, transformation of lens epithelial cells into fibroblasts with contractile elements, and collagen deposition.[25-30] The anterior lens epithelial cells proliferate onto the posterior capsule at the site of apposition of the anterior capsule flaps to the posterior capsule.[31] The

Figures and portions of the text were previously published in Steinert RF, Puliafito CA: *The Nd:YAG laser in Ophthalmology: principles and clinical applications of photodisruption*, Philadelphia, 1985, WB Saunders.

617

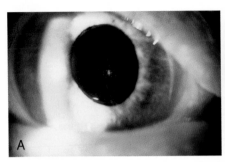 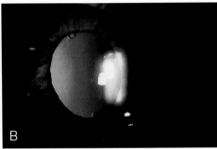 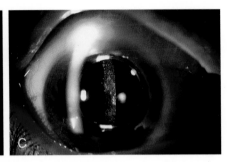

Figure 51-1 **A** and **B**, Fine fibrosis of the posterior capsule seen at the second postoperative examination represents cortical lamellae left at the time of surgery. The fibrosis is evident with oblique slit-lamp illumination (**A**) but is optically insignificant when viewed with a red reflex (**B**). **C**, Fine fibrosis may also develop months or years after cataract surgery on an initially clear capsule. This eye is shown 2.5 years after phacoemulsification cataract extraction with implantation of a one-piece polymethylmethacrylate intraocular lens (IOL) within the capsular bag. (From Steinert RF, Puliafito CA: *The Nd:YAG laser in ophthalmology: principles and clinical applications of photodisruption*, Philadelphia. Copyright Elsevier, 1985.)

contraction caused by the myoblastic features of the lens epithelial cells produces wrinkling of the posterior capsule.

Collagen deposition results in white fibrotic opacities. Mitotic inhibitors instilled into the anterior chamber after extracapsular cataract extraction have been shown to reduce capsular opacification dramatically, but pharmacologic inhibition of capsular opacification has yet to be successfully introduced into clinical practice.[32,33]

The finding that posterior capsule opacification results from lens epithelial cells proliferating onto the posterior capsule at the site of apposition of the anterior capsule flaps explains the inability of polishing the capsule at surgery to delay the onset or reduce the frequency of late capsular opacification,[4,6-8] because polishing the posterior capsule cannot remove the epithelial cells from the anterior capsule flaps. A peripheral ring in the capsular bag may reduce opacification, however.[34]

Additional clinical evidence that (1) a convex posterior chamber IOL can inhibit posterior capsule opacification and (2) close apposition of peripheral anterior and posterior capsule flaps leads to posterior capsule opacification was provided in an early study by Tan and Chee.[35] They reported an unusual form of early central posterior capsule fibrosis that occurred when a posteriorly vaulted biconvex optic IOL was positioned with the optic anterior to a capsulorrhexis opening smaller than the optic diameter. This positioning, usually with haptic fixation in the ciliary sulcus, allowed the anterior capsule flaps to be apposed to the posterior capsule and the IOL not to be in close apposition to the central posterior capsule. Migration of lens epithelial cells onto the posterior capsule then resulted in early central opacification.

The edge profile of the IOL is now generally regarded as the dominant factor in the rate of PCO.[36-65] Truncated edge design has been associated with reduced rates of PCO for both silicone and acrylic IOL optics. When the anterior capsulorrhexis edge overlies the optic for 360°, several studies have indicated that the PCO rate is lower,[43,66] but not all studies have shown this.[67] The presence of a sharp-edge truncated optic does increase the risk of undesirable optical phenomena after surgery, however.[68-70]

Clinically, optical degradation of initially clear posterior capsules takes several forms. Fibrosis connotes a gray-white band or plaque-like opacity that may be recognized in the early postoperative period or may occur later. Fibrosis that is present in the

first days to weeks postoperatively probably most often represents cortical lamellae left at the time of surgery (Figure 51-1). Fibrosis that develops months to years postoperatively is caused by migration of anterior lens epithelium, fibroblastic metaplasia, and collagen production.[31] Figure 51-2 shows a dense fibrinous plaque. Heavy fibrosis occurs frequently at the edge of a posterior chamber IOL placed in the bag with apposition of anterior and posterior capsules (Figure 51-3).

Formation of small Elschnig pearls and bladder cells (Figure 51-4), the second major form of opacity, occurs months to years after surgery. This type of opacity occurs from proliferating lens epithelial cells, which may form layers several cells thick.[31]

Capsular wrinkling can have two manifestations. Broad undulations of clear capsule are particularly common in the early postoperative period before the capsule becomes tense. Posterior chamber lens haptics may induce these broad wrinkles along the axis of the haptic orientation. Conversely, a posterior chamber lens may tend to flatten broad wrinkles if the optic body presses on the capsule. Fibrotic contraction can also induce wrinkles (Figure 51-5). Broad,

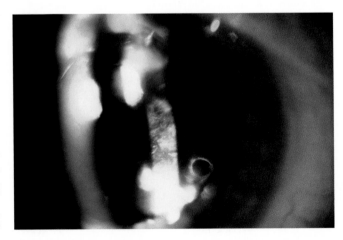

Figure 51-2 Heavy diffuse fibrosis of a posterior capsule behind a posterior chamber intraocular lens. (From Steinert RF, Puliafito CA: *The Nd:YAG laser in ophthalmology: principles and clinical applications of photodisruption*, Philadelphia. Copyright Elsevier, 1985.)

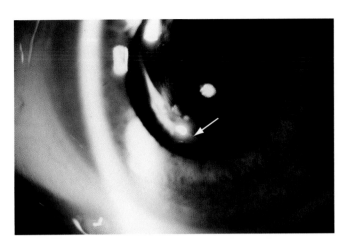

Figure 51-3 Dense fibrosis at the edge of a posterior chamber intraocular lens optic placed in the bag (arrow) in which an anterior capsular flap is apposed to the posterior capsule. (From Steinert RF, Puliafito CA: *The Nd:YAG laser in ophthalmology: principles and clinical applications of photodisruption*, Philadelphia. Copyright Elsevier, 1985.)

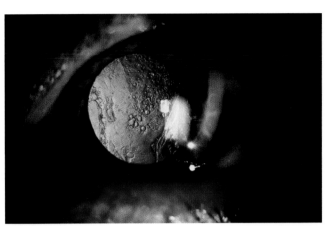

Figure 51-4 Red reflex view shows formation of multiple small epithelial pearls after anterior epithelial cells migrate centrally from peripheral areas of apposition of anterior capsular flaps to the posterior capsule. (From Steinert RF, Puliafito CA: *The Nd:YAG laser in ophthalmology: principles and clinical applications of photodisruption*, Philadelphia. Copyright Elsevier, 1985.)

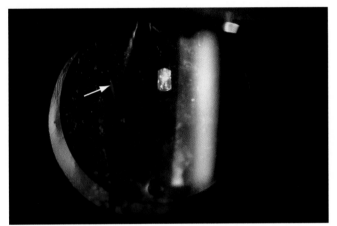

Figure 51-5 Broad wrinkles of the clear posterior capsule (arrow) are seen on red reflex, with numerous small epithelial pearls. (From Steinert RF, Puliafito CA: *The Nd:YAG laser in ophthalmology: principles and clinical applications of photodisruption*, Philadelphia. Copyright Elsevier, 1985.)

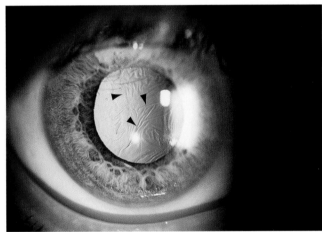

Figure 51-6 Fine wrinkles in the posterior capsule are evident on red reflex (arrowheads). These wrinkles alone can be visually disturbing and can reduce acuity by several lines or cause Maddox rod light streaks. (From Steinert RF, Puliafito CA: *The Nd:YAG laser in ophthalmology: principles and clinical applications of photodisruption*, Philadelphia. Copyright Elsevier, 1985.)

undulating wrinkles of clear capsule rarely are visually disturbing to the patient; an occasional patient may perceive linear distortion or shadows that correspond to the wrinkles and that are relieved by capsulotomy. In contrast, fine wrinkles or folds in the capsule caused by myoblastic differentiation may result in marked optical disturbance (Figure 51-6). These fine wrinkles are caused by myofibroblastic differentiation on the migrating lens epithelial cells, which acquire contractile properties.[31]

If the iris forms synechiae to the capsule, reactive pigment epithelial hyperplasia and migration onto the capsule may occur. Most often these adhesions occur if large amounts of cortex are left at the time of surgery, which is particularly common with traumatic cataracts. Figure 51-7 shows dense melanin deposition on a pupillary membrane after an old traumatic cataract.

Localized pigmented precipitates on the capsule and IOL can occur spontaneously or after hemorrhage or inflammation.

◼ POSTERIOR CAPSULOTOMY ◼

INDICATIONS

Nd:YAG laser capsulotomy is indicated for treatment of opacification of the posterior capsule resulting in decreased visual acuity or visual function, or both, for the patient. Careful assessment is necessary to be certain that the posterior capsule opacification is the cause of decreased visual acuity. Some patients may particularly complain of difficulty with glare despite what appears to be minimal capsular opacification. Glare testing can be helpful in validating these symptoms.[71]

POSTERIOR CAPSULOTOMY

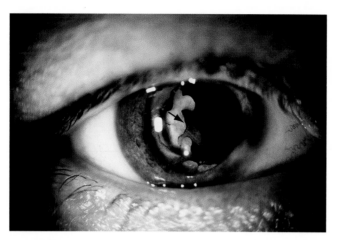

Figure 51-7 Pigment from proliferating uveal melanocytes has covered a large portion of this dense pupillary membrane, which formed after a traumatic cataract 40 years previously. The border of the pigment has a sharp scalloped configuration (arrow). (From Steinert RF, Puliafito CA: *The Nd:YAG laser in ophthalmology: principles and clinical applications of photodisruption*, Philadelphia. Copyright Elsevier, 1985.)

CONTRAINDICATIONS

Attempted Nd:YAG laser capsulotomy is contraindicated if corneal scars, irregularity, or edema preclude adequate visualization of the target aiming beam or degrade the Nd:YAG laser beam optics, preventing reliable and predictable optical breakdown. The procedure is also contraindicated if the patient proves unable or unwilling to fixate adequately, with the threat of inadvertent damage to adjacent intraocular structures.

The presence of a glass IOL, few of which remain, is a relative contraindication because of the possibility of causing a complete fracture in the glass optic.[72] The merits of surgical discission in this instance should be carefully weighed.

Known or suspected active cystoid macular edema (CME) is a relative contraindication, given evidence regarding a beneficial effect of the barrier function of an intact posterior capsule and rare cases of clinical CME that occur after Nd:YAG laser capsulotomy.[73] Conservative practice suggests avoidance of capsulotomy in an eye with active inflammation until the visual impairment becomes functionally unacceptable to the patient.

Nd:YAG laser posterior capsulotomy rarely may be complicated by a retinal tear or detachment. Despite a lack of clinical data establishing a correlation between the number or energy level of laser pulses and retinal detachment, prudence dictates that in eyes already at high risk for retinal detachment, the least amount of energy and the lowest possible number of shots should be used to accomplish the capsulotomy, and only a small opening should be made (Table 51-1). The alternative of repolishing the capsule may be considered in very high-risk patients.

TECHNIQUE

PREOPERATIVE ASSESSMENT

All patients require a complete ophthalmic history and examination before treatment, including notation of medical history and systemic medications, vision, intraocular pressure in both eyes, slit-lamp examination, and fundus examination. Judging the

Table 51-1 Contraindications to laser capsulotomy

Absolute contraindications
Corneal scars, irregularities, or edema that:
Interferes with target visualization
Makes optical breakdown unpredictable
Inadequate stability of the eye

Relative contraindications
Glass intraocular lens
Known or suspected cystoid macular edema
Active intraocular inflammation
High risk for retinal detachment

contribution of a capsular opacity to a patient's overall visual deficit may be difficult. Table 51-2 lists useful techniques. Some capsular opacities are impressive in oblique slit-lamp illumination but are insignificant when viewed against the red reflex. In general, these opacities cause little visual difficulty. The single most reliable technique for assessing capsular opacity is direct ophthalmoscopy because the surgeon's view of retinal details generally correlates with the patient's view of the world. Retinoscopy and the red reflex seen at the slit-lamp examination or with a direct or indirect ophthalmoscope also reveal significant optical disturbances. The fundus view with the Hruby lens or 90 diopter (D) lens may also allow accurate assessment of capsular clouding, whereas the indirect ophthalmoscope can penetrate significant capsular opacity.

The laser interferometer and the potential acuity meter should penetrate mild-to-moderate capsular opacity and be able to predict macular function. However, both instruments may give false-positive ("good") acuity prediction in the presence of CME,[74] which is the most common cause of postcataract visual impairment, besides capsular opacity itself. False-negative acuity predictions may also occur because of diffuse posterior capsule opacification, poor pupillary dilation, poor patient posture at the slit-lamp examination, communication problems, alphabet illiteracy, nystagmus, tremor, senility, poor patient cooperation, and fatigue.[75,76]

Unless the capsule is extremely dense, adequate visualization may be present for fluorescein angiography or angioscopy. Posterior segment optical coherence tomography (OCT) is possible in mild levels of PCO but more advanced levels of PCO may disrupt the scan to clinically unacceptable levels. In patients in

Table 51-2 Assessment of the significance of capsular opacity

Direct ophthalmoscopic visualization of fundus structures
Retinoscopy
Red reflex evaluation by:
Slit-lamp examination
Direct ophthalmoscopic examination
Indirect ophthalmoscopic examination
Hruby lens view of fundus
Laser interferometer evaluation
Potential acuity meter evaluation
Fluorescein angiography

whom the capsular opacity seems inadequate to explain the quality of vision, CME should be anticipated and documented so that unnecessary and possibly deleterious capsulotomy can be avoided.

PREPARATION OF THE PATIENT

The purpose and nature of the procedure should be explained to the patient and informed consent must be obtained beforehand. At the time of treatment, the patient usually is reassured by the familiar presence of the slit-lamp delivery system. The surgeon should remind the patient that the procedure is painless. The patient may hear small clicks or pops, but the patient must simply maintain steady fixation. The procedure is completed in a matter of minutes.

Brimonidine, apraclonidine, or a beta-blocking agent should be administered in the eye immediately on completion of the Nd: YAG laser posterior capsulotomy to minimize a postoperative intraocular pressure spike. If the administration of these agents is contraindicated, a topical or systemic carbonic anhydrase inhibitor, prostaglandin analogue, or, in a case of an extremely vulnerable optic nerve, oral hyperosmotic agent may be used to prevent or treat any intraocular pressure elevation following laser therapy.

Dilation of the pupil facilitates visualization of the capsule over a broad expanse. Except in cases of an iris-clip lens, dilation is helpful for a surgeon inexperienced with laser capsulotomy. In the absence of a miotic pupil, however, dilation may be omitted when an experienced surgeon is performing the procedure.

If the pupil is to be dilated, the landmarks of the pupillary zone of the capsule should be sketched beforehand. Pupils are often eccentric or may dilate eccentrically, as shown in Figure 51-8. Inattention to the pupillary zone may result in an eccentric capsulotomy and may necessitate a second session at the laser to induce the surgeon to perform an overly large capsulotomy to prevent this possibility. If the laser is available, the patient can be brought to the laser before dilation, and a single "marker" shot can be placed in the capsule near the middle of the pupillary axis. When the pupil is subsequently dilated, the marker shot accurately reminds the surgeon of the patient's true visual axis.

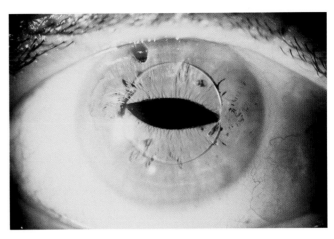

Figure 51-9 Iris capture of a ciliary sulcus-fixated planar haptic posterior chamber intraocular lens. This phenomenon can occur after wide dilation for posterior capsulotomy. If dilation is necessary at all, weak mydriatics and cycloplegics should be employed. (From Steinert RF, Puliafito CA: *The Nd:YAG laser in ophthalmology: principles and clinical applications of photodisruption*, Philadelphia. Copyright Elsevier, 1985.)

For routine dilation, we recommend only a single drop of 2.5% phenylephrine. If this is inadequate, a drop of 0.5% or 1% tropicamide may be added. Weak dilation is intended to prevent iris capture of a posterior chamber IOL (Figure 51-9), which may be difficult to properly reposition.

No anesthesia is generally required for capsulotomy unless a contact lens is used. In that case, a drop of topical anesthetic is applied to the cornea immediately before the beginning of the procedure. In rare circumstances, such as nystagmus, a retrobulbar injection to establish akinesia may be helpful. If a topical anesthetic is applied in advance of the procedure for examination or instillation of painful mydriatic and cycloplegic agents, the patient should be instructed to keep the eyes closed during the interval while waiting for the laser treatment to maintain the surface integrity and optical quality of the corneal epithelium.

The patient must be seated comfortably with properly adjusted stool, table, and chin rest heights and a footrest when

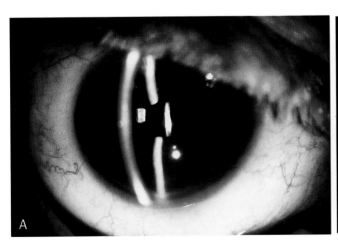

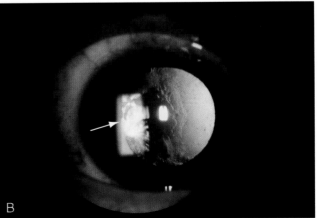

Figure 51-8 A, Typical capsular opacity before dilation. **B,** Capsulotomy appears eccentric because of uneven pupillary dilation caused by posterior synechia to the capsule (arrow). The capsular opening is properly centered for the undilated pupil. (From Steinert RF, Puliafito CA: *The Nd:YAG laser in ophthalmology: principles and clinical applications of photodisruption*, Philadelphia. Copyright Elsevier, 1985.)

Table 51-3 Preparation of the patient before the procedure

Before the treatment session

Preparation of the patient

Complete ophthalmic history and examination

Discussion of proposed procedure, including risks, benefits, and alternatives; signing of informed consent form

Apraclonidine or beta-adrenergic blocking agent

Pupillary dilation (optional)

Determination of visual axis and normal pupillary size: sketch and preliminary laser marker shot

Weak mydriatic and cycloplegic agents: 2.5% phenylephrine or 0.5% or 1% tropicamide

At the laser

Review of the procedure, the expected pop or click, and the importance of fixation

Application of topical anesthetic if contact lens is to be used

Adjustment of stool, table, chin rest, and footrest for optimal patient comfort

Application of head strap to maintain forehead position

Darkening of the room (optional)

Provision of fixation target for fellow eye

appropriate. A strap that passes from the headrest behind the patient's head is useful to counteract the tendency of many patients to move back during the course of the treatment. The surgeon's visualization of the target is usually improved in a darkened room. If a patient is expected to fixate with the other eye, however, an illuminated fixation target should be provided. Table 51-3 summarizes the steps in patient preparation.

PROCEDURE

A contact lens such as the Peyman or central Abraham lens may be used to stabilize the eye, improve the laser beam optics, and facilitate accurate focusing. The Abraham Nd:YAG laser increases the convergence angle to 24° from 16°, decreases the area of laser at the posterior capsule to 14 μm from 21 μm, and increases the beam diameter at both the cornea and the retina. The Abraham Nd:YAG laser lens must be used with care because it is a modified posterior pole lens; if the Nd:YAG laser is not sent through the lens button, but rather the peripheral "carrier" portion of the lens, the Nd:YAG laser may be focused on the retina and cause damage.[77]

The minimal amount of energy necessary to obtain breakdown and rupture the capsule is desired. With most lasers, a typical capsule can be opened by using 1–2 mJ/pulse.

The capsule is examined for wrinkles that indicate tension lines. Shots being placed across tension lines results in the largest opening per pulse because the tension causes the initial opening to widen.

Figure 51-10 shows an actual capsulotomy, photographed sequentially and drawn from the photographs, showing the opening as it develops and the location of the next laser shot. Table 51-4 outlines the basic technique. The usual strategy is to create a cruciate opening, beginning superiorly near the 12 o'clock position and progressing downward toward the 6 o'clock position. Unless a wide opening has already developed, shots are then placed at the edge of the capsule opening, progressing laterally toward the 3 and 9 o'clock positions. If any capsular flaps remain in the pupillary space, the laser is fired specifically at the flaps to cut them and cause them to retract and fall back to the periphery.

The goal is to achieve flaps based in the periphery inferiorly. Free-floating fragments should be avoided because they may remain and cause visual interference. Cutting in a circle ("can-opener" style) tends to create large fragments that may not sink from the visual axis or that may settle against the endothelium or angle structures. A large "vitreous floater" of residual capsule may bother the patient.

Beginning the cruciate opening in the superior periphery has several advantages. The initial shots are in the periphery so that if the patient becomes startled and an adjacent IOL is marked, the mark appears in the periphery. Both the patient and surgeon can have settled down before the more critical central area is treated. Furthermore, as the flaps develop, gravity aids in pulling them toward the inferior periphery. In contrast, it can be much more difficult to cause a flap that is hanging down from above to retract.

An IOL may be marked in the course of the capsulotomy. This is particularly true for posterior chamber lenses for which there is little or no separation of the capsule from the IOL. The issue of laser damage to the IOL is discussed under Complications. Figure 51-11 shows a capsulotomy without damage to an overlying posterior chamber IOL.

Visually significant pits and cracks can be minimized and avoided through careful techniques, as outlined in Table 51-5. The minimal amount of energy must be employed. With a typical capsule and careful focusing, 1–2 mJ is usually adequate. The capsule should be carefully examined for an area of separation from the IOL in which to begin the capsulotomy. Once the capsulotomy has begun, further areas of separation usually develop.

Following the usual strategy of beginning the capsulotomy in the 12 o'clock periphery gives an indication of the tendency for IOL marking in a noncritical area. If there is a tendency for unavoidable repeated marks, the usual cruciate pattern should be modified. Instead of progressing from the 12 o'clock to the 6 o'clock position across the visual axis, the cut should be made nasally and temporally, staying in the periphery of the optical zone. The capsule can then be opened in a "Christmas-tree" fashion, based inferiorly, without any shots in the central visual axis.

One other technique is very helpful in avoiding IOL marks. The laser can be intentionally focused posterior to the capsule, causing optical breakdown in the anterior vitreous. The shock wave then radiates forward and ruptures the capsule. Optical breakdown just at the capsule and IOL surface, with resultant IOL marking, is avoided. Because the breakdown threshold is higher in the anterior vitreous than at an optical interface like the capsule, higher energy is required to use this technique, usually a minimum of 2 mJ. Therefore, care must be taken to focus consistently at an area posterior to the capsule so that the breakdown is not allowed to come up to the back of the IOL, which would result in a larger mark. Because this technique traumatizes the vitreous, we prefer to reserve the deep focus technique for cases in which IOL marks are occurring with focus directly on the capsule.

In aphakic eyes, the reverse of a deep focus approach, namely, deliberate focus anterior to the capsule, has been advocated by some as a mechanism for opening the capsule while leaving the anterior hyaloid intact.

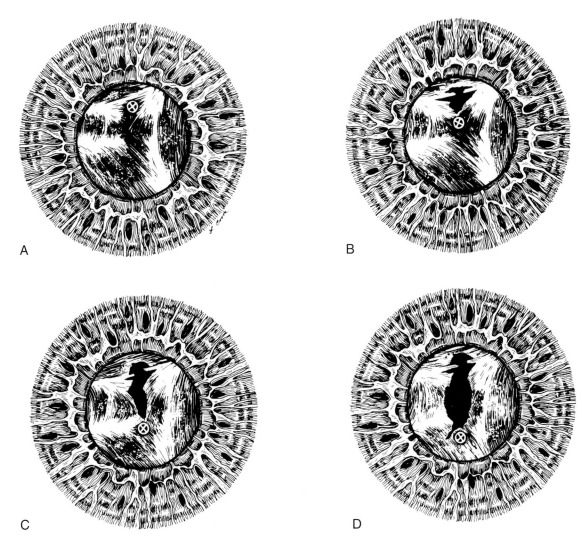

Figure 51-10 Artist drawing based on sequential capsulotomy photographs. The capsulotomy is developed in a cruciate pattern. **A,** The first shot is made superiorly in the location of some fine tension lines. **B,** The second shot is aimed inside the inferior edge of the initial opening. **C,** The next shot again is made at the 6 o'clock position of the capsulotomy border. **D,** The fourth shot is made across inferior tension lines to allow the capsulotomy to widen. Artist drawing based on sequential capsulotomy photographs. The capsulotomy is developed in a cruciate pattern.

(Continued)

CAPSULOTOMY SIZE

In the absence of a specific reason for a small opening, such as concern for a patient at high risk of retinal detachment, the capsulotomy should be as large as the pupil in isotopic conditions, such as driving at night, when glare from the exposed capsulotomy edge is most likely. A small opening in a dense membrane results in excellent optics, analogous to those of a small pupil (Figure 51-12). When the capsule is only hazy and transmits images to the retina, however, a small opening is an improvement but is still suboptimal. The hazy membrane continues to transmit a poor quality image that mixes at the retina with the image transmitted through the clear opening. The patient may experience symptoms of blur, glare, or decreased contrast sensitivity.

Figure 51-13 shows an example of a posterior capsulotomy performed without dilation. As the patient looks up, down, left, and right, the laser can be applied to capsular edges behind the sphincter so that the capsulotomy can be perfectly centered.

The slit-lamp illumination should be with a narrow beam, angled obliquely, to minimize miosis and indicate average pupillary size with ambient dim lighting.

Capsulotomies may also spontaneously enlarge postoperatively. Capone et al.[78] demonstrated that capsulotomies may increase in mean area by 32% within 6 weeks and that the capsular enlargement tended toward sphericity with capsular tag retention. Tension created by contractile properties of myofibroblastic lens epithelial cells or by IOL haptics, or both, may cause this alteration in capsulotomy contour.

A capsule with residual haze not only impairs vision under standard conditions but also produces glare. A clinical study of glare after extracapsular cataract extraction substantiated the deleterious effect of capsular opacification.[71] Steinert and Puliafito[79] demonstrated that glare and haze continue to be a problem for 1 and 2 mm capsular openings, decrease with a 3 mm opening, and fully resolve only with a 4 mm capsular opening.

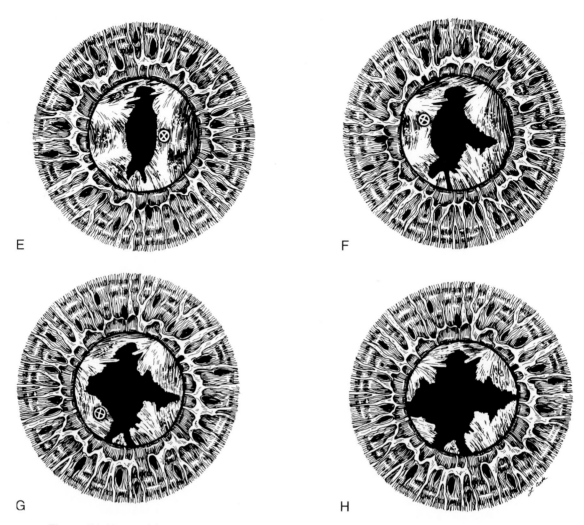

Figure 51-10, cont'd E, The opening is nearly 3 mm wide. It is widened by a shot at the 3 o'clock capsulotomy margin. F, The opening now needs to be directed to the left, with a shot at the 9 o'clock position. G, The cruciate opening has been accomplished, but a triangular flap extends into the pupillary space from the 7:30 region in the left inferior pupil. A shot is applied to the flap both to cut it and to push it toward the periphery. H, The capsulotomy is complete, and the pupil will be clear of capsule after the dilation wears off. (From Steinert RF, Puliafito CA: *The Nd:YAG laser in ophthalmology: principles and clinical applications of photodisruption*, Philadelphia. Copyright Elsevier, 1985.)

Table 51-4 Posterior capsulotomy technique
Use minimum energy: 1 mJ if possible
Identify and cut across tension lines

Perform a cruciate opening:
  Begin at the 12 o'clock position in the periphery
  Progress toward the 6 o'clock position
  Cut across at the 3 and 9 o'clock positions
  Clean up any residual tags
  Avoid freely floating fragments darkened

POSTOPERATIVE CARE

After Nd:YAG laser posterior capsulotomy in all patients, brimonidine, apraclonidine, or a beta-blocker should be administered topically to minimize any intraocular pressure increase. For high-risk patients, intraocular pressure may be measured again 1 h following laser treatment. If the patient has significant pre-existing glaucomatous disc damage or the intraocular pressure is increased 5 mm Hg or more at 1 h, the intraocular pressure should also be remeasured at 4 h.

An increased intraocular pressure may be treated with further brimonidine, apraclonidine, topical beta-adrenergic antagonists, prostaglandin analogue, topical pilocarpine, topical or systemic carbonic anhydrase inhibitor, or hyperosmotic agents. The patient's medical history, allergies, and current ocular therapy should be reviewed before determining the appropriate acute antiglaucoma therapy. If the intraocular pressure has increased following the posterior capsulotomy, antiglaucoma therapy should be continued for at least 1 week to prevent a delayed pressure elevation. Intraocular pressure should be measured again about 1 week after laser surgery and sooner if indicated by a pressure increase or pre-existing glaucomatous optic nerve damage or visual field loss.

Treatment following laser therapy (Table 51-6) with topical steroids and cycloplegic agents varies widely according to the individual surgeon's experience. Many patients may be managed easily with no therapy following laser treatment. Because a few

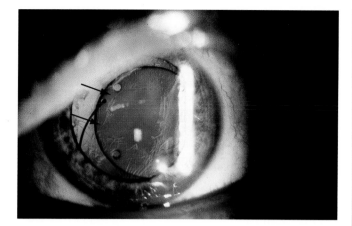

Figure 51-11 Posterior capsulotomy performed on a capsule in direct apposition to a lathe-cut posterior chamber intraocular lens. Figure 51-6 is the pretreatment photograph of the same eye. Note the eccentric location of the optic caused by the displacement of the inferior haptic in the bag and the superior haptic in the ciliary sulcus. The capsulotomy is properly located in the visual axis, but care is taken not to extend the opening beyond the edge of the optic to avoid vitreous herniation around the optic (arrow). (From Steinert RF, Puliafito CA: *The Nd:YAG laser in ophthalmology: principles and clinical applications of photodisruption*, Philadelphia. Copyright Elsevier, 1985.)

Table 51-5 Minimizing Intraocular Lens Laser Marks

Use minimum energy

Use a contact lens to:
   Stabilize the eye
   Improve laser beam optics
   Facilitate accurate focusing

Identify and areas of intraocular lens–capsule separation and begin treatment there
If lens making is occurring, make an opening in the shape of a Christmas tree from the 12 o'clock to the 4:30 position and from the 12 o'clock to the 7:30 position without placing any shots in the central optical zone

Use deep focus techniques:
   Optical breakdown occurs in the anterior vitreous
   The shock wave radiates forward and ruptures the capsule
   Higher energy (2 mJ or more) must be used

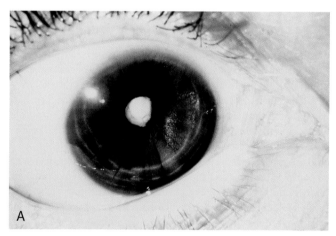
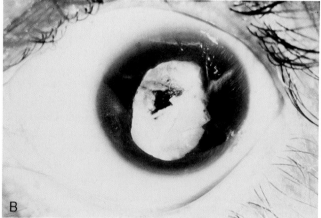

Figure 51-12 **A,** Dense retropupillary membrane after complicated extracapsular cataract extraction. **B,** An adequate membrane opening is well centered on the pupillary axis. (From Steinert RF, Puliafito CA: *The Nd:YAG laser in ophthalmology: principles and clinical applications of photodisruption*, Philadelphia. Copyright Elsevier, 1985.)

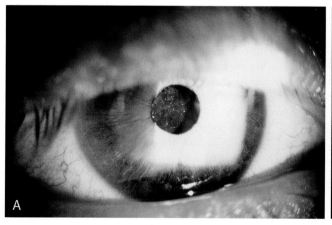
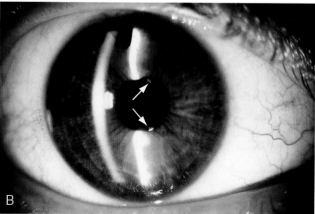

Figure 51-13 Posterior capsulotomy performed without pupillary dilation. **A,** Hazy capsule before treatment. **B,** After laser application, the pupillary zone is clear. Two tags of capsule at the edge of the pupil can be seen (arrows). These could be easily exposed to the laser by having the patient look up and down. (From Steinert RF, Puliafito CA: *The Nd:YAG laser in ophthalmology: principles and clinical applications of photodisruption*, Philadelphia. Copyright Elsevier, 1985.)

Table 51-6 Care following capsulotomy

Medication

Antiglaucoma medications:
  Apraclonidine immediately following capsulotomy
  Optional additional antiglaucoma therapy (beta-adrenergic antagonist, pilocarpine, carbonic anhydrase inhibitor, hyperosmotic agents) as needed for intraocular pressure control

Cycloplegics (optional)
  1% cyclopentolate at time of treatment

Steroids (optional)
  1% prednisolone or 0.1% dexamethasone four times a day tapered as needed

Minimal suggested follow-up protocol

1 to 4 h
Pressure rise to 5 mm Hg: treatment should be given

1 day
1 week
1 month
3 month
6 month

patients experience iritis, some surgeons favor topical steroids four times daily for one or more postoperative weeks. The topical steroids may usually be discontinued at that point, although some patients may require a tapered dosage.

RESULTS

Nd:YAG laser posterior capsulotomy results in improved visual acuity in 83–96% of eyes.[73,80–87] Failure of vision to improve following Nd:YAG laser posterior capsulotomy is often due to pre-existing ocular disease, including age-related macular degeneration, CME, other macular disease, retinal detachment, corneal edema, glaucoma, ischemic optic neuropathy, and amblyopia.

COMPLICATIONS

Complications of Nd:YAG laser posterior capsulotomy causing decreased vision are uncommon but include elevated extraocular pressure, CME, retinal detachment, IOL damage, endophthalmitis, iritis, vitritis, macular holes, and corneal edema.

INTRAOCULAR PRESSURE ELEVATION

Elevated intraocular pressure is recognized as the most common, although usually transient, complication following Nd:YAG laser capsulotomy. The frequency of intraocular pressure elevations greater than 10 mm Hg has been variably observed in 15–67% of eyes.[88–94] The intraocular pressure typically begins to rise immediately after the laser capsulotomy, peaks at 3–4 h, decreases but may remain elevated at 24 h, and usually returns to baseline at 1 week.[89] Rarely, the intraocular pressure may remain persistently

elevated, causing visual field loss[95,96] or requiring glaucoma surgery, or both. The acute intraocular pressure increase may also be high enough to cause loss of light perception vision.[97] The elevated intraocular pressure following Nd:YAG laser posterior capsulotomy has been associated with preexisting glaucoma,[89,90] capsulotomy size, lack of a posterior chamber IOL,[88,89,92–94] sulcus fixation of a posterior chamber IOL,[98] laser energy required for the capsulotomy,[89–91] myopia,[93] and pre-existing vitreoretinal disease.[93] Although not well studied, most surgeons believe that reliable in-the-bag fixation of posterior chamber IOLs has vastly reduced the incidence of clinically significant elevation of intraocular pressure after Nd:YAG laser capsulotomy.

Increased intraocular pressure following Nd:YAG laser capsulotomy is associated with a reduced facility for aqueous humor outflow.[89,99] This reduced facility has been attributed to capsular debris,[100] acute inflammatory cells, liquid vitreous,[93,101] and shock wave damage to the trabecular meshwork.[73] Laboratory studies have demonstrated pigment granules, erythrocytes, fibrin, lymphocytes, and macrophages within the trabecular meshwork after laser capsulotomy,[99] supporting the proposal that acute inflammatory cells and capsular debris are the cause of the increased intraocular pressure. Eyes with pre-existing glaucoma may have an increased frequency and magnitude of intraocular pressure elevation following laser treatment because the glaucomatous eyes already have a reduced outflow facility, and further obstruction of the trabecular meshwork results in a marked intraocular pressure increase.

Liquid vitreous as the cause of outflow obstruction has been supported by the clinical association between increased intraocular pressure following laser treatment and myopia,[93] pre-existing vitreoretinal disease,[93] lack of a posterior chamber IOL,[88,89,92–94] and sulcus-fixated posterior chamber IOLs.[98] A capsule-fixated posterior chamber IOL and a smaller capsulotomy may provide a barrier effect, preventing liquid vitreous from reaching the anterior chamber and trabecular meshwork. Experimentally, liquid vitreous injected into the anterior chamber in owl monkey eyes was found to increase intraocular pressure.[101]

Nd:YAG laser-induced shock waves causing increased intraocular pressure resulting in damage to the trabecular meshwork is supported clinically by the association between increased intraocular pressure and higher total laser energy used to create the capsulotomy.[89,91] However, photodisruption pulses in the aqueous of the midanterior chamber have not been associated with increased intraocular pressure,[101] nor has there been microscopic evidence of damage to the trabecular cords.[99]

Because increased intraocular pressure is a common complication following laser therapy and can result in permanent loss of vision, prevention of the intraocular pressure increase is appropriate. Apraclonidine,[102,103] brimonidine,[104] timolol,[94,105,106] levobunolol,[106,107] and pilocarpine[57] have been shown to decrease the frequency and magnitude of intraocular pressure increases following laser treatment, although apraclonidine is the most effective. Apraclonidine, timolol, levobunolol, or other beta-adrenergic antagonists are all administered 1 h before the Nd:YAG laser posterior capsulotomy and again following the procedure. Because of its miotic effect, pilocarpine should only be administered postoperatively. Patients at high risk for intraocular pressure elevation or those with vulnerable optic nerves should be carefully monitored following the laser capsulotomy because prophylactic therapy may not prevent late intraocular pressure increases.[94]

The intraocular pressure following Nd:YAG laser capsulotomy may also be elevated by vitreous obstruction of a sclerostomy,[108] the development of neovascular glaucoma,[109] or pupillary block glaucoma.[110,111]

Ge et al.[112] found evidence that the long-term intraocular pressure may remain elevated above precapsulotomy baseline in patients with existing glaucoma or for whom a high intraocular pressure developed acutely after capsulotomy.

CYSTOID MACULAR EDEMA

CME has been reported to develop in 0.55–2.5% of eyes following Nd:YAG laser posterior capsulotomy.[73,84–86,113–115] CME may occur between 3 weeks and 11 months after the capsulotomy.[115] One prospective study examined fluorescein angiography before and 4–8 weeks after Nd:YAG laser posterior capsulotomy in 136 patients and found no CME.[93] This study provides evidence that the incidence of new CME is low following laser capsulotomy, although some patients may acquire CME at a later date than the follow-up fluorescein angiograms performed in this study. Stark et al.[85] concluded that the risk of CME could be lowered by a longer interval between extracapsular cataract extraction and laser capsulotomy, although other studies have not confirmed this.[115] Treatment of CME following Nd:YAG laser posterior capsulotomy is identical to its treatment following cataract extraction and is discussed in Chapter 47.[116]

RETINAL DETACHMENT

Retinal detachment may complicate Nd:YAG laser posterior capsulotomy in 0.08–3.6% of eyes.[73,82,84–86,113–115,117,118] A retrospective analysis of Medicare claims found that the cumulative probability of retinal detachment over 36 months following cataract surgery was 1.6–1.9% in patients who had laser capsulotomy versus 0.8–1% in patients undergoing cataract surgery alone.[119] However, this retrospective study could not distinguish if the same or fellow eye had cataract surgery, capsulotomy, and retinal detachment, nor could it determine the sequence. A retinal detachment may occur early after the laser capsulotomy or more than 1 year later.[115] Asymptomatic retinal breaks were found at a rate of 2.1% within 1 month of posterior capsulotomy in one study.[120] Myopia,[121–124] a history of retinal detachment in the other eye,[123,125] younger age,[121,123] and male sex[88] are risk factors following Nd:YAG laser posterior capsulotomy.

In uncomplicated phacoemulsification and posterior-chamber IOL implantation, two series reported a rate of retinal detachment after laser capsulotomy of 0 to 0.4% over 1–8 years.[126,127] In one of these series, no retinal detachments occurred in eyes with axial lengths under 24 mm.[126] A case control study found no increased risk of retinal detachment after Nd-YAG laser capsulotiomy in eyes that did not have a posterior capsule tear at the time of cataract surgery.[128]

INTRAOCULAR LENS DAMAGE

Pitting of IOLs occurs in 15–33% of eyes during Nd:YAG laser posterior capsulotomy.[73,85] The pitting usually is not visually significant, although rarely the damage may cause sufficient glare and image degradation that the damaged IOL must be explanted.[129]

The type and extent of lens damage depend on the material used in the IOL. Glass IOLs may be fractured by the Nd:YAG laser.[72,130] PMMA IOLs sustain cracks and central defects with radiating fractures.[131] Molded PMMA IOLs are more easily damaged than higher-molecular-weight lathe-cut lenses.[132] Damage to silicone lenses is characterized by blistered lesions and localized pits surrounded by multiple tiny pits.[131,133]

The damage threshold is lowest for silicone, intermediate for PMMA, and highest for acrylic materials.[134,135] The frequency of the damage depends on the IOL style. IOLs designed with a ridge separating the posterior capsule from the IOL sustain less damage than lenses with a convex posterior surface and close apposition between the posterior chamber IOL and the posterior capsule.[134]

ENDOPHTHALMITIS

Several cases of propionibacterium acnes endophthalmitis have been reported following Nd:YAG laser posterior capsulotomy.[136–138] The patients were reported to have decreased vision caused by posterior capsular opacification and an otherwise quiet eye. Following the laser capsulotomy, the eyes developed significant uveitis and loss of vision. Presumably, the capsulotomy created an opportunity for the organisms sequestered within the capsule to reach the vitreous and develop into endophthalmitis.

OTHER COMPLICATIONS

Iritis persisting for 6 months after laser capsulotomy has been reported in less than 1% of eyes.[12,119] Macular holes have rarely been reported to develop after capsulotomy.[113,139] Specular microscopic studies have reported corneal endothelial cell loss of 2.3–7% following Nd:YAG laser posterior capsulotomy.[84,140,141]

References

[1] Aron-Rosa D, Aron JJ, Griesemann M, et al. Use of the neodymium-YAG laser to open the posterior capsule after lens implant surgery: a preliminary report. J Am Intraocul Implant Soc 1980;6:352.

[2] Aron-Rosa D, Griesemann JC, Aron JJ. Use of a pulsed neodymium-YAG laser (picosecond) to open the posterior lens capsule in traumatic cataract: a preliminary report. Ophthalmic Surg 1981;12:496.

[3] Fankhauser F, Lortscher J, Van der Zypen E. Clinical studies on high and low power laser radiation upon some structures of the anterior and posterior segments of the eye. Int Ophthalmol 1982;5:15.

[4] Wilhelmus KR, Emery JM. Posterior capsule opacification following phacoemulsification. In: Emery JM, Jacobson AC, editors. Current concepts in cataract surgery: selected proceedings of the Sixth Biennial Cataract Surgical Congress. St Louis: Mosby; 1980. p. 304–380.

[5] Baratz KH, Cook BE, Hodge DO. Probability of Nd:YAG laser capsulotomy after cataract surgery in Olmsted County, Minnesota. Am J Ophthalmol 2001;131:161–166.

[6] Emery JM, Wilhelmus KR, Rosenberg S. Complications of phacoemulsification. Ophthalmology 1978;85:141.

[7] Coonan P, Fung WE, Webster RG, et al. The incidence of retinal detachment following extracapsular cataract extraction: a ten-year study. Ophthalmology 1985;4:206.

[8] Sinskey RM, Cain W. The posterior capsule and phacoemulsification. J Am Intraocul Implant Soc 1978;4:206.

[9] Kraff MC, Sanders DR, Lieberman HL. Total cataract extraction through a 3 mm incision: a report of 650 cases. Ophthalmic Surg 1979;10:46.

[10] Wilhelmus KR, Emery JM. Posterior capsule opacification following phacoemulsification. Ophthalmic Surg 1980;11:264–267.

[11] Sterling S, Wood TO. Effect of intraocular lens convexity on posterior capsule opacification. J Cataract Refract Surg 1986;12:651.

[12] Downing JE. Long term discission rate after placing posterior chamber lenses with the convex surface posterior. J Cataract Refract Surg 1986;12:651.

[13] Frezzotti R, Caporossi A. Pathogenesis of posterior capsule opacification. Part I. Epidemiological and clinico-statistical data. J Cataract Refract Surg 1990;16:347.

[14] Born CP, Ryan DK. Effect of intraocular lens optic design on posterior capsular opacification. J Cataract Refract Surg 1990;16:188.

[15] Davidson MG, Morgan DH, McGahan MC. Effect of surgical technique on in vitro posterior capsule opacification. J Cataract Refract Surg 2000;26:1550–1554.
[16] Apple DA, Peng Q, Visessook N, et al. Eradication of posterior capsule opacification: documentation of a marked decrease in Nd:YAG laser posterior capsulotomy rates noted in an analysis of 5416 pseudophakic human eyes obtained postmortem. Ophthalmology 2001;108:505–518.
[17] Apple DA, Peng Q, Visessook N, et al. Surgical prevention of posterior capsule opacification. Part 1. Progress in eliminating this complication of cataract surgery. J Cataract Refract Surg 2000;26:180–187.
[18] Peng Q, Apple DA, Visessook N, et al. Surgical prevention of posterior capsule opacification. Part 2. Enhancement of cortical cleanup by focusing on hydrodissection. J Cataract Refract Surg 2000;26:188–197.
[19] Peng Q, Visessook N, Apple DA, et al. Surgical prevention of posterior capsule opacification. Part 3. Intraocular lens optic barrier effect as a second line of defense. J Cataract Refract Surg 2000;26:198–213.
[20] Hollick EJ, Spalton DJ, Ursell PG, et al. Posterior capsule opacification with hydrogel, polymethylmethacrylate, and silicone intraocular lenses: two-year results of a randomized prospective trial. Am J Ophthalmol 2000;129:577–584.
[21] Wang M-C, Woung L-C. Digital retroilluminated photography to analyze posterior capsule opacification in eyes with intraocular lenses. J Cataract Refract Surg 2000;26:56–61.
[22] Hollick EJ, Spalton DJ, Ursell PG, et al. The effect of polymethylmethacrylate, silicone, and polyacrylic intraocular lenses on posterior capsule opacification 3 years after cataract surgery. Ophthalmology 1999;106:49–55.
[23] Nishi O, Nishi K, Wickstrom K. Preventing lens epithelial cell migration using intraocular lenses with sharp rectangular edges. J Cataract Refract Surg 2000;26:1543–1549.
[24] Zaczek A, Zetterstrom C. Posterior capsule opacification after phacoemulsification in patients with diabetes mellitus. J Cataract Refract Surg 1999;25:233–237.
[25] Roy FH. After-cataract: clinical and pathological evaluation. Ann Ophthalmol 1971;3:1364.
[26] Hiles DA, Johnson BL. The role of the crystalline lens epithelium in postpseudophakos membrane formation. J Am Intraocul Implant Soc 1980;6:141.
[27] McDonnell PJ, Green WR, Maumenee AE, et al. Pathology of intraocular lenses in 33 eyes examined postmortem. Ophthalmology 1983;90:386.
[28] McDonnell PJ, Stark WJ, Green WR. Posterior capsule opacification: a specular microscopic study. Ophthalmology 1984;91:853.
[29] Cobo ML, Ohsawa E, Chandler D, et al. Pathogenesis of capsular opacification after extracapsular cataract extraction: an animal model. Ophthalmology 1984;91:851.
[30] Nishi O. Posterior capsule opacification. Part 1. Experimental investigations. J Cataract Refract Surg 1999;25:106–117.
[31] McDonnell PJ, Zarbin MA, Green WR. Posterior capsule opacification in pseudophakic eyes. Ophthalmology 1983;90:1548.
[32] Chan RY, Emery JM, Kretzer F. Mitotic inhibitors in preventing posterior lens capsule opacification. In: Emery JM, Jacobson AC, editors. Current concepts in cataract surgery: selected proceedings of the Seventh Biennial Cataract Surgical Congress. New York: Appleton-Century-Crofts; 1982. p. 217–224.
[33] Clark DS, Emery JM, Munsell MF. Inhibition of posterior capsule opacification with an immunotoxin specific for lens epithelial cells: 24 month clinical results. J Cataract Refract Surg 1998;24:1614–1620.
[34] Nishi O, Nishi K, Menapace R. Capsule-bending ring for the prevention of capsule opacification: a preliminary report. Ophthalmic Surg Lasers 1998;29:749–753.
[35] Tan DTH, Chee SP. Early central posterior capsular fibrosis in sulcus-fixated biconvex intraocular lenses. J Cataract Refract Surg 1993;19:471.
[36] Peng Q, Visessook N, Apple DJ, et al. Surgical prevention of posterior capsule opacification. Part 3: Intraocular lens optic barrier effect as a second line of defense. J Cataract Refract Surg 2000;26:198–213.
[37] Nishi O, Nishi K. Preventing posterior capsule opacification by creating a discontinuous sharp bend in the capsule. J Cataract Refract Surg 1999;25:521–526.
[38] Aasuri MK, Shah U, Veenashree MP, Deshpande P. Performance of a truncated-edged silicone foldable intraocular lens in Indian eyes. J Cataract Refract Surg 2002;28:1135–1140.
[39] Abhilakh Missier KA, Nuijts RM, Tjia KF. Posterior capsule opacification: silicone plate-haptic versus AcrySof intraocular lenses. J Cataract Refract Surg 2003;29:1569–1574.
[40] Buehl W, Findl O, Menapace R, et al. Effect of an acrylic intraocular lens with a sharp posterior optic edge on posterior capsule opacification. J Cataract Refract Surg 2002;28:1105–1111.
[41] Buehl W, Findl O, Menapace R, et al. Long-term effect of optic edge design in an acrylic intraocular lens on posterior capsule opacification. J Cataract Refract Surg 2005;31:954–961.
[42] Buehl W, Menapace R, Sacu S, et al. Effect of a silicone intraocular lens with a sharp posterior optic edge on posterior capsule opacification. J Cataract Refract Surg 2004;30:1661–1667.
[43] Daynes T, Spencer TS, Doan K, et al. Three-year clinical comparison of 3-piece AcrySof and SI-40 silicone intraocular lenses. J Cataract Refract Surg 2002;28:1124–1129.
[44] Findl O, Menapace R, Sacu S, et al. Effect of optic material on posterior capsule opacification in intraocular lenses with sharp-edge optics: randomized clinical trial. Ophthalmology 2005;112:67–72.
[45] Georgopoulos M, Menapace R, Findl O, et al. After-cataract in adults with primary posterior capsulorhexis: comparison of hydrogel and silicone intraocular lenses with round edges after 2 years. J Cataract Refract Surg 2003;29:955–960.
[46] Hayashi K, Hayashi H. Posterior capsule opacification after implantation of a hydrogel intraocular lens. Br J Ophthalmol 2004;88:182–185.
[47] Hayashi K, Hayashi H, Nakao F, Hayashi F. Changes in posterior capsule opacification after poly(methyl methacrylate), silicone, and acrylic intraocular lens implantation. J Cataract Refract Surg 2001;27:817–824.
[48] Heatley CJ, Spalton DJ, Kumar A, et al. Comparison of posterior capsule opacification rates between hydrophilic and hydrophobic single-piece acrylic intraocular lenses. J Cataract Refract Surg 2005;31:718–724.
[49] Hollick EJ, Spalton DJ, Ursell PG, et al. Posterior capsular opacification with hydrogel, polymethylmethacrylate, and silicone intraocular lenses: two-year results of a randomized prospective trial. Am J Ophthalmol 2000;129:577–584.
[50] Kruger AJ, Schauersberger J, Abela C, et al. Two year results: sharp versus rounded optic edges on silicone lenses. J Cataract Refract Surg 2000;26:566–570.
[51] Kucuksumer Y, Bayraktar S, Sahin S, Yilmaz OF. Posterior capsule opacification 3 years after implantation of an AcrySof and a MemoryLens in fellow eyes. J Cataract Refract Surg 2000;26:1176–1182.
[52] Kurosaka D, Kato K. Membranous proliferation of lens epithelial cells on acrylic, silicone, and poly(methyl methacrylate) lenses. J Cataract Refract Surg 2001;27:1591–1595.
[53] Mester U, Fabian E, Gerl R, et al. Posterior capsule opacification after implantation of CeeOn Edge 911A, PhacoFlex SI-40NB, and AcrySof MA60BM lenses: one-year results of an intraindividual comparison multicenter study. J Cataract Refract Surg 2004;30:978–985.
[54] Nejima R, Miyata K, Honbou M, et al. A prospective, randomised comparison of single and three piece acrylic foldable intraocular lenses. Br J Ophthalmol 2004;88:746–749.
[55] Ober MD, Lemon LC, Shin DH, et al. Posterior capsular opacification in phacotrabeculectomy: a long-term comparative study of silicone versus acrylic intraocular lens. Ophthalmology 2000;107:1868–1873, discussion 74.
[56] Pohjalainen T, Vesti E, Uusitalo RJ, Laatikainen L. Posterior capsular opacification in pseudophakic eyes with a silicone or acrylic intraocular lens. Eur J Ophthalmol 2002;12:212–218.
[57] Prosdocimo G, Tassinari G, Sala M, et al. Posterior capsule opacification after phacoemulsification: silicone CeeOn Edge versus acrylate AcrySof intraocular lens. J Cataract Refract Surg 2003;29:1551–1555.
[58] Rauz S, Stavrou P, Murray PI. Evaluation of foldable intraocular lenses in patients with uveitis. Ophthalmology 2000;107:909–919.
[59] Sacu S, Findl O, Menapace R, et al. Comparison of posterior capsule opacification between the 1-piece and 3-piece Acrysof intraocular lenses: two-year results of a randomized trial. Ophthalmology 2004;111:1840–1846.
[60] Sacu S, Menapace R, Buehl W, et al. Effect of intraocular lens optic edge design and material on fibrotic capsule opacification and capsulorhexis contraction. J Cataract Refract Surg 2004;30:1875–1882.
[61] Sacu S, Menapace R, Findl O, et al. Long-term efficacy of adding a sharp posterior optic edge to a three-piece silicone intraocular lens on capsule opacification: five-year results of a randomized study. Am J Ophthalmol 2005;139:696–703.
[62] Sundelin K, Shams H, Stenevi U. Three-year follow-up of posterior capsule opacification with two different silicone intraocular lenses. Acta Ophthalmol Scand 2005;83:11–19.
[63] Wang MC, Woung LC. Digital retroilluminated photography to analyze posterior capsule opacification in eyes with intraocular lenses. J Cataract Refract Surg 2000;26:56–61.
[64] Wejde G, Kugelberg M, Zetterstrom C. Posterior capsule opacification: comparison of 3 intraocular lenses of different materials and design. J Cataract Refract Surg 2003;29:1556–1559.
[65] Li N, Chen X, Zhang J, et al. Effect of Acrysof versus silicone or polymethyl methacrylate intraocular lens on posterior capsule opacification. Ophthalmology 2008;115:830–838.
[66] Wejde G, Kugelberg M, Zetterstrom C. Position of anterior capsulorhexis and posterior capsule opacification. Acta Ophthalmol Scand 2004;82:531–534.
[67] Vasavada AR, Raj SM. Anterior capsule relationship of the AcrySof intraocular lens optic and posterior capsule opacification: a prospective randomized clinical trial. Ophthalmology 2004;111:886–894.
[68] Farbowitz MA, Zabriskie NA, Crandall AS, et al. Visual complaints associated with the AcrySof acrylic intraocular lens(1). J Cataract Refract Surg 2000;26:1339–1345.
[69] Davison JA. Positive and negative dysphotopsia in patients with acrylic intraocular lenses. J Cataract Refract Surg 2000;26:1346–1355.
[70] Masket S. Truncated edge design, dysphotopsia, and inhibition of posterior capsule opacification. J Cataract Refract Surg 2000;26:145–147.
[71] Nadler DJ, Jaffee NS, Clayman HM, et al. Glare disability in eyes with intraocular lenses. Am J Ophthalmol 1984;97:43.
[72] Riggins J, Pedrotti LS, Keates RH. Evaluation of the neodymium:YAG laser for treatment of ocular opacities. Ophthalmic Surg 1983;14:675.
[73] Keates RH, Steinert RF, Puliafito CA, et al. Long-term follow-up of Nd-YAG laser posterior capsulotomy. J Am Intraocul Implant Soc 1984;10:164.
[74] Faulkner W. Laser interferometric prediction of postoperative visual acuity in patients with cataracts. Am J Ophthalmol 1983;95:626.
[75] Klein TB, Slomovic AR, Parrish II RK, et al. Visual acuity prediction before neodymium-YAG laser posterior capsulotomy. Ophthalmology 1986;93:808.
[76] Smiddy WE, Radulovic D, Yeo JH, et al. Potential acuity meter for predicting visual acuity after neodymium:YAG posterior capsulotomy. Ophthalmology 1986;93:397.
[77] Dickerson DE, Gilmore JE, Gross J. The Abraham lens with the neodymium-YAG laser. J Am Intraocul Implant Soc 1983;9:438.
[78] Capone A, Rehkopf PG, Warnicki JW, et al. Temporal changes in posterior capsulotomy dimensions following neodymium:YAG laser discission. J Cataract Refract Surg 1990;16:451.
[79] Steinert RF, Puliafito CA. Posterior capsulotomy and pupillary membranectomy. In: Steinert RF, Puliafito CA, editors. The Nd-YAG laser in ophthalmology: principles and clinical applications of photodisruption. Philadelphia: WB Saunders; 1985. p. 72–95.
[80] Aron-Rosa DS, Aron J-J, Cohn HC. Use of a pulsed picosecond Nd:YAG laser in 6,664 cases. J Am Intraocul Implant Soc 1984;10:35.
[81] Aron-Rosa DS. Posterior capsulotomy and picosecond pulsed YAG laser influence on eye pressure. Cataract 1983;1:13.
[82] Aron-Rosa DS. Pulsed picosecond pulsed and nanosecond YAG lasers: principles and uses. Cataract 1984;1:9.
[83] Terry AC, Apple DJ, Price FW, et al. Neodymium-YAG laser for posterior capsulotomy. Am J Ophthalmol 1983;96:716.
[84] Johnson SH, Kratz RP, Olson PF. Clinical experience with the Nd:YAG laser. J Am Intraocul Implant Soc 1984;10:452.
[85] Stark WJ, Worthen D, Holladay JT, et al. Neodymium:YAG lasers: an FDA report. Ophthalmology 1985;92:209.
[86] Bath PE, Fankhauser F. Long-term results of Nd:YAG laser posterior capsulotomy with the Swiss laser. J Cataract Refract Surg 1986;12:150.
[87] Wasserman EL, Axt JC, Sheets JH. Neodymium-YAG laser posterior capsulotomy. J Am Intraocular Implant Soc J 1985;11:245.
[88] Slomovic AR, Parrish II RK. Acute elevations of intraocular pressure following Nd:YAG laser posterior capsulotomy. Ophthalmology 1985;92:973.
[89] Richter CU, Arzeno G, Pappas H, et al. Intraocular pressure elevation following Nd:YAG laser posterior capsulotomy. Ophthalmology 1985;92:636.
[90] Flohr MJ, Robin AL, Kelley JS. Early complications following Q-switched neodymium:YAG laser posterior capsulotomy. Ophthalmology 1985;92:360.
[91] Chanell MM, Beckman H. Intraocular pressure changes after neodymium:YAG laser posterior capsulotomy. Arch Ophthalmol 1984;102:1024.
[92] Brown SVL, Thomas JV, Belcher CD, et al. Effect of pilocarpine in treatment of intraocular pressure following neodymium:YAG laser posterior capsulotomy. Ophthalmology 1985;392:354.
[93] Schubert HD. Vitreoretinal changes associated with rise in intraocular pressure after Nd:YAG laser capsulotomy. Ophthalmic Surg 1987;18:19.
[94] Migliori ME, Beckman H, Channell MM. Intraocular pressure changes after following neodymium:YAG laser capsulotomy in eyes pretreated with timolol. Arch Ophthalmol 1987;105:473.
[95] Demer JL, Koch DD, Smith JA, et al. Persistent elevation in intraocular pressure after Nd:YAG laser treatment. Ophthalmic Surg 1986;17:465.
[96] Kurata F, Krupin T, Sinclair S, et al. Progressive glaucomatous visual field loss after neodymium: YAG laser capsulotomy. Am J Ophthalmol 1984;98:632.
[97] Vine AK. Ocular hypertension following Nd-YAG laser capsulotomy: a potentially blinding complication. Ophthalmic Surg 1984;15:283.
[98] Gimbel HV, Van Westenbrugge JA, Sanders DR, et al. Effects of sulcus vs. capsular fixation on YAG-induced pressure rises following posterior capsulotomy. Arch Ophthalmol 1990;108:1126.

[99] Lynch MG, Quigley HA, Green WR, et al. The effect of neodymium:YAG laser capsulotomy on aqueous humor dynamics in the monkey eye. Ophthalmology 1986;93:1270.

[100] Altamirano D, Mermoud A, Pittet T, et al. Aqueous humor analysis after Nd:YAG laser capsulotomy with the laser flare-cell meter. J Cataract Refract Surg 1992;18:554.

[101] Schubert HD, Morris WJ, Trokel SL, et al. The role of the vitreous in the intraocular pressure rise after neodymium-YAG laser capsulotomy. Arch Ophthalmol 1985;103:1538.

[102] Pollack IP, Brown RH, Crandall AS, et al. Prevention of the rise in intraocular pressure following neodymium-YAG laser posterior capsulotomy using topical 1% apraclonidine. Arch Ophthalmol 1988;106:754.

[103] Rosenberg LF, Krupin T, Ruderman J, et al. Apraclonidine and anterior segment surgery: comparison of 0.5% vs 1.0% apraclonidine for prevention of postoperative intraocular pressure rise. Ophthalmology 1995;102:1312–1318.

[104] Gartaganis SP, Mela EK, Katsimpris JM, et al. Use of topical brimonidine to prevent intraocular pressure elevations following Nd:YAG laser posterior capsulotomy. Ophthalmic Surg Lasers 1999;30:647–652.

[105] Richter CU, Arzeno G, Pappas HR, et al. Prevention of intraocular pressure elevation following neodymium-YAG laser posterior capsulotomy. Arch Ophthalmol 1985;103:912.

[106] Rakofsky S, Koch DD, Faulkner JD, et al. Levobunolol 0.5% and timolol 0.5% to prevent intraocular pressure elevation after neodymium:YAG laser posterior capsulotomy. J Cataract Refract Surg 1997;23:1075–1080.

[107] Silverstone DE, Novack GD, Kelley EP, et al. Prophylactic treatment of intraocular pressure elevations after neodymium-YAG laser posterior capsulotomies and extracapsular cataract extractions with levobunolol. Ophthalmology 1988;95:713.

[108] Schrader CE, Belcher III CD, Thomas JV, et al. Acute glaucoma following Nd-YAG laser membranotomy. Ophthalmic Surg 1983;14:1015.

[109] Weinreb RN, Wasserstrom JP, Parker W. Neovascular glaucoma following neodymium-YAG laser posterior capsulotomy. Arch Ophthalmol 1986;104:730.

[110] Gstalder RJ. Pupillary block with anterior chamber lens following Nd:YAG laser capsulotomy. Ophthalmic Surg 1986;17:249.

[111] Ruderman JM, Mitchell PG, Kraff M. Pupillary block following Nd-YAG laser capsulotomy. Ophthalmic Surg 1983;14:1418.

[112] Ge J, Wand M, Chiang R, Paranhos A, et al. Long-term effect of Nd:YAG laser posterior capsulotomy on intraocular pressure. Arch Ophthalmol 2000;118:1334–1337.

[113] Winslow RL, Taylor BC. Retinal complications following YAG capsulotomy. Ophthalmology 1985;92:785.

[114] Chambless WS. Neodymium:YAG laser posterior capsulotomy results and complications. J Am Intraocul Implant Soc J 1985;11:31.

[115] Steinert RF, Puliafito CA, Kumar SR, et al. Cystoid macular edema, retinal detachment, and glaucoma after Nd:YAG laser posterior capsulotomy. Am J Ophthalmol 1991;112:373.

[116] Lewis H, Singer TR, Hanscom TA, et al. A prospective study of cystoid macular edema after neodymium:YAG laser posterior capsulotomy. Ophthalmology 1987;94:478.

[117] Liesegang TJ, Bourne WM, Ikstrup DM. Secondary surgical and neodymium:YAG laser discissions. Am J Ophthalmol 1985;100:510.

[118] Rickman-Barger L, Florine CW, Larson RS, et al. Retinal detachment after neodymium:YAG laser posterior capsulotomy. Am J Ophthalmol 1989;107:531.

[119] Javitt JC, Tielsch JM, Canner JK, et al. National outcomes of cataract extraction: increased risk of retinal complications associated with Nd:YAG laser posterior capsulotomy. Ophthalmology 1992;99:1487.

[120] Ranta P, Tommila T, Immonen I, Summanen P, et al. Retinal breaks before and after neodymium:YAG laser posterior capsulotomy. J Cataract Refract Surg 2000;26:1190–1197.

[121] Koch DD, Liu JF, Gill EP, et al. Axial myopia increases the risk of retinal complications after neodymium:YAG laser posterior capsulotomy. Arch Ophthalmol 1989;107:986.

[122] Dardenne MU, Gerten GJ, Kokkas K, et al. Retrospective study of retinal detachment following neodymium:YAG laser posterior capsulotomy. J Cataract Refract Surg 1989;15:676.

[123] Davison JA. Retinal tears and detachments after extracapsular cataract surgery. J Cataract Refract Surg 1988;14:624.

[124] Jacobi FK, Hessemer V. Pseudophakic retinal detachment in high axial myopia. J Cataract Refract Surg 1997;23:1096–1102.

[125] Shah GR, Gills JP, Durham DG, et al. Three thousand YAG lasers in posterior capsulotomies: an analysis of complications and comparing to polishing and surgical discission. Ophthalmic Surg 1986;17:473.

[126] Olsen G, Olson RJ. Update on a long-term, prospective study of capsulotomy and retinal detachment rates after cataract surgery. J Cataract Refract Surg 2000;26:1017–1021.

[127] Jahn CE, Richter J, Jahn AH, et al. Pseudophakic retinal detachment after uneventful phacoemulsification and subsequent neodymium: YAG capsulotomy for capsule opacification. J Cataract Refract Surg 2003;29:925–929.

[128] Tuft SJ, Minassian D, Sullivan P. Risk factors for retinal detachment after cataract surgery: a case-control study. Ophthalmology 2006;113:650–656.

[129] Bath PE, Hoffer KJ, Aron-Rosa D, et al. Glare disability secondary to YAG laser intraocular lens damage. J Cataract Refract Surg 1987;13:309.

[130] Fritch CD. Neodymium:YAG laser damage to glass intraocular lens. J Am Intraocul Implant Soc 1984;10:225.

[131] Joo C-K, Kim J-H. Effect of neodymium:YAG laser photodisruption on intraocular lenses in vitro. Am J Cataract Refract Surg 1992;18:562.

[132] Downing JE, Alberhasky JT. Biconvex intraocular lenses and Nd:YAG capsulotomy: experimental comparison of surface damage with different poly(methylmethacralate) formulations. J Cataract Refract Surg 1990;16:732.

[133] Keates RH, Sall KN, Kreter JK. Effect of the Nd:YAG laser on polymethylmethacrylate, HEMA copolymer, and silicone intraocular materials. J Cataract Refract Surg 1987;13:401.

[134] Fallor MK, Hoft RK. Intraocular lens damage associated with posterior capsulotomy: a comparison of intraocular lens designs and four different Nd:YAG laser instruments. J Am Intraocul Implant Soc J 1985;11:564.

[135] Newland TJ, McDermott ML, Eliott D, et al. Experimental neodymium:YAG laser damage to acrylic, poly(methylmethacrylate), and silicone intraocular lenses. J Cataract Refract Surg 1999;25:72–76.

[136] Tetz MR, Apple DJ, Price FW, et al. A newly described complication of neodymium:YAG laser capsulotomy: exacerbation of an intraocular infection. Arch Ophthalmol 1987;105:1324.

[137] Piest KL, Kincaid MC, Tetz MR, et al. Localized endophthalmitis: a newly described cause of the so-called toxic lens syndrome. J Cataract Refract Surg 1987;13:498.

[138] Carlson AN, Koch DD. Endophthalmitis following Nd:YAG laser posterior capsulotomy. Ophthalmic Surg 1988;19:168.

[139] Blacharski PA, Newsome DA. Bilateral macular holes after Nd:YAG laser posterior capsulotomy. Am J Ophthalmol 1988;105:417.

[140] Slomovic AR, Parrish II RK, Forster RK, et al. Neodymium-YAG laser posterior capsulotomy: central corneal endothelial cell density. Arch Ophthalmol 1986;104:536.

[141] Schrems W, Belcher III CD, Tomlinson CP. Changes in the human central corneal endothelium after neodymium:YAG laser surgery. Ophthalmic Laser Ther 1986;1:143.

POSTERIOR CAPSULOTOMY

Neodymium:Yttrium-Aluminum-Garnet Laser in the Management of Postoperative Complications of Cataract Surgery

Roger F. Steinert, MD

52

CONTENTS

CHAPTER HIGHLIGHTS

>> Uses of laser photodisruption

>> Treatment of vitreous strands and cystoid macular edema

>> Treatment of pupillary abnormalities

>> Treatment of anterior capsule phimosis

Photodisruption with the neodymium:yttrium-aluminum-garnet (Nd:YAG) laser can effectively treat a number of disorders arising after cataract surgery and intraocular lens (IOL) implantation. The pressure wave generated by optical breakdown of an Nd:YAG laser pulse allows the surgeon to cut and manipulate intraocular structures in a variety of postoperative disorders.

Portions of the text and figures have previously been published in Steinert RF, Puliafito CA: The Nd:YAG laser in ophthalmology: principles and clinical applications of photodisruption, Philadelphia, 1985, WB Saunders.

PUPILLARY BLOCK GLAUCOMA

Acute angle closure glaucoma in aphakia and pseudophakia may take several forms, as outlined in Table 52-1.[1,2] Corneal edema and haze, anterior chamber reaction, and iris congestion may make argon laser iridectomy impossible. Even if a patent iridectomy is formed, an argon laser iridectomy may not relieve the glaucoma because of the role of the vitreous. In many cases, the Nd:YAG laser can better treat these conditions and is the treatment of first choice.[3] The success of the Nd:YAG laser "anterior hyaloidotomy" in curing ciliovitreal block glaucoma, in which surgical and argon iridectomies have failed, demonstrates the pathophysiologic role of the anterior hyaloid face in many cases of pupillary block glaucoma.

Figure 52-1 illustrates a case of pupillary block in a patient who had an iridectomy and antibiotic therapy for endophthalmitis after complex extracapsular cataract extraction with an anterior-chamber IOL (AC IOL). The surgical iridectomy became occluded postoperatively, but an argon laser iridotomy succeeded in relieving the resultant iris bombé. Within weeks, the argon laser iridotomy closed, and the iris bombé recurred with an intraocular pressure of 50 mm Hg. The Nd:YAG laser at 4 mJ readily created several new iridotomies with permanent relief of the iris bombé and pressure elevation. The pupillary membrane also was cleared by the Nd:YAG laser.

The most common setting for pseudophakic block is after placement of an AC IOL, typically after complicated extracapsular cataract extraction or phacoemulsification. The risk of pupillary block is heightened when the surgeon fails to place a large surgical iridectomy. Even after a large anterior vitrectomy, further vitreous may prolapse and occlude the pupil against the optic of the AC IOL. A large surgical iridectomy may also be occluded by prolapsing vitreous, of course, as well as by capsular and cortical remnants.

The role of the hyaloid face in aphakic malignant glaucoma is clearly illustrated by the case shown in Figure 52-2. Three months after complicated cataract extraction and subsequent IOL removal in a patient who also had a large superior loss of iris, the chamber nevertheless became shallow, and the pressure rose to 34 mm Hg over several days, with the onset of deep pain. A thin, intact hyaloid face or inflammatory membrane was present. The patient was treated with the Nd:YAG laser, which was focused and fired

Table 52-1 Classification of acute aphakic and pseudophakic glaucoma

Pupillary block (iridovitreal block)
Absent, imperforate, or secluded peripheral iridectomies
Inflammatory adhesion of intact hyaloid face to iris
Anterior chamber hemorrhage and exudate
Aphakic malignant glaucoma (ciliovitreal block)
Posterior diversion of aqueous

at 3 mJ on the hyaloid face through the mild corneal edema despite less than 1 mm of residual anterior chamber depth. The anterior chamber deepened immediately.

TECHNIQUE FOR APHAKIC AND PSEUDOPHAKIC IRIDECTOMY AND ANTERIOR HYALOID VITREOLYSIS ■

PREPARATION OF THE PATIENT

In many cases, the patient will have been treated maximally with miotic agents. If not, application of a miotic agent such as pilocarpine 2% is advisable to place the iris on maximal stretch.

PROCEDURE

From 4 to 8 mJ is usually adequate to perforate the iris in one pulse. Corneal edema or an anterior-chamber reaction may necessitate higher energy to obtain the same optical breakdown cutting

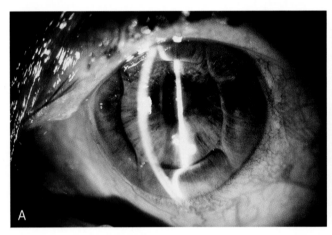

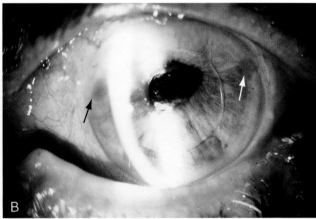

Figure 52-1 **A,** Recurrent pseudophakic pupillary block with iris bombé after endophthalmitis and closure of argon laser iridectomy. **B,** Nd:YAG laser at 4 mJ readily created several iridectomies (arrows) with permanent relief of the iris bombé. A pupillary membranectomy was also performed. (From Steinert RF, Puliafito CA: *The Nd:YAG laser in ophthalmology: principles and clinical application of photodisruption*, Philadelphia. Copyright Elsevier, 1985.)

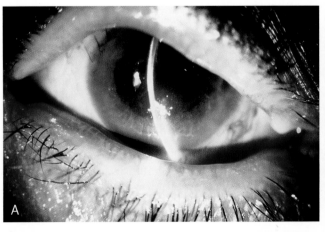

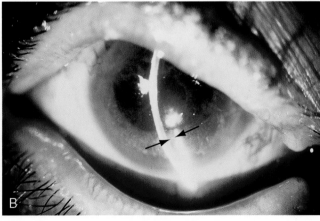

Figure 52-2 **A,** Aphakic malignant glaucoma with apposition of inferior iris to edematous cornea. **B,** Depth is restored to the anterior chamber immediately after Nd:YAG laser pulses have opened the anterior hyaloid face. Arrows show separation of iris and cornea, in comparison with part A. (From Steinert RF, Puliafito CA: *The Nd:YAG laser in ophthalmology: principles and clinical applications of photodisruption*, Philadelphia. Copyright Elsevier, 1985.)

power. In most cases, at least three iridotomies should be made to ensure full relief of aqueous entrapment, which may be localized into sectors around an AC IOL, and to increase the chance of maintaining at least one long-term patent iridotomy. Iridotomies tend to shrink as bombé is relieved, and the iris falls back. Inflammation also may close iridotomies postoperatively.

If the chamber is markedly shallow or flat, the haptic of an AC IOL, when present, usually provides a small area of clearance from the cornea. The first laser shots can be made immediately adjacent to such a haptic insertion to avoid corneal injury.

After the iridotomy has been completed or when a patent basal surgical iridectomy is already present, the Nd:YAG laser should be fired into the anterior vitreous through the iridectomy or the pupil. This procedure ruptures the hyaloid face and relieves any malignant glaucoma component caused by the intact hyaloid face.

POSTOPERATIVE CARE

Intense topical steroid therapy such as prednisolone acetate 1%, or dexamethasone 0.1%, is used at least four times daily and more often as inflammation requires. Inflammation and a tendency for synechia formation also require cycloplegia and mydriasis. Intraocular pressure must be monitored and treated appropriately

ANTERIOR VITREOLYSIS AND CYSTOID MACULAR EDEMA

Vitreous strands and bands to the wound may cause eccentric pupils and can be associated with cystoid macular edema (CME) (Irvine-Gass CME).[4,5] Iliff[6] first reported visual improvement after surgical section of such vitreous bands to the wound. He coined the term vitreous-tug syndrome; although no evidence was given that tugging on the vitreous body was, in fact, present or responsible for the visual loss.

Katzen, Fleischman, and Trokel[7] first reported the use of the Nd:YAG laser to lyse strands of vitreous to cataract wounds in their series. Vision improved by variable amounts in all 14 patients treated. However, the presence of CME was judged clinically, and the results of fluorescein angiography before and after laser treatment were not reported for 13 of the eyes.

Because of the unpredictable natural history of aphakic CME, with erratic response to anti-inflammatory agents and frequent spontaneous improvement,[8,9] small and controlled series cannot unequivocally prove the efficacy of a given technique. However, my clinical experience has confirmed a high rate of visual improvement after anterior segment vitreolysis, particularly in favorable cases.[10] In that series of 29 patients, 22 of the patients had fluorescein angiographic confirmation of the presence of CME before laser treatment. The interval between cataract extraction and treatment averaged 10 months, with a range of 1–42 months; average follow-up after laser vitreolysis was also 10 months, with a range of 3–27 months.

The change in best-corrected Snellen acuity is shown in Figure 52-3. No patient had loss of vision after laser vitreolysis. The visual acuity in 16 of the 29 patients (55%) improved by two or more lines, with stable acuity following treatments. Five (17%) patients' vision improved by at least two lines, but they experienced ongoing fluctuation of acuity. Vision in eight patients (28%) showed

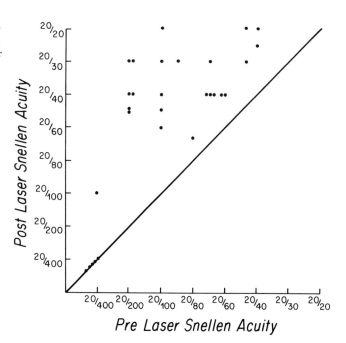

Figure 52-3 Scattergram of visual acuity level before and after Nd:YAG laser vitreolysis. Points above the diagonal line represent improvement. (From Steinert RF, Wasson PJ: Neodymium:YAG laser anterior vitreolysis for Irvine-Gass cystoid macular edema, *J Cataract Refract Surg* 15:304–307. Copyright Elsevier, 1989.)

less than two lines of improvement. Of these eight patients, two had progressive maculopathy in addition to the CME (one had an epiretinal membrane and one had progressive diabetic maculopathy), two had severe glaucoma with loss of central vision in addition to the CME, and two had persistent CME. Two other patients were lost to follow-up without documentation of the basis for persistent unimproved acuity. Of note, patients who did not respond to vitreolysis had the poorest pretreatment visual acuity measurements.

Postlaser fluorescein angiography was performed on nine eyes. Three eyes showed complete resolution of the CME, two showed improvement but persistent leakage, one showed no improvement in the appearance of the fluorescein angiographic leakage but still experienced improved acuity, and three had persistent CME and less than two lines of visual improvement.

TECHNIQUES FOR ANTERIOR VITREOLYSIS

PREOPERATIVE ASSESSMENT

The evaluation and medical treatment of CME are reviewed in detail in Chapter 54. A comprehensive examination including fluorescein angiography should be performed to establish a definitive diagnosis of CME.

Small vitreous strands may be missed on casual examination. The strand is usually best seen on slit-lamp examination with a narrow slit beam in a darkened room. Careful gonioscopy may be necessary to visualize the strand, particularly if the vitreous enters the anterior chamber through the area of a peripheral iridectomy. The most favorable cases for Nd:YAG laser vitreolysis are those with relatively discrete strands under tension. Broad bands are

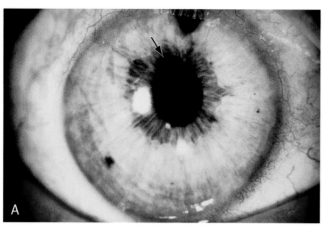
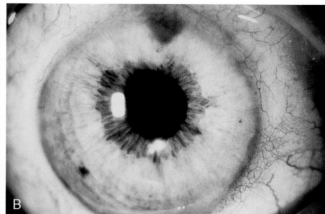

Figure 52-4 A, Fine vitreous strand caused mild peaking of the pupil (arrow). Gonioscopy showed a fine vitreous strand to the wound. **B,** After laser vitreolysis, less peaking is present, but chronic change in the sphincter prevents a completely normal pupillary contour. (From Steinert RF, Puliafito CA: *The Nd:YAG laser in ophthalmology: principles and clinical applications of photodisruption*, Philadelphia. Copyright Elsevier, 1985.)

most difficult to fully transect. Amorphous vitreous herniation is extremely difficult to cut with a laser approach. In general, the larger the amount of vitreous involvement, the more consideration should be given to pars plana vitrectomy for definitive removal of all pathologic vitreous.

Pupillary distortion may be subtle. Figure 52-4A shows mild peaking of a pupil, indicating a vitreous strand coming around the pupil. After vitreolysis, less peaking is present, although some permanent change has occurred in the sphincter, preventing complete rounding of the pupil, as seen in Figure 52-4B. Permanent changes in the iris stroma are frequent in cases of long duration. Figure 52-5 shows the decreased but persistent oval shape of the pupil after lysis of a vitreous strand. The iris stroma is partially depigmented locally, perhaps indicating chafing of the iris by the vitreous strand. The vitreous band may distort the pupil in

several ways, depending on the angle, direction, and number of vitreous strands under tension. Figure 52-6 shows a "hammock" effect by two separate strands.

PREPARATION OF THE PATIENT

The procedure should be explained beforehand and informed consent obtained. The patient should be told that the procedure often requires more than one session.

When the vitreous strand or band passes through the pupil, treatment is often facilitated by administration of pilocarpine 2% every 10 min for three or four drops preoperatively. Inducing stretch of the vitreous through miosis facilitates identification of the strand. Moreover, release of tension when the laser transects the strand is shown more definitively.

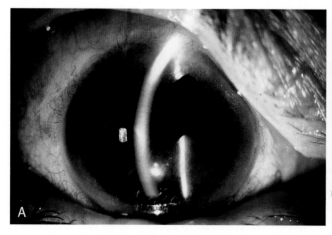
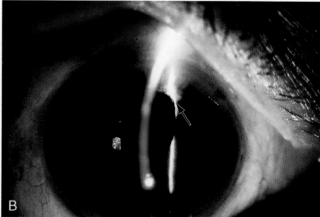

Figure 52-5 A, Eccentric pupil caused by a vitreous strand. **B,** After vitreolysis, depigmentation of the underlying iris stroma, present before the laser treatment, is more readily seen (arrow), and the pupil remains partially distorted. (From Steinert RF, Puliafito CA: *The Nd:YAG laser in ophthalmology: principles and clinical applications of photodisruption*, Philadelphia. Copyright Elsevier, 1985.)

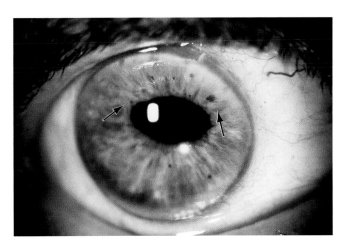

Figure 52-6 Pupillary distortion caused by two separate strands of vitreous to the wound (arrows). The pupil became round after treatment. Despite CME of 57 months' duration, vision improved from counting-fingers level to 20/50. (From Steinert RF, Puliafito CA: *The Nd:YAG laser in ophthalmology: principles and clinical applications of photodisruption*, Philadelphia. Copyright Elsevier, 1985.)

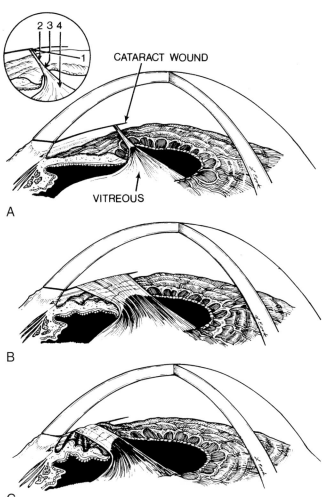

Figure 52-7 A, A narrow vitreous strand to a cataract wound. The inset shows possible laser pathways for vitreolysis: (1) a gonioscopic approach, directed at the cataract wound – the location at which the vitreous strand is often the most discrete; (2) a direct approach near the limbus; (3) a direct approach in the region of the collarette; and (4) a direct approach at the pupil. This last approach is rarely successful. **B,** A broad vitreous band at the wound. **C,** Iris pulled upward in a tentlike configuration and entrapped by the vitreous incarceration in the wound. (From Steinert RF, Puliafito CA: *The Nd:YAG laser in ophthalmology: principles and clinical applications of photodisruption*, Philadelphia. Copyright Elsevier, 1985.)

PROCEDURE

Figure 52-7 illustrates the three most common configurations of vitreous to the wound: (1) a small discrete strand, (2) a broad band, and (3) a band with either adhesions to the iris or iris entrapment behind the band.

The laser can be directed at a vitreous strand in four general areas (inset, Figure 52-7A). The most reliable landmark during vitreolysis is the cataract wound because the vitreous band or strand has to terminate at that location. The cataract wound is visualized with a gonioscopy lens (pathway 1 on the figure), and the laser can be fired at the wound area with a reasonable chance of successful vitreolysis. Because of the contact lens and mirror optics, the energy settings are usually in the 6–12 mJ range to obtain adequate cutting power. The disadvantages of this technique include the requirement of a gonioscopy lens, which involves some extra manipulation and positioning requirements, and the subsequent commitment to use a contact lens for the completion of the treatment session, even if a different approach is needed later in the session, because of the application of gonioscopy fluid to the cornea.

If the cornea is clear near the limbus and a vitreous strand can be visualized with some clearance from the iris stroma, direct cutting without a contact lens or with a peripheral button Abraham lens may be successful along pathway 2 (see Figure 52-7). Usually 4–8 mJ is required. In the course of dozens to hundreds of shots along this pathway, considerable pigment may be liberated from the underlying iris stroma, which will ultimately obscure the surgeon's view. Misfocused shots can cause local damage to the underlying or overlying stroma.

Occasionally the use of pathway 3 (see Figure 52-7), directed at the vitreous passing over the iris collarette, can be helpful. This is particularly true when the vitreous has formed adhesions to the collarette, pulling it forward in a tentlike formation. Close proximity of vitreous and iris makes damage to the underlying iris stroma likely, but this may be clinically tolerable.

The use of pathway 4 (see Figure 52-7), directed at the vitreous as it passes around the pupil, is tempting but rarely successful. Vitreous traction components are poorly defined as they come around the pupil. The shock wave is ineffective at rupturing vitreous strands except directly at the laser focal point. Firing the laser immediately adjacent to the pupillary border inevitably causes low-grade capillary hemorrhage, as well as the release of pigment, obscuring further visualization of the area.

Successful treatment releases the tension and converts a discrete strand or band to an amorphous gelatinous appearance. The observation of a change and any iris deformation is the best indicator of a successful release of tension. Hundreds of shots over several treatment sessions may be necessary to cut a large band.

POSTOPERATIVE CARE

Strong topical steroids such as prednisolone acetate 1% or dexamethasone 0.01% are given four times daily until visual improvement occurs, typically in 2 to 3 months. Topical nonsteroidal anti-inflammatory drugs may well be of further benefit alone or in conjunction with topical steroids. Typically, ketorolac or diclofenac drops are administered four times daily.

Intraocular pressure elevation following vitreolysis has not been well documented. A drop of a beta-blocker or brimonidine at the time of treatment probably provides adequate prophylaxis if desired.

In recalcitrant cases, the addition of a systemic nonsteroidal anti-inflammatory drug can be considered.

■ "PROPHYLACTIC" VITREOLYSIS ■

With the availability of laser vitreolysis, the surgeon may treat vitreous strands to the wound in the absence of CME in an effort to prevent its later development. Only a large, long-term randomized treatment trial can scientifically determine the usefulness of this approach, and such a study is unlikely. Certainly, some patients with vitreous strands to the wound never acquire CME.

In patients with vitreous to the wound and good visual acuity, a baseline fluorescein angiogram is recommended to document the macular status. If CME is detected, laser vitreolysis is probably indicated even in the presence of good acuity. If visual loss later develops in conjunction with the new onset of CME, the baseline angiogram will be a useful reference to further support therapeutic intervention.

■ COREOPLASTY ■

The Nd:YAG laser can cut through iris stroma or the pupillary sphincter to open an occluded visual axis. Indications for coreoplasty including pupillary enlargement for restoration of vision or improvement of the fundus view for examination and treatment. Synechialysis can also affect a pupillary configuration, as discussed in the next section.

Figure 52-8 illustrates a case in which the pupil became updrawn after intracapsular cataract extraction many years earlier. The upper lid covered the pupil. Unless the lid was elevated, vision was limited to counting fingers. The Nd:YAG laser cut through the sphincter with only a localized, self-limited hemorrhage. Vision improved to 20/70 and was limited only by preexisting maculopathy.

In Figure 52-9, postoperative inflammation has caused nearly complete seclusion of the pupil over a posterior-chamber IOL (PC IOL). Dense associated fibrosis was present with thickening of the iris stroma. The pupil was successfully enlarged by 6 mJ pulses directed through a central button Abraham lens with a resultant improvement in acuity from 20/80 to 20/30.

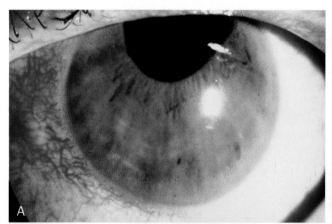

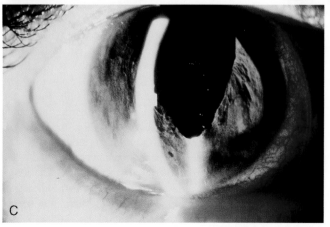

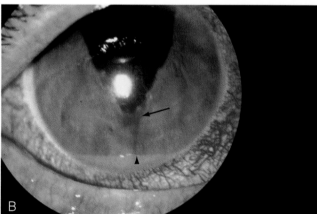

Figure 52-8 A, Updrawn pupil after intracapsular cataract extraction. **B,** Immediately after sphincterotomy, a candle wax-like trickle of blood was seen clotted at the inferior margin of the sphincterotomy (arrow). A light reflection from the lid margin gave an appearance similar to hypopyon (arrowhead), but no gross hemorrhage or inflammation occurred. **C,** One week later, the clot had cleared, and the central cornea was in the optical axis. (From Steinert RF, Puliafito CA: *The Nd:YAG laser in ophthalmology: principles and clinical applications of photodisruption*, Philadelphia. Copyright Elsevier, 1985.)

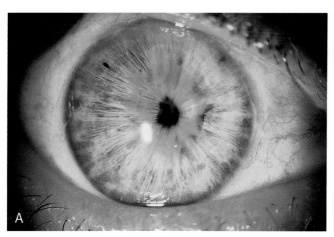
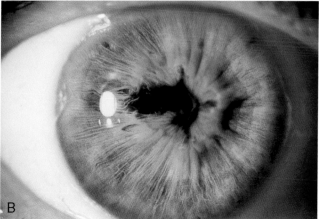

Figure 52-9 A, Nearly total seclusion of the pupil secondary to postoperative inflammation after extracapsular cataract extraction with posterior chamber intraocular lens implantation. **B,** Coreoplasty with the Nd:YAG laser resulted in little improvement superiorly, inferiorly, and nasally (to the right). However, in the temporal zone, to the left, the sphincter was successfully transected, and a clear visual axis was restored.

TECHNIQUE

PREPARATION OF THE PATIENT

In addition to a comprehensive eye examination and informed consent, information regarding the presence of bleeding abnormalities must be specifically elicited in the history because clotting abnormalities increase the risk of a large hyphema.

Preparatory thermal iris photocoagulation with an argon laser has not been necessary or helpful in most cases. Very heavy and extensive iris coagulation is necessary to prevent bleeding when the pulsed Nd:YAG laser is subsequently used. The pressure wave after optical breakdown radiates over several millimeters with enough shearing force to cause a capillary oozing. Thus, it is difficult to eliminate bleeding without widespread intense preparatory coagulation. An exception to this principle is a visible blood vessel whose patch cannot be avoided; it would be folly to cut such a vessel with the Nd:YAG laser without prior photocoagulation. Patients in whom preparatory laser coagulation has been performed generally state that the photocoagulation is more painful than the photodisruption.

PROCEDURE

The is usual setting is 6–10 mJ. Numerous shots are required to cut across 3–5 mm of sphincter and stroma.

The sphincter is the most difficult region to cut and, with the minor arterial circle, the most prone to hemorrhage. If the surgeon starts at the pupil and cuts across the sphincter first, gross hemorrhage and free red blood cells and fibrin in the anterior chamber may prevent completion of the treatment in one session. To avoid significant hemorrhage until nearly the end of the session, the treatment should begin in the peripheral iris stroma and progress toward the sphincter and pupil. Figure 52-10 illustrates a sequential sphincterotomy.

If bleeding begins without clotting and does not cease rapidly, pressure should be applied to the globe through a contact lens, if one is being used, by a finger through the eyelids, or with a cotton-tipped swab applied to the globe. Pressure adequate to stop the bleeding is maintained for several minutes until effective iris intravascular coagulation has time to occur.

Because the damage zone from optical breakdown ("plasma growth") occurs backward along the beam path toward the Nd:

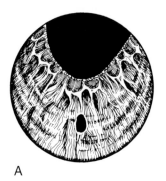
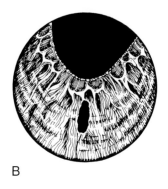
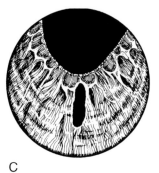
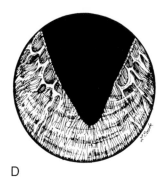

A   B   C   D

Figure 52-10 Technique for Nd:YAG laser sphincterotomy. **A,** Treatment is begun in the peripheral iris stroma. **B** and **C,** Progressive cutting is made toward the iris sphincter. **D,** Sphincter is cut last so that bleeding is minimized for as long as possible to increase the chance of completing the treatment in one session. (From Steinert RF, Puliafito CA: *The Nd:YAG laser in ophthalmology: principles and clinical applications of photodisruption*, Philadelphia. Copyright Elsevier, 1985.)

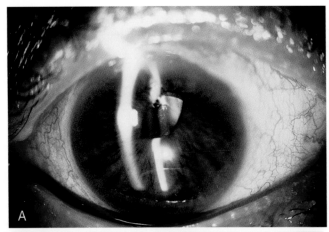

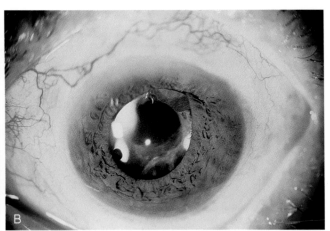

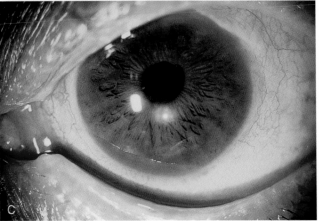

Figure 52-11 A, Iris capture of a posterior-chamber intraocular lens (IOL) secondary to iridocapsular adhesions in an undilated patient. B, Adhesion of the iris to the anterior capsular edge is seen clearly after dilation. C, IOL capture is released, and the pupil becomes round after Nd:YAG laser capsulotomy releases the iridocapsular adhesions.

YAG laser source, it is possible to perform sphincterotomy and coreoplasty over a PC IOL without damaging the underlying lens. However, it is not advisable to perform this procedure in a phakic patient. The pressure wave generated can rupture the anterior capsule of the natural crystalline lens, inducing immediate cataract formation.

POSTOPERATIVE CARE

A strong topical steroid (typically prednisolone acetate 1% or dexamethasone 0.1%) is given four times daily, initially, with the dosage tapered as inflammation subsides. Cycloplegia is usually unnecessary. Intraocular pressure elevation is monitored and treated appropriately.

■ SYNECHIALYSIS ■

Localized synechiae with associated pigment may be broken by photocoagulation with the argon laser. Generally, however, the Nd:YAG laser is more successful than the argon laser in synechialysis because pigmentation of the target is not required and forceful rupture of adhesions can be achieved.

The most common synechiae are to the anterior or posterior capsule, or both. Often a tag of anterior capsule, such as is typically present after a can-opener anterior capsulotomy, adheres to the underside of the iris. As progressive fibrosis and adhesion between the anterior and posterior capsule occur, the iris

adhesion is brought posteriorly. This process can exert sufficient force to bring the iris sphincter around the edge of a PC IOL, leading to iris capture of the IOL optic. In Figure 52-11A the iridocapsular adhesion has exposed the superior edge of the PC IOL. This is more evident after dilation. The adhesion is frozen and the posterior capsule in that area ruptured through the application of 2 mJ shots. Following treatment (Figure 52-11C), the iris sphincter is back in proper position anterior to the PC IOL.

Another cause of iridocapsular adhesion is a retained fragment of anterior capsule that becomes incarcerated in the cataract wound. The appearance will simulate a vitreous strand to the wound as shown in Figure 52-12A. Careful examination will disclose a typically grayish membrane resulting from fibrosis of the epithelial cells on the anterior capsule, distinctly different from the appearance of a vitreous strand. After dilation, the capsular origin can be seen (Figure 52-12B). The capsular fragment is disrupted with the laser at approximately 2–3 mJ if the laser is used and approximately 6 mJ if the laser is used gonioscopically. Extra energy is needed because of the thickened fibrotic nature of the capsule.

If the capsular fragment is not disrupted within several months postoperatively, however, additional adhesions may form because of the proliferation of the cells present on the anterior capsule fragment. In one case, shown in Figure 52-12C, the pupillary position has improved with photodisruption of the capsule strand incarcerated in the wound, but the pupil remains partially eccentric. The edge of the PC IOL is exposed and a source of functionally

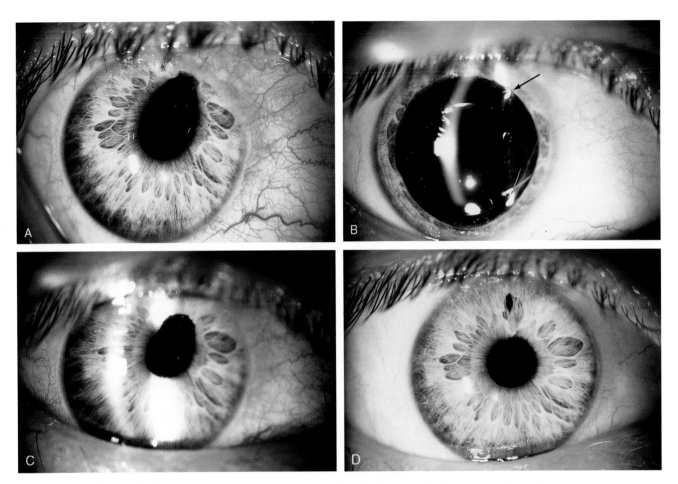

Figure 52-12 **A,** Iridocapsular adhesion simulating pupillary distortion seen with vitreous incarceration in the wound. **B,** After dilation, the iridocapsular adhesion is better seen (arrow). **C,** After lysis of the anterior capsular fragment, improvement in the pupillary position is seen compared with the preoperative photo (**A**), but the iris distortion continues to expose the edge of the intraocular lens optic, giving glare symptoms. **D,** After gonioscopic application of Nd:YAG laser pulses to the iridocapsular adhesions posterior to the iris, the pupil becomes central, and the glare symptoms are resolved.

significant glare for the patient. This was addressed with further Nd:YAG laser pulses to the epithelial pearl adhesion underlying the iris superiorly. This succeeded in further freeing the sphincter and resulting in a nearly round pupil (see Figure 52-12D).

■ REMOVAL OF THE INTRAOCULAR LENS PRECIPITATES ■

Inflammatory precipitates on the IOL surface are not usual. They may consist of both pigmented and nonpigmented, relatively round precipitates similar in appearance to keratic precipitates or the inflammation may cause the deposition of a more fibrinous gray sheet.

In some cases, these precipitates will respond to appropriate anti-inflammatory therapy. In some cases, however, visually significant precipitates will remain after the inflammation is quiet.

As shown in Figure 52-13A, a mixture of localized dense inflammatory precipitates and a sheetlike precipitate remain after a severe postoperative inflammation. Marked clearing of the IOL

optics is evident in Figure 52-13B, following Nd:YAG laser therapy.

To remove IOL precipitates, the Nd:YAG laser is set at an energy level adequate to create optical breakdown in the aqueous. This is typically about 2–3 mJ. The Nd:YAG laser aiming beams are first focused on the anterior IOL surface. The laser is then slightly defocused by withdrawing the laser slightly toward the beam origin and away from the beam target. The abrupt pressure wave generated by the subsequent optical breakdown in front of the IOL precipitate liberates inflammatory debris into the aqueous humor, leaving a cleaned IOL.

■ ANTERIOR CAPSULE ■

The lens anterior capsule becomes hazy postoperatively because of the epithelial cells present on the inner surface of the anterior capsule. Retained anterior capsule in the pupillary zone will invariably become opaque. Fortunately, the retained capsule does not strongly adhere to the underlying IOL.

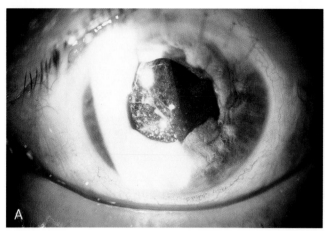
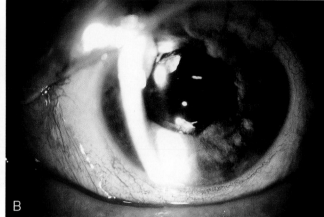

Figure 52-13 **A,** After complicated extracapsular cataract extraction with posterior-chamber intraocular lens (IOL) implantation and prolonged postoperative inflammation, fibrinous and cellular debris persist on the anterior IOL optic. **B,** Nd:YAG laser photodisruptive pulses have cleared most of the debris from the IOL surface.

In Figure 52-14A, a large remnant of anterior capsule remained after implantation of a PC IOL and significantly opacified. The pupillary zone was cleared with Nd:YAG laser photodisruptive pulses of 2–3 mJ. These pulses were applied beginning in the upper left corner and were then carried in the direction of the lower right corner (Figure 52-14B). The capsular membrane was not fully liberated but rather was left adherent at the lower right to curl up on itself. Damage to the underlying PC IOL is avoided by focusing on the anterior capsule and then withdrawing the laser focus slightly anterior to the target. The propagation of the laser plasma is toward the laser source. Accordingly, the damage to the underlying IOL can be avoided as long as the photodisruptive optical breakdown is not focused within the IOL itself.

Contracture of a continuous curvilinear capsulorrhexis may cause progressive blockage of an initially clear pupillary zone. This may be due to eccentric contracture of an anterior capsule, as shown in Figure 52-15A, or a more symmetric contracture, as shown in Figure 52-16A. This "capsule contraction syndrome"[11] or "capsular phimosis syndrome" is seen more commonly when the diameter of the original cataract surgical capsulorrhexis is 4 mm or smaller. It is attributed to contracture of the structurally strong round anterior capsule opening by the lens epithelial cells that have undergone myofibroblastic differentiation. In addition to causing pupillary obstruction, the capsular contracture stretches the peripheral zonules, with the risk of frank rupture of the zonules and potential weakening of the IOL support. Capsular contracture is best avoided by keeping the diameter of continuous curvilinear capsulorrhexis to 5 mm or greater.

As soon as the capsular contracture syndrome is recognized postoperatively, Nd:YAG laser photodisruption of the capsular margin should be undertaken. This will prevent further contraction of the capsule because the disrupted anterior capsule no longer has mechanical integrity. In addition, the pupillary zone is clear of the opaque capsule.

The technique typically consists of 2–3 mJ pulses at the edge of the capsulorrhexis, transecting the round capsulorrhexis edge into

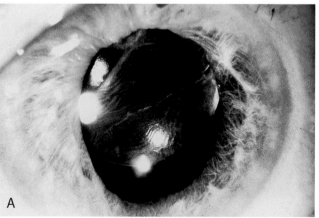
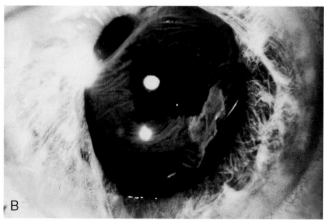

Figure 52-14 **A,** Anterior capsule was inadvertently retained after posterior-chamber intraocular lens (IOL) implantation. Opacification of the anterior capsule occurred rapidly. **B,** A window has been cut in the anterior capsule with the Nd:YAG laser, with a small amount of the anterior capsule remaining attached in the lower right to avoid a free-floating capsular remnant in the anterior chamber. No damage has occurred to the anterior IOL surface.

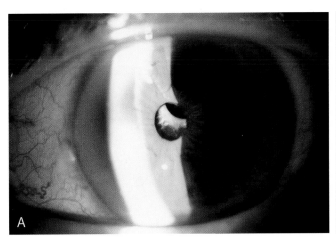
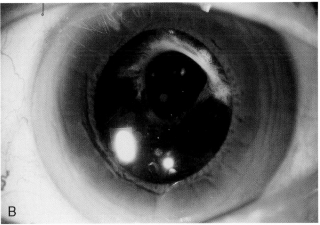

Figure 52-15 A, Contracture of the anterior capsule inferiorly has nearly occluded the optical zone. B, Nd:YAG laser cutting of the inferior capsule adhesion restores an adequate visual axis.

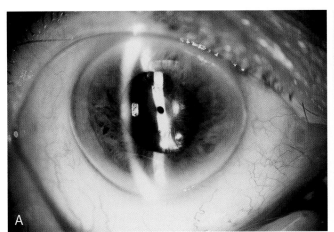
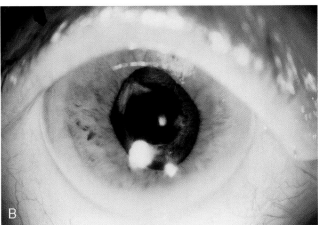

Figure 52-16 A, Symmetric contracture of the anterior capsulorrhexis leaves an inadequate visual axis. B, Photodisruption of the anterior capsulotomy edge restores an adequate visual axis.

at least four quadrants. The capsule will then contract and eventually resume a relatively round appearance with a much larger opening (see Figure 52-16B).

Damage to the underlying PC IOL is avoided by deliberate anterior defocusing of the laser beam, as described earlier, for removal of the IOL precipitates and opening of retained anterior capsule.

■ RETAINED CORTICAL MATERIAL ■

Occasionally, cortex is retained postoperatively. It may be unrecognized initially or may be deliberately left because of a defect in the posterior capsule or a difficult-to-reach location, particularly under the incision. Cortex will become hydrated in the hours after surgery, swelling and loosening its position. Occasionally, on the day after surgery the visual axis has been occluded by such hydrated retained cortical material (Figure 52-17A).

Retained cortex may slowly resorb, but this process is particularly slow when the cortex is trapped between the posterior capsule and the PC IOL anteriorly. With essentially no aqueous

turnover, the gradual clearing of this material can take a number of months. Moreover, rather than clearing fully, the retained material may slowly become a dense fibrotic sheet that is difficult to open with laser techniques and may require more invasive surgery.

In such a case, the hydrated opaque cortical material can be liquefied with photodisruptive laser pulses. A minimal amount of laser energy is used, just adequate to cause optical breakdown within the cortical material. A typical amount of energy would be 2 mJ. The pressure wave from Nd:YAG pulses within the cortex will emulsify the hydrated cortex, creating an appearance of a more uniform lens "milk." Within 24 h, this more liquefied material will usually clear, restoring a good visual zone (see Figure 52-17B).

The rapid liberation of lens protein through photodisruption may cause secondary inflammation and pressure elevation. Prophylactic antiglaucoma medical therapy is indicated, as is close monitoring of the patient. The surgeon should be prepared to surgically irrigate the retained cortical material if a clinically intolerable level of inflammation or pressure elevation occurs.

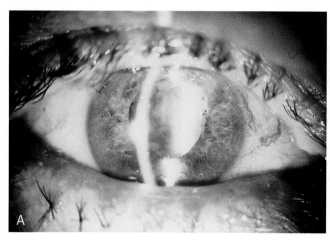
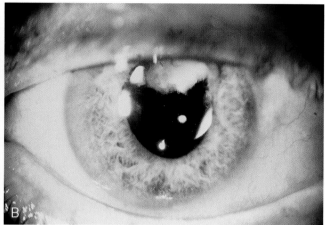

Figure 52-17 **A,** Retained cortex is hydrated but trapped behind the posterior chamber intraocular lens optic. **B,** Nd:YAG laser pulses have disrupted the retained cortex in the pupillary zone.

■ INTRAOCULAR LENS REPOSITIONING ■

In rare circumstances, Nd:YAG laser photodisruption can be used to manipulate the position of an IOL. The pressure wave from optical breakdown can shift an IOL optic if the optic is sufficiently mobile.

One special case is illustrated in Figure 52-18A. A previously well-centered ciliary sulcus-fixated PC IOL became captured in the pupil after pupillary dilation. The pupil could not be redilated beyond the border of the IOL optic. Mechanical manipulation of the IOL optic by placing the patient in the supine position or with pressure of a cotton-tipped applicator over the ciliary sulcus failed to cause the IOL optic to shift posteriorly.

A 6 mJ pulse from an Nd:YAG laser was then applied to the peripheral edge of the IOL. The laser was focused just anterior

to the anterior IOL surface. This anterior pressure wave caused the IOL optic to shift posteriorly, just behind the pupillary sphincter. The sphincter was then constricted with pilocarpine, successfully maintaining the PC IOL in the posterior chamber (see Figure 52-18B).

■ CONCLUSIONS ■

Nd:YAG laser photodisruption allows a surgeon to effectively reach inside the eye with a pair of microscissors delivered on a beam of light. In rare circumstances, photodisruptive laser energy can be constructively used to push and cut. Photodisruption, therefore, gives the surgeon a range of additional options for the correction of a wide range of complications following cataract surgery.

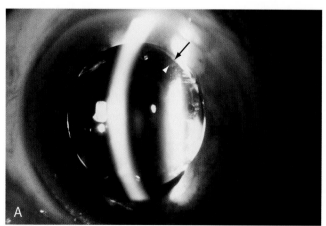
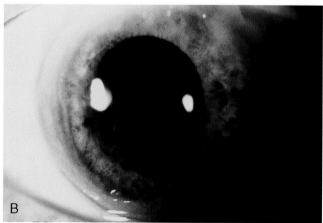

Figure 52-18 **A,** Iris capture of the optic of a posterior-chamber intraocular lens (IOL) (arrow). A single 6 mJ pulse focused at an area just anterior to the lens surface, approximately 1 mm centrally from the optic edge (arrowhead), retropulsed the optic behind the iris. **B,** IOL is now in proper position behind the iris. (From Steinert RF, Puliafito CA: *The Nd:YAG laser in ophthalmology: principles and clinical applications of photodisruption,* Philadelphia. Copyright Elsevier, 1985.)

References

[1] Shaffer RN. The role of vitreous detachment in aphakic and malignant glaucoma. Trans Am Ophthalmol Otolaryngol 1954;28:217–231.

[2] Shaffer RN. A suggested anatomic classification to define the pupillary block glaucomas. Invest Ophthalmol 1973;12:540–542.

[3] Epstein DL, Steinert RF, Puliafito CA. Neodymium-YAG laser therapy to the anterior hyaloid in aphakic malignant (ciliovitreal block) glaucoma. Am J Ophthalmol 1984;98:137–143.

[4] Irvine SR. A newly defined vitreous syndrome following cataract surgery. Am J Ophthalmol 1953;36:599–619.

[5] Gass JDM, Norton EWD. Cystoid macular edema and papilledema following cataract extraction. Arch Ophthalmol 1966;76:646–661.

[6] Iliff CE. Treatment of vitreous tug syndrome. Am J Ophthalmol 1966;162:856–859.

[7] Katzen LE, Fleischman JA, Trokel S. YAG laser treatment of cystoid macular edema. Am J Ophthalmol 1983;95:589–592.

[8] Gass JDM, Norton EWD. Follow-up study of cystoid macular edema following cataract extraction. Trans Am Acad Ophthalmol Otolaryngol 1969;73:665–682.

[9] Jacobson DR, Dellaporta A. Natural history of cystoid macular edema after cataract extraction. Am J Ophthalmol 1974;77:445–447.

[10] Steinert RF, Wasson PJ. Neodymium:YAG laser anterior vitreolysis for Irvine-Gass cystoid macular edema. J Cataract Refract Surg 1989;15:304–307.

[11] Davison JA. Capsule contraction syndrome. J Cataract Refract Surg 1993;19:582–589.

CONCLUSIONS

Ingrowths

Alex P. Hunyor, MB, BS, FRANZCO, FRACS and
C. Davis Belcher III, MD

CONTENTS

CHAPTER HIGHLIGHTS

>> Differential diagnosis of epithelial cysts, epithelial sheet ingrowth, and fibrous ingrowth

>> Technique for cyst destruction without triggering sheet ingrowth

Options in managing epithelial cysts and sheets

Epithelial and fibrous invasions into the anterior chamber have long been recognized as complications of cataract surgery, other anterior segment surgery, and trauma. These conditions, particularly the former, continue to pose a significant diagnostic and management problem for ophthalmic surgeons, despite their decreasing incidence resulting from advances in surgical technique.

◼ EPITHELIAL INVASION ◼

HISTORICAL PERSPECTIVE

In 1830 Mackenzie[1] described the occurrence of a posttraumatic iris inclusion cyst. Rothmund[2] in 1872 reported a study of 37 cases of epithelial cysts of the anterior chamber, with two occurring after cataract extraction and the remainder following trauma. He proposed that these cysts resulted from implantation of epithelium at the time of trauma or surgery. Collins and Cross[3] in 1892 demonstrated histopathologically the presence of epithelium in the anterior chamber in two cases of epithelial implantation cyst after cataract extraction. The work of Guaita[4] and Meller[5] emphasized poor wound healing in allowing entry of epithelial cells. Perera[6] in 1937 reviewed numerous reports, differentiating cystic epithelial lesions from sheetlike epithelial ingrowth, noting the importance of incarceration of iris or lens capsule and of hypotony in favoring epithelial invasion. He proposed a classification of epithelial invasion into (1) "pearl" tumors of the iris, (2)

epithelial (inclusion) cysts of the iris, and (3) epithelialization (also referred to as epithelial ingrowth or downgrowth) of the anterior chamber. This classification remains useful in differentiating these three entities with related etiologies but clearly different clinical course, treatment and outcome.

PEARL TUMORS

Pearl tumors (pearl cysts) are rare, opaque, cystic or solid "pearly" lesions that usually occur after trauma but have been described after intraocular surgery.[7] They result from traumatic implantation of skin or hair follicles into the anterior chamber and usually form a small, circumscribed lesion that is not connected with the entry site and confined to the iris (Figure 53-1). These lesions grow slowly and rarely exceed 2–3 mm in diameter. Histologically, they are encapsulated structures of cuboidal or stratified epithelial cells with a central mass of keratinized cells, cholesterol crystals, and necrotic debris; hair follicles and foreign bodies have also been found. In the uncommon instances that these cysts significantly enlarge or cause iridocyclitis, en bloc excision usually yields good results.

EPITHELIAL INCLUSION CYSTS

Of the two major forms of epithelial invasion resulting from implantation of surface epithelium into the anterior chamber, epithelial inclusion (or implantation) cysts tend to follow a more benign, although quite variable, clinical course.

INCIDENCE

There are no figures for the incidence of epithelial cyst as a separate entity. The overall incidence of cystic and sheetlike epithelial invasion after accidental and surgical penetration of the anterior segment has been estimated in early studies[8,9] at 0.06–0.11%, and cysts are considered the more common form.

PREDISPOSING FACTORS AND PATHOGENESIS

Epithelial inclusion cysts have been reported after cataract extraction, penetrating keratoplasty, and other forms of surgery and

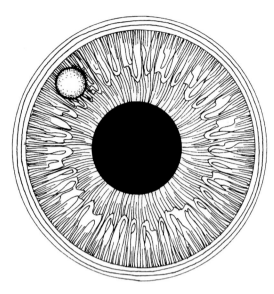

Figure 53-1 "Pearl" tumor of the iris.

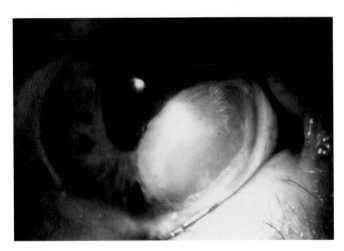

Figure 53-2 Epithelial inclusion cyst of the anterior chamber.

trauma to the anterior segment, as summarized by Farmer and Kalina.[10] In cases following cataract surgery, there is usually evidence of poor wound closure, often with incarcerated iris, lens matter, or vitreous. Rarely, cysts are discontinuous with the wound from their onset and are presumably due to implantation of surface epithelium by intraocular instruments, as discussed by Ferry.[11] Experimental evidence[12,13] points to contact with the iris and exposure to plasmoid aqueous (containing proliferative factors) as determinants of the development and size of epithelial cysts.

The factors regulating development of implanted or ingrowing epithelial cells into cysts, as opposed to sheetlike ingrowths, are unclear. The number of cells, initial morphology of the ingrowth (a bilayer or loop as opposed to a single layer), degree of attachment to iris and angle structures, vascular supply, and duration of exposure to plasmoid aqueous (a longer exposure favoring progressive sheetlike ingrowth) may all play a role. As discussed later on, in some cases epithelial cysts may be converted into sheetlike downgrowth if treated with surgery or laser.

PRESENTATION, CLINICAL FEATURES, AND DIAGNOSIS

Cysts may remain quiescent for many years before enlarging and/ or causing symptoms. Patients may seek treatment because of recognition or noticeable enlargement of an otherwise asymptomatic lesion, visual symptoms caused by extension into the visual axis, or symptoms of intraocular inflammation and secondary glaucoma that may accompany periods of cyst growth.

Epithelial inclusion cysts are typically translucent or gray in appearance and usually are associated with the anterior surface of the peripheral iris. There may be displacement of an iris pillar or distortion of the pupil (Figure 53-2). Cysts may grow through an iridotomy or peripheral iridectomy into the posterior chamber and appear to arise from the iris itself. For a review of the differential diagnosis of cystic lesions of the iris, see Shields, Sanborn, and Augsburger.[14] Signs of anterior uveitis, sometimes with secondary glaucoma, may be present. Sympathetic ophthalmia

associated with secondary glaucoma from cystic epithelial invasion of the anterior chamber has been reported,[15] as has mucogenic open-angle glaucoma resulting from a goblet cell cyst of the anterior chamber.[16] Subluxation of an anterior chamber intraocular lens (IOL) by a large epithelial cyst has also been noted.[17] Massive enlargement of cysts may cause corneal decompensation by extensive contact with the corneal endothelium.

The diagnosis of epithelial inclusion cyst is suggested by the history or signs of surgery or trauma; contact with the surgical or traumatic wound; characteristics of cystic lesions such as transillumination, occasionally mobility, and tremulousness; scant pigmentation; lack of vascularity; superficial relationship to the iris; and signs of associated uveitis.

HISTOPATHOLOGIC FEATURES

Cysts are typically thin-walled structures lined with squamous or cuboidal epithelium, sometimes including goblet cells (Figure 53-3). Electron microscopic studies[18] demonstrate epithelial cells with

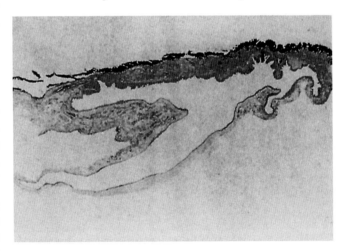

Figure 53-3 Light microscopy of an epithelial inclusion cyst, showing a clear lumen lined by nonkeratinized squamous epithelium. (Hematoxylin and eosin stain; ×40.) (From Orlin SE, Raber IM, Laibson PR et al: Epithelial downgrowth following the removal of iris inclusion cysts, *Ophthalmic Surg, Lasers & Imaging* 22:330-335, 1991. Reprinted with permission from SLACK Incorporated.)

a thin basal lamina, desmosomal junctions, cytoplasmic filaments, scant mitochondria, terminal bars, and apical microvilli, characteristic of ocular surface epithelium, most likely conjunctival. They contain straw-colored, turbid, or mucinous fluid. There may be pigmentation, particularly of the posterior portion of the cyst. Often there is evidence of contact between the cyst and the traumatic or surgical wound, which may be lost later in its development.

MANAGEMENT

Although some authors have advocated early surgical intervention for epithelial cysts, they follow a highly variable clinical course (from spontaneous regression[19] to rapid growth), and there is a well-established risk of conversion to sheetlike epithelial downgrowth after surgery and laser treatment. There is general agreement that the most appropriate management includes periodic observation at 3–4-month intervals with serial anterior segment photography and prompt intervention in cases in which vision is impaired by encroachment on the visual axis, uveitis, glaucoma, or corneal edema.

Various treatment modalities have been employed, including needle aspiration, injection with radioactive and sclerosing substances, diathermy, cryotherapy, electrolysis, radiotherapy, photocoagulation, numerous surgical approaches, and combinations of the preceding methods. In the absence of any large series, comparison of the efficacy of these techniques is difficult. The management of epithelial cysts of the anterior chamber remains a difficult balance between the need for elimination of the cyst with low risk of recurrence and minimization of complications of the treatment itself. As yet, no single treatment modality has provided this combination.

Radiotherapy, despite the initial enthusiasm of Perera[6] and others, has been abandoned because of variable results and lack of safety. Diathermy coagulation[20,21] has largely been supplanted by laser photocoagulation.

Ferry and Naghdi[22] successfully treated a large cyst by insertion of a cryostylet into the cyst (via a needle puncture), freezing it to −10° to 0° F for 15 s, and exteriorization and excision of the cyst and adherent iris tissue. Cyst aspirations with injection of astatine,[23] iodine,[24] and other sclerosing agents have also been reported, with varying degrees of success and safety. Cyst aspiration with laser photocoagulation and/or cryotherapy, and surgical techniques, are the mainstay of current therapy and will be discussed in more detail.

CURRENT TECHNIQUES

For small unpigmented cysts, aspiration followed by cryotherapy to the collapsed cyst is the authors' preferred treatment. For unpigmented cysts too large for cryotherapy and for all pigmented cysts, aspiration followed by argon laser photocoagulation is favored. Large unpigmented cysts, if fully aspirated and collapsed against the iris with the technique to be described, are usually successfully photocoagulated using the heat sink effect of the underlying iris pigment.

Aspiration and photocoagulation

Meyer-Schwickerath,[25] Okun and Mandell,[26] and others have described treatment of epithelial cysts with xenon arc photocoagulation. Multiple treatments were required, and cysts were collapsed

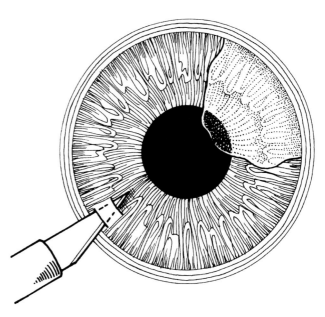

Figure 53-4 Initial anterior chamber paracentesis is performed well away from the cyst.

and fibrosed, preventing further growth. In 1975 L'Esperance and James[27] first described successful treatment of epithelial cysts by argon laser photocoagulation. The authors' preferred method of treatment for pigmented epithelial inclusion cysts and larger unpigmented cysts is argon laser photocoagulation, with a technique similar to that described by Thomas, Lederer, and Simmons,[28] as outlined next.

In a minor operating room under topical anesthesia (or peribulbar anesthesia in less cooperative patients), the affected eye is prepared as for cataract surgery with skin sterilization and draping, and a lid speculum is inserted. A first paracentesis through clear cornea is performed well away from the cyst with an angled 15° disposable blade (Figure 53-4). The second paracentesis is made into the cyst at its base, via its attachment to the anterior chamber angle where present (Figure 53-5), avoiding cyst puncture within the anterior chamber, which can potentially increase the risk of conversion to sheetlike ingrowth.

A 27-gauge intraocular cannula attached to a syringe is inserted into the cyst cavity via the second paracentesis, and the cyst contents are aspirated to collapse the cyst (Figure 53-6). Cytologic examination of the aspirated fluid (for epithelial cells) may be performed. The anterior chamber is re-formed with air, which promotes the collapse of the cyst against its posterior wall (Figure 53-7). Blunt dissection of the anterior cyst wall from the posterior cornea, with a spatula inserted via the first paracentesis, may also be required (Figure 53-8). Physiologic saline solution is then exchanged for the air in the anterior chamber. Routine postoperative topical antibiotics are instilled in the eye.

The patient is then taken to the argon laser, and with a sterile Goldmann 3-mirror contact lens the cyst is treated with a spot size of 200 μm, duration of 0.2 s, and power increasing from 200–1000 mW, as high as required to photocoagulate all visible epithelial tissue. Cyst epithelium extending into the angle of the anterior chamber should also be eradicated using the semicircular

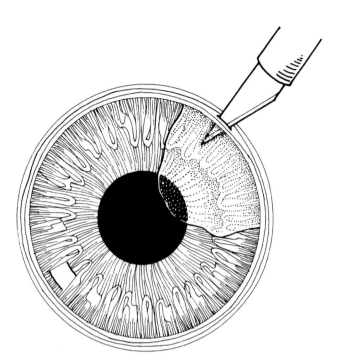

Figure 53-5 Second paracentesis enters the base of the cyst, avoiding cyst puncture that communicates with the anterior chamber.

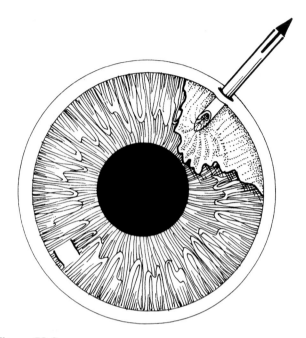

Figure 53-6 Cyst contents are aspirated with a 27-gauge intraocular cannula.

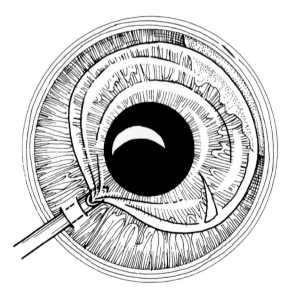

Figure 53-7 Anterior chamber is re-formed with air, promoting cyst collapse against the iris.

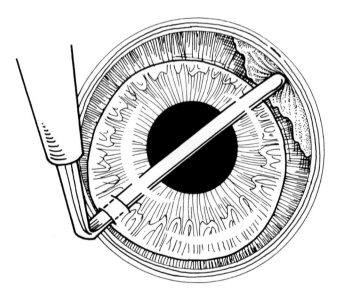

Figure 53-8 Blunt dissection of the cyst wall from the posterior cornea may be performed via the first paracentesis.

mirror of the Goldmann lens. Cycloplegic drops are instilled postoperatively, but topical steroids are generally avoided because the ensuing inflammatory response assists in fibrosis and contraction of cyst remnants. Further photocoagulation may be required if follow-up examination shows significant residual epithelial tissue. Cryotherapy to angle structures can also be used as an adjunct to photocoagulation. Figure 53-9 shows the appearance of the inclusion cyst in Figure 53-2 following the photocoagulation treatment described.

L'Esperance and James[27] reported shrinkage and disappearance of four cysts over a 6-week period following argon laser photocoagulation (without prior aspiration). Scholz and Kelly[29] and Sugar, Jampol, and Goldberg[30] reported successful eradication of epithelial cysts with the same technique. The authors prefer the technique outlined earlier, with aspiration before photocoagulation, because it facilitates more complete photocoagulation and theoretically reduces the likelihood of leaving a free epithelial edge, which may progress to sheetlike epithelial ingrowth.

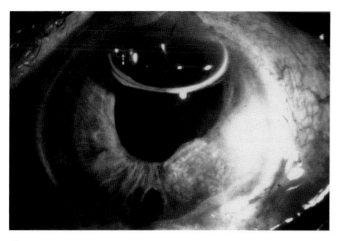

Figure 53-9 Appearance of the cyst from Figure 53-2 following aspiration and photocoagulation.

Honrubia, Brito, and Grijalbo[31] reported elimination of several epithelial cysts, with no recurrence or significant complications, using this technique.

The complications of photocoagulation include iritis, which may be marked; a transient rise in intraocular pressure resulting from outflow obstruction by protein and cellular debris, which usually responds to medical treatment and resolves within 2 weeks; corneal opacity from photocoagulation of cyst material adjacent or adherent to the posterior cornea (largely avoidable by posterior displacement of the cyst and angling of the laser beam); hemorrhage from iris vessels (rarely, hemorrhage into a cyst may facilitate argon laser absorption); cataract induction in the phakic eye; and conversion to sheetlike epithelial ingrowth.[32] Treatment of epithelial implantation cysts with the Nd:YAG laser is not recommended because without accompanying cryotherapy or photocoagulation to ensure fibrosis of cyst remnants, the risk of sheetlike ingrowth with such a procedure seems high. Recurrence of such cysts after Nd:YAG treatment is also likely.[33]

Surgery

Surgery for epithelial inclusion cysts has ranged from excision by iridectomy[10] following cryotherapy[22] or aspiration, including debridement or alcohol swabbing of the involved cornea,[34] to block excision with cryotherapy (with or without vitrectomy)[35] and more radical excision including lamellar corneal excision[36] or corneal and corneoscleral grafting.[37] A summary of surgical techniques is given in Table 53-1. Some authors still advocate en bloc excision as the treatment of choice for epithelial inclusion cysts. Surgical approaches, particularly more extensive procedures, carry considerable risks of complications, such as conversion to sheetlike ingrowth, glaucoma, corneal edema, vitreous loss and hemorrhage, and cystoid macular edema. Such procedures may often be avoided by thorough treatment with aspiration followed by cryotherapy with or without photocoagulation, depending on cyst size.

Regardless of technique, the aim of treatment should be complete eradication of the epithelial cells, as incomplete treatment carries a significant risk of conversion to sheetlike epithelial ingrowth. Early detection of treatment failures with more conservative techniques should allow consideration of more aggressive surgery, such as block excision, before ingrowth is too advanced. Long-term follow-up is required in all cases, as recurrences or conversion to sheetlike epithelial ingrowth may be detected years after initial apparently successful treatment.

Table 53-1 Chronology of surgical techniques for epithelial inclusion cyst*†

Year	Author(s)	Technique/Comments
1955	Maumenee, Shannon[34]	Eleven cases; subtotal/total cyst removal, large iridectomies, denudation of involved posterior cornea; no recurrence, complications, downgrowth
1955	Rizzuti[39]	Aspiration-excision by iridectomy-iridodialysis; postoperative VA, 20/30
1962	Sugar, Willenz[36]	Excision of cyst, involved iris, posterior corneoscleral lamella; VA 20/25
1974	Harbin, Maumenee[40]	Reported 6 cases of conversion to epithelial downgrowth after cyst excision; urged conservative management (cyst aspiration with cryotherapy to angle and photocoagulation to cyst remnants on iris)
1981	Bruner et al[35]	Closed-eye approach in aphakic patients: cyst aspiration/cryotherapy. Open-sky cyst excision/transscleral cryotherapy in phakic patients. Seven cases: 4 uncomplicated, 2 persistent CME, 1 sheetlike ingrowth, 1 persistent corneal edema; VA better than 20/60 in 43%
1981	Eiferman, Rodrigues[18]	Iridocyclectomy/penetrating keratoplasty; wound dehiscence and graft failure from unrelated cause (no recurrence)
1981	Farmer, Kalina[10]	Excision by iridectomy-iridodialysis; postoperative VA 20/20
1992, 1996	Naumann, Rummelt[37,38]	Forty-five cases; block excision by sector iridectomy with excision of cornea, sclera and ciliary body and tectonic corneoscleral grafting; 28% vitreous hemorrhage; 22% corneal decompensation; VA 20/60 or better in 43%; no recurrences; no conversion to sheetlike ingrowth

CME, Cystoid macular edema; PPV, pars plana vitrectomy; VA, visual acuity (postoperative).
*This table is a summary only. The reader should consult the appropriate sources as referenced.
†Single case reports unless otherwise indicated.

PROGNOSIS

The long-term outlook for eyes with epithelial inclusion cysts is far better than for sheetlike ingrowth; however, the visual results from published cases of surgical treatment of such cysts are generally poor. There is clearly considerable bias toward a poorer prognosis group in such reports, as the large numbers of epithelial cysts that require no intervention have not been included. Those eyes that develop complications of treatment (particularly sheet-like epithelial ingrowth and cystoid macular edema) and those with pre-existing poor visual acuity make up the majority of those with poor visual outcome. Corneal decompensation from causes other than sheetlike ingrowth is usually successfully treated with penetrating keratoplasty. Ideally, a large prospective study of such cysts, both treated and untreated, would give a more accurate assessment of the optimal treatment modality and overall prognosis.

EPITHELIAL INGROWTH

Since the 1800s, the grim visual prognosis of eyes with epithelial ingrowth, which almost always invariably progressed to intractable glaucoma and blindness, was recognized. This condition is also referred to as epithelial downgrowth, epithelialization of the anterior chamber, and diffuse or sheetlike epithelial ingrowth (to distinguish it from the cystic form described earlier). It may be difficult to diagnose, and despite the use of multiple therapies, including aggressive surgical approaches, its treatment remains challenging, and good visual outcomes are few.

INCIDENCE

The quoted clinical incidence of epithelial ingrowth has long been accepted as an underestimate, owing to lack of recognition and the difficulty of making the diagnosis on clinical, rather than pathologic, grounds. As mentioned earlier, the overall incidence of cystic and sheetlike epithelial invasion of the anterior segment after trauma and surgery in earlier studies[8,9] was 0.06% to 0.11% (up to 1.1% in one study[41]), and in a clinicopathologic review by Weiner et al.,[42] the incidence after cataract surgery was 0.12% overall from 1953 to 1983, dropping to 0.076% in the period 1973–1983.

More important than the incidence of this condition is its occurrence in eyes enucleated after cataract surgery – an average of 16% and 17%, respectively, in the large series compiled by Maumenee[43] and Jaffe et al.[44] A review of eyes enucleated more recently (1962–1976) by Merenmies and Tarkkanen[45] demonstrated epithelial ingrowth in 10.6% of eyes enucleated following cataract surgery; they noted that all cases of ingrowth occurred before 1969.

The decreasing incidence of epithelial ingrowth has been attributed to the use of the operating microscope; improvements in surgical technique (modern extracapsular and phacoemulsification surgery, with smaller incisions); and the use of finer, higher quality suture material. There are now several reports of epithelial ingrowth following sutureless small-incision cataract surgery, both with scleral tunnel and clear corneal incisions.[46–49] Despite the impression of a decreasing incidence of epithelial ingrowth, it is of significant concern that the proportion of cases that are clinically unrecognized appears to be increasing, which suggests a lower awareness by clinicians of this potentially devastating condition.[50]

PREDISPOSING FACTORS AND PATHOGENESIS

Epithelial ingrowth has most commonly been reported following intracapsular and extracapsular cataract surgery (with or without IOL implantation), trauma, and penetrating keratoplasty. In a series by Weiner et al.,[42] 15% of cases followed trauma, and 85% followed surgery (86% cataract surgery, 12% penetrating keratoplasty, 2% other). In a series of 207 histopathologically proven cases of epithelial ingrowth, Kuchle and Green found cataract surgery was the cause in 59.4% of cases.[50] Ingrowth has also been described after surgery for epithelial inclusion cyst (as discussed earlier), Nd:YAG laser treatment of inclusion cyst,[32] pterygium excision,[42] glaucoma filtration procedure,[9] transcorneal (McCannel) suture,[50] discission of posterior capsule,[51] and aspiration of aqueous.[52]

Predisposing factors

Factors predisposing to the development of epithelial ingrowth include technically difficult or complicated surgery (particularly with capsular rupture and vitreous loss); incomplete or delayed wound healing; hypotony; wound fistula; inadvertent filtering bleb; chronic inflammation; and incarceration of iris, vitreous, or lens remnants in the wound. Paufique and Hervouët[53] found that young, highly myopic or diabetic patients were at higher risk of developing ingrowth – the known poor wound healing of diabetics and the relative thinness of ocular tissues in young and highly myopic patients may account for these findings.

There is experimental evidence[54,55] that anticoagulants inhibit the formation of the usual fibrinous barrier to epithelial migration, and five of Weiner's 124 cases were in anticoagulated patients; however, the significance of these findings is unclear. No other medications have been proposed to influence ingrowth. Previous assertions that epithelial ingrowth was less likely with a limbus-based than a fornix-based flap, not supported in larger series,[42,56] are largely inconsequential in view of modern wound closure techniques. Similarly, corneoscleral sutures per se have been dismissed as a potential cause,[57] and catgut and silk sutures in cataract incisions (previously implicated in epithelial ingrowth) are essentially obsolete. In a considerable number of cases of epithelial ingrowth, surgery and the postoperative period appeared uneventful and no predisposing factors were identified.

Pathogenesis

Most attempts to further understand the pathogenesis of epithelial ingrowth, by the use of animal experimental models, have met with little success. For a review of experimental work in this area, which is beyond the scope of this chapter, see Burris, Nordquist, and Rowsey[58] and Regan.[13] Burris, Nordquist, and Rowsey[58–60] developed a cat model of epithelial ingrowth that correlates well both clinically and histologically with the features of the human condition. Despite its potential for evaluation of treatment modalities for epithelial ingrowth, we could find no reports of its use after 1986.[61]

It has generally been accepted that epithelial ingrowth largely results from suboptimal surgical technique, allowing a free edge of surface epithelium to proliferate into the anterior chamber. It is equally clear that implantation of epithelial cells alone will not produce ingrowth. The following factors are recognized as being significant in the pathogenesis of epithelial ingrowth; however, none are invariably present in cases of ingrowth, and, conversely, they may be present in the absence of ingrowth.

Poor wound healing, with or without a clinically evident fistula, may result from poor incision or suturing technique or incarceration of iris, vitreous, or lens remnants. Persistence of plasmoid or secondary aqueous, which contains proliferative factors not found in normal aqueous (which may not sustain the invading epithelium, let alone allow proliferation), appears important in establishing and maintaining ingrowth – its persistence may be due to hypotony or chronic inflammation. Approximation of iris tissue to the wound (even without incarceration) is frequently seen and provides a rich vascular bed for the epithelium. Damage to the underlying corneal endothelium may in part be a prerequisite for migration of the epithelial membrane (by loss of the usual cell contact inhibition) and to a larger extent may represent a cytotoxic effect of the extension of pseudopodia by the epithelial cells, causing disruption of the endothelial plasma membrane.[51,59]

Many features of the pathogenesis of epithelial ingrowth remain unclear, particularly how in some eyes there can be relentless progression of the epithelial membrane in the absence of a fistula, hypotony, or signs of inflammation.

PRESENTATION, CLINICAL FEATURES, AND DIAGNOSIS

Patients often present within weeks to months after surgery or trauma, but there are reports of presentations as early as 4 days[5] and as late as 38 years[50] following surgery. Weiner et al.[42] found the most common symptoms (in decreasing order of frequency) to be decreasing visual acuity, red eye, painful eye, tearing, photophobia, and foreign body sensation. Patients may have been labeled as having "uveitis" that failed to respond to topical corticosteroids.

The clinical signs at first presentation of epithelial ingrowth may individually be nonspecific (particularly in the absence of an obvious retrocorneal membrane), and a high index of suspicion is required to make an early diagnosis. A gaping wound, inadvertent filtering bleb, or an obvious wound fistula should arouse such suspicions.

The epithelial sheet (shown in Figure 53-10A) is most often seen as a retrocorneal membrane with a "gray line" at the leading edge (Figure 53-10B), sometimes with focal "pearl-like" regions resulting from clustering of epithelial cells. These features are best appreciated with retroillumination (Figure 53-11). The involved cornea is frequently clear, although there may be epithelial edema or prominent corneal vascularization. There is clinical evidence of stromal vascularization in approximately half of cases (which Calhoun[62] equated with more rapid progression of ingrowth) and histopathologic evidence in almost all (see further on). Burris, Nordquist, and Rowsey[58] identified pre-Descemet's vascularization as "a harbinger of occult epithelial downgrowth" in their cat model. Descemet's folds may be evident in hypotonous eyes, particularly those with corneal edema. Less common corneal findings include bullous keratopathy, band keratopathy, and a variable level of reduction in corneal sensation.

There may be signs of iridocyclitis, and the membrane may be visible on the surface of the iris. Often iris involvement is manifest as loss of the usual iris contour and mobility or pupillary distortion. Advancement of epithelial ingrowth is usually more rapid over the richly vascular iris than the posterior cornea, and thus progression or otherwise of the retrocorneal membrane is not a reliable indicator. Gonioscopy (Figure 53-12) often reveals peripheral anterior synechiae, a degree of epithelialization of the angle, or incarcerated iris, lens remnants, or vitreous. An epithelialized communication with a fistula or bleb may also be evident.

Intraocular pressure is abnormal in the majority of affected eyes, partly depending on the extent of disease on presentation. Hypotony is documented in up to one-third of cases and is highly suggestive of a wound fistula. A significant number of patients

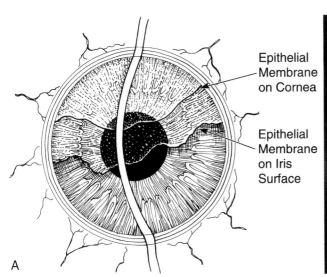
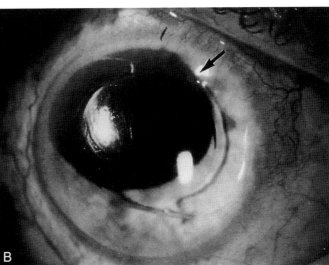

Epithelial Membrane on Cornea

Epithelial Membrane on Iris Surface

A

B

Figure 53-10 A, Ingrowing epithelial membrane on the posterior corneal surface. B, Ingrowing epithelial membrane. Arrow indicates the leading edge of the epithelium.

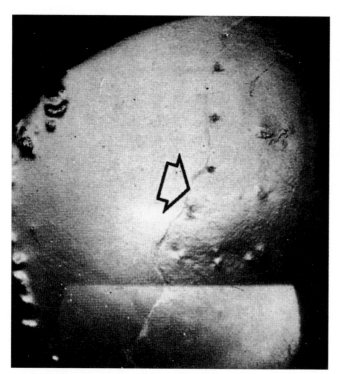

Figure 53-11 Retroillumination appearance of the epithelial sheet on the posterior corneal surface, with thickened and irregular leading edge (arrow). (From Stark WJ, Michels RG, Maumenee AE et al: Surgical management of epithelial ingrowth, *Am J Ophthalmol* 85:772-780, 1978. Copyright Elsevier, 1978.)

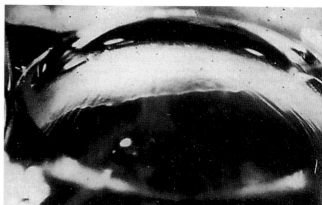

Figure 53-12 Gonioscopic view of the superior angle of the left eye, showing the ingrowing membrane throughout the entire view. A large strand of vitreous extends into the cataract incision at 12 o'clock. (From Zavala EY, Binder PS: The pathologic findings of epithelial ingrowth, *Arch Ophthalmol* 98:2007-2014, 1980. Copyright 1980, American Medical Association.)

with a clinically demonstrable fistula have normal intraocular pressures. Glaucoma is present in approximately half of cases and is almost invariably present in advanced epithelial ingrowth.

The epithelial membrane may extend over the pupil, vitreous face, ciliary body, and retina and may cause retinal detachment. Epithelial ingrowth has been reported, primarily involving the anterior and posterior lens capsule,[63] and proliferating over the surface of an IOL.[64–66] Cystoid macular edema may be present, particularly in eyes with long-standing inflammation. The use of topical steroid medications may temporarily ameliorate some of the symptoms and signs associated with epithelial ingrowth, sometimes delaying the diagnosis.

Diagnostic adjuncts

The diagnosis of epithelial ingrowth requires a combination of awareness of the condition, history and thorough examination for the clinical signs outlined earlier, and the use of additional diagnostic procedures.

Noninvasive procedures

Seidel's test

To perform Seidel's test, 2% fluorescein drops are instilled into the eye, and gentle pressure is applied to the globe. Using the slit lamp with the cobalt blue filter, aqueous flowing from a fistula appears as a lighter stream of fluid in the pool of green fluorescein. Up to one-third of eyes have a fistula demonstrable in this fashion on presentation, although presumably all have a fistula at some stage in the development of ingrowth.

Specular and confocal microscopy

At the level of the endothelium, a sharply defined border may be seen between areas of normal endothelium and the epithelial membrane[51,67] (Figure 53-13), and there is usually evidence of endothelial cell loss, reflected in the large size of the remaining endothelial cells, which also appear morphologically abnormal.[68] Confocal microscopy has also been used to identify epithelial ingrowth on the corneal endothelium.[69]

Argon laser photocoagulation

Application of a 500 μm spot size, 100–300 mW intensity burn for 0.1 s will produce a characteristic white fluffy appearance if invading epithelium is present on the iris, and a slight focal burn on normal iris (Figure 53-14).

Invasive procedures

Iris biopsy

First advocated by Verhoeff,[70] full-thickness biopsy of iris adjacent to the wound, which is invariably involved in ingrowth if present, may be performed to confirm the diagnosis.

Curettage of the posterior corneal surface

Calhoun[71] described curettage of the posterior corneal surface in a region of suspected downgrowth. He used a 1 mm serrated curette to procure a specimen for microscopy, which can easily differentiate between regular, evenly spaced endothelial cells and epithelial cells that are closely packed, spindled, and less regular and have denser cytoplasm. This technique is used infrequently.

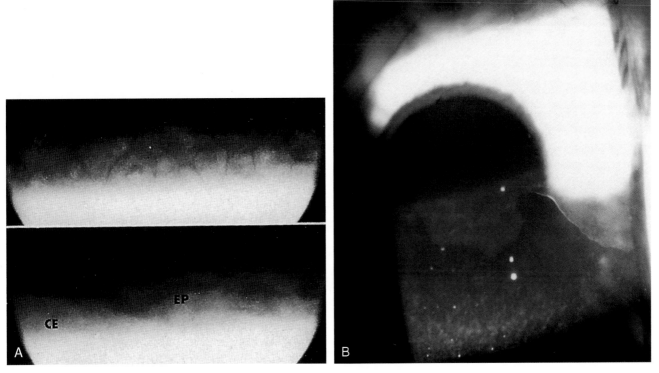

Figure 53-13 A, Specular microscopy of epithelial ingrowth (×400). Top, Specular micrograph of inferior central (clear) part of corneal endothelium. Cells are grossly enlarged and distorted, and nuclei are prominent. Cell count is 600 per mm². Bottom, Specular micrograph of leading edge of epithelial ingrowth. The membrane edge is sharp, and individual epithelial cells cannot be delineated in the area of epithelial ingrowth (EP). With careful focusing, individual enlarged, distorted corneal endothelial (CE) cells can be visualized. (From Zavala EY, Binder PS: The pathologic findings of epithelial ingrowth, *Arch Ophthalmol* 98:2007–2014, 1980. Copyright 1980, American Medical Association.) B, Leading edge of epithelium ingrowth clearly seen advancing over corneal endothelium. (Courtesy Ann M. Bajart, MD.)

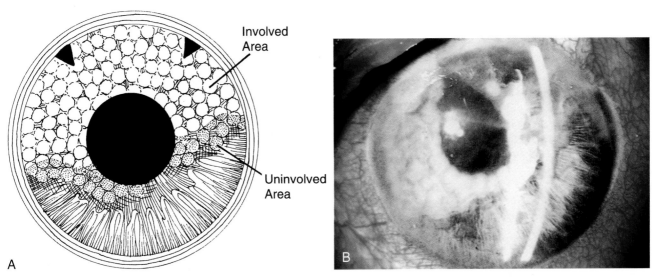

Figure 53-14 A, Argon laser photocoagulation produces characteristic fluffing of iris involved with epithelial ingrowth and a slight focal burn on normal iris. B, Argon laser photocoagulation of iris involved in epithelial ingrowth.

Anterior chamber paracentesis

This technique[72] along with cytologic examination of aqueous for epithelial cells has been used, but has a relatively poor yield, and it is unhelpful if negative.

Differential diagnosis

As outlined by Maumenee,[43] the differential diagnosis of epithelial ingrowth includes:

1. Reduplication of Descemet's membrane, which appears as a glassy membrane on the posterior cornea, anterior iris, and angle. This usually occurs in eyes with chronic iridocyclitis and is the condition most likely to resemble epithelialization, but photocoagulation does not produce the appearance described earlier.

2. Fibrous ingrowth, which may have a similar retrocorneal membrane but tends to be slower growing and display more prominent vascularity.

3. Vitreocorneal adhesions, which may appear grayish and may cause corneal edema; however, their slit-lamp appearance is characteristic, and they and do not progress in the same fashion as ingrowth.

4. Anterior shelved clear corneal or scleral tunnel incision.

5. Detachment of Descemet's membrane.

6. Peripheral corneal edema.

HISTOPATHOLOGIC FEATURES

Microscopic examination of tissue involved in epithelial ingrowth typically reveals 1 to 12 layers of irregularly arranged, stratified squamous ocular surface epithelium.[50] Goblet cells are sometimes seen, and even in their absence, the electron microscopic characteristics of the epithelium suggest conjunctiva rather than cornea as the source in many cases.[51,59,60,73]

The epithelium is usually present as a membrane of one to three cell layers over the posterior cornea, almost invariably with evidence of stromal vascularization, particularly along the tract of the wound or incision.[74] Weiner et al.[42] found concomitant stromal (fibrous) ingrowth in 55% of postsurgical cases of epithelial ingrowth. The "gray line" that may be seen clinically corresponds to heaped up epithelial cells at the margin of the epithelial sheet. At the leading edge there is a sloping appearance, as observed in epithelial wound healing[75] (Figure 53-15). The irregular arrangement of epithelial cells at the margin gives rise to the scalloped edge seen on slit-lamp examination.

In the majority of cases, there is extension of the membrane as a "more luxuriant" growth averaging three to five cell layers[42] on the anterior surface of the iris and angle (or false angle created by peripheral anterior synechiae). The membrane may extend over the posterior iris, anterior vitreous face, ciliary body, and retina. Fibrous contraction resulting from concomitant rubeosis may cause ectropion uveae. Ocular surface epithelium usually extends well into the surgical or traumatic wound, and fine sectioning of enucleated specimens often reveals continuity of the epithelial lining of the anterior chamber with the surface epithelium. There is often incarceration of iris, lens remnants, or vitreous in the wound.

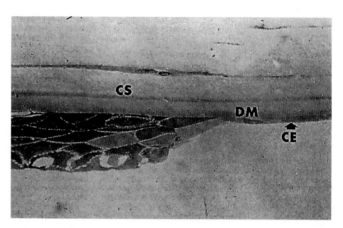

Figure 53-15 Light microscopy of ingrowing epithelium on the posterior corneal surface (corneal endothelium [CE]), with a tapered leading edge. The most superficial ingrowing cells are edematous and vacuolated. Descemet's membrane (DM) and the corneal stroma (CS) appear unaffected. (Basic fuchsin stain, ×400.) (From Zavala EY, Binder PS: The pathologic findings of epithelial ingrowth, *Arch Ophthalmol* 98:2007-2014, 1980. Copyright 1980, American Medical Association.)

The mechanisms of glaucoma in epithelial ingrowth, as discussed by Smith et al.,[76] include secondary angle closure by contraction of the epithelial and fibrous tissue lining the false angle; obstruction of outflow by epithelium lining the entire angle; pupillary block from occlusion by the epithelial sheet; obstruction of the trabecular meshwork by macrophages and desquamating epithelial cells; chronic uveal inflammation, leading to trabeculitis and decreased outflow; and the rare mucogenic glaucoma resulting from goblet cell secretion.[77] An infiltrate of chronic inflammatory cells is commonly seen in the ciliary body, iris, and episclera. Cystoid macular edema may also be present in eyes with long-term inflammation.

MANAGEMENT

Although surgical eradication of epithelial ingrowth is the only widely accepted therapeutic modality capable of curing this condition, the results are modest even in the most experienced of hands. A chronologic summary of surgical techniques used in the management of epithelial ingrowth is given in Table 53-2.

Radiotherapy was first used in 1924[78] but was abandoned by the late 1960s because of questionable efficacy, unclear guidelines regarding dosage, and its high potential for damage to ocular structures. Reports of success with radiotherapy were also criticized for the lack of a tissue diagnosis in many cases. Early experience with surgery was so discouraging that it was considered to accelerate the progression of the disease,[79] which (treated or untreated) resulted in blindness and often in enucleation.

There was renewed interest in surgical treatment of epithelial ingrowth in the 1950s[80–82] (see Table 53-2), and Maumenee[43] in 1964 was the first to publish a large series (26 cases) of surgically treated ingrowths. His technique involved identification and excision of any fistula; wide excision of all involved iris tissue; and treatment of the involved area of posterior cornea with curettage, debridement, or swabbing with 70% alcohol. Subsequent modifications to this technique by Maumenee and co-workers have resulted in the currently accepted surgical approach, as outlined here.

Table 53-2 Chronology of surgical techniques for epithelial ingrowth*

Year	Author(s)	Technique/Comments
1957	Maumenee[82]	Single case; alcohol/curettage of epithelium from posterior cornea; iridectomy/anterior vitrectomy; VA 20/20 at 2½ years, no recurrence
1958	Sullivan[81]	Four cases; corneoscleral excision/grafting; membrane excised from iris, ciliary body, vitreous; 1 enucleation; VA, 2 count fingers, one 20/100
1964	Maumenee[43]	Conjunctival flap; identify/excise any fistula; excision of all involved iris; involved posterior cornea curetted, debrided, swabbed with 70% alcohol; 26 cases; 3 enucleations, 3 RD, 13 CO, 6 VA 20/50 or better (23%)
1970	Maumenee et al[56]	Preceding technique with excision/cryotherapy of involved ciliary body, anterior vitrectomy, either cryotherapy/curettng or alcohol to involved cornea; 40 cases; 5 enucleations, 20 CE, 17 glaucoma, 5 hypotony (3 phthisis), 1 RD, 11 successes (27.5%)
1973	Brown[83]	Three cases (advanced ingrowth); modification of Maumenees technique, with deep lamellar scleral/angle excision; cryotherapy to involved cornea; 1 subsequent PK; no recurrences; all 3 had postoperative (controlled) glaucoma; all achieved ambulatory vision (best 20/80)
1977	Friedman[84]	Three cases; en bloc excision of cornea, sclera, iris, ciliary body, vitreous; repair with corneoscleral graft; VAs 20/50, 20/60, 20/100; no recurrence
1978	Stark et al[85]	Ten cases; argon laser to define iris involvement; surgical technique as described in text; 4 PKs; VA improved in 8/10; 4 successes† (40%)
1979	Brown[64]	Fourteen cases of advanced ingrowth; 9 cases, technique as preceding (1973); 4 PKs; 3 recurrences, 1 success†; 5 cases, cornea debrided (not cryotherapy); 2 PKs; 1 recurrence, 1 success†; 6 required cyclocryotherapy for glaucoma (not caused by recurrence)
1992	Naumann, Rummelt[37]	Four cases; excision cornea, sclera, iris, ciliary body; anterior vitrectomy; tectonic corneoscleral grafting; complications: VH, CE, glaucoma; VA, 2 patients 20/100, 2 patients LP
2002	Lai, Haller[88]	Fluid-gas exchange with intraocular 5-FU; 2 treatments; VA 20/200 with no recurrence at 8 months
2002	Shaikh et al[89]	Intraocular 5-FU mixed with sodium hyaluronate–viscodissection of retrocorneal epithelial membrane; no recurrence at 14 months

*This table is a summary only. Please consult the appropriate sources as referenced.
†Defined as VA 20/50 or better, normal intraocular pressure on topical or no medication, no recurrence. CE, Corneal edema; CO, corneal opacification; 5-FU, 5-fluorouracil; LP, light perception; PK, penetrating keratoplasty; RD, retinal detachment; SO, sympathetic ophthalmia; VA, visual acuity (postoperative); VH, vitreous hemorrhage.

In his 1970 series of 40 cases, Maumenee established stringent criteria for success in treating epithelial ingrowth:[56] postoperative visual acuity 20/50 or better, no recurrence of ingrowth, and intraocular pressure controlled on topical or no medication. Limited anterior vitrectomy was added to excision of involved iris and ciliary body, with cryotherapy to the involved posterior corneal surface becoming preferred to other methods of epithelial eradication. Success was achieved in 27.5% of cases, enucleation was required in 12.5%, and complications included corneal edema, hypotony, glaucoma, vitreous opacity, and retinal detachment.

Alterations to Maumenee's technique (see Table 53-2) have included deep lamellar excision of sclera and angle structures,[83] cryotherapy to suspected areas of angle/ciliary body involvement,[64] corneoscleral excision and grafting,[39,81,84] and the modifications of Stark et al.[85] (see further on). The more surgically destructive approaches, in an attempt to more thoroughly eradicate invading epithelium, have not achieved any higher success rates; however, they have included small numbers of patients or, in the case of Brown's series, involved more advanced cases of ingrowth (involving at least 50% of the cornea, iris, or both).

CURRENT TECHNIQUES

The most widely accepted surgical approach is the modification of Maumenee's technique by Stark et al.[85] Preoperative argon laser photocoagulation is used to delineate the extent of iris involvement. This is best performed within 24 h of surgery, as this degree of photocoagulation usually results in significant anterior-chamber inflammation.

Rectus muscle traction sutures are placed transconjunctivally after conjunctival peritomy. A limbal or fornix-based conjunctival flap is dissected to expose the superior corneoscleral limbus. A careful search for aqueous leakage from a fistula (which may not have been evident with Seidel's test at the slit-lamp examination) is performed, using 2% fluorescein and external pressure on the globe. If a fistula is found, it is excised and closed with sutures; or a scleral flap, hinged anteriorly, is prepared for later closure of larger fistulae. The leading edge of the epithelial sheet on the posterior surface of the cornea may be marked with a blade.

In cases where a pars plana vitrectomy approach is used, sclerotomies are performed 3–4 mm posterior to the limbus, and the

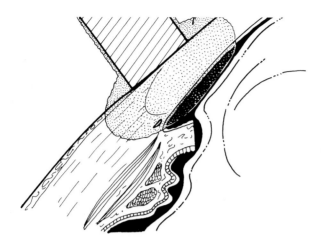

Figure 53-16 Transcorneal and transscleral cryotherapy is used to eliminate residual ingrowing epithelium.

vitrectomy instrument is used to excise involved iris and vitreous. Bleeding is controlled with bipolar diathermy or by transiently increasing intraocular pressure. Excised tissue is studied cytologically to confirm the diagnosis of epithelial ingrowth. As complete a vitrectomy as possible should be performed, to allow space for fluid–air exchange to enhance the effects of cryotherapy, and minimise the risk of vitreous prolapse or incarceration.

If a large fistula is present, its site is sealed by suturing the previously prepared scleral flap to the peripheral cornea. Indirect ophthalmoscopy with scleral indentation is performed, and any retinal tears are treated with cryotherapy, laser, and/or scleral buckling as required. After fluid–air exchange, transcorneal and transscleral cryotherapy is then performed to eliminate residual epithelium on the posterior cornea, angle, and ciliary body (Figure 53-16). Stark et al.[85] recommend that a single freeze is adequate if air insulation is used. Unless required for tamponade of retinal breaks, the air bubble is replaced with physiologic saline solution. Frequent topical corticosteroid drops are used postoperatively. The treated epithelium on the cornea usually sloughs after a few days.

Stark et al.[85] achieved impressive results in their report of 10 consecutive patients treated with this technique (average 23 months' follow-up), with improvement in visual acuity in 8 of 10 cases and four eyes with 20/40 or better vision. Four eyes required penetrating keratoplasty: one eye had residual epithelial cells on examination of the corneal button, and all grafts remained clear during the follow-up period. Brown,[64] who used a similar technique with more extensive excision of angle structures, also reported favorable results from keratoplasty in eyes treated for ingrowth. As emphasized by previous authors, patients with epithelial ingrowth must be observed for some years after treatment before recurrence can be ruled out.

Most contemporary cases of epithelial ingrowth that we have seen as a complication of cataract surgery have involved aphakic eyes with secondary anterior chamber IOLs. The IOL is usually removed as part of the surgical management of this condition, although there are no data to suggest the optimal surgical management in these circumstances. Experience with posterior-chamber IOLs is limited.

In eyes with extensive involvement from epithelial ingrowth not amenable to curative surgery, particularly in very elderly patients, it is reasonable to aim for control of intraocular pressure, preservation of some functional vision, and avoidance of enucleation. Fish et al.[86] reported nine cases in which Molteno implants were used for intractable secondary glaucoma caused by epithelial ingrowth, achieving control of intraocular pressure in seven, comfort in six, and maintenance of formed vision (at least 1/200) in five patients. The use of a Krupin-Denver valve for control of glaucoma in this condition has also been described.[87] Closure of a fistula is contraindicated if curative surgery is not possible because intraocular pressure will almost certainly become uncontrollable.

The most promising recent advance in the treatment of diffuse epithelial ingrowth is the use of intraocular 5-fluorouracil (5-FU).[88,89] Loane and Weinreb[90] reported the use of subconjunctival 5-FU, but this had only a temporary effect in halting the progress of the epithelial membrane, and the eye was ultimately enucleated. Lai and Haller[88] treated an aphakic patient with fluid-gas exchange and 500 μg of 5-FU injected into the anterior chamber, followed by face-down positioning to concentrate the 5-FU in the retrocorneal space. After a second injection of 5-FU, the epithelial membrane was no longer visible. There was no recurrence at 8 months' follow-up. Shaikh et al.[89] used 1 mg of 5-FU mixed with sodium hyaluronate to viscodissect an epithelial ingrowth membrane from the posterior corneal surface. Repeat penetrating keratoplasty was required for graft failure, but no recurrence was observed at 14 months' follow-up.

The use of 5-FU (and possibly other antimetabolites) may offer a less invasive approach, or act as a useful adjunct to surgical intervention, for management of these challenging cases. Even if corneal endothelial toxicity and corneal decompensation occurs, penetrating keratoplasty has a reasonable chance of success if the ingrowth has been eliminated. Further experience and long-term follow-up are required to establish the role of this treatment modality.

PROGNOSIS

Even if clinically recognized and surgically treated, epithelial ingrowth carries a poor prognosis. Patients with fistulae were recognized by Maumenee[43] as having a worse outcome. Even in patients with ultimately poor visual acuity, surgery improves outcome in terms of comfort and avoidance of enucleation, compared with medical management (topical antibiotics and steroids) or no treatment. In the series by Weiner et al.,[42] 52% of patients with epithelial ingrowth after surgery eventually required enucleation; only 19% of patients treated with iridectomy and surgical excision had enucleations, compared with all patients treated medically and 95% of those not treated.

FIBROUS INGROWTH

In contrast to epithelial ingrowth, there has been relatively little attention given to fibrous ingrowth in the ophthalmic literature. It is often an incidental pathologic finding and infrequently behaves in the aggressive, almost malignant fashion of epithelial ingrowth. Alternative expressions for fibrous ingrowth include fibrous overgrowth, fibrous metaplasia, fibrocytic ingrowth, fibroblastic ingrowth, stromal ingrowth, and stromal overgrowth. Some authors also use the term retrocorneal membrane interchangeably with fibrous ingrowth, particularly in cases following penetrating keratoplasty.

HISTORICAL PERSPECTIVE

Early in the twentieth century, fibrous ingrowth was included in discussions of the complications of cataract surgery, with Henderson[91] emphasizing the role of incarceration of iris, lens capsule, or lens debris in allowing entry of connective tissue to the anterior chamber, paralleling epithelial invasion, and Collins[92] asserting that fibrous ingrowth was invariably a result of infection. In 1947, Levkoieva[93] highlighted the incidence of fibrous ingrowth in eyes enucleated after penetrating injury. He and others have debated the likely source of the ingrowing fibrous tissue (see Predisposing Factors and Pathogenesis)

INCIDENCE

Fibrous ingrowth is usually diagnosed on pathologic grounds, and estimates of its clinical incidence have not been reported. Its incidence in enucleated eyes after cataract surgery is as high as 36% in some series[94] and has generally been found to be more common than epithelial ingrowth. Despite this, fibrous ingrowth is a less frequent cause of enucleation than is epithelial ingrowth. Weiner et al.[42] found concomitant fibrous ingrowth in 55% of cases of epithelial ingrowth following cataract surgery.

PREDISPOSING FACTORS AND PATHOGENESIS

Similar factors predispose to fibrous ingrowth as those discussed earlier under epithelial ingrowth, namely technically difficult or complicated surgery (particularly with capsular rupture and vitreous loss); incomplete or delayed wound healing; hypotony; uveitis; and incarceration of iris, vitreous, or lens remnants in the wound. Swan[95] emphasizes recurrent hemorrhage as a predisposing factor to fibrous ingrowth and states that more posterior incisions, which may damage the deep scleral plexus, are more likely to cause hemorrhage. The importance of incarceration of material in the cataract wound was emphasized by findings of McDonnell, de la Cruz, and Green:[96] 84% of cases with vitreous incarceration after cataract surgery studied histopathologically showed evidence of fibrous ingrowth. Swan[95] noted that ingrowth along incarcerated tissue is unlikely if the outer wound edges are in good apposition.

The exact source of fibroblasts in fibrous ingrowth remains a contentious issue. Swan[95] confirmed the observations of Henderson[91] that subepithelial connective tissue is most likely the major source of fibroblasts that invade the anterior chamber in fibrous ingrowth (rather than being overgrowth of corneal, scleral, or limbal stroma, as is often stated). He also observed that the usual physiologic degree of fibroblastic ingrowth, as part of wound healing, may extend further than usual if the endothelium (which usually bridges the inner wound margin) has been damaged. This is supported by the studies of Brown and Kitano[97] in rabbits. The degree of perforation of Descemet's membrane (which may determine the likelihood of invasion of fibrous tissue) has been highlighted by some authors[98,99] as an important pathogenetic factor.

Blood-derived mononuclear cells[95] and metaplastic endothelial cells have also been proposed as sources of fibroblasts. Retrocorneal/posterior corneal membranes resulting from fibrous metaplasia of endothelial cells, such as those following penetrating keratoplasty and clear corneal cataract incisions, differ in histologic appearance to those of fibrous ingrowth from limbal incisions and should be considered separately. One report[100] describes a "double membrane" composed of an anterior, vascularized fibrous ingrowth, apparently arising from subepithelial connective tissue, and a posterior, relatively amorphous and acellular layer, which appeared to arise from fibroblastic transformation of endothelial cells. Production of extracellular matrix by endothelial cells in response to disease and injury is well established and has been discussed in detail by Waring et al.[101–103] Their classification of abnormal collagenous tissue in the region of the posterior cornea into three types of "posterior collagenous layer of the cornea" is a useful and more accurate method of describing this fibrous tissue, regardless of its cell(s) of origin.

PRESENTATION, CLINICAL FEATURES, AND DIAGNOSIS

Fibrous ingrowth has been observed following penetrating anterior segment trauma, cataract surgery, glaucoma filtering surgery, and penetrating keratoplasty. It has some features in common with epithelial ingrowth, but as a rule runs a self-limiting course, and the ingrowing membrane has a different appearance (Figure 53-17).

The clinical course of fibrous ingrowth is highly variable and depends on extent of the factors promoting ingrowth. Frequently, it runs an insidious course with little discomfort, and if the condition is diagnosed clinically, the membrane is often noted as an incidental finding. Less commonly, patients present with decreased visual acuity caused by the fibrous membrane or symptoms related to uveitis, glaucoma, or (rarely) retinal detachment.

Typically, the membrane of fibrous ingrowth is gray or white and has a less well-defined border than that of epithelial ingrowth. It is well described by Swan[104] as an interlacing meshwork of fine fibers, with the appearance of woven cloth, and fine tonguelike strands of fibrous tissue extending from the leading edge. Any extension over the angle, iris, and vitreous is usually identifiable as a thick fibrous membrane. It may also appear as a fine gray sheet over the vitreous face, resembling the membrane associated with postoperative iridocyclitis or hyphema. In cases associated with recurrent hyphema, the membrane may be straw colored as a result of blood pigment deposition. The membrane on the posterior cornea may also be translucent, with a relatively well-defined margin and a similar appearance to the membrane of epithelial ingrowth, especially in regions of stripping of Descemet's membrane, or vitreous touch.

There is usually corneal edema overlying the affected area of cornea, and bullous keratopathy is also common. An updrawn pupil resulting from contraction of fibrous tissue may be evident. Glaucoma is a frequent finding and may be due to overgrowth of the anterior chamber angle or peripheral anterior synechiae associated with chronic inflammation. The degree of inflammation tends to parallel the behavior of the fibrous proliferation, from self-limited fibrous ingrowth with minimal inflammation to extensive proliferation of fibrous tissue, which may be

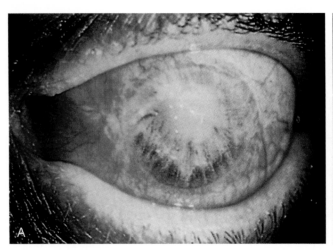
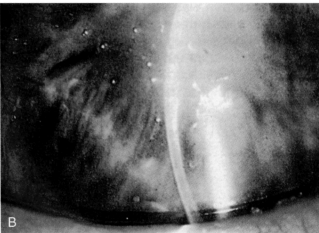

Figure 53-17 A, Marked corneal opacity resulting from fibrous ingrowth. **B,** Magnified view demonstrating the irregular serrated margin of the fibrous membrane. (From Bloomfield SE, Jakobiec FA, Iwamoto T: Fibrous ingrowth with retrocorneal membrane, *Ophthalmology* 88:459-465, 1981. Copyright Elsevier, 1981.)

accompanied by marked uveitis. As noted by Duke-Elder,[105] there may be an absence of marked inflammatory changes if the uveal structures are enveloped in fibrous tissue. Subsequent contraction of this tissue may result in retinal detachment, hypotony, and phthisis bulbi. Conversely, fibrous ingrowth is a common finding in phthisical eyes enucleated after cataract surgery.[99]

The diagnosis of fibrous ingrowth should be made on the basis of the preceding clinical features and awareness of the factors predisposing to the development of fibrous ingrowth in the setting of previous anterior segment surgery or trauma. There are no specific recommended diagnostic adjuncts, although if there is sufficient suspicion of epithelial ingrowth on clinical grounds, the further tests recommended earlier may be useful. The differential diagnosis of fibrous ingrowth corresponds to that of epithelial ingrowth, as detailed earlier. Clearly, if surgery is performed for one of the complications mentioned previously, a histopathologic diagnosis should be made on examination of the excised tissue.

HISTOPATHOLOGIC FEATURES

Externally there may be evidence of poor apposition of wound edges. Similar inadequate apposition internally is reflected in a larger gap between the cut edges of Descemet's membrane, filled with advancing fibrous tissue. The source of this fibrous tissue (subepithelial connective tissue, corneal/limbal stroma, or metaplastic endothelium) is usually not apparent. The corneal stroma may show deep vascularization and a chronic inflammatory cell infiltrate. There may be evidence of suture-related inflammation, and poorly placed or improperly tensioned sutures, resulting in poor wound coaptation, may be seen.

There is usually damage to the endothelium and stripping of Descemet's membrane adjacent to the wound. The anterior chamber angle may be closed by peripheral anterior synechiae or a fibrocellular sheet; the trabecular meshwork in eyes with long-standing fibrous ingrowth appears atrophic or sclerotic. There may be incarceration of iris, lens capsule, lens cortical remnants,

or vitreous, as discussed earlier. A pupillary membrane may be present, and contraction of fibrous tissue may lead to pupillary distortion, or, in cases of extensive ingrowth, retinal detachment (Figure 53-18). Wound fistulae appear less common in cases of fibrous ingrowth (without concomitant epithelial ingrowth) than in epithelial ingrowth alone.

MANAGEMENT

As for epithelial ingrowth, modern surgical technique has led to a reduction in the risk factors for development of fibrous ingrowth. Prevention of these conditions is far more effective than attempts at cure. Treatment of the underlying ingrowth itself is not nearly

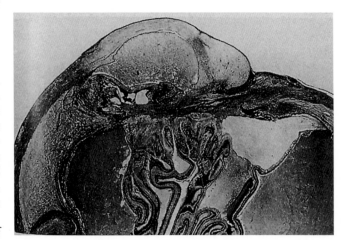

Figure 53-18 Light microscopy of massive fibrous ingrowth through a cataract incision forming a dense secondary membrane and causing retinal detachment. (Hematoxylin and eosin stain; ×10.) (From Allen JC: Epithelial and stromal ingrowth, *Am J Ophthalmol* 65:179-182, 1968. Copyright Elsevier, 1968.)

so important in fibrous as in epithelial ingrowth; as many eyes remain stable or progress little over the years, treatment is usually confined to managing specific sequelae of ingrowth. This may include treatment for corneal edema or uveitis (although it is generally accepted that topical steroids will not halt progression of membrane itself); retrocorneal membrane excision with or without penetrating keratoplasty; surgical or Nd:YAG cutting of pupillary membranes; release of vitreous and retinal traction, which may require vitrectomy and scleral buckling; and management of secondary glaucoma. Viscoelastic displacement of a retrocorneal membrane due to fibrous ingrowth has also been recently described.[106] Although Friedman and Henkind[107] proposed radiotherapy in progressive fibrous ingrowth, there are no clinical reports of its use.

PROGNOSIS

In the absence of any large clinical series of cases of fibrous ingrowth, the prognosis of this condition is based largely on anecdotal experience. The overall outlook is considerably better than that of epithelial ingrowth, because many cases of fibrous ingrowth are self-limited. Eyes with more extensive or progressive forms of fibrous ingrowth have a poor prognosis, similar to that of epithelial ingrowth, and surgery may be of benefit in treatment of specific complications, although results are modest at best.

References

[1] Mackenzie W. A practical treatise on the diseases of the eye. London: Longman, Rees, Orme, Brown and Green; 1830.
[2] Rothmund A. Ueber cysten der regenbogenhaut. Klin Monatsbl Augenheilkd 1872;10:189–223.
[3] Collins ET, Cross FR. Two cases of epithelial implantation cyst in the anterior chamber after extraction of cataract. Trans Ophthalmol Soc UK 1892;12:175.
[4] Guaita M. Proliferation de l'endothélium cornéen sur l'iris et le champ pupillaire après l'extraction de la cataracte. Arch d'Ophth 1893;13:507.
[5] Meller J. Ueber epitheleinsenkung und cystenbildung im auge. Arch F Ophth 1901;52:436.
[6] Perera CA. Epithelium in the anterior chamber of the eye after operation and injury. Trans Am Acad Ophthalmol Otolaryngol 1937;42:142–164.
[7] Sitchevska O, Payne BF. Pearl cysts of the iris. Am J Ophthalmol 1951;34:833–839.
[8] Terry TL, Chisholm JF, Schonberg AL. Studies on the surface-epithelium invasion of the anterior segment of the eye. Am J Ophthalmol 1939;22:1083–1110.
[9] Theobald GD, Haas JS. Epithelial invasion of the anterior chamber follow ing cataract extraction. Trans Am Acad Ophthalmol Otolaryngol 1948;52:470–485.
[10] Farmer SG, Kalina RE. Epithelial implantation cyst of the iris. Ophthalmology 1981;88:1286–1289.
[11] Ferry AP. The possible role of epithelial-bearing surgical instruments in pathogenesis of epithelialization of the anterior chamber. Ann Ophthalmol 1971;3:1089–1093.
[12] Cogan DG. Experimental implants of conjunctiva into the anterior chamber. Am J Ophthalmol 1955;39:165–172.
[13] Regan EF. Epithelial invasion of the anterior chamber. Arch Ophthalmol 1958;60:907.
[14] Shields JA, Sanborn GE, Augsburger JJ. The differential diagnosis of malignant melanoma of the iris: a clinical study of 200 patients. Ophthalmology 1983;90:716.
[15] Schwartzenberg T, Cahnita M. Sympathetic ophthalmitis associated with cystic epithelial invasion of the anterior chamber: a clinical case. J Fr Ophtalmol 1982;5:831–837.
[16] Layden WE, Torczynsk E, Font RL. Mucogenic glaucoma and goblet cell cyst of the anterior chamber. Arch Ophthalmol 1978;96:2259–2263.
[17] Ruiz-Moreno T, Cortes-Valdes E, Zazurca-Muinos J. Luxation of an anterior chamber lens caused by secondary serous epithelial cyst. J Fr Ophtalmol 1989;12:313–315.
[18] Eiferman RA, Rodrigues MM. Squamous epithelial implantation cyst of the iris. Ophthalmology 1981;88:1281.
[19] Winthrop SR, Smith RE. Spontaneous regression of an anterior chamber cyst: a case report. Ann Ophthalmol 1981;13:431–432.
[20] Vail D. Treatment of cysts of the iris with diathermy coagulation. Trans Am Ophthalmol Soc 1953;51:371–383.
[21] Hogan MJ, Goodner EK. Surgical treatment of epithelial cysts of the anterior chamber. Arch Ophthalmol 1960;64:286–291.
[22] Ferry AP, Naghdi MR. Cryosurgical removal of epithelial cyst of iris and anterior chamber. Arch Ophthalmol 1967;77:86–87.
[23] Shaffer RN. Alpha Irradiation: effect of astatine on the anterior segment and on an epithelial cyst. Trans Am Ophthalmol Soc 1952;50:607.
[24] Fralick FB. Management of complications after cataract extraction. Trans Pac Coast Otoophthalmol Soc 1951;32:42–53.
[25] Meyer-Schwickerath G. Light coagulation. St Louis: Mosby; 1960.
[26] Okun E, Mandell A. Photocoagulation treatment of epithelial implantation cysts following cataract surgery. Trans Am Ophthalmol Soc 1974;72:170–183.
[27] L'Esperance FA, James WA. Argon laser photocoagulation of iris abnormalities. Trans Am Acad Ophthalmol Otolaryngol 1975;79:321–339.
[28] Thomas JV, Lederer CM, Simmons RJ. Photocoagulation for epithelial ingrowth and cysts of the anterior chamber. In: Belcher CD, Thomas JV, Simmons RJ, editors. Photocoagulation in glaucoma and anterior segment disease. Baltimore: Williams & Wilkins; 1984. p. 196–205.
[29] Scholz RT, Kelly JS. Argon laser photocoagulation treatment of iris cysts following penetrating keratoplasty. Arch Ophthalmol 1982;100:926–927.
[30] Sugar J, Jampol LM, Goldberg MF. Argon laser destruction of anterior chamber implantation cysts. Ophthalmology 1984;91:1040–1044.
[31] Honrubia FM, Brito C, Grijalbo MP. Photocoagulation of iris cyst. Trans Ophthalmol Soc UK 1982;102:184–186.
[32] Orlin SE, Raber IM, Laibson PR, et al. Epithelial downgrowth following the removal of iris inclusion cysts. Ophthalmic Surg 1991;22:330–335.
[33] Cahane M, Rosner M, Avni I, et al. Nd-YAG laser treatment of anterior chamber implantation cysts. Metab Syst Pediatr Ophthalmol 1988;11:47–49.
[34] Maumenee AE, Shannon CR. Epithelial invasion of the anterior chamber. Trans Pac Coast Otoophthalmol Soc 1955;36:107–135.
[35] Bruner WE, Michels RG, Stark WJ, et al. Management of epithelial cysts of the anterior chamber. Ophthalmic Surg 1981;12:279–285.
[36] Sugar HS, Willenz AL. Posterior lamellar resection of the cornea for epithelial implantation cyst in the anterior chamber. Am J Ophthalmol 1962;54:800–803.
[37] Naumann GOH, Rummelt V. Block excision of cystic and diffuse epithelial ingrowth of the anterior chamber. Arch Ophthalmol 1992;110:223–227.
[38] Rummelt V, Naumann GO. Block excision with tectonic corneoscleroplasty for cystic and/or diffuse epithelial invasion of the anterior eye segment: report of 51 consecutive patients (1980–1996). Klin Monatsbl Augenheilkd 1997;211:312–323.
[39] Rizzuti AB. Traumatic implantation cysts of the iris with special emphasis on surgical aspects. Am J Ophthalmol 1955;39:13–20.
[40] Harbin TS, Maumenee AE. Epithelial downgrowth after surgery for epithelial cyst. Am J Ophthalmol 1974;78:1–4.
[41] Christensen L. Epithelialization of the anterior chamber. In: Transactions of the New Orleans academy of ophthalmology: symposium on cataracts. St Louis: Mosby; 1965.
[42] Weiner MJ, Trentacoste J, Pon DM, et al. Epithelial downgrowth: a 30-year clinicopathological review. Br J Ophthalmol 1989;73:6–11.
[43] Maumenee AE. Treatment of epithelial downgrowth and intraocular fistula following cataract extraction. Trans Am Ophthalmol Soc 1964;62:153–166.
[44] Jaffe NS, Jaffe MS, Jaffe GF. Epithelial invasion of the anterior chamber. In: Cataract surgery and its complications. 5th ed. St Louis: Mosby; 1989. p. 582–613.
[45] Merenmies L, Tarkkanen A. Causes of enucleation following cataract extraction. Acta Ophthalmol 1977;55:47–352.
[46] Holliday JN, Buller CR, Bourne WM. Specular microscopy and fluorophotometry in the diagnosis of epithelial downgrowth after a sutureless cataract operation. Am J Ophthalmol 1993;116:238–240.
[47] Knauf HP, Rowsey J, Margo C. Cystic epithelial downgrowth following clear-corneal cataract extraction. Arch Ophthalmol 1997;115:668–669.
[48] Lee BL, Gaton DD, Weinreb RN. Epithelial downgrowth following phacoemulsification through a clear cornea. Arch Ophthalmol 1999;117:283.
[49] Vargas LG, Vroman DT, Solomon KD, Holzer MP, Escobar-Gomez M, Schmidbauer JM, et al. Epithelial downgrowth after clear cornea phacoemulsification: report of 2 cases and review of the literature. Ophthalmology 2002;109:2331–2335.
[50] Kuchle M, Green WR. Epithelial ingrowth: a study of 207 histopathologically proven cases. German J Ophthalmol 1996;5:211–223.
[51] Abbott RL, Spencer WH. Epithelialization of the anterior chamber after transcorneal (McCannel) suture. Arch Ophthalmol 1978;96:482–484.
[52] Zavala EY, Binder PS. The pathologic findings of epithelial ingrowth. Arch Ophthalmol 1980;98:2007–2014.
[53] Paufique L, Hervouët F. L'invasion épithéliale de la chambre antérieure après opération de cataracte. Am J Ophthalmol 1997;105–129.
[54] Binder R, Binder H. Experimentelle Untersuchungen über den Einfluss von Anticoagulatien auf die Heilung von Hornhautschnittwunden. Graefes Arch Ophthalmol 1954;155:337–344.
[55] Bick MN. Heparinization of the eye. Am J Ophthalmol 1949;32:663–670.
[56] Maumenee AE, Paton D, Morse PH et al. Review of 40 histologically proven cases of epithelial downgrowth following cataract extraction and suggested surgical management. Am J Ophthalmol 1970;69:598–603.
[57] Allen JC, Duehr PA. Sutures and epithelial downgrowth. Am J Ophthalmol 1968;66:293–294.
[58] Burris TE, Nordquist RE, Rowsey JJ. Model of epithelial downgrowth. I. Clinical correlations and light microscopy. Cornea 1983;2:277–287.
[59] Burris TE, Nordquist RE, Rowsey JJ. Model of epithelial downgrowth. II. Scanning and transmission electron microscopy of corneal epithelialization. Cornea 1984;3:141–151.
[60] Burris TE, Nordquist RE, Rowsey JJ. Model of epithelial downgrowth. III. Scanning and transmission electron microscopy of iris epithelialization. Cornea 1985;4:249–255.
[61] Burris TE. Cryopexy of epithelial downgrowth. Cornea 1986;5:173–180.
[62] Calhoun Jr FP. The clinical recognition and treatment of epithelialization of the anterior chamber following cataract extraction. Trans Am Ophthalmol Soc 1949;47:498–553.
[63] Bruner WE, Green WR, Stark WJ. A case of epithelial ingrowth primarily involving the lens capsule. Ophthalmic Surg 1986;17:483–485.
[64] Brown SI. Results of excision of advanced epithelial downgrowth. Ophthalmology 1979;86:321–328.
[65] Samples JR, Van Buskirk EM. Epithelial ingrowth on an intraocular lens. Ophthalmic Surg 1984;15:869–870.
[66] Schaeffer AR, Nalbandian RM, Brigham DW, et al. Epithelial downgrowth following wound dehiscence after extracapsular cataract extraction and posterior chamber lens implantation: surgical management. J Cataract Refract Surg 1989;15:437–441.
[67] Smith RE, Parrett C. Specular microscopy of epithelial downgrowth. Arch Ophthalmol 1978;96:1222–1224.
[68] Laing RA, Sandstrom MM, Leibowitz HM, et al. Epithelialization of the anterior chamber: clinical investigation with the specular microscope. Arch Ophthalmol 1979;97:1870.
[69] Chiou AGY, Kaufman SC, Kaz K, et al. Characterisation of epithelial downgrowth by confocal microscopy. J Cataract Refract Surg 1999;25:1172–1174.
[70] Verhoeff A. In discussion of Vail D: Epithelial downgrowth into the anterior chamber following cataract extraction arrested by radiation treatment. Trans Am Ophthalmol Soc 1935;33:306.
[71] Calhoun FP. An aid to the clinical diagnosis of epithelial downgrowth into the anterior chamber following cataract extraction. Am J Ophthalmol 1966;61:1055–1059.
[72] Verrey F. Cytologie de l'humeur aqueuse et invasion épitheliale de la chambre antérieure. Ophthalmologica 1967;154:310.
[73] Iwamoto T, Srinivasan BD, DeVoe AG. Electron microscopy of epithelial downgrowth. Ann Ophthalmol 1977;9:1095–1110.

[74] Bernadino VB, Kim JC, Smith TR. Epithelialization of the anterior chamber after cataract extraction. Arch Ophthalmol 1969;82:742–750.

[75] Matsuda H, Smelser GK. Electron microscopy of corneal wound healing. Exp Eye Res 1976;16:427–442.

[76] Smith P, Stark WJ, Maumenee AE, et al. Epithelial, fibrous, and endothelial proliferation. In: Ritch R, Shields MB, Krupin T, editors. The glaucomas. St Louis: Mosby; 1989. p. 1299–1335.

[77] Küchle M, Naumann GOH. Mucogenic secondary open-angle glaucoma in diffuse epithelial ingrowth treated by block-excision. Am J Ophthalmol 1991;111:230–234.

[78] Handmann M. Disparition complète d'un Kyste traumatique de l'iris après roentgenthérapie. Klin Monatsld Augenheilkd 1924;72:111.

[79] Pincus MH. Epithelial invasion of the anterior chamber following cataract extraction: effect of radiation therapy. Arch Ophthalmol 1950;43:509.

[80] Maumenee AE. Epithelial invasion of the anterior chamber. Trans Am Acad Ophthalmol Otolaryngol 1957;61:51–57.

[81] Sullivan GL. Epithelization of the anterior chamber following cataract extraction: a new approach to treatment. Trans Am Ophthalmol Soc 1958;56:606–654.

[82] Long JC, Tyner GS. Three cases of epithelial invasion of the anterior chamber treated surgically. Arch Ophthalmol 1957;58:396–400.

[83] Brown SI. Treatment of advanced epithelial downgrowth. Trans Am Acad Ophthalmol Otolaryngol 1973;77:618–622.

[84] Friedman AH. Radical anterior segment surgery for epithelial invasion of the anterior chamber: report of three cases. Trans Am Acad Ophthalmol Otolaryngol 1977;83:216–223.

[85] Stark WJ, Michels RG, Maumenee AE, et al. Surgical management of epithelial ingrowth. Am J Ophthalmol 1978;85:772.

[86] Fish LA, Heuer DK, Baerveldt G, et al. Molteno implantation for secondary glaucomas associated with advanced epithelial ingrowth. Ophthalmology 1990;97:557–561.

[87] Bacin F, Kantelip B. Tentative de traitement des complications de l'invasion epitheliale par la valve de Krupin-Denver. Bull Soc Ophthalmol Fr 1983;83:519–521.

[88] Lai MM, Haller JA. Resolution of epithelial ingrowth in a patient treated with 5-fluorouracil. Am J Ophthalmol 2002;133:562–564.

[89] Shaikh AA, Damji KF, Mintsioulis G, et al. Bilateral epithelial downgrowth managed in one eye with intraocular 5-fluorouracil. Arch Ophthalmol 2002;120:1396–1398.

[90] Loane ME, Weinreb RN. Glaucoma secondary to epithelial downgrowth and 5-fluorouracil. Ophthalmic Surg 1990;21:704–706.

[91] Henderson T. A histological study of the normal healing of wounds after cataract extraction. Ophthalmol Rev 1907;26:127.

[92] Collins ET. Discussion on post-operative complications of cataract extractions. Trans Ophthalmol Soc UK 1914;34:18–44.

[93] Levkoieva E. The regeneration of wounds of external membrane of the eye in the light of new pathologicoanatomical results. Br J Ophthalmol 1947;31:336–361.

[94] Allen JC. Epithelial and stromal ingrowths. Am J Ophthalmol 1968;65:179–182.

[95] Swan KC. Fibroblastic ingrowth following cataract extraction. Arch Ophthalmol 1973;89: 445–449.

[96] McDonnell PJ, de la Cruz ZC, Green WR. Vitreous incarceration complicating cataract surgery. Ophthalmology 1986;93:247.

[97] Brown SI, Kitano S. Pathogenesis of the retrocorneal membrane. Arch Ophthalmol 1966;75:518–525.

[98] Sherrard ES, Rycroft PV. Retrocorneal membranes. I. Their origin and structure. Br J Ophthalmol 1967;51:379–386.

[99] Bettman JW. Pathology of complications of intraocular surgery. Am J Ophthalmol 1969;68:1037–1050.

[100] Bloomfield SE, Jakobiec FA, Iwamoto T. Fibrous ingrowth with retrocorneal membrane. Ophthalmology 1981;88:459–465.

[101] Waring GO, Laibson PR, Rodrigues M. Clinical and pathologic alterations of Descemet's membrane: with emphasis on endothelial metaplasia. Surv Ophthalmol 1974;18:325.

[102] Waring GO. Posterior collagenous layer of the cornea: ultrastructural classification of abnormal collagenous tissue posterior to Descemet's membrane in 30 cases. Arch Ophthalmol 1982;100:122–134.

[103] Waring GO, Bourne WM, Edelhauser HF, et al. The corneal endothelium: normal and pathologic structure and function. Ophthalmology 1982;89:531–590.

[104] Swan KC. Some contemporary concepts of scleral disease. Arch Ophthalmol 1951;45:630–644.

[105] Duke-Elder S. A system of ophthalmology. vol. XIV, injuries, St Louis: Mosby; 1958. p. 335.

[106] Mandelcorn M, Men G. Viscoelastic displacement of fibrous ingrowth: a new surgical approach to retrocorneal membranes. Can J Ophthalmol 2001;36:341–343.

[107] Friedman AH, Henkind P. Corneal stromal overgrowth after cataract extraction. Br J Ophthalmol 1970;54:528–534.

Macular Causes of Poor Postoperative Vision: Cystoid Macular Edema, Epiretinal Fibrosis, and Age-Related Macular Degeneration

Raja Narayanan, MD and Baruch D. Kuppermann, MD, PhD

CONTENTS

- Cystoid Macular Edema
- Diabetic Macular Edema
- Epiretinal Membrane
- Retinal Vein Occlusion
- Macular Hole
- Macular Degeneration
- Photic Injury
- Conclusions

Great advancements in the field of cataract surgery have been made over the past 2 decades, with fewer rates of complications and better surgical outcomes. However, for good visual outcome after cataract surgery, a fully functional, healthy macula is necessary. Every surgeon who has performed cataract surgery has encountered disappointing cases of poor visual outcome in spite of a successful cataract surgery, where the problem lies in the macula. Additionally, when complications during cataract surgery do occur, the outcomes can be adversely affected due to secondary macular issues.

In advanced cataracts with inadequate visualization of the macula, macular pathologies may be undetected until the postoperative period. Similarly, there are no investigative modalities that give a precise estimate of the macular function in such cases. A few of the macular disorders, such as cystoid macular edema (CME) and epiretinal membrane formation, occur postoperatively, both in cases associated with complications as well as in uncomplicated surgery. It is important for the anterior segment surgeon to remain alert to these conditions, and this chapter deals with a few important macular conditions causing poor postoperative visual acuity. Some of the important macular disorders associated with poor visual acuity are listed in Table 54-1.

CYSTOID MACULAR EDEMA

Macular edema as a complication of cataract surgery causing a reduction in central vision was first recognized by Irvine in 1953.[1] Also known as Irvine–Gass syndrome, cystoid macular edema (CME) after cataract surgery is characterized by multiple cyst-like (cystoid) areas of fluid in the macula. The incidence of Irvine–Gass syndrome is variable depending on the type of surgical procedure performed and the clinical series reported. Overall, the incidence of angiographic CME is approximately 50% after intracapsular cataract extraction,[2] and 20% after extracapsular cataract extraction (ECCE),[3] and 19% after phacoemulsification,[4] but the overall incidence of clinically evident CME is much less. Various studies have reported that the occurrence of clinically significant CME varies between 1.5 and 2.3%.[5] Postoperative CME in one eye is associated with an increased risk of CME developing in the other eye. Fortunately, however, most patients recover their vision with treatment.

The condition may be divided into CME based on biomicroscopic examination and angiographic CME based on fluorescein angiography. Angiographic CME does not necessarily reduce the visual acuity.[6] Multiple remissions and exacerbations of macular edema or persistent macular edema may result in photoreceptor damage and foveal atrophy with permanent impairment of central vision.

PATHOPHYSIOLOGY

Leaking perifoveal capillaries lead to accumulation of fluid in Muller cells, [7] or in the loosely arranged outer plexiform layer of Henle,[8] the fibers of which are arranged horizontally. This produces a petalloid pattern on fluorescein angiography. Breakdown of the inner blood retinal barrier leading to CME has many possible etiologies. The most popular theory implicates intraocular inflammation. Inflammatory mediators, such as prostaglandins and leukotrienes have been implicated in the pathogenesis. In the prostaglandin pathway, inflammation causes the enzyme phospholipase to release arachidonic acid from cell walls. Subsequently, cyclooxygenase converts the arachidonic acid to prostaglandins. Steroids inhibit the enzyme phospholipase, and nonsteroidal anti-inflammatory drugs (NSAIDs) inhibit the cyclo-oxygenase pathway. Leukotrienes account for an alternate pathway where the enzyme lipoxygenase converts arachidonic acid to leukotrienes, which are chemotactic agents. However, the exact role of leukotrienes in CME remains unclear.

In Irvine–Gass syndrome, light toxicity originating from the operating microscope or postoperative inflammation may contribute

Table 54-1 Common macular diseases causing poor postoperative vision after cataract surgery

1. Cystoid macular edema
2. Epiretinal membrane
3. Diabetic macular edema
4. Vitreo-macular traction
5. Macular hole
6. Retinal vein occlusions
7. Age-related macular degeneration
8. Photic Injury

Table 54-3 Clinical signs of cystoid macular edema

| Prominence of yellow xanthophyll pigment dot |
| Multiple cysts in the fovea |
| Perifoveal splinter hemorrhages |
| Macular thickening |
| Disc edema |
| Vitreous cells |

to free radical release with subsequent prostaglandin synthesis. Vitreoretinal traction to the macula may also contribute to postoperative CME.[9] Vitreous incarcerated in the surgical wound and pulling on the retina at points of vitreo-retinal attachment have been found to be associated with an increased risk of CME.[10]

SYMPTOMS

Although complicated surgery accounts for most cases of CME (Table 54-2), this condition may also occasionally occur after uneventful surgery. Vision ranges from 20/25 to 20/400 depending on the severity of the edema. Patients may also experience metamorphopsia. The natural history of CME is variable. Pseudophakic CME often resolves spontaneously, and 90% of eyes improve to 20/40 or better visual acuity in cases with a posterior-chamber (PC) intraocular lens (IOL). However, remissions and exacerbations of macular edema can result in photoreceptor damage with permanent impairment of central vision.

HISTORY

Patients presenting with Irvine–Gass syndrome often have a history of prior intraocular surgery. Risk factors may be present in the affected eye. The patient presents with gradually decreasing vision, usually 1 to 3 months after cataract surgery.

EXAMINATION

Clinical examination of the anterior segment can provide important clues. Peaked pupil, poorly positioned IOL, anterior-chamber (AC) IOL, and anterior-chamber inflammation may be found in cases of CME. Biomicroscopic examination reveals the characteristic cystic spaces in the foveal region (Table 54-3).

Table 54-2 Surgical factors that may contribute to cystoid macular edema

| Posterior capsule rupture |
| Vitreous prolapse |
| Repeated iris prolapse |
| Prolonged surgery |
| Improper positioning of IOL causing iris tuck |
| Vitreous or iris incarceration in the wound |

Subtle CME can be highlighted by the technique of light scattering. Retro-illumination by focusing the slit beam of illumination at the edge of the fovea delineates the cystic spaces. These cysts may coalesce into a macular cyst and which may then progress to form a hole. CME may also be associated with perifoveal hemorrhages.

IMAGING STUDIES

FLUORESCEIN ANGIOGRAPHY

In the early and mid phases of the fluorescein angiogram, parafoveal retinal capillary leakage occurs in most cases. In the late phases of the fluorescein angiogram, a petaloid pattern of leakage in the macula and leakage on or around the optic disc occurs.[11] However, visual acuity is not predicted by the amount of leakage.[12]

OPTICAL COHERENCE TOMOGRAPHY

Optical coherence tomography (OCT) is an important modality in confirming the diagnosis and in monitoring the course of the disease. OCT demonstrates well-defined cystic spaces in the fovea and increased foveal thickness.[13]

MANAGEMENT

PHARMACOLOGIC TREATMENT

Most cases of pseudophakic CME resolve spontaneously within several weeks to a few months. However, 20% of cases are evident angiographically for more than 5 years after onset. When other conditions cause CME, treatment often entails managing the underlying problem. Corticosteroids inhibit the enzyme phospholipase and have a primary role in the treatment of CME secondary to uveitis. Corticosteroids can be administered topically, orally, injected in the sub-Tenon space or intravitreally. Intravitreal triamcinolone has been shown to improve visual acuity that may be sustained for an extended period.[14] NSAIDs inhibit the enzyme cyclooxygenase and can be highly effective in the treatment of CME.[15–17] In a prospective, double-masked, multicenter study of ketorolac versus placebo in the treatment of patients with chronic aphakic or pseudophakic CME, statistically significant improvement in visual acuity occurred in patients that received ketorolac after 30, 60, and 90 days of therapy.[18] This remained significant 1 month after cessation of treatment. Preoperative use of ketorolac for 3 days has been shown to be effective in preventing postoperative CME.[19] The Italian Diclofenac Study

Group reported a prospective, randomized, double-blind, multicenter study of diclofenac versus fluorometholone in the treatment of CME after ECCE with PC IOL placement.[20] At both 36 and 140 days postoperatively, angiographic CME was lower in patients treated with diclofenac compared with the control group. A newer non-steroidal agent, nepafenac, is being studied in clinical trials. Early reports suggest that it is more efficacious than the traditional non-steroidal agents that have been used until now.

SURGICAL TREATMENT

In select cases, YAG laser may be a preferable option to cut adherent strands of vitreous and relieve traction.[21] When vitreous traction contributes to CME, surgical vitrectomy can lessen the CME and improve vision.[22] Vitrectomy is effective through the following mechanisms:

a. Remove inflammatory mediators

b. Remove retained lens fragments

c. Reposition a dislocated or malpositioned IOL

d. A greater penetration of topical and oral corticosteroids into the posterior segment occurs after pars plana vitrectomy (PPV).

■ DIABETIC MACULAR EDEMA ■

In the Wisconsin Epidemiologic Study, macular edema was present in 2–6% of patients with background, diabetic retinopathy; 20–63% in pre-proliferative diabetic retinopathy; and 70–74% in proliferative diabetic retinopathy. The prevalence of macular edema also increased with the duration of diabetes mellitus. Diabetic macular edema (DME), defined as retinal thickening within one disc diameter of the macula, is often aggravated by cataract surgery. In a recent study, the incidence of preoperative macular edema as determined by OCT in diabetics undergoing cataract surgery was 22%. Eyes with no pre-existing diabetic retinopathy did not develop any significant increase in central foveal thickness, whereas patients with moderate-to-severe diabetic retinopathy had an increase of 145 μm in the central foveal thickness 1 month after cataract surgery. This was associated with a less than two line improvement in visual acuity after cataract surgery.[23] Rupture of the posterior capsule often increases the macular edema. Over the previous few decades, there have been a few large-scale trials that have influenced the management of diabetic complications in the eye. The Early Treatment Diabetic Retinopathy Study (ETDRS) identified macular edema as a study objective. To date, the ETDRS has presented the most comprehensive and detailed directives in the management of diabetic macular edema.[24] More recently, the Diabetic Retinopathy Clinical Research network (DRCR.net) has initiated a series of trials assessing laser, surgical, and pharmacological treatments of DME.

PATHOPHYSIOLOGY

DME is the result of retinal microvascular changes that occur in patients with diabetes.[25–27] Thickening of the basement membrane and reduction in the number of pericytes is believed to lead to increased permeability and incompetence of retinal vasculature.[28] This compromise of blood–retinal barrier leads to the leakage of plasma constituents in the surrounding retina, resulting in retinal edema. Focal retinal thickening is almost always caused by leaking microaneurysms. Diffuse retinal thickening is usually caused by a generalized breakdown of the inner and outer blood–retinal barriers. Macular ischemia may sometimes be the cause of significant visual loss.

HISTORY

- *Diabetic history:* Specific inquiry should be made into risk factors for the development of diabetic retinopathy.
- *Type of diabetes:* After 20 years of disease, nearly all patients with type I and 60% of patients with type II have some degree of retinopathy.
- *Duration of the diabetes:* Increased risk of diabetic retinopathy
- *Diabetic control:* The Diabetes Control and Complication Trail (DCCT) has clearly demonstrated that tighter control of blood sugar is associated with reduced incidence of diabetic retinopathy.[29]
- *Renal disease:* Proteinuria is a good marker for the development of diabetic retinopathy; thus, patients with diabetic nephropathy should be observed more closely.
- *Systemic hypertension:* Increased risk of retinopathy (diabetic retinopathy with superimposed hypertensive retinopathy).
- *Triglycerides and lipids*: Normalization of lipid levels reduces retinal leakage and exudate deposition.

EXAMINATION

Fundus evaluation under stereopsis and high magnification should be performed on every patient with diabetes, to assess DME and diabetic retinopathy. DME is defined as retinal thickening within two disc diameters of the center of the macula. Focal edema is associated with hard exudate rings resulting from leakage from microaneurysms. Diffuse edema results from breakdown of blood–retinal barrier with leakage from microaneurysms, retinal capillaries, and arterioles.

Clinically significant macular edema (CSME), as defined by the ETDRS (Table 54-4), exists when any of the following conditions exist:

1. Retinal thickening within 500 μm of the center of the fovea

2. Hard, yellow exudates within 500 μm of the center of the fovea with adjacent retinal thickening

3. At least one disc area of retinal thickening, any part of which is within one disc diameter of the center of the fovea.

Table 54-4 Clinically significant macular edema

Definition
1. Retinal thickening at or within 500 μm of the center of macula
2. Hard exudates at or within 500 μm from the center of the macula with associated thickening of the adjacent retina
3. Retinal thickening at least 1 disc diameter in size, any part of which lies within 1 disc diameter of the center of the macula

Visual acuity is an important parameter in following the progression of CSME, although it does not aid in the diagnosis of CSME because patients may have a visual acuity of 20/20 with co-existing CSME. The status of the posterior hyaloid, if detached, taut, thickened should also be noted.

MANAGEMENT

The goal of treatment is to decrease retinal edema which may result in visual gain in some patients. It is important to treat any pre-existing CSME prior to cataract surgery, as cataract surgery may aggravate the macular edema. Cataract surgery can be performed after the macular edema resolves. However, if there is significant cataract which precludes adequate examination or treatment with focal photocoagulation of macular edema, it may still be possible to obtain a pre-operative OCT to determine if central macular edema is present. If so, off-label pharmacotherapy with intravitreal triamcinolone or bevacizumab as per below can be initiated prior to cataract surgery. Pre- and postoperative management options for CSME are listed below and can be used simultaneously.

SYSTEMIC TREATMENT

Hypertension, renal failure, congestive heart failure may worsen DME. Control of blood pressure and diuresis may decrease retinal capillary perfusion pressure with reduction of macular edema.

PHOTOCOAGULATION

Macular photocoagulation is indicated for clinically significant macular edema and despite recent off-label use of pharmacotherapy remains the gold standard. Photocoagulation is performed for macular thickening, and not fluorescein angiographic leakage, which can often be seen without clinical evidence of thickening.

Photocoagulation is beneficial for both diffuse and focal retinal thickening, though the benefit appears greater for focal retinal thickening. The Early Treatment Diabetic Retinopathy Study group showed that macular photocoagulation is beneficial in treating macular edema and stabilizing the vision.[30] Photocoagulation decreases the risk of significant visual loss, defined as doubling of the visual angle, by about 50% at the end of 3 years. This benefit was seen regardless of the baseline vision or angiographic characteristics. However, these reports stress that laser treatment does not necessarily improve vision. Patients should be reviewed 2–3 months after macular photocoagulation to assess the need for additional macular laser if macular edema persists.

PHARMACOLOGIC TREATMENT

Various steroids and anti-vascular endothelial growth factors (VEGF) are in clinical trials for use in DME. The anti-VEGF agents pegaptanib (Macugen) and ranibizumab (Lucentis), which are USFDA approved for the treatment of age-related macular degeneration, are under evaluation for the treatment of DME.[31,32] Triamcinolone acetonide has been found to be useful in reducing macular edema, but the need for repeated injections and the risks of cataract and glaucoma have been concerning factors. However, the success of intravitreal triamcinolone acetonide as well as bevacizumab in reducing macular edema has been such that, despite the lack of data from randomized controlled clinical trials, off-label pharmacotherapy has been adopted by many retina specialists as a key element in the management of CSME. The Diabetic Retinopathy Clinical Research network has completed enrollment in a study that compares triamcinolone acetonide to laser photocoagulation for the treatment of CSME but as of this date no results are available. Other steroids that are being evaluated in clinical trials are delivered in drug-delivery implants in the hopes of providing more durable control. They include Posurdex, a dexamethasone based injectable biodegradable drug delivery system (Allergan Pharmaceuticals),[33] Medidur, a fluocinolone acetonide injectable non-biodegradable implant (Alimera Sciences),[34] and I-vation, a triamcinolone acetonide helical coil implant (Surmodics),[35] all of which are in phase 3 clinical trial testing for CSME.

SURGICAL MANAGEMENT

Occasionally, the cause of CSME may be due to vitreomacular traction or taut posterior hyaloid. Evaluation with OCT is beneficial in this setting. When either condition is encountered, and is felt to be the main cause of vision loss, pars plana vitrectomy with removal of vitreo-retinal attachments and the posterior hyaloid is indicated.[36]

■ EPIRETINAL MEMBRANE ■

In early stages, epiretinal membrane (ERM) may be asymptomatic, or it may create only a minor reduction in acuity. Its progression may cause metamorphopsia and lead to severe visual impairment. The incidence of mild ERM may almost double within 1 year of cataract surgery, although this may not cause significant visual impairment.[37]

PATHOPHYSIOLOGY

ERM formation occurs as a result of retinal glial cell proliferation along the surface of the internal limiting membrane (ILM). Small, focal defects in the ILM allow these cells to "break through" to the retinal–vitreous interface and reproduce, creating a thin veil of tissue. ERMs have been found in association with retinal vascular diseases, retinal breaks and detachments, ocular trauma, uveitis, and following retinal cryopexy, laser photocoagulation, and intraocular surgery.[38] Often, the membranes occur idiopathically in patients over 50 years of age.[39]

EXAMINATION

The ophthalmoscopic picture of ERM varies from a fine, glistening membrane overlying the macula (cellophane maculopathy), to a thick opaque scar that obscures the underlying vasculature.

As the ERM progresses, traction at the macula creates a puckering effect that may be seen as retinal folds radiating outward from the macula. Vision in eyes with ERM may be reduced through various causes that may include full-thickness retinal folds, foveal ectopia, macular edema or a dense opaque membrane. Early identification of ERM requires careful inspection with a slit-lamp fundus lens (78 diopter (D), 90 D or Goldmann lens). Both OCT and fluorescein angiography are useful for confirming the presence of ERMs. Typical fluorescein patterns in

ERM show "corkscrew" distortion and dragging of the retinal vessels at the posterior pole, with a characteristic diminishing of the foveal avascular zone. OCT findings including macular edema, ERM with macular pucker, vitreomacular traction, and cystic changes are readily visible on the OCT scans.

MANAGEMENT

Most patients suffer only a minimal reduction of acuity or slight metamorphopsia. Reassurance as to the nature of the disorder and follow-up periodically, using an Amsler grid for home monitoring of progression, is all that may be required. In severe cases, vision may drop to 20/50 or worse, and this may indicate the need for vitrectomy and surgical peeling of the membrane.

■ RETINAL VEIN OCCLUSION ■

SIGNS AND SYMPTOMS

The patient will usually be elderly, often with a history of systemic diseases such as diabetes and hypertension. The patient may be asymptomatic, but often will complain of sudden painless unilateral loss of vision and/or visual field, and may complain of a sudden onset of floating spots or flashing lights. Acuity may range anywhere from 20/20 to finger counting. If vision loss is severe, there may be a relative afferent pupillary defect.

Ophthalmoscopically, in central retinal vein occlusion (CRVO), there will be retinal edema, intraretinal hemorrhages in all four quadrants, disc swelling, cotton wool spots, and tortuous and dilated retinal veins. A hemi-central retinal vein occlusion will involve only the superior or inferior half of the retina. A branch retinal vein occlusion will present with findings in only one quadrant, usually supero-temporal, with the apex of the hemorrhages at an arteriovenous crossing.

The hemorrhaging may be so severe that all features of the underlying retina are obscured. Multiple cotton wool spots indicate retinal ischemia and capillary non-perfusion. Anterior and posterior segment neovascularization may occur later in the disease.

PATHOPHYSIOLOGY

The etiology of central and hemi-central retinal vein occlusion is an obstruction of the central retinal vein, or one of the vein's two trunks, as it constricts through the lamina cribrosa.[40] The cause is obscure, but may involve abnormal blood flow or blood constituents, atherosclerosis, vessel anomalies or a combination of these factors.

The etiology of a branch retinal vein occlusion is an arteriolosclerotic arteriole crossing and constricting the underlying venule.[41] This will result in leakage from the capillary beds draining into these vessels. The capillary beds may be irreversibly damaged by this leakage, resulting in perpetual non-perfusion of the retinal tissue. If a significant area of capillary non-perfusion is present, then the occlusion is considered ischemic. Loss of retinal capillary beds with subsequent retinal non-perfusion will lead to retinal hypoxia and the subsequent release of vasoproliferative substance. Vasoproliferative factors will then stimulate the proliferation of neovascularization from nearby viable capillary beds.

In branch and hemi-central occlusions, neovascularization will most often form on the optic disc or adjacent retina and can lead to vitreous hemorrhage and tractional retinal detachment. In central retinal vein occlusions, the closest viable capillary network from which neovascularization will form is typically the posterior iris. This can lead to rubeosis irides and neovascular glaucoma. In all cases of venous occlusion, the main cause of vision impairment is macular edema, which is caused by the increased venous pressure. However, if retinal capillary non-perfusion involves the perifoveal region, then vision is dramatically and irreversibly lost.

MANAGEMENT

Fluorescein angiography, which was long held to be the gold standard in assessing retinal vascular disease, is not indicated initially, as the fresh hemorrhage will block transmission and reveal no useful information. Later in the course of the disease, it can provide useful information about retinal capillary perfusion and whether or not the occlusion is ischemic, and also about any areas of retinal neovascularization. OCT is useful in quantitating and monitoring the course of macular edema. Ischemic central retinal vein occlusions do not benefit from prophylactic panretinal photocoagulation and it is best to withhold this procedure until the patient develops frank neovascularization of the iris, disc or retina. These patients also do not benefit from grid photocoagulation for macular edema.[42] Intravitreal triamcinolone and anti-VEGF agents may be useful in treating the macular edema and improving the vision, although evidence from large prospective randomized studies is not available.

Patients need to be monitored monthly with serial ophthalmoscopy, fundus photography and gonioscopy until the neovascularization resolves. If the patient has a hemi-central or branch retinal vein occlusion and vision is below 20/40 due to macular edema, the patient may benefit from focal laser photocoagulation anywhere between three and 18 months after the occlusion's onset.[43] Since vein occlusions have an association with systemic disease, it is essential to have an internist evaluate the patient. Tests to be ordered include blood pressure, fasting blood glucose, lipid and cholesterol studies.

■ MACULAR HOLE ■

SIGNS AND SYMPTOMS

Idiopathic or senile macular holes are typically encountered in patients older than 60, and occur slightly more often in women than in men. Presenting symptoms include decreased central acuity, a central scotoma and/or metamorphopsia. The various stages of macular hole include: foveal detachments (stage I), partial-thickness holes (stage II), and full-thickness holes (stage III). A stage IV macular hole is an advanced full-thickness hole, with vitreous separation from the optic disc and macula.[44] Depending on the stage, vision may range from 20/20 to <20/400, although in full-thickness macular holes, the visual acuity is generally 20/80 to 20/200. Patients usually report blurring of central vision or metamorphopsia in one eye when they cover the other eye.

The best way to examine the macula is with a contact fundus lens. For suspected macular holes that appear equivocal, the Watzke-Allen test can be useful. A vertical beam of light is projected at the fovea, using a slit-lamp beam with a fundus lens or a direct ophthalmoscope. The patient is asked if the line is uniform or broken in the center. Patients with full-thickness macular hole will report a broken line. A full-thickness macular hole clinically appears as a round, brick-colored lesion in the center of the macula, usually one-third to two-thirds of a disc diameter. The surrounding retinal tissue appears gray and elevated, and often there are small yellow deposits within the hole (Klein's tags), reminiscent of drusen. Foveal detachments and partial-thickness holes do not appear red, but rather present as a loss of the foveolar depression with the development of a central yellow spot or ring. Stage II holes are accompanied by a red, crescent-shaped retinal break at the lesion's edge. OCT is the confirmatory test to be performed in patients with suspected macular hole. Fluorescein angiography reveals an RPE "window defect" with early-stage hyperfluorescence.

PATHOPHYSIOLOGY

Controversy surrounds the etiology of idiopathic macular holes. Diverse mechanisms have been proposed, including systemic vascular disease, hormonal variations, cystic retinal degeneration, anterior vitreoretinal traction, and tangential vitreoretinal tractional forces.[45] Currently, the most widely held theory proposes that pre-foveal vitreal shrinkage induces tangential traction on the fovea, eventually promoting hole formation. As contraction ensues, the tangential tugging at the fovea induces a separation of the sensory retina from the underlying RPE. Ultimately, the sensory retina atrophies, forming a break and progressing to a full-thickness hole. Macular holes may also result from chronic macular edema, solar retinopathy and blunt ocular trauma.

MANAGEMENT

Untreated 50% of stage I holes will progress to stage II, and 70% of stage II holes will progress to stage III. Pars plana vitrectomy, excision of the attached cortical vitreous with or without peeling of the internal limiting membrane and fluid–gas exchange with perfluropropane is the standard of care. Candidates for surgical intervention usually have 20/50 visual acuity or worse. OCT is a useful guide to determine the dimensions of a full-thickness hole which can help guide in surgical decision making.

▮ MACULAR DEGENERATION ▮

Age-related macular degeneration (AMD) is the leading cause of blindness in individuals over the age of 50 years in developed countries.[46–48] Early manifestations of AMD include focal drusen associated with minor visual complaints, but the later stages of the disease result in severe vision loss. The nonexudative or dry form of AMD is approximately 10 times more prevalent than the exudative form, but the latter is the leading cause of blindness from AMD.

Examination of the other eye may give a very important clue if the fundus of the eye to be operated can not be visualized preoperatively.

PREVALENCE

The prevalence of exudative AMD in the Framingham Eye Study was 1.5%, while the dry type of AMD accounted for 90% of all cases.[49] The Beaver Dam Eye Study defined early age-related maculopathy (ARM) as the presence of any drusen (except for hard, distinct drusen) with degeneration of the retinal pigment epithelium (RPE) or increased pigment in the macular area. It defined late ARM or AMD as the presence of geographic atrophy or exudative disease or both. The prevalence of late ARM was 1.6% in the Beaver Dam eye study,[50] and exudative maculopathy in at least one eye was present in 1.2% of the population. The prevalence of late ARM was 7.1% in subjects older than 75 years.

RISK FACTORS

DEMOGRAPHIC FACTORS

All studies indicate that both the prevalence and the incidence of all forms of AMD increase with age. The Framingham Study found a 17-fold increased risk of AMD when comparing the oldest to the youngest age group.[49] Several studies indicate a genetic factor in the pathogenesis of the disease.[51] Those examining the concordance of AMD in monozygotic and dizygotic twins strongly support the role of genetics in the pathogenesis of AMD.[52]

LIFESTYLE FACTORS

Most of the epidemiological evidence indicates a strong positive association between dry and wet AMD with smoking.[53] Supplementation with zinc and vitamins A, C, and E helped prevent wet AMD as well as advance atrophic AMD in the Age-Related Eye Diseases Study (AREDS).[54]

Excessive exposure to light can damage the retina. In the Beaver Dam Eye Study, participants exposed to the summer sun for more than 5 h a day during their teens, in their 30s, and at the baseline examination were at a higher risk of developing increased retinal pigmentation and early ARM by 10 years than those exposed less than 2 h per day during the same periods.[55] The shorter wavelengths of light pose the greatest hazard to the retinal photoreceptors, because they contain more energy. Exposure to these wavelengths has been called the *blue–light hazard*, because they appear blue to the human eye. It has also been suggested that the removal of the natural lens, as in cataract surgery, should be followed by replacement with a tinted IOL to restore the eye's natural barrier to light radiation.[56] (See Chapter 41 for a full discussion of spectral factors and vision)

CARDIOVASCULAR FACTORS

High cholesterol, especially HDL cholesterol[57,58] and oxidized LDL,[59] as well as hypertension,[60,61] have been associated with a higher incidence of AMD. In the Macular Photocoagulation Study, there was an increased risk of exudative AMD associated with hypertension in the second eye of individuals with exudative AMD in one eye at baseline.

OCULAR RISK FACTORS

The Macular Photocoagulation Study group described the risk factors for a patient's developing choroidal neovascularization (CNV) in his fellow eye when his opposite eye already has

CNV. They include five or more drusen, focal hyperpigmentation, one or more large drusen (>63 μm), and systemic hypertension.[62] Based on the follow-up of patients with juxtafoveal CNV, the 5-year incidence rate for the development of CNV was 87% if all four risk factors were present. Lanchoney et al reported that the 10-year risk of developing CNV in patients with bilateral soft drusen ranged from 8.6% to 15.9%.[63] Hyperopia has a higher association with AMD, whereas darker irides may be protective against AMD.[64,65]

PROTECTIVE MECHANISMS IN THE RETINA AND CRYSTALLINE LENS

Carotenoids, including the xanthophyllic yellow pigments lutein and zeaxanthin, protect the macula from damaging blue light because of their maximum absorption spectrum at the lower wavelengths. When molecules within the retinal pigment epithelium (RPE) absorb blue light, however, the formation of free radicals ensues, leading to cellular injury.[66] The crystalline lens is the major protective barrier to near-UV radiation (between 300 and 400 nm). Yellowing of the natural crystalline lens results in a greater absorbance of light of lower wavelengths such as blue light.[67]

Data from the Framingham Eye Study showed that nuclear cataracts were associated with a slightly reduced incidence of mild-to-severe macular changes compared with cortical cataracts.[68] Recent analysis of data from the AREDS showed no correlation between cataract surgery and the development of advanced neovascular AMD, although there was a possible risk of advancing geographic atrophy.[69] In a subset analysis of patients in the AREDS who underwent cataract surgery, the risk for developing exudative (neovascular) AMD after cataract surgery was only 1% greater when compared with subjects who did not undergo cataract surgery, but the risk for developing advanced geographic atrophy was 47% greater in patients who underwent cataract surgery. Recently, Alcon Laboratories, Inc. (Fort Worth, TX), began marketing the Acrysof Natural lens, an IOL that blocks both UV radiation and blue light.[70] Researchers have demonstrated that yellow-tinted IOLs reduce the death of RPE laden with the lipofuscin fluorophore A2E.[71] Moreover, the incidence of CNV in patients with bilateral drusen and pigmentary changes was much higher in eyes that received untinted IOLs than in phakic fellow eyes.[72] However, the use of blue-blocking IOLs has been controversial. Blue-blocking IOLs may affect color and scotopic vision especially in the elderly,[73] but no studies to date have been conducted to prove this hypothesis.

PHOTODYNAMIC THERAPY

In photodynamic therapy (PDT), tissues treated with photosensitizers (verteporfin) are exposed to low-intensity light exposure to produce a photochemical effect. It causes selective destruction of CNV with preservation of the overlying neurosensory retina (Table 54.5).

The efficacy and safety of Verteporfin therapy were studied in the treatment of AMD with photodynamic therapy (TAP) investigation. In the total population, the treatment benefit was sustained at month 24, with fewer verteporfin-treated patients (47%) having moderate vision loss compared with patients given placebo (62%).[74]

Table 54-5 Treatment options for choroidal neovascular membrane (CNVM) in exudative age-related macular degeneration

Lesion	Treatment
Extrafoveal	Thermal laser
Juxtafoveal	Thermal laser, ranibizumab or bevacizumab, pegaptanib, or PDT (with or without steroid adjuvant
Subfoveal, predominantly classic	Ranibizumab, bevacizumab, PDT (with steroid), pegaptanib
Subfoveal, minimally classic, less than 4 MPS disc area	Ranibizumab, bevacizumab, PDT (with steroid), pegaptanib
Subfoveal, minimally classic, greater than four MPS disc area	Ranibizumab, bevacizumab, pegaptanib
Subfoveal, occult only with no classic	Ranibizumab, bevacizumab, PDT (with steroid), pegaptanib

PDT: Photodynamic therapy; MPS: macular photocoagulation study

The Verteporfin in Photodynamic Therapy (VIP) trial, another large-scale, double-masked, placebo-controlled, randomized clinical trial, investigated the efficacy of verteporfin therapy in a different group of patients from those in the TAP Investigation. The study mainly included patients with occult with no classic CNV with presumed recent disease progression, and patients with AMD who had classic CNV and visual acuity better than an approximate Snellen equivalent of 20/40.[75] At 24 months, the risk of moderate and severe vision loss was significantly reduced in verteporfin-treated patients compared with patients given placebo. The treatment benefit of verteporfin therapy was greater for patients with occult with no classic CNV who presented with *either* smaller lesions (= 4 MPS disc areas), *or* lower levels of visual acuity ($\leq 20/50^{-1}$ approximate Snellen equivalent). PDT helps prevent severe visual loss, but improvement of visual acuity is rare.

PHARMACOLOGIC INTERVENTION

The recent approval of ranibizumab (Lucentis, Genentech) as well as the off-label use of bevacizumab (Avastin, Genentech) has for the first time provided an effective treatment for choroidal neovascularization associated with AMD that results in improvement in vision in a significant number of patients. Pharmacotherapy not only avoids laser-induced damage to the overlying retina, but also may serve as either an adjunct or sole treatment of poorly defined lesions, occult lesions, and may prevent recurrences. At present the therapies are based on either inhibition of vascular endothelial growth factor (VEGF) or use of various formulations of steroids to control the inflammatory response associated with CNV.

Rosenfeld and colleagues published a case report in July 2005 describing encouraging results with off-label use of intravitreal bevacizumab (the monoclonal antibody to vascular endothelial growth factor, VEGF) for exudative AMD.[76] The suggestion of the potential clinical efficacy of intravitreal bevacizumab, coupled with the impressive results from two phase 3 clinical trials of intravitreal ranibizumab (the Fab fragment to the VEGF monoclonal antibody) in patients with choroidal neovascularization due to AMD had led to the widespread use of intravitreal bevacizumab for AMD.

Bevacizumab (Avastin™) is an anti-VEGF antibody approved by FDA in USA and Europe for use in treatment of metastatic colorectal cancers and is reported to bind to all known isoforms of VEGF. Spaide and colleagues reported a retrospective study of 266 patients treated with bevacizumab for ARMD and observed improvement in visual acuity, macular thickness.[77] No significant ocular or systemic side effects were observed.

Ranibizumab (Lucentis™) is a monoclonal antibody fragment against VEGF-A that has been affinity matured to provide stronger binding. In the MARINA study at 12 months, 94.6% of those given ranibizumab 0.5 mg lost fewer than 15 letters, as compared with 62.2% of patients receiving sham injections.[78] Visual acuity improved by 15 or more letters in 33.8% of the 0.5 mg group, as compared with 5.0% of the sham-injection group. Mean increases in visual acuity was 7.2 letters in the 0.5 mg group, as compared with a decrease of 10.4 letters in the sham-injection group. The benefit in visual acuity was maintained at 24 months.

Pegaptanib sodium (Macugenä, anti-VEGF$_{165}$ aptamer) is an FDA approved anti-VEGF agent. Aptamers are oligonucleotides that are designed to bind to specific molecular targets. This agent is a polyethylene glycol (PEG)-conjugated oligonucleotide that binds specifically to the VEGF165 isoform.[79] Pegaptanib is administered intravitreally every 6 weeks. The 2-year efficacy results of the VEGF inhibition study in ocular neovascularization (V.I.S.I.O.N.) trial have been published recently,[80] and has shown that patients who continued to receive pegaptanib injections were less likely to lose = 15 letters than those who discontinued treatment at 1 year ($P<0.05$). The number of patients who gained more than three lines of visual acuity at 54 weeks was not impressive.

It has been demonstrated that intravitreal triamcinolone acetonide could re-establish the blood–retinal barrier and down-regulate the inflammatory markers.[81] However, Triamcinolone Acetonide seems to be ineffective as monotherapy in the treatment of CNV.[82] It may be potentially effective as an adjunct to PDT,[83,84] but it is associated to numerous side effects, such as elevated intraocular pressure (25–30%), cataract formation or progression (25–75%), infectious (0.87% range 0–2.3%) or presumed noninfectious endophthalmitis.[85,86]

PHOTIC INJURY

Photic injury of the macula is an uncommon condition and the exact incidence is not known. Clinical features include blurring of vision, paracentral scotoma and a round to oval hypopigmented lesion at the macula due to RPE atrophy. Although there is no known treatment, it can be prevented by using the minimum possible intensity of illumination during surgery, especially after placing the IOL, and using a filter to block the central light from the microscope whenever possible.

CONCLUSIONS

Various macular disorders may affect complete recovery of vision after cataract surgery. All patients planned for cataract surgery should have preoperative evaluation of the fundus. This will not only help in prognosticating as well as adequate management of the condition prior to cataract surgery when possible, but also give the patient a realistic expectation of postoperative recovery of vision. All patients with poor postoperative vision should have a retinal evaluation to rule out any macular causes of poor postoperative vision. Many of the macular diseases can be treated and may help in the visual rehabilitation of the patient.

References

[1] Irvine SR. A newly described vitreous syndrome following cataract surgery, interpreted according to recent concepts of the structure of the vitreous. AJO 1953;36:599–619.

[2] Hitchings RA, Chisholm IH. Incidence of aphakic macular edema: a prospective study. Br J Ophthalmol 1975;59:444–450.

[3] Wright PL, Wilkinson CP, Balyeat HD, et al. Angiographic cystoid macular edema after posterior chamber lens implantation. Arch Ophthalmol 1988;106:740–744.

[4] Ursell PG, Spalton DJ, Whitcup SM, Nussenblatt RB. Cystoid macular edema after phacoemulsification: relationship to blood–aqueous barrier damage and visual acuity. J Cataract Refract Surg 1999;25:1492–1497.

[5] Stark WJ, Maumenee AE, Fagadau W, et al. Cystoid macular edema in pseudophakia. Surv Ophthalmol 1984;28:442–451.

[6] Wright PL, Wilkinson CP, Balyeat HD, Popham J, Reinke M. Angiographic cystoid macular edema after posterior chamber lens implantation. Arch Ophthalmol 1988;106:740–744.

[7] Fine BS, Brucker AJ. Macular edema and cystoid macular edema. Am J Ophthalmol 1981;92:466–481.

[8] Gass JDM. Stereoscopic atlas of macular diseases. 3rd ed. St. Louis: Mosby; 1987.

[9] Tolentino FI, Schepens CL. Edema of the posterior pole after cataract extraction: a biomicroscopic study. Arch Ophthalmol 1965;74:781–786.

[10] Schepens CL, Avila MP, Jalkh AE, et al. Role of the vitreous in cystoid macular edema. Surv Ophthalmol 1984;28:499–504.

[11] Jaffe NS, Luscombe SM, Clayman HM. A fluorescein angiographic study of cystoid macular edema. AJO 1981;92:775–780.

[12] Nussenblatt RB, Kaufman SC, Palestine AG, et al. Macular thickening and visual acuity: measurement in patients with cystoid macular edema. Ophthalmology 1987;94:1134–1139.

[13] Voo I, Mavrofrides EC, Puliafito CA. Clinical applications of optical coherence tomography for the diagnosis and management of macular diseases. Ophthalmol Clin North Am 2004;17:21–31.

[14] Konstantopoulos A, Williams CP, Luff AJ. Outcome of intravitreal triamcinolone acetonide in postoperative cystoid macular oedema. Eye 2008;22:219–222. Epub 2006 Sep 29.

[15] Sivaprasad S, Bunce C, Wormald R. Non-steroidal anti-inflammatory agents for cystoid macular oedema following cataract surgery: a systematic review. Br J Ophthalmol 2005;89:1420–1422.

[16] Flach AJ, Stegman RC, Graham J, Kruger LP. Prophylaxis of aphakic cystoid macular edema without corticosteroids. Ophthalmology 1990;97:1253–1258.

[17] Jampol LM. Pharmacologic therapy of aphakic and pseudopakic cystoid macular edema. Ophthalmology 1984;92:807–810.

[18] Flach AJ, Jampol LM, Weinberg D, et al. Improvement in visual acuity in chronic aphakic and pseudophakic cystoid macular edema after treatment with topical 0.5% ketorolac tromethamine. Am J Ophthalmol 1991;112:514–519.

[19] Donnenfeld ED, Perry HD, Wittpenn JR, Solomon R, Nattis A, Chou T. Preoperative ketorolac tromethamine 0.4% in phacoemulsification outcomes: pharmacokinetic-response curve. J Cataract Refract Surg 2006;32:1474–1482.

[20] Group Italian Diclofenac Study. Efficacy of diclofenac eyedrops in preventing postoperative inflammation and long-term cystoid macular edema. J Cataract Refract Surg 1997;23:1183–1189.

[21] Steinert RF, Wasson PJ. Neodymium:YAG laser anterior vitreolysis for Irvine-Gass cystoid macular edema. J Cataract Refract Surg 1989;15:304–307.

[22] Fung WE. Vitrectomy for chronic aphakic cystoid macular edema. Ophthalmology 1985;92:1102–1111.

[23] Kim SJ, Equi R, Bressler NM. Analysis of macular edema after cataract surgery in patients with diabetes using optical coherence tomography. Ophthalmology 2007;114:881–889, Epub 2007 Feb 1.

[24] Early Treatment Diabetic Retinopathy Study Research Group. Photocoagulation for diabetic macular edema: relationship of treatment effect to retinal angiographic and retinal characteristics at baseline. ETDRS report no. 19. Arch Ophthalmol 1995;113:1144–1155.

[25] Frank RN, Keirn RJ, Kennedy A, Frank KW. Galactose-induced retinal capillary basement membrane thickening: prevention by sorbinil. IOVS 1983;24:1519–1524.

[26] Wallow IHL, Engeman RL. Permeability and patency of retinal blood vessels in experimental diabetes. IOVS 1977;16:447–461.

[27] Pino RM, Essner E. Permeability of rat choriocapillaris to hemoproteins: restriction of tracers by a fenestrated endothelium. Cogan DG, Toussaint D, and Kuwabara T. Retinal vascular patterns. IV. Diabetic Retinopathy. Arch Ophthalmol 1961;66:366–378.

[28] Cogan DG, Toussaint D, Kuwabara T. Retinal vascular patterns. IV. Diabetic retinopathy. Arch Ophthalmol 1961;66:366–378.

[29] Control Diabetes, Group Complications Trial Research. Perspectives in diabetes: the absence of a glycemic threshold for the development of long-term complications: the perspective of the Diabetes Control and Complications Trial. Diabetes 1996;45:1289–1298.

[30] Early Treatment Diabetic Retinopathy Study Research Group. Photocoagulation for diabetic macular edema, ETDRS report No. 1. Arch Ophthalmol 1985;103:1796–1806.

[31] Cunningham ET Jr, Adamis AP, Altaweel M, Aiello LP, Bressler NM, D'Amico DJ, et al. Macugen Diabetic Retinopathy Study Group. A phase II randomized double-masked trial of pegaptanib, an anti-vascular endothelial growth factor aptamer, for diabetic macular edema. Ophthalmology 2005;112:1747–1757.

[32] Chun DW, Heier JS, Topping TM, Duker JS, Bankert JM. A pilot study of multiple intravitreal injections of ranibizumab in patients with center-involving clinically significant diabetic macular edema. Ophthalmology 2006;113:1706–1712.

[33] Narayanan R, Kuppermann BD. Anti-VEGF agents for macular edema secondary to retinal vascular disorders. Retinal Physician March 2006.

[34] Ober MD, Klais CM, Cunningham ET Jr. Management options for macular edema. Review of Ophthalmology October 2005.

[35] Callanan DG. Novel intravitreal fluocinolone acetonide implant in the treatment of chronic non-infectious posterior uveitis. Expert Review of Ophthalmology 2007;2:33–34.

[36] Pournaras CJ, Kapetanios AD, Donati G. Vitrectomy for traction macular edema. Doc Ophthalmol 1999;97:439–447.

[37] Jahn CE, Minich V, Moldaschel S, et al. Epiretinal membranes after extracapsular cataract surgery (1). J Cataract Refract Surg 2001;27:753–760.

[38] Appiah AP, Hirose T. Secondary causes of premacular fibrosis. Ophthalmology 1989;96:38–392.

[39] McDonald HR, Aaberg TM. Idiopathic epiretinal membranes. Semin Ophthalmol 1986;1:89–95.

[40] Green WR, Chan CC, Hutchins GM, Terry JM. Central retinal vein occlusion: a prospective histopathologic study of 29 eyes in 28 cases. Retina 1981;1:27–55.

[41] Zhao J, Sastry SM, Sperduto RD, Chew EY, Remaley NA. Aretrovenous crossing patterns in branch retinal vein occlusion: They Eye Disease Case Control Study Group. Ophthalmology 1993;100:423–428.

[42] Group The Central Vein Occlusion Study. Natural history and clinical management of central retinal vein occlusion. Arch Ophthalmol 1997;115:486–491.

[43] Group Branch Vein Occlusion Study. Argon laser photocoagulation for macular edema in branch retinal vein occlusion. Am J Ophthalmol 1984;98:271–282.

[44] Gass JD. Reappraisal of biomicroscopic classification of stages of development of macular hole. Am J Ophthalmol 1995;119:752–759.

[45] Gass JDM. Stereoscopic atlas of macular diseases: diagnosis and treatment. 3rd ed. St Louis: Mosby; 1987.

[46] Kahn HA, Moorhead HB. Statistics on blindness in the model reporting areas 1969–1970. United States Department of Health, Education and Welfare (NIH). Washington, DC: US Government printing office; 1973.

[47] Wormald R. Assessing the prevalence of eye disease in the community. Eye 1995;9:674–676.

[48] Bird AC. Age-related macular disease. Br J Ophthalmol 1996;80:1–2.

[49] Leibowitz HM, Krueger DE, Maunder LR, et al. The Framingham Eye Study monograph: an ophthalmological and epidemiological study of cataract, glaucoma, diabetic retinopathy, macular degeneration, and visual acuity in a general population of 2631 adults, 1973–1975. Surv Ophthalmol 1980;24:335–610.

[50] Klein R, Klein BE, Linton KL. Prevalence of age-related maculopathy. The Beaver Dam Eye Study. Ophthalmology 1992;99:933–943.

[51] Piguet B, Wells JA, Palmvang IB, et al. Age-related Bruch's membrane change: a clinical study of the relative role of heredity and environment. Br J Ophthalmol 1993;77:400–403.

[52] Seddon JM, Cote J, Page WF, Aggen SH, Neale MC. The US twin study of age-related macular degeneration: relative roles of genetic and environmental influences. Arch Ophthalmol 2005;123:321–327.

[53] Age-Related Eye Disease Study Research Group. Risk factors associated with age-related macular degeneration. A case-control study in the age-related eye disease study: Age-Related Eye Disease Study report number 3. Ophthalmology 2000;107:2224–2232.

[54] Age-Related Eye Disease Study Research Group. A randomized, placebo-controlled, clinical trial of high-dose supplementation with vitamins C and E, beta carotene, and zinc for age-related macular degeneration and vision loss: AREDS report no. 8. Arch Ophthalmol 2001;119:1417–1436.

[55] Tomany SC, Cruickshanks KJ, Klein R, et al. Sunlight and the 10-year incidence of age-related maculopathy: the Beaver Dam Eye Study. Arch Ophthalmol 2004;122:750–757.

[56] Okuno T, Saito H, Ojima J. Evaluation of blue-light hazards from various light sources. Dev Ophthalmol 2002;35:104–112.

[57] Tomany SC, Wang JJ, Van Leeuwen R, et al. Risk factors for incident age-related macular degeneration: pooled findings from 3 continents. Ophthalmology 2004;111:1280–1287.

[58] Van Leeuwen R, Klaver CC, Vingerling JR, et al. Cholesterol and age-related macular degeneration: is there a link? Am J Ophthalmol 2004;137:750–752.

[59] Ikeda T, Obayashi H, Hasegawa G, et al. Paraoxonase gene polymorphisms and plasma oxidized low-density lipoprotein level as possible risk factors for exudative age-related macular degeneration. Am J Ophthalmol 2001;132:191–195.

[60] Age-Related Eye Disease Study Research Group. Risk factors associated with age-related macular degeneration. A case-control study in the age-related eye disease study: Age-Related Eye Disease Study report number 3. Ophthalmology 2000;107:2224–2232.

[61] Klein R, Peto T, Bird A, Vannewkirk MR. The epidemiology of age-related macular degeneration. Am J Ophthalmol 2000;137:486–495.

[62] Macular photocoagulation study group. Risk factors for choroidal neovascularization in the second eye of patients with juxtafoveal or subfoveal choroidal neovascularization secondary to age-related macular degeneration. Arch Ophthalmol 1997;115:741–747.

[63] Lanchoney DM, Maguire MG, Fine SL. A model of the incidence and consequences of choroidal neovascularization secondary to age-related macular degeneration. Comparative effects of current treatment and potential prophylaxis on visual outcomes in high-risk patients. Arch Ophthalmol 1998;116:1045–1052.

[64] Age-Related Eye Disease Study Research Group. Risk factors associated with age-related macular degeneration. A case-control study in the age-related eye disease study: Age-Related Eye Disease Study Report Number 3. Ophthalmology 2000;107:2224–2232.

[65] Sandberg MA, Gaudio AR, Miller S, Weiner A. Iris pigmentation and extent of disease in patients with neovascular age-related macular degeneration. Invest Ophthalmol Vis Sci 1994;35:2734–2740.

[66] Sparrow JR, Zhou J, Ben Shabat S, et al. Involvement of oxidative mechanisms in blue-light-induced damage to A2E-laden RPE. Invest Ophthalmol Vis Sci 2002;43:1222–1227.

[67] Mellerio J. Yellowing of the human lens: nuclear and cortical contributions. Vision Res 1987;27:1581–1587.

[68] Sperduto RD, Hiller R, Seigel D. Lens opacities and senile maculopathy. Arch Ophthalmol 1981;99:1004–1008.

[69] Guttman C, Ferris FL. No link between cataract surgery, AMD, study shows, Ophthalmology Times 2003;28. Available: www.Ophthalmologytimes.com. [http://www.Ophthalmologytimes.com/Ophthalmologytimes/article/articleDetail.jspfiid=47063].

[70] Niwa K, Yoshino Y, Okuyama F, et al. Effects of tinted intraocular lens on contrast sensitivity. Ophthalmic Physiol Opt 1996;16:297–302.

[71] Sparrow JR, Miller AS, Zhou J. Blue light-absorbing intraocular lens and retinal pigment epithelium protection in vitro. J Cataract Refract Surg 2004;30:873–878.

[72] Pollack A, Marcovich A, Bukelman A, et al. Age-related macular degeneration after extracapsular cataract extraction with intraocular lens implantation. Ophthalmology 1996;103:1546–1554.

[73] Mainster MA. Intraocular lenses should block uv radiation and violet but not blue light. Arch Ophthalmol 2005;123:550–555.

[74] The Treatment of Age-Related Macular Degeneration with Photodynamic Therapy (TAP) Study Group. Photodynamic therapy of subfoveal choroidal neovascularization in age-related macular degeneration with verteporfin: two-year results of 2 randomized clinical trials-TAP report #2. Arch Ophthalmol 2001;119:198–207.

[75] The Verteporfin in Photodynamic Therapy (VIP) Study Group. Verteporfin therapy of subfoveal choroidal neovascularization in age-related macular degeneration: two-year results of a randomized clinical trial including lesions with occult no classic choroidal neovascularization-VIP report # 2. Am J Ophthalmol 2001;131:541–560.

[76] Rosenfeld PJ, Moshfeghi AA, Puliafito CA. Optical coherence tomography findings after an intravitreal injection of bevacizumab (avastin) for neovascular age-related macular degeneration. Ophthalmic Surg Lasers Imaging 2005;36:331–335.

[77] Spaide RF, Laud K, Fine HF, et al. Intravitreal bevacizumab treatment of choroidal neovascularization secondary to age-related macular degeneration. Retina 2006;26:383–390.

[78] Rosenfeld PJ, Brown DM, Heier JS, Boyer DS, Kaiser PK, Chung CY, et al. MARINA Study Group: Ranibizumab for neovascular age-related macular degeneration. N Engl J Med 2006;355:1419–1431.

[79] Group The Eyetech Study. Preclinical and phase IA clinical evaluation of an anti-VEGF pegylated aptamer (EYE001) for the treatment of exudative age-related macular degeneration. Retina 2002;22:143–152.

[80] Gragoudas ES, Adamis AP, Cunnigham Jr ET, et al. VEGF inhibition study in ocular neovascularization clinical trial group. Pegaptanib for neovascular age-related macular degeneration. N Engl J Med 2004;351:2805–2816.

[81] Penfold PL, Wen L, Madigan MC, et al. Triamcinolone acetonide modulates permeability and intercellular adhesion molecule-1 (ICAM-1) expression of the ECV304 cell line: implications for macular degeneration. Clin Exp Immunol 2000;121:458–465.

[82] Gillies MC, Simpson JM, Luo W, et al. A randomized clinical trial of a single dose of intravitreal triamcinolone acetonide for neovascular age-related macular degeneration: one-year results. Arch Ophthalmol 2003;121:667–673.

[83] Spaide RF, Sorenson J, Maranan L. Combined photodynamic therapy with verteporfin and intravitreal triamcinolone acetonide for choroidal neovascularization. Ophthalmology 2003;110:1517–1525.

[84] Rechtman E, Danis RP, Pratt LM, Harris A. Intravitreal triamcinolone with photodynamic therapy for subfoveal choroidal neovascularisation in age related macular degeneration. Br J Ophthalmol 2004;88:344–347.

[85] Roth DB, Chieh J, Spirn MJ, et al. Noninfectious endophthalmitis associated with intravitreal triamcinolone injection. Arch Ophthalmol 2003;121:1279–1282.

[86] Nelson ML, Tennant MT, Sivalingam A, et al. Infectious and presumed noninfectious endophthalmitis after intravitreal triamcinolone acetonide injection. Retina 2003;23:686–691.

Postoperative Endophthalmitis

David A. Eichenbaum, MD, Robert I. Park, MD
and Trexler M. Topping, MD

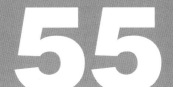

CONTENTS

CHAPTER HIGHLIGHTS

>> Clinical signs and symptoms

>> Differential diagnosis

>> Lessons from the Endophthalmitis Vitrectomy Study

>> Treatment protocols

Postoperative endophthalmitis is a rare but much feared complication of cataract surgery. The potential sequelae of untreated or late treated endophthalmitis include loss of vision, severe ocular damage, and, in some cases, phthisis bulbi or enucleation. However, early detection and treatment of endophthalmitis may limit damage, and patients may regain good vision. Early identification and prompt treatment or referral of endophthalmitis cases are thus crucial factors in salvaging a patient's vision.

This chapter addresses the issue of post-cataract extraction endophthalmitis and should not be directly extrapolated to cases of trauma or glaucoma filtration-related endophthalmitis because the mode of infection and the causative organisms are very different. Emphasis is placed on the results of the Endophthalmitis Vitrectomy Study (EVS), a randomized, prospective, multicenter trial evaluating the treatment of endophthalmitis following cataract surgery (see later description).

EPIDEMIOLOGY

A number of retrospective studies have been undertaken to define the incidence of endophthalmitis following cataract extraction.[1–7] The overall results appear in Table 55-1. The incidence of endophthalmitis has been reported to be between 0.04 and 0.22%.[1–5] It is worthy to note that incidences have been decreasing since the early 1990s, and in the more recent series, the majority of the surgeries have been performed using small-incision phacoemulsification. The most comprehensive review was performed by Javitt et al.,[4] who reviewed billing records for approximately 50% of all Medicare beneficiaries over the age of 65 who underwent cataract extraction in 1984. The incidence of endophthalmitis was found to be 0.17% for intracapsular cataract extraction and 0.12% for extracapsular cataract extraction. The primary criticism of Javitt's study is that it was based on a review of Medicare billing records. Although the results are likely to be unbiased, clinical information about each case was limited; that is, no data regarding the organisms or culture positivity or negativity were available. Although the exact incidence of endophthalmitis varied from study to study, all reported the incidence of endophthalmitis to be well below 0.5% following cataract surgery.

A number of factors that increase the risk of postoperative endophthalmitis have been identified. Diabetes mellitus, chronic alcoholism, complicated surgery, wound complications, intracapsular vs. extracapsular cataract extraction, capsular rupture, amount and duration of instrumentation, history of prior surgery, vitreous loss, and intraocular lens (IOL) type have been implicated with regard to the increased rate of endophthalmitis.[11–15] An interesting finding from Miller's recent study is that an increased incidence of endophthalmitis was found in right-eye surgery performed by right-handed surgeons through a temporal approach. This finding implicates an inferior incision location as an additional risk factor. Of particular note are data from

Table 55-1 Incidence of endophthalmitis after cataract surgery

Year	Author	Number of Charts	Overall Incidence	Culture (+) Incidence	Location
2004	Wong et al	44,804	0.076%	0.040	Singapore
2005	Miller et al	15,920	0.04%	0.03%	Miama, FL
1998	Aaberg et al[1]	41,654	0.082%	NA	Miami, FL
1991	Menikoff et al[2]	24,105	0.22%	0.17%	New York, NY
1991	Kattan et al[3]	30,002	0.089%	0.072%	Miami, FL
1991	Javitt et al[4]	338,141	0.13%	NA	Medicare database
1974	Allen and Mangiaracine[5]	36,000	NA	0.086	Boston, MA

NA, Not applicable.

Javitt's review of the Medicare database in 1991, which demonstrated that the incidence of endophthalmitis after cataract extraction with anterior vitrectomy was significantly higher than for cataract surgery alone (0.58% for cataract extraction with anterior vitrectomy vs. 0.13% for cataract surgery alone, $P < 0.0001$). Javitt's conclusion that complicated surgery increases the risk of infection has been supported in subsequent studies.[4,7–9]

CLINICAL PRESENTATION

A high level of clinical suspicion must be maintained during the examination of postoperative patients. A detailed history including the time course of onset of symptoms and a careful examination may increase the rate of early detection of endophthalmitis. The circumstances of the surgery and any intraoperative complications should be known to the examiner. Patients should be well informed of the signs of possible infection on the day of surgery, as well as during the postoperative visit, and should be instructed to contact the surgeon's office immediately should they develop postoperative problems. Early detection by patients may give the best hope for a good outcome. The surgeon should not fear overdiagnosis, because the sequelae of a missed diagnosis are severe.

SYMPTOMS

Blurred vision, a red eye, and pain are common complaints of patients developing endophthalmitis. Counterintuitively, blurred vision and a red eye were more common than pain as the presenting symptom in the EVS.[16] Table 55-2 summarizes the presenting symptoms in the EVS.

Table 55-2 Patients presenting with type of symptom in Endophthalmitis Vitrectomy Study[11]

Symptom	Percentage
Blurred vision	94.3%
Red eye	82.1%
Pain	74.3%
Swollen lid	34.5%

Table 55-3 Patients presenting at given periods after cataract extraction in Endophthalmitis Vitrectomy Study

Number of Days Post-cataract Extraction	Percentage of Endophthalmitis Patients
0–3 days	24%
4–7 days	37%
8–13 days	17%
2–6 weeks	22%

Data from Endophthalmitis Vitrectomy Study Group: Results of the endophthalmitis vitrectomy study: a randomized trial of immediate vitrectomy and of intravenous antibiotics for the treatment of postoperative bacterial endophthalmitis, *Arch Ophthalmol* 113:1479–1496, 1995.

The median time to presentation in the EVS was 6 days after cataract extraction, with a majority presenting within 2 weeks of cataract extraction. However, a significant number of patients (22%) presented after 2–6 weeks. Table 55-3 shows the distribution of time to presentation in the EVS.

Other studies demonstrate a similar time course, with a majority presenting between 3 and 10 days of surgery and 88% presenting within 6 weeks of surgery.[6,7,17,18] Late-onset endophthalmitis is discussed later in the chapter.

EXAMINATION

A thorough ocular examination should be performed. Common presenting signs in the EVS are listed in Table 55-4. Anterior segment examination may reveal conjunctival injection or chemosis, significant anterior segment inflammation, a hypopyon, an afferent pupillary defect, and a loss of red reflex. Corneal ring ulcers may be present in infections with streptococci, clostridia, and bacilli; in rare cases of *Clostridium endophthalmitis*, a gas bubble may be seen in the anterior chamber. Any abnormalities of the surgical wound(s) should be noted. Wound gape, vitreous wick, wound leaks, or torn or broken sutures, because they have been found to be associated with endophthalmitis. The wound should always be checked with a Seidel test.[19–23] Examination

Table 55-4 Incidence of ocular signs in Endophthalmitis Vitrectomy Study

Sign	Incidence
Hypopyon	85.7%
Red eye	82.1%
No view of retinal vessel	79.1%
Loss of red reflex	68.0%
Corneal infiltrate or ring ulcer	4.8%

Data from Endophthalmitis Vitrectomy Study Group: Results of the endophthalmitis vitrectomy study: a randomized trial of immediate vitrectomy and of intravenous antibiotics for the treatment of postoperative bacterial endophthalmitis, *Arch Ophthalmol* 113:1479–1496, 1995.

of the retina should be performed to assess the clarity of the ocular media and to determine the status of the retina. If no view of the retina is possible, ultrasound examination should be performed to assess for retinal detachment, retained lens fragments, choroidal thickening, or vitreous membranes.

■ DIFFERENTIAL DIAGNOSIS ■

A number of conditions may present with clinical findings similar to endophthalmitis, and a distinction between early endophthalmitis and other entities may be difficult to find. Retained nuclear fragments or a posteriorly displaced lens nucleus may cause severe intraocular inflammation.[24] The surgeon is generally aware of dislocation of any lens fragments; however, in the case of inadvertent lens particle dislocation, intraocular pressure may be useful in distinguishing lens particle inflammation from endophthalmitis. The intraocular pressure is more often elevated with lens particle retention than with endophthalmitis. Careful examination of the retina and vitreous for retained lens fragments, either by visualization or ultrasound, must be performed. Other causes of intraocular inflammation must be considered. Severe anterior segment inflammation and a hypopyon may accompany corneal ulcers without endophthalmitis (Figure 55-1).

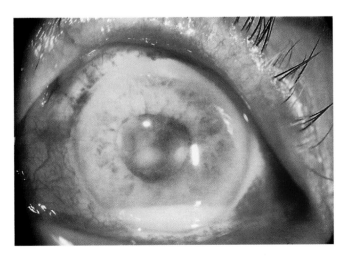

Figure 55-1 Hypopyon in patient with postoperative endophthalmitis.

Incarceration of vitreous in the surgical wound may cause an intraocular inflammation that is generally less severe than endophthalmitis but may be mistaken for early endophthalmitis. Intraocular blood may be mistaken for inflammation. Reaction to IOL materials and processing chemicals is rare today but must be considered; during the early days of IOLs, reactions to residual polishing compounds and sterilizing agents were reported.[25,26]

Alternative sources of endophthalmitis must also be considered during history taking. Concurrent infections, including dental abscesses, and previous surgery, especially glaucoma filtration surgery, are potential sources of seeding of bacteria into the eye and have broad implications regarding the infecting organism and potential clinical course.

Unfortunately, there is no specific combination of signs and symptoms that a surgeon may use to definitively diagnose endophthalmitis, especially early cases. It is especially imperative not to disregard inflammation following complicated surgery with posterior capsule rupture and lens particle loss as non-infectious, since data support complicated surgery as being a significant risk factor for infectious endophthalmitis.[4,7–9] Given the severity of the damage that may be inflicted by endophthalmitis, questionable cases should be treated empirically as endophthalmitis.

■ ENDOPHTHALMITIS VITRECTOMY STUDY ■

The EVS[16] was a National Eye Institute-funded multicenter, prospective, randomized trial evaluating the effectiveness of immediate vitrectomy and intravenous antibiotics in the treatment of postoperative bacterial endophthalmitis. Specifically, the EVS looked at 420 cases of endophthalmitis occurring after cataract extraction. Patients were randomized to either pars plana vitrectomy or vitreous needle biopsy, and intravenous antibiotics or no intravenous antibiotics. Study end-points were media clarity and visual acuity. All patients received the following:

1. Intravitreal vancomycin (1 mg/0.1 mL) and amikacin (0.4 mg in 0.1 mL)

2. Subconjunctival vancomycin (25 mg/0.5 mL), ceftazidime (100 mg/0.5 mL), and dexamethasone sodium phosphate (6 mg in 0.25 mL). Subconjunctival amikacin (25 mg/ 0.1 mL) was substituted for ceftazidime if the patient was allergic to penicillin

3. Topical vancomycin, 50 mg/mL; amikacin, 20 mg/mL; cycloplegic; and prednisolone acetate 1%

4. Oral prednisone, 30 mg bid, for 5–10 days.

Patients randomized to the intravenous antibiotic arm received the following:

1. Ceftazidime, 2 g q8 h, or ciprofloxacin, 750 mg PO bid, if allergic to penicillin

2. Amikacin, 7.5 mg/kg IV loading dose and then 6 mg/kg every 12 h. Doses were adjusted to keep peak and trough levels within an acceptable level.

The EVS demonstrated several important points:

1. There was no difference in final visual acuity or media clarity whether or not intravenous antibiotics were used. The findings were consistent across all subsets of patients.

2. Patients with light perception vision who received pars plana vitrectomy had a threefold increase in the likelihood of achieving 20/40, a twofold chance of achieving 20/100 vision, and a 50% decrease in the likelihood of severe visual loss as compared with patients receiving vitreous needle biopsy.

3. Patients with hand-motions vision or better demonstrated no significant difference in final visual acuity or media clarity whether or not immediate vitrectomy was performed.

The EVS should be used as a general guide to the care of postoperative endophthalmitis patients. Clinical judgment should, however, be used to determine care on a case-by-case basis. Coverage of the details of the EVS is beyond the scope of this chapter; for more information, see EVS journal articles.[16,27–33]

ORGANISMS

Identification of the infectious organism has been reviewed in a number of studies. The distribution of organisms causing endophthalmitis in the EVS appears in Table 55-5.[27] Microbiologic culture growth was demonstrated in 69.3% of samples, and Gram-positive coagulase-negative organisms predominated.

Although the exact percentages of organisms causing endophthalmitis varies through other smaller studies, the trends seen in the EVS are upheld.[6,7,10,18,19,37,38] Gram-positive, coagulase-negative bacteria, *Staphylococcus aureus*, and *Streptococcus* species are reported to be the three leading infecting organisms in post-cataract extraction endophthalmitis. The vast majority of culture-positive infections yield a single organism.[10]

Late-onset endophthalmitis associated with glaucoma filtration surgery presents a very different microbiologic spectrum. Several studies have reported a predominance of *Streptococcus* and Gram-negative bacteria in bleb-associated endophthalmitis.[38–41] Because of the virulence of the causative organisms, patients with bleb-associated endophthalmitis carry a much poorer visual prognosis than early post-cataract extraction endophthalmitis. The virulence of the causitive organisms for bleb associated endophthalmitis leads to poorer visual results, and evidence supports more aggressive intervention for patients with bleb-associated endophthalmitis, with patients receiving prompt pars plana vitrectomy having better visual outcomes.[40] Fungal endophthalmitis is generally uncommon but must be considered as a potential cause.

Table 55-5 Incidence of inciting organisms in Endophthalmitis Vitrectomy Study

Organism	Incidence
Gram positive, coagulase negative (*Staphylococcus epidermidis*)	70.0%
Staphylococcus aureus	9.9%
Streptococcus	9.0%
Miscellaneous Gram-positive	3.1%
Enterococcus	2.2%
Gram-negative	5.9%

Data from Han DP, Wisniewski SR, Wilson LA et al: Spectrum and susceptibilities of microbiologic isolates in the Endophthalmitis Vitrectomy Study, *Am J Ophthalmol* 122:1–17, 1996.

INVESTIGATIONS

Once the clinical diagnosis of endophthalmitis has been made, anterior-chamber and vitreous samples should be obtained for Gram staining and culture because the results from the vitreous and anterior chamber biopsies will guide antibiotic selection during postoperative treatment. Vitreous samples have been demonstrated to show growth at a greater rate than anterior-chamber samples.[42] However, in early cases of endophthalmitis with an intact capsule and posterior-chamber (PC) IOL, anterior-chamber biopsies have been found to show growth even with no growth from vitreous biopsies.[43]

The EVS guidelines should be followed, although with some caveats. Patients presenting with hand-motions vision or better may receive anterior chamber and vitreous needle biopsy with an injection of intravitreal antibiotics. Patients with light perception or nonlight perception vision should receive an anterior-chamber biopsy with pars plana vitrectomy and intravitreal antibiotics. Clinical judgment, however, must be used to temper the decision to perform or not perform pars plana vitrectomy. Patients with a rapidly worsening clinical picture should be considered for immediate vitrectomy because the etiologic organism may be extremely virulent. A low threshold for vitrectomy should be used for diabetic and immunocompromised patients. In the EVS, diabetic patients with endophthalmitis demonstrated a nonstatistically significant trend toward better outcome with pars plana vitrectomy than with needle biopsy.[32] The samples size, however, was small; a larger study is required to further investigate this trend.

COLLECTION AND ANTIBIOTIC INJECTION

NEEDLE BIOPSY

Needle biopsy samples may be taken in the operating room or in the office setting if the appropriate equipment is available. Virtually all samples may be taken under local anesthesia; only in rare cases of severe periorbital inflammation is general endotracheal anesthesia required. Occasionally, a retrobulbar or subconjunctival block with 2% lidocaine is performed, although subconjuctival anesthesia with 2% lidocaine is usually adequate. The eye is then prepared in the usual sterile fashion, and a lid speculum is placed. Conjunctival cultures are generally not taken. Next, several drops of 5% povidone-iodine are instilled into the fornices, and the eye is not disturbed for several minutes to allow antimicrobial action by the povidone-iodine.

Table 55-6 lists the steps taken in obtaining samples. A 27- or 30-gauge needle is inserted into the anterior chamber through the peripheral clear cornea, and 0.1 mL of fluid is aspirated into a tuberculin syringe. Care is taken to avoid any previous surgical incisions. If a capsule or PC IOL is present, a pars plana needle biopsy may be obtained by passing a 25-gauge needle 3.5 mm posterior to the limbus into the midvitreous. In either case, 0.2–0.3 mL should be gently aspirated. If a sample cannot be aspirated with a 25-gauge needle, a 23-gauge needle passed in the same location can be used. If no sample can be obtained during needle-tap vitreous biopsy, the patient should receive a standard three-port pars plana vitrectomy. Otherwise, antibiotics should be injected into the midvitreous through a 25-gauge, $^1/_2$-inch needle placed 3.5 mm posterior to the limbus. The intraocular pressure is checked, and a second anterior chamber paracentesis can be performed if the pressure is elevated. The anterior chamber and vitreous samples are sent for Gram staining and culture.

PARS PLANA VITRECTOMY

Pars plana vitrectomy should be performed in the operating room under local or general anesthesia. Generally, a retrobulbar block with 2% lidocaine and 0.75% bupivacaine is performed. The eye is then prepared in the usual sterile fashion, and a lid speculum is placed. Conjunctival cultures are not routinely taken. Table 55-6 lists the steps taken in obtaining samples.

The eye is prepared for a standard three-port vitrectomy. A 6 mm infusion cannula is placed because the view into the vitreous is often very poor. To obtain anterior-chamber samples, a 25- or 27-gauge needle is inserted into the anterior chamber at the limbus, and 0.1 mL of fluid is aspirated into a tuberculin syringe. Care is taken to avoid any previous surgical incisions. The pars plana vitrectomy is performed. On initiation of the pars plana vitrectomy, prior to turning on the infusion, 0.2–0.3 mL of undiluted vitreous fluid is withdrawn. This fluid is often manually

---

Table 55-6 Treatment of endophthalmitis: anterior chamber and vitreous biopsy and injection of antibiotics

Needle biopsy

Anterior chamber
1. Insert 30-gauge needle attached to a tuberculin syringe. Avoid previous surgical incisions.
2. Withdraw 0.1 ml aqueous solution.

Vitreous chamber
1. Insert a 25-gauge, $^1/_2$-inch needle into the midvitreous chamber through a point 3.5 mm posterior to the limbus.
2. Gently withdraw 0.2–0.3 mL fluid.
3. Use a 23- or 22-gauge needle if there is no vitreous aspirated with moderate suction. If the yield continues to be poor, proceed to three-port vitrectomy.
4. Otherwise, inject antibiotics through a 30-gauge, $^1/_2$-inch needle into the midvitreous through a point 3.5 mm posterior to the limbus.
5. Check intraocular pressure and repeat anterior chamber paracentesis to relieve pressure, if necessary.

Pars plana vitrectomy

Prepare a three-port pars plana vitrectomy using a 6-mm infusion cannula.

Anterior chamber
1. Insert 30-gauge needle attached to a tuberculin syringe. Avoid previous surgical incisions.
2. Withdraw 0.1 mL aqueous solution.

Vitreous chamber
1. Perform a core vitrectomy.
2. Close two of three sclerotomies.
3. Inject antibiotics and then close final sclerotomy.
4. Check intraocular pressure and perform anterior chamber paracentesis, if necessary, to relieve pressure.

---

aspirated into a syringe connected to the infusion line. The infusion is then opened, and the core vitrectomy is carried out. Two of the three sclerotomies are closed, and antibiotics are injected before closure of the final sclerotomy. All surgical wound abnormalities from the initial surgery, including wound gape, exposed sutures, vitreous wick, and so on, should be corrected before antibiotic injection and closure. In addition to the anterior-chamber and vitreous sample, the vitrectomy cassette is sent for concentration, culture, and Gram staining.

Other surgical techniques have been explored for managing postoperative endophthalmitis. Use of intraocular endoscopy has been reported as an adjunct in surgery.[34] There is limited literature that performing more aggressive procedures, including scleral buckling, at the time of initial vitrectomy decrease the incidence of additional procedures.[35] Small-gauge vitrectomy, which is theoretically a less-traumatic procedure with better preservation of the conjunctive, has been described for treatment in this setting.[36] Our recommendation is to limit surgical intervention to standard pars plana vitrectomy at the time of initial surgery unless more evidence emerges supporting the facility of more aggressive surgery.

CULTURE

Specimens obtained from anterior-chamber aspiration and vitreous needle biopsy or pars plana vitrectomy should be cultured and stained separately. Cassette washings from pars plana vitrectomy should be concentrated by centrifuge or filtration before culture and staining. Samples should be plated on blood agar, chocolate agar, Sabouraud, and thioglycolate broth and should be cultured in aerobic and anaerobic conditions. Samples should be placed on slides and stained using Gram and Giemsa stains. A positive culture result is defined as growth on two or more media or confluent growth on one solid medium at the site of inoculation.

■ TREATMENT ■

INITIAL TREATMENT

Initial treatment is directed toward the sterilization of the eye using intravitreal, topical, and oral antibiotics. Most vitreoretinal surgeons agree that intravitreal antibiotics are crucial for maximizing chances for a good outcome. The authors choose to inject two antibiotics: vancomycin (1 mg in 0.1 mL) and ceftazidime (2.5 mg in 0.1 mL). In cases of penicillin or cephalosporin allergy, we inject vancomycin (1 mg in 0.1 mL) and amikacin (0.4 mg in 0.1 mL). Table 55-7 summarizes the combination of medications recommended.

Dilutions must be performed carefully, especially in the case of amikacin, because higher concentrations may be toxic to the eye or may cause systemic complications. Although dilutions can be performed by the surgeon, intraocular antibiotics may be safer when performed by the pharmacist.

CHOICE OF ANTIBIOTICS

Controversy exists regarding the choice of antibiotics for intravitreal injection. The EVS used a combination of antibiotics, including intravitreal vancomycin and amikacin, subconjunctival

Table 55-7 Initial therapeutic regimen for endophthalmitis

Intravitreal injection for endophthalmitis
1. Vancomycin 1 mg in 0.1 mL normal saline
2. Ceftazidime 2.5 mg in 0.1 mL normal saline
3. Dexamethasone 400 μg in 0.1 mL normal saline is reasonable to consider as an adjunct.
4. Substitute amikacin 0.4 mg in 0.1 mL water for ceftazidime in patients allergic to penicillin or cephalosporin

Topical regimen
1. Vancomycin 25–50 mg/mL with Gentamicin 11–14 mg/mL hourly if the patient has been receiving fourth-generation quinolones
2. Consider topical gatifloxacin 0.3% or topical moxifloxacin 0.5% hourly in lieu of fortified antibiotics if the patient has not received fourth-generation fluoroquinolones
3. Scopolamine 0.25% twice daily
4. Prednisolone acetate 1% hourly

Oral regimen
Moxifloxacin or Gatifloxacin 400 mg once each day

vancomycin, ceftazidime (amikacin if patients were allergic to penicillin or cephalosporin), and dexamethasone, and topical vancomycin and amikacin postoperatively. The EVS's empiric choice to use multiple antibiotics has been shown to be best in clinical evaluation. In a review of culture-proven endophthalmitis cases, it was confirmed that no single antibiotic covered all microbes isolated.[44]

Vancomycin is very effective in the treatment of endophthalmitis for a number of reasons. First, vancomycin has been found to be active against most Gram-positive organisms found in endophthalmitis. Second, vancomycin is cleared from the eye anteriorly, resulting in a long half-life. Data from rabbit studies demonstrated a vitreal half-life of 20–40 h in uninfected rabbit eyes and 38–54 h in infected rabbit eyes.[44,45–47]

Vancomycin appears to be well tolerated by ocular structures.

The choice of an agent for coverage of Gram-negative organisms remains controversial. Although the EVS used amikacin, an aminoglycoside, a number of vitreoretinal surgeons have advocated the use of other antibiotics. The potential benefits of amikacin include a good Gram-negative spectrum of coverage, a long half-life, a synergistic effect with vancomycin against Gram-positive cocci, and concentration-dependent bactericidal activity.[48] Potential problems are ocular toxicity (including macular infarction), ototoxicity, and nephrotoxicity.[50]

Intravitreal ceftazidime (a beta-lactam) has also been used for treatment of endophthalmitis. Ceftazidime has a similar spectrum of coverage and a similar half-life as amikacin.[52] Although ceftazidime does not have the synergistic effect with vancomycin against Gram-positive cocci that amikacin has, neither does it carry the potential risk of ocular and systemic toxicity. Additionally, the high intravitreal concentration of each individual intravitreal antibiotic decreases the importance of antibiotic synergy.[51]

Fluoroquinolones have been considered for intravitreal injection. Ciprofloxacin has a similar spectrum of coverage to amikacin and ceftazidime, but several problems preclude its use in intravitreal injection. Doses higher than 100 μg injected into rabbit vitreous have been demonstrated to cause retinal and corneal toxicity,[53] and the half-life of ciprofloxacin is short (~2 h in the rabbit).[54] Intravitreal moxifloxacin, a fourth-generation fluoroquinolone, has also been studied in animal eyes. It shows similar pharmacokinetics as ciprofloxacin.[49]

On the basis of the preceding evidence, the authors' choice is to inject vancomycin and ceftazidime. The authors do not routinely treat for fungal endophthalmitis and limit antifungal agents to culture-proven cases.

INTRAVITREAL STEROID INJECTION

Controversy exists concerning the use of intravitreal injection of steroids. A number of studies have been performed in animal models, as well as in humans. Some studies demonstrate an improvement in clinical inflammation and visual outcome with concurrent intravitreal injection of steroids and antibiotics,[57–60] whereas others demonstrate worsened inflammation and visual outcome.[61–65] Histopathologic studies have shown similarly contradictory results for intravitreal steroids.[57,58,61] The study designs, including type of antibiotic, dose of steroid injected, and type of bacterium injected (in the animal models), were not consistent across studies; therefore, comparison of results is difficult. Intravitreal triamcinolone has been shown to exhibit a beneficial effect for postoperative endophthalmitis when combined with intravitreal antibiotics.[66] On the basis of the existing studies, the authors do not support the injection of intravitreal steroids at the time of antibiotic injection but await a comprehensive evaluation of the efficacy of intravitreal steroids in endophthalmitis.

ADJUVANT TREATMENT

The EVS used subconjunctival antibiotics for eradication of any anterior segment infection and many surgeons advocate their use in the treatment of endophthalmitis. The authors believe that the application of subconjunctival antibiotics is redundant when an aggressive postoperative topical antibiotic regimen is planned and do not generally use subconjunctival antibiotics or steroids.

Our recommendations for postoperative treatment with topical antibiotics is the use of fortified medications, with the EVS trial as a guiding principal, if the patient presents with an apparent infection while taking fourth-generation fluoroquinolones topically, as they are often prescribed in the postoperative regimen. Topical fortified vancomycin (25 or 50 mg/mL) is used to treat any Gram-positive infection, whereas topical fortified amikacin (20 mg/mL) or ceftazidime (100 mg/mL) are good choices to treat any Gram-negative organisms. Although unused in the EVS, topical fortified gentamicin (11 or 14 mg/mL) is also a reasonable choice for Gram-negative coverage. If a patient has not received a topical fourth-generation quinolone, one may be started as treatment for both Gram-positive and Gram-negative coverage following intravitreal antibiotics. Both aqueous and vitreous penetration of these topical fluoroquinolones has been reported.[62,63]

Oral administration of fourth-generation fluoroquinolones have also been shown to achieve high intravitreal concentrations in the noninflamed eye. Following oral administration, both gatifloxacin and moxifloxacin have been shown to penetrate the vitreous of the non-inflamed eye within hours, exceeding MIC therapeutic levels gains a wide range of both Gram-positive and Gram-negative organisms causative of endophthalmitis.[55,56] Oral fourth-generation fluoroquinolones certainly represent a significant advance in endophthalmitis treatment, and we recommend prescribing them at the time of diagnosis.

On the basis of EVS data, no intravenous antibiotics are recommended.

Aggressive postoperative administration of prednisolone acetate 1% is started 1 day after surgery. The EVS utilized oral prednisone at 30 mg/day. This dose may be started if the patient has no contraindications to steroid use, but the authors rarely use it. Cycloplegic drops are used postoperatively to relieve discomfort and synechiae formation.

CLINICAL COURSE

The clinical course varies on a case-by-case basis. Often, the clinical appearance is worse 1 day after surgery than on the day of surgery. Generally speaking, 2 days after surgery, the eye should appear clinically improved, although a hypopyon and media opacities may be present. Although the eye may be sterilized, aggressive anti-inflammatory therapy is imperative to prevent late sequelae. It is important to evaluate and reevaluate the anterior and posterior segments for development of complications such as posterior synechiae with iris bombé, vitreous membranes, retinal traction, and retinal detachment. As long as the media is hazy, the posterior segment should be followed with ultrasound. The surgeon should not hesitate to bring the patient back to the operating room should further complications develop or should a persistent infection be suspected.

PROGNOSIS

The final outcome depends on a number of factors, including appearance at presentation, the inciting organism, and the baseline medical condition. Patients infected with coagulase-negative Staphylococcus generally have the best outcome, whereas those with streptococcal infections have a worse prognosis. Gram-negative endophthalmitis carries a poor prognosis. Recent data from the EVS demonstrate a trend toward worsened outcomes for diabetic patients; the surgeon should consider earlier, more aggressive intervention for diabetics.[67] Some surgeons advocate vitrectomy following injection of antibiotics if media haze persists and examination continues to reveal vitreous haze and membranes, despite vision better than LP. Early detection and treatment may be the best hope for a good outcome.

PREVENTION

Evidence exists that the use of topical 5% povidone-iodine applied to the ocular surface preoperatively decreases the incidence of culture-positive endophthalmitis,[68] and the authors advocate its use. There has been a recent trend toward the use of antibiotics within the irrigating solution. Studies involving animal models and retrospective chart reviews have not definitively demonstrated a benefit to the use of antibiotics within irrigating solutions during cataract surgery, but a recent large multicenter study showed a fivefold reduction in the risk of endophthalmitis following cataract surgery with intracameral cefuroxime. Based upon the emerging risk-reduction data, it is the authors' recommendation to consider adding intracameral cefuroxime to cataract surgery.[69–73]

CHRONIC POSTOPERATIVE ENDOPHTHALMITIS

Although most of this chapter has focused on early postoperative endophthalmitis, the surgeon should be aware of the signs of chronic postoperative endophthalmitis. A number of weakly virulent organisms may produce a late, chronic infection that may mimic a chronic uveitis. Organisms that have been reported to produce such a reaction include *Propionibacterium acnes*, *Staphylococcus epidermidis*, and fungi, such as *Candida* species.

P. acnes is a commensal anaerobic diphtheroid bacterium that is found on the skin. *P. acnes* endophthalmitis has been reported to present with an equatorial white plaque on the lens capsule after extracapsular cataract extraction, low-grade chronic inflammation, granulomatous keratic precipitates, fibrin strands or beaded infiltrates in the anterior vitreous, and an intermittent hypopyon. The inflammation associated with *P. acnes* infection often responds to steroid treatment, but recurs once treatment is withheld.[74–76] The authors' experience has been that *P. acnes* generally produces a chronic low-grade inflammation with a white plaque seen within the capsular bag but without hypopyon or other changes. Patients have often been treated chronically with steroids, which may mask the development of classic findings.

A number of treatments for patients with *P. acnes* endophthalmitis have been used, including various combinations of topical, intravenous, and intraocular antibiotics with or without vitrectomy.[76] Data have supported treating *P. acnes* infection with vitrectomy, capsulectomy, and IOL extraction with intravitreal antibiotics to yield the greatest chance of cure. However, if less aggressive intervention fails, studies do not show that visual acuity decreases as more aggressive steps are taken. It is the authors' recommendation to consider initial intervention with vitrectomy, posterior capsulectomy, and injection of antibiotics, whereas consideration of IOL removal is reasonable if primary intervention fails.[77,78] A planned secondary IOL placement after complete resolution of inflammation is reasonable. In all cases, the vitreous washings and capsular remnant are sent for culture and staining.

A patient with suspected chronic late endophthalmitis that is not believed to be *P. acnes* or has not proven culture-positive for the organism is treated with a pars plana vitrectomy, anterior chamber biopsy, and injection of intravitreal antibiotics. The authors elect to use intravitreal vancomycin, 1 mg in 0.1 mL, and ceftazidime, 2 mg in 0.1 mL. Coagulase-negative staphylococcal species can mimic *P. acnes*, and often respond to this treatment regimen without IOL removal. Postoperatively, patients receive anti-inflammatory drops, cycloplegics, and fourth-generation fluoroquinolone drops supplemented by an oral fourth-generation quinolone. The authors do not start antifungal therapy until cases are culture proven, although one can consider submission of the posterior capsule for fungal culture in cryptic cases of chronic endophthalmitis.[79]

■ CONCLUSION ■

Postoperative endophthalmitis is a greatly feared complication of cataract surgery with potentially devastating results. However, early diagnosis and prompt treatment of endophthalmitis can result in the preservation of good vision. Surgeons should remain vigilant during their evaluation of the postoperative patient and should treat or refer the patient for immediate treatment if endophthalmitis is suspected.

References

[1] Aaberg TM, Flynn HW, Schiffman J, et al. Nosocomial acute-onset postoperative endophthalmitis survey: a 10-year review of incidence and outcomes. Ophthalmology 1998;105:1004–1010.

[2] Menikoff JA, Speaker MG, Marmor M, et al. A case-control study of risk factors for postoperative endophthalmitis. Ophthalmology 1991;98:1761–1768.

[3] Kattan HM, Flynn HW, Pflugfelder SC, et al. Nosocomial endophthalmitis survey: current incidence of infection after intraocular surgery. Ophthalmology 1991;98:227–238.

[4] Javitt JC, Vitale S, Canner JK, et al. National outcomes of cataract surgery: endophthalmitis following inpatient cataract surgery. Arch Ophthalmol 1991;109:1085–1089.

[5] Allen HF, Mangiaracine AB. Bacterial endophthalmitis after cataract extraction. II. Incidence in 36,000 consecutive operations with special reference to topical preoperative antibiotics. Arch Ophthalmol 1974;91:3–7.

[6] Miller JJ, Scott IU, Flynn HW, Smiddy WE, Newton J, Miller D. Acute-onset endophthalmitis after cataract surgery (2000–2004): incidence, clinical settings, and visual acuity outcomes after treatment. Am J Ophthalmol 2005;139:983–987.

[7] Wong TY, Chee SP. The epidemiology of acute endophthalmitis after cataract surgery in an Asian population. Ophthalmology 2004;111:699–705.

[8] Norregaard JC, Thoning H, Bernth-Petersen P, Andersen TF, Javitt JC, Anderson GF. Risk of endophthalmitis after cataract extraction: results from the International Cataract Surgery Outcomes study. Br J Ophthalmol 1997;81:102–106.

[9] Menikoff JA, Speaker MG, Marmor M, Raskin EM. A case-control study of risk factors for postoperative endophthalmitis. Ophthalmology 1991;98:1761–1768.

[10] Ng JQ, Morlet N, Pearman JW, Constable IJ, McAllister IL, Kennedy CJ, et al. Management and outcomes of postoperative endophthalmitis since the endophthalmitis vitrectomy study: the Endophthalmitis Population Study of Western Australia (EPSWA)'s fifth report. Ophthalmology 2005;112:1199–1206.

[11] Haiman MH, Burton TC, Brown CK. Epidemiology of retinal detachment. Arch Ophthalmol 1982;100:289–292.

[12] Wilkinson CP, Anderson LS, Little JH. Retinal detachment following phacoemulsification. Ophthalmology 1978;85:151–156.

[13] Smith PW, Stark WJ. Maumenee et al. Retinal detachment after extracapsular cataract extraction with posterior chamber intraocular lens. Ophthalmology 1987;94:495–504.

[14] Javitt JC, Vitale S, Canner JK, et al. National outcomes of cataract extraction. I. Retinal detachment after inpatient surgery. Ophthalmology 1991;98:895–902.

[15] Steinert RF, Puliafito CA, Kumar SR, et al. Cystoid macular edema, retinal detachment, and glaucoma after Nd:YAG laser posterior capsulotomy. Am J Ophthalmol 1991;112:373–380.

[16] Group Endophthalmitis Vitrectomy Study. Results of the endophthalmitis vitrectomy study: a randomized trial of immediate vitrectomy and of intravenous antibiotics for the treatment of postoperative bacterial endophthalmitis. Arch Ophthalmol 1995;113:1479–1496.

[17] Rowsey JJ, Jensen H, Sexton DJ. Clinical diagnosis of endophthalmitis. Int Ophthalmol Clin 1987;27:82–88.

[18] Weber DJ, Hoffman KL, Thoft RS, et al. Endophthalmitis following intraocular lens implantation: a report of 30 cases and review of the literature. Rev Infect Dis 1986;8:12–20.

[19] Driebe WT, Mandelbaum S, Forster RK, et al. Pseudophakic endophthalmitis: diagnosis and management. Ophthalmology 1986;93:442–448.

[20] Lindstrom RL, Doughman DJ. Bacterial endophthalmitis associated with vitreous wick. Ann Ophthalmol 1979;11:1775–1778.

[21] Gelender H. Infectious endophthalmitis following cutting of sutures after cataract surgery. Am J Ophthalmol 1982;94:528–533.

[22] Stonecipher KG, Parmley VC, Jensen H, et al. Infectious endophthalmitis following sutureless cataract surgery. Arch Ophthalmol 1991;109:1562–1563.

[23] Cinfino J, Brown SI. Bacterial endophthalmitis associated with exposed monofilament sutures following corneal transplantation. Am J Ophthalmol 1985;99:111–113.

[24] Irvine WE, Flynn HW, Murray TG, et al. Retained lens fragments after phacoemulsification manifesting as marked inflammation with hypopyon. Am J Ophthalmol 1992;114:610–614.

[25] Meltzer DW. Sterile hypopyon following intraocular lens surgery. Arch Ophthalmol 1980;98:100–104.

[26] Stark WJ, Rosenblum P, Maumenee AE, et al. Postoperative inflammatory reactions to intraocular lenses sterilized with ethylene oxide. Ophthalmology 1980;87:385–389.

[27] Han DP, Wisniewski SR, Wilson LA, et al. Spectrum and susceptibilities of microbiologic isolates in the Endophthalmitis Vitrectomy Study. Am J Ophthalmol 1996;122:1–17.

[28] Johnson MW, Doft BH, Kelsey SF, et al. The Endophthalmitis Vitrectomy Study: relationship between clinical presentation and microbiologic spectrum. Ophthalmology 1997;104:261–272.

[29] Barza M, Pavan PR, Wisniewski SR, et al. Evaluation of the microbiological diagnostic techniques in postoperative endophthalmitis in the Endophthalmitis Vitrectomy Study. Arch Ophthalmol 1997;115:1142–1150.

[30] Doft BH, Kelsey SF, Wisniewski SR, the EVS Study Group: Additional procedures after the initial vitrectomy or tap-biopsy in the Endophthalmitis Vitrectomy Study. Ophthalmology 1998;105:707–716.

[31] Han DP, Wisniewski SR, Kelsey SF, et al. Microbiologic yields and complication rates of vitreous fine needle aspiration vs mechanized vitreous biopsy in the Endophthalmitis Vitrectomy Study. Retina 1999;19:98–102.

[32] Doft BH, Wisniewski SR, Kelsey SF, et al. Diabetes and postoperative endophthalmitis in the Endophthalmitis Vitrectomy Study. Arch Ophthalmol 2001;119:650–656.

[33] Doft BH, Wisniewski SR, Kelsey SF, Groer-Fitzgerald S. Endophthalmitis Vitrectomy Study Group. Diabetes and postcataract extraction endophthalmitis. Curr Opin Ophthalmology 2002;13:147–151.

[34] De Smet MD, Carlborg EA. Managing severe endophthalmitis with the use of an endoscope. Retina 2005;25:976–980.

[35] Kaynak S, Oner FH, Kocak N, Cingil G. Surgical management of postoperative endophthalmitis: comparison of 2 techniques. [see comment]. J Cataract Refract Surg 2003;29:966–969.

[36] Yanyali A, Celik E, Horozoglu F, Oner S, Nohutcu AF. 25-gauge sutureless transconjunctival vitrectomy. Eur J Ophthalmol 2006;16:141–147.

[37] Stern GA, Engel HM, Driebe WT. The treatment of postoperative endophthalmitis: results of differing approaches to treatment. Ophthalmology 1989;96:62–67.

[38] Puliafito CA, Baker AS, Haaf J, et al. Infectious endophthalmitis: review of 36 cases. Ophthalmology 1982;89:921–929.

[39] Ciulla TA, Beck AD, Topping TM, et al. Blebitis, early endophthalmitis, and late endophthalmitis after glaucoma filtering surgery. Ophthalmology 1997;115:986–995.

[40] Busbee BG, Recchia FM, Kaiser R, Nagra P, Resenblatt B, Pearlman RB. Bleb associated endophthalmitis clinical characteristics and visual outcomes. Ophthalmology 2004;111:1496–1503.

[41] Mandelbaum S, Forster RK, Gelender H, et al. Late onset endophthalmitis associated with filtering blebs. Ophthalmology 1985;92:964–972.

[42] Mandelbaum S, Forster RK. Postoperative endophthalmitis. Int Ophthalmol Clin 1987;27:95–106.

[43] Beyer TL, O'Donnell RE, Goncalves V, et al. Role of posterior capsule in the prevention of postoperative bacterial endophthalmitis: experimental primate studies and clinical implications. Br J Ophthalmol 1985;69:841–846.

[44] Benz MS, Scott IU, Flynn Jr HW, Unonius N, Miller D. Endophthalmitis isolates and antibiotic sensitivities: a 6-year review of culture-proven cases. Am J Ophthalmol 2004;137:38–42.

[45] Homer P, Peyman GA, Koziol J, et al. Intravitreal injection of vancomycin in experimental staphylococcal endophthalmitis. Acta Ophthalmol 1975;53:311–320.

[46] Smith MA, Sorensen JA, Lowy FD, et al. Treatment of experimental methicillin resistant Staphylococcus epidermidis endophthalmitis with intravitreal vancomycin. Ophthalmology 1986;93:1328–1335.

[47] Smith MA, Sorenson JA, Smith C, et al. Effects of intravitreal dexamethasone on concentration of intravitreal vancomycin in experimental methicillin resistant Staphylococcus epidermidis endophthalmitis. Antimicrob Agents Chemother 1991;35:1298–1302.

[48] Doft BH, Barza MB. Optimal management of postoperative endophthalmitis and results of the Endophthalmitis Vitrectomy Study. Curr Opin Ophthalmol 1996;7:84–94.

[49] Iyer MN, He F, Wensel TG, Mieler WF, Benz MS, Holz ER. Clearance of intravitreal moxifloxacin. Invest Ophthalmol Vis Sci 2006;47:317–319.

[50] Campochiaro PA, Lim JI. Aminoglycoside toxicity in the treatment of endophthalmitis (the Aminoglycoside Toxicity Study Group). Arch Ophthalmol 1994;112:48–53.

[51] Roth DB, Flynn Jr HW. Antibiotic selection in the treatment of endophthalmitis: the significance of drug combinations and synergy. Surv Ophthalmol 1997;41:395–401.

[52] Meridith TA. Antimicrobial pharmacokinetics in endophthalmitis treatment: studies of ceftazidime. Trans Am Ophthalmol Soc 1993;91:653–699.

[53] Stevens SX, Fouraker BD, Jensen HG. Intraocular safety of ciprofloxacin. Arch Ophthalmol 1991;109:1737–1743.

[54] Pearson PA, Hainsworth DP, Ashton P. Clearance and distribution of ciprofloxacin after intravitreal injection. Retina 1993;13:326–330.

[55] Harispaad SM, Mieler WF, Holz ER. Vitreous and aqueous penetration of orally administered gatifloxacin in humans. Arch Ophthalmol 2003;121:345–350.

[56] Hariprasad SM, Shah GK, Mieler WF, Feiner L, Blinder KJ, Holekamp NM, et al. Vitreous and aqueous penetration of orally administered moxifloxacin in humans. Arch Ophthalmol 2006;124:178–182.

[57] Meredith TA, Aguilar HE, Trabelsi A, et al. Comparative treatment of experimental Staphylococcus epidermidis endophthalmitis. Arch Ophthalmol 1990;108:857–860.

[58] Maxwell DP, Brent BD, Diamond JG, et al. Effect of intravitreal dexamethasone on ocular histopathology in a rabbit model of endophthalmitis. Ophthalmology 1991;98:1370–1376.

[59] Park SS, Samly N, Ruoff K, et al. Effect of intravitreal dexamethasone in treatment of pneumococcal endophthalmitis in rabbits. Arch Ophthalmol 1995;113:1324–1329.

[60] Jett BD, Jensen HG, Atkuri RV, et al. Evaluation of therapeutic measures for treating endophthalmitis caused by isogenic toxin producing and non-toxin producing Enterococcus faecalis strains. Invest Ophthalmol Vis Sci 1995;36:9–15.

[61] Meredith TA, Aguilar HE, Drews C, et al. Intraocular dexamethasone produces a harmful effect on treatment of experimental Staphylococcus aureus endophthalmitis. Trans Am Ophthalmol Soc 1996;XCIV:241–252.

[62] Kim DH, Stark WJ, O'Brien TP, Dick JD. Aqueous penetration and biological activity of moxifloxacin 0.5% ophthalmic solution and gatifloxacin 0.3% solution in cataract surgery patients. Ophthalmology 2005;112:1992–1996.

[63] Costello P, Bakri SJ, Beer PM, Singh RJ, Falk NS, Peters GB, et al. Vitreous penetration of topical moxifloxacin and gatifloxacin in humans. Retina 2006;26:191–195.

[64] Das T, Jalali S, Gothwal VK, et al. Intravitreal dexamethasone in exogenous bacterial endophthalmitis: results of a prospective randomized study. Br J Ophthalmol 1999;83:1050–1055.

[65] Shah GK, Stein JD, Sharma S, et al. Visual outcomes following the use of intravitreal steroids in the treatment of postoperative endophthalmitis. Ophthalmology 2000;107:486–489.

[66] Falk NS, Beer PM, Peters 3rd GB. Role of intravitreal triamcinolone acetonide in the treatment of postoperative endophthalmitis. Retina 2006;26:545–548.

[67] Doft BH, Wisniewski SR, Kelsey SF, Groer-Fitzgerald S. Endophthalmitis Vitrectomy Study Group. Diabetes and postcataract extraction endophthalmitis. Curr Opin Ophthalmol 2002;13:147–151.

[68] Speaker MG, Menikoff JA. Prophylaxis of endophthalmitis with topical povidone-iodine. Ophthalmology 1991;98:1769–1775.

[69] Beigi B, Westlake W, Chang B, et al. The effect of intracameral, per-operative antibiotics on microbial contamination of anterior chamber aspirates during phacoemulsification. Eye 1998;12:390–394.

[70] Gritz DC, Cevallos AV, Smolin G, et al. Antibiotic supplementation of intraocular irrigating solutions: an in vitro model of antibacterial action. Ophthalmology 1996;103:1204–1208.

[71] Adenis JP, Robert PY, Mounier M, et al. Anterior chamber concentrations of vancomycin in the irrigation solution at the end of cataract surgery. J Cataract Refract Surg 1997;23:111–114.

[72] Feys J, Salvanet-Bouccara A, Edmond JP, et al. Vancomycin prophylaxis and intraocular contamination during cataract surgery. J Cataract Refract Surg 1997;23:894–897.

[73] Barry P, Seal DV, Gettinby G, Lees F, Peterson M, Revie CW. ESCRS Endophthalmitis Study Group. ESCRS study of prophylaxis of postoperative endophthalmitis after cataract surgery: preliminary report of principal results from a European multicenter study. J Cataract Refract Surg 2006;32:407–410.

[74] Meisler DM, Palestine AG, Vastine DW, et al. Chronic *Propionibacterium acnes* endophthalmitis after extracapsular cataract extraction and intraocular lens implantation. Am J Ophthamol 1986;102:733–739.

[75] Meisler DM, Mandelbaum S. *Propionibacterium acnes* associated endophthalmitis after extracapsular cataract extraction: review of reported cases. Ophthalmology 1989;96:54–61.

[76] Zambrano W, Flynn HW, Pflugfelder SC, et al. Management options for *Propionibacterium acnes* endophthalmitis. Ophthalmology 1989;96:1100–1105.

[77] Clark L, Kaiser P, Flynn H. Treatment strategies and visual acuity outcomes in chronic postoperative *Propionibacterium acnes* endophthalmitis. Ophthalmology 1999;106:1665–1670.

[78] Aldave AJ, Stein JD, Deramo VA, Shah GK, Fischer DH, Maguire JI. Treatment strategies for postoperative *Probionibacterium acnes* endophthalmitis. Ophthalmology 1999;106:2395–2401.

[79] Pflugfelder SC, Flynn HW, Zwickey TD, Forster RK, Tsiligianni A, Culbertson WW, et al. Exogenous fungal endophthalmitis. Ophthalmology 1988;95:19–30.

CONCLUSION

Management of Postoperative Complications: Retinal Detachment

56

Jay S. Duker, MD

CONTENTS

CHAPTER HIGHLIGHTS

>> Guidelines for preoperative prophylactic treatment

>> Recognition of peripheral retinal pathology in the presence of cataract

>> Current treatment options

INTRODUCTION

Retinal detachment (RD) represents the physical separation of the neurosensory retina from its underlying retinal pigment epithelium (RPE) by an accumulation of fluid. This separation results in dysfunction of the photoreceptors and is clinically manifested by a scotoma corresponding to the area of detached retina.

Generally speaking, RD can be divided into three varieties on the basis of etiology: rhegmatogenous (RRD), exudative RD, and tractional RD. It is the first type, RRD, that is pathophysiologically related to cataract surgery and, therefore, pseudophakic RRD will be the focus of this chapter.

With current techniques, most RRD (>95%) can be eventually repaired, i.e. the retina returned to its normal anatomic position, juxtaposed to the RPE. However, visual recovery does not necessarily mirror anatomic appearance. Since the presence or absence of sub-macular fluid is the most important preoperative factor correlating to visual recovery, early diagnosis and prompt therapy prior to macular detachment can preserve sight. In this regard, education of the post-cataract patient concerning the symptoms of retinal detachment with instructions to seek immediate attention if symptoms should develop is paramount.

PATHOPHYSIOLOGY

The current understanding of the pathophysiology of primary RRD hinges on the basic tenet that a posterior vitreous detachment (PVD) is the inciting event in most, if not all, acute symptomatic primary RRD.[1,2] In susceptible individuals, the PVD creates one or more retinal tears via associated abnormal vitreoretinal traction. These tears, in turn, allow for the passage of vitreous fluid into the subretinal space and eventual RRD. The relationship between RRD and cataract surgery can, therefore, be reduced to a study of the relationship between cataract surgery and the induced alterations in the vitreous gel that eventually culminate in PVD. Barring rare instances of direct surgical trauma to the posterior segment resulting in a secondary retinal detachment (e.g. globe perforation from the anesthetic needle), it is currently believed that cataract surgery is a risk factor for retinal detachment only so far as cataract surgery is a risk factor for earlier onset PVD. When a PVD ensues, pseudophakic eyes do not appear to be at any more risk than age-matched and axial length-matched phakic eyes for retinal tears (Table 56-1).

Following the removal of the crystalline lens by any method, structural changes in the vitreous have been documented to occur. Loss of hyaluronic acid, increased vitreous gel mobility, and progressive vitreous syneresis result, together, in the development of PVD. These alterations occur sooner in aphakic and pseudophakic globes than in eyes in which the crystalline lens remains intact.

The status of the posterior capsule is also important. Laboratory and epidemiologic data suggest that the presence of an intact posterior capsule delays the onset of these vitreous changes compared to eyes with open posterior capsules. While the hyaluronic acid concentration in the vitreous cavity is reduced in aphakic eyes, in eyes in which the posterior capsule is intact show minimal loss of hyaluronic acid.[3] PVD has been noted to occur more

Table 56-1 Non-modifiable risk factors for pseudophakic retinal detachment

Increased axial length
Younger age
Male sex
Lattice degeneration
Family history

commonly in aphakic eyes when compared to phakic eyes.[4] In aphakic or pseudophakic eyes with intact posterior capsules, however, the rate of PVD appears to be less than when the posterior capsule is interrupted.[5] When PVD does develop, aphakic eyes do not appear to be any more susceptible to retinal tear formation than are phakic eyes.[6]

Controversy exists over whether anterior manipulation of the vitreous results in earlier PVD. RRD does appear to be more common in eyes that have undergone cataract surgery complicated by vitreous loss. Improperly performed vitrectomy with undue traction on the vitreous base or aggressive intraoperative traction on the vitreous base in the setting of dislocated nuclei and intraocular lenses (IOL) can certainly cause direct trauma to the retina, resulting in a secondary RRD. Fortunately, this is rare.

INCIDENCE, TIMING, AND RISK FACTORS

Over 40% of all patients presenting with acute RRD are either pseudophakic or aphakic. Therefore, previous cataract surgery represents the most important risk factor for patients undergoing surgical repair of RRD.[7] Other risk factors are well known: high myopia, lattice degeneration, blunt trauma, familial history of retinal detachment, and certain systemic diseases, such as Stickler's syndrome and Marfans disease (Table 56-2).

In pseudophakic eyes operated on with an extracapsular technique, the overall incidence of subsequent retinal detachment is between 1 and 2%.[8–10] In one large retrospective series of Medicare recipients re-hospitalized for retinal detachment over a 4-year period following cataract surgery, the incidence following extracapsular surgery was found to be 0.9% while it was 1.55% for intracapsular surgery.[10] In this study, initial vitrectomy increased the risk of retinal detachment to 5%. Other authors have documented a higher rate of RRD in complicated cases that were associated with vitreous loss. Wilkerson found an incidence between 7 and 14%.[8] In such eyes, persistent anterior traction on the vitreous base due to vitreous adherence to the wound,

Table 56-2 Prevention and prophylaxis of pseudophakic retinal detachment

Keep posterior capsule intact
Careful preoperative dilated fundus examination prior to both cataract surgery and Nd:YAG laser capsulotomy
Frequent dilated fundus examinations in the first year after surgery
Patient education

intraocular lens (IOL), or anterior segment structures may result in an increased risk for traction-induced peripheral retinal tears.

As already stated above, the status of the posterior capsule is an important determinant of the onset of PVD, and, therefore, the risk of RRD. Any maneuver that interrupts the posterior capsule is likely to accelerate the loss of hyaluronic acid and culminate in premature PVD. With the advent of neodymium (Nd):YAG laser capsulotomy, extracapsular surgery rapidly became the method of choice for cataract extraction. Nd:YAG laser, however, increases the risk of RRD compared to eyes with intact posterior capsules.[11–13] The incidence of RRD following capsulotomy with the Nd:YAG laser has been estimated to be between 0.1 and 3.6%. In another large retrospective study of Medicare patients undergoing laser capsulotomy following cataract surgery, the incidence of subsequent retinal detachment was 1.6%,[14] and was 0.8% for those who did not require capsulotomy. Younger age, male sex, and white race all were increased risk factors for RRD. This study was flawed, however, in that it did not differentiate between eyes. Therefore, patients suffering rehospitalization for RRD in a contralateral eye were counted as an RRD after capsulotomy. Axial myopia appears to increase the risk of RRD following laser capsulotomy as well. Neither the size of the capsulotomy, nor the amount of energy delivered appears to be significant risk factors for RRD.[11] It is not believed that the Nd:YAG laser produces retinal tears directly.

Most pseudophakic RRD occur within 1 year of the cataract removal.[8,9] Following laser capsulotomy, the typical time for RRD is within 6 months of the procedure.[14,15] It is rare for RRD to be seen in the immediate postoperative period following cataract surgery. A recent retrospective review of 215 aphakic and pseudophakic RRD found that only 13% occurred with 3 months of cataract surgery.[16] Presumably, this time course pattern is due to the timing of PVD following cataract surgery. A recent study suggests that the cumulative risk of RRD in eyes following extracapsular cataract surgery continues to increase for at least 20 years after surgery, with the risk at 20 years estimated to be 1.79%.[17]

EXAMINATION TECHNIQUES

Retinal tear and/or RRD are clinical diagnoses made with the indirect ophthalmoscope when the media is clear. Scleral depression should be used as an adjunct. Although other posterior-segment viewing systems (direct ophthalmoscopy, non-contact slit lamp lenses) can also be employed to diagnose RRD, none give the wide field, stereoscopic view obtained with the binocular indirect ophthalmoscope. With the addition of scleral depression, none of the other techniques can match indirect ophthalmoscopy for the examination of the ora serrata region either.

Indirect ophthalmoscopy should be performed preoperatively on all patients scheduled for cataract surgery. In the commonly encountered scenario in which the lens opacity precludes adequate view to the anterior retina, repeat indirect examination as soon as it is practical following cataract surgery should be performed.

In the postoperative period, the onset of flashes, floaters, visual field loss, or any unexplained drop in central visual acuity should prompt an immediate posterior segment examination through a pharmacologically dilated pupil. Up to 50% of patients with acute RRD will not complain of previous flashes and floaters prior to presentation for detached retina.

If the media is not clear, ultrasonography is invaluable to rule out the presence of RRD. When the media is too cloudy secondary to the cataract to obtain an adequate view to the posterior pole, B scan ultrasonography should be performed prior to cataract surgery. This examination is sensitive and specific for retinal detachment but is less helpful in the identification of occult retinal breaks.

In the post-cataract surgery patient who complains of acute flashes, floaters or other symptoms of PVD/RRD, the presence of pigment granules in the anterior vitreous (tobacco dust) in the setting of an intact posterior capsule is suggestive that a retinal break is present. Similarly the finding of vitreous hemorrhage with a symptomatic PVD implies a greater than 70% chance a retinal tear is present. Acute flashes and floaters in an eye that lacks any pigment or red blood cells in the vitreous is associated with an acute retinal tear in less than 5% of cases.

PROPHYLACTIC TREATMENT

Whenever possible, retinal lesions that represent a significant risk for RRD should be identified and treated prior to cataract surgery and/or laser capsulotomy. Although controversy still exists concerning the appropriateness of prophylactic treatment for certain lesions (e.g. asymptomatic lattice degeneration without breaks in the fellow eye of an individual whose contralateral eye had a RRD), all agree that more worrisome lesions should be treated with retinopexy (Table 56-3).

The same guidelines for prophylactic treatment hold true for patients about to undergo Nd:YAG capsulotomy. In fact, some authors believe that laser capsulotomy carries anywhere from two to four times a greater risk for subsequent RRD than does uncomplicated extracapsular cataract surgery alone. In contrast, another recent study suggests that unmodifiable risk factors, such as axial length, patient age and male sex, exert a greater effect on the risk of pseudophakic RRD than do modifiable risk factors, such as intraoperative complications or YAG capsulotomy.[18]

In the asymptomatic patient about to undergo cataract surgery or Nd:YAG laser capsulotomy the following lesion ought to be considered for prophylactic treatment: (1) any tear with significant subretinal fluid (more than one disc diameter), (2) horseshoe or flap tears in the contralateral eye of a patient who already

suffered a RRD, (3) lattice degeneration with holes and/or subretinal fluid in the contralateral eye of a patient who already suffered RRD.[19]

Asymptomatic flap tears with pigment, round holes, and atrophic holes probably do not need prophylactic treatment. Asymptomatic lattice degeneration does not require prophylactic treatment.

TREATMENT OF SYMPTOMATIC LESIONS

If the patient is symptomatic with evidence of ongoing vitreous traction, then the threshold for the treatment of observed retinal pathology should be lowered. Attention should be directed especially to the superior retina, since approximately 80% of pseudophakic retinal tears will be found in the superior clock hours.[20] In about 50% of eyes, PVD-induced tears will be multiple. In acutely symptomatic eyes, flap or horseshoe tears, operculated tears, and atrophic holes with fluid may all be considered for retinopexy.

Laser or cryotherapy retinopexy should be performed within 24–48 h of the identification of symptomatic retinal tears. The decision as to which modality to use is based on the size of tear, its location, and the availability. There is no direct clinical evidence that one is preferential. Theoretically, laser retinopexy is preferred whenever possible, since an immediate, albeit incomplete, adhesion is obtained and fewer RPE cells are liberated.[21,22] Laser indirect ophthalmoscope units, both argon and diode, have revolutionized the treatment of postoperative eyes since a non-contact lens laser treatment can be performed.

Patients requiring retinopexy for symptomatic retinal lesions need careful post-treatment follow-up. Up to 22% may require additional treatment and 5% will need treatment in the fellow eye.[23]

DIFFERENTIAL DIAGNOSIS

In the setting of an acute visual field defect with an examination showing a corresponding area of retinal elevation accompanied by an open retinal tear, the diagnosis of RRD is confirmed. When the view to the posterior segment is poor due to media opacity or a small pupil, or no open break can be found, than the diagnosis may be less clear. In this case, certain ancillary testing can be helpful.

The most likely entity to be confused with RRD in the immediate postoperative period is localized choroidal detachment and/or choroidal hemorrhage. Usually seen in the setting of hypotony, choroidal detachment appears as a dark, solid multi-lobular mass or masses. Its development may be delayed by hours or days after surgery and may be heralded by the onset of acute pain. Often the ora serrata is elevated, allowing for its visualization without scleral depression. Associated findings to rule out include a leaking wound, filtering bleb, or posterior perforation from the anesthetic needle or bridle suture. Exudative RD may develop overlying the choroidal detachment. This usually resolves spontaneously. B scan ultrasonography is often diagnostic for choroidal detachment.

Central serous chorioretinopathy can result in a serous RD involving the posterior pole. Rarely, such an RD can extend into the interior retina. No open retinal break will be visible and

Table 56-3 Treatment of suspicious retinal lesions
Asymptomatic
Any tear with greater than one disc diameter of fluid (subclinical RRD)
Horseshoe or flap tears with fluid
Horseshoe or flap tear in contralateral eye of patients with previous RRD
Symptomatic
Any tear with greater than one disc diameter of fluid (subclinical RRD)
All horseshoe or flap tears
Most operculated tears
Atrophic holes in contralateral eye of patients with previous RRD

retinal pigment epithelial alterations in the posterior pole may be apparent. Intravenous fluorescein angiography (IVFA) will usually confirm the diagnosis.

Cystoid macular edema (CME) is one of the most common causes of decreased vision in the post-cataract patient. Rarely, it may be confused with RRD.[24] It may result in clinical thickening of the central macula, but is not associated with significant subretinal fluid. Optical coherence tomography (OCT) and/or IVFA will confirm the diagnosis.

A variety of underlying choroidal, retinal, or scleral disorders may result in secondary exudative retinal detachment. Differentiation from RRD often represents a daunting clinical challenge. Shifting fluid that pools inferiorly, the absence of fixed folds, the lack of a full-thickness retinal tear, the presence of intraocular inflammation, and/or scleral, choroidal or retinal inflammatory, infiltrative, or tumorous lesions will all point toward an exudative RD.

IMMEDIATE MANAGEMENT OF RETINAL DETACHMENT

If an acute RRD is diagnosed with the macula threatened, all efforts should be made to repair the retina as soon as possible. If a delay is unavoidable, bedrest with bilateral patching can slow the accumulation of subretinal fluid. Pseudophakic RRD remains a vision-threatening occurrence with only half of patients recovering to 20/40 or better visual acuity.[25] Once the macula is involved with subretinal fluid, the timing of surgical intervention is less critical. Recent evidence suggests that macula-off RRD repaired within 5–7 days has no different visual outcome than those operated within 1–2 days.[26] In addition, the length of time of macular detachment appears to have no prognostic significance for final visual acuity following repair for durations of macular-off status of up to 30 days.[27] If the macula has been off for a longer interval, elective surgery is appropriate.

SURGICAL MANAGEMENT

Pars plana vitrectomy (PPV), with or without scleral buckling, has become the preferred surgical choice for pseudophakic RRD, supplanting scleral buckling alone.[28] Aside from improved anatomic outcome, vitrectomy alone carries one major advantage over scleral buckling in pseudophakic RRD; it is a refractive neutral procedure. PPV is also less painful, less likely to result in diploplia and does not carry the risks of buckle extrusion or infection. In addition, vitrectomy usually reduces or eliminates the prominent vitreous floaters that often accompany retinal tears and RRD. The addition of an encircling scleral buckle in conjunction with vitrectomy is advocated by some surgeons, while others choose to use a buckle rarely, if ever. Two studies suggest that the addition of the scleral buckle adds little to the final outcome in pseudophakic RRD repair.[29,30]

PPV can be employed with either endolaser or external cryotherapy to seal the tears. Most surgeons use a long-acting gas tamponade (SF6 or C3F8), or, on occasion, silicone oil. One recent study employed PPV, laser and aqueous tamponade without gas with good anatomic results.[31] In addition, some advocate internal drainage of the subretinal fluid in all cases, either through a peripheral break or through a deliberate retinotomy. Alternatively,

intraoperative perfluorocarbon liquid can be temporarily employed to evacuate subretinal fluid from pre-existing breaks. Many RRD, especially with superior breaks, can be successfully treated with gas tamponade alone, without intraoperative drainage of subretinal fluid.

In one large (294 eyes), prospective, non-randomized trial, PPV with fluid-gas exchange and endolaser without scleral buckling reattached pseudophakic RRD 88% of the time with one operation.[32]

Scleral buckling surgery alone can be used for many pseudophakic RRD. Most surgeons advocate encirclement of the entire globe via a circumferential buckling element in eyes that have undergone previous cataract surgery to reduce the risk of failure due to new or missed retinal breaks. Data exist suggesting that the addition of an encircling element may reduce the risk of reoperation by 3%.[33]

Regardless of technique at least 85% of all pseudophakic RRD can be fixed with one operation.[34] The ultimate rate of retinal reattachment is 98%.

Pneumatic retinopexy can be used for RRD following cataract surgery but the success rate is less than in phakic eyes. New or missed breaks account for most of the failed cases. Proliferative vitreoretinopathy (PVR) does not appear to be any greater in eyes treated with pneumatic retinopexy.

SUMMARY

RRD subsequently develops in 1–2% of all patients undergoing cataract extraction by an extracapsular or phacoemulsification technique. Interruption of the posterior capsule either intraoperatively or postoperatively increases the risk for RRD. Prior to both cataract extraction and Nd:YAG laser capsulotomy, a dilated examination should be performed to identify lesions at risk. Since the majority of RRD occur within 1 year following cataract extraction, patients should be screened relatively frequently with dilated examinations during this time period. Most importantly, all post-cataract patients must be educated to the signs and symptoms of RRD and instructed to seek medical attention immediately if any such changes develop.

References

[1] Michels RG, Wilkinson CP, Rice TA. Retinal detachment. St. Louis: C.V. Mosby; 1990.
[2] Benson WE. Retinal detachment. Diagnosis and management. Philadelphia: J. B. Lippincott; 1988.
[3] Kangro M, Osterlin S. Hyaluronate concentration in the vitreous of the pseudophakic eye. Invest Ophthalmol Vis Sci 1985;26:28.
[4] Heller MD, Straatsma BR, Foos RY. Detachment of the posterior vitreous in phakic and aphakic eyes. Mod Probl Ophthalmol 1972;10:23–26.
[5] McDonnell PJ, Patel A, Green WR. Comparison of intracapsular and extracapsular cataract surgery. Histopathologic study of eyes obtained postmortem. Ophthalmology 1985;92:1208–1225.
[6] Friedman Z, Neumann E. Posterior vitreous detachment after cataract surgery in non-myopic eyes and the resulting retinal lesions. Br J Ophthalmol 1975;59:451–454.
[7] Haiman MH, Burton TC, Brown CK. Epidemiology of retinal detachment. Arch Ophthalmol 1982;100:289–292.
[8] Wilkinson CP, Anderson LS, Little JH. Retinal detachment following phacoemulsification. Ophthalmology 1978;85:151–156.
[9] Smith PW, Stark WJ, Maumenee AE, et al. Retinal detachment after extracapsular cataract extraction with posterior chamber intraocular lens. Ophthalmology 1987;94:495–504.
[10] Javitt JC, Vitale S, Canner JK, et al. National outcomes of cataract extraction I. Retinal detachment after in patient surgery. Ophthalmology 1991;98:895–902.
[11] Steinert RF, Puliafito CA, Kumar SR, et al. Cystoid macular edema, retinal detachment, and glaucoma after Nd:YAG laser posterior capsulotomy. Am J Ophthalmol 1991;112:373–380.
[12] Ober RR, Wilkinson CP, Fiore JV, et al. Rhegmatogenous retinal detachments after neodymium-YAG laser capsulotomy in aphakic and pseudophakic eye. Am J Ophthalmol 1986;101:81–87.
[13] Rickman-Barger L, Florine CW, Larson RD, et al. Retinal detachment after neodynium-YAG laser posterior capsulotomy. Am J Ophthalmol 1989;107:531–536.
[14] Javitt JC, Tielsch JM, Canner JK, et al. National outcome of cataract extraction. Increased risk of retinal complications associated with Nd:YAG laser capsulotomy. Ophthalmology 1992;99:1486–1498.

[15] Yoshida A, Ogasawara H, Jalkh AE, et al. Retinal detachment after cataract surgery. Ophthalmology 1992;99:453–459.

[16] Duker JS, Sabates NR, Thomas GJ, et al. Retinal detachment following recent cataract extraction Unpublished data.

[17] Erie JC, Raecker BA, Baratz KH, et al. Risk of retinal detachment after cataract extraction, 1980–2004. Ophthalmology 2006;113:2026–2032.

[18] Tuft S, Minassian D, Sullivan P. Risk factors for retinal detachment after cataract surgery. Ophthalmology 2006;113:650–656.

[19] Preferred practice pattern. Retinal detachment. San Francisco: American Academy of Ophthalmology; 1990.

[20] Jungschaffer OH. Retinal detachment after intraocular lens implants. Arch Ophthalmol 1977;95:1203–1204.

[21] Yoon YH, Marmor MF. Rapid enhancement of retinal adhesion by laser photocoagulation. Ophthalmology 1988;95:1385–1388.

[22] Campochiaro PA, Kaden IH, Vidaurri-Leal J, Glaser BM. Cryotherapy enhances intravitreal dispersion of viable retinal pigment epithelial cells. Arch Ophthalmol 1985;103:434–436.

[23] Smiddy WE, Flynn HW, Nicholson DH, et al. Results and complications in treated retinal breaks. Am J Ophthalmol 1991;112:623–631.

[24] Lakhanpal V. Schocket SS Pseudophakic and aphakic retinal detachment mimicking cystoid macular edema. Ophthalmology 1987;94:785–791.

[25] Haddad WM, Monin C, Morel C, et al. Retinal detachment after phacoemulsification: a study of 114 cases. Am J Ophthalmol 2002;133:630–638.

[26] Ross WH, Kozy DW. Visual recovery in macula-off rhegmatogenous retinal detachments. Ophthalmology 1998;105:2149–2153.

[27] Salicone A, Smiddy WE, Venkatraman A, Feuer W. Visual recovery after scleral buckling procedure for retinal detachment. Ophthalmology 2006;113:1934–1942.

[28] Arya AV, Emerson JW, Engelbert M, et al. Surgical management of pseudophakic retinal detachments. A meta-analysis. Ophthalmology 2006;113:1924–1933.

[29] Weichel ED, Martidis A, Fineman M, et al. Pars plana vitrectomy versus combined pars plana vitrectomy-scleral buckle for primary repair of pseudophakic retinal detachment. Ophthalmology 2006;113:2033–2040.

[30] Stangos AN, Petropoulos IK, Brozou CG, et al. Pars-plana vitrectomy alone vs vitrectomy with scleral buckling for primary rhegmatogenous pseudophakic retinal detachment. Am J Ophthalmol 2004;138:952–958.

[31] Martinez-Castillo V, Zapata MA, Boixadera A, et al. Pars plana vitrectomy, laser retinopexy, and aqueous tamponade for pseudophakic rhegmatogenous retinal detachment. Ophthalmology 2007;114:297–302.

[32] O'Malley P, Swearingen K. Scleral buckling with diathermy for simple retinal detachments. Ophthalmology 1992;99:269–277.

[33] Greven CM, Sanders RJ, Brown GC, et al. Pseudophakic retinal detachments. Ophthalmology 1992;99:257–262.

[34] Campo RV, Sipperley JO, Sneed SR, et al. Pars plana vitrectomy without scleral buckle for pseudophakic retinal detachments. Ophthalmology 1999;106:1811–1816.

SUMMARY

Prolonged Intraocular Inflammation

Michael B. Raizman, MD

CONTENTS

- Recognition of Abnormal Inflammation
- Causes of Prolonged Inflammation
- Examination of the Eye
- Management
- *Propionibacterium* and Other Chronic Endophthalmitis

CHAPTER HIGHLIGHTS

>> Causes of prolonged postoperative inflammation

>> Key elements in examining for causes

>> Treatment

>> Late-onset inflammation

The most feared and severe form of inflammation after cataract surgery is acute endophthalmitis. Occurring within days of surgery, acute endophthalmitis often results in rapid loss of vision (see Chapter 55). Bacteria usually cause acute endophthalmitis but since 2005, toxic anterior segment syndrome (TASS) has become more prevalent (see Chapter 48). This chapter concentrates on a more insidious form of postoperative inflammation. Chronic inflammation may begin weeks, months, or even years after cataract surgery and can last as long as endophthalmitis. This inflammation is often caused by infection with organisms of low virulence that are sequestered in the capsular bag. However, other causes must also be considered, including the lens implant, retained lens material, and coincidental uveitis unrelated to the surgery.[1] This chapter reviews the practical aspects of diagnosis and management of prolonged intraocular inflammation after cataract surgery.

The incidence and degree of inflammation after cataract surgery have decreased significantly in recent years. Modern instrumentation, better surgical techniques, and improved intraocular lens (IOL) designs are all responsible for this advance. Perhaps more important is the common use of surgical techniques that minimize iris manipulation and reduce the amount of transected vascular tissue. The elimination of iridectomy and the use of smaller incisions

in the cornea and/or sclera are good examples of such techniques. Placement of the IOL in the capsular bag certainly reduces contact with the vascularized and pigmented ocular tissues. Phacoemulsification contributes to the ability to minimize ocular manipulation; hence, it reduces inflammation. With phacoemulsification it is usually possible to avoid contact with the iris. Although manual expression of the nucleus can be performed with minimal iris manipulation in most cases (and with minimal resultant inflammation), some stretching of the iris is unavoidable.

Fortunately, improvements in IOL design have also reduced inflammation. Early versions of IOLs incited inflammation in a variety of ways. A few lenses were contaminated during manufacture or packaging with substances toxic to the eye. Some lenses were poorly finished, with rough surfaces that induced inflammation. Others, such as closed-loop anterior-chamber IOLs, caused inflammation because of their shape and design. Any lens that led to increased contact with the iris or cocoons of uveal tissue around haptics was liable to induce inflammation. The uveitis-glaucoma-hyphema (UGH) syndrome is rarely encountered today because of improved lens design.

A better understanding of the tolerance and physiology of ocular tissues led to the development of better irrigating solutions, intraocular viscosurgical agents, and intraocular medications. Together these limit the amount of inflammation induced by the cataract-extraction procedure. It is interesting to note that little development of new pharmacologic agents for the treatment of postoperative inflammation has occurred, although our understanding of the application of existing medications has proved beneficial. The Retisert fluocinolone steroid implant (Bausch & Lomb) is rarely needed in this type of inflammation, since it provides sustained drug levels for over 2 years. Shorter acting implantable sustained-release drug delivery systems may be useful after cataract extraction in the future.[2-5]

RECOGNITION OF ABNORMAL INFLAMMATION

Acute endophthalmitis and TASS in the first week after cataract surgery are discussed in Chapters 48 and 55. Many of the conditions discussed in this chapter may also cause acute inflammation and should be considered in that context. Abnormal chronic inflammation is cellular activity in the eye of a greater degree and a longer duration than generally expected. Some inflammation is inevitable after any cataract extraction. After routine phacoemulsification and lens implantation, there is often remarkably little inflammation. Many of these eyes would probably do well without postoperative anti-inflammatory therapy, although few surgeons would be willing to take this risk, considering the current medico-legal atmosphere. With low-dose topical corticosteroids or topical nonsteroidal anti-inflammatory agents, most of these eyes have little inflammation after 1 or 2 weeks and are free of inflammation after 2 to 3 weeks. On the other side of the spectrum, a case of complicated manual expression of a nucleus, with iris sphincterotomies, peripheral iridectomy, and vitreous loss, may cause inflammation for 6–8 weeks. Therefore, inflammation lasting more than 3–8 weeks, depending on the clinical setting, should raise concerns about infection or other causes of abnormal inflammation. Of equal concern is inflammation that does not respond to aggressive topical corticosteroids, the development of a hypopyon at any time, and an increase in vitreous cellular infiltrate.

■ CAUSES OF PROLONGED INFLAMMATION ■

Patients with preoperative uveitis are at an increased risk of excessive postoperative inflammation (see Chapter 25). Diabetics usually display more inflammation, and some surgeons in the Far East believe that Asians are more prone to inflammation, especially from retained lens epithelium. Children's eyes typically have more inflammation than adults, even after routine intraocular surgery. (Some surgeons suggest routine use of heparin in the infusion during cataract surgery on children, although there may be an increased risk of hemorrhage.[6–10] This strategy has not been routinely employed.) As mentioned previously, intraoperative factors such as manipulation of the iris, vitrectomy, and prolonged surgical times may contribute to increases in postoperative vascular leakage and inflammation. Residual cortical material induces inflammation in many cases by inducing attempts by phagocytes to clear the material and perhaps by stimulating cytokine release in the anterior chamber, with subsequent recruitment of inflammatory cells. Cortical material may also harbor organisms that induce an inflammatory response (Figure 57-1). Retained nuclear material commonly causes inflammation and elevated intraocular pressure. Iris to the wound is especially likely to induce inflammation and cystoid macular edema (CME).

Debate continues about the role of lens materials in inducing inflammation. Polymethylmethacrylate seems to induce less complement activation than polypropylene (Prolene),[11] but the clinical relevance of this finding is not certain. Epidemiological studies suggest the Prolene haptics are more often associated with endophthalmitis than are polymethylmethacrylate haptics,[12] perhaps because of differences in bacterial adhesion. Surface modification of lens implants with heparin may reduce postoperative inflammation.[13] As noted previously, improvements in lens design over the past 15 years have dramatically reduced the incidence of excessive postoperative inflammation.

When the IOLs are responsible for prolonged inflammation, it is generally their misplacement that is to blame. Anterior-chamber

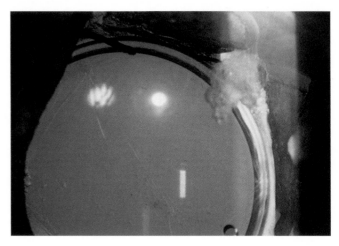

Figure 57-1 Cortical material, shown adjacent to the posterior-chamber intraocular lens, may harbor bacteria and incite postoperative inflammation.

lenses are most likely to induce inflammation because they necessarily contact the angle structures. This is rarely a problem unless the lens is too long (causing pressure or even erosion), too short (leading to excessive movement), anteriorly displaced (inducing corneal endothelial damage), or posteriorly displaced (causing iris trauma, iris tuck, or cocooning). Posterior-chamber IOLs (PC IOLs) that are placed in the capsular bag rarely cause inflammation. One or both haptics in the sulcus are almost always well tolerated. On occasion, haptics may abrade or erode uveal tissue, producing inflammation and recurrent hemorrhage.[14–17] Capture of the lens optic by the pupil is often associated with iritis and with deposition of inflammatory cells and debris on the optic surface from repeatedly traumatized iris tissue (Figure 57-2) or continuous contact of the IOL with the vascular iris.

Uveitis unrelated to the surgery may present for the first time any time after cataract surgery. This coincidental appearance can cause a delay in diagnosis. Sympathetic ophthalmia after modern cataract extraction is exceedingly rare.[18] The prostaglandin analogs used to treat glaucoma (latanoprost, bimatoprost, and travoprost) can induce intraocular inflammation and CME.[19] Miotic agents and other glaucoma medications can do the same.

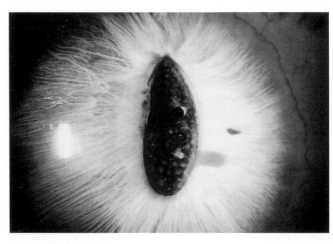

Figure 57-2 Deposits coat the optic of this pupil-captured intraocular lens. Repeated neodymium:yttrium-aluminum-garnet laser cleaning of the lens optic surface provided only transient effect.

■ EXAMINATION OF THE EYE ■

The examination should be directed at those conditions outlined previously. The patient should be asked about localized pain, which may suggest an offending IOL haptic contacting uveal tissue. Keratic precipitates (Figure 57-3) and anterior chamber cell and flare should be quantified to allow accurate comparisons from one visit to the next. A widely dilated pupil should allow better visualization of the implant to determine IOL position, of the capsular bag to visualize residual cortex and abscesses (Figure 57-4), and of the posterior capsule to detect plaques of anaerobic organisms (Figure 57-5). Gonioscopy is useful to view the angle for synechiae, iris to the wound, and haptic position; the mirror also assists in the posterior-chamber evaluation. Gonioscopy can allow visualization of a greater portion of the peripheral capsule and PC IOL. The vitreous should be examined at the slit-lamp examination to grade any vitreous infiltrate. CME is best seen with a contact lens or with a 78 or 90 diopter (D) lens at the slit-lamp examination. Indirect ophthalmoscopy allows visualization of retained lens material and inflammation in the vitreous. Ultrasound biomicroscopy (UBM) is useful for evaluating those

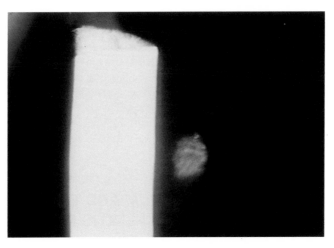

Figure 57-5 Posterior capsular plaque in a case of presumed *Propionibacterium acnes* endophthalmitis. In this case, vitreous culture revealed no organisms, but Gram-positive rods were found on the capsule in the region of the plaque.

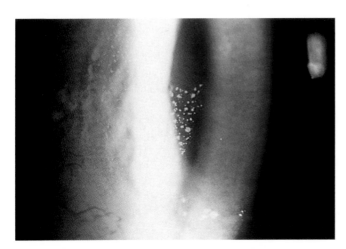

Figure 57-3 Granulomatous keratic precipitates in a case of chronic postoperative endophthalmitis from *Propionibacterium acnes*.

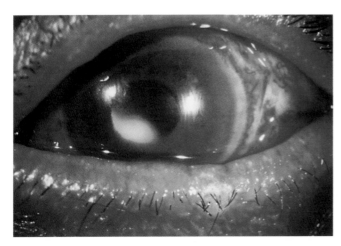

Figure 57-4 Posterior capsular abscess containing *Staphylococcus epidermidis* developed in this case about 1 year after cataract extraction.

portions of the posterior chamber not visible on slit-lamp examination. In particular, UBM can evaluate the position of the IOL haptics relative to the iris and ciliary body.

■ MANAGEMENT ■

Any obvious cause of excessive inflammation should be corrected where possible and when indicated. Some low-grade inflammation from IOL misplacement may not reduce vision or cause discomfort and may be controllable with low doses of corticosteroids. Such cases may be followed without surgical intervention. Inflammation may disappear weeks or months later. If glaucoma therapy is suspected as a contributing factor to the inflammation, the drops should be stopped as a trial. Eyes with visual loss (usually below 20/40), uncontrollable inflammation, glaucoma, hyphema, or CME may require appropriate surgical intervention, that is, lens reposition or exchange, removal of residual cortex from the anterior chamber, or release of iris from the wound. The presence of an abscess or plaque on the capsule suggests endophthalmitis and requires antibiotic and/or surgical therapy, as discussed in Chapter 55.

In many cases, no obvious cause of inflammation is apparent, or the inflammation may be considered consistent with operative trauma. In such cases, topical corticosteroids may be given frequently, up to every hour. A significant reduction in inflammation should be seen. If little or no response is noted, it is often helpful to try an intraorbital injection (through the lower lid and orbital septum) of triamcinolone (Kenalog), 40 mg in 1 mL. If little or no response is seen following the injection, endophthalmitis must be seriously considered. On occasion, the inflammation responds nicely but relapses when corticosteroids are tapered. Failure to control the inflammation by these techniques should raise suspicions of the possibility of chronic endophthalmitis.

Several series of cases have been published on the use of subconjunctival or intraocular injection of tissue plasminogen activator (tPA). TPA is a naturally occurring enzyme that induces fibrinolysis by converting plasminogen into plasmin; plasmin is responsible for the degradation of fibrin. TPA seems to be a safe method of reducing or eliminating fibrin clots in situations where this must be accomplished quickly (e.g., obstructed filtering blebs or pupillary block glaucoma). The ideal dose has not been determined, but current formulations of tPA, created for other clinical and laboratory uses, need to be diluted. The cost is quite high, and the use of tPA for treating ocular fibrin must be considered experimental pending the performance of larger-scale studies.[20–23] Topical use of tPA is ineffective.[24]

■ *PROPIONIBACTERIUM* AND OTHER CHRONIC ENDOPHTHALMITIS ■

When all noninfectious causes of chronic postoperative inflammation have been addressed and ruled out, infection with *Propionibacterium* species or other organisms must be presumed. Chronic endophthalmitis may present in many ways, but characteristic features have been recognized: chronic, often mild granulomatous or nongranulomatous uveitis; white plaques on the lens capsule; and onset of inflammation months (or, rarely, years) after surgery. Cases appearing after neodymium: yttrium-aluminum-garnet capsulotomy suggest that organisms may be sequestered in the capsular bag. Patients may or may not complain of pain. Blurry vision is a common symptom. Conjunctival hyperemia, keratic precipitates, hypopyon, and vitritis are variable signs. In unusual cases of *Propionibacterium acnes* endophthalmitis, the onset of severe inflammation may be acute. The average time to onset is about 4 months after cataract extraction. The inflammation may respond transiently to topical corticosteroids. Although most cases are caused by the Gram-positive anaerobic *P. acnes* rod, other offending organisms include *Staphylococcus* species, *Actinomyces*, *Achromobacter*, *Corynebacterium*, *Propionibacterium granulosum*, and fungi.[25–26]

All suspected cases deserve at least a culture of the vitreous and injection of vancomycin (1 mg in 0.1 mL) into the vitreous cavity. Some cases of successful treatment with systemic and/or topical (but no intraocular) antibiotics suggest that this may be a feasible alternative, but the literature contains multiple cases of failure with such an approach.[27–30] Recurrence of endophthalmitis after simple culture and injection of vancomycin has been reported, prompting some investigators to recommend more aggressive surgery. Among the additional interventions needed in some cases are partial capsulectomy and total capsulectomy with lens explantation.[31–34]

Based on the literature, the following guidelines are suggested: the combined techniques of pars plana vitrectomy with culture; partial capsulectomy, including removal of capsule-containing plaques or abscesses; and injection of vancomycin. Cases with extensive areas of capsular infection probably require full capsulectomy. If inflammation recurs after partial capsulectomy, then removal of the entire capsule is recommended. This usually necessitates removal of any PC IOL. Concurrent IOL exchange is reasonable in most cases, with a replacement IOL either sutured in the posterior chamber or placed in the anterior chamber. Removal of the capsular bag may be facilitated by the use of chymotrypsin. Iris hooks or pupil expanders may aid visualization when pupillary dilation is inadequate.

In addition to the routine culture, vitreous specimens should be cultured under anaerobic conditions for 14 days to increase the chances of recovering the *P. acnes* organisms. Culture-negative cases of chronic inflammation may represent infections that failed to grow in the laboratory. It has been suggested that culturing the vitrectomy cassette contents may be more rewarding than culturing an initial vitreous aspirate.[35] It is probably prudent to do both. It may also be helpful to stain and culture the excised portion of the posterior capsule, as this may demonstrate organisms when vitreous cultures do not (see Figure 57-5). *P. acnes* DNA may be detected by polymerase chain reaction on the IOL and in the aqueous humor.[34]

As with all rare conditions, suspicion is the key to diagnosis. All cases of chronic inflammation after cataract extraction should be considered infectious until proven otherwise. The rewards of such a diagnosis are great because good vision is the rule after appropriate treatment.[37]

References

[1] Berrocal AM, Davis JL. Uveitis following intraocular surgery. Ophthalmol Clin North Am 2002;15:357–364.

[2] Tan DTH, Chee SP, Lim L, et al. Randomized clinical trial of a new dexamethasone drug delivery system (Surodex) for treatment of post-cataract surgery inflammation. Ophthalmology 1999;106:223–231.

[3] Chang DF, Garcia IH, Hunkeler JD, et al. Phase II results of an intraocular steroid delivery system for cataract surgery. Ophthalmology 1999;106:1172–1177.

[4] Wadood AC, Armbrecht AM, Aspinal PA, et al. Safety and efficacy of a dexamethasone anterior segment drug delivery system in patients after phacoemulsification. J Cataract Refract Surg 2004;30:761–768.

[5] Siqueira RC, Filho ER, Fialho SL, et al. Pharmacokinetic and toxicity investigations of a new intraocular lens with a dexamethasone drug delivery system: a pilot study. Ophthalmologica 2006;220:338–342.

[6] Kohnen T, Dick B, Hessemer V, et al. Effect of heparin in irrigating solution on inflammation following small incision cataract surgery. J Cataract Refract Surg 1998;24:237–243.

[7] Bayramlar H, Totan Y, Borazan M. Heparin in the intraocular irrigating solution in pediatric cataract surgery. J Cataract Refract Surg 2004;30:2163–2169.

[8] Rumelt S, Stolovich C, Sega ZI, et al. Intraoperative enoxaparin minimizes inflammatory reaction after pediatric cataract surgery. Am J Ophthalmol 2006;141:433–437.

[9] Wilson Jr ME, Trevedi RH. Low molecular-weight heparin in the intraocular irrigating solution in pediatric cataract and intraocular lens surgery. Am J Ophthalmol 2006;141:537–538.

[10] Zarei R, Azimi R, Moghimi S, et al. Inhibition of intraocular fibrin formation after infusion of low-molecular-weight heparin during combined phacoemulsification-trabeculectomy surgery. J Cataract Refract Surg 2006;32:1921–1925.

[11] Mondino BJ, Nagata S, Glovsky MM. Activation of the alternative complement pathway by intraocular lenses. Invest Ophthalmol Vis Sci 1985;26:905–908.

[12] Menikoff JA, Speaker MG, Marmor M, et al. A case-control study of risk factors for post-operative endophthalmitis. Ophthalmology 1991;98:1761–1768.

[13] Trocme SD, Li H. Effect of heparin-surface-modified intraocular lenses on postoperative inflammation after phacoemulsification: a randomized trial in a United States patient population: Heparin-Surface-Modified Lens Study Group. Ophthalmology 2000;107:1031–1037.

[14] Percival SP, Das SK. UGH syndrome after posterior chamber lens implantation. J Am Intraocul Implant Soc 1983;19:200–201.

[15] Van Liefferinge T, Van Oye R, Kestelyn P. Uveitis-glaucoma-hyphema syndrome: a late complication of posterior chamber lenses. Bull Soc Belge Ophthalmol 1994;252:61–66.

[16] Aounuma H, Matsushita H, Nakajima K, et al. Uveitis-glaucoma-hyphema syndrome after posterior chamber intraocular lens implantation. Jpn J Ophthalmol 1997;47:98–100.

[17] Masket S. Pseudophakic posterior iris chafing syndrome. J Cataract Refract Surg 1986;12:252–256.

[18] Lubin JR, Albert DM, Weinstein M. Sixty-five years of sympathetic ophthalmia: a clinicopathologic review of 105 cases (1913–1978). Ophthalmology 1980;87:109.

[19] Miyaki K, Ota I, Maekubo K, et al. Latanoprost accelerates disruption of the blood brain barrier and the incidence of angiographic cystoid macular edema in early postoperative pseudophakia. Ophthalmology 1999;117:34–40.

[20] Snyder RW, Lambrou FH, Williams GA. Intraocular fibrinolysis with recombinant human tissue plasminogen activator. Arch Ophthalmol 1987;105:1277–1280.

[21] Piltz JR, Starita RJ. The use of subconjunctivally administered tissue plasminogen activator after trabeculectomy. Ophthalmic Surg 1994;25:51–53.

[22] Wedrich A, Menapace R, Ries E, et al. Intracameral tissue plasminogen activator to treat severe fibrinous effusion after cataract surgery. J Cataract Refract Surg 1997;23:873–877.

[23] Helingenhaus A, Steinmetz B, Lapuente R, et al. Recombinant tissue plasminogen activator in cases with fibrin formation after cataract surgery: a prospective randomized multicentre study. Br J Ophthalmol 1998;82:810–815.

[24] Zwaan J, Latimer WB. Topical tissue plasminogen activator appears ineffective for the clearance of intraocular fibrin. Ophthalmic Surg Lasers 1998;29:476–483.

[25] Meisler DM, Mandelbaum S. Propionibacterium-associated endophthalmitis after extracapsular cataract extraction: review of reported cases. Ophthalmology 1989;96:54–61.

[26] Scott IU, Flynn HW, Miller D. Delayed-onset endophthalmitis following cataract surgery caused by *Acremonium strictum*. Ophthalmic Surg Lasers Imaging 2005;36:506–507.

[27] Meisler DM, Zakov ZN, Bruner WE, et al. Endophthalmitis associated with sequestered intraocular *Propionibacterium acnes*. Am J Ophthalmol 1987;104:428–429. [letter].

[28] Brady SE, Cohen EJ, Fischer DH. Diagnosis and treatment of chronic postoperative bacterial endophthalmitis. Ophthalmic Surg 1988;19:580–584.

[29] Sawusch MR, Michels RG, Stark WJ, et al. Endophthalmitis due to *Propionibacterium acnes* sequestered between IOL optic and posterior capsule. Ophthalmic Surg 1989;20:90–92.

[30] Pellegrino FA, Wainberg P, Schalen A, et al. Oral clarithromycin as a treatment option in chronic post-operative endophthalmitis. Arch Soc Esp Oftalmol 2005;80:339–344.

[31] Winward KE, Pflugfelder SC, Flynn HW, et al. Postoperative *Propionibacterium* endophthalmitis: treatment strategies and long-term results. Ophthalmology 1993;100:447–451.

[32] Clark WL, Kaiser PK, Flynn Jr HW, et al. Treatment strategies and visual acuity outcomes in chronic post-operative *Propionibacterium acnes* endophthalmitis. Ophthalmology 1999;106:1665–1670.

[33] Aldave AJ, Stein JD, Deramo VA, et al. Treatment strategies for postoperative *Propionibacterium* endophthalmitis. Ophthalmology 1999;106:2395–2401.

[34] Srinivasan S, Kumar BV, Prasad S, et al. Partial posterior capsulotomy through an anterior approach: an intraocular lens retaining technique in the management of presumed *Propionibacterium acnes* endophthalmitis. Eye 2006;20:382–384.

[35] Donahue SP, Kowalski RP, Jewart BH, et al. Vitreous cultures in suspected endophthalmitis: biopsy or vitrectomy. Ophthalmology 1993;100:452–455.

[36] Lai JY, Chen KH, Lin YC et al. *Propionibacterium acnes* endophthalmitis DNA from an explanted intraocular lens detected by polymerase chain reaction in a case of chronic pseudophakic endophthalmitis. J Cataract Refract Surg 2006;32:522–525.

[37] Zambano W, Flynn HW, Pflugfelder SC, et al. Management options for *Propionibacterium acnes* endophthalmitis. Ophthalmology 1989;96:1100–1105.

part viii

INNOVATIONS AND FUTURE TRENDS FOR CATARACT SURGERY

Cataract Surgery: Future Predictions   **695**

Cataract Surgery: Future Predictions

58

Robert H. Osher, MD

CHAPTER HIGHLIGHTS

>> Personal perspectives from Dr. Robert Osher

>> Phaco and intraocular lens technology directions

>> Regulatory and reimbursement challenges

When I was invited to write a brief closing chapter on the future of cataract surgery, I knew there would be inevitable advances that did not require a crystal ball to predict. The machines will get better, the incisions will get smaller, and the lenses will outperform even our wildest expectations! Having demonstrated my clairvoyance, this chapter could now be concluded, although I could also safely predict that another invitation to re-write this chapter in the future would never be forthcoming.

So let's begin our glimpse into the future by exploring patient qualifications necessary for cataract surgery. Virtually every person will become a candidate as refractive lens replacement becomes a birthright. Ironically, it is likely that cataract surgery will become an infrequent operation when the transparent crystalline lens is routinely removed for the correction of refractive errors. Spherical, cylindrical, and presbyopic "tune-ups" will become highly accurate, quick, and enormously successful procedures that will ultimately eliminate glasses and contact lenses. Similar to the economics of goods and services, satisfaction will rise but expensive pricing will decline. The biggest winner of all will be Medicare since the government will no longer foot the bill for millions of cataract surgeries each year. Hospitals will be the big losers as ophthalmologists continue to distance themselves from institutional medicine and the rest of the medical community.

In the near future, cataract removal and subsequently clear lens removal will be achieved through smaller and smaller incisions. Phaco-ersatz was a concept developed by Jean Marie Parel, Henry Gelender, MD, and Edward Norton, MD in the early 1980s whereby the lens content was removed through a tiny opening in the capsule and injectable material was used to reform the lens.[1] Okihiro Nishi, MD has continued this intriguing work in Japan while many surgeons have already embraced sleeveless bimanual micro phacoemulsification or microcoaxial phacoemulsification through incisions 2 mm or less.[2] Amar Agarwal, MD

and his colleagues from India were the first to crack the 1 mm barrier with phaconit.[3] While phacoemulsification has withstood the test of time, 40 years is almost forever on the technology timeline. Innovations such as torsional ultrasound may improve efficiency but eventually alternative technologies for lens removal will emerge, introducing failsafe thermal and capsular protection. Virtual media textbooks will no longer contain chapters on the management of intraoperative complications. When the patient asks, what is the worst thing that can happen during surgery, the surgeon will be able to smile and respond, "For me to die . . . other than that, nothing!"

With respect to the future of intraocular lenses (IOLs), newer materials with preloaded injection devices will allow insertion through tiny incisions. Every lens will have the capability to correct all types of pre-existing refractive errors and higher-order aberrations. Technology will become available for confirming that the ideal intraocular lens has been implanted at the conclusion of surgery, also conquering the challenge of IOL accuracy in an epidemic of patients who have undergone previous refractive surgery. Should an inadvertent residual refractive error occur, adjustment of the lens will be possible, a concept introduced by Calhoun Vision with their proprietary method of changing the shape of the IOL by postoperative irradiation. It may be possible to incorporate electronic features into the lens that offer telescopic imaging at distance and macroscopic magnification at near. Moreover, the lens of the future will contain pharmacologic agents that empower the IOL with anti-inflammatory, antibiotic, hypotensive, and posterior capsule opacification-inhibiting characteristics. Frenchman, Gilbert Serpin, MD has already introduced an IOL that leaches out Diclofenac over a 15-day interval.[4] and Guy Kleinmann and colleagues have published preliminary results with a hydrophilic lens that delivers antibiotics.[5] Intracameral drug delivery will stimulate a variety of devices that will be used for glaucoma and other disorders. Since 1993, I have predicted that a CTR was a viable candidate to serve as a reservoir and drug-delivery system, which will cause present-day issues of penetration and compliance to vanish.

The IOL will become a vehicle capable of providing other solutions for ocular disease. There will be improved optical systems that will address the severe disability of age-related macular degeneration without compromising peripheral vision, and it is likely that pressure-sensing devices may be incorporated into the IOL design for continuous monitoring of the glaucoma patient. The lens may even serve to monitor blood sugar in diabetics and other chemistries like the creatinine and BUN in the patient with renal failure. I will volunteer to be the first with a "signature" IOL that will confirm my identity and allow me to pass quickly through the airport security lines!

I will offer one final word about the regulatory process in the future. Innovation in ophthalmology has been restrained by the US Food and Drug Administration, which has established nearly insurmountable hurdles that often keep new products and devices from gaining approval in a timely and affordable fashion. More than 11 years were required for the approval of the capsular tension ring since Robert Cionni, MD and I implanted the first rings in the United States in 1993. Kenneth Rosenthal, MD was the first American to implant the twin inter-digitating prosthetic iris devices in 1996 and I quickly followed with the full-size iris and the sector device manufactured by Morcher. Even though the prosthetic irides are the only effective method of reducing intolerable glare in patients with severe iris loss, these devices are still not approved in the USA. This is to our national shame.

At some point there will be an outcry from either the public or, more likely, the politicians in Washington that will expedite the review process and make it affordable for start-up companies to gain product approvals. Moreover, there will also be a backlash from the years and years of drastic cuts in the reimbursement from Medicare and from private carriers that have driven many of our more innovative physicians into other specialties where their ideas are financially rewarded. The industry will continue to consolidate since these severe reductions limit the dollars available for research and development. However, by sidestepping Medicare and the traditional payment systems, it is likely that the highly competent, refractive lens surgeon will be fairly compensated for his or her wonderful contribution to society. One final prediction is certain: the future for the compassionate and adaptable anterior-segment surgeon committed to excellence will continue to be exciting and enormously satisfying.

References

[1] Parel J, Gelender H, Trefers W, et al. Phaco-Ersatz: Cataract surgery designed to preserve accommodation. Graefes Arch Clin Exp Ophthalmol 1986;224:165–173.
[2] Nishi O, Nishi K, Mano C, Ichihara M, Honda T. Lens refilling with injectable silicone in rabbit eyes. J Cataract Refract Surg 1998;24:975–982.
[3] Agarwal A. Microphakonit. In: Agarwal's A, editor. Phaco nightmares: conquering cataract catastrophes. Thorofare, NJ: Slack Inc, USA; 2007. p. 395–405.
[4] Serpin G. Loaded IOL: a new anti-inflammatory delivery system. Vid J Cataract Refract Surg 2004;XX.
[5] Kleinmann G, Apple DJ, Chew J, Hunter B, Stevens S, Larson S, et al. Hydrophilic acrylic intraocular lens as a drug-delivery system for fourth-generation fluoroquinolones. J Cataract Refract Surg 2006;32:1717–1721.

Note: Page numbers in *italics* refer to figures and page numbers in **bold** refer to tables.